COMPLETE GUIDE TO

SYMPTOMS, ILLNESS & SURGERY

Revised Fifth Edition

By H. Winter Griffith, M.D.

Revised and updated by
Stephen Moore, M.D.
and
Kenneth Yoder, M.D.

Surgical Illustrations
by Mark Pederson

A Perigee Book

THE BERKLEY PUBLISHING GROUP
Published by the Penguin Group
Penguin Group (USA) Inc.
375 Hudson Street, New York, New York 10014, USA
Penguin Group (Canada), 90 Eglinton Avenue East, Suite 700, Toronto, Ontario M4P 2Y3, Canada
(a division of Pearson Penguin Canada Inc.)
Penguin Books Ltd., 80 Strand, London WC2R 0RL, England
Penguin Group Ireland, 25 St. Stephen's Green, Dublin 2, Ireland (a division of Penguin Books Ltd.)
Penguin Group (Australia), 250 Camberwell Road, Camberwell, Victoria 3124, Australia
(a division of Pearson Australia Group Pty. Ltd.)
Penguin Books India Pvt. Ltd., 11 Community Centre, Panchsheel Park, New Delhi—110 017, India
Penguin Group (NZ), Cnr. Airborne and Rosedale Roads, Albany, Auckland 1310, New Zealand
(a division of Pearson New Zealand Ltd.)
Penguin Books (South Africa) (Pty.) Ltd., 24 Sturdee Avenue, Rosebank, Johannesburg 2196,
South Africa

Penguin Books Ltd., Registered Offices: 80 Strand, London WC2R 0RL, England

While the author has made every effort to provide accurate telephone numbers and Internet addresses at the time of publication, neither the publisher nor the author assumes any responsibility for errors, or for changes that occur after publication. Further, publisher does not have any control over and does not assume any responsibility for author or third-party websites or their content.

COMPLETE GUIDE TO SYMPTOMS, ILLNESS & SURGERY, REVISED 5TH EDITION

PRINTING HISTORY
First Perigee edition / July 1995
Fifth Perigee edition / March 2006
Text copyright © 1985, 1995, 2000, 2006 by Penguin Group (USA) Inc.
Surgical illustrations copyright © 1985, 1995, 2000, 2006 by Mark Pederson.

Fifth Perigee edition ISBN: 0-399-53321-4

The Library of Congress has cataloged the fourth Perigee edition as follows:

Griffith, H. Winter (Henry Winter), 1926–1993
    Complete guide to symptoms illness & surgery / H. Winter Griffith ;
surgical illustrations by Mark Pederson.—4th ed.
    p.
    Includes index.
    ISBN 0-399-52610-2
    1. Medicine, Popular—Handbooks, manuals, etc.
2. Symptoms—Handbooks, manuals, etc. 3. Surgery—
RC81.G834   2000
616—dc21   00-036049
ISBN 0-399-52609-9

PRINTED IN THE UNITED STATES OF AMERICA

10 9 8 7 6 5 4 3 2

PUBLISHER'S NOTE: Neither the publisher nor the author is engaged in rendering professional advice or services to the individual reader. The ideas, procedures, and suggestions contained in this book are not intended as a substitute for consulting with your physician. All matters regarding your health require medical supervision. Neither the author nor the publisher shall be liable or responsible for any loss or damage allegedly arising from any information or suggestion in this book.

Preface

I first came across Winter Griffith's name when asked to take over the U.S. Food and Drug Administration's patient information program. When reviewing correspondence from the 1960s, I found a letter from a Florida doctor asking if there was any problem in distributing written drug information to patients.

As far as I know, no one had previously thought of providing specific written information to patients. This was Dr. Griffith's idea and goal, and it became his lifelong mission.

Until the 1970s, patient education consisted of doctors patting patients on their heads and telling them to call if they had problems. Doctors did not discuss risks and side effects of drugs for fear of how patients would react.

Some doctors still have this attitude. But most doctors and patients recognize that information about risks and benefits of drug treatment is not only a patient's right, it is a patient's responsibility. Taking care of oneself means active participation in treatment decisions. Promoting participation between doctors and patients is the purpose of this book.

Winter Griffith is the godfather of patient education. His first books were compilations of simple instruction sheets that doctors hand out to patients. The sheets contained information the doctor wanted patients to know about illness and treatment. These instruction sheets are still copied an average of 16 million times a year and distributed to patients.

Dr. Griffith's later books have evolved to contain information the patient wants to know! Over the years, Dr. Griffith has come to understand people's needs for accurate, understandable information.

Some doctors think patients want to make their own decisions about health care, so they try to control the amount of information patients receive. Dr. Griffith understands that people want to decide with their doctors about treatment and other decisions affecting their health.

This book is a patient-advocate bible. It provides the information people want about symptoms, illnesses and surgeries.

The beauty of this book is that it explains what happens to the patient, why it happens, what risks are involved, what to expect in diagnosis and treatment, and how to monitor treatment.

The book is chock-full of usable information. Dr. Griffith has mastered the art of transmitting technical information. There is no medical jargon—just solid, helpful facts.

Louis A. Morris, Ph.D.
Head, Patient Education, Research, and Labeling Branch
U.S. Food and Drug Administration

Take Care of Yourself

YOUR ROLE

As a patient, you can and should share responsibility with your health care provider for your medical care. Knowing the "what," "why," and "how" of a medical problem enables you to get maximum benefit from your medical treatment.

Many thoughtful and assertive patients wish to be more involved with their medical care. They don't want to be passive and powerless in matters that affect their own bodies. They don't want instructions or advice that is incomplete or lacking in credibility. They seek—and sometimes demand—enough information so they can think for themselves and participate in important medical decisions affecting them.

A patient who is well educated about his or her illness or a recommended surgical procedure is more likely to have a greater satisfaction with their medical care. The educated patient will have a better understanding and fewer surprises about the treatment steps, the expected outcome and possible complications.

THE INFORMATION GAP

Somehow, and sometimes for justifiable reasons, a health care provider's medical information does not get explained, translated or transmitted into usable form for the most important member of the health-care team—the patient.

Even when information *is* competently conveyed to the patient by a doctor, nurse or other health professional, the patient has no follow-up written checklist to remind and reinforce what he or she has learned. This book is intended to provide patients and their families with the missing checklist and to supplement information you have received from your health care provider.

SIMPLE, CONCISE INFORMATION

Condensing the available mass of medical and surgical knowledge into one volume has required much simplification. We have tried not to omit major facts and concepts, but of necessity, many details have been left out.

It is impossible to include all the factors and circumstances that affect each individual's health. Thus, your health care provider may take into account other factors not included here when he or she makes a precise diagnosis and recommends treatment for you.

The information in this book barely scratches the surface of all the information available about various medical subjects. It is supplemental to the knowledge doctors and other medical professionals have acquired. In addition to a medical education, most doctors have extensive clinical experience—and ideally, a great deal of wisdom and compassion.

WHAT YOU CAN FIND IN THIS BOOK

This book contains three major sections: Symptoms, Illnesses and Disorders, and Surgeries. Information for each is organized in chart form. The three chart formats vary somewhat, and each format is explained in detail in the following pages.

The book contains an appendix section to supplement information in the charts. The appendix entries cover a variety of topics that do not fit into the chart format used in the other sections. The topics include: a number of special diets; suggestions to reduce stress; instructions for breast, skin and testicle self-exams; guidelines for safe drug use; information about sexually transmitted diseases as well as other subjects.

A special feature of the book is a list of resources for additional information. If you want more, in-depth information about symptoms, illnesses, surgeries or other medical problems discussed in this book, the list provides a starting place to find that type of information. The resource list contains names, addresses telephone numbers, and, where available, websites of organizations and government health agencies devoted to specific disorders.

A glossary section of medical-related terms is also included. This includes definitions of medical tests and medical terms that are used throughout the book. In addition, it will give a brief description of some rare illnesses and disorders that are not covered in the other sections due to lack of space.

WHAT YOU CAN'T FIND IN THIS BOOK

This book will not help you diagnose or treat your own illnesses in most cases. It can be a valuable starting point. Printed words cannot replace the knowledge and expertise that your health care provider provides.

This book does not replace the services of doctors and other health care providers. It is not a substitute for communication between you and your health care provider. Only he or she knows your medical history and special circumstances about your health. Only you know the intensity and exact quality of your symptoms. The printed page cannot capture or convey the *feelings* that accompany illness.

HOW YOU WILL BENEFIT

Yet, armed with introductory knowledge about symptoms, illness and surgical procedures discussed in this book, you benefit in the following ways:
• You can better understand the nature of your illness.

• You can more easily recognize circumstances when medical help is necessary.
• You can learn useful facts about how to prevent disease and injury.
• You can confirm, refresh your memory and help your family learn and understand the facts regarding your illness.
• You can review a checklist of ways to make yourself better if you are ill.
• You can ask questions if treatment steps mentioned in the book differ greatly from what your health care provider advises. Recognize that medical professionals may have differing opinions, ideas or practices on the course of treatment for a particular illness. Plus, newer and improved methods of treatment continue to be developed.

You should feel free to ask questions and discuss your concerns about treatment options with your health care provider. He or she should welcome and answer your questions. If not, you may want to consult another health care provider.

Your best chance to achieve and maintain optimal health is to participate fully in taking care of yourself. This book provides a tool to help you reach that goal.

Guide to Symptom Charts

The symptom charts are designed to suggest one or more illnesses and disorders that a specific symptom might indicate. Each chart focuses on one common symptom as shown on the list at the beginning of the section. The chart for *excessive sweating* appears on the facing page.

These charts do not include every possible *sign* or *symptom* the human body can exhibit, but they represent the most familiar and easily recognizable ones. *Signs* are observed. *Symptoms* are felt or experienced. A sign may be observed by the patient or by someone else. Symptoms are feelings only the patient can describe.

The charts provide a guide for how serious symptoms are. They give you clues as to what symptoms can mean. They refer you to other sections of the book for further information. *However, they are not intended as self-diagnosis charts*. No book should replace a competent doctor's diagnosis! The charts are only to help you decide how to proceed when you or someone else develops symptoms.

Refer to the numbers on the sample chart for an explanation of each heading described below.

1—SYMPTOM NAME

Charts are titled and arranged alphabetically by the name that is most common or that best describes the symptom (**SWEATING, EXCESSIVE**).

In cases where the symptom name is ambiguous, or the symptom can apply to several parts of the body, the body part is part of the title. For example,

SWELLING (a symptom) appears as separate charts titled: **ABDOMINAL SWELLING; ANKLES, SWOLLEN; SWELLING OR LUMP**; and **TESTICLES OR PENIS, PAINFUL OR SWOLLEN**. One chart is alphabetized by the symptom name, **SWELLING OR LUMP**. The rest are alphabetized by the body part the swelling affects.

If you can't find your symptom under its own name, refer to the list at the start of the section and check alphabetically for the main part of the body it affects.

2—SYMPTOMS & FACTORS

The main symptom is grouped in the first column with other symptoms or factors that frequently accompany it. Each group represents one or more separate illnesses or disorders that the symptom can indicate.

For instance, excessive sweating can mean many things, depending on what other symptoms appear with it. When accompanied by chest pain, excessive sweating can be a sign of heart attack. When accompanied instead by weight loss, coughing with blood, fever and fatigue, it can be a strong indication of serious lung disorders. Another entry relating to a disorder of the thyroid gland presents yet another possibility.

Often, none of the symptom groups will match your present problem. Your doctor knows your medical history and can perform a physical examination and use laboratory tests to diagnose your condition.

SWEATING, EXCESSIVE

SYMPTOMS & FACTORS	POSSIBLE PROBLEM	WHAT TO DO*
• Excessive sweating. • Anxiety or excitement.	Normal occurrence with stress.	• See Anxiety Disorder, Generalized. • See Stress.
• Excessive sweating. • Overweight.	Effect of excess weight.	See Obesity & Overweight.
• Excessive sweating in woman older than 38. • Irregular menstrual periods.	Hormone changes; end of menstrual cycles approaching.	See Menopause.
• Excessive sweating in woman during menstrual period. OR • Excessive sweating due to tension or apprehension. OR • Excessive sweating following coffee consumption.	No underlying disorder.	Nothing.
Excessive sweating in teenager.	Normal occurrence during adolescence.	Nothing.
• Sweating. • Palpitations; tremors; flushing. • Symptoms of anxiety when exposed to, or thinking of, a particular stimulus.	Fears.	See Phobias.
• Excess sweating. • Unpleasant body odor.	Several disorders.	See Hyperhidrosis.
• Skin is cool and moist. • Prolonged exposure to hot temperature.	Excessive fluid loss.	See Heatstroke or Heat Exhaustion.
• Excessive sweating. • Chest pain.	Heart attack.	• Call doctor now! • See Heart Attack. • See Coronary Artery Disease.
• Excessive sweating at night. • Weight loss. • Persistent cough with blood in sputum. • Fever. • Fatigue.	• Lung inflammation or infection. • Cancer.	• See Tuberculosis. • See Hodgkin's Disease. • See Lung Cancer.
• Excessive sweating, plus 2 or more of following: • Weight loss. • Increased appetite. • Anxiety. • Sleeping problems.	Overactive thyroid gland.	See Hyperthyroidism.
• Excessive sweating. • Use of prescription, nonprescription or illegal drug.	Adverse reaction or side effect of drug.	• Consult doctor about prescription drug. • Discontinue use of nonprescription or illegal drug.
• Excessive sweating. • Fever.	Normal occurrence with fever.	See Fever charts (in Symptoms section).

*All references are to Illness section unless noted otherwise.

—POSSIBLE PROBLEM

The center column provides a short description of what a symptom group can indicate and may briefly define the illness or disorder to which you are referred in the third column.

In some cases, a group of symptoms can indicate more than one illness—sometimes they are totally unrelated. In that event, each description is listed next to an editor's bullet. For instance, one group of symptoms that we have discussed can indicate lung inflammation or infection, *or* cancer.

No attempt has been made to include every possible illness or disorder signaled by a symptom group. The identifications are based on illnesses that are *more obvious, most common or most serious*. For similar reasons, some rare illnesses described on illness charts in this book may not be referred to on symptom charts.

4—WHAT TO DO

The more serious medical problems that require immediate help are usually preceded by directions to call your doctor *now*. Below that, you will often be directed to the illness chart in this book that explains the problem. For instance, one entry has the instructions:

• Call doctor now.
• See Heart Attack.
• See Coronary Artery Disease.

All "See ..." instructions refer to illness charts. Exceptions to this rule will be noted on the symptom chart.

If the chart says "Call doctor now," don't waste precious time looking up the illness in this book. Wait to read more about it when the crisis has passed. Call your doctor immediately!

If anyone develops dramatic symptoms that you think represent life-threatening danger, call for *emergency help*. Dial 911 and report your address or location (with directions if needed).

In extreme situations, render what first aid you can, such as giving cardiopulmonary resuscitation (CPR). Yell for help from anyone within range.

Additional emergency information appears on the pages just before the index.

Guide to Illness & Disorder Charts

The information about illnesses and disorders is organized in 570 condensed, easy-to-read charts. They cover the majority of illnesses (diseases or disorders) and some injuries that can affect humans.

Each one is described in a one-page format shown in the sample chart, **HYPERTHYROIDISM**.

Major sections of the chart format are numbered and explained in the next few pages.

Most of the charts in this section refer to an illness. In some cases, however, charts refer to disorders, injuries or problems that are not really illnesses. The chart, **TEETHING**, is not about a disease—or even a disorder. It deals with a normal process that all people experience. It would be a disorder only if it did *not* occur.

But teething can be a medical problem. It often affects an infant's sense of well-being, and it may require treatment. Because teething is so common, and because some treatments for it are appropriate and others are not, it is included with illness charts.

1—CHART NAME

Charts are arranged alphabetically by the most-common name for the illness, disorder or medical problem. Other names or terms for these appear in parentheses below the main heading. Hyperthyroidism may also be referred to as thyrotoxicosis; toxic goiter or Graves' disease.

All names in this book, including alternate names, are listed in the index. To find information about a medical problem, check for its name in the index.

2—GENERAL INFORMATION

This section includes seven topics: *Definition; Body Parts Involved; Sex or Age Most Affected; Signs and Symptoms; Causes; Risk Increases With;* and *How to Prevent.* Each is discussed separately.

3—DEFINITION

A short definition of the problem or disease is provided. Sometimes the definition must include information from other categories, such as causes, body parts involved and others. The definition may also include information of general interest, such as how common a disease is, or whether it is contagious, cancerous or inherited.

4—BODY PARTS INVOLVED

This is usually a list of specific body parts or organs, such as bones, skin or liver. Sometimes general body systems, such as central nervous system, genitourinary system or gastrointestinal system, will be listed. The list usually includes body parts affected at the beginning of the disease, as many diseases spread to other body parts as they progress.

Of course, some illnesses involve all body cells—even from the beginning. Then the words "Total body" appear.

5—SEX OR AGE MOST AFFECTED

Some medical problems affect specific population groups only. Others affect all ages and both sexes indiscriminately. This section explains whether the medical problem occurs more often in males or females, or whether the incidence is about equal in either sex. It also lists the age group usually affected. These are generalizations, and variations can occur with specific individuals.

Sometimes labels, such as "newborns" or "adolescents," are used to describe age ranges. These labels are arbitrary names for specific ages, but they are commonly used in medical texts. Following are the age classifications:
• Newborns (0 to 2 weeks)
• Infants (2 weeks to 1 year)
• Young children (1 to 5 years)
• Older children (5 to 12 years)
• Adolescents (12 to 20 years)
• Young adults (20 to 40 years)
• Middle-aged adults (40 to 60 years)
• Older adults (over 60 years).

6—SIGNS AND SYMPTOMS

Signs are observed. *Symptoms* are felt or experienced.

A sign may be observed by the patient or by someone else, or it may represent physical findings determined by laboratory tests, x-rays and other diagnostic measures. Symptoms are feelings only the patient can describe.

Refer to the chart. The first item under this heading—hyperactivity—is a sign. It can be observed by the patient and others around him or her. The next three items— feeling warm or hot all the time, tremors and sweating—are signs *and* symptoms. They can be observed by others and they can be felt by the patient. The fifth— itching skin—is a symptom that only the patient can feel and describe.

Signs and symptoms are listed together in this book; no attempt is made to separate the two. On most charts, a wide range of possible signs and symptoms are listed. *It is unlikely that any patient will have all, or even most, of the possible signs and symptoms.* The presence or absence of signs and symptoms may vary according to:
• The age and sex of the patient.
• Extent of the illness.
• The stage of the illness.
• Medical and family history.
• Current state of health.

7—CAUSES

Many times the cause of a disorder is unknown. Causes for most medical problems include the following:
• Inherited (congenital) defects.
• Infections from bacteria, viruses, parasites, yeasts or fungi. All of these are sometimes referred to as "germs," but most people associate "germs" with bacteria only.
• Physical injury.
• Toxins (poisons) from a wide range of sources, such as contaminated food, environmental pollution and bites from poisonous snakes or insects.
• Allergies.
• Tumors. These may be benign or malignant. Benign tumors do not spread to adjacent or distant organs and threaten life. Malignant (cancerous) tumors can.
• Endocrine disorders. This means too many or too few hormones are produced from the pituitary gland, thyroid gland, parathyroid gland, pancreas, adrenal glands, ovaries, testicles or thymus gland.
• Mental or emotional disorders, such as anxiety, depression or schizophrenia.
• Diseases caused by defects in the body's immune system. These include disorders of hypersensitivity, such as rheumatic fever, rheumatoid arthritis, systemic lupus erythematosus and many others.

HYPERTHYROIDISM (Thyrotoxicosis; Goiter; Graves' Disease; Overactive Thyroid)

GENERAL INFORMATION

DEFINITION—Hyperthyroidism means the thyroid gland is overactive and produces too much thyroid hormone. The most common form of hyperthyroidism is called Graves' disease. The thyroid hormone is used by the body for metabolism (producing energy).

BODY PARTS INVOLVED—Thyroid gland and most other body organs, especially the endocrine system, which includes the pituitary gland, parathyroid glands, pancreas, adrenal glands, and ovaries or testicles.

SEX OR AGE MOST AFFECTED—Adults between ages 20 and 50, mostly women.

SIGNS & SYMPTOMS
* Anxiety, nervousness, and restlessness.
* Feeling warm or hot all the time.
* Sweating.
* Heart palpitations.
* Weight loss, even though appetite increases.
* Sleeplessness.
* Fatigue and weakness.
* Frequent bowel movements.
* Women may have less menstrual flow.
* Eyes appear to bulge out. There is swelling around the eyes. Vision changes may occur.
* Goiter (visibly enlarged thyroid) may occur.
* Hair loss.
* Tremor of the hands.

CAUSES—Graves' disease is an autoimmune disorder. In these disorders, the immune system by mistake attacks the body itself in different ways. In Graves' disease, abnormal antibodies from the immune system cause the thyroid to produce more hormone. Other causes of hyperthyroidism may be due to thyroid disorders.

RISK INCREASES WITH
* Thyroid nodules or tumors.
* Thyroiditis (inflammation of thyroid gland).
* Personal or family history of thyroid or autoimmune diseases.
* Radiation treatment.
* Females more than males.
* Excess iodine intake.
* Stress may be a contributing factor.

HOW TO PREVENT—No specific preventive measures.

WHAT TO EXPECT

DIAGNOSTIC MEASURES
* Your health care provider will do a physical exam.
* Medical tests include blood studies for thyroid levels. Radioactive iodine studies may be done.

APPROPRIATE HEALTH CARE
* Treatment usually involves drugs to reduce thyroid hormone levels. Permanent treatment involves use of radioactive iodine or surgery. With these two treatments, thyroid hormone production is decreased. Sometimes, hypothyroidism (too little thyroid hormone) occurs, which will need to be treated.
* Radioactive iodine treatment is usually done as an outpatient. The iodine (taken by mouth) causes the thyroid gland to shrink over a period of months.
* Surgery to remove part of the thyroid (called a thyroidectomy) may be advised. It is usually done in a hospital with a general anesthetic.
* For eye symptoms, an exam and follow-up by an eye specialist (ophthalmologist).

POSSIBLE COMPLICATIONS
* Thyroid eye disease. This includes blurred and double vision, difficulty in seeing, tearing, and light sensitivity.
* Heart problems.
* Dermopathy (a skin disorder).
* Hypothyroidism (low thyroid hormone levels).
* Surgery complications (infection or bleeding).

PROBABLE OUTCOME—Treatment is effective in controlling the disorder. It may take 6 months for thyroid levels to return to normal.

HOW TO TREAT

GENERAL MEASURES—It is important for your doctor to monitor the treatment. Be sure to keep follow-up appointments.

MEDICATION
* Antithyroid drugs to depress thyroid activity are usually prescribed. Follow-up blood tests are done to adjust the dosage until thyroid hormone levels are normal.
* Beta blockers to treat the heart and nervous system symptoms may be prescribed.
* Thyroid replacement drugs if the thyroid gland becomes underactive due to treatment.
* Avoid drugs or supplements containing iodine. Iodine may interfere with treatment drugs.

ACTIVITY—Usually no limits in otherwise healthy persons. In older persons or those with heart problems, decrease activity until thyroid levels are normal.

DIET—No special diet.

CALL YOUR DOCTOR IF

* You or a family member has symptoms of hyperthyroidism.
* Symptoms worsen, or new, unexplained symptoms develop during treatment.

8—RISK INCREASES WITH

Many disorders have known risk factors that can trigger the problem, make it more likely to occur or increase its duration and intensity. The most common risk factors include:
• Age, especially older persons or newborns and infants.
• Stress—either physical or emotional.
• Anxiety, depression and other mental or emotional problems.
• Fatigue or overwork.
• Poor nutrition due to improper diet or disease.
• Obesity.
• Recent or chronic illness that can lower resistance to other diseases.
• Recent surgery or injury.
• Genetic factors, such as family or ethnic tendency toward a disease.
• Use of drugs, such as alcohol, tobacco, caffeine, narcotics, psychedelics, hallucinogens, marijuana, sedatives, hypnotics or cocaine.
• Use of medications, whether prescription or nonprescription. Even necessary drugs cause adverse reactions and side effects that can complicate treatment and outcome of medical problems.
• Exposure to allergens, environmental pollutants or poisons.
• Geographic areas.
• Crowded or unsanitary living conditions.
• Socioeconomic factors (e.g., income, poverty, social class and education).

9—HOW TO PREVENT

Prevention can be of two types—prevention of the initial disease or prevention of a relapse or recurrence after recovery.

Prevention of any medical problem is the *best treatment*. Researchers continue to discover ways to prevent, delay or diminish some illness, pain, disability and

untimely deaths. These are included whenever available.

The causes and risk factors for a disease often provide the best clues for prevention. Many diseases, however, cannot be prevented at present.

10—WHAT TO EXPECT

This section includes four topics: *Diagnostic Measures; Appropriate Health Care; Possible Complications;* and *Probable Outcome.* Each is discussed separately below.

11—DIAGNOSTIC MEASURES

Your own observation of symptoms is usually the first—and often, most important—diagnostic measure. It is the first step toward medical treatment. For that reason, it is listed under this heading on almost all illness charts. Exceptions are made for a few medical problems, such as those that are signaled by unconsciousness, in which case self-observation is impossible.

A medical history and physical exam by a health care provider are also almost universal requirements before treatment for any disorder can begin. Even if a medical problem is usually treated at home, a history and exam will be necessary if complications develop that require medical treatment.

Additional diagnostic measures include laboratory studies and other medical tests. The most-common include:
• Studies of body fluids, such as blood, serum, plasma or spinal fluid.
• Microscopic and chemical examination of excreted material, such as urine or stools.
• CAT (computerized axial tomography) scans or x-rays of the affected body part.
• ECG (electrocardiogram), EEG (electroencephalogram) and EMG (electromyogram).

• Therapeutic trial of medication. This is used sometimes for a critically ill patient without a specific diagnosis while awaiting laboratory results.

You may not undergo every diagnostic test listed on the chart, and conversely, you may undergo tests not listed. Some tests are performed only if previous tests have not provided enough information. Others are performed only when complications develop. All medical diagnostic tests mentioned in this book are defined in the Glossary.

12—APPROPRIATE HEALTH CARE

Self-care or home care is sometimes listed as the first form of appropriate health care. It is an important part of care for many disorders. Sometimes total self-care suffices if you have previous experience with a medical problem and a source to review important points in treatment.

Usually, however, a medical problem should be diagnosed by a doctor before you attempt self-care. Once your doctor diagnoses an illness and outlines a treatment program, self-care or home care is often important. Treatment measures outlined in this book are designed to guide you, whether you are caring for yourself or taking care of someone else.

Effective self-care includes maintaining a positive attitude about yourself and being determined to improve or heal. During illness, a sense of humor and a positive outlook are helpful in addition to the medication or other treatments.

Medical care is often necessary, not only to diagnose and prescribe treatment for a medical problem, but to supervise self-care (or hospitalization, when necessary) and to provide additional medical treatment such as surgery.

In addition, even the simplest medical problems sometimes develop complications and require a doctor's care. In those cases, a doctor's treatment can be appropriate even though it applies to a small fraction of cases.

Find a personal physician who communicates well with you and with whom you can establish a good rapport and mutual respect.

Psychotherapy, counseling or biofeedback training may be the only useful health care for a medical problem caused mainly by stress or emotional problems.

Counseling and therapy are also helpful in providing personal and family support, especially with illnesses that are terminal or represent major lifestyle adjustments.

Rehabilitation is often helpful for illnesses or injuries that cause temporary or permanent disability. Rehabilitation may be provided by trained physical therapists or physiatrists (medical doctors who specialize in physical therapy). If rehabilitation is mentioned as appropriate health care, ask your doctor for information specific to your disability.

13—POSSIBLE COMPLICATIONS

Complications are additional medical problems triggered by or as a result of the original illness. Complications sometimes occur, despite accurate diagnosis and competent treatment. Some are preventable, a few are inevitable—but most are rare.

14—PROBABLE OUTCOME

Outcome (or prognosis) is a very important concern of the patient (and the family) in any illness. "What is going to happen to me? Is there a cure? How will this disease or injury affect my life?"

No one can completely predict the outcome of an illness or accident. The predicted or expected outcome information in this section is based on averages.

Patients and doctors work toward optimal results, but medicine is an inexact science. Response to treatment depends on many variables, and there are many unanswered questions about health and disease.

Some illnesses are considered incurable at present. The term "incurable" is a general one that includes everything from insignificant conditions that are mere annoyances to fatal diseases that bring certain death in a short time. For that reason, additional information about life expectancy is sometimes included for incurable illnesses. Again, individual variations are common, but the predictions are an attempt to answer a patient's most important questions. They help you adopt optimistic but realistic expectations.

In almost all cases—no matter how serious the illness—symptoms can be relieved or controlled to minimize pain and discomfort.

15—HOW TO TREAT

This section provides the checklist mentioned earlier that reminds you of instructions your doctor has given you. The information should not replace your doctor's instructions, because treatments vary a great deal between individuals.

If the instructions don't seem to fit your problem, ask your doctor or nurse for answers that apply uniquely to you.

The four major headings include: *General Measures; Medication; Activity;* and *Diet.*

16—GENERAL MEASURES

The instructions under this heading apply to home treatment. They cover common matters, such as soaks for skin problems, use of crutches, appropriate clothing, bandages or bathing.

They are not complete and may not apply to everybody, but they provide a good review of general measures helpful for most patients.

17—MEDICATION

Information under this heading is generally of two types—drugs your doctor may prescribe, and nonprescription drugs you can take safely.

Prescription drugs are named by generic name or drug class. A brief description of a drug's purpose and effect is given. For more information about a specific drug, see the Glossary. It contains entries for generic drugs and drug classes mentioned in this book.

Additionally, you may refer to the book, *Complete Guide to Prescription and Nonprescription Drugs.*

For general instructions about safe use of medicine, see the Appendix section.

18—ACTIVITY

Patients are often confused about whether they must stay in bed during an illness. They are often concerned with returning to work or school, and whether activity will be restricted after recovery. General answers to these questions are found under this heading.

In some topics, guidelines are given for resuming sexual relations—an important area that patients are sometimes reluctant to mention. If the illness has been life-threatening, as with a heart attack, or if it involves abdominal or genital organs, this is particularly pertinent information.

Exercise references are often included,

and when not specified otherwise, references to regular physical exercise mean an *aerobic* exercise such as walking.

19—DIET

Diet information can vary from "no special diet" to references to special diets. Some of these special diets are included in the Appendix section.

For additional specialized diets, consult your doctor or a dietitian.

20—CALL YOUR DOCTOR IF

For most medical problems, a phone call or visit to your doctor is recommended to establish a diagnosis.

After diagnosis, when the course of an illness differs from what is expected, your doctor wants to know. Many developing complications can be averted with prompt medical treatment. Specific symptoms are often listed that indicate complications.

Of course, if any other symptoms begin that you believe are related to your illness or the drugs you take, call your doctor about them, too.

Guide to Surgery Charts

The information about common surgeries, procedures or medical tests is organized in charts with a format similar to that for illness and disorder charts (see sample chart on facing page).

Generally, topics discussed in this section are those commonly performed as treatment for a disorder, such as thyroid-gland removal, or as a diagnostic procedure, such as dilatation and curettage. The topics may be about a minor procedure such as a toenail removal, or a major lifesaving procedure such as a heart transplant.

Sometimes a surgery is mentioned on an illness chart as part of treatment for that disorder. For instance, thyroid-gland removal is mentioned on the chart for hyperthyroidism (the previous sample chart) as a treatment for patients whose disorder does not respond to other treatment.

Each major heading on the surgery charts is numbered in the sample chart, and the numbered sections are explained in the next few pages.

1—NAME OF SURGERY

Charts are arranged alphabetically by the name that most simply describes the surgical procedure. In some cases, medical professionals refer to the surgery by a more technical name. The technical name may appear in parentheses below the main title.

Thyroid-gland removal is clearly understood by everyone, but your surgeon may refer to it as *thyroidectomy*. Both names are included on the chart, and the surgery appears in the index under both names.

2—GENERAL INFORMATION

This section contains four topics: *Definition; Body Parts Involved: Reasons for Surgery* and *Surgical Risk Increases With*. Each topic is discussed separately.

3—DEFINITION

A short definition of the surgery may include information about how common the procedure is and whether or not the medical problem requiring surgery is caused by congenital defects or is the result of disease or injury.

4—BODY PARTS INVOLVED

Body parts can refer to specific organs, such as the brain, or to body systems, such as the central nervous system.

Body parts are often defined in the text, if space permits. If you are not familiar with the body parts involved in a procedure, and the parts are not defined in text, refer to the Glossary for information.

5—REASONS FOR SURGERY

This section lists the most common reasons for a surgical procedure. (Of course, it cannot include *all* possible reasons.)

If the medical problems listed are unfamiliar to you, refer to the index. Some have separate illness charts, and the rest may be explained in the Glossary.

6—SURGICAL RISK INCREASES WITH

Risk factors make a surgery more complicated or delay healing. Following are common risk factors for most surgeries:

THYROID GLAND REMOVAL (Thyroidectomy)

GENERAL INFORMATION

DEFINITION—Removal of part or all of the thyroid gland.

BODY PARTS INVOLVED—Thyroid gland, the organ in the neck below the Adam's apple that controls the body's metabolism; lymph nodes in the neck.

REASONS FOR SURGERY
- Hyperthyroidism.
- Benign or cancerous tumors of the thyroid.
- Goiter (see Glossary).

SURGICAL RISK INCREASES WITH
- Adults over 60.
- Obesity; poor nutrition.
- Smoking.
- Untreated hyperthyroidism (see Glossary).
- Diabetes.
- Use of some prescription and nonprescription drugs. Inform your doctor of any drugs, medications, or vitamin and herb supplements you are using or have used in the last month.

WHAT TO EXPECT

WHO OPERATES—General surgeon.

WHERE PERFORMED—Hospital.

DIAGNOSTIC TESTS
- Before surgery: Blood studies; ultrasound; CT scan; needle biopsy; radioactive-iodine uptake and scan (see Glossary for all).
- After surgery: Blood studies.

ANESTHESIA—General anesthesia by injection and inhalation with an airway tube placed in the windpipe.

DESCRIPTION OF OPERATION
- An incision is made in the neck following natural skin lines.
- Neck muscles are cut or retracted.
- Blood supply to the thyroid gland is clamped.
- The thyroid gland is cut free and removed, and a drain is left in place. In certain cases, some normal thyroid gland tissue is left intact.
- If cancer is present, some lymph nodes may be removed around the thyroid.
- The muscles are closed and the skin is closed with sutures or clips, which can usually be removed in 2 to 10 days after surgery.

POSSIBLE COMPLICATIONS
- Hoarseness or loss of voice, if vocal-cord nerves are damaged during surgery.
- Hypothyroidism (see Glossary).
- Hypoparathyroidism (see Glossary).
- Excessive bleeding.
- Surgical-wound infection.

AVERAGE HOSPITAL STAY—0 to 3 days.

PROBABLE OUTCOME—Underlying problem cured in most patients. Cancer that is present but has not spread may require radiation treatment. Allow about 6 weeks for recovery from surgery.

POSTOPERATIVE CARE

GENERAL MEASURES
- A hard ridge should form along the incision. As it heals, the ridge will gradually recede.
- Use an electric heating pad, a heat lamp or a warm compress to relieve incisional pain.
- Shower as usual. You may wash the incision gently with mild, unscented soap. After showering, replace any wet dressings with clean, dry ones.

MEDICATION
- Your doctor may prescribe:
  - Pain relievers. Don't take prescription pain medication longer than 4 to 7 days. Use only as much as you need.
  - Thyroid hormones.
  - Antibiotics to fight or prevent infection.
- You may use nonprescription drugs, such as acetaminophen, for minor pain. Avoid aspirin.

ACTIVITY
- Return to daily activities and work as soon as possible to promote healing.
- Resume driving 2 weeks after you return home.
- Resume sexual relations when able.

DIET—No special diet.

CALL YOUR DOCTOR IF

- Pain, swelling, redness, drainage or bleeding increases in the surgical area.
- You develop signs of infection, including headache, muscle aches, dizziness or a general ill feeling and fever.
- You develop symptoms of hypothyroidism, including excessive weakness, fatigue, intolerance to cold, menstrual irregularities, constipation, or dry and coarse skin and hair.
- You develop symptoms of hypoparathyroidism (see Glossary), including dry hair, brittle fingernails; dry, scaly skin or irregular heartbeat.
- New, unexplained symptoms develop. Drugs used in treatment may produce side effects.

- Poor nutrition from any cause.
- Chronic illness.
- Recent illness, surgery or injury.
- Genetic factors.
- Obesity.
- Smoking.
- Alcoholism.
- Age, especially newborns and infants or older adults.
- Stress, anxiety, depression or other emotional problems.
- Use of drugs of abuse, such as narcotics, psychedelics, hallucinogens, marijuana, sedatives, hypnotics or cocaine.
- Use of some drugs or medications, whether prescription or nonprescription. Medicines most likely to increase surgical risk include antihypertensives, muscle relaxants, tranquilizers, sleep inducers, insulin, sedatives, cortisone, beta-adrenergic blockers, calcium-channel blockers and antibiotics.

These same drugs, of course, are lifesaving for some serious illnesses, but they can complicate treatment and outcome of other medical or surgical problems.

7—WHAT TO EXPECT

This section includes eight topics: *Who Operates; Where Performed; Diagnostic Tests; Anesthesia; Description of Operation; Possible Complications; Average Hospital Stay;* and *Probable Outcome*. Each topic is discussed separately.

8—WHO OPERATES

A routine surgery is often performed by a general surgeon or by a doctor who specializes in the body system involved. For instance, either a general surgeon or an obstetrician-gynecologist might remove an ovarian cyst.

Highly complicated surgeries, such as a heart transplant, are usually done by surgeons with additional specialized training.

We have included the type of surgeon most likely to perform the procedure, but variations can occur. In many communities general surgeons perform operations that are customarily performed elsewhere by a surgical subspecialist.

Your surgeon should not be uneasy about discussing with you before surgery his or her previous experience and education. Most competent surgeons welcome and sometimes recommend a second opinion when the surgery to be performed is elective rather than an emergency.

9—WHERE PERFORMED

A surgical procedure may be performed in any of the following places:
- A doctor's office.
- An independent, outpatient surgical facility.
- A hospital outpatient surgical facility.
- The operating room of a hospital.
- An emergency room.

10—DIAGNOSTIC TESTS

Diagnostic tests related to surgery can occur before, during or after the surgical procedure.

Laboratory studies are helpful in diagnosis and in providing necessary anatomical information prior to surgery. Many tests are the same as those discussed earlier in diagnosis of illnesses.

Some tests are especially useful in surgery. Examples include:
- Special x-ray studies of the gastrointestinal tract (upper GI series or lower GI series).
- Intravenous studies of the kidney and urinary tract (intravenous pyelogram and retrograde pyelogram).
- Coronary angiography (x-ray studies of the coronary arteries performed during a

cardiac catheterization procedure).
• Biopsy (microscopic study of tissue) before surgery to establish a diagnosis prior to extensive surgery (usually for cancer) and biopsy afterward of tissue removed during the surgical procedure.

11—ANESTHESIA

Anesthesia makes surgery possible without pain. Prior to giving anesthesia, most surgeons prescribe preoperative medications. These generally consist of:
• Tranquilizers or sedatives to help reduce apprehension.
• Pain relievers (frequently a narcotic drug such as morphine). This medication also reduces apprehension and decreases the amount of anesthesia needed.
• An anticholinergic drug, such as scopolamine or atropine, to decrease secretions from the nose, throat and lungs during the operation.

The type of anesthesia used depends on the surgical problem, the age and general condition of the patient, and sometimes on the availability of personnel to administer the anesthesia.

If an operation can be performed with any of several types of anesthesia, you have a right to know the advantages and disadvantages of each. If you wish, you have the right to participate in the selection. Don't hesitate to ask questions.

Before you have any anesthesia, tell your doctor or dentist about any allergic responses you have had to anesthesia in the past. Also inform him or her about any prescription or nonprescription drugs you take, and about any cardiovascular disease, heartbeat irregularities or peripheral vascular disease you have.

If a chart lists several anesthesia options for a surgery, you will have one of them, but not all.

The various types of anesthesia include:

Local Anesthesia—This is usually an injectable form of a drug ending in "caine," such as novocaine or lidocaine.

Local anesthesia is frequently injected into an injury site, such as a fracture, and bleeding from the injury disperses the anesthetic to all pain-sensitive parts of the injury. Local anesthesia may also be used to block a specific nerve bundle, allowing a pain-free procedure such as a tooth extraction.

Regional Anesthesia—This is used when it is desirable for the patient to remain conscious during the operation. Regional anesthesia works only on the part of the body upon which surgery is performed. Types of regional anesthesia includes: Spinal or epidural anesthesia.

Spinal anesthesia involves an injection of local anesthetic into the spinal canal, above the level of the surgery site. It relieves pain satisfactorily for many procedures below the waist, such as surgery of the rectum, genitourinary tract or lower extremities.

A special type of low-spinal anesthesia is called caudal anesthesia or "saddle block" (it affects the body area that comes into contact with a horse saddle).

Epidural anesthesia involves an injection of local anesthetic into the extradural (epidural) space in the lower back. It is used to block pain for the abdominal region.

General Anesthesia—This form of anesthesia is generally administered by inhalation or injection, or a combination of the two.

A short-acting hypnotic or sedative is injected into a vein, followed by a muscle relaxer. This quickly produces light sleep and allows placement of an airway tube (endotracheal tube) without discomfort. The tube is connected to hoses that lead to gas machines.

The anesthesiologist controls the flow

of anesthesia gases and monitors many body functions, such as blood pressure, breathing rate, pulse and ECG, while the patient sleeps.

When you awaken, the endotracheal tube may still be in place or may have been removed. Unless your respiration needs continued machine support, the endotracheal tube is usually removed in the recovery room.

The tube will make your throat sore for about 24 hours. This is normal and requires no treatment.

12—DESCRIPTION OF OPERATION

The surgical procedure is described in brief, nontechnical terms. Individual surgeons may use slightly varying techniques, but the basic steps are included and only details vary.

If you want additional information, your surgeon can give more details. An Internet search can also help you find resource materials with fuller descriptions and explanations. Be sure the website is a reliable one (such as those provided by the government, a university or hospital).

During some surgeries of the gastrointestinal tract, a hollow tube (Levin tube) is passed through your nose into your stomach after you are asleep. The tube will probably be in place when you awaken in the recovery room. The purpose of the tube is to keep the stomach empty to prevent vomiting or aspiration of material while you are asleep. It also keeps the stomach decompressed until normal muscular movement of the gastrointestinal tract can resume after surgery. An empty stomach is more comfortable and helps prevent complications that may arise if the stomach becomes distended with air or gas.

The average time in surgery and in the recovery room are left out because variations are too great. Factors that affect the time limits depend upon:
• The exact techniques chosen.
• The experience and preference of the surgeon.
• The availability and experience of assistants and operating room personnel.
• The presence or absence of complications during surgery.
• The age and condition of the patient prior to surgery.

Don't hesitate to ask your surgeon to estimate the time your operation will require.

13—POSSIBLE COMPLICATIONS

Complications are additional medical problems related to the surgery that occur during or after the procedure. They sometimes happen despite accurate diagnosis, skillful surgery, competent assistance and well-equipped operating rooms. Some complications are preventable, and some occur frequently— but most are rare.

14—AVERAGE HOSPITAL STAY

This estimate is based on an average. It varies according to how healing and recuperation progress and whether complications develop before, during or after surgery. It is also influenced by the amount insurance companies will allow as reimbursement of specific procedures.

15—PROBABLE OUTCOME

This heading relates to the surgery's effect on the underlying disorder and the average length of time required to recover from surgery. Estimates are based on the assumption that complications do not occur and healing proceeds normally. Complications can alter the course of healing dramatically. A positive outlook following surgery is an important factor in good outcome and rapid healing.

16—POSTOPERATIVE CARE

This section generally provides instructions for self-care during recuperation after hospitalization. It should serve as a reminder for instructions given you by your surgeon. It does not replace your doctor's instructions.

The section has four major topics: *General Measures; Medication; Activity;* and *Diet.*

17—GENERAL MEASURES

Some questions are almost universal following surgery. Most patients are unsure how to care for a surgical wound. They have questions about pain, bathing, stitches, clothing and other matters. These questions are answered in this section.

18—MEDICATION

Drugs usually prescribed after surgery are described, along with brief instructions for their use.

See Safe Use of Medicine (in Appendix) for general instructions.

19—ACTIVITY

Resumption of activity is a strong area of concern for postsurgical patients. Guidelines may be provided for when to return to school or work, when to resume driving, when to resume sexual relations and what types of exercise are appropriate. Again, it should serve as a reminder for instructions given you by your surgeon; it should not replace specific medical instructions.

20—DIET

During surgery with general anesthesia, the gastrointestinal tract is kept empty. After the patient awakens, clear liquids are usually provided until the gastrointestinal tract begins to function again. When appropriate, this information is included in the surgery charts. Additional diet instructions often refer to special diets in the Appendix section.

21—CALL YOUR DOCTOR IF

Call your doctor if healing and recuperation after surgery don't follow the usual course of events. Excessive bleeding and general or surgical-wound infection are common dangers after most surgical procedures, and these are always mentioned on surgery charts when appropriate.

Other reasons listed can serve as reminders of possible complications. If you develop symptoms you believe are related to your illness—even if they don't appear on the chart—call your doctor about them.

Symptoms

Symptom Charts

Find your main symptom on this list and then look at that chart for additional symptoms you may have. Remember, if you have symptoms that cause concern consult a health care provider

Abdominal Pain, Recurrent Attacks
Abdominal Pain, Sudden Attack
Abdominal Swelling
Ankle Pain
Ankles, Swollen
Anxiety and Nervousness
Appetite Loss
Arm or Hand Pain
Backache
Behavioral or Emotional Changes
Bleeding, Rectal
Bowel, Lack of Control
Breast Pain or Lumps
Breath, Bad
Breathing Difficulty
Bruising or Blood Spots Under the Skin,
    Unexplained
Burping or Gas
Chest Pain
Confusion (Person Over Age 65)
Confusion (Person Under Age 65)
Constipation
Cough
Cough With Blood
Coughing In Children
Crying, Excessive (Infant 0 To 6 Months)
Depression
Diarrhea (Infant 0 To 6 Months)
Diarrhea (Person Over 6 Months)
Dizziness
Ear, Ringing or Buzzing Sounds
Earache
Eye Pain; Swelling; Dryness; Itching;
    Tearing
Face Pain
Facial Skin Problems
Faintness or Fainting
Fatigue or Tiredness
Fever (Child 0 To 2 Years)
Fever (Child Over 2 Years)
Fever (Person Over Age 12)
Foot Problems
Genital Sores, Blisters, Warts or Boils
Hair Growth In Women, Excessive
Hair Loss
Headache
Hearing Loss
Heartbeat Irregularity

Impotence, Male Sexual
Itching
Knee Pain
Leg Pain
Memory Problems
Menstrual Periods, Late or Absent
Menstrual Periods, Painful or Heavy
Mouth, Sore; Tingling; Dry
Muscle Cramp; Ache; Weakness
Neck Pain
Nose, Stuffy or Runny
Numbness, Tingling or Prickling
Sexual Intercourse, Painful For Man
Sexual Intercourse, Painful For Woman
Shoulder Pain
Skin, Bumps on
Skin Problems (Child Under Age 2)
Skin Problems (Person Over Age 2)
Skin Rash With Fever
Skin Rash Without Fever
Sleeping Problems
Speaking Difficulty
Stool, Abnormal Appearance
Swallowing Difficulty
Sweating, Excessive
Swelling or Lump
Testicles or Penis, Painful or Swollen
Throat, Sore
Tongue, Sore
Toothache
Trembling or Twitching
Urination, Frequent
Urination, Lack of Control
Urination, Painful
Urine, Abnormal Color
Vaginal Bleeding, Unexpected
Vaginal Discharge, Abnormal
Vaginal Itching
Vision Disturbance or Loss
Voice Loss or Hoarseness
Vomiting (Infant 0 To 6 Months)
Vomiting, Recurrent Attacks
Vomiting, Sudden Attack
Weight Gain
Weight Gain, Slow (Child 0 To 5 Years)
Weight Loss
Wheezing

ABDOMINAL PAIN, RECURRENT ATTACKS

SYMPTOMS & FACTORS	POSSIBLE PROBLEM	WHAT TO DO*
• Recurrent pain in upper right abdomen that may spread to chest, back or shoulders. • No fever.	Gallbladder disorder.	See Gallstones.
• Recurrent pain in lower abdomen. • Nausea. • Recurrent diarrhea. • General ill feeling. • Fever during attacks. • Blood or mucus in stool.	Inflammatory disease of large intestine.	See Colitis, Ulcerative.
• Pain or cramping in the upper abdomen. • Appetite loss. • Weight loss.	• Inflammation. • Peptic-ulcer disease.	• See Gastritis. • See Ulcer, Peptic.
• Cramping pain in lower left abdomen (male). • Constant urge to have a bowel movement.	Rectum inflammation.	See Proctitis.
• Recurrent pain in upper abdomen. • Poor appetite. • Unexplained weight loss.	• Tumor. • Disorder of pancreas.	• See Stomach Cancer. • See Pancreatitis. • See Pancreatic Cancer.
• Recurrent pain in lower abdomen. • No fever. • Recurrent diarrhea, usually without blood.	• Inflammation of large intestine. • Tumor.	• See Diverticular Disease. • See Large Intestine Cancer.
• Recurrent pain in lower abdomen. • Recurrent diarrhea, usually without blood or mucus in stool. • General ill feeling. • Fever during attacks.	Inflammation of small intestine.	See Crohn's Disease.
• Recurrent pain in upper right abdomen. • Vomiting. • Fever during attacks.	Gallbladder inflammation.	See Cholecystitis or Cholangitis.
• Recurrent pain in lower abdomen. • Alternating diarrhea and constipation. • Recurrent, burning pain in upper abdomen, especially if bending forward or lying down.	• Disorder of muscle contractions in colon. • Stomach acid in esophagus.	• See Irritable Bowel Syndrome. • See Gastroesophageal Reflux Disease.
• Pain in upper abdomen. • Loss of appetite and weight loss. • Tender mass in upper right abdomen.	Cancer.	See Liver Cancer.
Pain in the pelvic, lower stomach and back areas.	Chronic pain.	See Chronic Pelvic Pain.

*All references are to Illness section unless noted otherwise.

ABDOMINAL PAIN, SUDDEN ATTACK (continued on next page)

SYMPTOMS & FACTORS	POSSIBLE PROBLEM	WHAT TO DO*
Abdominal pain following excessive consumption of alcohol or food.	Stomach inflammation.	• See Indigestion. • See Gastritis.
• Abdominal pain. • Diarrhea. • Vomiting.	• Infections of digestive tract. • Food poisoning.	• See Gastroenteritis. • See Food Poisoning. • See Salmonella Infections.
• Abdominal pain. • Diarrhea. • Flatulence and bloating.	Reaction to swallowed substance.	See Food Allergy.
• Abdominal pain that began in small of back, spreading to genital area. • Fever. • Frequent, painful, occasionally bloody urination.	Infection in urinary tract.	• See Bladder Infection, Female. • See Kidney Infection, Acute.
• Mild pain in lower abdomen. • Constipation or gas. • Recent diet change, such as adding more fiber.	Intestinal disturbance caused by diet change.	Consult doctor if discomfort persists longer than 3 hours.
• Severe abdominal pain, plus any of following: • Temperature of 100°F (37.8°C) or higher. • Constipation. • Abdominal swelling. • Vomiting.	Serious abdominal disorder.	• Call doctor now. • See Intestinal Obstruction. • See Appendicitis. • See Aneurysm. • See Peritonitis.
• Severe abdominal pain. • Menstrual period late 4 or more weeks. • Shoulder pain. • Abdominal pain that began in small of back, spreading to genital area. • No fever at onset of pain. • Smoky or bloody urine.	• Pregnancy developing outside uterus. • Kidney colic.	• See Ectopic Pregnancy. • See Kidney Stones.
• Pain in lower abdomen in woman. • Green-yellow, heavy or bad-smelling vaginal discharge.	Infection of reproductive organs.	• See Pelvic Inflammatory Disease. • See Ovarian Tumor, Benign.
• Burning pain of abdominal skin with tenderness along pain route. • Skin blisters.	Virus infection of sensory nerves.	See Herpes Zoster.
• Pain in upper right abdomen that may spread to chest, back or shoulders. • Nausea or vomiting.	• Gallbladder disorder. • Heart problem.	• See Gallstones. • See Pancreatitis. • See Heart Attack.

*All references are to Illness section unless noted otherwise.

ABDOMINAL PAIN, SUDDEN ATTACK
(continued from previous page)

SYMPTOMS & FACTORS	POSSIBLE PROBLEM	WHAT TO DO*
• Pain in lower abdomen in females. • Unexplained vaginal bleeding.	Several disorders.	See Vaginal Bleeding, Unexpected (in Symptoms section).
Recurrent abdominal pain for 1 week or more.	Several disorders.	See Abdominal Pain, Recurrent (in Symptoms section).
• Abdominal cramps. • Intermittent diarrhea. • Gas and abdominal bloating.	Parasitic infection.	See Amebiasis.

*All references are to Illness section unless noted otherwise.

ABDOMINAL SWELLING

SYMPTOMS & FACTORS	POSSIBLE PROBLEM	WHAT TO DO*
• Lower abdominal swelling that is slowly increasing. • No signs of pregnancy. • Persistent constipation.	• Intestinal disorder. • Tumor.	• See Constipation. • See Ovarian Tumor, Benign.
Abdominal swelling in woman 1 to 5 days before or during menstrual period.	Fluid retention caused by hormone changes.	• See Premenstrual Syndrome. • See Premenstrual Dysphoric Disorder.
• Abdominal swelling; bloated and full feeling. • Gas or belching. • Abdominal pain or discomfort.	• Heartburn. • Stones in gallbladder.	• See Indigestion. • See Gallstones.
• Abdominal swelling in last 24 hours. • Severe abdominal pain. • Fever. • Diarrhea or constipation. • Vomiting.	Serious abdominal disorder.	• Call doctor now. • See Intestinal Obstruction.
• Abdominal swelling. • Swollen ankles. • Breathing difficulty, especially at night.	Fluid in abdomen and other body parts caused by heart condition.	• Consult doctor. • See Congestive Heart Failure.
• Abdominal swelling. • Puffy ankles that hold a dent when pressed with finger. • Decreased urination.	Kidney disorder.	• Consult doctor. • See Glomerulonephritis. • See Wilms' Tumor (children only).
• Abdominal swelling. • Yellow skin and eyes.	Liver disorder.	• Consult doctor. • See Cirrhosis of the Liver.
• Abdominal swelling. • Overweight.	Effect of excess weight.	See Obesity & Overweight.
• Abdominal swelling in woman of childbearing age. • Tender, enlarged breasts. • Morning nausea. • No menstrual period for 2 months or longer.	Pregnancy.	Consult doctor to confirm pregnancy.
• Swollen abdomen in an infant. • Weight loss or slow weight gain. • Loose, pale, bad-smelling stools.	Gluten intolerance.	See Celiac Disease.

*All references are to Illness section unless noted otherwise.

ANKLE PAIN

SYMPTOMS & FACTORS	POSSIBLE PROBLEM	WHAT TO DO*
• Severe pain in ankle following injury. • Ankle can't move or bear weight. • Ankle swells rapidly and turns blue.	• Severe injury. • Broken bone.	• See Sprains & Strains. • See Bone Fracture.
• Pain in ankles or other joints, such as knees or fingers. • Affected joints red, warm, swollen. • No fever.	• Joint inflammation. • Degenerative condition of joints.	• See Arthritis, Rheumatoid. • See Arthritis, Juvenile Rheumatoid (children only). • See Gout. • See Osteoarthritis.
• Moderate pain in ankle following injury. • Ankle can move and bear weight.	Mild ligament injury.	See Sprains & Strains.
• Pain in ankle. • Ankle swollen, red and hot. • Fever. • Recent infection, such as gonorrhea.	Joint infection.	See Arthritis, Infectious.
• Pain in ankles or other joints. • Affected joints red, warm, swollen. • Fever. • General ill feeling. • Recent illness, such as sore throat or skin infection.	Complication of prior streptococcal infection.	• Consult doctor. • See Rheumatic Fever.
• Acute attack of swelling and pain in one or more joints. • Attacks may last for 2 or more days.	Joint disorder.	See Pseudogout.

*All references are to Illness section unless noted otherwise.

ANKLES, SWOLLEN

SYMPTOMS & FACTORS	POSSIBLE PROBLEM	WHAT TO DO*
• Swollen ankle. • Injury to ankle in last 4 months.	Normal swelling following injury.	If ankle becomes painful, consult doctor.
• Swollen ankles. • Recent confinement for several hours, such as car, bus, train, airplane. • No pain.	Normal occurrence.	• Elevate legs. When possible, avoid prolonged sitting or standing—move around frequently. • If swelling persists more than 48 hours, consult doctor.
Swollen, painful ankle.	Several disorders.	See Ankle Pain (in Symptoms section).
• Swollen ankles. • Use of prescription or nonprescription drug.	Adverse reaction or side effect of drug.	• Consult doctor about prescription drug. • Discontinue use of nonprescription drug.
• Swollen ankles. • Menstrual period due in a few days.	Fluid retention caused by hormone changes or excess salt intake.	See Premenstrual Syndrome.
Swollen or distended veins in ankles.	Dilated, twisted or blocked veins.	• See Varicose Veins. • See Thrombophlebitis, Superficial.
• Swollen ankles. • Pregnancy.	Common occurrence during pregnancy, but may be sign of high blood pressure.	See Preeclampsia & Eclampsia.
• Swollen ankle. • Calf of swollen leg is tender. • Pain when flexing ankle.	Blood clot in deep vein.	• Call doctor now. • See Thrombosis, Deep-Vein.
• Swollen ankles. • Chronic breathing difficulty that is worsening. • Cough that is worse when lying down.	Fluid in lungs and other body parts caused by heart condition.	• See Congestive Heart Failure. • See Glomerulonephritis.
• Swollen ankles. • Use of oral contraceptives, cortisone drugs or nonsteroidal anti-inflammatory drugs.	• Adverse reaction or side effect of drug. • Blood clot in deep vein.	• Consult doctor. • See Thrombosis, Deep-Vein.

*All references are to Illness section unless noted otherwise.

ANXIETY AND NERVOUSNESS
(continued on next page)

SYMPTOMS & FACTORS	POSSIBLE PROBLEM	WHAT TO DO*
• Anxiety, plus any of following: • Inability to listen attentively and remember. • Clinging dependency. • Cold or hot flashes. • Cool, sweaty hands. • Abdominal cramps. • Diarrhea or constipation. • Dizziness. • Dry mouth. • Lack of concentration. • Faintness. • Rapid heartbeat. • Impotence in men. • Low frustration level. • Muscle tension and pain (backache, neck ache, headache). • Painful menstruation. • Painful sexual intercourse. • Pale or flushed skin. • Restlessness. • Tightness in chest. • Frequent urination.	Effect of stress or unrecognized fear.	• See Anxiety Disorder, Generalized. • See Stress.
Anxiety about any of following: enclosed spaces, airplanes, crowds, heights, "going crazy," infection; or death.	Psychological disorder.	See Phobias.
• Anxiety, plus 2 or more of following: • Weight loss. • Bulging eyes. • Excessive sweating. • Fatigue. • Rapid or irregular heartbeat.	Overactive thyroid gland.	See Hyperthyroidism.
Persistent anxiety without other symptoms.	Effect of stress.	See Anxiety Disorder, Generalized.
• Anxiety. • Dizziness or lightheadedness. • Rapid breathing. • Frequent sighing.	Decreased carbon dioxide in blood.	See Panic Disorder.
• Anxiety. • Use of prescription or nonprescription drug.	Adverse reaction or side effect of drug.	• Consult doctor about prescription drug. • Discontinue use of nonprescription drug if symptoms persist.
• Nervousness and irritability in a female. • Menstrual period is due.	Hormone fluctuation.	• See Premenstrual Syndrome. • See Premenstrual Dysphoric Disorder.

*All references are to Illness section unless noted otherwise

ANXIETY AND NERVOUSNESS
(continued from previous page)

SYMPTOMS & FACTORS	POSSIBLE PROBLEM	WHAT TO DO*
• Anxiety. • Recent withdrawal from tobacco, alcohol or drug, such as sleeping pills.	Withdrawal symptom.	• Consult doctor about drug withdrawal. • See Substance Abuse. • See Alcoholism.
• Anxiety behavior in a child. • Restlessness; inability to be still. • Unable to pay attention to directions.	Psychological disorder.	See Attention Deficit Hyperactivity Disorder.
• Anxiety involving recurrent, intrusive and distressing recollection of an event. • Reliving of an event.	Psychological disorder.	See Post-Traumatic Stress Disorder.

*All references are to Illness section unless noted otherwise.

APPETITE LOSS (continued on next page)

(continued on next page)

SYMPTOMS & FACTORS	POSSIBLE PROBLEM	WHAT TO DO*
• Appetite loss. • Nausea and vomiting. • Fever.	Irritation or infection of digestive tract.	See Gastroenteritis.
• Appetite loss. • Use of vitamins or prescription or nonprescription drug, especially: anticancer drugs; digitalis; aminophylline; narcotics; antihistamines; ephedrine; methylphenidate; diphenyl-hydantoin; or amphetamines.	Adverse reaction or side effect of drug.	• Consult doctor about prescription drug. • Discontinue use of nonprescription drugs.
• Appetite loss, plus 2 or more of following: • Fever. • Sore throat. • Headache. • Painful swelling in neck, armpit or groin. • Fatigue. • Jaundice (yellow skin and eyes). • Pain in upper right abdomen.	Virus infection.	See Mononucleosis, Infectious.
• Appetite loss. • Pain or pressure in stomach. • Excessive consumption of alcohol or food.	Stomach inflammation caused by alcohol or spices.	See Gastritis.
• Appetite loss. • Depression or anxiety.	Effect of stress.	• See Depression. • See Anxiety Disorder, Generalized. • See Anorexia Nervosa. • See Stress.
• Decrease in appetite (especially in a child). • Low-grade fever. • Runny nose and cough.	Virus infection.	See Respiratory Syncytial Virus.
• Appetite loss. • Emotional upset such as grief.	Temporary emotional situation.	Appetite will return in time. Drink plenty of fluids.
• Appetite loss (sudden). • Headache. • Nausea or vomiting. • Bloody, decreased urine. • Puffy face.	Kidney disorder.	See Glomerulonephritis.
• Appetite loss. • Nausea at sight of food, plus 2 or more of following: • Jaundice (yellow skin and eyes). • Vomiting. • Tenderness over liver area. • Fever. • Weakness and fatigue.	Liver disorder.	• See Hepatitis, Viral. • See Cirrhosis of the Liver.
• Appetite loss. • Weight loss. • Vague feeling of illness or fatigue.	Early signs of cancer or other disorder.	Consult doctor.

*All references are to Illness section unless noted otherwise.

APPETITE LOSS
(continued from previous page)

SYMPTOMS & FACTORS	POSSIBLE PROBLEM	WHAT TO DO*
• Appetite loss. • Fatigue. • Weight loss. • Hair loss. • Craving for salt. • Skin that darkens. • Dizziness on standing.	Inadequate cortisone hormone.	See Addison's Disease.
• Appetite loss with weight gain. • Loss of energy, fatigue. • Puffy face. • Decreased sex drive. • Dry skin and hair. • Constipation. • Low voice.	Underactive thyroid gland.	See Hypothyroidism.
• Appetite loss. • Excessive alcohol consumption.	Vitamin deficiency caused by alcohol.	See Alcoholism.
• Appetite loss. • Weight loss, plus 2 or more of following: • Paleness. • Sore, red, smooth, burning tongue. • Yellowish skin.	Vitamin B-12 and folic-acid deficiency.	See Anemia, Pernicious.
• Gradual appetite loss in woman 45 or older. • Fatigue. • Menstrual changes.	Normal occurrence with the decreasing estrogen level of menopause.	See Menopause.
• Appetite loss. • Fluid retention. • Reduced urine production.	Kidney disease.	See Nephrotic Syndrome.
• Appetite loss in child. • Irritability. • Paleness.	Disorder of red-blood cells.	See Anemia, Iron Deficiency.
• Appetite loss. • Nausea. • Pregnancy or possible pregnancy.	Effect of hormone change during pregnancy.	Eat small, frequent meals.
Appetite loss in child around age 2.	Normal occurrence caused by slowed growth rate.	Nothing. Appetite will return when growth accelerates.
• Poor appetite. • Sleeping problems. • Lack of energy. • Feelings of hopelessness; self-pity.	Chronic mild depression.	See Dysthymia.
• Appetite loss and weight loss. • Tender mass in upper right abdomen. • Pain in upper right abdomen.	Cancer.	See Liver Cancer.

*All references are to Illness section unless noted otherwise.

ARM OR HAND PAIN

SYMPTOMS & FACTORS	POSSIBLE PROBLEM	WHAT TO DO*
• Pain in elbow, wrist or finger joint when bending arm or hand. • No redness or swelling.	Tendon inflammation.	• See Tendinitis. • See Tennis Elbow.
• Pain in arm or hand. • Numbness or tingling in arm or hand, especially at night. • No recent injury.	Pressure on nerves in wrist.	See Carpal Tunnel Syndrome.
• Severe pain in arm after injury. • Arm not misshapen.	Muscle or ligament injury.	See Sprains & Strains.
• Severe pain in arm after injury. • Arm misshapen.	Broken bone.	• Call doctor now. • See Bone Fracture.
• Pain in arm during exercise. • Feeling of pressure in chest.	Temporary lack of oxygen to heart.	• Call doctor if pain lasts longer than 5 minutes. • See Angina Pectoris. • See Coronary Artery Disease.
• Pain in elbow, wrist or finger joint. • Affected joint red and swollen. • Fever and general ill feeling.	Bone or joint infection.	• Consult doctor. • See Osteomyelitis. • See Arthritis, Infectious.
• Pain in elbow, wrist or finger joints. • Joints are red, warm, swollen. • Fever. • Recent illness, such as sore throat, gonorrhea or skin infection.	Complication of prior streptococcal infection.	See Rheumatic Fever.
• Discomfort in fingers. • Fingers turn pale, then bluish, then red, when exposed to cold.	Circulation disorder.	See Raynaud Disease & Phenomenon.
• Pain in elbow, wrist or finger joint. • Affected joint red, warm, swollen.	Joint inflammation.	• See Osteoarthritis. • See Arthritis, Rheumatoid. • See Arthritis, Juvenile Rheumatoid (children only). • See Bursitis. • See Gout. • See Psoriatic Arthritis.
• Pain in arm or hand. • Numbness or tingling in arm or hand. • Stiff neck and cracking sound with neck movement.	Pressure on nerves in neck.	See Cervical Spondylosis.
Pain around fingernails.	Tissue inflammation.	See Paronchia.
• Redness, swelling, warmth around a nail. • Sudden pain around the nail.	Herpes infection of the skin.	See Herpetic Whitlow.
• Arm or leg pain (may be burning or aching) and swelling. • Changes in skin color.	Unknown.	See Reflex Sympathetic Dystrophy.

*All references are to Illness section unless noted otherwise.

BACKACHE
(continued on next page)

SYMPTOMS & FACTORS	POSSIBLE PROBLEM	WHAT TO DO*
• Sudden backache. • Recent fall or injury to back. • Pain only at injury site.	Muscle injury or muscle spasm.	• See Sprains & Strains. • See Back Pain, Low. • See Disk, Ruptured.
• Sudden sharp pain down back of leg. • Recent heavy lifting or strenuous exercise.	Pressure on large nerve in leg.	See Back Pain, Low.
• Sudden backache in person over age 60. • Sharp pain in one place over the spine. OR • Recent confinement to bed or wheelchair.	Bone damage caused by softening of bones.	• Consult doctor. • See Osteoporosis.
• Backache. • Fever. • Painful urination.	• Kidney infection. • Virus infection.	• See Kidney Infection, Acute. • See Influenza.
• Backache in person older than 60. • Pain in other joints.	Degenerative condition.	See Osteoarthritis.
• Backache. • Overweight plus any of the following: • Use of chair too high or too low for desk. • Recent heavy lifting or strenuous exercise. • Recent use of jackhammer or other heavy equipment.	Strain of back muscle or ligament.	• See Back Pain, Low. • See Obesity &. Overweight.
• Chronic backache. • Numbness or tingling in extremities that is worsening.	Pressure on spinal cord.	See Spinal-Cord Tumor.
• Sudden backache. • Recent fall or injury to back, plus any of following: • Difficulty moving arm or leg. • Loss of bladder or bowel control. • Numbness or tingling in extremities.	Damaged spinal cord.	• Call doctor now. • Don't move injured person.
• Backache in female. • Wearing high heels.	Poor weight distribution.	Wear lower heels.
• Chronic backache. • Repetitive work such as computer use or typing.	Poor posture, incorrect chair or desk height.	• Correct problem with posture or equipment. • See Back Pain, Low.
Backache that is worse in morning.	• Lack of adequate back support during sleep. • Chronic inflammation.	• Sleep on back or side. • Use mattress that is neither too firm or too soft. • See Spondylitis, Ankylosing.

*All references are to Illness section unless noted otherwise.

BACKACHE
(continued from previous page)

SYMPTOMS & FACTORS	POSSIBLE PROBLEM	WHAT TO DO*
• Backache that worsens with lifting. • Lump in back or front of the vagina or projecting outside of it.	Fallen uterus.	See Uterine Prolapse.
• Pain in bones in back. • Weight loss. • Symptoms of anemia.	Cancer.	See Multiple Myeloma.
• Back pain in female. • Pain with sexual intercourse. • Blood in the urine.	Disorder of the uterus.	See Endometriosis.
• Back pain. • Visible curving of the upper body.	Curvature of the spine.	See Scoliosis.

*All references are to Illness section unless noted otherwise.

BEHAVIORAL OR EMOTIONAL CHANGES (continued on next page)

SYMPTOMS & FACTORS	POSSIBLE PROBLEM	WHAT TO DO*
• Behavior that involve thoughts of failure, inadequacy and negative thoughts. • Lack of energy. • Sleeping problems. • Poor appetite.	Mild or clinical depression.	• See Dysthymia. • See Depression.
• Behavioral changes. • Use of a prescription or nonprescription drug.	Adverse reaction or side effect of drug.	• Consult doctor about prescription drug. • Discontinue nonprescription drug.
Obsessions and/or compulsive behaviors that consume more than an hour a day.	Psychological disorder.	See Obsessive Compulsive Disorder.
Anxiety symptoms when exposed to, or thinking of, a particular stimulus.	Psychological disorder.	See Phobias.
• Recurrent, intrusive and distressing recollection of an event. • Reliving of an event.	Psychological disorder.	See Post-Traumatic Stress Disorder.
• Start of winter season. • Depression. • Irritability. • Tiredness.	Lack of light.	See Seasonal Affective Disorder.
• Fear of going crazy. • Fear of dying. • Sense of terror or doom. • Palpitations. • Rapid heartbeat.	Severe anxiety.	See Panic Disorder.
• Behavioral changes in a female. • Week to 14 days before menstrual period. OR • Beginning of menopause.	Hormone fluctuations.	• See Premenstrual Syndrome. • See Premenstrual Dysphoric Disorder. • See Menopause.
• Young child. • Easily distracted. • Squirms in seat.	Behavioral problem.	See Attention Deficit Hyperactivity Disorder.
• Irritability. • Paleness, fatigue, lethargy. • Abdominal discomfort. • Headache. • Tremor.	Inhalation or ingestion of lead.	See Lead Poisoning.
Behavioral changes in an elderly person.	Mental deterioration.	• See Alzheimer's Disease. • See Dementia.

*All references are to Illness section unless noted otherwise.

BEHAVIORAL OR EMOTIONAL CHANGES
(continued from previous page)

SYMPTOMS & FACTORS	POSSIBLE PROBLEM	WHAT TO DO*
• Behavioral changes. • Recent withdrawal from tobacco, alcohol or drug, such as sleeping pills.	Withdrawal symptom.	• Consult doctor about drug withdrawal. • See Substance Abuse. • See Alcoholism.
• Behavioral or personality changes. • Stiff neck. • General ill feeling. • Headache; vomiting; fever.	Brain inflammation.	See Encephalitis, Viral.
• Confusion. • Restlessness and anxiety. • Weakness. • Muscle cramps.	Electrolyte disorder.	See Sodium Imbalance.
In infant: Restlessness, poor sleep habits, profuse sweating, delayed motor skills.	Vitamin deficiency.	See Vitamin Deficiencies.
• Behavior changes. • Stressful life event (sometimes called a stressor).	Reaction to an event.	See Adjustment Disorders.
Child is not behaving, talking, playing, or learning new skills as expected for their age group.	Developmental problem.	See Autism.
Child's behavior changes (avoiding family or friends, sleeping problems, school problems, emotional upsets).	Possible child abuse.	See Child Abuse.
• Behavior includes: delusions (fixed false, unreal beliefs) and hallucinations (hearing voices or seeing things that are not there). • Becomes more withdrawn.	Mental disorder.	See Schizophrenic Disorders.

*All references are to Illness section unless noted otherwise.

BLEEDING, RECTAL

SYMPTOMS & FACTORS	POSSIBLE PROBLEM	WHAT TO DO*
• Bright red bleeding. • Rectal pain and itching.	Dilated rectal and anal veins.	See Hemorrhoids.
• Rectal bleeding. • Pain with bowel movements. • Discomfort when cleaning after bowel movements.	Tear in the skin or sphincter muscle surrounding the rectum.	See Anal Fissure.
Bright red rectal bleeding following injury, insertion of foreign object in the rectum, or anal sex.	Traumatic tear in the skin or sphincter muscle surrounding the rectum.	Consult doctor immediately.
• Rectal bleeding. • Abdominal cramps. • Severe abdominal pain. • Vomiting.	• Intestinal adhesions. • Intestinal tumors and cancers. • Twisted bowel.	See Intestinal Obstruction.
Rectal bleeding in a child with severe abdominal pain.	Telescoping of intestine into itself.	See Intussusception.
Rectal bleeding plus unexplained bleeding from other body orifices.	Bleeding disorder.	• See Renal Failure, Acute. • See Anemia, Aplastic. • See Leukemia, Acute.
• Blood in stool. • Vomiting blood.	Ulceration of stomach lining.	See Gastric Erosion.
• Bloody diarrhea with mucus. • Abdominal pain.	Inflammation of bowel.	See Colitis, Ulcerative.
• Blood, mucus or pus in stool. • Diarrhea and abdominal cramps. • Fever.	Bacteria infection.	See Dysentery, Bacillary.
Blood in stool that is mixed with feces and appears black or dark red.	Bleeding from an abnormality in the stomach, duodenum or colon.	• Consult doctor. • See Stomach Cancer. • See Ulcer, Peptic. • See Diverticular Disease. • See Large Intestine Polyp. • See Crohn's Disease. • See Large Intestine Cancer. • See Small Intestine Tumor.
• Mucous discharge, sometimes tinged with blood. • Sense of fullness in abdomen or rectal area. • Tissue mass that can be felt after bowel movement.	Rectal tissue disorder.	See Rectal Prolapse.

*All references are to Illness section unless noted otherwise.

BOWEL, LACK OF CONTROL

SYMPTOMS & FACTORS	POSSIBLE PROBLEM	WHAT TO DO*
• Lack of bowel control, plus any of following: • Recent childbirth with episiotomy. • Recent surgery of vagina. • History of rectal surgery. • Anal fissure or fistula. • Hemorrhoids.	Rectal or anal abnormalities caused by any of several factors.	Consult doctor.
• Lack of bowel control. • Convulsions or unconsciousness.	Brain abnormality, such as tumor or stroke.	Call doctor now.
• Lack of bowel control. • Lump just inside anus.	Rectal tumor.	See Large Intestine Cancer.
• Lack of bowel control, plus any of following: • Slurred speech. • Weakness or paralysis of any part of body. • Unconsciousness. • Blurred vision.	• Decreased blood supply to brain. • Pressure on spinal cord.	• See Stroke. • See Spinal-Cord Tumor.
• Lack of bowel control. • Acute diarrhea.	Powerful, uncontrollable bowel function.	See Diarrhea, Acute.
• Frequent leakage of small amounts of stool. • Chronic constipation, especially in child or person over 65.	Stretched anus caused by constipation.	See Fecal Impaction.
Lack of bowel control in a young child who once was toilet-trained.	• Regressive behavior. • Emotional disturbance caused by factors such as: new siblings; change in home or school; divorce of parents; parental withdrawal, neglect or abuse.	See Encopresis.
• Lack of bowel control. • Mental retardation.	Failure to achieve control due to intellectual deficit.	Continue attempts to toilet train. Place person on toilet at regular times. Provide rewards for success.

*All references are to Illness section unless noted otherwise.

BREAST PAIN OR LUMPS

SYMPTOMS & FACTORS	POSSIBLE PROBLEM	WHAT TO DO*
Breast pain or lump that can be felt or seen.	• Cyst. • Tumor.	• Consult doctor. • See Fibrocystic Breast Changes. • See Breast Cancer.
• Pain or tenderness in breasts before menstrual periods. • Irregular periods. • Woman over age 38.	Thickening of gland tissue in breasts caused by hormonal changes.	See Menopause.
• Throbbing pain in breast of new mother. • Hard, tender, red lump on breast, or inflamed nipple. • Fever.	Breast infection.	See Mastitis.
• Breast pain. • Use of estrogen medications.	Adverse reaction or side effect of drug.	Consult doctor.
• Pain or tenderness in breasts. • Possible pregnancy.	Common sensitivity during pregnancy.	Wear a support bra as breasts enlarge.
Swollen, tender, hard breasts within 4 days of delivering baby.	Engorgement of breast tissue with milk.	Consult doctor.
• Sore nipples in woman who is breast-feeding. OR • Sharp pain in nipple of nursing mother when breast-feeding baby. • No fever. • No other symptoms related to breast.	Cracked or sore nipples. Common occurrence during first weeks of breast-feeding.	• Wash nipples and apply lanolin cream after breast-feeding. • Consult doctor if fever develops.
• Pain or tenderness in breasts. • Menstrual period due in a few days.	Discomfort caused by hormone changes.	• See Premenstrual Syndrome. • See Premenstrual Dysphoric Disorder.
• Breast pain. • Breast is tender, red or hard. • Fever and chills. • Tenderness in the area under the arm.	Bacterial infection.	See Breast Abscess.

*All references are to Illness section unless noted otherwise.

BREATH, BAD

SYMPTOMS & FACTORS	POSSIBLE PROBLEM	WHAT TO DO*
• Bad breath. • Bleeding gums. OR • Aching teeth and gums when eating hot, cold or sweet foods.	Gum inflammation.	• See Gingivitis. • See Periodontitis.
• Bad breath. • Dentures.	Food particles trapped in dentures.	Consult dentist if home-cleaning techniques fail.
• Bad breath. • No visit to dentist in last 6 months or poor dental hygiene.	Tooth decay or plaque deposits.	• Consult dentist. • See Tooth Decay.
• Bad breath. • Recent consumption of garlic, onions or alcohol.	Metabolism of these substances.	Nothing. Breath will return to normal.
• Bad breath. • Cold or sore throat.	Symptom of infection.	Nothing. Breath will return to normal.
• Bad breath caused by dry mouth. • Use of drugs causing dry mouth, such as diuretics, antihistamines, some drugs for high-blood pressure, cancer and angina.	Effects of dry mouth on odor control.	• Drink plenty of water or citrus juices; chew sugarless gum or suck on hard candies. • Consult doctor if problem is causing concern.
• Bad breath. • Persistent cough with bad-smelling sputum.	Chronic lung infection.	• See Bronchiectasis. • See Lung Abscess.
• Bad breath. • Fever.	Common occurrence with fever and illness.	See Fever charts (in Symptoms section).
• Bad breath that smells like ammonia. • Kidney disease.	Kidney failure.	• See Renal Failure, Acute. • See Renal Failure, Chronic.
• Bad breath. • Sore mouth or tongue.	Infection or sores in mouth or tongue.	See Sore Mouth (in Symptoms section).

*All references are to Illness section unless noted otherwise.

BREATHING DIFFICULTY (continued on next page)

SYMPTOMS & FACTORS	POSSIBLE PROBLEM	WHAT TO DO*
• Breathing difficulty. • Fever. • Cough with green-yellow or brownish sputum.	Infection of breathing passages.	• See Pneumonia (all charts). • See Bronchitis, Acute.
• Breathing difficulty. • Lightheadedness. • Numbness or tingling in hands and feet. • Stress, fear or anxiety.	Decreased carbon dioxide in blood.	• See Panic Disorder. • See Anxiety Disorder Generalized.
• Mild breathing difficulty. • Noisy breathing.	Spasm of bronchial tubes.	See Wheezing (in Symptoms section).
• Chronic breathing difficulty that is worsening. • Persistent cough with sputum. • Dusty working conditions.	Lung inflammation.	• See Pneumoconiosis. • See Silicosis. • See Asbestosis.
• Chronic breathing difficulty that is worsening. • Persistent cough with sputum. • No dusty working conditions.	Chronic inflammation or infection of breathing passages.	• See Bronchitis, Chronic. • See Chronic Obstructive Pulmonary Disease. • See Bronchiectasis. • See Emphysema.
• Shortness of breath. • Chest pain. • Shock.	Lung collapse.	See Atelectasis.
• Shortness of breath. • Ascent to high altitude. • Headache; nausea.	Lack of oxygen.	See Altitude Illness.
• Trouble breathing. • Dizziness. • Headache. • Nausea and vomiting.	Gas inhalation.	See Carbon Monoxide Poisoning.
• Difficult breathing in child under 6. • Barking cough. OR • Wheezing with rapid, shallow breathing.	Inflammation or infection.	• See Croup. • See Bronchiolitis.
• Shortness of breath. • Tiredness and weakness. • Paleness.	Lack of red blood cells.	See Anemia (all charts).
• Shortness of breath. • Fatigue. • Irregular heartbeat.	Heart inflammation.	See Myocarditis.
• Difficult breathing. • Tingling or numbness. • Sneezing, wheezing or itching.	Allergic reaction.	• Call doctor now or seek emergency help. • See Anaphylaxis.

*All references are to Illness section unless noted otherwise.

BREATHING DIFFICULTY
(continued from previous page)

SYMPTOMS & FACTORS	POSSIBLE PROBLEM	WHAT TO DO*
• Rapid breathing. • Dull or sharp pain in front of chest. • Cough; fever; chills.	Heart inflammation.	See Pericarditis.
• Sudden breathing difficulty. • Severe chest pain spreading to jaw, neck or arms.	Heart attack or other heart problem.	• Call doctor now. • See Heart Attack. • See Coronary Artery Disease. • See Heart Rhythm Irregularity. • See Heartbeat, Rapid.
• Sudden breathing difficulty. • Sharp chest pain that worsens with inhalation.	• Blood clot in lung. • Collapsed lung.	• Call doctor now. • See Pulmonary Embolism. • See Pneumothorax.
• Sudden breathing difficulty. • Chest pain.	Temporary lack of oxygen to heart.	See Angina Pectoris.
• Chronic breathing difficulty that is worsening. • Swollen ankles.	Fluid in lungs and other body parts caused by heart condition.	See Congestive Heart Failure.
• Extreme shortness of breath. • Congestive heart failure.	Lack of oxygen in blood.	• Call doctor now. • See Pulmonary Edema.
• Rapid, shallow breathing. • Chest pain. • Chills and fever.	Severe lung infection.	See Empyema.

*All references are to Illness section unless noted otherwise.

BRUISING OR BLOOD SPOTS UNDER THE SKIN, UNEXPLAINED

SYMPTOMS & FACTORS	POSSIBLE PROBLEM	WHAT TO DO*
• Unexplained blood spots under skin. • Fever. • Pain in affected area. • Headache. • Weakness. • General ill feeling.	Bacterial, viral or parasitic infection.	Consult doctor.
• Unexplained bruising or blood spots under skin. • Use of prescription or nonprescription drug, such as: anticoagulants; aspirin; sulfa drugs; Digitoxin; quinine; quinidine; antihistamines; phenothiazines; antidepressants; local anesthetics; penicillin; mercury; bismuth; cortisone drugs; or anticonvulsants.	Adverse reaction or side effect of drug.	Consult doctor.
Unexplained bruising in healthy child.	Possible child abuse.	See Child Abuse.
• Unexplained bruising or blood spots under skin. • Swollen gums that bleed occasionally.	Poor nutrition.	• Consult doctor. • See Vitamin Deficiencies.
Unexplained blood spots under skin following violent coughing, vomiting or choking.	Raised pressure in blood vessels of head and neck.	Consult doctor.
• Unexplained bruising in newborn. • Jaundice (yellow skin and eyes).	Blood disorder.	See Rh Isoimmunization.
• Unexplained bruising or blood spots under skin. • Recent virus infection.	Blood disorder.	• Call doctor now. • See Thrombocytopenia.
• Unexplained bruising on lower extremities. • Abdominal pain. • Red, swollen and tender joints.	Allergic disorder.	See Purpura, Allergic.
• Frequent bruises. • Painful, swollen joints. • Excessive bleeding from minor cuts.	Blood disorder.	See Hemophilia.
• Unexplained bruising or blood spots under skin. • Kidney or liver disorder.	Abnormal platelet function.	See Renal Failure, Chronic.
• Easy bruising and spontaneous bleeding. • Fever; tiredness; paleness. • General ill feeling.	Cancer.	See Leukemia, Acute.

*All references are to Illness section unless noted otherwise.

BURPING OR GAS

SYMPTOMS & FACTORS	POSSIBLE PROBLEM	WHAT TO DO*
• Burping. • Discomfort and fullness after eating.	Air swallowed while eating.	• See Indigestion. • See Heartburn.
• Burping that worsens after eating fatty foods. • Pain in upper right abdomen that may spread to back.	Gallbladder disorder.	See Gallstones.
• Gas or bloating. • Consumption of cow's milk or other dairy product.	Inability to digest lactose.	See Lactose Intolerance.
• Gas. • Pale, bad-smelling stool. • Unexplained weight loss.	Poor digestion.	See Malabsorption.
Burping that worsens when bending or lying down.	Stomach acid in esophagus.	See Gastroesophageal Reflux Disease.
Burping excessively plus any of the following: drinking carbonated beverages; eating too quickly; not chewing food properly; chewing gum or sucking hard candies.	Swallowed air.	Change eating habits. Avoid causative agent.
• Gas. • Alternating constipation and diarrhea. • Lower abdominal pain that is relieved by passing gas or bowel movements.	Disorder of muscle contractions in colon.	See Irritable Bowel Syndrome.
• Burping. • Discomfort and fullness after eating. • Nausea; poor appetite.	Tumor.	See Stomach Cancer.
• Gas. • High-fiber diet or consumption of gas-causing foods.	Effect of diet.	Nothing. Improves eventually.
• Indigestion symptoms (burping). • Pain in upper abdomen. • Pain comes and goes.	Ulcer.	See Ulcer, Peptic.
• Gas and abdominal bloating. • Abdominal cramps. • Intermittent diarrhea.	Parasitic infection.	See Amebiasis.

*All references are to Illness section unless noted otherwise.

CHEST PAIN
(continued on next page)

SYMPTOMS & FACTORS	POSSIBLE PROBLEM	WHAT TO DO*
• Severe chest pain beneath breastbone, spreading to jaw, neck or arms. • Sweating. • Anxious feeling. • Sudden breathing difficulty. • Nausea, vomiting.	Life-threatening heart attack.	• Call doctor now. • See Heart Attack. • See Heartbeat, Rapid. • See Coronary Artery Disease.
• Chest pain. • Sudden breathing difficulty. • Recent surgery. OR • Recent injury or illness requiring bed confinement.	Blood clot from leg or pelvis that has lodged in lung.	• Call doctor now. • See Pulmonary Embolism. • See Atelectasis.
• Severe chest pain, spreading to jaw, neck or arms. • No other symptoms.	• Temporary lack of oxygen to heart. • Life-threatening heart damage.	• Call doctor now. • See Angina Pectoris. • See Coronary Artery Disease.
• Sharp chest pain that worsens with inhalation. • Sudden breathing difficulty. • No other factors.	Collapsed lung.	• Call doctor now. • See Pneumothorax.
• Chest pain. • Shortness of breath. • Cough. • Fever.	• Lung infection. • Inflammation of membranes around lungs. • Fungal infection.	• See Pneumonia (all charts). • See Pleurisy. • See Empyema. • See Blastomycosis.
• Chest pain on one side. • Burning feeling at pain site. • Pain unaffected by breathing. • Skin rash at pain site.	Virus infection of sensory nerves.	See Herpes Zoster.
• Chest pain. • Cough with green or gray-yellow sputum.	Infection of bronchial tubes.	See Bronchitis, Acute.
• Chest pain on one side. • Recent chest injury, chest surgery or severe cough.	Pulled muscle or broken rib.	• See Sprains & Strains. • See Bone Fracture.
• Pain in the chest or upper abdomen. • Heartburn.	Digestive disorder.	• See Indigestion. • See Gastroesophageal Reflux Disease. • See Heartburn. • See Hiatal Hernia.
Chest pain that worsens when swallowing.	Several disorders.	See Swallowing Difficulty (in Symptoms section).
• Pain in chest wall. • Affected area sensitive to touch.	Cartilage inflammation.	See Costochondritis.
• Chest pain (sharp, dull or pressing). • Fatigue, shortness of breath. • Dizziness; anxiety.	Heart disorder.	See Mitral Valve Prolapse.

*All references are to Illness section unless noted otherwise.

CHEST PAIN
(continued from previous page)

SYMPTOMS & FACTORS	POSSIBLE PROBLEM	WHAT TO DO*
• Chest pain; palpitations. • Rapid heartbeat. • Shortness of breath. • Numbness or tingling around mouth, hands or feet. • Emotional changes.	Severe anxiety.	See Panic Disorder.
• Dull or sharp pain in front of chest. • Rapid breathing. • Cough; fever; chills.	Heart inflammation.	See Pericarditis.
• Burning pain in the center of the chest and upper abdomen. • Pregnant.	Pregnancy symptom.	See Heartburn During Pregnancy.
Chest pain without symptoms or factors listed on this chart.	Many disorders, including stress and anxiety.	Consult doctor. Chest pain should never be ignored.

*All references are to Illness section unless noted otherwise.

CONFUSION (PERSON OVER AGE 65)

SYMPTOMS & FACTORS	POSSIBLE PROBLEM	WHAT TO DO*
• Confusion. • Use of drugs, including: antihistamines; appetite suppressants; muscle relaxants; pain killers; sedatives; tranquilizers; or mind-altering drugs, such as marijuana, cocaine, LSD and heroin.	• Adverse reaction or side effect of drug. • Drug interaction.	Consult doctor.
• Confusion. • Slurred speech. • Weakness in extremities.	Decreased blood supply to brain.	• Call doctor now. • See Stroke. • See Transient Ischemic Attack.
• Sudden confusion. • Unusually long time since eating. OR • Use of insulin or oral hypoglycemic drug.	Low blood sugar.	Drink sweet drink or eat sweet snack. If confusion lasts longer than 10 minutes, call doctor.
• Confusion appearing over several weeks. • Fall or head injury in last 2 months.	Effect of injury.	• Call doctor now. • See Subdural Hemorrhage & Hematoma.
• Sudden confusion. • Signs of physical illness, such as fever, cough or loss of bladder control.	Effect of illness.	Call doctor now.
• Sudden confusion. • Cold abdomen. • Recent chill.	Drop in body temperature.	See Hypothermia.
• Sudden confusion. • Use of prescription drug. OR • Use of mind-altering drugs, such as marijuana or cocaine.	Adverse reaction or side effect of drug.	Consult doctor.
• Confusion appearing over several weeks, plus 2 or more of following: • Inability to remember recent events. • Decline in attention to personal appearance or cleanliness. • Personality change.	• Poor nutrition. • Mental deterioration.	• See Vitamin Deficiencies. • See Dementia. • See Alzheimer's Disease.
• Confusion. • Dehydrated. • Poor diet; lack of fluid intake.	Electrolyte imbalance.	• See Fluid & Electrolyte Disorders. • See Dehydration.

*All references are to Illness section unless noted otherwise.

CONFUSION (PERSON UNDER AGE 65)

SYMPTOMS & FACTORS	POSSIBLE PROBLEM	WHAT TO DO*
• Confusion. • Use of drugs, including: antihistamines; appetite suppressants; muscle relaxants; pain killers; sedatives; tranquilizers; or mind-altering drugs, such as marijuana, cocaine, LSD and heroin.	• Adverse reaction or side effect of drug. • Drug interaction.	Consult doctor.
• Confusion, plus any of following: • Blurred vision. • Dizziness. • Numbness or tingling in any part of body. • Speaking difficulty. • Weakness in extremities.	Decreased blood supply to brain.	• Call doctor now. • See Stroke. • See Transient Ischemic Attack.
• Confusion in a child. • Lethargy; weakness; paralysis in an arm or leg. • Personality changes.	Brain and liver infection.	See Reye's Syndrome.
• Confusion. • Alcohol consumption either alone or with drug.	• Adverse reaction or side effect of alcohol. • Drug interaction.	• Consult doctor. • Stop drinking alcohol.
• Sudden confusion. • Recent head injury.	Brain injury.	• Call doctor now. • See Head Injury.
• Confusion. • Excessive dieting.	Vitamin deficiency.	Consult doctor for proper method of weight control.
• Confusion in a woman of childbearing age. • Sudden fever of 101°F (38.3°C) or higher. • Vomiting. • Skin rash.	Infection.	• Call doctor now. • See Toxic Shock Syndrome.
• Confusion. • Fever of 103°F (39.4°C) or higher.	Effect of fever.	• Call doctor now. • See Fever of Unknown Origin.
• Confusion, plus any of following: • Heart disease. • Lung disease. • Diabetes.	Complication of underlying disorder.	Call doctor now.
• Confusion, plus any of following: • Agitation. • Delirium. • Disorientation. • Inability to recognize others. • Hallucinations.	• Mental illness. • Sugar in the urine. • Bleeding inside skull. • Tumor.	• Call doctor now. • See Diabetes Type 1. • See Diabetes Type 2. • See Diabetes Hypoglycemia. • See Subdural Hemorrhage & Hematoma. • See Brain Tumor.
• Confusion. • Dehydrated. • Poor diet; lack of fluid intake.	Electrolyte imbalance.	• See Fluid & Electrolyte Disorders. • See Dehydration.

*All references are to Illness section unless noted otherwise.

CONSTIPATION

SYMPTOMS & FACTORS	POSSIBLE PROBLEM	WHAT TO DO*
• Constipation. • Pain with bowel movements. • Occasional blood in stool.	• Varicose veins in anus. • Split in skin around anus.	• See Hemorrhoids. • See Constipation.
• Constipation. • Use of prescription or nonprescription drug.	Adverse reaction or side effect of drug.	• Consult doctor about prescription drug. • Discontinue use of nonprescription drug.
• Constipation. • Pain in lower abdomen within last week.	Inflammation of large intestine.	• See Diverticular Disease. • See Intestinal Obstruction. • See Large Intestine Cancer.
• Chronic constipation. • Recurrent pain in lower abdomen.	Disorder of muscle contractions in colon.	See Irritable Bowel Syndrome.
• Constipation, plus 2 or more of following: • Fatigue. • Unexplained weight gain. • Dry skin or hair. • Decreased tolerance to cold.	Underactive thyroid gland.	See Hypothyroidism.
• Chronic tendency toward constipation. • Frequent suppression of urge for bowel movement. OR • Regular laxative use.	Poor bowel reflexes.	See Constipation.
Constipation while dieting.	Lack of adequate water or fiber in diet.	Include more fiber in your diet.
• Chronic tendency toward constipation. • No other symptoms.	Lack of adequate water or fiber in diet.	See Constipation.
• In male, constant urge to have a bowel movement when little or no stool present. • Rectal pain. • Cramping pain in lower abdomen.	Rectum inflammation.	See Proctitis.
• Chronic constipation or chronic diarrhea. • Gas and bloating. • Laxative use.	Excess laxative use.	See Laxative Abuse.

*All references are to Illness section unless noted otherwise.

COUGH
(continued on next page)

SYMPTOMS & FACTORS	POSSIBLE PROBLEM	WHAT TO DO*
• Recent cough. • Stuffy or runny nose. • Sore throat.	Virus infection.	See Cold, Common.
• Recent cough. • Fever.	Inflammation or infection of breathing passages.	• See Bronchitis, Acute. • See Influenza.
• Persistent cough following cold or flu. • History of persistent cough during previous cold or flu seasons.	Chronic inflammation or infection.	• See Bronchitis, Chronic. • See Sinusitis.
• Persistent cough with sputum. • Chronic breathing difficulty that is worsening. • No dusty working conditions.	Chronic inflammation or infection of breathing passages.	• See Chronic Obstructive Pulmonary Disease. • See Emphysema.
• Chronic cough. • Smokers in the home.	Effect of second-hand smoke.	Encourage smoker to quit or stop smoking inside the house.
• Recent cough with green-yellow or rusty sputum. • Fever. • Breathing difficulty.	Lung infection.	• See Pneumonia (all charts). • See Histoplasmosis. • See Coccidioidomycosis. • See Psittacosis.
• Persistent cough with sputum that is worsening. • Fever. • Unexplained weight loss. • Fatigue. • Excessive sweating at night.	Lung infection or inflammation.	• See Tuberculosis. • See Bronchiectasis. • See Lung Abscess.
• Sudden cough without sputum. • Inhalation of irritating substance or fumes such as smog.	Irritation of breathing passages.	Avoid exposure to chemicals, dust and cigarettes.
• Recent cough without sputum. • Hoarseness or voice loss.	Inflammation of vocal cords.	See Voice Loss or Hoarseness (in Symptoms section).
• Cough. • Chest pain. • Chills; fever; sweats. • Shortness of breath.	Fungal infection.	See Blastomycosis.
• Sudden violent cough. • Inhalation of foreign object.	Normal coughing to expel object from lungs.	Consult doctor if cough lasts longer than 1 hour.
Persistent cough without sputum.	• Tumor. • Heart disorder. • Spasm of bronchial tubes. • Irritation of bronchial tubes from smoking.	• Request chest X-ray. • See Lung Cancer. • See Congestive Heart Failure. • See Asthma.

*All references are to Illness section unless noted otherwise.

COUGH
(continued from previous page)

SYMPTOMS & FACTORS	POSSIBLE PROBLEM	WHAT TO DO*
• Cough. • Shortness of breath.	Several disorders.	See Breathing Difficulty (in Symptoms section).
• Slow onset of dry, nonproductive cough. • Fever. • Shortness of breath. • Immune disorder such as HIV or AIDS.	Protozoan infection.	See *Pneumocystis Jiroveci* Pneumonia.
• Cough; sore throat; increased saliva. • Fatigue; slight fever. • Recent animal bite.	Virus infection.	See Rabies.

*All references are to Illness section unless noted otherwise.

COUGH WITH BLOOD

SYMPTOMS & FACTORS	POSSIBLE PROBLEM	WHAT TO DO*
• Cough with blood. • Recent surgery. OR • Recent bed confinement because of illness or injury.	Blood clot in lung.	• Call doctor now. • See Pulmonary Embolism.
• Cough with blood. • Persistent cough following recent cold or flu.	Bleeding in breathing passages.	Call doctor now.
• Persistent cough with blood for several weeks. • Fever of 100°F (37.8°C) or higher. • Unexplained weight loss. • Fatigue. • Excessive sweating at night.	• Bacterial inflammation or infection of lung. • Tumor.	• Call doctor now. • See Tuberculosis. • See Lung Cancer. • See Lung Abscess.
• Cough with blood or frothy pink or brownish sputum. • Breathing difficulty. • History of high blood pressure or heart disorder.	Fluid in lungs.	• Consult doctor. • See Pulmonary Edema.
• Cough with blood or brownish sputum. • Fever of 102°F (38.9°C) or higher.	Lung infection.	• Call doctor now. • See Pneumonia (all charts).

*All references are to Illness section unless noted otherwise.

COUGHING IN CHILDREN

SYMPTOMS & FACTORS	POSSIBLE PROBLEM	WHAT TO DO*
• Cough. • Fever.	Virus infection.	• See Cold, Common. • See Influenza.
• Cough, sometimes with wheezing. • Runny nose. • Low grade fever. • Decrease in appetite. • Lethargy. • Infant or child may refuse to eat. • Ear ache.	Virus infection.	See Respiratory Syncytial Virus.
• Cough. • Severe breathing difficulty. • Wheezing. OR • Bluish face or fingertips.	• Spasm of bronchial tubes. • Swelling in vocal cords.	• Call doctor now. • See Asthma. • See Croup.
• Cough. • Use of prescription or nonprescription drug.	Adverse reaction or side effect of drug.	• Consult doctor about prescription drug. • Discontinue use of non prescription drug.
• Cough. • Fever. • Rapid or difficult breathing.	Infection of breathing passages.	• Call doctor now. • See Bronchitis, Acute. • See Bronchiolitis. • See Pneumonia (all charts).
• Severe uncontrollable cough. • Noisy "whooping" gasps for air following cough.	Bacterial lung infection.	See Whooping Cough.
• Cough. • Noisy breathing with wheezing. • Possible inhalation of small foreign object, such as peanut.	Coughing to expel object from lung.	Call doctor now or seek emergency help.
• Cough. • Sore throat.	Several disorders.	See Throat, Sore (in Symptoms section).
• Persistent cough in an infant. • Abdominal swelling. • Frequent, bad-smelling stools.	Inherited disorder.	See Cystic Fibrosis.
• Cough. • Chronic runny or stuffy nose.	Enlarged adenoids.	Consult doctor.
• Cough. • Adult smokers in house or child may have smoked.	Irritation caused by tobacco smoke.	• Adult smokers should smoke outside. • Talk to child about hazards of smoking.
• Sudden "barking" cough. • Sore throat; fever. • Odd head posture.	Bacterial infection.	See Epiglottitis, Acute.

*All references are to Illness section unless noted otherwise.

CRYING, EXCESSIVE (INFANT 0 TO 6 MONTHS)

SYMPTOMS & FACTORS	POSSIBLE PROBLEM	WHAT TO DO*
• Excessive crying. • Irritability. • Lethargy. • Poor appetite. • Fever.	Infection.	• Consult doctor. • See Fever (Child 0 to 2 Years) in Symptoms section.
• Excessive crying. • Irritability. • Lethargy. • Poor appetite.	Minor illness.	Consult doctor if symptoms persist longer than 1 day.
Excessive crying in infant younger than 3 months usually after feeding.	Irritation of digestive tract.	See Colic in Infants.
• Excessive crying. • Crying stops after feeding. • Crying resumes less than 2 hours after feeding.	• Inadequate nourishment. • Thirst.	• If breast-feeding, feed on demand and increase sucking time. • If bottle-feeding, increase amount offered. • Offer water between feedings. • See Colic in Infants.
• Excessive crying. • Rash in diaper area.	Chemical skin irritation.	See Diaper Rash.
Crying until picked up.	Boredom or loneliness.	• Touch and talk to infant more. • Place infant within sight of you.
• Crying. • Cool or chilly environment.	Cold.	• Dress infant warmly. • Move infant into warm room.
Crying in infant younger than 3 months before falling asleep.	Muscle jerks and twitches when falling asleep.	Wrap infant firmly in blanket before putting to bed.
• Crying and other fussy behavior. • Excess saliva and drooling.	Eruption of new teeth.	See Teething.

*All references are to Illness section unless noted otherwise.

DEPRESSION

SYMPTOMS & FACTORS	POSSIBLE PROBLEM	WHAT TO DO*
• Depression. • Chronic illness, especially rheumatoid arthritis, multiple sclerosis and chronic heart disease.	Any illness, severe or mild, can cause significant depression.	• Consult doctor. • See Depression. • See chart in Illness section for the particular disorder.
• Depression. • Use of prescription or nonprescription drug. OR • Excessive alcohol consumption.	Adverse reaction or side effect of drug or alcohol.	• Consult doctor. • See Alcoholism.
• Depression. • Recent virus infection with fever such as flu, infectious mononucleosis or hepatitis.	Common occurrence following infection.	Consult doctor if depression worsens or lasts longer than 2 weeks.
Depression following traumatic or sad event, such as death in family.	Normal occurrence for 3 to 6 months following such experiences.	Feelings are a normal part of mourning and will gradually improve over time. Seek medical help if depression worsens.
Depression experienced at the start of winter season.	Lack of light.	See Seasonal Affective Disorder.
Chronic depressive mood.	Mild depression.	See Dysthymia.
Depression in a woman following childbirth.	Common occurrence for several weeks after delivery.	See Postpartum Mood Disturbance.
• Depression. • Persistent fatigue over the last 6 months.	Unknown cause.	See Chronic Fatigue Syndrome.
• Depression and anxiety. • Sadness, numbness, pain or anger.	Emotional reaction following loss of a loved one or other significant loss.	See Grief.

*All references are to Illness section unless noted otherwise.

DIARRHEA (INFANT 0 TO 6 MONTHS)

SYMPTOMS & FACTORS	POSSIBLE PROBLEM	WHAT TO DO*
• Diarrhea. • Fever. • Vomiting.	Infection of digestive tract.	• See Gastroenteritis. • See Diarrhea, Acute. • See Dehydration.
• Diarrhea. • Baby content, alert and feeding well. • Baby taking nonprescription drug.	Adverse reaction or side effect of drug.	• Consult doctor. • Discontinue use of drug unless recommended by doctor.
• Diarrhea. • Baby taking prescription drug for some other disorder.	Adverse reaction or side effect of drug.	Consult doctor. Dose may need adjustment, substitution or discontinuation.
• Diarrhea. • Itching at night. OR • Worms in stool.	Parasites.	• See Pinworms. • See Roundworms.
• Diarrhea. • Recent addition of solids to diet.	Baby too young to digest solid food.	• Consult doctor. • Wait until age 4 months before trying solids.
• Diarrhea. • Pulling at the ear.	Ear infection.	See Ear Infection, Middle.
• Diarrhea. • Baby seems content, alert and feeds well on bottle feedings. • Sugar added to any formula or water. OR • Less than recommended amount of water added to baby's orange juice. OR • Fruit juice sweetened with sugar.	Upset digestion due to excess sugar.	• Consult doctor. • Don't add sugar to baby's food. • Use recommended amounts of water to dilute juice.
Chronic, frequent loose stools in young child.	Intestinal problem.	See Diarrhea, Chronic, Non-Specific of Childhood.
• Diarrhea. • Abdominal pain. • Flatulence and bloating.	Reaction to a swallowed substance.	• See Food Allergy. • See Lactose Intolerance.
• Diarrhea. • Vomiting.	Several disorders.	See Vomiting (Infant 0 to 6 months) (in Symptoms section).
• Loose, pale, bad-smelling stools. • Weight loss or slow weight gain. • Swollen abdomen; abdominal pain.	Gluten intolerance.	See Celiac Disease.

*All references are to Illness section unless noted otherwise.

DIARRHEA (PERSON OVER 6 MONTHS)

SYMPTOMS & FACTORS	POSSIBLE PROBLEM	WHAT TO DO*
• Diarrhea. • Nausea or vomiting.	Viral, bacterial or parasitic infection of digestive tract.	• See Gastroenteritis. • See Dysentery, Bacillary. • See Diarrhea, Acute.
• Diarrhea for 24 hours or longer. • Vomiting. • Abdominal pain. • Consumption of spoiled food or contaminated food or water.	Effect of toxins in food.	• See Food Poisoning. • See Salmonella Infections. • See Typhoid.
• Recurrent attacks of diarrhea. • Pain in lower abdomen.	• Intestinal parasites. • Several disorders.	• See Amebiasis. • See Giardiasis. • See Recurrent Abdominal Pain (in Symptoms section).
• Diarrhea. • Use of prescription or nonprescription drug.	Adverse reaction or side effect of drug.	• Consult doctor about prescription drug. • Discontinue use of nonprescription drug.
• Diarrhea. • Blood in stool.	Inflammation of large intestine.	See Colitis, Ulcerative.
Recurrent attacks of diarrhea during periods of stress.	Effect of stress.	• See Anxiety Disorder, Generalized. • See Irritable Bowel Syndrome. • See Stress.
• Diarrhea. • Use of sorbitol, a common sweetener found in many diet products.	The sugar is not absorbed by the small intestine.	Discontinue use of the product with sorbitol.
• Diarrhea. • Abdominal pain. • Flatulence and bloating.	Reaction to a swallowed substance.	See Food Allergy.
• Explosive diarrhea. • Weakness and faintness. • Recent stomach surgery.	Intestinal disorder.	See Dumping Syndrome.
• Chronic diarrhea. or chronic constipation. • Gas and bloating. • Laxative use.	Excess laxative use.	See Laxative Abuse.

*All references are to Illness section unless noted otherwise.

DIZZINESS

SYMPTOMS & FACTORS	POSSIBLE PROBLEM	WHAT TO DO*
• Dizziness. • Use of prescription or nonprescription drug.	Adverse reaction or side effect of drug.	• Consult doctor about prescription drug. • Discontinue use of nonprescription drug.
• Dizziness. • Decreased hearing. • Noises in ear. OR • Earache.	Infection or disorder of inner ear.	• See Labyrinthitis. • See Meniere's Disease.
Dizziness when turning head in person over age 50.	Pressure on nerves in neck.	See Cervical Spondylosis.
Dizziness when standing suddenly.	• Temporary drop in blood pressure. • Red blood cell disorder. • Inner ear problem.	• Avoid rising suddenly. • See Anemia, Iron Deficiency. • See Benign Paroxysmal Positional Vertigo.
• Dizziness. • Stress or anxiety.	Hyperventilation.	• See Anxiety Disorder, Generalized. • See Panic Disorder. • See Phobias. • See Stress.
Dizziness (spinning sensation).	• Travel by air, sea or motor vehicle. • Inner ear problem.	• See Motion Sickness. • See Benign Paroxysmal Positional Vertigo.
• Dizziness. • Headache. • Faintness. • Nausea, vomiting.	Toxic gas inhalation.	See Carbon Monoxide Poisoning.
• Dizziness. • Excess sun or heat exposure.	Body overheated.	See Heatstroke or Heat Exhaustion.
• Dizziness, plus any of following: • Speaking difficulty. • Blurred vision. • Numbness or tingling in any part of body. • Weakness or paralysis in extremities.	Decreased blood supply to brain.	• Call doctor now. • See Stroke. • See Transient Ischemic Attack. • See Subarachnoid Hemorrhage.
• Dizziness. • Recurrent morning headache. • Nausea or vomiting.	• Bleeding inside skull. • Tumor.	• Call doctor now. • See Subdural Hemorrhage & Hematoma. • See Brain Tumor.
• Dizziness. • Irregular heartbeat.	Heart rhythm disorder.	• See Atrial Fibrillation. • See Heart Rhythm Irregularity. • See Heart Block.

*All references are to Illness section unless noted otherwise.

EAR, RINGING OR BUZZING SOUNDS

SYMPTOMS & FACTORS	POSSIBLE PROBLEM	WHAT TO DO*
• Ear noises. • Use of prescription or nonprescription drug.	Adverse reaction or side effect of drug.	• Consult doctor about prescription drug. • Discontinue use of nonprescription drug.
• Ear noises. • Hearing loss.	Damaged auditory nerve.	See Hearing Impairment or Loss.
• Noises in the ear. • Dizziness.	Fluid in the ear.	See Meniere's Disease.
• Strange, loud ear noises. • Severe, uncomfortable tickling in ear.	Insect in outer-ear canal.	Consult doctor.
Ear noises after airplane flight.	Middle-ear problem caused by change in air pressure.	See Barotitis Media.
Noise in ear (ringing, buzzing, roaring, whistling or hissing).	Damaged auditory nerve.	See Tinnitus.
• Ringing in ear. • Slow, progressive hearing loss.	Abnormal bone growth in middle ear.	See Otosclerosis.

*All references are to Illness section unless noted otherwise.

EARACHE

SYMPTOMS & FACTORS	POSSIBLE PROBLEM	WHAT TO DO*
• Earache. • Sticky, green-yellow discharge from ear canal or middle ear.	Infection of outer-ear.	• See Ear Infection, Outer. • See Ear Infection, Middle. • See Eardrum, Ruptured.
• Earache. • Fever.	Infection of middle ear.	See Ear Infection, Middle.
• Earache. • Stuffy nose.	Common occurrence with cold or allergy.	See Ear Infection, Middle.
Earache that worsens when earlobe is pulled.	Infection of outer-ear canal.	See Ear Infection, Outer.
• Earache. • Pain in tooth or jaw.	• Tooth or gum infection. • Inflammation of joint in jaw.	• Consult dentist. • See Tooth Abscess. • See Temporomandibular Joint Syndrome.
• Earache. • Blocked feeling in ear that cannot be cleared by swallowing. • Diminished hearing.	Wax in ear canal.	See Earwax Blockage.
• Earache that began during airplane flight. • Blocked feeling in ear that cannot be cleared by swallowing.	Middle-ear damage caused by change in air pressure.	See Barotitis Media.

*All references are to Illness section unless noted otherwise.

EYE PAIN; SWELLING; DRYNESS; ITCHING; TEARING (continued on next page)

SYMPTOMS & FACTORS	POSSIBLE PROBLEM	WHAT TO DO*
• Eye pain. • Eye injury without visible damage.	Minor injury.	See Eye Contusion or Laceration.
• Pain behind eye. • Area of tenderness over nose or cheekbones. • Pain that worsens when bending forward. • Recent cold or nasal allergies.	Sinus infection.	See Sinusitis.
• Itching, watery eyes. • Frequent sneezing; stuffy nose; with clear discharge.	Allergy.	See Hay Fever.
• Eye pain. • Watery, red eye.	Foreign object in eye.	See Eye, Foreign Body in.
• Eye pain. • Red, swollen bump on eyelid. • Red eye.	Infection of hair follicle on eyelid.	See Stye.
• Eye pain. • Red eye. • Gritty feeling in eye. • Stickiness around eye.	Infection of eye membrane.	See Conjunctivitis.
• Eye pain. • Red eye. • Gritty feeling in eye.	Inadequate tear production.	Use nonprescription artificial tears. Consult doctor if discomfort lasts longer than 2 days.
• Eye pain. • Eyelid curls inward. • Red eyelid and eye.	Disorder of eyelid.	See Entropion and Ectropion.
Swelling on eyelid.	Eye infection.	See Chalazion.
• Redness and greasy scales on the eyelid edges. • Eyelashes that fall out.	Infection.	See Blepharitis.
• Pain around eye. • Sudden onset of headache. • Headache appears at same time on consecutive days.	Chronic headache disorder.	See Headache, Cluster.
• Eye pain. • Sensitivity to light. • Tearing.	Inflammation of the cornea.	See Keratitis.
• Eye pain. • Purple-red inflamed area in one or more areas of the white of the eye.	Eye inflammation.	See Scleritis.
• Bulging eyes. • Double vision.	Tissue swelling.	See Exophthalmos.

*All references are to Illness section unless noted otherwise.

SYMPTOMS & FACTORS	POSSIBLE PROBLEM	WHAT TO DO*
• Dryness of eyes. • Foreign body sensation. • Dryness of mouth. • Parotid gland enlargement (chipmunk look).	Autoimmune disorder.	See Sjögren's Syndrome.
Sudden appearance of blood in the white of the eye.	Spontaneous bleeding.	See Subconjunctival Hemorrhage.
• Persistent tearing of one or both eyes. • Drainage of mucous and pus from tear duct.	Obstructed tear duct.	See Tear Duct Infection or Blockage.
• Severe eye pain. • Recent eye injury with visible damage. • Loss of vision.	Serious injury.	Call doctor now.
• Pain behind eye. • Tenderness in temple on affected side.	Inflammation of arteries in temples.	• Call doctor now. • See Polymyalgia Rheumatica or Temporal Arteritis.
• Pain behind eye, plus any of following: • Eyes sensitive to light. • Lethargy. • Confusion. • Pain that worsens when bending head forward. • Severe headache.	• Inflammation of membranes around brain. • Bleeding in membrane around brain.	• Call doctor now. • See Meningitis, Aseptic. • See Meningitis, Bacterial. • See Subarachnoid Hemorrhage.
• Eye pain. • Blurred vision.	• Excess pressure in eye. • Inflammation in eye. • Eye injury.	• See Glaucoma, Angle-Closure. • See Iritis. • See Corneal Abrasion & Ulcer.
• Eye pain. • Sensitivity to light. • Eye redness. • Tears, blurred vision. • Smaller pupil in affected eye.	Infection.	See Iritis.

*All references are to Illness section unless noted otherwise.

FACE PAIN

SYMPTOMS & FACTORS	POSSIBLE PROBLEM	WHAT TO DO*
• Pain on one side of face or all over head. • Tight feeling around head.	Headache.	• See Headache, Migraine. • See Headache, Tension.
• Pain or tenderness around eyes and cheekbones that worsens when bending head forward. • Recent cold or nasal allergies.	Sinus infection.	See Sinusitis.
Throbbing pain on one side of face that worsens at night, when eating or when touching a particular tooth.	Infection around tooth.	Consult doctor or dentist.
• Aching pain over or around jaw joint. • Jaw that sometimes clicks when opening. • Frequent headaches.	Inflammation of joint in jaw.	See Temporomandibular Joint Syndrome.
• Pain around ear. • Sudden paralysis on one side of face.	Facial paralysis.	See Bell's Palsy.
• Parotid gland enlargement (chipmunk look). • Dryness of eyes and mouth.	Autoimmune disorder.	See Sjögren's Syndrome.
• Face pain. • Recent rash at site of pain.	Virus infection of sensory nerves.	See Herpes Zoster.
• Frequent contractions of muscles on the side of the face. • Tooth-grinding noises at night.	Tooth problem.	See Tooth Grinding.
• Severe pain on one side of face over eye. • Redness of white of eye. • Blurred vision.	Excess pressure in eye.	See Glaucoma, Angle-Closure.
Sharp pain on one side of face when face is touched or when chewing.	Damaged nerve.	See Trigeminal Neuralgia.
• Sudden, throbbing pain in temple. • General ill feeling. • Tender scalp.	Inflammation of arteries in temples.	See Polymyalgia Rheumatica or Temporal Arteritis.
• Face pain, plus any of following: • Chest pain. • Neck pain. • Shoulder pain. • Arm pain.	Heart attack.	• Call doctor now. • See Heart Attack. • See Coronary Artery Disease. • See Atherosclerosis.
• Pain and swelling of parotid gland or sublingual salivary gland. • Dry mouth. • May be hard to open mouth wide.	Gland infection.	See Salivary Gland Infection.

*All references are to Illness section unless noted otherwise.

FACIAL SKIN PROBLEMS

SYMPTOMS & FACTORS	POSSIBLE PROBLEM	WHAT TO DO*
• Any of following conditions on face: • Painful, red bumps. • Bumps with white or yellow centers. • Blackheads.	Skin disorder beginning after puberty.	See Acne.
• Flushed face that may last minutes or hours to several days. • Facial tenderness.	Disorder of tiny blood vessels.	See Acne Rosacea.
Blister or red, rough or painful area around mouth.	Virus infection.	See Herpes Simplex.
Sore on face or lip that doesn't heal in 3 weeks.	Skin cancer.	• See Skin Cancer, Basal-Cell. • See Skin Cancer, Squamous-Cell.
• Blister-like rash on one side of face. • Painful, burning sensation at site 1 or 2 days before rash appears.	Virus infection of sensory nerves.	See Herpes Zoster.
Blisters that burst and become crusty.	Skin infection.	See Impetigo.
Red, itching, scaling rash on face.	Allergic reaction.	See Dyshidrotic Eczema.
• Rash (usually on the cheeks). • Fatigue. • Fever. • Joint pain.	Autoimmune disorder.	See Lupus Erythematosus, Systemic.
Red bumps on cheeks, on either side of nose and on scalp (sometimes).	Autoimmune disorder.	See Lupus Erythematosus, Discoid.
• Rough, red patch on cheek, nose or forehead. • Person over age 35.	Skin damage caused by sun exposure.	• See Sunburn. • See Keratosis, Actinic.
Patch of skin on face that is lighter or darker than surrounding skin.	Disorder of skin pigment.	See Vitiligo.
• Rash (especially in children) starting on cheeks, then spreading to other body parts. • Slight tiredness or fatigue.	Virus infection.	See Erythema Infectiosum.
• Change in face mole's size, color or sensitivity. OR • A new mole or lump on face.	Skin cancer.	See Melanoma.

*All references are to Illness section unless noted otherwise.

FAINTNESS OR FAINTING
(continued on next page)

SYMPTOMS & FACTORS	POSSIBLE PROBLEM	WHAT TO DO*
Fainting.	No underlying disorder.	See Fainting.
* Faintness when standing suddenly. OR * Faintness following bed confinement.	Temporary drop in blood pressure.	Avoid rising suddenly.
* Faintness. * Breathing deeply, rapidly or sighing before faintness.	Effect of stress. No underlying disorder.	* See Panic Disorder. * See Anxiety Disorder, Generalized. * Consult doctor if happens repeatedly.
* Faintness. * Use of drug for high blood pressure.	Adverse reaction or side effect of drug.	Consult doctor.
* Faintness. * Dizziness.	Several disorders.	See Dizziness (in Symptoms section).
* Faintness or fainting. * Feeling that heart speeds or slows before faintness. * Known heart disease.	Heart rhythm disorder.	* Call doctor now. * See Heart Block. * See Heart Rhythm Irregularity. * See Atrial Fibrillation. * See Cardiac Arrest.
* Faintness, plus any of following: * Blurred vision. * Speaking difficulty. * Confusion. * Numbness or tingling in any part of body. * Weakness or paralysis in extremities.	Decreased blood supply to brain.	* Call doctor now. * See Transient Ischemic Attack. * See Stroke.
* Fainting. * Seizure disorder.	Minor seizure.	See Epilepsy.
Faintness after several hours in strong sunshine or hot environment.	Excess heat exposure.	* Call doctor now. * See Heatstroke or Heat Exhaustion.
* Faintness. * Diabetes.	Low blood sugar.	* Drink sweetened juice or beverage or eat something sugary or starchy. * See Diabetes Hypoglycemia.
* Faintness. * Fatigue. * Shortness of breath. * Person older than 50.	* Heart disease. * Disorder of red blood cells.	* See Congestive Heart Failure. * See Anemia, Pernicious.
Faintness when turning head (in person older than 50).	Pressure on nerves in neck.	See Cervical Spondylosis.

*All references are to Illness section unless noted otherwise.

FAINTNESS OR FAINTING
(continued from previous page)

SYMPTOMS & FACTORS	POSSIBLE PROBLEM	WHAT TO DO*
• Fainting. • Shortness of breath before faintness. • Recent strenuous exercise.	Temporary change in blood chemistry.	Consult doctor if happens repeatedly.
• Fainting and weakness. • Sweating; irregular heartbeat. • Recent stomach surgery. • Diarrhea.	Intestinal disorder.	See Dumping Syndrome.
• Faintness. • Headache; dizziness; nausea and vomiting.	Toxic gas inhalation.	See Carbon Monoxide Poisoning.
• Fainting and weakness. • Sweating, headache, confusion. • Excessive hunger.	Low blood sugar.	See Hypoglycemia, Functional.

*All references are to Illness section unless noted otherwise.

FATIGUE OR TIREDNESS
(continued on next page)

SYMPTOMS & FACTORS	POSSIBLE PROBLEM	WHAT TO DO*
• Fatigue. • Appetite loss. • Weight loss.	• Cancer. • Disorder of red blood cells.	• Consult doctor. • See Anemia (all charts).
• Fatigue, plus 2 or more of following: • Appetite loss. • Fever. • Headache. • Painful swelling in neck, armpit or groin. • Jaundice (yellow skin and eyes). • Sore throat.	Virus infection.	See Mononucleosis, Infectious.
• Fatigue. • Use of prescription or nonprescription drug.	Adverse reaction or side effect of drug.	• Consult doctor about prescription drug. • Discontinue use of nonprescription drug.
• Fatigue. • Coarse skin and hair. • Low voice. • Loss of sex drive. • Puffy face.	Underactive thyroid gland.	See Hypothyroidism.
• Fatigue. • Fever. • Headache, plus any of following: • Nausea, vomiting or diarrhea. • Drowsiness. • Cough. • Sore throat. • Pain in neck. • Aches in bones or joints. • Skin rash. • Pain in back. • Painful urination.	Bacterial or viral infection.	Consult doctor.
• Fatigue in woman at menopause. • Appetite loss.	Normal occurrence with decreasing estrogen level of menopause.	See Menopause.
• Fatigue. • Pregnancy. • Shortness of breath.	Dietary deficiency of pregnancy, particularly of protein, calcium, vitamins or iron.	• Consult doctor. • Eat extra protein foods. • Drink 2 extra glasses of skim milk daily. • Take iron supplement and prenatal vitamin supplement.
• Fatigue. • Depression or anxiety.	Effect of stress.	• See Depression. • See Anxiety Disorder, Generalized. • See Stress.
• Ongoing fatigue for several months. • Numerous other symptoms.	Unknown infection or problem.	See Chronic Fatigue Syndrome.

*All references are to Illness section unless noted otherwise.

FATIGUE OR TIREDNESS
(continued on next page)

SYMPTOMS & FACTORS	POSSIBLE PROBLEM	WHAT TO DO*
• Fatigue. • Chest discomfort with exertion that is relieved by rest.	Narrowing of coronary arteries.	• Consult doctor. • See Atherosclerosis. • See Coronary Artery Disease. • See Heart Valve Disease.
• Tiredness. • Depression. • Increased appetite. • Beginning of winter.	Lack of light.	See Seasonal Affective Disorder.
• Fatigue and weakness. • Intermittent fever, chills, sweating. • Weight loss.	Heart valve or heart lining infection.	See Endocarditis.
• Fatigue. • Fever; rash (usually on the cheeks). • Joint pain.	Autoimmune disorder.	See Lupus Erythematosus, Systemic.
• Fatigue. • Appetite loss. • Weight loss. • Hair loss. • Craving for salt. • Skin that darkens.	Inadequate cortisone hormone.	See Addison's Disease.
• Fatigue. • Cough. • Fever. • Weight loss. • Shortness of breath.	• Lung infection. • Tumor.	• See Tuberculosis. • See Bronchiectasis. • See Pneumonia (all charts). • See Influenza. • See Lung Cancer.
• Fatigue. • Headache and nausea. • Recent travel to foreign country.	Parasite infection.	See Malaria.
• Fatigue. • Shortness of breath. • Irregular heartbeat.	Heart inflammation.	See Myocarditis.
• Fatigue, slight fever. • Restlessness and irritability. • Cough; sore throat; increased saliva. • Animal bite.	Virus infection.	See Rabies.
• Fatigue. • Chills; fever; sweating. • Tenderness along spine.	Bacterial infection.	See Brucellosis.

*All references are to Illness section unless noted otherwise.

FATIGUE OR TIREDNESS
(continued from previous page)

SYMPTOMS & FACTORS	POSSIBLE PROBLEM	WHAT TO DO*
• Fatigue and lethargy. • Paleness. • Behavioral changes. • Abdominal discomfort.	Inhalation or ingestion of lead.	See Lead Poisoning.
• Tiredness. • Fever. • Swollen lymph glands.	Protozoan infection.	See Toxoplasmosis.
• Fatigue and weakness. • Tingling sensation in arms, hands, legs and feet. • Urinary frequency.	Endocrine disorder.	Hyperaldosteronism.
• Lethargy; weakness; paralysis in an arm or leg (in a child). • Confusion. • Personality changes.	Brain and liver infection.	See Reye's Syndrome.
• Fatigue in a child who fails to grow normally. • Shortness of breath. • Blueness under fingernails.	Congenital heart disease.	Consult doctor.
• Fatigue. • Appetite loss. • Nausea at sight of food, plus 2 or more of following: • Jaundice (yellow skin and eyes). • Vomiting. • Tenderness over liver. • Fever. • Weakness.	Liver disorder.	• See Hepatitis, Viral. • See Cirrhosis of the Liver.
• Fatigue. • Sleep disturbances, malaise. • Loss of concentration.	Disturbance in the body's physiological processes.	See Jet Lag.
• Tiredness and weakness. • Low fever, chills, and sweating. • Anemia (pale skin, fatigue). • General ill feeling. • Easy bruising or bleeding or cuts that heal slowly. • Pin-head size spots on the skin.	Cancer.	See Leukemia, Chronic.

*All references are to Illness section unless noted otherwise.

FEVER (CHILD 0 TO 2 YEARS)

SYMPTOMS & FACTORS	POSSIBLE PROBLEM	WHAT TO DO*
• Fever. • Runny nose. • Recent exposure to contagious disease, such as measles, mumps or chickenpox.	Early stage of contagious illness.	Consult doctor.
• Fever. • Diarrhea.	Infection of digestive tract.	• Consult doctor. • See Gastroenteritis.
• Fever. • Runny nose.	Virus infection.	• See Cold, Common. • See Respiratory Syncytial Virus. • Consult doctor if temperature rises.
• Fever. • Infant overdressed. • Hot weather or environment.	Overheating.	• Remove some of infant's clothing. • Offer water to drink. • Give cool sponge bath.
• Fever. • Crying as if in pain. • Pulling at ear.	Infection of middle ear.	• Consult doctor. • See Ear Infection, Middle.
• Fever. • Convulsions.	Effect of high fever.	• Call doctor now. • See Febrile seizure.
• Fever. • Infant of 3 months or younger.	Many possibilities. Signs of illness at this age require prompt medical evaluation.	Consult doctor.
• Fever. • Rash.	Several disorders.	See Rash with Fever (in Symptoms section).
• Fever. • Noisy breathing.	Swelling in vocal cords.	• Consult doctor. • See Croup.
• Fever. • Rapid or difficult breathing.	Infection of breathing passages.	• Call doctor now. • See Bronchitis, Acute. • See Bronchiolitis. • See Pneumonia (all charts).

*All references are to Illness section unless noted otherwise.

FEVER (CHILD OVER 2 YEARS)

SYMPTOMS & FACTORS	POSSIBLE PROBLEM	WHAT TO DO*
• Fever. • Diarrhea.	Infection of digestive tract.	See Gastroenteritis.
• Fever. • Earache. • Child pulls at ear.	Infection of middle ear.	See Ear Infection, Middle.
• Fever. • Cough. • Runny nose.	Virus infection.	• See Cold, Common. • See Influenza. • See Respiratory Syncytial Virus. • Consult doctor if temperature rises.
• Fever. • Convulsions.	Several disorders.	• Call doctor now. • See Febrile seizure.
• Fever of 102°F (38.9°C) or higher. • No other symptoms.	Infection.	Consult doctor.
• Fever. • Cough. • Rapid or difficult breathing.	Infection of breathing passages.	See Pneumonia (all charts).
• Fever. • Rash.	Several disorders.	See Rash with Fever (in Symptoms section).
• Fever. • Abdominal pain.	Several disorders.	See Abdominal Pain, Sudden Attack (in Symptoms section).
• Fever. • Swelling between ear and jaw.	Virus infection.	See Mumps.
• Fever. • Sore throat or hoarseness.	Infection of upper respiratory tract.	• See Tonsillitis. • See Pharyngitis. • See Laryngitis.
• Fever. • Runny nose. • Recent exposure to contagious disease, such as measles, mumps or chickenpox.	Early stage of contagious illness.	Consult doctor.
• Fever. • Child seems very ill, plus any of following: • Stiff neck. • Pain when bending head forward. • Eyes sensitive to light. • Headache. • Vomiting.	Infection of membranes around brain.	• Call doctor now. • See Meningitis, Aseptic.
• Fever. • Chills; muscle aches, cough. • Listlessness. • Exposure to field mice or other rodents.	Virus infection.	See Hantavirus.

*All references are to Illness section unless noted otherwise.

FEVER (PERSON OVER AGE 12)
(continued on next page)

SYMPTOMS & FACTORS	POSSIBLE PROBLEM	WHAT TO DO*
• Fever. • Cough. • Headache. • Aches in bones or joints. • Stuffy or runny nose.	Virus infection.	• See Cold, Common. • See Influenza.
• Fever for 24 hours without other symptoms. OR • Recurrent fever with normal temperature between fevers.	Several disorders.	• Consult doctor. • See Fever of Unknown Origin.
• Fever. • Nausea or vomiting. • Diarrhea.	Infection of digestive tract.	See Gastroenteritis.
• Fever. • Pain in back below last rib.	Infection of urinary tract.	See Kidney Infection, Acute.
Fever after several hours in strong sunshine or hot environment.	Excess heat exposure.	• See Heatstroke or Heat Exhaustion. • See Sunburn.
• Fever. • Cough. • Shortness of breath, even when resting.	Lung infection.	See Pneumonia (all charts).
• Fever. • Cough with gray-yellow sputum. OR • Wheezing.	Infection of bronchial tubes.	See Bronchitis, Acute.
• Fever. • Use of prescription or nonprescription drug.	Adverse reaction or side effect of drug.	• Consult doctor about prescription drug. • Discontinue use of nonprescription drug.
• Fever. • Painful urination. • Frequent urination.	Urinary-tract infection.	• See Bladder Infection, Female. • See Bladder Infection, Male. • See Kidney Infection, Acute.
• Fever. • Sore throat.	Infection.	• See Tonsillitis. • See Pharyngitis. • See Agranulocytosis.
• Fever. • Rash.	Several disorders.	See Rash with Fever (in Symptoms section).
• Sudden high fever. • Vomiting and watery diarrhea. • Rash resembling sunburn.	Blood poisoning.	See Toxic Shock Syndrome.

*All references are to Illness section unless noted otherwise.

FEVER (PERSON OVER AGE 12) (continued from previous page)

SYMPTOMS & FACTORS	POSSIBLE PROBLEM	WHAT TO DO*
• Fever. • Other symptoms similar to cold (cough, tiredness, chills).	Fungal infection or tick caused disorder.	• See Blastomycosis. • See Coccidioidomycosis. • See Histoplasmosis. • See Lyme Disease. • See Rocky Mountain Spotted Fever.
• Fever. • Headache, plus any of following: • Pain bending forward. • Lethargy. • Confusion. • Nausea or vomiting.	Infection of membranes around brain.	• Call doctor now. • See Meningitis, Aseptic.
• Intermittent fever and chills. • Fatigue and weakness. • Weight loss. • Vague aches and pains.	Heart valve or lining infection.	See Endocarditis.
• Fever and sometimes, chills. • General ill feeling. • Headache. • Muscle ache.	Bacterial or viral infection.	• See Legionnaire's Disease. • See Encephalitis, Viral. • See West Nile Virus.
• Low-grade fever. • Weight loss. • Recurrent respiratory and skin infections.	Virus infection.	See HIV & AIDS.
• Fever (rapid temperature rise). • Shaking chills. • Pounding heartbeat. • General ill feeling.	Severe bacterial infection.	See Blood Poisoning.
• Intermittent fever. • Chills. • Marked fatigue. • Enlarged lymph glands.	Bacterial infection.	See Brucellosis.
• Fever. • Chills; muscle aches, cough. • Exposure to field mice or other rodents.	Virus infection.	See Hantavirus.
• Fever. • Tiredness. • Swollen lymph glands.	Protozoan infection.	See Toxoplasmosis.
• Low fever, chills, and sweating. • Tiredness and weakness. • Anemia (pale skin, fatigue). • General ill feeling. • Easy bruising or bleeding or cuts that heal slowly. • Pin-head size spots on the skin.	Cancer.	See Leukemia, Chronic.
• Fever over 100.4°F (38.0°C). • Headache, overall feeling of discomfort, and body aches. • Foreign travel (possibly).	Viral infection.	See Severe Acute Respiratory Syndrome.

*All references are to Illness section unless noted otherwise.

FOOT PROBLEMS
(continued on next page)

SYMPTOMS & FACTORS	POSSIBLE PROBLEM	WHAT TO DO*
Excessively sweaty feet.	No underlying disorder.	• Wash and dry feet twice a day. Apply talcum powder. • Wear cotton socks.
• Foot pain. • Big toe turned inward.	Bony protrusion.	See Bunion.
Small blisters on toes or soles.	Effect of stress.	See Dyshidrotic Eczema.
Pain in foot following injury.	• Broken bone. • Ligament injury.	• See Bone Fracture. • See Sprains & Strains.
• Pain and tenderness in the sole of the foot under the heel. • Pain often occurs after resting or after rising in the morning.	Tissue inflammation.	• See Heel Pain. • Plantar Fasciitis.
• Pain in foot joint, especially big toe. • Affected joint red, warm, swollen.	Joint inflammation.	See Gout.
• Pain on bottom of foot. • Small growth or area on sole that hurts when walking.	Skin growth caused by virus.	See Warts.
• Itching foot. • Skin between toes red, soft and peeling.	Fungus infection.	See Athlete's Foot.
Pain in foot after walking or running.	• Circulatory disorder. • Bone injury.	• See Atherosclerosis. • See Buerger's Disease.
• Pain on bottom of foot. • Red, swollen area on sole.	Infection caused by a penetrating wound or splinter.	Consult doctor. You may need tetanus protection.
• Pain in toe joints. • Affected joints red, warm, swollen.	Inflammatory disease of joints.	See Arthritis, Rheumatoid.
• Pain or tenderness in foot joint, especially big toe. • Affected joint red, warm, swollen. • Use of prescription drug to prevent fluid retention (diuretic).	Adverse reaction or side effect of diuretic drug.	• Consult doctor. • See Gout.
• Aching feet. • Significantly overweight.	Effect of excess weight.	See Obesity & Overweight.
• Pain in toe joints, ankles, knees or hips. • Person over age 50.	Degenerative condition of joints.	See Osteoarthritis.

*All references are to Illness section unless noted otherwise.

FOOT PROBLEMS
(continued from previous page)

SYMPTOMS & FACTORS	POSSIBLE PROBLEM	WHAT TO DO*
Numbness, hardness or paleness in skin exposed to subfreezing temperatures.	Tissue injury.	See Frostbite.
• Tingling and numbness in feet or hands. • Shooting pain that may worsen at night.	Nerve disorder.	See Peripheral Neuropathy.
• New sores or ulcers on the foot that take a long time to heal. • Diabetes.	Foot infection.	See Diabetes Feet & Skin Problems.
• Pain in toe joints. • Affected joints red, warm, swollen. • Fever. • Recent illness, such as sore throat or skin infection.	Complication of prior streptococcal infection.	See Rheumatic Fever.

*All references are to Illness section unless noted otherwise.

GENITAL SORES, BLISTERS, WARTS OR BOILS

SYMPTOMS & FACTORS	POSSIBLE PROBLEM	WHAT TO DO*
• Scaling patches on the skin of the groin, thighs, and buttocks. armpit, or groin. • Patches have well-defined edges.	Fungal infection.	See Tinea Cruris.
Painless blister on genitals.	Sexually transmitted disease.	See Granuloma Inguinale.
• Painless red sore on genitals. • Enlarged lymph glands in neck, armpit, or groin. • Headache. • Rash on skin.	Sexually transmitted disease.	See Syphilis.
• Small flesh colored bumps or tiny cauliflower like bumps. • Warts may produce no symptoms, or cause itching, burning, tenderness or pain.	Sexually transmitted disease.	See Warts, Genital.
Genital sores on a child.	Possible child abuse.	See Child Abuse.

*All references are to Illness section unless noted otherwise.

HAIR GROWTH IN WOMEN, EXCESSIVE

SYMPTOMS & FACTORS	POSSIBLE PROBLEM	WHAT TO DO*
• Excessive hair growth over 4 or 5 months. • Unexplained weight gain. • Menstrual changes or absent periods. • Deep voice.	Disorder or tumor of ovaries or adrenal gland.	• See Ovarian Tumor, Benign. • See Ovarian Cancer. • See Cushing's Syndrome. • See Polycystic Ovarian Syndrome.
• Excessive hair growth over 2 months or less. • Use of prescription drug, such as hormones, cortisone drugs or anticonvulsants.	Adverse reaction or side effect of drug.	Consult doctor.
• Excessive hair on face or body that developed before age 20. • Similar hairiness in other female family members.	Genetic causes; no underlying disorder.	Consult cosmetologist for removal of unwanted hair.
Excessive hair growth, especially on face, in woman who has had ovaries removed or is over age 40.	Normal occurrence with decreasing estrogen level of menopause.	• Consult doctor. • Consult cosmetologist for removal of unwanted hair.
Excessive hair growth during pregnancy.	Hormone changes of pregnancy.	Nothing. Hair growth decreases after delivery.
• Excessive hair growth on the face and body of a woman. • Irregular or no menstruation. • Acne.	Excessive production of male hormones.	See Hirsutism.

*All references are to Illness section unless noted otherwise.

HAIR LOSS

SYMPTOMS & FACTORS	POSSIBLE PROBLEM	WHAT TO DO*
• Hair loss. • Use of prescription drug or radiation therapy, especially for cancer or circulatory disorders.	Adverse reaction or side effect of drug.	Consult doctor.
Sudden hair loss in patches on head.	Skin disorder.	• See Lichen Planus. • See Alopecia Areata. • See Ringworm. • See Telogen Effluvium.
Hair thinning in a woman within 2 to 3 months following childbirth.	Effect of hormonal changes.	Nothing. Hair growth will return to normal.
Gradual hair loss in women, especially thinning of hair on top of head.	Normal occurrence with aging.	See Baldness, Pattern.
Receding front hairline or thinning of hair on top of head in men.	Hereditary baldness occurring in men at any age.	See Baldness, Pattern.
• Hair loss. • Frequent use of any of following hair-care products or styles: permanent waves; dyes; bleaches; curling irons or hot rollers; straighteners; tight braids; ponytails; or cornrows.	Hair damage.	• Change hair style; avoid damaging products or styles. • Consult doctor if hair loss persists.
Hair loss in 2 to 3 months following serious illness.	Temporary effect of illness and high fever.	Nothing. Hair should return to normal within few months.
Pulling out of hair.	Psychological disorder called trichotillomania.	Consult doctor.

*All references are to Illness section unless noted otherwise.

HEADACHE
(continued on next page)

SYMPTOMS & FACTORS	POSSIBLE PROBLEM	WHAT TO DO*
• Headache. • Use of prescription or nonprescription drug.	Adverse reaction or side effect of drug.	• Consult doctor about prescription drug. • Discontinue use of nonprescription drug.
• Severe headache. • Fever.	Common occurrence with infection.	See Fever charts (in Symptoms section).
• Headache. • Recent head injury. • No other symptoms.	Common occurrence after head injury.	See Head Injury.
• Headache. • Vision disturbance before headache. • Nausea or vomiting.	Severe vascular headache.	See Headache, Migraine.
• Headache in forehead or back of head. • Tense, stressed feeling. • Sleeping difficulty.	Effect of stress.	• See Anxiety Disorder, Generalized. • See Headache, Tension. • See Depression. • See Stress.
• Sudden onset of headache. • Pain around eyes. • Headache occurs at same time every day.	Chronic headache disorder.	See Headache, Cluster.
• Pain or tenderness around eyes and cheekbones that worsens when bending head forward. • Recent cold or nasal allergies.	Sinus infection.	See Sinusitis.
• Headache without pain around eyes and cheekbones. • Runny or stuffy nose.	Virus infection.	See Cold, Common.
• Headache. • Decreased consumption of caffeine-containing beverages (coffee, colas, cocoa, tea).	Caffeine withdrawal.	• Reduce consumption of caffeine gradually. • Use a nonprescription pain reliever, such as acetaminophen.
• Headache, plus any of following: • Unusually long time since eating. • Excessive alcohol consumption. • Stuffy, smoky or noisy room. • Exposure to strong sunlight.	Circumstantial headache. No underlying disorder.	Use a nonprescription pain reliever, such as acetaminophen.
• Headache after excessive alcohol consumption. • Nausea or vomiting.	"Hangover."	Use a nonprescription pain reliever, such as acetaminophen.

*All references are to Illness section unless noted otherwise.

HEADACHE
(continued from previous page)

SYMPTOMS & FACTORS	POSSIBLE PROBLEM	WHAT TO DO*
• Severe headache that worsens when bending head forward. • Eyes sensitive to light. • Lethargy. • Confusion. • No recent head injury.	Bleeding in membrane around brain.	• Call doctor now. • See Subarachnoid Hemorrhage. • See Brain or Epidural Abscess.
• Headache that worsens when bending head forward. • Fever. • Eyes sensitive to light.	Infection of membranes around brain.	• Call doctor now. • See Meningitis, Aseptic. • See Meningitis, Bacterial.
• Headache. • Eye pain. • Blurred vision. • Nausea or vomiting. • No injury to eye.	Excess pressure in eye.	• Call doctor now. • See Glaucoma, Angle-Closure.
• Habitual headache on waking; no excessive alcohol consumption. • Double vision. • Nausea or vomiting.	• High blood pressure. • Brain tumor.	• See Hypertension. • See Brain Tumor.
Headache after reading or straining to see.	Strain on neck muscles (not strain on eyes).	See Headache, Tension.
• Headache; nausea; vomiting. • Ascent to higher altitude.	Lack of oxygen.	See Altitude Illness.
• Headache. • Dizziness. • Nausea; vomiting. • Faintness.	Gas inhalation.	See Carbon Monoxide Poisoning.
• Headache. • Stiff neck. • Fever.	Fungal infection.	See Cryptococcosis.
• Headache. • General ill feeling. • Chills and fever. • Muscle aches.	Bacterial infection.	See Legionnaire's Disease.
• Headache. • Fatigue and nausea. • Travel to foreign country.	Parasite infection.	See Malaria.
• Headache. • General ill feeling. • Fever and sometimes, chills. • Muscle ache.	Bacterial or viral infection.	• See Legionnaire's Disease. • See Encephalitis, Viral. • See West Nile Virus.

*All references are to Illness section unless noted otherwise.

HEARING LOSS

SYMPTOMS & FACTORS	POSSIBLE PROBLEM	WHAT TO DO*
• Hearing loss. • Use of prescription or nonprescription drug.	Adverse reaction or side effect of drug.	• Consult doctor about prescription drug. • Discontinue use of nonprescription drug.
• Hearing loss. • Sticky, green-yellow discharge from ear.	• Infection of outer-ear canal or middle ear. • Injury to eardrum.	• See Ear Infection, Outer. • See Ear Infection, Middle. • See Eardrum, Ruptured.
• Hearing loss. • Dizziness.	Disorder or infection of inner ear.	• See Labyrinthitis. • See Meniere's Disease.
• Hearing loss, especially of high-pitched sounds. • Exposure to excessive noise, such as a jackhammer.	Damage caused by exposure to harmful noise levels.	See Hearing Impairment or Loss.
• Hearing loss. • Earache.	Infection or blockage.	See Earache (in Symptoms section).
Gradual hearing loss in person over age 60.	Common occurrence with aging.	Consult doctor.
• Gradual hearing loss over several weeks or months. • History of similar hearing loss in other family members.	Poor function of middle-ear bones.	See Otosclerosis.
• Hearing loss. • Recent cold or sore throat.	Blockage of canal between middle ear and back of throat (eustachian tube).	• See Cold, Common. • Consult doctor if hearing loss lasts longer than 3 days.
Gradual hearing loss over several weeks or months without other symptoms.	Earwax blockage.	See Earwax Blockage.
Noise in ear (ringing, buzzing, roaring, whistling or hissing).	Acoustic nerve disorder.	See Tinnitus.
• Hearing loss. • Plugged feeling in ear. • Change in air pressure (flying, diving).	Ear damage.	See Barotitis Media.

*All references are to Illness section unless noted otherwise.

HEARTBEAT IRREGULARITY

SYMPTOMS & FACTORS	POSSIBLE PROBLEM	WHAT TO DO*
• Irregular heartbeat. • General ill feeling. • History of heart disease.	Disorder of heart rate or rhythm.	• Call doctor now. • See Atrial Fibrillation. • See Heart Rhythm Irregularity. • See Heart Block. • See Heartbeat, Rapid. • See Potassium Imbalance. • See Aneurysm. • See Heart Valve Disease. • See Calcium Imbalance. • See Idiopathic Hypertrophic Subaortic Stenosis.
• Irregular heartbeat. • Use of prescription or nonprescription drugs, such as: thyroid medication; digitalis preparations; diuretics; diet pills; stimulants; caffeine; decongestants; cold remedies, including nasal sprays; illegal drugs, including marijuana, cocaine, psychedelics, amphetamines.	Adverse reaction or side effect of drug.	• Consult doctor about prescription drug. • Discontinue use of nonprescription or illegal drug.
• Irregular heartbeat. • Unexplained weight loss. • Anxiety. • Excessive sweating. • Fatigue.	Overactive thyroid gland.	See Hyperthyroidism.
• Rapid or irregular heartbeat. • Recent tension or worry.	Effect of stress.	• See Anxiety Disorder, Generalized. • See Panic Disorder. • See Phobias. • See Stress.
• Irregular heartbeat. • Excessive smoking. OR • Excessive consumption of caffeine-containing beverages such as coffee, cola, tea or cocoa.	Effect of nicotine or caffeine.	Decrease nicotine or caffeine use.
• Rapid or irregular heartbeat. • Fever.	Infection.	See Fever charts (in Symptoms section).
• Heartbeat irregularity. • Shortness of breath. • Fatigue.	Heart inflammation.	See Myocarditis.
• Rapid heartbeat following exercise, emotional upset or exposure to cold. • Tremors and nervousness. • Feelings of doom.	Adrenal tumor.	See Pheochromocytoma.

*All references are to Illness section unless noted otherwise.

IMPOTENCE, MALE SEXUAL (Erectile Dysfunction)

SYMPTOMS & FACTORS	POSSIBLE PROBLEM	WHAT TO DO*
• Sexual impotence. • Use of prescription or nonprescription or mood-altering drugs, such as: antihypertensives; narcotics; cocaine; antidepressants; antihistamines; antiulcer medicines; diuretics; hormones including birth-control pills; beta-adrenergic blockers; tranquilizers; reserpine; marijuana; digitalis; skeletal-muscle relaxants; sedatives; hypnotics; or phenothiazines.	Adverse reaction or side effect of drug.	• Consult doctor about prescription drug. • Discontinue use of nonprescription drug.
• Sexual impotence. • Chronic illness.	• Low level of testosterone (male sex hormone). • Diminished blood circulation to genitals.	• Consult doctor. • See Atherosclerosis. • See Diabetes Type 1. • See Diabetes Type 2. • See Cirrhosis of the Liver. • See Hypothyroidism. • See Multiple Sclerosis. • See Prostatic Hypertrophy, Benign. • See Pituitary Gland, Underactive.
• Sexual impotence. • Excessive alcohol consumption.	Effect of alcohol.	See Alcoholism.
• Sexual impotence. • Anxiety or depression.	Effect of stress.	• See Anxiety Disorder, Generalized. • See Depression. • See Stress.
• Sexual impotence. • History of sexually transmitted disease.	Scarring or other effect of infection.	• See Syphilis. • See Gonorrhea. • See Urethritis. • See HIV & AIDS. • See Herpes, Genital. • See Reiter's Syndrome. • See Warts, Genital. • See Lymphogranuloma Venereum.
• Sexual impotence. • History of premature ejaculation or other sexual dysfunction.	Psychosexual problem.	• See Impotence. • See Premature Ejaculation.
• Sexual impotence. • Acute illness with fever.	Temporary effect of illness.	Nothing. Sexual function will return when illness subsides.

*All references are to Illness section unless noted otherwise.

ITCHING

SYMPTOMS & FACTORS	POSSIBLE PROBLEM	WHAT TO DO*
• Itching hands. • Hands are frequently wet or exposed to chemicals.	Effect of chemicals or moisture.	See Dermatitis, Contact.
• Itching on head or between toes. • Small bald patches on scalp.	Fungus infection.	• See Ringworm. • See Athlete's Foot.
• Itching on head. • Tiny white spots on hair that won't come off.	Parasites.	See Lice.
• Itching. • Insect bite or sting.	Reaction.	See Insect Bites & Stings.
• Itching or bleeding around anus. • Painful bowel movements.	• Varicose veins in anus. • Split in skin around anus.	• See Hemorrhoids. • See Anal Fissure.
Itching around anus following severe diarrhea.	Normal response to irritation.	Apply ointment containing zinc oxide.
• Itching. • Diarrhea. • Abdominal pain. • Flatulence and bloating. • Rash.	Reaction to a swallowed substance.	See Food Allergy.
• Intense itching and burning. • Bright red skin rash. • Contact with poisonous plant.	Allergic reaction to plant.	See Poison Ivy, Oak, Sumac.
• Itching. • Fluid-filled blisters. • Skin disorder elsewhere on body.	Allergic reaction.	See Id Reaction.
• Itching. • Yellow skin and eyes.	• Liver disorder. • Blood disorder.	Call doctor now.
• Itching. • General ill feeling.	• Blood disorder. • Kidney disorder. • Overactive thyroid gland. • Adverse reaction or side effect of drug. • Cancer.	• Consult doctor. • See Polycythemia. • See Renal Failure, Acute. • See Hyperthyroidism. • See Drug Hypersensitivity.
• Itching. • Rash.	Several skin disorders.	See Rash without Fever (in Symptoms section).
Itching in genital area in females.	Irritation or infection.	See Vaginal Itching (in Symptoms section).
Itching around anus, especially at night.	• Parasites. • Several causes.	• See Pinworms. • See Pruritus Ani.
• Itching. • Wheezing; coughing; sneezing. • Swelling around face and hands. • Difficult breathing.	Allergic reaction.	• Call doctor now. • See Anaphylaxis.

*All references are to Illness section unless noted otherwise.

KNEE PAIN

SYMPTOMS & FACTORS	POSSIBLE PROBLEM	WHAT TO DO*
• Pain in knee. • Knee "catches" or won't bear weight.	Injured knee cartilage.	See Sprains & Strains.
• Pain in knee following injury. • Knee won't bear weight. • Knee misshapen.	Broken bone or dislocation.	• Call doctor now. • See Bone Fracture. • See Dislocation or Subluxation.
• Pain in knee. • Knee red, warm, swollen. • Fever. • General ill feeling.	Bone or joint infection.	See Osteomyelitis.
• Pain in knee and other joints. • Affected joints red, warm, swollen. • Fever. • Recent illness such as sore throat, gonorrhea or skin infection.	Complication of prior infection.	• See Rheumatic Fever. • See Arthritis, Infectious.
• Pain in knee or other joints. • Affected joints red, warm, swollen. • No fever.	Joint inflammation.	• See Bursitis. • See Gout. • See Arthritis, Rheumatoid. • See Arthritis, Juvenile Rheumatoid (children only). • See Osgood-Schlatter Disease (older children and adolescents only). • See Psoriatic Arthritis.
• Chronic pain in knee. • Knee sometimes "catches" or won't support weight. OR • Persistent discomfort in knee, fingers or other joints without other symptoms.	Degenerative joint disease.	See Osteoarthritis.
• Pain in knee in child under 12. • Hip pain. • Limp.	• Degenerative condition of hip joint in children. • Inflammation.	• See Legg-Perthes Disease. • See Transient Synovitis of the Hip.
• Acute attack of swelling and pain in the knee. • Attack lasts for 2 or more days.	Joint disorder.	See Pseudogout.

*All references are to Illness section unless noted otherwise.

LEG PAIN

SYMPTOMS & FACTORS	POSSIBLE PROBLEM	WHAT TO DO*
• Leg pain. • Back pain.	Muscle strain or sciatica.	See Back Pain, Low.
• Leg pain following strenuous exercise or following injury. • Leg can bear weight.	Muscle, tendon, ligament, or bone problem.	• See Sprains & Strains. • See Shin Splints.
• Leg pain. • Restricted movement, swelling and tenderness around a tendon.	Tendon inflammation.	See Tendinitis.
• Leg pain following injury. • Leg won't bear weight.	Broken bone.	• Call doctor now. • See Bone Fracture.
Sharp pain down back of leg, especially when coughing, sneezing or laughing hard.	Pressure on large nerve in leg.	• See Disk, Ruptured. • See Backache (in Symptoms section).
• Leg pain. • Muscles tighten briefly—usually while asleep—then return to normal.	Several disorders.	See Muscle Cramp, Ache or Weakness (in Symptoms section).
• Leg ache, especially after standing a long time. • Prominent veins in legs.	Disorder of veins.	See Varicose Veins.
• Shooting pain in leg. • Tingling and numbness that begins in hands or feet. • Gradual muscle weakness.	Nerve disorder.	See Peripheral Neuropathy.
• Pain in calf. • One vein red, hot and hard.	Blood clot in superficial vein.	See Thrombophlebitis, Superficial.
• Pain in calf when flexing ankle. • Swollen, tender calf.	Blood clot in deep vein.	• Call doctor now. • See Thrombosis, Deep Vein.
• Persistent pain in part of leg. • Fever. • General ill feeling.	• Bone infection. • Cancer.	• See Osteomyelitis. • See Multiple Myeloma.
• Pain in calf after walking. • Pain disappears with rest.	Circulatory disorder.	• See Atherosclerosis. • See Buerger's Disease. • See Claudication. • See Thrombosis & Embolus, Arterials.
• Leg pain. • Painful or stiff hip on same side.	• Degenerative condition of joints (in adult). • Inflammation (in child).	• See Osteoarthritis. • See Transient Synovitis of the Hip.
• Leg pain along sciatic nerve. • Recurrent low backache. • Stiffness.	Joint disease.	See Spondylitis, Ankylosing.
• Leg or arm pain (may be burning or aching) and swelling. • Changes in skin color.	Pain syndrome.	See Reflex Sympathetic Dystrophy.
• Leg sensations (may be painful) • Sensations occur while resting.	Movement disorder.	See Restless Legs Syndrome.

All references are to Illness section unless noted otherwise.

MEMORY PROBLEMS

SYMPTOMS & FACTORS	POSSIBLE PROBLEM	WHAT TO DO*
Gradual decline over past 10 years in ability to remember everyday things in person over age 50.	Common occurrence with aging; no underlying disorder.	• Consult doctor at next appointment. • Write lists to help your memory. This is not the beginning of serious mental decline.
• Inability to remember everyday things, such as location of keys, pens, glasses, or forgetting items on shopping list. • Depression or tension.	Effect of stress.	• See Depression. • See Anxiety Disorder, Generalized. • See Stress.
• Inability to remember a period of time. • Use of prescription or nonprescription drug, especially for sleeping difficulty.	Adverse reaction or side effect of drug.	Consult doctor.
Total memory loss.	Psychological disorder.	Consult doctor.
• Inability to remember a period of time. • Recent head injury.	Brain injury.	• Call doctor now. • See Head Injury.
Inability to remember episodes of excessive-alcohol consumption.	Effect of alcohol.	• Consult doctor. • See Alcoholism.
• Inability to remember recent events while remembering long-ago events, plus 2 or more of following: • Poor attention span in conversations or with instructions. • Decline in attention to personal appearance or cleanliness. • Personality change. • Decline in ability to cope with everyday matters.	Mental deterioration.	• See Dementia. • See Vitamin Deficiencies. • See Alzheimer's Disease.
• Inability to remember a period of time, plus events surrounding any of the following: • Epileptic seizure. • Diabetic coma. • Period before and after surgery. • Severe, feverish, illness such as meningitis or pneumonia.	Common occurrence following these situations.	Nothing.
• Memory problems and confusion. • Inability to speak or move part of body. OR • Low body temperature.	• Decrease in blood supply to brain. • Prolonged exposure to cold, especially in the elderly.	• Call doctor now. • See Stroke. • See Hypothermia.
• Memory loss. • Headaches; vomiting. • Vision changes.	Tumor.	• Call doctor now. • See Brain Tumor.
• Memory problems. • Recent surgical procedure with general anesthetic.	Often occurs.	Memory should return to normal.

*All references are to Illness section unless noted otherwise.

MENSTRUAL PERIODS, LATE OR ABSENT

SYMPTOMS & FACTORS	POSSIBLE PROBLEM	WHAT TO DO*
• Menstrual periods absent. AND • Eating disorder. OR • Current participation in strenuous exercise or activity. OR • Chronic illness. OR • Tension or worry. OR • Change in lifestyle such as new job or new home. OR • Menstrual periods absent since discontinuing use of oral contraceptives. OR • Obesity. OR • Other symptoms.	• Hormone changes. • Effect of stress. • Chronic illness. • Result of surgery. • Endocrine problem. • Disordered eating.	• See Amenorrhea, Secondary. • See Female Athlete Triad.
Menstrual periods have never started.	Hormone changes of puberty have not occurred.	• Consult doctor if older than 16. • See Amenorrhea, Primary.
• Menstrual period late by 2 or more weeks. • Sexual intercourse within last month.	Pregnancy.	• Consult doctor to confirm pregnancy. • Take home pregnancy test.
• Menstrual periods absent. • Use of prescription drug.	Adverse reaction or side effect of drug.	• Consult doctor. • See Amenorrhea, Secondary.
Menstrual periods absent in woman over age 38.	Normal menstrual irregularities at this age.	See Menopause.
Menstrual periods absent since delivery of baby.	Normal occurrence caused by hormone changes following childbirth.	• If bottle-feeding, consult doctor if periods do not resume within 8 weeks after delivery. • If breast-feeding, consult doctor if periods do not resume within 4 weeks after weaning.
• Menstrual periods absent. • Round face, puffy eyes. • Abnormal hairiness.	Hormone imbalance.	See Cushing's Syndrome.
• Irregular menstrual periods. • Discomfort or pain in lower abdomen. OR • Pain with intercourse. OR • Bleeding with intercourse. OR • Abnormal hairiness.	Cancer (possibly).	• See Ovarian Cancer. • See Uterine Malignancy.

*All references are to Illness section unless noted otherwise.

MENSTRUAL PERIODS, PAINFUL OR HEAVY

SYMPTOMS & FACTORS	POSSIBLE PROBLEM	WHAT TO DO*
• Excessive menstrual flow. • Menstrual period lasts more than 7 days.	Menstrual irregularity.	See Menorrhagia.
Menstrual period more painful or heavier than usual, especially during last days of period.	Disorder of lining of pelvic organs.	• See Endometriosis. • See Dysmenorrhea.
• Current menstrual period more painful or heavier than usual. • Period arrived one week or more late.	• Early pregnancy and miscarriage. • Pregnancy outside uterus.	• Consult doctor. • See Miscarriage. • See Ectopic Pregnancy.
Menstrual periods more painful or heavier since receiving intrauterine contraceptive device (IUD).	Common side effect of using IUD.	Consult doctor.
• Menstrual periods more painful or heavier than usual. • No other pelvic or genital symptoms.	Benign growth in uterus.	See Uterine Fibroids.
Menstrual periods painful or heavy since discontinuing use of oral contraceptives.	Hormone changes caused by discontinuing pill.	Consult doctor.
• Menstrual periods painful. • Periods began within last 3 years. • Healthy otherwise.	No disease.	See Dysmenorrhea.
Menstrual period heavy in woman who has recently. delivered a baby.	Normal occurrence during first 2 menstrual periods following childbirth.	Consult doctor if heavy periods persist.
Menstrual flow always heavy.	No underlying disorder.	Consult doctor for blood test for anemia.
• Heavy menstrual flow. • Bleeding between normal menstrual periods.	Excessive estrogen.	See Endometrial Hyperplasia.
Painful, prolonged or irregular bleeding through the vagina.	Several causes.	See Uterine Bleeding, Dysfunctional.
• Menstrual periods more painful or heavier than usual. • Bad-smelling vaginal discharge. • Fever.	Infection of reproductive organs.	• Call doctor now. • See Pelvic Inflammatory Disease.

*All references are to Illness section unless noted otherwise

MOUTH, SORE; TINGLING; DRY (continued on next page)

SYMPTOMS & FACTORS	POSSIBLE PROBLEM	WHAT TO DO*
• Sore mouth. • Blisters or red, rough or painful areas on lips or in mouth.	Virus infection.	• See Herpes Simplex. • See Hand, Foot & Mouth Disease.
• Sore mouth. • Creamy-white patches in mouth or tongue.	Fungus infection.	See Thrush.
Mouth sores that are shallow, usually red, and may have a white coating over them.	Inflammation.	See Stomatitis (Canker Sore).
• Dry mouth. • Use of prescription or nonprescription medication.	Adverse reaction or side effect of medication.	• Consult doctor about prescription drug. • Discontinue nonprescription drug if dry mouth is causing problems.
• Sore mouth. • Fever. • Sores in mouth. • Use of prescription or nonprescription drugs.	Adverse reaction or side effect of drug.	Call doctor now.
• Sore mouth. • Red, painful gums that bleed easily. • Bad breath.	Bacterial infection.	See Trench Mouth.
• Sore mouth. • Painful ulcers in the mouth.	Infection or inflammation.	See Canker Sores.
• Sore mouth. • Use of new cosmetics.	Allergic reaction caused by chemical.	Discontinue use of new cosmetic.
• Dry mouth. • Stress or apprehension.	Normal occurrence.	Dry mouth will disappear when stress is diminished.
Small white patch in the mouth that feels firm, rough and stiff.	Several causes.	See Leukoplakia, Oral.
• Small bumps or sores in the mouth. • Sores form an irregular whitish line in the mouth.	Infection.	See Lichen Planus.
• Dry mouth. • Decreased urination. • Severe thirst.	Electrolyte disorder.	See Dehydration.
• Sore mouth. • Rough or split corners of mouth.	Vitamin or mineral deficiency.	• See Vitamin Deficiencies • See Anemia, Folic Acid Deficiency. • See Anemia, Aplastic.
• Bleeding from the gums. • Easy bruising. • Tiredness; low fever; anemia.	Cancer.	See Leukemia, Acute.

*All references are to Illness section unless noted otherwise.

MOUTH, SORE; TINGLING; DRY (continued from previous page)

SYMPTOMS & FACTORS	POSSIBLE PROBLEM	WHAT TO DO*
• Pale, painless lump in mouth. • Lump may enlarge, ulcerate and bleed.	Cancer.	See Oral Cancer.
• Mouth tingling. • Sneezing, coughing, wheezing. • Watery eyes. • Difficult breathing.	Allergic reaction.	• Call doctor now. • See Anaphylaxis.
• Dryness of mouth. • Dryness of eyes. • Parotid gland enlargement (chipmunk face).	Autoimmune disorder.	See Sjögren's Syndrome.
• Numbness and tingling around the mouth. • Palpitations; rapid heartbeat. • Shortness of breath. • Emotional fears.	Severe anxiety.	See Panic Disorder.
• Soft or firm mass in the in the floor of the mouth or jaw. • There may be pain or swelling.	Tumor.	See Salivary Gland Tumor.

*All references are to Illness section unless noted otherwise.

MUSCLE CRAMP; ACHE; WEAKNESS
(continued on next page)

SYMPTOMS & FACTORS	POSSIBLE PROBLEM	WHAT TO DO*
Muscle cramp while relaxed or resting in bed. OR • Muscle cramp in arm or leg during or after exercise. OR • Muscle cramp after sitting in awkward position.	Common occurrence; usually no underlying disorder.	• Massage muscle and use heat to relieve pain. • See Sprains & Strains. • See Tendinitis.
Recurrent leg cramps when walking.	Circulatory disorder.	• See Atherosclerosis. • See Buerger's Disease. • See Thrombosis & Embolus, Arterial. • See Claudication.
Muscle cramp following exposure to heat.	Heat exhaustion.	See Heatstroke or Heat Exhaustion.
Pain, tenderness and limited movement in muscle.	Inflammation.	See Bursitis.
• Recurrent muscle cramps. • Tender nodules on skin. • Stiffness and weakness.	Inflammation of connective tissue.	See Fibromyalgia.
• Muscle cramp. • Use of diuretic drug for high blood pressure or heart disorder.	Adverse reaction or side effect of drug.	Consult doctor.
• Muscle cramp. • Numbness, tingling in arms or legs. • Irregular heartbeat.	Electrolyte disorder.	See Calcium Imbalance.
• Muscle aches. • Chills; fever; cough. • Exposure to field mice or other rodents.	Virus infection.	See Hantavirus.
• Muscle aches. • Fever; tiredness. • Exposure to cats; cat litter or dirt soiled by cats.	Protozoan disorder.	See Toxoplasmosis.
• Muscle weakness in hands, feet and arms. • Weakness spreads within 72 hours. • Shock.	Inflammatory nerve condition.	See Guillain-Barré Syndrome.
• Weakness. • Ducklike gait. • Falling; difficulty in getting up after falling.	Muscle deterioration.	See Muscular Dystrophy.
• Weakness in the pelvic or shoulder muscles. • Skin rash on the face, shoulders, arms, and over joints.	Connective tissue disorder.	See Polymyositis.

*All references are to Illness section unless noted otherwise.

MUSCLE CRAMP; ACHE; WEAKNESS
(continued from previous page)

SYMPTOMS & FACTORS	POSSIBLE PROBLEM	WHAT TO DO*
• Muscle cramps (usually in the legs). • Confusion; restlessness; anxiety. • Weakness.	Electrolyte disorder.	See Sodium Imbalance.
• Muscle weakness or cramps (in infants). • Swelling of ankles, abdomen and face. • Anemia in premature infant.	Vitamin deficiency.	See Vitamin Deficiencies.
• Weakness of arm and leg muscles. • Weakness of facial muscles.	Autoimmune disorder.	See Myasthenia Gravis.
• Muscle pain, aches, soreness, stiffness, and/or swelling. • New or changed exercise or activity.	Excess exercise or activity.	See Delayed Onset Muscle Soreness.
• Muscle ache. • General ill feeling. • Headache. • Fever and sometimes, chills.	Bacterial or viral infection.	• See Legionnaire's Disease. • See Encephalitis, Viral. • See West Nile Virus.

*All references are to Illness section unless noted otherwise.

NECK PAIN

SYMPTOMS & FACTORS	POSSIBLE PROBLEM	WHAT TO DO*
• Stiffness or severe neck pain on waking. • No pain before going to bed.	Uncomfortable sleeping position.	Consult doctor if pain lasts longer than 24 hours.
• Sudden, severe neck pain. • Injury to neck.	Muscle injury.	See Sprains & Strains.
• Neck pain. • Stressful situation.	Muscle tension.	Take a hot shower or have someone massage your neck muscles to relieve tension.
• Severe neck pain. • Sharp pain in shoulders or arms when moving head.	• Slipped disk in neck. • Neck-muscle injury.	• See Disk, Ruptured. • See Whiplash. • See Torticollis.
• Neck and shoulder pain. • Working at computer or other repetitive task for many hours.	Muscle spasm.	• Be sure computer screen is at proper eye level and chair is at correct height. • Take a break every hour.
• Sudden neck pain, especially when bending head forward, plus any of following: • Lethargy. • Confusion. • Eyes sensitive to light. • Nausea or vomiting. • Severe headache.	Infection or bleeding in membrane around brain.	• Call doctor now. • See Meningitis, Aseptic. • See Subarachnoid Hemorrhage.
• Sudden, severe neck pain. • Recent strong jolt. • Difficulty controlling arms or legs. • Loss of bowel or bladder control.	Damaged spinal cord.	Call doctor now.
• Stiff neck. • Behavioral or personality changes. • General ill feeling. • Headache; vomiting; fever.	Brain inflammation.	See Encephalitis, Viral.
Swelling or lump in neck.	Several disorders.	See Swelling or Lump (in Symptoms section).
• Chronic neck pain that is worsening. • Numbness or tingling in arm or hand. • Person over age 40.	Pressure on nerves in neck.	See Cervical Spondylosis.

*All references are to Illness section unless noted otherwise.

NOSE, STUFFY OR RUNNY

SYMPTOMS & FACTORS	POSSIBLE PROBLEM	WHAT TO DO*
• Stuffy or runny nose (clear, watery discharge) plus any of following: • Fever. • Cough. • Headache. • Aches in bones or joints. • Sore throat.	Virus infection.	• See Cold, Common. • See Influenza.
• Stuffy or runny nose (clear, watery discharge). • Itching eyes. • Sneezing.	Nasal allergy.	See Hay Fever.
• Runny nose. • Low-grade fever. • Decrease in appetite. • Cough; lethargy.	Virus infection.	See Respiratory Syncytial Virus.
• Stuffy or runny nose (thick, cloudy, yellow-green discharge). • Pain or tenderness around eyes and cheekbones that worsens when bending head forward.	Sinus infection.	See Sinusitis.
• Chronic "stuffy nose" feeling. • Impaired sense of smell. • Feeling of fullness in the face.	Growth in nasal cavity.	See Nasal Polyps.
• Obstruction of air through the nostrils. • Nasal discharge.	Septum problem.	See Nasal Septum, Deviated.
• Chronic "stuffy nose" feeling. • Use of nasal decongestants for more than 3 days.	Decongestant is suddenly withdrawn after extended use or they are overused.	Consult doctor.

*All references are to Illness section unless noted otherwise.

NUMBNESS, TINGLING OR PRICKLING (continued on next page)

SYMPTOMS & FACTORS	POSSIBLE PROBLEM	WHAT TO DO*
• Numbness or tingling in feet or hands after sitting in one position a long time or waking from deep sleep. • No underlying disorder.	• Stretching of, or pressure on, a nerve. • Temporary decrease in blood supply to a nerve.	Nothing. Feeling returns in a few minutes.
• Numbness or tingling in any part of body. • Use of prescription drug.	Adverse reaction or side effect of drug.	Consult doctor.
• Numbness or tingling in hands and fingers, especially at night. • Sharp pain in hand or arm, especially at night. • Weak grip.	Pressure on nerves in wrist.	See Carpal-Tunnel Syndrome.
• Numbness and tingling in injured area of the skin. • Formation of scar tissue.	Normal occurrence.	Nothing.
• Numbness or tingling on one side of body, plus any of following: • Weakness in extremities. • Dizziness. • Confusion. • Blurred vision. • Speaking difficulty.	Decreased blood supply to brain.	• Call doctor now. • See Stroke. • See Transient Ischemic Attack.
• Numbness or tingling in an arm or leg. • Weakness in the affected side. • Recent heavy lifting or strenuous exercise.	Pressure on nerves.	See Disk, Ruptured.
• Numbness or tingling in fingers or toes. • Blue fingers or toes in cold weather. • Redness and pain when numbness subsides and feeling returns.	Disorder of blood circulation in fingers and toes.	See Raynaud Disease & Phenomenon.
• Numbness or tingling in hands. • Stiff neck. • Person over age 35.	Pressure on nerves in neck.	• See Cervical Spondylosis. • See Thoracic-Outlet-Syndrome.
• Numbness or tingling in hands and face, especially around lips. • Dizziness.	Decreased carbon dioxide in blood.	See Panic Attack.
• Numbness, tingling in arms or legs. • Muscle cramps. • Irregular heartbeat.	Electrolyte disorder.	See Calcium Imbalance.

*All references are to Illness section unless noted otherwise.

NUMBNESS, TINGLING OR PRICKLING
(continued from previous page)

SYMPTOMS & FACTORS	POSSIBLE PROBLEM	WHAT TO DO*
• Numbness and tingling that begins in hands and feet. • Shooting pain that may worsen at night.	Nerve disorder.	See Peripheral Neuropathy.
• Fatigue and weakness. • Tingling sensation in arms, hands, legs and feet. • Frequent urination.	Endocrine disorder.	See Hyperaldosteronism.
• Tremors and nervousness. • Rapid heartbeat following exercise, emotional upset or exposure to cold. • Feelings of doom.	Adrenal tumor.	See Pheochromocytoma.

*All references are to Illness section unless noted otherwise.

SEXUAL INTERCOURSE, PAINFUL FOR MAN

SYMPTOMS & FACTORS	POSSIBLE PROBLEM	WHAT TO DO*
• Pain during ejaculation. • Burning when urinating. • Discharge from penis.	Infection of urethra or prostate gland.	• See Urethritis. • See Prostatitis. • See Gonorrhea.
• Pain in penis during intercourse. • Red, swollen, tender bumps or sores on skin or tip of penis.	Skin inflammation or infection.	• See Herpes, Genital. • See Balanitis.
• Pain in penis during intercourse. • Partner tense, difficult to arouse or uncomfortable during intercourse.	Lack of lubrication in partner's vagina.	• See Dyspareunia. • See Vaginismus.
• Pain in tip of penis after intercourse. • Use of latex condom. OR • Partner uses contraceptive cream or douching solution.	Allergic reaction to cream, solution or condom.	See Dyspareunia.
• Pain in penis before, during or after intercourse. • No other symptoms or factors.	Psychosexual problem.	• See Dyspareunia. • See Impotence.
A prolonged, painful, tender erection unaccompanied by sexual arousal.	Penis disorder.	• Call doctor now or seek emergency care. • See Priapism.

*All references are to Illness section unless noted otherwise.

SYMPTOMS

SEXUAL INTERCOURSE, PAINFUL FOR WOMAN

SYMPTOMS & FACTORS	POSSIBLE PROBLEM	WHAT TO DO*
• Painful intercourse only when partner penetrates vagina deeply. • Heavy, painful periods.	Disorder of lining of pelvic organs.	See Endometriosis.
• Painful intercourse. • Abnormal vaginal discharge.	Several disorders.	• See Abnormal Vaginal Discharge (in Symptoms section). • See Vaginitis.
• Painful intercourse. • Tenderness over bladder. • Frequent, painful urination.	Bladder inflammation.	See Bladder Infection, Female.
Painful intercourse in woman past menopause or over age 45.	Normal occurrence caused by decreased vaginal secretions.	• See Vaginismus. • See Dyspareunia. • See Menopause.
• Painful intercourse. • Recent childbirth.	Inflammation or scarring caused by a stretched or torn vagina or episiotomy repair.	• Wait at least 3 weeks before resuming sexual relations after childbirth. • Consult doctor if pain lasts longer than 8 weeks.
• Painful intercourse. • Vaginal itching.	Several disorders.	See Vaginal Itching (in Symptoms section).
• Painful intercourse. • Vagina seems too tight.	Muscle spasm.	• See Vaginismus. • See Dyspareunia.
• Painful intercourse. • Recent start or increase in sexual activity.	No underlying disorder.	• Wait 2 to 3 days for symptoms to disappear before resuming sex. • See Vaginismus. • See Dyspareunia.
• Dryness of vagina causing painful intercourse. • Dryness of eyes and mouth.	Autoimmune disorder.	See Sjögren's Syndrome.
• Pain with intercourse. • Bad smelling vaginal discharge. • Frequent, painful urination.	Infection.	See Pelvic Inflammatory Disease.
• Pain with intercourse. • Lump in back of the vagina or projecting outside of it. • Vague backache.	Fallen uterus.	See Uterine Prolapse.
• Painful intercourse. • Swelling without pain in lower abdomen or severe abdominal pain. • Stinging or burning with urination.	Cysts.	See Polycystic Ovarian Syndrome.
• Painful intercourse. • No other symptoms or factors.	• Vaginal malformation. • Lack of experience and education.	Consult doctor.

*All references are to Illness section unless noted otherwise.

SHOULDER PAIN

SYMPTOMS & FACTORS	POSSIBLE PROBLEM	WHAT TO DO*
• Pain in shoulder following injury. • Shoulder misshapen. • Bruising in affected area. • Inability to move shoulder.	Broken bone or dislocation.	• Call doctor now. • See Bone Fracture. • See Dislocation or Subluxation.
• Pain in shoulder following injury. • Shoulder appearance normal. • Shoulder movement uncomfortable.	Injury to shoulder-cuff muscle or ligament.	• See Sprains & Strains. • See Tendinitis.
• Pain in shoulder, especially when moving arm. • No other symptoms.	Shoulder inflammation.	See Bursitis.
• Pain in shoulder and other joints. • Affected joints red, warm, swollen.	Inflammatory disease of joints.	• See Arthritis, Rheumatoid. • See Psoriatic Arthritis.
• Sudden pain in shoulder. • No fever.	Shoulder inflammation.	• See Gout. • See Pseudogout.
• Shoulder and neck pain. • Working at computer or typing for many hours.	Muscle spasm.	• Be sure computer screen is at proper eye level and chair is at correct height. • Take a break every hour.
• Sudden pain in shoulder or other joint. • Affected joint red, warm, swollen. • Fever. • Recent illness, such as sore throat or skin infection.	Complication of prior streptococcal infection.	See Rheumatic Fever.
• Pain in shoulder when moving arm. • Stiffness and severity of pain increasing.	Severe shoulder inflammation.	See Shoulder, Frozen.
• Pain between shoulder blades. • Tightness, pressure, squeezing, or mild ache in the chest. • Heart disorder.	Lack of blood to heart.	• Consult doctor. • See Angina Pectoris.

*All references are to Illness section unless noted otherwise.

SKIN, BUMPS ON
(continued on next page)

SYMPTOMS & FACTORS	POSSIBLE PROBLEM	WHAT TO DO*
Thickened bump on toe.	Skin thickening caused by pressure.	See Corn or Callus.
Bumps on skin that are cysts, blisters, scaly patches, white patches or sores.	Several disorders.	See Skin Problems (in Symptoms section).
Rough, hard bump on hand or foot with tiny black dots in bump.	Skin growth caused by virus.	See Warts.
Painful, red bump with white or yellow center in part of body with hair.	Infected hair follicle.	See Boils.
• Small raised bumps that are firm, white and have a dry sandpaper feel. • Bumps are in clusters in hair follicles.	Common skin disorder.	See Keratosis Pilaris.
• Bumps or rash. • Fever.	Several disorders.	See Rash with Fever (in Symptoms section).
• Papules (small, raised bumps) that are flat-topped with well-defined borders. • Papules don't itch or hurt.	Inflammatory skin disorder.	See Keratoses, Seborrheic.
• Nodules under the skin that are dome-shaped. • Nodules feel "doughy," smooth and are easily movable.	Benign fat-cell tumors.	See Lipomas.
Rough, small bumps on skin of anus, vagina or penis.	Skin growth caused by virus.	See Warts, Genital.
• Light-red bumps with raised edges. • Severe itching.	Allergic reaction.	See Hives.
• Dark, slow-growing lump. OR • Change in mole size or color. • Borders of mole become irregular. • Bleeding or pain in mole.	Skin cancer or precancerous lesion.	• See Melanoma. • See Dysplastic Nevi.
Single lump that grows.	• Skin growth caused by virus. • Skin cancer, especially if center is an open sore. • Spread of cancer from other body parts.	• Consult doctor. • See Skin Cancer, Basal-Cell. • See Skin Cancer, Squamous-Cell.
Red bumps on cheeks, on either side of nose and on scalp.	Autoimmune disorder.	See Lupus Erythematosus, Discoid.
• Skin symptoms that vary. • Use of latex product, such as rubber gloves.		See Latex Allergy.

*All references are to Illness section unless noted otherwise.

SKIN, BUMPS ON
(continued from previous page)

SYMPTOMS & FACTORS	POSSIBLE PROBLEM	WHAT TO DO*
• Nodules in the armpit. • Nodules are firm, tender and domed.	Blocked glands.	See Hidradenitis Suppurativa.
• Small red, raised bumps (papules) on the skin of the thighs, buttocks or armpits. • Followed by other symptoms: muscle aches, fatigue, chills, fever, stiff neck, headache, backache, nausea and vomiting.	Tick bite.	See Lyme Disease.
• Small, raised bumps (papules) on the skin. • Bumps are firm, smooth, domed with a central pit, and skin-colored or white.	Virus infection of the skin.	See Molluscum Contagiosum.

*All references are to Illness section unless noted otherwise.

SKIN PROBLEMS (CHILD UNDER AGE 2)

SYMPTOMS & FACTORS	POSSIBLE PROBLEM	WHAT TO DO*
Rash in diaper area.	Chemical skin irritation.	See Diaper Rash.
• Rash or blotches. • Hot weather or environment.	Sweat retention.	• Remove excess clothing. • Consult doctor if rash lasts longer than 24 hours or child seems ill. • See Prickly Heat.
Greasy, scaling, crusty patches on scalp.	Cradle cap.	Use half-strength coal-tar cream on affected areas. Your pharmacist can provide this. Cradle cap usually disappears when hair grows.
• Rash. • Fever.	Several disorders.	See Rash with Fever (in Symptoms section).
Rash, spots, blisters or discoloration in infant 3 months or younger.	Several disorders.	Consult doctor.
Inflamed skin with itching, flaking patches.	Allergic skin disorder.	See Dyshidrotic Eczema.
Blisters on face that burst and become crusty.	Skin infection.	See Impetigo.
Patch of skin that is lighter or darker than surrounding skin.	• Disorder of skin pigment. • Inherited skin lesion.	• See Pityriasis Alba. • See Skin Lesions, Benign.
• Small, itching blisters, usually in a thin line. • Broken blisters leave scratch marks.	Disease of the skin.	See Scabies.
Dark red or purple spots that don't fade when skin is pressed or stretched.	Allergic disorder.	• Call doctor now. • See Purpura, Allergic.
• Small raised bumps on the skin (often on the face). • Bumps don't hurt or itch.	Virus infection.	See Molluscum Contagiosum.
• Small, raised itch bumps. • Bumps swell and produce pink or red lesions (wheals). • Wheals form larger areas of redness.	Allergic disorder.	See Hives.

*All references are to Illness section unless noted otherwise.

SKIN PROBLEMS (PERSON OVER AGE 2) (continued on next page)

SYMPTOMS & FACTORS	POSSIBLE PROBLEM	WHAT TO DO*
• Red, circular, flat, scaling lesions. • May be on the scalp, skin, nails and bearded area of the face.	Fungal infection.	See Ringworm.
• Rash. • Use of prescription or nonprescription drug.	Adverse reaction or side effect of drug.	• Call doctor now about prescription drug. • Discontinue use of nonprescription drug.
Red skin areas covered with silvery scales.	Chronic skin disorder.	See Psoriasis.
Flaking, white scales over reddish patches on the skin where hair grows.	Dandruff or cradle cap.	See Dermatitis, Seborrheic.
Painful, red bump with white or yellow center in part of body with hair.	Infected hair follicle.	See Boils.
Patch of skin that is lighter or darker than surrounding skin.	• Disorder of skin pigment. • Yeast infection of skin.	• See Vitiligo. • See Pityriasis Alba. • See Tinea Versicolor.
Yellow or greenish-yellow tint to the skin (jaundice).	Numerous disorders or drugs.	Call doctor now.
• Yellow-orange tint to the skin. • Consumption of large amounts of carrots or yellow vegetables.	Excess of carotene in the system.	Stop eating offending food for 2 to 6 weeks. Resume eating it in moderation.
• A new mole or dark lump. OR • Change in a mole or skin lesion.	Skin cancer or precancerous lesion.	• See Melanoma. • See Dysplastic Nevi.
• Dome-shaped cyst. • Cyst is whitish or skin-colored.	Infected cyst.	See Sebaceous Cyst.
• Blister-like rash. • Burning sensation at site 1 or 2 days before rash appears.	Virus infection of sensory nerves.	See Herpes Zoster.
Small blisters on fingers, toes, palms and soles.	Bacterial or fungal skin infection.	See Folliculitis.
Reddish, scaly, oval patches on chest, back or abdomen without fever or other symptoms.	Inflammatory skin disorder.	See Pityriasis Rosea.
• Skin symptoms that vary. • Use of latex product, such as rubber gloves.		See Latex Allergy.
Itching rash without fever.	Several disorders.	See Rash Without Fever (in Symptoms section).

*All references are to Illness section unless noted otherwise.

SYMPTOMS & FACTORS	POSSIBLE PROBLEM	WHAT TO DO*
• Redness, swelling and tenderness in skin. • Fever. • General ill feeling.	Skin infection.	See Cellulitis.
• Skin lesions (blue-red nodules) on face, arms and trunk. • HIV infection.	Skin cancer.	See Kaposi Sarcoma.
Numbness, hardness or paleness in skin exposed to subfreezing temperature.	Tissue injury.	See Frostbite.
• Painless blister on genitals that ulcerates and heals quickly. • Enlarged lymph glands in the groin that form large, red, tender masses.	Sexually transmitted disease.	See Lymphogranuloma Venereum.
Pain, redness, and tenderness at the base of the spine.	Infected cyst.	See Pilonidal Disease.
• Small, movable, nontender nodule that appears under the skin of the finger. • The nodule enlarges and becomes pink and ulcerates.	Fungal infection.	See Sporotrichosis.
New scars on the skin that arise in an area of injury, burn or other skin problem.	Defective healing process.	See Keloids.
• Clusters of small, itching blisters. • Clusters appear on both sides of the body in the same place.	Inflammation of skin.	See Dermatitis, Herpetiformis.
• Sudden appearance of warm, painful or tender nodules (usually start on front of leg). • Color changes from pink to red to blue to brown.	Inflammatory skin disease.	See Erythema Nodosum.
• Small, raised bumps on the skin in the shape of a ring. • Pink or violet color with a dome or slightly flat shape.	Chronic benign skin disorder.	See Granuloma Annulare.
• Small raised bumps on the skin that appear first as pinhead size, but grow rapidly. • Bumps bleed easily if injured.	Skin disorder of unknown cause.	See Granuloma, Pyogenic.
• Redness, swelling, warmth around a nail. • Sudden pain around the nail.	Herpes infection of the skin.	See Herpetic Whitlow.
• New sores or ulcers that take a long time to heal. • Diabetes.	Skin infection.	See Diabetes Feet & Skin Problems.

*All references are to Illness section unless noted otherwise.

SYMPTOMS & FACTORS	POSSIBLE PROBLEM	WHAT TO DO*
• Rash. • Fever.	Several disorders.	See Rash with Fever (in Symptoms section).
Skin problems in child under 2.	Several disorders.	See Skin Problems (Person Under Age 2) (in Symptoms section).
Skin problem on feet.	Several disorders.	See Foot Problems (in Symptoms section).
Skin problem on face.	Several disorders.	See Facial Skin Problems (in Symptoms section).
Itching without change in skin appearance.	Several disorders.	See Itching (in Symptoms section).
Bumps on skin.	Several disorders.	See Skin, Bumps on (in Symptoms section).
• Plaques (flat areas with the following characteristics): • Bright red patches with poorly defined borders. • Some are weeping or oozing. • Skin appears moist or crusted. • Severe itching.	Yeast infection of the skin.	See Candidiasis of Skin.

*All references are to Illness section unless noted otherwise.

SKIN RASH WITH FEVER
(continued on next page)

SYMPTOMS & FACTORS	POSSIBLE PROBLEM	WHAT TO DO*
• Raised, red, itching bumps that become blisters on face, trunk and genitals. • Fever.	Virus infection.	See Chickenpox.
• Red rash. • Fever. • Swelling on both sides of neck or at base of skull.	Virus infection.	See Rubella.
• Rash starting on cheeks and then spreading. • Fever. • Young child.	Virus infection.	See Erythema Infectiosum.
• Rash in child age 1-3. • Fever. • Irritability.	Childhood disorder.	See Roseola Infantum.
• Red spots or blotches on face or trunk. • Fever, plus 2 or more of following: • Dry cough. • Sore, red eyes. • Runny nose. • Sore throat. • Headache.	• Virus infection. • Rickettsia infection.	• See Measles. • See Hand, Foot & Mouth Disease. • See Rocky Mountain Spotted Fever.
• Painful red, blister-like rash on body. • Fever. • General ill feeling.	Virus infection.	See Herpes Zoster.
• Purple spots, plus 2 or more of following: • Fever. • Headache. • Pain when bending head forward. • Eyes sensitive to light. • Vomiting.	Infection of membranes around brain.	• Call doctor now. • See Meningitis, Bacterial.
• Red rash in woman of childbearing age. • Fever of 101°F (38.3°C) or higher. • Rapid heartbeat. • Fatigue and weakness. • Excessive thirst.	Bacterial infection.	• Call doctor now. • See Toxic Shock Syndrome.
• Purple rash. • Fever.	Allergic disorder.	• Call doctor now. • See Purpura, Allergic.

*All references are to Illness section unless noted otherwise.

SKIN RASH WITH FEVER
(continued from previous page)

SYMPTOMS & FACTORS	POSSIBLE PROBLEM	WHAT TO DO*
• Red rash. • Paleness around mouth. • Fever of 102°F (38.9°C) or higher. • Bright red, sore throat. • Swollen tonsils. • Enlarged glands in neck.	Complication of preceding streptococcal infection.	• Call doctor now. • See Scarlet Fever.
• Mild skin rash on chest, back and abdomen. • Fever; fatigue and paleness. • Pain caused by joint inflammation.	Complication of preceding streptococcal infection.	See Rheumatic Fever.
• Red rash or spots that begins on palms, soles, arms and legs. • Rash develops into blisters. • Fever (sometimes).	Inflammatory disorder.	See Erythema Multiforme.

*All references are to Illness section unless noted otherwise.

SKIN RASH WITHOUT FEVER
(continued on next page)

SYMPTOMS & FACTORS	POSSIBLE PROBLEM	WHAT TO DO*
• Light-red bumps with raised edges. • Severe itching.	Allergic reaction.	See Hives.
• Itching rash. • Use of prescription or nonprescription drug.	Adverse reaction or side effect of drug.	• Call doctor now. • See Drug Hypersensitivity.
Itching, red, scaling or moist rash under cosmetics, jewelry or new clothing.	Allergic reaction.	See Dermatitis, Contact.
Itching, red, scaling or moist rash, especially on hands.	Skin disorder aggravated by stress.	See Dermatitis, Atopic.
• Itching, red, scaling or moist rash, plus: • Recent contact with plant, such as poison ivy, poison oak, poison sumac, primrose or mango. OR • Recent contact with irritating detergents or other chemicals.	Allergic reaction.	• See Poison Ivy, Oak, Sumac. • See Dermatitis, Contact.
• Itching rash around genitals or anus. • No other symptoms or factors.	• Sugar in urine. • Vaginal infection.	• See Diabetes Type 1. • See Diabetes Type 2. • See Vulvovaginitis, Candidiasis.
Red bumps in a small area without other symptoms.	Insect bites.	See Insect Bites & Stings.
• Red rash. • Rash is located in areas of heavy perspiration.	Obstruction of sweat glands.	See Prickly Heat.
• Red rash scattered over body. • Severe itching at night. • Gray lines or red, sore spots between fingers or on wrists.	Parasites.	See Scabies.
• Rash that consists of small, white blisters with pus inside. • Blisters are located in hair follicles of the skin.	Bacterial or fungal skin infection.	See Folliculitis.
Red, scaling patch that spreads into a ring.	Fungus infection.	See Ringworm.
Rash without fever in child under 2.	Several disorders.	See Skin Problems (Child Under Age 2) (in Symptoms section).
• Red rash that begins on palms, soles, arms and legs. • Rash develops into blisters.	Inflammatory disorder.	See Erythema Multiforme.

*All references are to Illness section unless noted otherwise.

SKIN RASH WITHOUT FEVER
(continued from previous page)

SYMPTOMS & FACTORS	POSSIBLE PROBLEM	WHAT TO DO*
• Red, raised rash or skin lesions. • Rash appears on cheeks in a "butterfly" appearance.	Autoimmune disorder.	• See Lupus Erythematosus, Discoid. • See Lupus Erythematosus, Systemic.
• Rash starting on cheeks then spreading. • Slight tiredness or fatigue. • Young child.	Virus infection.	See Erythema. Infectiosum.
• Skin rash, progressing to thin, raised lines on the skin. • Contact with soil or sand.	Hookworm infestation.	See Larva Migrans Cutaneous.
• Skin rash (that may itch) on face, shoulders, arms and over joints. • Weakness in the pelvic or shoulder muscles.	Connective tissue disorder.	See Polymyositis.
• Red skin rash, sometimes with small blisters. • A burning reaction similar to those that follow prolonged sun exposure. • Dizziness, nausea, vomiting. • Brief sun exposure.	Sensitivity to sun.	See Photosensitivity.
• Scaling patches on the skin of the groin, thighs, and buttocks. armpit, or groin. • Patches have well-defined edges.	Fungal infection.	See Tinea Cruris.

*All references are to Illness section unless noted otherwise.

SLEEPING PROBLEMS
(continued on next page)

SYMPTOMS & FACTORS	POSSIBLE PROBLEM	WHAT TO DO*
Sleep disturbance (difficulty falling asleep, staying asleep or remaining asleep).	Many causes.	• See Insomnia. • See Sleep Disorders.
• Sleeping problems (sleepiness or insomnia). • Use of prescription or nonprescription drug, such as appetite suppressants, decongestants or diuretics.	Adverse reaction or side effect of drug.	Consult doctor.
Sleeping problems following late, heavy dinner or consumption of 3 or more alcoholic beverages at night.	Common occurrence.	• Eat lighter or earlier dinner. • Decrease alcohol consumption.
• Sleeping problems. • Use of caffeine-containing beverage or drug.	Stimulant effect of caffeine.	Decrease use of caffeine, especially during late afternoon or evening.
• Sleeping problems. • Sedentary lifestyle.	Common occurrence.	Begin an exercise program. Consult your doctor first if you have any chronic illness or are at risk for heart disease.
Change in sleep pattern in person over age 60.	Normal occurrence; less sleep may be needed with aging.	Nothing.
• Inability to fall asleep. • Daytime tension.	Effect of stress.	• See Anxiety Disorder, Generalized. • See Stress.
• Wakefulness during night, plus 2 or more of following: • Reduced sex drive. • Inability to concentrate. • Lowered self-esteem. • Feelings of guilt, worthlessness, self-reproach. • Fatigue. • Loss of pleasure in usual activities. • Poor appetite or overeating.	Depression.	See Depression.
• Sleeping problems. • Recent withdrawal from narcotics, sleeping pills, tranquilizers or alcohol.	Withdrawal symptom.	Nothing. Normal sleep pattern should return within several weeks.
• Sleeping problems. • Use of illegal drug.	Adverse reaction or side effect of drug.	• Discontinue use of drug. • See Substance Abuse.

*All references are to Illness section unless noted otherwise.

SLEEPING PROBLEMS
(continued from previous page)

SYMPTOMS & FACTORS	POSSIBLE PROBLEM	WHAT TO DO*
• Sleeping problems, plus 2 or more of following: • Excessive sweating. • Unexplained weight loss. • Increased appetite. • Anxiety. • Rapid or irregular heartbeat.	Overactive thyroid gland.	See Hyperthyroidism.
• Sleep problems. • Poor appetite. • Self-pity and pessimism.	Chronic mild depression.	See Dysthymia.
Sleep attacks that may occur up to 10 times a day.	Sleep disorder.	See Narcolepsy.
• Sleepiness. • Constipation. • Decreased tolerance for hot or cold.	Underactive thyroid gland.	See Hypothyroidism.
• Fitful sleep. • Shortness of breath when awake.	Fluid in lungs caused by heart condition.	See Congestive Heart Failure.
• Long periods of not breathing when asleep. • Choking while sleeping. • Snoring.	Breathing problem.	See Sleep Apnea.
• Poor sleep habits in infants, such as restlessness and profuse sweating. • Delayed motor skills.	Vitamin deficiency.	See Vitamin Deficiencies.
• Difficulty in remaining asleep. • Stiffness and weakness. • Sudden, painful muscular spasms.	Muscle inflammation.	See Fibromyalgia.
• Child has sleepless nights. • Child is restless during day.	Behavior disorder.	See Attention Deficit Hyperactivity Disorder.

*All references are to Illness section unless noted otherwise.

SPEAKING DIFFICULTY

SYMPTOMS & FACTORS	POSSIBLE PROBLEM	WHAT TO DO*
• Speaking difficulty. • Use of prescription or nonprescription drug.	Adverse reaction or side effect of drug.	Consult doctor.
• Inability to complete words without repeating first consonants. OR • Inability to speak when ready to say something.	Stammering or stuttering in children, and stress in adults.	Consult doctor or speech therapist.
• Expressionless speech with abnormal tone and phrasing. • Trembling that is worse at rest. • Shuffling walk.	Disorder of central nervous system.	See Parkinson's Disease.
Normal pronunciation, but confused words or ideas in person under age 45.	Psychiatric disorder.	Consult doctor.
• Normal pronunciation but confused words or ideas, plus 1 or more of following: • Poor attention span with conversations or instructions. • Decline in attention to personal appearance or cleanliness. • Personality changes.	Mental deterioration.	• See Alzheimer's Disease. • See Dementia.
Speaking difficulty because of inability to move muscles on one side of face.	Disorder of facial nerves.	See Bell's Palsy.
• Speaking difficulty. • Vague eye problems. • Weakness; difficulty in walking and balance.	Nervous system disorder.	See Multiple Sclerosis.
Speaking difficulty because of pain in mouth or tongue.	Infection or sores in mouth or tongue.	See Mouth, Sore; Tingling; Dry (in Symptoms section).
• Speaking difficulty, plus any of following: • Blurred vision. • Numbness or tingling in any part of body. • Weakness in extremities. • Dizziness.	Decreased blood supply to brain.	• Call doctor now. • See Stroke. • See Transient Ischemic Attack. • See Aneurysm. • See Thrombosis & Embolism, Arterial.

*All references are to Illness section unless noted otherwise.

STOOL, ABNORMAL APPEARANCE

SYMPTOMS & FACTORS	POSSIBLE PROBLEM	WHAT TO DO*
• Stool that is very dark, black or contains black material, plus any of following: • Recent consumption of green, leafy vegetables; licorice; chocolate; grapes, raisins and cranberries. • Current use of iron-supplement tablets. • Recent use of Pepto-Bismol.	No underlying disorder.	Nothing. If discoloration continues, consult doctor.
• Red-looking stools. • Recent consumption of beets, tomatoes, red-colored drinks or cereal, cherry-flavored medicines.	Stools are reddish due to something you ate or drank.	Nothing. If discoloration continues, consult doctor.
• Dark or black stool. • Use of prescription or nonprescription drug.	Adverse reaction or side effect of drug.	• Consult doctor about prescription drug. • Discontinue use of nonprescription drug.
Light colored or almost white stool.	• Jaundice. • May be a symptom of numerous disorders.	Consult doctor.
• Blood in stool. OR • Stool has a black or dark-red color.	Several disorders.	See Bleeding, Rectal (in Symptoms section).
Worms in stool.	Parasitic infection.	• Call doctor now. • See Pinworms. • See Roundworms.
• Pale stool. • Yellow skin and eyes (jaundice).	Gallbladder or liver disorder.	• Call doctor now. • See Cholecystitis or Cholangitis. • See Hepatitis, Viral.
• Pale, foamy, bulky, bad-smelling stool. • No jaundice.	Poor digestion.	See Malabsorption.

*All references are to Illness section unless noted otherwise.

SWALLOWING DIFFICULTY

SYMPTOMS & FACTORS	POSSIBLE PROBLEM	WHAT TO DO*
• Swallowing difficulty. • Sensation that food is stuck high in chest. • Occasional chest pain, especially when bending forward or lying down.	Discomfort in upper digestive tract.	See Gastroesophageal Reflux Disease.
Normal swallowing with sensation that food is stuck.	Effect of stress.	• Increase fluid intake when eating. • See Anxiety Disorder, Generalized.
• Swallowing difficulty. • Sore throat. • Fever.	Throat infection.	• Request throat culture. • See Strep Throat. • See Tonsillitis. • See Pharyngitis. • See Herpangina. • See Diphtheria.
• Swallowing difficulty. • Recent swallowing of foreign object, such as fish bone. • Sore throat.	Object stuck in throat.	Call doctor now.
• Swallowing difficulty that is chronic or worsening. • Sensation that food is stuck high in chest.	Esophagus muscle disorder.	• See Hiatal Hernia. • See Dysphagia.
• Swallowing difficulty. • Pain with swallowing. • Bloody mucus regurgitation.	Tumor or esophagus disorder.	• See Esophagus Cancer. • See Esophageal Stricture.
• Swallowing difficulty. • Drooping eyelids. • Arm and leg weakness.	Autoimmune disorder.	See Myasthenia Gravis.
• Severe swallowing difficulty. • Muscle pain and spasms. • Fever. • Difficulty in using chest muscles to breathe.	Infection in a wound or injury site.	See Tetanus.
• Swallowing difficulty. • Hardening and thickening of the skin of the fingers and face.	Connective tissue disease.	See Scleroderma.
• Swallowing difficulty. • Muscle weakness of neck, chest and extremities. • Drooping eyelids. • Double vision. • No fever.	Toxin from contaminated food.	• Call doctor now. • See Botulism.
Swallowing difficulty that started with solid foods and now liquids.	Cancer.	See Esophageal Stricture.
• Swallowing difficulty. • Rapid weight loss.	Cancer.	See Esophagus Cancer.

*All references are to Illness section unless noted otherwise.

SWEATING, EXCESSIVE

SYMPTOMS & FACTORS	POSSIBLE PROBLEM	WHAT TO DO*
• Excessive sweating. • Anxiety or excitement.	Normal occurrence with stress.	• See Anxiety Disorder, Generalized. • See Stress.
• Excessive sweating. • Overweight.	Effect of excess weight.	See Obesity & Overweight.
• Excessive sweating in woman older than 38. • Irregular menstrual periods.	Hormone changes; end of menstrual cycles approaching.	See Menopause.
• Excessive sweating in woman during menstrual period. OR • Excessive sweating due to tension or apprehension. OR • Excessive sweating following coffee consumption.	No underlying disorder.	Nothing.
Excessive sweating in teenager.	Normal occurrence during adolescence.	Nothing.
• Sweating. • Palpitations; tremors; flushing. • Symptoms of anxiety when exposed to, or thinking of, a particular stimulus.	Fears.	See Phobias.
• Excess sweating. • Unpleasant body odor.	Several disorders.	See Hyperhidrosis.
• Skin is cool and moist. • Prolonged exposure to hot temperature.	Excessive fluid loss.	See Heatstroke or Heat Exhaustion.
• Excessive sweating. • Chest pain.	Heart attack.	• Call doctor now! • See Heart Attack. • See Coronary Artery Disease.
• Excessive sweating at night. • Weight loss. • Persistent cough with blood in sputum. • Fever. • Fatigue.	• Lung inflammation or infection. • Cancer.	• See Tuberculosis. • See Hodgkin's Disease. • See Lung Cancer.
• Excessive sweating, plus 2 or more of following: • Weight loss. • Increased appetite. • Anxiety. • Sleeping problems.	Overactive thyroid gland.	See Hyperthyroidism.
• Excessive sweating. • Use of prescription, nonprescription or illegal drug.	Adverse reaction or side effect of drug.	• Consult doctor about prescription drug. • Discontinue use of non-prescription or illegal drug.
• Excessive sweating. • Fever.	Normal occurrence with fever.	See Fever charts (in Symptoms section).

*All references are to Illness section unless noted otherwise.

SWELLING OR LUMP
(continued on next page)

SYMPTOMS & FACTORS	POSSIBLE PROBLEM	WHAT TO DO*
Firm swelling in groin that does not disappear when pressed.	• Infection in leg or genitals. • Protruding intestinal tissue.	• Consult doctor. • See Hernia.
• Nodule or bump under the skin. • Nodule feels "doughy," smooth and easily movable.	Benign fat-cell tumor.	See Lipomas.
• Painful, red lump or swelling. • Recent injury to area.	Bleeding under skin.	• See Sprains & Strains. • See Tendinitis.
Lump in breast.	• Benign changes. • Cancer.	• Consult doctor. • See Fibrocystic Breast Changes. • See Breast Cancer.
Soft lump or swelling in groin or near navel that disappears when pressed or enlarges with cough.	Protruding intestinal tissue.	See Hernia.
Swelling between ear and jaw.	• Virus infection of glands. • Infection around tooth. • Disorder or tumor of salivary gland.	• See Mumps. • See Tooth Abscess. • See Salivary Gland Infection.
• Lump or swelling in neck, armpit or groin. • Fever.	Virus infection.	See Mononucleosis, Infectious.
Swelling or lump in child 3 months or younger.	Several disorders.	Consult doctor.
• Swelling on both sides of neck, toward front. • Sore throat.	Bacterial or viral infection.	• See Tonsillitis. • See Pharyngitis. • See Mononucleosis, Infectious.
• Swelling at both sides of back of neck. • Pink rash. • Fever.	Virus infection.	See Rubella.
• Tender swelling in armpit, groin, elbow or base of neck. • Sore, cut or bite on hand, arm, leg or shoulder on same side as swelling.	Infected bite or wound.	Consult doctor.
Tender or hard lump in neck just below Adam's apple.	Inflammation or tumor of thyroid.	• See Thyroiditis. • See Thyroid Nodule.
• Tender lump on elbow or in armpit. • Fever. • Exposure to cats.	Virus infection.	See Cat-Scratch Disease.
Swelling in front of neck with movement when swallowing.	Thyroid goiter.	Consult doctor.

*All references are to Illness section unless noted otherwise.

SWELLING OR LUMP
(continued from previous page)

SYMPTOMS & FACTORS	POSSIBLE PROBLEM	WHAT TO DO*
• Swelling in neck, armpit or groin. • Recent vaccination, such as tetanus or typhoid.	Swelling caused by vaccination.	Consult doctor.
Painless swelling near joint that is overused.	Ganglion cyst.	Consult doctor.
• Mass in abdomen that can be felt, especially in young child. • Cramping abdominal pain.	Intestinal obstruction.	• Call doctor now. • See Intussusception.
Lump or swelling in neck, armpit or groin without other symptoms or factors.	• Infection. • Tumor.	• See Hodgkin's Disease. • See Lymphoma, Non-Hodgkin's.
• Lump or swelling in neck, armpit or groin. • Use of prescription drug, especially for epilepsy or thyroid disorder.	Adverse reaction or side effect of drug.	Consult doctor.
• Swollen lymph nodes. • Low-grade fever. • Weight loss. • Recurrent respiratory and skin infections.	Virus infection.	See HIV & AIDS.
• Hard mass in right, upper abdomen. • Unexplained weight loss and appetite loss. • Bleeding tendency.	Liver tumor.	• See Hepatoma. • See Liver Cancer.
• Swelling in superficial abscesses. • Rectal redness. • Throbbing pain. • Pain during bowel movement.	Swelling caused by bacteria or fungus.	See Anorectal Abscess.

*All references are to Illness section unless noted otherwise.

TESTICLES OR PENIS, PAINFUL OR SWOLLEN

SYMPTOMS & FACTORS	POSSIBLE PROBLEM	WHAT TO DO*
Painless swelling of testicles.	• Fluid accumulation. • Enlarged veins in testicle. • Protruding intestinal tissue.	• Consult doctor. • See Hernia.
• Sudden, painful swelling in testicle. • Recent injury to genital area.	Internal injury.	Call doctor now.
• Sudden, painful swelling in testicle. • No injury to genital area.	• Twisted testicle. • Infection of glands in testicle.	• Call doctor now. • See Testicular Torsion. • See Epididymitis.
Swelling or lump on one testicle.	Cyst or tumor.	• Consult doctor. • See Testicular Cancer.
• Pain in testicles. • Painless, rubbery strands extending up scrotum. • No injury to testicles.	Enlarged veins in testicle.	Consult doctor.
• Pain in testicles or penis. • Forceful blow, injury or wound in lower abdomen or genitals.	Injury to genitourinary tract.	See Genitourinary Injury.
• Pain in testicles. • Swelling between ear and jaw. • Fever.	Virus infection of glands.	• Consult doctor. • See Mumps.
• Ache (and sometimes pain) in the testicle. • Feeling of heaviness or dragging in the scrotum (the pouch of skin that contains the testicles).	Varicose veins.	See Varicocele.

*All references are to Illness section unless noted otherwise.

THROAT, SORE

SYMPTOMS & FACTORS	POSSIBLE PROBLEM	WHAT TO DO*
• Sore throat. • Fever. • Swelling on both sides of neck toward front. • Red, swollen tonsils with specks of pus on surface.	Bacterial or viral infection.	• Request throat culture. • See Tonsillitis. • See Strep Throat. • See Diphtheria. • See Mononucleosis, Infectious.
• Sore throat. • Excessive smoking or alcohol consumption. OR • Smoke-filled environment.	Throat irritation or inflammation.	See Pharyngitis.
• Sore throat. • Dripping nose. • Itching eyes.	Allergic reaction.	See Hay Fever.
• Sore throat. • Hoarseness or voice loss.	Several disorders.	• See Laryngitis. • See Voice Loss or Hoarseness (in Symptoms section).
• Sore throat. • Fever, plus any of following: • Aches in bones or joints. • Cough. • Headache. • Stuffy or runny nose.	Virus infection.	• See Cold, Common. • See Influenza.
• Sore throat. • Fever. • Swelling or tenderness between ear and jaw.	Virus infection of glands.	See Mumps.
• Sore throat. • Sudden "barking" cough. • Young child.	Bacterial infection of epiglottis.	See Epiglottitis, Acute.
• Sudden sore throat with redness, inflammation and painful swallowing. • Fever. • General ill feeling.	Virus infection.	See Herpangina.
• Sore throat. • Cough; chills; fever. • Muscle and joint aches. • Skin rash.	Fungal infection.	See Coccidioidomycosis.

*All references are to Illness section unless noted otherwise.

TONGUE, SORE

SYMPTOMS & FACTORS	POSSIBLE PROBLEM	WHAT TO DO*
• Sore tongue. • Use of prescription or nonprescription drugs.	Adverse reaction or side effect of drug.	Consult doctor.
• Sore tongue. • Discomfort confined to one spot.	Abrasion from denture or irregular tooth.	Consult dentist.
• Sore tongue. • Pain one one side of face.	Nerve inflammation or damage.	See Trigeminal Neuralgia.
• Sores on tongue. • Sores are small, very painful and shallow.	Several causes.	See Canker Sores.
• Sore tongue. • Hard lump on tongue or in mouth.	• Infection. • Tumor.	• Call doctor now. • See Mouth or Tongue Tumor, Benign. • See Oral Cancer.
• Sore tongue. • Diarrhea with loose, bulky, bad-smelling stool. • Retarded growth.	Poor digestion.	See Malabsorption.
• Sore tongue. • Discomfort involves whole tongue.	• Anemia. • Inflammation or infection.	• See Anemia, Pernicious. • See Anemia, Iron-Deficiency. • See Anemia During Pregnancy. • See Tongue Inflammation.
• Sore tongue. • Cracked, fissured, red tongue. • Mouth ulcers.	Poor nutrition.	• Consult doctor. • See Vitamin Deficiencies.

*All references are to Illness section unless noted otherwise.

TOOTHACHE

SYMPTOMS & FACTORS	POSSIBLE PROBLEM	WHAT TO DO*
• Toothache, plus any of following: • Fever. • Swollen face or gums. • Continual pain that interferes with sleep.	• Advanced tooth decay. • Infection around tooth.	• Call dentist now. • See Tooth Decay. • See Tooth Abscess.
• Toothache over several teeth. • Red, swollen, bleeding gums.	Gum infection.	• See Gingivitis. • See Periodontitis.
• Recurrent toothache. • No other symptoms.	Tooth decay.	• Consult dentist. • See Tooth Decay.
• Toothache when biting food. • Recent tooth filling.	• Common occurrence following a filling. • Filling not level.	Consult dentist if pain lasts longer than 1 week.
• Cheek pain that resembles a toothache. • Nasal condition. • Feeling of pressure inside the head.	Sinus infection.	See Sinusitis.
• Gnawing pain in lower teeth and neck. • Chest discomfort beneath breastbone. • Shoulder or arm pain. • Sweating.	Insufficient oxygen to heart.	• Call doctor now. • See Angina Pectoris. • See Coronary Artery Disease.

*All references are to Illness section unless noted otherwise.

TREMBLING OR TWITCHING

SYMPTOMS & FACTORS	POSSIBLE PROBLEM	WHAT TO DO*
• Trembling or twitching, especially of tongue and face muscles. • Use of prescription or non-prescription drug, especially phenothiazine.	Adverse reaction or side effect of drug.	• Consult doctor about prescription drug. • Discontinue use of nonprescription drug.
Trembling in one part of body, especially when affected part is at rest.	Movement disorder.	• See Parkinson's Disease. • See Essential Tremor.
• Trembling. • Alcohol withdrawal.	Withdrawal symptom.	See Alcoholism.
• Trembling. • Excessive consumption of coffee or tea. OR • Use of nonprescription drug containing caffeine.	Adverse effect of caffeine.	Decrease use of caffeine.
• Trembling, plus 2 or more of following: • Weight loss. • Fatigue. • Excessive sweating.	Overactive thyroid gland.	See Hyperthyroidism.
• Painful twitching on side of face. • Pain is triggered by stroking or touching the face.	Nerve disorder.	See Trigeminal Neuralgia.
Twitching in one small part of body, such as eyelid.	Fatigue or tension. Usually no underlying disorder.	• Nothing. • Consult doctor if you feel ill or if muscles seem weak.
Trembling in any part of body without other symptoms or factors.	Inherited tendency to tremble, especially from anxiety or stress.	Consult doctor to confirm diagnosis.
• Leg twitching or leg sensations (uncomfortable, to irritating, to painful). They may come and go. • Lying down and trying to relax causes the symptoms.	Movement disorder.	See Restless Legs Syndrome.
Unexpected body jerks when falling asleep.	Involuntary muscle spasms. No underlying disorder.	Nothing.

*All references are to Illness section unless noted otherwise.

URINATION, FREQUENT
(continued on next page)

SYMPTOMS & FACTORS	POSSIBLE PROBLEM	WHAT TO DO*
• Frequent urination, especially at night. • Increased urine production. • Excessive consumption of tea, coffee, cola or alcohol.	Effect of caffeine or alcohol.	Decrease consumption of caffeine or alcohol.
• Frequent urination, especially at night. • Increased urine production. • Use of diuretic drug for heart disease or high blood pressure.	Effect of diuretic drug.	Consult doctor if uneasy.
• Frequent urination. • Anxiety or excitement. OR • Cold weather.	Normal occurrence.	Nothing.
• Frequent urination. • Burning and stinging on urination. • Increased urge to urinate.	Bladder infection.	• See Bladder Infection, Female. • See Bladder Infection, Male.
• Frequent urination. • Painful urination. • Blood in urine.	Stones.	See Kidney Stones.
• Frequent urination. • Possible pregnancy.	Normal occurrence during first 3 months and last 3 months of pregnancy.	Consult doctor to confirm pregnancy.
• Frequent urination. • Pain with urination.	Several disorders.	See Urination, Painful (in Symptoms section).
• Frequent urination, especially at night. • Increased urine production, plus 2 or more of following: • Increased hunger and thirst. • Itching around genitals or anus. • Fatigue. • Weight loss.	Sugar in urine.	• See Diabetes Type 1. • See Diabetes Type 2.
• Frequent urination in man older than 50, plus 2 or more of following: • Involuntary urine leak after urination. • Weak urinary stream. • Difficulty starting urination. • Increased waking at night to urinate.	Disorder of prostate gland.	• See Prostatic Hypertrophy, Benign. • See Prostatitis.
• Frequent urination in a woman. • Intense urge to urinate followed quickly by uncontrollable urine leak.	Incontinence problem.	See Incontinence, Urge.
• Frequent urination. • Difficulty controlling bladder.	Several disorders.	See Urination, Lack of Control (in Symptoms section).

*All references are to Illness section unless noted otherwise.

URINATION, FREQUENT
(continued from previous page)

SYMPTOMS & FACTORS	POSSIBLE PROBLEM	WHAT TO DO*
• Frequent urination. • Discharge from urethra. • Small ulcers on mouth, tongue and tip of penis.	Inflammatory disease.	See Reiter's Syndrome.
• Passage of large amounts of urine. • Colorless urine. • Excessive thirst.	Hormone disorder.	See Diabetes Insipidus.
• Frequent urination. • Pelvic pain and pressure. • Sensation of incomplete emptying of bladder. • Pain during intercourse. • Burning on urination.	Inflammation in area of bladder.	See Interstitial Cystitis.
Decreased urination in males.	Prostate problem.	• See Prostatic Hypertrophy, Benign. • Prostate cancer.
• Decreased urine. • Smoky or slightly red urine.	Kidney infection.	See Glomerulonephritis.
Decreased urine even though urinating more frequently.	Infection, stone, or inflammation.	• Bladder Infection, Female. • See Bladder Infection, Male. • See Kidney Stones. • See Urethritis.
• Decreased urine. • Nausea, vomiting, appetite loss, diarrhea, mental changes.	Kidney conditions.	See Renal Failure, Acute.

*All references are to Illness section unless noted otherwise.

URINATION, LACK OF CONTROL

SYMPTOMS & FACTORS	POSSIBLE PROBLEM	WHAT TO DO*
Small urine leak in female when coughing, sneezing, laughing or running.	Incontinence problem.	See Incontinence, Stress.
• Lack of urinary control. • Use of prescription drug.	Adverse reaction or side effect of drug.	Consult doctor.
• Lack of urinary control. • Cloudy, bad-smelling urine.	Infection of urinary tract.	• See Bladder Infection, Female. • See Bladder Infection, Male. • See Urethritis.
Dribbling of urine after urination in male over age 50.	• Disorder of prostate gland. • Inflammation of urethra.	• See Prostatic Hypertrophy, Benign. • See Urethritis.
• Lack of urinary control. • Lack of bowel control.	Decreased blood supply to brain.	• Call doctor now. • See Stroke.
• Lack of urinary control. • Constipation for longer than 1 week.	Pressure on bladder from fecal impaction.	See Fecal Impaction.
• Lack of urinary control in person over age 60, plus 2 or more of following: • Inability to remember recent events. • Decline in attention to personal appearance or cleanliness. • Personality change.	• Poor nutrition. • Mental deterioration.	• See Vitamin Deficiencies. • See Alzheimer's Disease. • See Dementia.
Lack of urinary control in child over age 3-1/2.	Several causes.	See Bed-Wetting.
• Lack of urinary control. • Chronic illness.	Several disorders.	• Call doctor now. • See Multiple Sclerosis. • See Syphilis. • See Disk, Ruptured.

*All references are to Illness section unless noted otherwise.

URINATION, PAINFUL

SYMPTOMS & FACTORS	POSSIBLE PROBLEM	WHAT TO DO*
• Painful urination. • Pain in one side of back, between waist and last rib. • Fever.	Kidney infection.	See Kidney Infection, Acute.
• Painful urination. • Frequent urination.	Bladder inflammation.	• See Bladder Infection, Female. • See Bladder Infection, Male.
• Painful urination. • Painful blisters on genitals. • Fever.	Sexually-transmitted virus infection.	See Herpes, Genital.
• Painful urination in female. • Green-yellow or white discharge from vagina. • Itching around genitals.	Vaginal infection.	• See Vulvovaginitis, Candidiasis. • See Trichomoniasis.
• Painful urination in man. • Thick, yellow-green discharge from penis.	Sexually-transmitted infection.	• See Gonorrhea. • See Urethritis.
• Painful urination in woman. • Bad-smelling vaginal discharge. • Pain or tenderness in lower abdomen. • Fever.	Sexually-transmitted infection.	• See Gonorrhea. • See Urethritis.
• Painful urination in man. • Heavy feeling or dull pain between scrotum and anus. • Fever.	Infection of prostate gland.	See Prostatitis.
• Burning urination. • Blood in urine. • Pain in pelvic area.	Abnormal growth in bladder.	See Bladder Tumor.
• Painful urination or inability to urinate. • Forceful blow, injury or wound in lower abdomen or genitals.	Injury to genital tract.	See Genitourinary Injury.
• Discomfort on urinating. • Vaginal discharge (female). • Urethral discharge (male).	Infection.	See Chlamydia Infection.
• Discomfort with urination (male). • Painless sore or lesion on penis.	Cancer.	See Penis Cancer.

*All references are to Illness section unless noted otherwise.

URINE, ABNORMAL COLOR

SYMPTOMS & FACTORS	POSSIBLE PROBLEM	WHAT TO DO*
• Pink, red, smoky-brown or other color change in urine. • Use of new prescription drug in last 24 hours.	Side effect of drug.	Consult doctor if color change not expected.
• Dark yellow or orange urine. • Recent use of laxatives containing senna. OR • Recent consumption of rhubarb.	Effect of chemicals in these substances.	Nothing.
• Pink, red or smoky-brown urine. • Recent consumption of beets, blackberries or other red food.	Effect of natural or artificial color.	Nothing.
Pink, red or smoky-brown urine.	Disorder of urinary tract.	• Consult doctor. • See Bladder Infection, Female. • See Bladder Infection, Male. • See Prostatic Hypertrophy, Benign. • See Bladder Tumor. • See Tuberculosis. • See Kidney Stones. • See Kidney Infection (both Acute and Chronic). • See Wilms' Tumor (children only). • See Hypernephroma. • See Glomerulonephritis.
• Clear, dark-brown urine. • Pale stool. • Yellow skin and eyes.	Liver disorder.	• Call doctor now. • See Hepatitis, Viral.
• Dark yellow or orange urine. • Fever. OR • Very hot weather. OR • Decreased fluid intake.	Concentrated urine.	• See Fever charts (in Symptoms section). • See Heatstroke or Heat Exhaustion. • See Dehydration. • Increase fluid intake.
• Dark yellow or orange urine. • Vomiting. • Diarrhea.	Concentrated urine.	• See Vomiting, Recurrent Attacks (in Symptoms section). • See Diarrhea (in Symptoms section).
Green or blue urine.	Effect of artificial color in food or drug.	Nothing.
• Colorless urine. • Excessive thirst. • Passage of large amounts of urine.	Hormone disorder.	See Diabetes Insipidus.

*All references are to Illness section unless noted otherwise.

VAGINAL BLEEDING, UNEXPECTED

SYMPTOMS & FACTORS	POSSIBLE PROBLEM	WHAT TO DO*
Vaginal bleeding during first 3 months of pregnancy.	Spontaneous abortion.	• Call doctor now. • See Miscarriage.
Vaginal bleeding during 4th to 9th month of pregnancy.	Abnormal location of placenta.	• Call doctor now. • See Placenta Previa. • See Abruptio Placenta.
• Unexpected vaginal bleeding. • Severe abdominal pain. • Pregnancy possible. OR • Current use of intrauterine contraceptive device (IUD).	Pregnancy developing outside uterus.	• Call doctor now. • See Ectopic Pregnancy.
• Unexpected vaginal bleeding in woman over age 45. • Last menstrual period more than 6 months ago.	• Hormone changes. • Tumor or cancer.	• See Menopause. • See Postmenopausal Bleeding. • See Uterine Malignancy. • See Cervical Cancer. • See Ovarian Cancer. • See Vagina or Vulva Cancer.
• Unexpected vaginal bleeding in woman over age 45. • Use of prescription drug for hormone replacement therapy.	Breakthrough bleeding.	Consult doctor.
• Unexpected vaginal bleeding. • Vaginal discharge.	• Several disorders. • Cancer.	• See Cervical Polyps. • See Cervical Erosion. • See Cervical Cancer. • See Uterine Malignancy. • See Vagina or Vulva Cancer.
• Unexpected vaginal bleeding. • Pain in lower abdomen.	• Uterine fibroids. • Cancer.	• See Cervical Polyps. • See Uterine Bleeding, Dysfunctional. • See Uterine Fibroids. • See Ovarian Cancer. • See Uterine Malignancy.
• Unexpected vaginal bleeding. • Recent insertion of intrauterine contraceptive device (IUD).	Complications caused by IUD.	Consult doctor.
• Unexpected vaginal bleeding. • Use of oral contraceptives.	Breakthrough bleeding; common occurrence in women taking pill.	Consult doctor.
• Excessive menstrual flow. • Menstrual period lasts more than 7 days.	Menstrual irregularity.	See Menorrhagia.
• Menstrual disorders. • Course skin. • Sleepiness.	Underactive thyroid gland.	See Hypothyroidism.
• Unexpected vaginal bleeding. • Insertion of foreign object into vagina.	Vaginal injury.	Consult doctor.

*All references are to Illness section unless noted otherwise.

VAGINAL DISCHARGE, ABNORMAL

SYMPTOMS & FACTORS	POSSIBLE PROBLEM	WHAT TO DO*
• Heavy vaginal discharge. • Vaginal pain.	Irritation or infection of cervix.	See Cervicitis.
• Foul-smelling, frothy discharge that is most apparent several days after a menstrual period. • Vaginal itching and pain. • Pain with intercourse.	Vaginal parasitic infection.	See Trichomoniasis.
Discharge has a "fishy" smell.	Vaginal bacterial infection.	See Vaginosis. Bacterial.
• Heavy vaginal discharge that is normal in color and consistency. • Vaginal itching or soreness.	Irritation or infection.	See Vaginal Itching (in Symptoms section).
White, curd-like vaginal discharge.	Vaginal fungus infection.	See Vulvovaginitis, Candidiasis.
• Green-yellow, bad-smelling vaginal discharge. • Tampon, diaphragm or cervical cup left in vagina.	Vaginal infection.	• Remove tampon, diaphragm or cup if you can. • If not, consult doctor.
• Heavy vaginal discharge that is normal in color and consistency. • Use of oral contraceptives. OR • Possible pregnancy.	Normal occurrence caused by hormone changes.	Consult doctor to confirm pregnancy.
Heavy vaginal discharge that is normal in color and consistency during ovulation occurring during middle days between periods.	Normal occurrence.	Nothing.
• Vaginal discharge. • Reddening of vagina.	Vaginal infection.	• See Chlamydia Infection. • See Vaginitis.
• Vaginal discharge, which may or may not smell bad. • Redness, itching around genital area. • Young girl (before puberty).	Infection.	See Vulvovaginitis Before Puberty.
• Red or brown vaginal discharge. • Occasional spotting of blood between menstrual periods.	Several disorders.	• See Cervical Polyps. • See Vaginal Bleeding, Unexpected (in Symptoms section).
• Green-yellow, bad-smelling vaginal discharge. • Pain in lower abdomen. • Frequent or painful urination.	Infection of reproductive organs.	• See Pelvic Inflammatory Disease. • See Gonorrhea.
• Heavy, bad-smelling vaginal discharge 2 or more days after childbirth. • Fever. • Abdominal pain.	Infection of uterus.	See Puerperal Infection.

*All references are to Illness section unless noted otherwise.

VAGINAL ITCHING

SYMPTOMS & FACTORS	POSSIBLE PROBLEM	WHAT TO DO*
• Vaginal itching. • Unusual vaginal discharge.	Several disorders.	• See Vulvovaginitis Before Puberty. • See Vaginitis. • See Pruritus Vulvae. • See Vaginal Discharge, Abnormal (in Symptoms section).
• Vaginal itching. • Use of antibiotics.	Vaginal infection.	See Vulvovaginitis, Candidiasis.
• Vaginal itching. • Use of chemical spray, ointment, cream, douche or contraceptive foam.	Irritation caused by chemical or drug.	Discontinue use of possible irritant.
Vaginal itching in woman over age 38.	Decreasing level of estrogens at menopause.	See Pruritus Vulvae.
• Vaginal itching, plus 2 or more of following: • Unexplained weight loss. • Increased hunger and thirst. • Frequent urination. • Fatigue.	Sugar in urine.	• See Diabetes Type 1. • See Diabetes Type 2.

*All references are to Illness section unless noted otherwise.

VISION DISTURBANCE OR LOSS (continued on next page)

SYMPTOMS & FACTORS	POSSIBLE PROBLEM	WHAT TO DO*
• Sensitivity to light. • Discharge from eye. • Pain in eye.	Infection.	See Conjunctivitis.
• Blurred vision. • Person over age 50.	• Clouding of eye lens. • Decreased blood supply to back of eye.	See Cataract.
• Blurred vision in past 2 days. • Eye pain.	Inflammation of iris.	See Iritis.
• Blurred vision or sensitivity to light. • Use of prescription drug.	Adverse reaction or side effect of drug.	Consult doctor.
• Loss of peripheral vision in small areas. • Blurred vision on one side.	Excess pressure in eye.	See Glaucoma, Open-Angle.
• Blurred or fuzzy vision. • Squinting to see objects that aren't close to you. OR • Unable to see objects that are right in front of you.	Uncorrected vision problem.	Have an eye examination.
• Flashes of light or wavy spots in vision. • Severe headache. • Nausea and vomiting.	Severe vascular headache.	See Headache, Migraine.
• Sensitivity to light. • Eye pain. • Tears.	Infection.	See Keratitis.
Uncoordinated eye movements that may cause vision problems.	Eye muscle disorder.	See Strabismus.
• Double vision. • Bulging eyes.	• Overactive thyroid gland. • Tumor. • Inflammation of tissue behind eye.	• Consult doctor. • See Hyperthyroidism. • See Exophthalmos.
• Vision disturbance. • Recent head injury.	Bleeding inside skull.	• Call doctor now. • See Subdural Hemorrhage & Hematoma.
Sudden, partial or total loss of vision in one or both eyes.	• Decreased blood supply to back of eye or brain. • Disorder of central nervous system.	• Call doctor now. • See Stroke. • See Transient Ischemic Attack. • See Brain Tumor. • See Multiple Sclerosis.

*All references are to Illness section unless noted otherwise.

VISION DISTURBANCE OR LOSS
(continued from previous page)

SYMPTOMS & FACTORS	POSSIBLE PROBLEM	WHAT TO DO*
• Blurred vision in one eye. • Flashing lights. • Floating spots. • No pain.	Disorder of blood vessels and structures in back of eye.	See Retinal Detachment.
• Double vision. • Drooping eyelids. • Swallowing difficulty.	Autoimmune disorder.	See Myasthenia Gravis.
• Blurred vision. • Diabetes.	Diabetic retinopathy (retina injury).	Consult doctor.
• Poor night vision. • Dry, inflamed eyes. • Rough skin. • Loss of appetite.	Lack of vitamin A.	See Vitamin Deficiencies.
• Changes in vision. • Headache; nausea; vomiting. • Seizures. • Excessive thirst.	Tumor.	See Pituitary Tumor.
• Blurred vision. • Dizziness.	Inner ear problem.	See Benign Paroxysmal Positional Vertigo.

*All references are to Illness section unless noted otherwise.

VOICE LOSS OR HOARSENESS

SYMPTOMS & FACTORS	POSSIBLE PROBLEM	WHAT TO DO*
Hoarseness following excessive smoking or alcohol consumption.	Inflammation of vocal cords caused by alcohol or tobacco.	• Decrease smoking or alcohol consumption. • See Laryngitis.
• Hoarseness following excessive use of voice. OR • Exposure to tobacco smoke or toxic fumes.	Inflammation of vocal cords caused by overuse or exposure.	If hoarseness doesn't disappear in a few days, consult doctor.
• Hoarseness, plus 2 or more of following: • Dry skin or hair. • Decreased tolerance for cold. • Fatigue. • Unexplained weight gain.	Underactive thyroid gland.	See Hypothyroidism.
• Voice loss or hoarseness. • Tender or hard lump in neck just below Adam's apple.	Tumor of thyroid.	See Thyroid Nodule.
Hoarseness following cold, cough or sore throat.	Inflammation of vocal cords caused by nasal drainage.	See Laryngitis.
• Hoarseness. • Recent tension or depression.	Effect of stress.	See Anxiety Disorder, Generalized.
• Voice loss or hoarseness for longer than 1 week. OR • Recurrent attacks of hoarseness or voice loss in last 6 months.	• Inflammation of vocal cords. • Tumor.	• See Vocal-Cord Nodules. • See Larynx Cancer. • See Oral Cancer. • See Lung Cancer.

*All references are to Illness section unless noted otherwise.

VOMITING (INFANT 0 TO 6 MONTHS)

SYMPTOMS & FACTORS	POSSIBLE PROBLEM	WHAT TO DO*
• Vomiting. • Diarrhea.	Infection of digestive tract.	See Gastroenteritis.
• Vomiting. • Infant appears healthy. • No other symptoms.	• Single episode—no underlying disorder. • More than one episode—several disorders, such as food allergies or milk intolerance.	• Consult doctor if vomiting lasts longer than 6 hours. • Consult doctor for repeated vomiting. • See Food Allergy. • See Lactose Intolerance.
• Vomiting. • Recent playful bouncing. OR • Travel by airplane, boat or motor vehicle.	Disturbed equilibrium.	• Don't bounce after feedings. • See Motion Sickness.
• Vomiting. • Fever.	Infection.	See Fever (child 0 to 2 years) (in Symptoms section).
• Vomiting. • Cough or runny nose.	Virus infection.	Consult doctor if vomiting lasts longer than 6 hours.
• Vomiting. • Use of prescription drug.	Adverse reaction or side effect of drug.	Call doctor now.
• Forceful vomiting. • Possible accidental ingestion of drug, household cleaning supply or poison. OR • Recent head injury.	• Chemical irritation of stomach and toxic effect of chemical on brain. • Internal bleeding.	• Call doctor now or go to emergency room. • See Head Injury.
• Vomiting. • Fever of 101°F (38.3°C) rectally or higher, plus any of following: • Lethargy. • Eyes sensitive to light. • General ill appearance. • Crying with urination.	• Infection in membranes around brain. • Urinary-tract infection.	Call doctor now.
• Vomiting. • Swelling or lump in groin or testicle.	Protruding intestinal tissue.	See Hernia.
• Infant vomits forcefully after each feeding. • Infant appears healthy. • Infant is male and younger than 4 months.	Constriction in outlet to stomach.	See Pyloric Stenosis, Congenital.
• Vomiting. • Recurrent attacks of screaming or crying, as if in great pain.	Blockage in intestines.	• Call doctor now. • See Intussusception. • See Intestinal Obstruction.
• Vomiting. • Failure to gain weight. • Withdrawn affect.	Emotional deprivation from lack of touching or attention.	See Failure to Thrive.

*All references are to Illness section unless noted otherwise.

VOMITING, RECURRENT ATTACKS

SYMPTOMS & FACTORS	POSSIBLE PROBLEM	WHAT TO DO*
• Recurrent vomiting. • Burning sensation in chest or upper abdomen, especially when bending forward or lying down.	Stomach acid in esophagus.	See Gastroesophageal Reflux Disease.
• Recurrent vomiting. • Occasional pain or tenderness in upper right abdomen. • No fever.	Gallbladder disorder.	See Gallstones.
• Recurrent vomiting. • Occasional pain or tenderness in upper right abdomen. • Fever.	Gallbladder inflammation.	See Cholecystitis or Cholangitis.
• Recurrent vomiting. • Poor appetite. • Jaundice (yellow skin and eyes).	Gallbladder or liver disorder.	• See Gallstones. • See Hepatitis, Viral.
• Recurrent vomiting. • Use of prescription or nonprescription drug.	Adverse reaction or side effect of drug.	Consult doctor.
• Recurrent vomiting. • Pain or tenderness in center of upper abdomen. • Discomfort relieved by vomiting.	Peptic-ulcer disease.	See Ulcer, Peptic.
Vomiting within hours after drinking alcohol.	Stomach inflammation.	See Gastritis.
Recurrent, self-induced vomiting.	Psychological disorder.	See Bulimia.
• Vomiting. • Extreme dizziness. • Loss of balance.	Inner ear disorder.	See Labyrinthitis.
• Recurrent vomiting. • Poor appetite. • Constant pain in upper abdomen.	Tumor.	See Stomach Cancer.
• Recurrent vomiting without nausea. • Recurrent headaches, especially in morning.	• Bleeding inside skull. • Tumor.	• Consult doctor. • See Subdural Hemorrhage & Hematoma. • See Brain Tumor.
• Bloody vomit. • Bleeding from several body parts.	Blood-clotting problem.	See Disseminated Intravascular Coagulation.
• Vomiting. • Extreme abdominal pain, swelling and gas.	Disorder of the pancreas.	See Pancreatitis.
Nausea with or without vomiting.	Pregnancy.	See Nausea & Vomiting in Pregnancy.

*All references are to Illness section unless noted otherwise.

VOMITING, SUDDEN ATTACK
(continued on next page)

SYMPTOMS & FACTORS	POSSIBLE PROBLEM	WHAT TO DO*
• Vomiting. • Diarrhea. • Fever.	Infection of digestive tract.	See Gastroenteritis.
• Vomiting. • Feelings of nervousness and apprehension (such as before going on stage).	Emotional upset.	• Vomiting should stop when emotions calm down. • See Anxiety Disorder, Generalized. • See Panic Attack.
• Vomiting. • Headache.	Headache disorder.	See Headache, Migraine.
• Vomiting. • Use of prescription or nonprescription drug.	Adverse reaction or side effect of drug.	• Consult doctor about prescription drug. • Discontinue use of nonprescription drug.
• Vomiting. • Jaundice (yellow skin or eyes).	Gallbladder or liver disorder.	• Consult doctor. • See Hepatitis, Viral. • See Gallstones.
Recent, recurrent vomiting attacks.	Several disorders.	See Vomiting, Recurrent (in Symptoms section).
• Vomiting. • Consumption of spoiled, contaminated or improperly prepared food.	Effect of toxins in food.	• See Food Poisoning. • See Salmonella Infections. • See Botulism. • See Trichinosis.
• Vomiting. • Dizziness.	Infection or disorder of inner ear.	• See Labyrinthitis. • See Meniere's Disease.
• Vomiting. • Excessive consumption of alcohol or rich food.	Stomach inflammation.	See Gastritis.
Vomiting of blood or dark "coffee ground" material.	Bleeding in stomach.	• Call doctor now. • See Ulcer, Peptic. • See Gastric Erosion.
• Vomiting. • Severe abdominal pain. • No pain relief from vomiting.	Several disorders.	• Call doctor now. • See Appendicitis.
• Vomiting. • Dizziness; headache; faintness.	Gas inhalation.	See Carbon Monoxide Poisoning.
• Vomiting. • Headache, plus any of following: • Eyes sensitive to light. • Drowsiness or confusion. • Pain when bending head forward.	Infection or bleeding in membranes around brain.	• Call doctor now. • See Meningitis, Aseptic. • See Meningitis, Bacterial. • See Subarachnoid Hemorrhage.
• Vomiting. • Headache. • Head injury in last 24 hours.	Brain injury.	• Call doctor now. • See Head Injury.

*All references are to Illness section unless noted otherwise.

VOMITING, SUDDEN ATTACK
(continued from previous page)

SYMPTOMS & FACTORS	POSSIBLE PROBLEM	WHAT TO DO*
• Vomiting. • Abdominal pain or swelling. • Inability to have bowel movement.	Blockage in intestines.	• Call doctor now. • See Intestinal Obstruction.
• Vomiting. • Eye pain. • Blurred vision.	Excess pressure inside eye.	• Call doctor now. • See Glaucoma, Angle-Closure.
• Vomiting and watery diarrhea. • Sudden high fever. • Rash that resembles sunburn.	Blood poisoning.	See Toxic Shock Syndrome.

*All references are to Illness section unless noted otherwise.

WEIGHT GAIN

SYMPTOMS & FACTORS	POSSIBLE PROBLEM	WHAT TO DO*
• Weight gain. • Change from active to sedentary lifestyle.	Calorie intake too high for current activity level.	Decrease food consumption and increase physical activity.
• Weight gain. • No other symptoms.	More calories consumed than burned.	• See Obesity & Overweight. • See Childhood Obesity.
• Weight gain. • Depression.	Compensatory overeating.	See Depression.
• Weight gain. • Feeling of depression and tiredness. • Start of, or during, winter season.	Lack of light.	See Seasonal Affective Disorder.
• Weight gain. • Use of prescription or nonprescription drug that causes fluid retention, such as steroids, cortisone drugs, oral contraceptives or nonsteroid anti-inflammatory drugs.	Adverse reaction or side effect of drug.	Consult doctor.
• Weight gain. • Decreased tolerance for cold. • Dry skin or hair. • Fatigue. • Constipation.	Underactive thyroid gland.	See Hypothyroidism.
• Weight gain. • Recently discontinued smoking.	Normal occurrence.	Weight gain will soon stop. But be careful about what you eat. Get plenty of exercise.
• Rapid weight gain during pregnancy. • Puffiness in the face, hands and feet that is worse in the morning.	Complication of pregnancy.	See Preeclampsia & Eclampsia.
• Weight gain. • High blood pressure or history of heart, kidney or liver disease.	Fluid retention caused by disorder of blood vessels, heart, liver or kidney.	• See Hypertension. • See Congestive Heart Failure. • See Nephrotic Syndrome. • See Cirrhosis of the Liver.
• Weight gain with accumulation of fat over upper back and trunk. • Round face and puffy eyes.	Endocrine disorder.	See Cushing's Syndrome.
Weight gain due to fluid retention.	Several disorders.	• See Ankles, Swollen (in Symptoms section). • See Abdominal Swelling (in Symptoms section).

*All references are to Illness section unless noted otherwise.

WEIGHT GAIN, SLOW (CHILD 0 TO 5 YEARS)

SYMPTOMS

SYMPTOMS & FACTORS	POSSIBLE PROBLEM	WHAT TO DO*
• Weight gain slow in young child. • Child appears healthy and content. • Birth weight low (less than 5-1/2 pounds). OR • Parent smaller than average.	Genetic causes; no underlying disorder.	Consult doctor if worried.
• Weight gain slow in breast-fed infant younger than 1 year. • Feeding schedule rigid or allows little sucking time.	Inadequate nourishment.	• Consult doctor. • Feed on demand. • Increase sucking time.
• Weight gain slow in bottle-fed infant younger than 1 year. • Too much water added to powdered formula, or water added to ready-to-feed formula.	Inadequate nourishment.	• Prepare formula according to directions. • Do not dilute ready-to-feed formula.
• Weight gain slow in bottle-fed infant younger than 1 year. • Child empties every bottle of formula.	Inadequate nourishment.	• Tell doctor at next visit. • Increase amount offered.
• Weight gain slow in young child. • Use of cortisone drugs.	Adverse reaction or side effect of drug.	Consult doctor.
• Weight gain slow in young child. • Loose, pale, bulky, bad-smelling stool.	Digestive disorder.	• See Celiac Disease. • See Lactose Intolerance.
• Weight gain slow in infant younger than 6 months. • Infant vomits after feedings.	Several disorders.	See Vomiting (Infant 0 to 6 Months) (in Symptoms section).
• Weight gain slow in young child. • Withdrawn personality. • Slow mental, physical and emotional development.	Effect of abuse or neglect.	• Consult doctor. • See Failure to Thrive.

*All references are to Illness section unless noted otherwise.

Symptoms 121

WEIGHT LOSS
(continued on next page)

SYMPTOMS & FACTORS	POSSIBLE PROBLEM	WHAT TO DO*
• Weight loss, plus 2 or more of following: • Increased hunger. • Increased thirst. • Fatigue. • Family history of diabetes. • Frequent urination. • Itching rash in genital area.	Sugar in urine.	• See Diabetes Type 1. • See Diabetes Type 2.
• Weight loss, plus 2 or more of following: • Bulging eyes. • Excessive sweating. • Fatigue. • Anxiety. • Rapid heartbeat.	Overactive thyroid gland.	See Hyperthyroidism.
• Weight loss. • Anxiety, stress, or depression.	• Effect of stress. • Psychological disorder.	• See Anxiety Disorder. Generalized. • See Depression. • See Anorexia Nervosa. • See Bulimia. • See Stress.
• Weight loss. • Current use of prescription drug.	Adverse reaction or side effect of drug.	Consult doctor.
• Weight loss. • Recurrent diarrhea or constipation. • Recurrent pain in lower abdomen. • Black stool.	• Inflammation of intestine. • Tumor.	• See Crohn's Disease. • See Large Intestine Cancer.
• Weight loss. • Recurrent pain in upper abdomen.	• Peptic-ulcer disease. • Tumor. • Stress or emotional conflicts. • Intestinal inflammatory disorder.	• See Ulcer, Peptic. • See Stomach Cancer. • See Irritable Bowel Syndrome. • See Colitis, Ulcerative. • See Crohn's Disease.
• Weight loss, plus 2 or more of following: • Excessive sweating at night. • Fever. • Fatigue. • Persistent cough with blood in sputum.	Lung inflammation or infection.	• See Tuberculosis. • See Bronchitis, Chronic. • See Bronchiectasis.
• Weight loss. • Recurrent diarrhea. • Pale, bulky, bad-smelling stool.	Poor digestion.	See Malabsorption.
• Weight loss. • Increased physical activity.	Normal occurrence.	Consult doctor if weight loss is not expected and continues longer than 2 weeks.

*All references are to Illness section unless noted otherwise.

WEIGHT LOSS
(continued from previous page)

SYMPTOMS & FACTORS	POSSIBLE PROBLEM	WHAT TO DO*
• Weight loss. • Recurrent respiratory and skin infections.	Virus infection.	See HIV & AIDS.
• Unexplained weight and appetite loss. • Abdominal discomfort. • Hard mass in upper right abdomen.	Liver tumor.	See Hepatoma.
• Weight loss. • Fatigue (sometimes). • Not having monthly periods or periods that are not regular. • Female.	Harmful eating behavior.	See Female Athlete Triad.

*All references are to Illness section unless noted otherwise.

WHEEZING

SYMPTOMS & FACTORS	POSSIBLE PROBLEM	WHAT TO DO*
• Wheezing. • Fever.	Infection of bronchial tubes.	• See Bronchitis, Acute. • See Asthma. • See Bronchiolitis (young children only).
• Wheezing. • Breathing difficulty.	Spasm of bronchial tubes.	• Call doctor now. • See Asthma.
• Wheezing with a "barking" cough in an infant or young child. • Difficulty in breathing.	Bacterial or viral infection.	See Croup.
• Wheezing. • Possible inhalation of foreign object, such as peanut.	Foreign object in larynx or bronchial tubes.	Call doctor now.
• Persistent, mild wheezing. • Cough (may have gray or green-yellow sputum).	Chronic infection of breathing passages.	• See Bronchitis, Chronic. • See Bronchiectasis. • See Chronic Obstructive Pulmonary Disease. • See Emphysema.
• Wheezing. • Cough with frothy pink, brownish or white sputum.	Fluid in lungs.	• Call doctor now. • See Pulmonary Edema.
• Wheezing. • Breathing difficulty. • Swelling in face or hands. • Itching all over; hives.	Allergic reaction.	• Call doctor now or seek emergency help. • See Anaphylaxis.
• Symptoms similar to asthma (wheezing). • Flushed skin on the head and neck. • Diarrhea.	Tumors.	See Carcinoid Syndrome.

*All references are to Illness section unless noted otherwise.

Illness & Disorders

ABRUPTIO PLACENTA

GENERAL INFORMATION

DEFINITION—The placenta (also called the after-birth) separates from the uterine wall. The placenta carries all nutrients and oxygen to the fetus. A separation can cause complications for the mother and the fetus. With a small separation, there may be no or few symptoms. Larger separations usually cause symptoms.

BODY PARTS INVOLVED—Uterus.

SEX OR AGE MOST AFFECTED—Females.

SIGNS & SYMPTOMS
* Bleeding may be external (vaginal bleeding) or it may be concealed (bleeding remains in the uterus).
* Mild pain or discomfort, or there may be severe pain in the lower abdomen or back.
* Decreased fetal movement.
* Hard, tender abdomen.
* Uterine contractions.

CAUSES—The cause is unknown. Certain risk factors do exist.

RISK INCREASES WITH
* High blood pressure (hypertension).
* Smoking.
* Women over age 35 or younger than 20.
* Women who have had more than 4 or 5 pregnancies.
* A previous pregnancy with placental separation.
* Pregnancy with more than one fetus.
* Excess amniotic fluid (polyhydramnios).
* Chronic disorder (such as diabetes) or renal infection.
* Injury from motor vehicle accident, falls, or abuse.
* Short umbilical cord.
* Abnormal uterus or tumor.
* Premature rupture of the membranes (water breaks before delivery).
* Use of alcohol or drugs of abuse (such as cocaine).

HOW TO PREVENT
* There is no sure way to prevent the problem.
* Avoid risk factors such as smoking, alcohol, or cocaine use. Get treatment for high blood pressure.

WHAT TO EXPECT

DIAGNOSTIC MEASURES
* Your own observation of symptoms.
* Your obstetric provider will do a physical exam and ask questions about your symptoms.
* Medical tests will include blood studies and blood clotting tests. An ultrasound (see Glossary) may be done.

APPROPRIATE HEALTH CARE
* Treatment depends on the severity of the separation, the condition of the fetus, and the duration of the pregnancy. Hospital care is usually needed (except for mild cases) so the mother can be observed for any complications. If the placenta separation is slight, you may be able to return home for bed rest and close observation.
* In the hospital, fluids may be given through a vein (IV). A blood transfusion may be needed.
* Labor may be induced, if the pregnancy is at term or if there are signs of fetal distress.
* Surgery to deliver the unborn child by cesarean section, or vaginal delivery (sometimes).

POSSIBLE COMPLICATIONS
* Premature delivery of the child. This may lead to other complications for the newborn.
* Intrauterine growth restriction (IUGR) of the fetus.
* Shock or life-threatening bleeding in the mother.
* Blood clotting problems for the mother (disseminated intravascular coagulopathy or DIC).
* Risk of abruptio placentae in a future pregnancy.
* Uncontrolled bleeding after delivery may lead to an emergency hysterectomy.
* Death of child and/or mother.

PROBABLE OUTCOME
When the separation is less severe and with immediate medical care, the outlook for mother and fetus is good.

HOW TO TREAT

GENERAL MEASURES—Abruptio placentae requires emergency medical care, but there is usually time to obtain advice by telephone and arrange safe transportation to the hospital.

MEDICATION—A drug to induce labor may be used if immediate delivery is required.

ACTIVITY—Whether you are in the hospital or have been able to return home, follow all medical instructions about any activity limits.

DIET
* A liquid-only diet may be prescribed until it is decided if surgery will be needed.
* If you are resting at home, continue with regular diet.

CALL YOUR DOCTOR IF

* You have bleeding (anything more than slight spotting) during pregnancy. This is an emergency!
* You have any other new symptoms.

ACNE
(Acne Vulgaris)

GENERAL INFORMATION

DEFINITION—A common skin condition. It can last a few months, or years or for an entire lifetime.

BODY PARTS INVOLVED—It usually affects the skin on the face, chest, and back.

SEX OR AGE MOST AFFECTED—Acne has affected almost all people at some point during their lives. In teenagers, it is more common in males than in females. In adults, it is more common in women than men.

SIGNS & SYMPTOMS
* Mild acne usually causes blackheads (black spots the size of a pinhead) or whiteheads (white spots similar to blackheads).
* Pimples (also called zits). These are skin pores that have become pus-filled (clogged and infected).
* Severe acne produces many pimples.
* Redness and inflammation around pimples.
* Cysts (larger, firm swellings in the skin).

CAUSES—Glands in the skin make an oily substance called sebum. Sebum usually empties onto the skin surface through a pore (small opening) and causes no problems. With acne, the sebum becomes plugged up in the pore. Why this occurs is unclear. Sex-hormone changes during the teen years play a role. Contrary to commonly accepted myth, acne is not caused by dirt or foods.

RISK INCREASES WITH
* Teenagers and young adults.
* Endocrine disorders.
* Use of some drugs, such as cortisone.
* Family history of acne.

HOW TO PREVENT
* Acne cannot be prevented. Certain factors can cause a flare up. Avoid them if possible.
* A flare up of acne can be caused by some make-up and lotions, certain foods, sunlight, friction (tight clothes, bicycle helmets), and hormone changes in females before their periods.

WHAT TO EXPECT

DIAGNOSTIC MEASURES
* Your own observation of symptoms.
* Medical history and a skin exam by a health care provider.

APPROPRIATE HEALTH CARE
* Treatment will depend on the severity of the acne, any infection or inflammation, and if you are a female who may become pregnant.

* Removal of comedones (blackheads) may be done by your health care provider.
* Treatment may include drugs (both for topical use or taken by mouth).
* Cosmetic surgery (dermabrasion) may be done to remove scars after acne heals.
* Removal or drainage of a cyst may be done.

POSSIBLE COMPLICATIONS
* Poor self-image, depression and emotional stress.
* Facial scars or pitting of the skin.

PROBABLE OUTCOME
* Most cases respond well to treatment. It may take several months. Acne tends to disappear after teen years.
* Despite treatment, acne may flare up.

HOW TO TREAT

GENERAL MEASURES
* Wash face with a mild soap once or twice a day and after exercising. Clean skin gently; don't scrub. An antibacterial soap may help. Rinse soap off completely.
* Shampoo hair daily, especially if it is oily. Don't let hair hang in the face. Use dandruff-preventing shampoo if needed.
* Avoid oil-based cosmetics. Use thinner, lotion-style, water-based products.
* Don't squeeze, scratch, pick, or rub the skin. Acne heals better without damage to the skin.

MEDICATION
* Use nonprescription cream or lotion products to treat the acne. These may contain benzyl peroxide, sulfur, salicylic acid or resorcinol.
* Antibiotic may be prescribed for bacteria infection.
* For more severe cases, topical or oral retinoids (a form of vitamin A), hormone drugs, or stronger acne drugs may be prescribed. Some drugs may increase your sensitivity to sunlight and increase the risk of sunburn.
* Caution: If you are pregnant or planning a pregnancy, tell your health care provider before using acne drugs.

ACTIVITY—No limits.

DIET—Foods don't cause acne, but some foods may make it worse. To find any food problems, stop eating foods that you think may make the acne worse. Then reintroduce them one at a time. If acne flares up 2 to 3 days after a food is eaten, leave that food out of your diet.

CALL YOUR DOCTOR IF

* You or a family member has acne and self-care is not helping.
* Acne recurs despite treatment.

ACNE ROSACEA
(Rosacea; Adult Acne)

GENERAL INFORMATION

DEFINITION—Chronic inflammation of skin of the nose, cheeks, forehead, and chin. Rarely, the neck, chest, ears, or scalp may be affected. Extensive nose involvement, mostly in men, is called rhinophyma.

BODY PARTS INVOLVED—Face, especially the nose, and surrounding areas.

SEX OR AGE MOST AFFECTED—Acne rosacea tends to start between ages 30 and 50. It is more common in women, but more severe in men.

SIGNS & SYMPTOMS
* Symptoms vary from person to person and sometimes in the same person. They may be mild or more severe.
* Flushing or blushing.
* Persistent redness.
* Unsightly red, thickened skin on the nose and cheeks. Small blood vessels are visible on the skin surface.
* Papules (small raised bumps) and pustules (small, white blisters with pus) on the affected skin.
* Burning, stinging, itching, swelling, dryness, or tightness of affected skin.
* Eyes may be red, burning, watery or irritated.

CAUSES—Unknown.

RISK INCREASES WITH
* Fair skinned people.
* Family history of acne rosacea.

HOW TO PREVENT—Cannot be prevented. Flare-ups may be triggered by hot liquids, spicy foods, alcohol, emotional stress, some skin care products, sun exposure, hot and cold weather, heavy exercise, and hot baths.

WHAT TO EXPECT

DIAGNOSTIC MEASURES
* Your own observation of symptoms.
* Your health care provider can diagnose the condition by an exam of the affected skin area. Medical tests are usually not needed.

APPROPRIATE HEALTH CARE
* Treatment will depend on each individual's needs and severity of the symptoms. Treatment may include drugs and skin treatments.
* Steroid-induced rosacea is treated first by stopping the steroid drug.
* Surgery (such as laser therapy) may be recommended for visible blood vessels, to reduce redness, or to remove excess tissue from the nose.

* Psychotherapy or counseling, if disfigurement causes distress.

POSSIBLE COMPLICATIONS
* Emotional problems (such as lack of self confidence and low self-esteem).
* Eye complications.
* Scarring may occur, but it is rare.

PROBABLE OUTCOME—There is no cure. Symptoms can be controlled with treatment and self-care. Acne rosacea is a disease of remissions and frequent flare-ups.

HOW TO TREAT

GENERAL MEASURES
* Learn what factors cause flare-ups for you and avoid them. Keep a day-to-day diary of your activities and flare-ups to identify your trigger factors.
* Wash your face with a mild soap once or twice a day and after exercising. Clean skin gently; don't scrub. An antibacterial soap may help. Rinse soap off completely.
* Don't squeeze, scratch, pick, or rub the skin.
* Reduce stress in your life if possible. Counseling may help if the condition is adding to your stress.
* See How to Cope With Stress in Appendix.
* To learn more: National Rosacea Society, 800 S. Northwest Hwy., Suite 200 Barrington, IL 60010; (888) NO-BLUSH (662-5874);website www.rosacea.org.

MEDICATION
* Antibiotics (for the skin or taken by mouth) may be prescribed.
* Topical or oral retinoids (a form of vitamin A) or other drugs may be prescribed depending on the symptoms. Caution: If you are pregnant or planning a pregnancy, tell your health care provider before using acne drugs.
* Don't use nonprescription cortisone creams or lotions without medical advice. They may cause the condition to worsen.

ACTIVITY—Limit time spent in sunny, windy, very hot, or cold weather. Use a sunscreen (SPF 15 or higher).

DIET—No special diet. Avoid spicy foods, alcohol or anything that causes the face to flush.

CALL YOUR DOCTOR IF

You have symptoms of acne rosacea. This condition can be helped with treatment.

ADDISON'S DISEASE
(Adrenal Insufficiency)

 ## GENERAL INFORMATION

DEFINITION—A rare disease that leads to failure of the adrenal glands. The adrenal glands produce hormones (cortisol and aldosterone) that affect almost every body organ and tissue. These hormones help the body respond to stress, maintain blood pressure, help heart and blood vessel function, and are involved in metabolism.

BODY PARTS INVOLVED—Adrenal glands (located over the kidneys).

SEX OR AGE MOST AFFECTED—Addison's can occur in all age groups. It affects men and women equally.

SIGNS & SYMPTOMS
• Symptoms may develop slowly over months or years. Symptoms are caused by low levels of hormones produced by the adrenal glands.
• Weakness and fatigue.
• Nausea, vomiting, stomach pain, diarrhea, and appetite and weight loss.
• Low blood pressure causing faintness and dizziness.
• Brownish skin (looks suntanned) with white patches.
• Darkening of freckles, scars, and nipples.
• Hair loss.
• Feeling cold all the time.
• Behavior or mood changes, including aggression or depression.

CAUSES
• The cause is usually unknown, but is believed to be an autoimmune disorder.
• It also may be a result of tuberculosis, cancer, pituitary disease, or AIDS.
• Use of oral cortisone drugs for other conditions. When cortisone is stopped, normal adrenal function sometimes does not return.

RISK INCREASES WITH
• Other autoimmune diseases.
• Disorders mentioned in causes.

HOW TO PREVENT—No specific preventive measures.

 ## WHAT TO EXPECT

DIAGNOSTIC MEASURES
• Your own observation of symptoms.
• Your health care provider will do a physical exam and ask questions about your symptoms. Medical tests may include blood and urine studies, tests to measure adrenal function, and CT or MRI (see Glossary for both).

APPROPRIATE HEALTH CARE
• Treatment involves replacing the hormones the adrenal glands are not making.
• Hospitalization for an adrenal crisis (see Possible Complications).

POSSIBLE COMPLICATIONS
• Adrenal crisis caused by injury or illness. Symptoms may include pain, weakness, low blood pressure, high or low temperature, fainting.
• Increased risk of infections.

PROBABLE OUTCOME—The disease can be controlled with hormone-replacement. A normal lifestyle can be expected.

 ## HOW TO TREAT

GENERAL MEASURES
• Advise any doctor or dentist who treats you that you have Addison's disease.
• If you live or travel where medical care is not readily available, you may be given instructions on giving yourself cortisone injections in case of emergency.
• Wear a medical alert type bracelet or tag to indicate you have Addison's disease and the name of the drug and dosage that you take.
• Stay up-to-date on vaccines, such as those for influenza and pneumonia.
• To learn more: National Adrenal Diseases Foundation, 505 Northern Blvd, Great Neck, NY 11021, (516) 487-4992 (not toll free); website: www.medhelp.org/nadf.

MEDICATION—Drugs to replace the hormones cortisol and aldosterone will be prescribed as needed. Never change or stop taking your drugs without medical advice.

ACTIVITY—No limits.

DIET—Special diet may be prescribed (e.g., one to maintain proper balance of sodium and potassium).

 ## CALL YOUR DOCTOR IF

• You or a family member has symptoms of Addison's disease.
• After diagnosis, infection, injury, or dehydration develops. Drugs may need a dosage change.
• Swollen ankles, weight gain, or new symptoms occur.

ILLNESS & DISORDERS

ADJUSTMENT DISORDERS

GENERAL INFORMATION

DEFINITION—A person's response to a stressful life event (sometimes called a stressor) is out of proportion to what would be a normal reaction. The person is unable to adjust and this causes problems in both social and work (or school) situations or other functions of daily living.

BODY PARTS INVOLVED—Nervous system.

SEX OR AGE MOST AFFECTED—Both sexes, usually in adults.

SIGNS & SYMPTOMS
• Symptoms or behavior changes occur within three months of onset of the stressor. They usually last no more than six months after the end of the stressor.
• Symptoms vary from person to person. They are often more severe in teens and the elderly.
• Changes in sleeping and eating patterns.
• Withdrawal (avoids social activities and friends).
• Fearful about the future.
• Low self-esteem and feeling emotionally numb.
• Feeling tense, anxious and depressed.
• Feelings of fear, rage, guilt or shame.
• Denial of the stressful event (acting as if it never occurred).

CAUSES—A disruption in the normal process of adapting to a stressful event. Everyone reacts differently to an event. It depends on its importance and the intensity of the event. It depends on the person's personality, temperament, age, and well-being.

RISK INCREASES WITH
• The degree of undesired change a stressor causes.
• Whether the stressor was sudden or expected.
• The importance of the stressor in the person's life.
• Lack of support systems (e.g., family, friends, religious, cultural, and social ties).
• How well a person responds to stressful life events.

HOW TO PREVENT—No specific preventive measures known.

WHAT TO EXPECT

DIAGNOSTIC MEASURES
• Your own or other's observation of symptoms.
• Your health care provider will do a physical exam and ask questions about your symptoms and the changes that are going on in your life.

• It is important to identify the stressor that has led to the symptoms. It can be anything that is important to you. The stressor may be only one event or a string of events. It may seem minor to some, but is important to you.

APPROPRIATE HEALTH CARE
• Treatment may include self-care, counseling, and in some cases, drug therapy. This depends on severity of symptoms and impact on your lifestyle.
• Counseling or psychotherapy may be recommended. Several therapy methods are effective and are often needed for a brief period. Family therapy (including marital counseling) may be recommended for some.

POSSIBLE COMPLICATIONS
• Difficulty maintaining relationships or jobs.
• Lingering problems in teenagers.
• Self-treatment using alcohol or drugs to overcome un-desired symptoms and feelings.
• Chronic anxiety and depression.

PROBABLE OUTCOME—It usually clears up on its own by the person adapting to the changed situation, or the stressor ends. Treatment can help in other cases. These disorders are common and are often only temporary.

HOW TO TREAT

GENERAL MEASURES
• Learn to cope with stress. Keeping a journal about your stressors and feelings, talking to a friend, or joining a support group may help.
• Take good care of your physical health (diet, exercise, and sleep).

MEDICATION—Since adjustment disorders are usually of short duration, drugs are normally not needed. A drug may be prescribed short term for insomnia or for other specific symptoms, depending on their severity.

ACTIVITY—No limits. A routine physical exercise program is recommended. Physical activity helps reduce anxiety and stress.

DIET—Eat a well-balanced diet to maintain good health.

CALL YOUR DOCTOR IF

• You or a family member has symptoms of an adjustment disorder.
• Symptoms continue to worsen after treatment begins.

AGRANULOCYTOSIS
(Granulocytopenia; Neutropenia)

GENERAL INFORMATION

DEFINITION—Reduction in the normal number of circulating white blood cells (granulocytes or neutrophils) in the bloodstream. These cells are the first to attack bacterial infections. It is not contagious.

BODY PARTS INVOLVED—Blood and bone marrow.

SEX OR AGE MOST AFFECTED—Both sexes; all ages.

SIGNS & SYMPTOMS
* Fever, sometimes with chills.
* Aching, weakness or discomfort.
* Sore throat.
* Ulcers (especially in the mouth and throat), which do not produce pus.
* Any sign of infection in someone who has had agranulocytosis in the past. This may signal a recurrence.

CAUSES—Increased destruction or impaired production of granulocytes (white blood cells). It can be caused by a variety of risk factors.

RISK INCREASES WITH
* Autoimmune disorders.
* Chemotherapy (anticancer drugs).
* Radiation therapy.
* Disorders that damage the bone marrow.
* Some hereditary disorders.
* Certain medications (such as carbamazepine or clozapine).
* Exposure to certain toxic chemicals.

HOW TO PREVENT—No specific preventive measures.

WHAT TO EXPECT

DIAGNOSTIC MEASURES
* Your own observation of symptoms.
* A health care provider will do a physical exam and ask questions about your medications and family medical history.
* Medical tests may include blood and urine studies and bone marrow biopsy.
* Genetic testing may be done if a hereditary disorder is suspected.

APPROPRIATE HEALTH CARE
* Possible hospital care for intensive treatment and isolation to avoid infections.
* Stopping any medication that may be the cause. Sometimes this provides a cure.
* Other treatments may include bone marrow transplant, stem cell transplants, and treatment to stimulate the production of granulocytes.

POSSIBLE COMPLICATIONS
* Dangerous, sometimes fatal infections (bacterial, fungal, viral or others)—even with vigorous treatment.
* Chronic infections that can cause organ damage and other problems.
* Adverse effects of the treatment.

PROBABLE OUTCOME—Depending on cause, usually curable with intensive treatment.

HOW TO TREAT

GENERAL MEASURES—The following are helpful until blood counts are normal:
* Be extra careful about personal cleanliness.
* Keep the mouth clean by rinsing frequently with warm salt water (1 teaspoon salt to 8 oz. water) or gargling with hydrogen peroxide.
* Pay particular attention to oral hygiene. Brush teeth gently with a very soft brush, avoiding irritation of the gums.
* Avoid contact with harmful materials, such as cleaning chemicals, glue, insecticide, fertilizer and paint remover.
* Avoid contact with large crowds or people with infections.

MEDICATION
* You may be prescribed intravenous and oral antibiotics if the white blood cell count is very low.
* Drugs to stimulate bone marrow to produce more granulocytes may be prescribed.
* Stopping use of any drug that is suspected of causing agranulocytosis.

ACTIVITY
* Rest or limit activity during the acute stage. Resume normal activities gradually after symptoms subside.
* Avoid overexercising until blood counts are normal.

DIET—No special diet.

CALL YOUR DOCTOR IF

* You or a family member has symptoms of agranulocytosis.
* The following occurs after treatment:
  - Any sign of infection, especially fever.
  - Swelling of the feet and ankles.
  - Painful urination or decreased urine output in one day.
* New, unexplained symptoms develop. Drugs used in treatment may produce side effects.

ALCOHOLISM

GENERAL INFORMATION

DEFINITION—A chronic, progressive disease that involves dependence on, or an addiction to, alcohol. It involves:
* Craving. A strong need or urge to drink.
* Loss of control. Not being able to stop drinking once drinking has begun.
* Physical dependence. Withdrawal symptoms, such as upset stomach, sweating, shakiness, and anxiety after stopping drinking.
* Tolerance. The need to drink greater amounts of alcohol to get "high."

BODY PARTS INVOLVED—Brain; central nervous system; liver; heart.

SEX OR AGE MOST AFFECTED—Both sexes, but occurs 4 times more often in men than women. The incidence of alcoholism in children is increasing.

SIGNS & SYMPTOMS
* Need for alcohol at the start of the day.
* Use of alcohol to relieve stress or forget problems.
* Insomnia and nightmares.
* Vision, hearing, perception and alertness problems.
* Monday-morning hangovers. Lost work days.
* Promises to limit or stop drinking, but fails.
* Lies about drinking. Sneaks drinks at work or school.
* Anger and guilt when asked about drinking.
* Blackouts, personality and mood changes, confusion, memory loss, depression, anxiety, and fatigue.
* Tremors, violent shakes, hallucinations, or convulsions when no alcohol is in the body.
* Poor nutrition and poor hygiene. Bad breath.
* Lack of sexual interest and loss of potency.
* Money, work, or family problems.

CAUSES—Not fully understood. It appears to be a combination of genetic, environmental, and personality factors.

RISK INCREASES WITH
* Family history of alcoholism.
* Personal history of other substance abuse.
* Genetic factors. May affect the way people's bodies process and respond to alcohol.
* Personality factors, such as needing a lot of praise and reassurance, feeling inadequate or unsure, low frustration level, being impulsive or aggressive.
* Cultural factors. Some ethnic groups have high alcoholism rates.
* Factors such as alcohol being available, affordable, and socially acceptable.
* Having an emotional or psychiatric disorder.

HOW TO PREVENT—Avoid or limit use of alcohol. Women - no more than one drink a day and men - no more than two drinks a day.

WHAT TO EXPECT

DIAGNOSTIC MEASURES—Your health care provider will do a physical exam and ask about your symptoms. You may be asked verbal questions or to fill out a written form about your alcohol use. These help identify problem drinking. Medical tests may include blood and urine studies.

APPROPRIATE HEALTH CARE
* Treatment depends on the severity of the alcohol problem, other illnesses (physical, emotional, or mental), and how motivated you are to change. Treatment usually involves withdrawal of alcohol and detoxification, and long-term support to help you remain sober.
* Specific treatment steps include counseling (may be all that is needed), drugs (in some cases), inpatient care at a hospital or treatment center, or referral to a health care provider who treats addiction problems.

POSSIBLE COMPLICATIONS
* Brain, liver, heart, and other organ damage.
* Problems in children born to alcoholic mothers.
* Without treatment, alcoholism can be fatal.
* Suicide or fatal motor vehicle accidents.

PROBABLE OUTCOME—Treatment has varying success rates. Some people are able to quit on their own. Relapse is somewhat common, but many people have a full recovery.

HOW TO TREAT

GENERAL MEASURES
* The first and most difficult step of treatment is admitting the problem exists.
* Join a local Alcoholics Anonymous or other support group and attend regularly.
* Reassess your lifestyle to identify and alter factors that encourage drinking.

MEDICATION
* Drugs may be prescribed:
  - That reduce the craving for alcohol.
  - That cause unpleasant physical symptoms when alcohol is consumed.
  - That reduce the pleasure of alcohol.
  - For withdrawal symptoms, as needed.

ACTIVITY—Exercise daily. It helps to maintain your physical and mental well-being.

DIET—Normal, well-balanced diet, vitamin supplements may be recommended.

☎ CALL YOUR DOCTOR IF

* You or a family member has symptoms of alcoholism. It is an illness that can be treated.
* You have a relapse after recovery.

ALOPECIA AREATA

GENERAL INFORMATION

DEFINITION—Sudden hair loss in circular patches on the scalp. The hair loss does not occur with other visible evidence of scalp disease. It can involve hair on the scalp, eyebrows, eyelashes, genital area, or sometimes underarms.

BODY PARTS INVOLVED—Hair; scalp; eyebrows; eyelashes; beard; genital area; underarm (sometimes).

SEX OR AGE MOST AFFECTED—Alopecia can occur at any age, from birth to older adults. Many cases start before age 20.

SIGNS & SYMPTOMS
* Sudden hair loss in sharply defined circular patches. In rare cases, body hair loss may be total (alopecia universalis).
* Pain and itching may occur in some cases.
* Nails may be affected, such as pitting, in more severe cases.

CAUSES—Unknown. It is thought to be one of a group of autoimmune disorders. In these disorders, the immune system by mistake attacks the body itself. Heredity and emotional stress or psychiatric disorders may play a role.

RISK INCREASES WITH
* Family history of alopecia areata.
* Stressful life event preceding the hair loss may be a factor.
* Certain medical disorders may occur along with alopecia, but do not appear to be a cause or a risk factor.

HOW TO PREVENT—Cannot be prevented at present.

WHAT TO EXPECT

DIAGNOSTIC MEASURES
* Your own observation of symptoms.
* Your health care provider will do a physical exam of the affected scalp area. Medical tests are usually not needed unless some underlying disorder is suspected.

APPROPRIATE HEALTH CARE
* In a simple, self-limited case where the alopecia is not noticeable, no treatment may be needed. In other cases, drugs may be used for treatment depending on amount of hair loss and age of patient. No one treatment helps everyone with the disorder.
* For loss of eyebrow hair, dermatography may help. Small dots of colored pigment are injected into eyebrow area.

POSSIBLE COMPLICATIONS
* Loss of all hair.
* Slow or incomplete regrowth.
* Treatment may not be effective in extensive hair loss.
* Disorder frequently recurs.

PROBABLE OUTCOME—The outcome varies depending on the amount of hair loss. There is no permanent cure and the disorder may come and go. Most people have only a few areas of alopecia and regrowth occurs in about a year.

HOW TO TREAT

GENERAL MEASURES
* A change in hair-style may cover the affected area.
* Consider wearing a hairpiece or wig until the hair grows in again.
* Continue to bathe and shampoo as usual. The disorder is not contagious. Don't tug on normal hair close to areas of hair loss.
* Seek counseling if coping with the hair loss is causing emotional problems. Support groups are also available.
* To learn more: National Alopecia Areata Foundation, P.O. Box 150760, San Rafael, CA 94915; (415) 472-3780 (not toll free); website: www.naaf.org.

MEDICATION
* Topical steroids or topical anthralin may be prescribed. Follow instructions carefully.
* Topical minoxidil (a drug used for hair growth) may help. Its effectiveness is highly variable.
* In some cases, you may have injections of steroids into affected areas.
* Oral cortisone drugs may be recommended.
* Topical immunotherapy may be recommended. This involves producing a skin reaction to help hair growth.
* Photochemotherapy with PUVA may be recommended. It combines the use of a drug that sensitizes the skin along with a controlled dose of ultraviolet light.

ACTIVITY—No limits.

DIET—No special diet.

CALL YOUR DOCTOR IF

* You or a family member has symptoms of alopecia areata.
* The following occurs during treatment:
 - Hair loss increases or hair loss doesn't improve.
 - Areas show signs of infection (redness, swelling, tenderness, warmth) after injection treatment.

ALTITUDE ILLNESS

GENERAL INFORMATION

DEFINITION—Altitude illness results from travel to higher than normal altitudes. It can affect anyone, no matter what their age or how healthy they are. Types include:
* Acute mountain sickness (AMS); the most common.
* High-altitude pulmonary edema (HAPE) and high-altitude cerebral edema (HACE). These are less common.

BODY PARTS INVOLVED—These illnesses affect most body systems, especially the brain, heart, lungs, gastrointestinal tract, circulatory system and electrolytes.

SEX AND AGE MOST AFFECTED—Young adults of both sexes.

SIGNS & SYMPTOMS
* Mild symptoms may begin when you climb or travel to around 7,000 to 8,000 feet.
  - Headache, feeling lightheaded and weak.
  - Nausea or vomiting.
  - Sleeping problems.
* As you go higher, more severe symptoms may occur.
  - Cough and trouble with breathing.
  - Unsteady walk.
  - Confusion; hallucinations (seeing things that aren't there).
  - Coma (person cannot be aroused).

CAUSES—There is less oxygen in the air at higher altitudes. Symptoms start to develop when the body tries to adjust to having less oxygen than it normally has. People who live at high altitudes have adapted to these lower oxygen levels and do not get sick.

RISK INCREASES WITH
* Some people are more susceptible. It is unclear why certain people get sick while others do not. At 14,000 feet, most people will have at least mild symptoms.
* People with severe heart or lung disease or people with sickle-cell anemia.
* Going too high too quickly.

HOW TO PREVENT
* Educate yourself before your trip. Find out how high the altitude will be. Know the symptoms of altitude illness. Find out if medical help will be handy.
* Ask your health care provider for advice about high altitude travel for children, for pregnant women, and for people with chronic health problems. The travel may be considered safe, but find out for sure.
* While on the trip, slowly adjust to the change in altitude. Rest for a day or two at each 1,000 to 2,000 feet. Take it easy, don't overdo, drink fluids, but not alcohol.

WHAT TO EXPECT

DIAGNOSTIC MEASURES—Your health care provider will ask about your symptoms, may do a physical exam, and have medical tests performed to check on your heart, lungs, and other body systems.

APPROPRIATE HEALTH CARE
* Treatment steps will depend on your symptoms. You may be advised to go to a lower altitude. This is the most important and only sure treatment step.
* For more severe symptoms, you will need to go to a lower altitude immediately. You may need pure oxygen breathed in through a mask for a period of time. A hospital stay may be necessary until you recover.

POSSIBLE COMPLICATIONS—Serious outcomes, including death, are rare. They are only likely to occur if the person is unable to go down to a lower level, or is not able to get medical help.

PROBABLE OUTCOME—Most cases are mild and do not need medical treatment. Recovery takes only one to a few days.

HOW TO TREAT

GENERAL MEASURES
* If mild symptoms occur, rest for a day or two at that altitude. You may want to go back down (to descend) to a lower altitude. Do not travel higher (to ascend) until the symptoms resolve or get much better.
* Symptoms should improve in a few days if you rest, drink plenty of fluids, don't drink alcohol, and avoid heavy exercise.

MEDICATION
* Ask your health care provider's advice before you travel about drugs that can help prevent or treat symptoms. Drugs do have side effects, so be cautious.
* For mild symptoms, such as headache, you may use pain relievers, such as ibuprofen or naproxen.
* In severe cases, drugs will be given to treat complications and help speed recovery.

ACTIVITY—Resume daily activities gradually upon returning to your normal altitude.

DIET—Increase fluid intake, avoid alcohol, eat small meals.

CALL YOUR DOCTOR IF

You or a family member has altitude illness symptoms, or wants to discuss symptoms that occurred on a trip.

ALZHEIMER'S DISEASE
(Presenile Dementia)

 GENERAL INFORMATION

DEFINITION—Alzheimer's disease (AD) is a brain disorder that involves gradual mental deterioration. The more gradual form, with slow progress of symptoms, begins around ages 65 to 70. A rapidly progressive form begins around ages 36 to 45.

BODY PARTS INVOLVED—Brain.

SEX OR AGE MOST AFFECTED—Both sexes, usually beginning in middle age or older adults.

SIGNS & SYMPTOMS
Early stages:
• Forgetful of recent events.
• Increasing difficulty doing mental tasks, such as usual work, balancing a checkbook, or maintaining a household.
• Personality changes, including poor impulse control and poor judgment.
Later stages:
• Difficulty doing simple tasks, such as choosing clothing, solving problems.
• Failure to recognize familiar persons.
• Lack of interest in personal hygiene or appearance.
• Difficulty feeding self.
• Belligerence and denial that anything is wrong.
• Loss of usual sexual inhibitions.
• Wandering away.
• Anxiety and insomnia.
Advanced stages:
• Complete loss of memory, speech, muscle function, and bladder and bowel control.

CAUSES—Damage to or loss of brain cells for unknown reasons.

RISK INCREASES WITH
• Family history of Alzheimer's disease.
• Other genetic factors.
• Aging.
• Research shows that factors related to blood circulation may be involved (such as those causing heart disease or stroke).

HOW TO PREVENT—None specific; research continues. A healthy lifestyle may help.

 WHAT TO EXPECT

DIAGNOSTIC MEASURES
• Your own or other's observation of symptoms.
• Your health care provider will do a physical exam and ask questions about the symptoms. No specific test can diagnose Alzheimer's.
• Medical tests may include cognitive tests (answering questions). Blood, urine, and spinal fluid studies, heart studies, CT, MRI, PET scans (see Glossary), help rule out other disorders.

• Certain genetic tests help to identify inherited forms of Alzheimer's.

APPROPRIATE HEALTH CARE
• Treatment will depend on the stage of the disease. Different drugs are available that can help slow the progress of the disease.
• Drugs to treat the behavior symptoms can help make a patient more comfortable and make their care easier.
• Those with end-stage disease often need the care provided in an assisted living facility that handles Alzheimer's patients.

POSSIBLE COMPLICATIONS
• Infections. They are a major cause of death in Alzheimer's patients.
• Final stages of the disease will lead to death.

PROBABLE OUTCOME—There is no cure. Treatment helps slow the progress and helps relieve symptoms. Patients may progress from onset of symptoms to end-stage disease in 8 to 10 years. This varies from person to person.

 HOW TO TREAT

GENERAL MEASURES
• A diagnosis of Alzheimer's is overwhelming, both for the patient and the family. Educate yourselves as much as possible about what to expect and how to plan for it. With early diagnosis, the patient can take part in making decisions for the future.
• Caring for a family member with Alzheimer's is a difficult task. Caregivers need to take care of themselves. Joining a support group for caregivers may be helpful.
• To learn more: Alzheimer's Association, 225 N. Michigan Ave., Flr. 17, Chicago. IL 60601; (800) 272-3900; website: www.alz.org.

MEDICATION
• Drugs that slow the progress of the disease for a limited time are usually prescribed.
• Drugs as needed to help control behavior symptoms (insomnia, agitation, wandering, depression, anxiety, and others) will be prescribed.

ACTIVITY—As the condition progresses, all activity will eventually require supervision.

DIET—Regular diet. Feeding assistance will eventually be needed.

 CALL YOUR DOCTOR IF

• You or a family member has symptoms of Alzheimer's disease.
• Caregivers have questions or concerns about the patient, the symptoms, the treatment or signs of infection occur, or if you need support.

AMEBIASIS
(Amebic Dysentery; Entamebiasis)

 GENERAL INFORMATION

DEFINITION—A parasitic infection of the intestines (bowels). Amebiasis is found worldwide, but occurs most often in developing countries. In the United States, the disease is fairly rare in the general population. Amebic dysentery is a rare, more severe form.

BODY PARTS INVOLVED—Intestinal tract, especially the colon; liver.

SEX OR AGE MOST AFFECTED—Both sexes; all ages.

SIGNS & SYMPTOMS
* Only about 1 in 10 persons with the infection will have symptoms. Symptoms occur when the parasites (amoebas) invade the walls of the intestine.
* Diarrhea with bad-smelling stools. Constipation may alternate with diarrhea.
* Gas and stomach bloating, cramps, and tenderness.
* Amebic dysentery may cause bloody stools, stomach pain, chills, and fever.

CAUSES—A parasite, *Entamoeba histolytica*. The infection starts when someone swallows amoeba cysts (they can't be seen) that contaminate food or water. The cysts travel to the intestines and can live there without causing symptoms. Then, for unknown reasons, the amoebas invade the intestine wall. When this happens, symptoms occur. Symptoms usually begin one to four weeks after exposure, but can take a few days or a year.

RISK INCREASES WITH
* Immigrants from developing countries.
* Travel to a foreign country. In developing countries, the drinking water may be contaminated. In addition, some places use human feces for fertilizer.
* Male homosexuals.
* Living in institutions where there are poor sanitary conditions.

HOW TO PREVENT
* No specific preventive steps. No vaccine is available.
* Wash hands often to prevent spread of any germs.
* Travelers to countries where there is a risk of infection need to take proper precautions regarding food and drink.
* Avoid sexual practices that increase risk of infection.

 WHAT TO EXPECT

DIAGNOSTIC MEASURES
* Your own observation of symptoms.
* Your health care provider will do a physical exam and ask about your symptoms and recent travels.
* Medical tests may include blood and stool studies. If liver involvement is a concern, other tests may be done.

APPROPRIATE HEALTH CARE
* Home care.
* Treatment is with drugs. A stool sample may be rechecked after treatment is complete to be sure the infection is cleared up.
* In severe cases of dysentery, hospital care may be needed. Fluid replacement may be necessary to manage dehydration due to diarrhea.

POSSIBLE COMPLICATIONS—The amoebas can travel through the blood stream to other parts of the body and cause infection in different organs. This can lead to an amebic liver abscess (pus-filled area) or brain abscess.

PROBABLE OUTCOME—In most cases, amebiasis is curable in three weeks with treatment.

 HOW TO TREAT

GENERAL MEASURES—Amebiasis is contagious. Be extra careful about personal cleanliness. Bathe frequently. Wash hands with warm water and soap after each bowel movement and before handling food.

MEDICATION—Antibiotic drugs to treat amebiasis are usually prescribed. These are most often taken by mouth, but in some cases may be injected.

ACTIVITY—Get extra rest until diarrhea and other symptoms improve.

DIET—No special diet. Be sure to drink plenty of fluids to help prevent dehydration.

 CALL YOUR DOCTOR IF

* You or a family member has symptoms of amebiasis.
* The following occur during treatment:
  - Abdominal (stomach) cramps continue longer than 24 hours.
  - Diarrhea or blood in stool increases.
  - Vomiting begins.
  - Pain begins over liver or jaundice (yellow skin or eyes) occurs.
  - A skin rash appears.

AMENORRHEA, PRIMARY

 ## GENERAL INFORMATION

DEFINITION—Complete absence of menstruation in a young woman who is at least 16 years old, or at age 14 with a lack of normal growth or absence of secondary sexual development. It is a rare disorder, as over 95% of girls have their first menstrual period by age 15. Most girls begin menstruating by age 14. The average age is 12 years, 8 months.

BODY PARTS INVOLVED—Endocrine system; reproductive system.

SEX OR AGE MOST AFFECTED—Young females.

SIGNS & SYMPTOMS—Lack of menstrual periods after puberty.

CAUSES—A failure of certain complex body functions that normally result in menstruation. There are a number of disorders or health problems that can lead to the failure.

RISK INCREASES WITH
* Delayed puberty.
* Congenital abnormalities, such as the absence or abnormal formation of female organs (vagina, uterus, and ovaries).
* Intact hymen (membrane covering the vaginal opening) has no opening to allow passage of menstrual flow.
* Disorders (tumors, infections or other problems) of the endocrine system, including the pituitary, hypothalamus, thyroid, parathyroid, adrenal, and ovarian glands.
* Chromosome disorders.
* Chronic illness.
* Polycystic ovarian syndrome (Stein-Leventhal syndrome).
* Rarely, prior gynecological surgery.
* Severe nutritional or physical stressors such as anorexia or competitive sports.
* Use of drugs, including oral contraceptives, anticancer drugs, barbiturates, narcotics, cortisone drugs, chlordiazepoxide, and reserpine.
* Family tendency to start menstruation late.
* Excessive dieting or weight loss.
* Extreme obesity.

HOW TO PREVENT—No specific preventive measures. Avoid risk factors where possible.

 ## WHAT TO EXPECT

DIAGNOSTIC MEASURES
* Your health care provider will do a physical exam and a pelvic exam.
* Medical tests may include urine and blood studies, hormone levels, liver, thyroid, and adrenal function studies. Other tests may be done to diagnose an underlying disorder.

APPROPRIATE HEALTH CARE
* Treatment may involve hormone replacement therapy.
* Treatment for amenorrhea not related to hormone deficiency depends on the cause.
* Counseling may help if amenorrhea is related to stress, results from an eating disorder, or if a young woman has emotional concerns about sexual development.
* Surgery to correct abnormalities of the reproductive system or for cysts may rarely be needed.

POSSIBLE COMPLICATIONS
* Emotional stress about sexual development.
* May lead to infertility.
* Other complications may occur, depending on the underlying cause.

PROBABLE OUTCOME
* The absence of menstruation is not a health risk in itself, but the cause should be found.
* Amenorrhea is often curable with hormone treatment or treatment of the underlying cause. Treatment may be delayed to age 18, unless the cause can be identified and treated safely.
* Causes that sometimes cannot be corrected include chromosome disorders and abnormalities of the reproductive system.

 ## HOW TO TREAT

GENERAL MEASURES
* Seek help in resolving emotional stress.
* Don't use mood-altering, mind-altering stimulants or sedative drugs.

MEDICATION
* Hormones may be prescribed if there is a hormone imbalance. They may correct the problem.
* Birth control pills may be prescribed for polycystic ovary syndrome.
* Bromocriptine may be prescribed for pituitary tumor.

ACTIVITY—Exercise regularly, but not to excess. Reduce exercise or athletic activities if they are too strenuous.

DIET—If overweight or underweight, a change in diet to correct the problem may bring on a period.

 ## CALL YOUR DOCTOR IF

* You or a family member is 16 years old and has never had a period.
* Periods don't begin within 6 months, despite treatment.

AMENORRHEA, SECONDARY

GENERAL INFORMATION

DEFINITION—Absence of menstruation in a woman who has previously menstruated.

BODY PARTS INVOLVED—Endocrine system; reproductive system.

SEX OR AGE MOST AFFECTED—Females over age 16.

SIGNS & SYMPTOMS
• No menstrual periods for at least 3 to 6 months.
• Other symptoms may include infertility, acne, excess hair growth (hirsutism) or hair loss, obesity, galactorrhea (breasts produce milk when not breast-feeding), headaches, and vaginal dryness.

CAUSES—A stopping of certain complex body functions that normally result in menstruation. There are a number of conditions or health problems that can lead to the failure. Pregnancy is one of the most common causes.

RISK INCREASES WITH
• Breast-feeding an infant.
• Discontinuing use of or changes in hormone drugs or birth-control pills.
• Menopause (if a woman is over 35 and not pregnant).
• Emotional stress or psychological disorder.
• Surgical removal of the ovaries or uterus, or complications as a result of gynecological surgery.
• Disorder of the endocrine system, including the pituitary, hypothalamus, thyroid, parathyroid, adrenal, and ovarian glands.
• Hormone imbalance.
• Chronic illness, such as diabetes or tuberculosis.
• Obesity or eating disorders (anorexia or bulimia).
• Strenuous program of physical exercise, such as long-distance running, gymnastics or ballet.
• Use of certain drugs (sedatives, narcotics, or barbiturates).

HOW TO PREVENT—Not always preventable. To reduce risk, maintain a healthy lifestyle.

WHAT TO EXPECT

DIAGNOSTIC MEASURES
• Your health care provider will do a physical exam and a pelvic exam.
• Medical tests may include a pregnancy test, blood studies of hormone levels, and a Pap smear.
• Surgical diagnostic procedures such as laparoscopy or hysteroscopy may be recommended. These procedures use a special instrument to see inside the body's organs.

APPROPRIATE HEALTH CARE
• Treatment may include lifestyle changes, drugs, treatment of underlying disorder (if one is diagnosed), and surgery (sometimes).
• Dilatation and curettage, often referred to as D & C (dilation of the cervix and a scraping out of the uterus with a curette), may be performed.
• Counseling may help if amenorrhea is related to stress or other emotional problems.

POSSIBLE COMPLICATIONS
• None likely, if there is no serious underlying cause.
• May experience estrogen deficiency symptoms, such as hot flashes and vaginal dryness.
• May affect fertility.

PROBABLE OUTCOME
• Amenorrhea is not a threat to health. Whether it can be corrected varies with the cause.
• If from pregnancy or breast-feeding, periods will resume when these conditions cease.
• If from discontinuing use of oral contraceptives, periods should begin in 2 months to 2 years.
• If from menopause, periods will become less frequent or may never resume. Hysterectomy also ends menstruation permanently.
• If from endocrine disorders, hormone replacement usually causes periods to resume.
• If from eating disorders, successful treatment of that disorder will help menstruation to resume.
• If from diabetes or tuberculosis, menstruation may never resume.
• If from strenuous exercise, periods usually resume when exercise is decreased.

HOW TO TREAT

GENERAL MEASURES—Keep a record of menstrual cycles to aid in early detection of recurrent amenorrhea.

MEDICATION
• Progesterone and/or estrogen may be prescribed. If bleeding occurs after progesterone is withdrawn, the reproduction system is functional.
• Drugs to treat an underlying disorder may be prescribed.

ACTIVITY—Exercise regularly, but not to excess. Reduce exercise or athletic activities if they are too strenuous.

DIET—If overweight or underweight, a change in diet to correct the problem may be helpful.

CALL YOUR DOCTOR IF

• You or a family member has amenorrhea.
• Periods don't resume within 6 months.

AMYOTROPHIC LATERAL SCLEROSIS (ALS; Lou Gehrig's Disease)

GENERAL INFORMATION

DEFINITION—A progressive breakdown of the cells of the spinal cord. This results in gradual loss of muscle function.

BODY PARTS INVOLVED—Central nervous system; muscle system, especially in the hands, forearms, legs, head and neck.

SEX OR AGE MOST AFFECTED—It usually affects people ages 40 to 60 years, and occurs more often in men than women.

SIGNS & SYMPTOMS
* Muscle twitching and weakness. It begins in the hands and spreads to the arms and legs. The weakness then begins to affect muscles that control breathing and swallowing.
* Muscle cramps.
* Stiffening and spasticity of muscle groups.
* Weight loss.
* Slurring of speech.
* Mental function is rarely affected.
* Sudden involuntary bursts of laughter or crying.

CAUSES—Unknown. Research suggests that there may be more than one cause.

RISK INCREASES WITH
* Age over 40.
* Family history of ALS.
* Smoking.

HOW TO PREVENT—Cannot be prevented at present.

WHAT TO EXPECT

DIAGNOSTIC MEASURES
* Your own observation of symptoms.
* Your health care provider will do a physical exam and ask questions about your symptoms. No one test diagnoses ALS.
* Medical tests will include nerve studies such as electromyography and nerve conduction velocity (see Glossary for both). Other tests may include blood and urine studies and x-rays.

APPROPRIATE HEALTH CARE
* There is no specific treatment. Supportive care is provided to relieve symptoms and for complications.
* Counseling may be helpful in finding ways for both the patient and the family to cope.
* Surgery for tracheostomy is usually required once breathing difficulties develop.
* In later stages of the disease, the patient will require complete nursing care.
* Patient and family may benefit from hospice care.

POSSIBLE COMPLICATIONS
* The disorder affects the patient's personal relationships, career, income, muscle coordination, sexuality, and energy.
* Progressive inability to walk and to do things involved with daily living, such as being able to feed oneself.
* Wheelchair use is needed.
* Pressure sores or skin infections due to being bedridden or in a wheelchair.
* Pneumonia due to swallowing difficulty and choking.
* The disorder is eventually fatal due to respiratory muscle weakness.

PROBABLE OUTCOME
* This condition is currently considered incurable. It is usually fatal in 2 to 5 years, but 20% of patients survive 5 years and 10% survive 10 years.
* Medical research into causes and treatment continues. There is hope for effective treatment.

HOW TO TREAT

GENERAL MEASURES
* Aids for helping with daily living, maintain some function and quality of life.are available.
* Learn to do self-suction in order to handle increased amount of secretions in the lungs.
* Take special care to prevent pressure sores.
* To learn more: ALS Association, 27001 Agoura Rd., Suite 150, Calabasas Hills, CA 91301; (800) 782-4747; website: www.alsa.org.

MEDICATION
* Riluzole may be prescribed. It can help delay the progress of ALS for a few months.
* Antibiotics may be prescribed for infections.
* Drugs to help help reduce spasticity and to decrease excess saliva are often prescribed.

ACTIVITY
* Stay as active as possible. Weakness will gradually limit movement. A physical therapy program can help to maintain independence as long as possible.
* Obtain equipment that will aid in mobility, such as a walker or wheelchair.

DIET—If swallowing is difficult, eat soft, easy-to-swallow foods. (See Soft Diet in Appendix.)

CALL YOUR DOCTOR IF

* You or a family member has symptoms of ALS.(amyotrophic lateral sclerosis).
* After diagnosis, symptoms occur that cause concern.

ANAL FISSURE

GENERAL INFORMATION

DEFINITION—A laceration, tear, or crack in the lining of the anus.

BODY PARTS INVOLVED—Anus.

SEX OR AGE MOST AFFECTED—All ages, It is most common in infants, young children, adults over 60, and women more than men.

SIGNS & SYMPTOMS
• Sharp pain with passage of a hard or bulky stool. The pain may last up to an hour, and returns with the next bowel movement.
• Pain when sitting on a hard surface.
• Streaks of blood on the toilet paper, underwear, or diaper.
• Itching around the rectum.
• Refusal to have a bowel movement (in children).

CAUSES—The exact cause is unknown. Symptoms usually occur after the stretching of the anus from a large, hard stool.

RISK INCREASES WITH
• Constipation or prolonged diarrhea.
• Multiple pregnancies.
• Crohn's disease.
• Medical disorders of the body's immune system.

HOW TO PREVENT
• Avoid constipation by:
 - Drinking plenty of water each day.
 - Eating a diet high in fiber.
 - Using stool softeners, if needed.
• Don't strain when having a bowel movement.
• Avoid anal intercourse.

WHAT TO EXPECT

DIAGNOSTIC MEASURES
• Your own observation of symptoms.
• Your health care provider will do a physical exam of the anus and rectum to confirm the diagnosis. Other medical tests are usually not needed.

APPROPRIATE HEALTH CARE
• Home care.
• Health care provider's treatment.
• Minor surgery may be needed to remove the fissure if conservative treatment is not successful. (See Anal-Fissure Removal and Anal Sphincterectomy in Surgery section.)

POSSIBLE COMPLICATIONS—Fissure may become chronic and fail to heal.

PROBABLE OUTCOME—Most fissures heal on their own. Others can be corrected with surgery. Most infants and young children recover after the stool is softened.

HOW TO TREAT

GENERAL MEASURES
• Gently clean the anus with soap and water after each bowel movement.
• To relieve muscle spasms and pain around the anus, apply a warm towel to the area.
• Sitz baths also relieve pain. Use 8 inches of warm water in the bathtub, 2 or 3 times a day for 10 to 20 minutes.

MEDICATION
• For minor pain, use nonprescription drugs, such as acetaminophen or topical anesthetics.
• Zinc oxide ointment or petroleum jelly applied to the anal opening may help prevent any burning sensation.
• Bulk stool softeners will help to avoid the pain occurring with hard bowel movements.
• Lidocaine ointment may be recommended.
• Botulinum (Botox) injections may be prescribed to help relax the sphincter muscles.

ACTIVITY—No limits. Physical activity reduces the likelihood of constipation.

DIET—Eat a high-fiber diet and drink extra fluids to help prevent constipation.

CALL YOUR DOCTOR IF

• You or a family member has symptoms of an anal fissure.
• Pain continues despite treatment.

ANAL FISTULA

GENERAL INFORMATION

DEFINITION—A very small tube or tract that leads from the anal canal (the last part of the rectum) to the skin near the anal opening. Watery pus drains through this opening and causes irritation to the skin.

BODY PARTS INVOLVED—Anus.

SEX OR AGE MOST AFFECTED—Both sexes, usually in adults.

SIGNS & SYMPTOMS
* Discharge from the anus.
* Can feel a firm and tender lump.
* Pain during or after bowel movement.
* Color change of the skin surrounding fistula.

CAUSES
* Infection from a tear in the anal canal lining.
* May be due to an injury, rectal infection (including chlamydia), cancer, and radiation therapy.
* Tissue damage because of an abscess (a pocket of pus).

RISK INCREASES WITH
* Puncture wound in anal canal lining (e.g., from eating an eggshell or fishbone) or injury from an enema tip.
* Injection treatment for internal hemorrhoids.
* Inflammatory bowel disease.
* Acute appendicitis or diverticulitis.

HOW TO PREVENT—No specific preventive steps.

WHAT TO EXPECT

DIAGNOSTIC MEASURES
* Your own observation of symptoms.
* Your health care provider will do a physical exam of the anal area to confirm the diagnosis.

APPROPRIATE HEALTH CARE
* Home care.
* Health care provider's treatment.
* If it does not heal on its own, minor surgery can correct the fistula. It is usually done with local anesthetic on an outpatient basis. Follow your health care provider's instructions for after surgery care. See Anal Fistula Repair in Surgery Section.

POSSIBLE COMPLICATIONS
* Constipation.
* Fistula may recur.

PROBABLE OUTCOME—Some fistulas heal on their own. In others, surgical repair may be necessary and the results are usually excellent.

HOW TO TREAT

GENERAL MEASURES
* Gently clean the anus with soap and water after each bowel movement.
* Sitz baths help relieve discomfort. Sit in a tub of warm water (not hot) for 10 to 15 minutes several times a day. Dry the area carefully and completely after bathing.

MEDICATION
* Stool softeners may be prescribed to prevent constipation.
* Antibiotics may be prescribed if infection is present.

ACTIVITY—Resume work and normal activity as soon as possible.

DIET—No special diet.

CALL YOUR DOCTOR IF

* You or a family member has any symptoms of an anal fistula.
* Symptoms recur after treatment.

ILLNESS & DISORDERS

ANAPHYLAXIS
(Allergic Shock)

GENERAL INFORMATION

DEFINITION—A life-threatening allergic response to drugs or any other allergy-causing substance. Reactions that happen the fastest are often the worst.

BODY PARTS INVOLVED—Blood vessels throughout the body; heart; lungs; skin.

SEX OR AGE MOST AFFECTED—Both sexes; all ages.

SIGNS & SYMPTOMS—Any of the following can happen within seconds or a few minutes after being exposed to something that you are very allergic to:
* Tingling or numbness around the mouth.
* Sneezing, coughing, or wheezing.
* Swelling around the face or hands.
* Feeling anxious.
* Weak, rapid pulse.
* Stomach cramps, vomiting, and diarrhea.
* Itching all over. Hives often appear.
* Watery eyes.
* Chest feels tight; trouble breathing.
* Swelling or itching in the mouth or throat.
* Pounding heartbeat.
* Faintness; loss of consciousness.
* Not all symptoms occur. Seek help for any of them.

CAUSES—Sometimes the body overreacts when it tries to rid itself of the material it is allergic to. This can be life-threatening. Things that most often cause reactions:
* Drugs of all types, especially penicillin. Shots are a bigger risk than eyedrops or drugs taken by mouth.
* Stings or bites from insects, such as bees, wasps, hornets, biting ants and some spiders.
* Vaccines.
* Pollen.
* Injected chemicals used in some types of x-ray studies.
* Foods, especially eggs, beans, seafood, and fruit.

RISK INCREASES WITH
* A previous mild allergy to things listed above.
* A history of rashes, hay fever, or asthma.

HOW TO PREVENT—If you have an allergic history:
* Tell your health care provider before you begin taking any new drugs. Before you are given a shot, ask what it is. Always remain in a medical office 15 minutes after receiving a shot.
* Keep a special kit, such as Ana-Kit or EpiPen, with you at all times. Be sure your family knows how to use the kit if you need it.
* If you are allergic to insect stings, wear clothing that covers all of your body when you are outside.
* Wear a medical alert type bracelet or necklace showing that you have allergies.
* Ask your health care provider about allergy therapy that can make you less allergic.
* People with previous severe reaction to insect stings should consider immunization (allergy shots) as a preventive measure.

WHAT TO EXPECT

DIAGNOSTIC MEASURES—Skin tests to determine sensitivities.

APPROPRIATE HEALTH CARE
* Health care provider's treatment.
* Long-term treatment may involve steps to make your body less sensitive to things to which you are allergic.

POSSIBLE COMPLICATIONS—If not treated quickly, anaphylaxis can cause shock, cardiac arrest, and/or death.

PROBABLE OUTCOME—Full recovery (if treated quickly).

HOW TO TREAT

GENERAL MEASURES
* If you see signs of anaphylaxis in someone and they stop breathing:
  - Call 911 (emergency) for medical help.
  - Begin mouth-to-mouth breathing right away.
  - If their heart is not beating, give CPR (cardiopulmonary resuscitation).
  - Don't stop CPR until help arrives.
* Be aware that a reaction may happen when taking any medicine. Be ready to respond quickly if symptoms develop. If you have had a severe allergic reaction in the past, always carry your anaphylaxis kit.

MEDICATION
* Epinephrine shots are the immediate treatment for this condition.
* Other drugs may be given after epinephrine that will help prevent the return of symptoms.

ACTIVITY—Resume your normal activities as soon as symptoms improve after an attack. Stay under someone's observation for 24 hours in case symptoms recur.

DIET—Avoid foods to which you are allergic.

CALL YOUR DOCTOR IF

You or a family member has symptoms of anaphylaxis. This is an emergency!

ANEMIA, APLASTIC

GENERAL INFORMATION

DEFINITION—A serious disease that involves decreased bone-marrow production of white and red blood cells and platelets.

BODY PARTS INVOLVED—Bone marrow; lymphatic system; blood.

SEX OR AGE MOST AFFECTED—Both sexes; all ages.

SIGNS & SYMPTOMS
* Paleness.
* Weakness, tiredness, faintness and breathlessness.
* Frequent infections.
* Spontaneous bleeding from the nose, mouth, rectum, vagina, gums and other sites—including the central nervous system.
* Red dots of bleeding under the skin.
* Unexplained bruising.
* Ulcers in the mouth, throat and rectum.

CAUSES—Bone marrow contains stem cells that develop into red blood cells, white blood cells or platelets. These are all important in maintaining functions of the body. Stem cells can be damaged due to known or unknown factors and the cells do not develop properly. The bone marrow then fills up with fat. This leads to aplastic anemia.

RISK INCREASES WITH
* Airplane glue inhalation.
* Exposure to certain chemicals (such as benzene and pesticides).
* Inherited or genetic factors.
* Use of certain drugs, especially immunosuppressive drugs, anticancer drugs, or chloramphenicol.
* Pregnancy.
* Radiation therapy.
* Recent viral illness.

HOW TO PREVENT
* Avoid prolonged exposure to toxic compounds, such as benzene, that are used in many industrial chemicals.
* Don't use drugs that cause aplastic anemia if substitute drugs are available.

WHAT TO EXPECT

DIAGNOSTIC MEASURES
* Your own observation of symptoms.
* A health care provider will do a physical exam and ask questions about your medications and exposure to chemicals.
* Medical tests usually include blood studies and for some, a bone marrow biopsy.

APPROPRIATE HEALTH CARE
* Hospital care with isolation until the body can resist infection.
* Blood transfusions if necessary.
* Surgery to transplant bone marrow for some patients.
* Other therapy as determined by the cause.

POSSIBLE COMPLICATIONS—Poor response to treatment, resulting in uncontrollable infections and bleeding. Complications are fatal in 50% to 70% of those with severe aplastic anemia.

PROBABLE OUTCOME—If the cause can be identified and treated successfully, the disorder is curable. Anemia caused by immuno-suppressive drugs usually improves spontaneously when drugs are withdrawn. Full recovery often requires 6 to 8 months.

HOW TO TREAT

GENERAL MEASURES—The following are helpful until blood counts are normal:
* Be extra careful about personal cleanliness.
* Pay particular attention to oral hygiene. Brush teeth gently with a very soft brush, avoiding irritation of the gums.
* Avoid contact with harmful materials, such as cleaning chemicals, glue, insecticide, fertilizer and paint remover.
* Avoid contact with large crowds or people with infections.

MEDICATION
* Immunosuppressive drugs will be prescribed to prevent rejection, if a bone-marrow transplant is necessary.
* Antibiotics to prevent or treat infection may be prescribed.
* Medicated mouthwash to suppress fungus infections may be recommended.

ACTIVITY
* Rest in bed during the acute stage. Resume normal activities gradually after symptoms subside.
* Avoid overexercising until blood counts are normal.

DIET—No special diet. You may be prescribed iron and vitamin supplements.

CALL YOUR DOCTOR IF

* You or a family member have symptoms of aplastic anemia.
* Any sign of infection or other symptoms occur during treatment.

ANEMIA DURING PREGNANCY

 ## GENERAL INFORMATION

DEFINITION—A low level of red cells and hemoglobin in the blood during pregnancy. Hemoglobin is the protein inside red blood cells that carries oxygen to body tissues. Common anemias in pregnancy include iron-deficiency anemia and folic-acid deficiency. Other anemias are glucose-6-phosphate dehydrogenase (G6PD) deficiency, thalassemia, and sickle-cell anemia.

BODY PARTS INVOLVED—Blood cells.

SEX OR AGE MOST AFFECTED—Pregnant females.

SIGNS & SYMPTOMS
* Usually no symptoms are apparent.
* Shortness of breath.
* Fatigue, weakness, or fainting.
* Pale skin, gums, eyes, and nailbeds.
* Palpitations (awareness of the heartbeat).
* Inflamed, sore tongue.
* Nausea.
* Headache.
* Jaundice (yellow skin or eyes).
* Cravings for ice, paint, or dirt (pica).

CAUSES
* Poor diet with not enough iron.
* Folic-acid deficiency.
* Loss of blood from bleeding hemorrhoids or internal bleeding.
* Even if iron and folic-acid intake are sufficient, a pregnant woman may become anemic.

RISK INCREASES WITH
* Poor nutrition, including not enough vitamins.
* Excess alcohol use, leading to poor nutrition.
* History of any disorder that reduces absorption of nutrients.
* Pregnancy with multiple babies (e.g., twins).
* Use of drugs for seizures.
* Genetic risk for some anemias.

HOW TO PREVENT
* Eat foods rich in iron, such as liver, beef, dried beans, whole-grain breads and cereals, eggs, or dried fruit.
* Eat foods high in folic acid, such as wheat germ, beans, peanut butter, oatmeal, mushrooms, collards, broccoli, beef liver, and asparagus.
* Eating foods high in vitamin C, such as citrus fruits and fresh, raw vegetables.
* Take prenatal vitamin and mineral supplements, if they are prescribed.
* Get tested for certain anemias if you are at risk. Your obstetric provider will discuss the details.

 ## WHAT TO EXPECT

DIAGNOSTIC MEASURES
* Your own observation of symptoms.
* Your obstetric provider will do blood studies during your pregnancy. These can help diagnose anemia.

APPROPRIATE HEALTH CARE—Medical care will involve treatment for any underlying cause. Supplements are needed for most anemias.

POSSIBLE COMPLICATIONS
* Premature labor, intrauterine growth restriction (IUGR), low birth weight. Folic-acid deficiency may cause birth defects (neural tube defects).
* Blood loss during labor may require blood transfusion.
* Higher risk for mother of infection after childbirth.

PROBABLE OUTCOME—Usually curable with iron and folic-acid supplements, or other treatment if needed.

 ## HOW TO TREAT

GENERAL MEASURES
* If the tongue is red and sore, rinse with warm salt water 3 or 4 times a day. Mix one-half teaspoon salt in one cup of warm water.
* Brush teeth with a soft toothbrush.

MEDICATION
* Iron, folic acid, and other supplements may be prescribed. Take iron supplements 1 hour before eating or between meals. Iron will turn bowel movements black, and often causes constipation. Iron sometimes may be taken with meals if it has caused an upset stomach.
* If you are taking a calcium supplement in addition to an iron supplement, take them at different times of day, as calcium will interfere with iron absorption.

ACTIVITY—Rest often until the anemia improves.

DIET—Eat a healthy pregnancy diet and take prescribed supplements.

 ## CALL YOUR DOCTOR IF

* You or a family member has symptoms of anemia during pregnancy.
* You have diarrhea, nausea, abdominal pain, or constipation during pregnancy.
* You experience unexplained bleeding during pregnancy.

ANEMIA, FOLIC-ACID DEFICIENCY

 ## GENERAL INFORMATION

DEFINITION—Anemia that is caused by a deficiency of folic acid. It is often occurs along with iron-deficiency anemia.

BODY PARTS INVOLVED—Blood cells, which transport oxygen to all body parts.

SEX OR AGE MOST AFFECTED—Both sexes, but most common in women over 30.

SIGNS & SYMPTOMS
* Fatigue and weakness.
* Red, sore tongue.
* Mouth ulcers.
* Pale skin, gums, eyes, and nailbeds.
* Shortness of breath.
* Irritability.
* Nausea, vomiting and diarrhea (rare).
* Numbness and tingling of fingers and toes.

CAUSES
* Complication of pregnancy. A woman's body needs eight times more folic acid than usual with pregnancy.
* Not enough intake or absorption of foods with a high folic-acid content. These include meat, poultry, fish, cheese, milk, eggs, green vegetables, and yeast.
* Excess alcohol use.
* Over-cooking foods, which destroys folic acid.
* Deficiency of vitamin B-12 or vitamin C.

RISK INCREASES WITH
* Adults over 60.
* Pregnancy.
* Recent surgery.
* Illness such as tropical sprue, psoriasis, acne rosacea, eczema, or dermatitis herpetiformis.
* Fad diets or general poor nutrition.
* Chronic illness.
* Surgical removal of a portion of the stomach.
* Smoking, which decreases vitamin C absorption. Vitamin C is needed for folic-acid absorption.
* Use of some drugs, such as anticonvulsants, oral contraceptives, methotrexate, triamterene, or sulfasalazine.

HOW TO PREVENT
* Don't drink alcohol.
* Have regular medical checkups during pregnancy. Take prenatal vitamin supplements, if they are prescribed.
* Eat well. Include fresh vegetables, meat, and other animal proteins. Avoid fad diets. Don't over-cook food.
* Don't smoke. Smoking increases vitamin requirements.

 ## WHAT TO EXPECT

DIAGNOSTIC MEASURES
* Your own observation of symptoms.
* Your health care provider may do a physical exam.
* Medical tests may include blood studies, a Schilling test to measure vitamin B-12 levels and a trial of taking vitamin B-12.

APPROPRIATE HEALTH CARE—Medical treatment consists of folic acid supplements and treating any underlying causes.

POSSIBLE COMPLICATIONS
* Infertility.
* Increased risk of infections.
* Congestive heart failure (severe cases only).
* Can increase the risk of conceiving a child with a neural tube defect.

PROBABLE OUTCOME—Usually curable in three weeks with an adequate folic-acid intake.

 ## HOW TO TREAT

GENERAL MEASURES
* If you smoke, find a way to quit.
* If you take oral contraceptives, consider using another form of contraception.

MEDICATION
* Folic-acid supplements will be prescribed.
* Iron supplements to take orally will be prescribed.

ACTIVITY—Anemia does cause fatigue. Schedule regular rest periods until you are able to resume normal activity.

DIET—Eat foods daily that are high in folic acid. The liver can store folic acid for a limited time only. Foods include asparagus spears, beef liver, broccoli spears, collards (cooked), mushrooms, oatmeal, peanut butter, red beans, and wheat germ.

 ## CALL YOUR DOCTOR IF

* You or a family member has symptoms of anemia.
* Symptoms don't improve in two weeks, despite treatment.
* Symptoms of infection (fever, chills, and muscle aches) occur during treatment.

ILLNESS & DISORDERS

ANEMIA, HEMOLYTIC

GENERAL INFORMATION

DEFINITION—An anemia that is due to red blood cells being destroyed faster than the bone marrow can produce them. In the intrinsic type, the destruction is due to a defect in the red blood cells themselves. In the extrinsic type, healthy red blood cells are produced, but are destroyed in the spleen.

BODY PARTS INVOLVED—Blood; bone marrow; and the spleen.

SEX OR AGE MOST AFFECTED—Both sexes; all ages.

SIGNS & SYMPTOMS
* Sometimes there are no symptoms. Anemia may be diagnosed on a routine health exam.
* Fatigue and weakness.
* Pale skin, eyes, and fingernails.
* Shortness of breath.
* Irregular heartbeat.
* Jaundice (yellow skin and eyes, dark urine).

CAUSES—Bone marrow cannot produce red blood cells fast enough to make up for those being destroyed. This is a process known as hemolysis. More than 200 causes for hemolysis exist. Some are due to inherited disorders and some are acquired disorders. Sometimes, the cause is unknown.

RISK INCREASES WITH
* Inherited disorders. These include hereditary spherocytosis, glucose-6-phosphate dehydrogenase (G6PD) deficiency, sickle cell anemia, or thalassemia.
* Infections such as hepatitis, cytomegalovirus, Epstein-Barr virus, typhoid fever, streptococcus, or *Escherichia coli (E. coli)*.
* Leukemia or lymphoma.
* Use of certain drugs, such as penicillin, antimalarials, sulfa, or acetaminophen.
* Various tumors.
* Family history of hemolytic anemia.

HOW TO PREVENT
* Don't take any drugs that have previously caused hemolytic anemia.
* Seek genetic counseling before having children if you have a family history of hemolytic anemia (inherited forms).

WHAT TO EXPECT

DIAGNOSTIC MEASURES
* Your own observation of symptoms.
* Your health care provider will do a physical exam and ask questions about your symptoms.
* Medical tests include blood and urine studies. Other tests may be done to help diagnose an underlying cause for anemia.

APPROPRIATE HEALTH CARE
* Treatment depends on the specific hemolytic problem.
* Treatment may include drugs, blood transfusions, stopping drugs, or surgery.
* Blood transfusion therapy may be needed.
* Surgical removal of the spleen may be recommended.

POSSIBLE COMPLICATIONS
* Varies depending on the cause of the anemia.
* It may cause existing heart or lung disease to worsen.

PROBABLE OUTCOME
* If hemolytic anemia is acquired, it can usually be cured when the cause, such as a drug, is stopped.
* If it is due to an underlying disorder, the outcome depends on the course of the primary disease.
* If hemolytic anemia is inherited, it is currently considered incurable. However, symptoms can be relieved or controlled.

HOW TO TREAT

GENERAL MEASURES—If removal of the spleen is required, see Spleen Removal in Surgery section for an explanation of surgery and postoperative care.

MEDICATION
* Drugs will be prescribed depending on the specific cause of anemia. These may include corticosteroids, immune globulin, folic acid, iron therapy, and others.
* Drugs that are causing the anemia will be stopped.

ACTIVITY—No limits, except those caused by the symptoms.

DIET—No special diet. Fava beans should be avoided in certain patients (you will be advised).

CALL YOUR DOCTOR IF

* You or a family member has symptoms of hemolytic anemia.
* Fever, cough, sore throat, swollen joints, muscle aches, or bloody urine occur during treatment.
* Signs of infection (e.g., redness, pain, swelling, fever) occur in any part of the body.
* New, unexplained symptoms develop. Drugs used in treatment may produce side effects.

ANEMIA, IRON-DEFICIENCY

GENERAL INFORMATION

DEFINITION—An anemia caused by inadequate amounts of iron, which is required to meet the body's needs. Iron is present in all cells and has several vital functions.

BODY PARTS INVOLVED—Blood, which affects all body cells.

SEX OR AGE MOST AFFECTED—The anemia can affect any age and both sexes. It is more common in women of childbearing age.

SIGNS & SYMPTOMS
* There may be no symptoms. It may be diagnosed on a routine health exam.
* Fatigue and weakness.
* Pale skin, eyes, and fingernails.
* General feeling of discomfort.
* Being more sensitive to cold.
* Shortness of breath.
* Dizziness.
* Restless leg syndrome (odd sensations in the legs).

CAUSES—Iron is involved with red blood cell production. When iron stores are low, fewer red blood cells are produced and this leads to anemia.

RISK INCREASES WITH
* Rapid growth spurts in children and young teens.
* Heavy menstrual bleeding.
* Pregnancy.
* Not getting enough iron in the diet.
* Internal bleeding, such as from ulcers or colon polyps.
* Problems of the body in utilizing or absorbing iron.
* Kidney disease.
* Folic acid or vitamin B-12 deficiency.

HOW TO PREVENT
* Adequate iron intake with a well-balanced diet.
* Correct problems causing excess blood loss.

WHAT TO EXPECT

DIAGNOSTIC MEASURES
* Your own observation of symptoms.
* Your health care provider will do a physical exam and ask questions about your symptoms and diet
* Medical tests may include blood, urine, and stool studies. Other tests may be done to diagnose disorders that could be the cause of the anemia.

APPROPRIATE HEALTH CARE
* Iron deficiency can be treated with iron supplements. Other treatment will depend on the underlying cause. The cause needs to be treated so the iron deficiency does not recur.
* Internal bleeding problems may require surgery.

POSSIBLE COMPLICATIONS
* Complications are rare in mild anemia.
* If the anemia is more severe, heart complications can occur. Children may have developmental problems.

PROBABLE OUTCOME—Usually curable with treatment. It may take 2 months for the iron levels to return to normal. Some outcomes will also depend on the underlying cause.

HOW TO TREAT

GENERAL MEASURES
* The most important part of treatment for iron-deficiency anemia is to correct the underlying cause.
* Avoid risk of infections.

MEDICATION
* Oral iron supplements (always follow your health care provider's instructions):
  - Take iron on an empty stomach (at least 1/2 hour before meals) for best absorption. If it upsets your stomach, take it with a small amount of food (except milk).
  - If you take other drugs, wait at least 2 hours after taking iron before taking them. Antacids and tetracyclines especially interfere with iron absorption.
  - Iron supplements may cause black bowel movements, diarrhea, or constipation.
  - Too much iron is dangerous. A bottle of iron tablets can poison a child. Keep iron supplements out of the reach of children.
* In some cases, the iron supplement may be given by injection.

ACTIVITY—You may need to reduce activities until symptoms of fatigue are gone.

DIET
* Adults should limit milk to 1 pint a day. Milk interferes with iron absorption.
* Eat iron-rich foods, including meat, fish, poultry, beans, raisins, egg yolks, and leafy green vegetables.
* Increase dietary fiber to prevent constipation.

CALL YOUR DOCTOR IF

* You or a family member has symptoms of anemia.
* Nausea, vomiting, fever, stomach pain, severe diarrhea, or constipation occur during treatment.

ANEMIA, PERNICIOUS
(B-12 Deficiency Anemia)

 GENERAL INFORMATION

DEFINITION—An anemia that results from the failure of the digestive tract to absorb vitamin B-12. Vitamin B-12 (also called cobalamin) is needed for making red blood cells and keeping the nervous system functioning.

BODY PARTS INVOLVED—Blood, which affects all body cells; stomach.

SEX OR AGE MOST AFFECTED—Adults of both sexes, between ages 40 and 70.

SIGNS & SYMPTOMS
* Symptoms develop slowly and take time to notice.
* Weakness, especially in the arms and legs.
* Sore tongue.
* Nausea, appetite loss, and weight loss.
* Numbness or tingling in the hands and feet.
* Difficulty maintaining proper balance.
* Pale lips, tongue, and gums.
* Yellow eyes and skin.
* Bleeding gums.
* Shortness of breath.
* Depression, confusion, poor memory, and dementia.
* Headache.
* Ringing in the ears (tinnitus).

CAUSES
* Pernicious anemia is due to a lack of intrinsic factor. This is a substance made by cells in the stomach that makes it possible to absorb vitamin B-12. The reason for the lack of intrinsic factor is unknown. It may be an autoimmune reaction, a genetic factor, or both.
* Other vitamin B-12 deficiency-caused anemia may be due to a variety of factors.

RISK INCREASES WITH
* Stomach surgery or cancer, or gastritis.
* Diabetes and autoimmune disorders.
* Myxedema, Graves' disease, other thyroid disorders.
* Genetic factors (as in people of Northern European ancestry); rare in blacks and Asians.
* Family history of pernicious anemia.
* Age over 40.
* Strict vegetarian diet or infants breast-fed by a mother on a strict vegetarian diet.
* Lack of stomach acid in older adults.
* Parasitic infections and intestinal diseases.
* Drugs such as H2 blockers, proton pump inhibitors, colchicine, neomycin, and aminosalicylic acid.
* Alcoholism.

HOW TO PREVENT—Pernicious anemia cannot be prevented. In other anemias, avoiding risk factors, where possible, may help.

 WHAT TO EXPECT

DIAGNOSTIC MEASURES
* Your own observation of symptoms.
* Your health care provider will do a physical exam and ask questions about symptoms and your diet.
* Medical tests include blood tests for vitamin B-12 levels, to check for antibodies to the intrinsic factor, and to measure the body's ability to absorb vitamin B-12.

APPROPRIATE HEALTH CARE
* Treatment usually involves vitamin B-12 replacement. Lifetime treatment is needed for pernicious anemia. Some symptoms should start to clear up in a few days after treatment begins, while others may take several months.
* Any underlying disorder (such as thyroid problems) will be treated also.

POSSIBLE COMPLICATIONS
* Congestive heart failure.
* Nerve damage that cannot be reversed.
* Gastric cancer.

PROBABLE OUTCOME
* For pernicious anemia, lifelong vitamin B-12 therapy helps symptoms and prevents complications.
* For vitamin B-12 deficiency-caused anemia, vitamin B-12 therapy or diet changes can prevent deficiency.

 HOW TO TREAT

GENERAL MEASURES—Stop drinking if alcoholism led to the vitamin B-12 deficiency.

MEDICATION
* Vitamin B-12 replacement will be prescribed. Some patients are given injections (they can be self-administered). For other patients (or in addition to injections), the vitamin may be taken by mouth or as a nasal gel.
* Iron supplements may be prescribed.
* Avoid taking high amounts of folic acid.

ACTIVITY—Activity may be limited short term.

DIET
* Eat a well-balanced diet.
* Those on strict vegetarian diet can change the diet or take lifelong vitamin B-12 supplements.

 CALL YOUR DOCTOR IF

* You or a family member has symptoms of pernicious anemia.
* Symptoms don't improve with treatment.

ANEURYSM

GENERAL INFORMATION

DEFINITION—A ballooning or bulge in the wall of a blood vessel (almost always an artery). It can affect the arteries in the chest, abdomen, brain, legs, or heart wall. Aneurysms have thin, weak walls and have a tendency to rupture (burst) and cause hemorrhage (bleeding).

BODY PARTS INVOLVED—Arteries. Aneurysms occur most often in the aorta (major artery in the chest and abdomen), arteries that supply the brain or legs, or heart wall.

SEX OR AGE MOST AFFECTED—Adults of both sexes, usually over age 50.

SIGNS & SYMPTOMS
• Usually, there are no symptoms unless the aneurysm ruptures. Symptoms that occur depend on the artery affected.
• Thoracic (chest) aneurysm produces pain in the chest, neck, back, and abdomen. The pain may be sudden and sharp.
• Cerebral aneurysm in a brain artery produces headache (often throbbing), weakness, paralysis or numbness, pain behind the eye, vision change, partial blindness, and eye pupils of different sizes.
• Abdominal aneurysm produces back pain (sometimes severe), abdomen, and groin pain.
• Peripheral aneurysm in a leg artery causes poor circulation in the leg, with weakness and paleness or swelling, and bluish color.
• Ventricular aneurysm in the wall of the heart causes irregular heartbeat, shortness of breath, and chest pain.

CAUSES—Arterial walls become weak due to defect, disease, or injury. This may be due to an acquired condition or it may be congenital (present at birth).

RISK INCREASES WITH
• Adults over 55.
• Family history of aneurysms.
• Atherosclerosis (hardening of the arteries).
• High blood pressure.
• Congenital weak artery.
• Polycystic disease or connective tissue disorder.
• Complications of blood infections.
• Fibromuscular dysplasia.
• Injury (trauma).
• Cigarette smoking.

HOW TO PREVENT—No specific way to prevent aneurysms. Get medical care for risk factors where possible.

WHAT TO EXPECT

DIAGNOSTIC MEASURES—See Appropriate health Care.

APPROPRIATE HEALTH CARE
• Emergency treatment is needed for persons with symptoms of a ruptured aneurysm. Once the aneurysm is diagnosed, surgery may be performed. This is done to stop any bleeding and to prevent the aneurysm from recurring. Treatments called endovascular procedures can be done to plug or clog the blood vessel.
• Unruptured aneurysms may be diagnosed when a person has no symptoms. Sometimes they are found when medical tests are done for other reasons. The decision to treat or not treat these aneurysms with surgery is difficult. Both options carry risks. Your health care provider will discuss the risks and benefits of each with you. The size of the aneurysm, its location, the patient's symptoms, age, health status, and preferences must all be considered.
• Sometimes, the aneurysm can be removed and replaced with a graft (artificial blood vessel), or wrapped with a protective sleeve to prevent rupturing. See Aneurysm Repair in Surgery Section.

POSSIBLE COMPLICATIONS
• Stroke.
• Rupture of the aneurysm.

PROBABLE OUTCOME
• Diagnosed, unruptured aneurysms may or may not be treated. You may be followed up with regular medical exams to watch for complications.
• Outcome of a ruptured aneurysm varies. Some persons are treated and recover with little or no damage. Others die before, during, or after treatment.

HOW TO TREAT

GENERAL MEASURES—None specific.

MEDICATION
• After surgery, anticoagulants to prevent blood clots and pain relievers are usually prescribed.
• Antibiotics to prevent infection may be prescribed.

ACTIVITY—If surgery is done, you will be advised of any limits.

DIET—No special diet.

CALL YOUR DOCTOR IF

• You or a family member has symptoms of an aneurysm, especially a pulsating mass in the abdomen or leg, or chest or abdominal pain. This is an emergency! Call for help and rest in bed.
• You have had a heart attack and develop heartbeat irregularity or symptoms of congestive heart failure.
• After surgery, any symptoms return.

ANGINA PECTORIS

GENERAL INFORMATION

DEFINITION—Chest pain or discomfort due to a decrease in the blood (and oxygen) supply to the heart muscle (myocardium). Angina may be stable (symptoms are predictable), or unstable (symptoms are unexpected and usually occur while at rest).

BODY PARTS INVOLVED—Coronary arteries.

SEX OR AGE MOST AFFECTED—Men over age 35 and postmenopausal women.

SIGNS & SYMPTOMS
* Tightness, squeezing, pressure, fullness, ache, or pain in the center of the chest.
* Chest pain similar to indigestion.
* Discomfort or pain may also occur in the neck, jaw, shoulder, arm, or back.
* Symptoms may occur with exercise, strong emotions, heavy meals, or with temperature extremes. Some persons have angina while resting.

CAUSES
Angina occurs when the heart needs more blood and oxygen and it is unable to get what it requires. This is called ischemia. Most often it is due to coronary heart disease. With heart disease, one or more of the arteries that supply blood to the heart is narrowed or blocked. Angina also occurs if the blood does not carry enough oxygen, such as in severe anemia or carbon monoxide poisoning.

RISK INCREASES WITH
* Coronary or valvular heart disease.
* Hypertrophic cardiomyopathy (enlarged heart).
* Anemia.

HOW TO PREVENT—Prevention involves preventing the coronary heart disease that leads to angina. Don't smoke. Get treatment for chronic disorders such as diabetes, high blood pressure, and obesity. Reduce high cholesterol with diet or drugs.

WHAT TO EXPECT

DIAGNOSTIC MEASURES
* Your own observation of symptoms.
* Your health care provider will do a physical exam and ask questions about your symptoms.
* A number of medical tests will be done to assess heart function and to diagnose any underlying disorder.

APPROPRIATE HEALTH CARE
* Treatment usually involves drug therapy to relieve angina symptoms, slow the progress of heart disease, and prevent complications.
* If drugs cannot control the angina, there are other treatment options. They include balloon angioplasty to open blocked coronary arteries, stenting (a tiny metal tube or coil is placed in the artery to keep it open), or surgery to bypass severely blocked coronary arteries.

POSSIBLE COMPLICATIONS—Heart attack, unstable angina, and/or death.

PROBABLE OUTCOME—Minor angina can be relieved with rest and use of nitroglycerin and other drugs. Other treatment may be needed to correct underlying diseases.

HOW TO TREAT

GENERAL MEASURES
* Don't smoke. Find a way for you to quit.
* Avoid angina triggers, if possible, that add to the heart's workload, such as anger, sudden bursts of activity, temperature extremes, or high altitude (except in commercial airline flights).
* To learn more: American Heart Association, local branch listed in telephone directory. Call (800) 242-8721 or check website: www.americanheart.org.

MEDICATION
* Nitroglycerin relieves acute symptoms of angina or it can be used before activities. It does not affect symptoms of other disorders. It can work within seconds to relieve pain. Always keep it with you for immediate use.
* Drugs to prevent blood clots will be given after procedures such as balloon angioplasty or stenting.
* Other drugs for coronary disease, such as aspirin, beta-blockers, cholesterol-lowering drugs, ACE inhibitors, or calcium channel blockers may be prescribed. If they are, it is important to follow the prescribed drug regimen.

ACTIVITY
* Adjust activities to lessen angina attacks.
* Don't use angina as an excuse not to exercise. A regular moderate exercise routine (determined by your health care provider) can help to control symptoms.

DIET
* A low-fat, low-cholesterol diet may be helpful.
* Weight loss diet if overweight.

CALL YOUR DOCTOR IF

* You or a family member has symptoms of angina pectoris.
* Angina pain lasts longer than 10 to 15 minutes, despite rest and treatment with nitroglycerin.
* You wake from sleep with chest pain that does not go away with 1 nitroglycerin tablet. If these attacks continue, report them, even if nitroglycerin relieves them.

ANIMAL BITES

GENERAL INFORMATION

DEFINITION—Bite wounds to humans from dogs, cats, or other animals (including humans).

BODY PARTS INVOLVED—Usually the hands, face or legs.

SEX OR AGE MOST AFFECTED—All ages and both sexes, but more often occurs in children and males.

SIGNS & SYMPTOMS
* Bite wounds can be tears, punctures, scratches, ripping, or crushing injuries.
* Dog bites usually involve the hands, face, or the legs and feet.
* Cat bites usually involve the hands, followed by legs, feet, face, and trunk.

CAUSES
* Most bite wounds are from a domestic pet known to the victim. Large dogs are the most common source.
* Human bites are often the result of one person striking another in the mouth with a clenched fist.

RISK INCREASES WITH—Exposure to domestic pets or wild animals.

HOW TO PREVENT
* Education on how to avoid animal bites, for children as well as adults.
* Avoid stray animals.

WHAT TO EXPECT

DIAGNOSTIC MEASURES
* Your own observations.
* Doctor's examination.
* Culture of wound fluids, x-rays (if wound is near a bone or joint), exploratory surgery sometimes to determine extent of injuries.

APPROPRIATE HEALTH CARE
* Self-care.
* Call a health care provider, or take the patient to an emergency department if the wound is severe, it won't stop bleeding, or the bite was from a wild animal or one behaving strangely.
* Wound cleaning.
* Surgical closure if needed.
* Wound will usually be left open to heal to lessen risk of infection.
* Splint hand if it is injured.
* Human bite wounds on the hands should not be primarily closed due to the high risk of infection.

POSSIBLE COMPLICATIONS—Infection, extensive soft tissue injuries with scarring, hemorrhage, rabies, and sometimes death.

PROBABLE OUTCOME
* Wounds should steadily improve and close over within 7 to 10 days.
* Dog bites rarely become infected. Cat bites and human bites frequently become infected.

HOW TO TREAT

GENERAL MEASURES
* Elevate the injured extremity to prevent swelling.
* If the wound is bleeding, apply pressure to the area with clean towel or cloth until bleeding stops. Clean wound with soap and water, then dry the area and cover it with sterile gauze or clean cloth. Do not apply antiseptic or other medicine.
* Contact the local health department and consult with them about the prevalence of rabies in the species of animal involved.
* If possible the animal that caused the bite should be held and checked for rabies.

MEDICATION
* Preventive antibiotic treatment may be prescribed.
* Antitetanus injection may have to be given.
* Sometimes, an antirabies vaccine or serum may have to be given.

ACTIVITY—No limits, except those caused by the injury.

DIET—No special diet.

CALL YOUR DOCTOR IF

* You or a family member suffers from an animal bite.
* The bite does not begin to heal within 2 to 3 days.
* New or unexplained symptoms develop. Drugs used in treatment may produce side effects.

ILLNESS & DISORDERS

ANORECTAL ABSCESS

GENERAL INFORMATION

DEFINITION—An abscess (collection of pus due to infection) that develops in the area around the anus and rectum. They may occur on the edge of the anal opening or deep in the rectum and are also common in people with digestion problems.

BODY PARTS INVOLVED—Anus; rectum.

SEX OR AGE MOST AFFECTED—Both sexes; all ages. They are more common in men.

SIGNS & SYMPTOMS
* Swelling around the rectum.
* Redness around the rectum.
* Dull or throbbing pain around the rectum.
* Difficulty or pain with bowel movement.
* Unable to sit comfortably.
* Fever.
* Bleeding or discharge if abscess ruptures.

CAUSES—Bacterial infection. It may occur in the glands inside the rectum that produce mucus. Bacteria in the stool can also infect a scratch or cut in the skin or in the rectum.

RISK INCREASES WITH
* Food such as egg shell or fish bone or swallowed object such as a paperclip. They can cut the skin as they pass in a stool.
* Constipation.
* Hemorrhoids, or an injection to treat them.
* Use of enemas. Enema tips can damage skin.
* Foreign objects in the rectum.
* Anal sex.
* Diseases of the bowel.
* Weak immune system due to illness or drugs.

HOW TO PREVENT—Cannot always be prevented. Avoid risk factors where possible.

WHAT TO EXPECT

DIAGNOSTIC MEASURES
* Your own observation of symptoms.
* Your health care provider can diagnose the abscess with a physical exam of the affected area.
* Medical tests are usually not needed, but may include an x-ray or internal exam of the rectum with a special instrument.

APPROPRIATE HEALTH CARE
* Treatment most often involves outpatient surgery to open and drain the abscess.
* For an abscess deeper in the rectum, the patient may need hospital care.

POSSIBLE COMPLICATIONS
* An extra opening (fistula) may develop between the anus and the outside of the body.
* Abscess may return if the cause is not corrected.
* Incontinence of stool (unable to control bowel movements).

PROBABLE OUTCOME—With treatment, complete healing in 6 months (if no complications).

HOW TO TREAT

GENERAL MEASURES
* Follow your health care provider's instructions for changing bandages and other care after surgery. Keep that area of the body clean.
* Sitz baths every 2 to 4 hours after surgery. Sit in a bathtub with 6 to 8 inches of warm water for 20 minutes.
* Use warm compress as needed for pain.
* Have a bowel movement when you need to, even though you may anticipate pain.

MEDICATION—Drugs may be prescribed for pain, infection, and to help prevent constipation.

ACTIVITY—Move legs often as you recover from surgery. Return to normal activities as soon as possible after surgery.

DIET—An increase in fiber in the diet may help lower the risk of constipation. Drink plenty of fluids.

CALL YOUR DOCTOR IF

* You or a family member has symptoms of anorectal abscess.
* New or unexplained symptoms develop after surgery.

ANOREXIA NERVOSA

 GENERAL INFORMATION

DEFINITION—Anorexia nervosa is a type of eating disorder. A person refuses to eat enough to maintain a normal weight for height and age. It develops over time.

BODY PARTS INVOLVED—All body cells.

SEX OR AGE MOST AFFECTED—It can occur in both sexes. It most often affects young females ages 12 to 25.

SIGNS & SYMPTOMS
- Weight loss of at least 15% of ideal body weight.
- Continues to diet when not overweight. May restrict food intake or binge on food and then purge.
- Person feels fat even when extremely thin.
- Intense fear of becoming fat.
- Obsessed with food, but denies being hungry.
- Excess exercising.
- Stopping of menstrual periods or never starting.
- Uses diuretics, laxatives, emetics and amphetamines.
- Depressed, moody, irritable, withdrawn, ritual or odd behaviors, and insomnia.
- Hair loss, dry skin, feeling cold, brittle nails, low blood pressure, and poor blood circulation.

CAUSES—Unknown. There are many theories. It involves using food and weight to deal with emotional problems, such as issues of self-worth and control for the patient.

RISK INCREASES WITH
- Young females.
- Starting a normal weight-loss diet. The person refuses to stop dieting once they begin the diet.
- Some personality traits such as perfectionism, obsessiveness, or low self-esteem.
- Family history of eating disorders.
- Family influence (overprotective or placing too much value on physical appearance).
- Society, cultural and peer pressure to be thin.
- Emotional stress.
- Athletes, ballet dancers, cheerleaders, or models.

HOW TO PREVENT—No specific preventive measures. Early treatment may help keep it from progressing.

 WHAT TO EXPECT

DIAGNOSTIC MEASURES
- Your health care provider can usually diagnose anorexia with a physical exam and by asking questions about your symptoms, eating habits and weight concerns. There is no one test to diagnose anorexia.
- Medical tests may be done to check for possible underlying disorder, physical problems, or complications.

APPROPRIATE HEALTH CARE
- Treatment may involve psychotherapy (treatment of emotional and mental problems), self-care, and drugs.
- Treatment may include counseling for the patient and the family, nutrition counseling, and drug therapy if needed. Hospital care may be required if the weight is extremely low or there are life-threatening symptoms.
- A dental exam is usually recommended.
- Counseling focuses on the misconceptions that patients have of themselves (physically, mentally, and emotionally).

POSSIBLE COMPLICATIONS—Electrolyte imbalance, irregular heartbeat, esophagitis, gastritis, lack of menstrual periods, nerve disorders, anemia and weakness, infertility, osteoporosis, or suicide.

PROBABLE OUTCOME
- Treatable if the patient recognizes the problem, wants help, and follows treatment.
- Therapy may continue over several years. Relapses are common, especially when stressful situations occur.
- About 40% make a good recovery in 5 years, 40% have symptoms, but function fairly well, and 20% have severe, ongoing symptoms.

 HOW TO TREAT

GENERAL MEASURES
- Denial of the severity or even the existence of a problem is common in patients. Patients resist treatment and behavioral change at first. Some want a quick and easy cure and that is unlikely.
- The goal is for the patient to establish healthy eating patterns to regain normal weight.
- Support groups may help some patients.
- To learn more: Anorexia Nervosa and Related Eating Disorders, PO Box 5102, Eugene, OR 97405; (503) 344-1144 (not toll free); website: www.anred.org.

MEDICATION—Antianxiety drugs or antidepressants may be prescribed.

ACTIVITY—No limits, but avoid overexertion.

DIET—A dietitian will help you plan healthy meals that are not rigid, but provide food choices. Calories will be slowly increased over time to reach your individual needs.

 CALL YOUR DOCTOR IF

- You have symptoms of anorexia nervosa or observe them in a family member.
- Weight loss continues, despite treatment.

ANXIETY DISORDER, GENERALIZED

GENERAL INFORMATION

DEFINITION—An illness that involves constant worry even though nothing is wrong. A person feels tense most of the time and always expects the worst to happen. They may worry about health, money, family, work, or an unknown or unspecified threat. The symptoms may be severe and interfere with daily living. Attempts to avoid the anxiety lead to more anxiety.

BODY PARTS INVOLVED—Central nervous system; endocrine system.

SEX OR AGE MOST AFFECTED—Anxiety usually comes on slowly and can start in childhood, adolescence, or as an adult. It is more common in women.

SIGNS & SYMPTOMS
* Feeling that something undesirable or harmful is about to happen.
* Constant worry about things (big and small).
* Aches and pains for unknown reasons.
* Feeling tired.
* Unable to relax.
* Muscle tension, headaches, backache.
* Trouble falling or staying asleep.
* Dry mouth, swallowing difficulty, or hoarseness.
* Twitching or trembling.
* Unable to focus or concentrate.
* Feeling irritable or grouchy.
* Nausea, diarrhea, weight loss.
* Sweating or hot flashes.
* Easily startled.

CAUSES—It is most likely a combination of hereditary factors, environmental factors (such as childhood experiences), and chemical disturbances in the brain.

RISK INCREASES WITH
* Women.
* Stressful events or crisis in one's life.
* Family history of anxiety disorders.
* Other emotional or mental illness (depression, panic disorder, phobias, or dysthymia).
* Alcohol or substance abuse.
* Lack of social connections.
* Certain personality factors (being shy or a worrier).
* Living in poverty, in a minority group, or immigrants.

HOW TO PREVENT—There are no specific preventive measures.

WHAT TO EXPECT

DIAGNOSTIC MEASURES
* Your own observation of symptoms.
* Your health care provider will do a physical exam and ask questions about your symptoms.

* A mental health test may be done. There is no specific test to diagnose anxiety.
* Medical tests may be done to rule out other medical disorders.

APPROPRIATE HEALTH CARE
* Treatment may involve psychotherapy (treatment of emotional and mental problems), self-care, and drug therapy.
* Cognitive-behavior therapy (CBT) is often recommended. Cognitive therapy teaches how to change thoughts, behaviors, or attitudes. Behavior therapy teaches ways to reduce anxiety with deep breathing and muscle relaxation.

POSSIBLE COMPLICATIONS
* Impaired social and work functioning.
* Depression, panic disorder, or social phobia.
* Dependence on drugs or alcohol.

PROBABLE OUTCOME—Anxiety can be controlled with treatment. Overcoming anxiety often results in a richer, more satisfying life.

HOW TO TREAT

GENERAL MEASURES
* Self-care steps may include:
 - Talking to a friend or family member about your feelings. This sometimes defuses your anxiety.
 - Keep a journal about your anxious thoughts or emotions. Consider the causes and possible solutions.
 - Join a self-help group.
 - Learn relaxation techniques. For some people, meditation is effective.
 - Reduce stress in your life where possible.
* To learn more:
 - National Institute of Mental Health; 6001 Executive Blvd, Bethesda, MD 20892-9663; (800) 647-2642; website: www.nimh.nih.gov.
 - Anxiety Disorders Association of America, 8730 Georgia Ave., Suite 600, Silver Spring, MD 20910; (240) 485-1001; website: www.adaa.org.

MEDICATION
* Antianxiety drugs may be prescribed.
* Antidepressants may be prescribed.

ACTIVITY—Stay active. Physical exertion helps reduce anxiety.

DIET—No special diet. Avoid caffeine and other stimulants and alcohol.

CALL YOUR DOCTOR IF

* You or a family member has symptoms of anxiety and self-treatment has failed.
* Symptoms recur after treatment begins.

APPENDICITIS

GENERAL INFORMATION

DEFINITION—Inflammation of the appendix. The appendix is a small tubelike pouch that is part of the large intestine. The appendix has no known function, but it can become diseased. Symptoms vary widely.

BODY PARTS INVOLVED—Appendix; cecum; peritoneum (membrane covering the intestinal tract).

SEX OR AGE MOST AFFECTED—All ages, but rare in children under 2. The incidence peaks between ages 15 and 24.

SIGNS & SYMPTOMS
* Pain that frequently begins close to the navel and moves toward the right lower abdomen. Pain becomes persistent. It worsens with moving, breathing deeply, coughing, sneezing, walking, or being touched.
* Nausea and sometimes vomiting.
* Constipation and inability to pass gas.
* Diarrhea (occasionally).
* Low fever (begins after other symptoms).
* Abdominal swelling (late stages).

CAUSES—The exact cause is unknown. The appendix may be blocked with feces from the intestinal tract which leads to infection. When infected, the appendix becomes swollen, inflamed and filled with pus.

RISK INCREASES WITH
* Viral or bacterial infection of the gastrointestinal tract.
* Family history of appendicitis.
* Cystic fibrosis.
* Diet that is low in fiber.

HOW TO PREVENT—No specific preventive measures.

WHAT TO EXPECT

DIAGNOSTIC MEASURES
* Your own observation of symptoms.
* Your health care provider will do a physical exam and ask questions about your symptoms.
* Medical tests may include blood and urine studies, x-ray, CT, or ultrasound. Oher tests may be done to help confirm the diagnosis.

APPROPRIATE HEALTH CARE
* Treatment involves surgery to remove the appendix (appendectomy). Because appendicitis can be hard to diagnose, surgery may be delayed until symptoms and signs progress enough to confirm the diagnosis.
* Surgery may be done with a laparoscope (a tube-like instrument with a light on the end). Small incisions (3 to 4) are made in the abdomen. The appendix is removed using instruments inserted into the incisions.

* Open surgery may be done. This involves one larger incision in the abdomen to remove the appendix. This type of surgery is done if the appendix has ruptured (burst).
* If an abscess has formed, surgery may be delayed until the abscess is drained and has time to heal.
* See Appendectomy in Surgery Section.

POSSIBLE COMPLICATIONS
* Rupture of the appendix, abscess (pus-filled area), and peritonitis. This is more common in older persons.
* Wound infection or other surgery complications.
* Bowel obstruction.

PROBABLE OUTCOME—Curable with surgery. People can live a normal life without their appendix.

HOW TO TREAT

GENERAL MEASURES
* Don't take any laxatives, enemas, or drugs for pain prior to diagnosis. Laxatives may lead to rupture, and pain or fever reducers make diagnosis more difficult.
* For an explanation of surgery and postoperative care, see Appendectomy in Surgery section.

MEDICATION
* Antibiotics for infection and drugs for pain are usually prescribed after surgery.
* Stool softeners to prevent constipation may be recommended.

ACTIVITY
* Rest in a bed or chair until surgery.
* Resume normal activities gradually after surgery.

DIET
* Don't eat or drink anything until appendicitis has been diagnosed. Anesthesia for surgery is much safer if the stomach is empty. If you are very thirsty, wash your mouth out with water.
* After surgery, a liquid diet is used for a short time. A regular diet may be resumed as the intestinal tract returns to normal.

CALL YOUR DOCTOR IF

* You or a family member has symptoms of appendicitis.
* The following occur after surgery:
  - Fever of 101.5°F (38.6°C) or higher.
  - Increased redness, swelling, or pain at the incision site or if the site has drainage.
  - Vomiting or diarrhea occurs.

ILLNESS & DISORDERS

ARTHRITIS, INFECTIOUS
(Septic Arthritis)

 GENERAL INFORMATION

DEFINITION—Inflammation in a joint resulting from infection. This is one of the few forms of arthritis that is curable.

BODY PARTS INVOLVED—Any joint, but most common in larger ones, such as the hip, or those subject to trauma, such as the knee or joints in the hands.

SEX OR AGE MOST AFFECTED—Both sexes; all ages.

SIGNS & SYMPTOMS
* Chills and fever (sometimes high).
* Redness, swelling, tenderness and pain (often throbbing) in the affected joint. Pain sometimes spreads to other joints. It worsens with movement.
* Pain in the buttocks, thighs or groin (sometimes).

CAUSES—Entry into a joint by bacteria (streptococci, staphylococci, gonococci, hemophilus or tubercle bacillus), virus (hepatitis or mumps),or fungus (more rare). Germs gain entry from:
* Infection elsewhere in the body, as with gonorrhea or tuberculosis.
* Infection next to the joint, as with skin boils, cellulitis or bone infection.
* Injury to the joint, including puncture wounds and skin abrasions.

RISK INCREASES WITH
* Adults over 60.
* Illness that has lowered resistance.
* Sexually transmitted diseases.
* Diabetes, rheumatoid arthritis, or liver disease.
* Weak immune system due to illness or drugs.
* Joint surgery or injections into joints.
* Excess alcohol use.
* Many sexual partners.
* Use of mind-altering drugs, especially those that are injected.
* Poor hygiene.
* Prosthetic (artificial) joint.
* The use of aspirin and other nonsteroidal anti-inflammatory drugs for other disorders may suppress signs of joint inflammation, delaying diagnosis.

HOW TO PREVENT
* Protect exposed joints, such as the knee, during activities involving injury risks.
* Obtain prompt medical treatment for infections elsewhere in the body.
* Protect yourself from sexually transmitted diseases.

 WHAT TO EXPECT

DIAGNOSTIC MEASURES
* Your own observation of symptoms.
* A health care provider will do a physical exam and ask questions about illnesses or any contact with infected persons.
* Medical tests may include blood counts, blood culture, culture of fluid from the infected joint and x-rays of affected joints.

APPROPRIATE HEALTH CARE
* Hospital care is often required for complete rest and intravenous (IV) antibiotics.
* Surgery to drain fluid or remove foreign material introduced by an injury.
* Physical therapy after recovery.

POSSIBLE COMPLICATIONS
* Misdiagnosis as gout or another noninfectious condition, delaying antibiotic treatment.
* Blood poisoning.
* Permanent joint damage.

PROBABLE OUTCOME—Usually curable with early diagnosis and treatment. Recovery may take weeks or months. Treatment delay or severe infections may result in a badly damaged joint and loss of movement, requiring joint replacement.

 HOW TO TREAT

GENERAL MEASURES
* Apply heat or cold (whichever feels better) to painful joints.
* Follow medical instructions for self-care after the infection clears up.

MEDICATION
* Antibiotics (often intravenous) or other drugs to treat the infection will be prescribed.
* Drugs may be prescribed for a short time to relieve pain.

ACTIVITY—Splints or casts may be necessary to rest the affected joint. Movement delays healing. After cure, physical therapy is often necessary to restore joint function. Resume activities gradually as symptoms improve.

DIET—No special diet.

 CALL YOUR DOCTOR IF

* You or a family member has symptoms of joint infection. Call immediately.
* The following occurs during the illness:
  - Fever rises to 103°F (39.4°C).
  - Fatigue, headache, muscle aches and sweating.

ARTHRITIS, JUVENILE RHEUMATOID

GENERAL INFORMATION

DEFINITION—A chronic inflammatory disease of the joints that affects children. Symptoms vary from mild to severe. Major types are:
• Pauciarticular (limited to a few joints; 40% to 50% of cases).
• Polyarticular (5 or more joints involved; 35% of cases).
• Systemic-onset (involves at least 1 joint and involves inflammation of internal organs; 10% to 20% of cases).

BODY PARTS INVOLVED—Joints, usually knees, elbows, ankles and neck. It may also involve adjacent muscles, cartilage and membranes lining the joints.

SEX OR AGE MOST AFFECTED—It often starts at 2 to 5 years and occurs more frequently in girls.

SIGNS & SYMPTOMS
• The first symptoms are often noticed with physical or emotional stress. Symptoms may occur often or rarely.
• Stiffness in the morning or after a nap.
• Swelling, warm, painful or aching joints. Children may not complain about joint pain.
• Limping. The child may refuse to walk without being able to explain why.
• Clumsiness.
• Fevers that come and go.
• Rashes that come and go.
• Poor appetite and weight loss.
• Swelling of lymph nodes.
• Eye pain and redness.

CAUSES—Unknown. It is probably caused by an autoimmune disorder in which the body's immune system attacks its own normal tissues. Infection may also be a factor.

RISK INCREASES WITH—A family history of JRA.

HOW TO PREVENT—Cannot be prevented at present.

WHAT TO EXPECT

DIAGNOSTIC MEASURES
• Your own observation of symptoms.
• Your child's health care provider will do a physical exam and ask questions about the symptoms.
• Medical tests may include blood and joint fluid studies and x-rays of the involved joints. No one test is available to diagnose JRA.

APPROPRIATE HEALTH CARE
• Treatment involves relieving symptoms, preserving joint function, preventing complications, and to help the child live as normal a life as possible.

• Treatment includes drug therapy, physical therapy, occupational therapy, and emotional help. You and your child's health care provider will decide on a treatment plan depending on your child's special needs.
• Surgery may (rarely) be needed for joint problems.
• Eye exams at least twice a year will help detect any eye complications. Dental exams are also important.

POSSIBLE COMPLICATIONS
• Eye complications.
• Permanent joint damage.

PROBABLE OUTCOME—Some cases are mild and may disappear at puberty. In other cases, it becomes a progressive, crippling arthritis. Symptoms can be helped with treatment.

HOW TO TREAT

GENERAL MEASURES
• Children should attend regular school on a daily basis. Where needed, the school system should provide extra services to accommodate the child's needs.
• Learning special techniques to control pain may help.
• Help morning stiffness with a warm bath or shower, sleeping in a sleeping bag, doing range-of-motion exercises, or use a heating pad or cold pack (if it feels better).
• Encourage the child to be as independent as possible.
• To learn more: American Juvenile Arthritis Organization, PO Box 7669, Atlanta, GA 30357; (800) 283-7800; website: www.arthritis.org.

MEDICATION
• Nonsteroidal anti-inflammatory drugs will be prescribed for inflammation and pain.
• Other drugs are usually prescribed to help alter the progress of the disease and delay and prevent joint damage.

ACTIVITY
• Physical therapy exercises will be prescribed. Some the child can do alone. Some the parents will perform for the child. It is important that the child does the exercises.
• Splints may be used to help the joints.
• In general, contact sports should be avoided. The child should be encouraged to participate in other sports and recreational activities.

DIET—Provide a healthy diet.

CALL YOUR DOCTOR IF

• Your child has symptoms of juvenile rheumatoid arthritis.
• Chest pain, fever. appetite loss.or new, unexplained symptoms develop with treatment.

ARTHRITIS, RHEUMATOID

GENERAL INFORMATION

DEFINITION—A chronic, inflammatory disease that mainly affects the joints.

BODY PARTS INVOLVED—Joints, including cartilage, synovial membranes, muscles and ligaments; blood vessels; eyes.

SEX OR AGE MOST AFFECTED—It often begins between ages 25 and 50, and is more common in women than in men.

SIGNS & SYMPTOMS
- Redness, pain, warmth, and tenderness in the affected joints. They may be in the hands and wrists (most often), elbows, shoulders, feet, and ankles.
- Morning stiffness.
- Muscle aches, weakness, fever, and weight loss.
- Feeling generally unwell.
- Nodules (bumps) under the skin (sometimes).

CAUSES—Unknown. It is probably caused by an autoimmune disorder in which the body's immune system attacks its own normal tissues. Infection may also be a factor.

RISK INCREASES WITH
- Family history of rheumatoid arthritis or other autoimmune disorders.
- Genetic factors.
- Women.
- Native Americans (occurs more often in this group).

HOW TO PREVENT—No specific preventive measures.

WHAT TO EXPECT

DIAGNOSTIC MEASURES
- Your own observation of symptoms.
- Your health care provider will do a physical exam and ask questions about the symptoms.
- No one test is available to diagnose arthritis. Medical tests may include blood and joint fluid studies. CT, MRI (see Glossary for both), or x-rays of the involved joints.

APPROPRIATE HEALTH CARE
- Treatment involves steps to relieve symptoms, to preserve joint function, to prevent complications, and help the person live as normal a life as possible.
- Treatment steps include drug therapy, physical therapy, occupational therapy, surgery, and lifestyle changes. A treatment plan is based on your special needs.
- Occupational therapy helps with activities of daily life.
- Options for treatment (to help symptoms such as pain) include relaxation techniques, counseling, meditation, stress reduction,

biofeedback, and support groups. Flare-ups may be triggered by emotional stress.
- Surgery may be recommended for joint problems. It may involve joint replacement, tendon reconstruction, joint realignment, or removing inflamed tissue. See Knee Replacement; Hip Replacement; and Arthroplasty, Shoulder in Surgery Section.

POSSIBLE COMPLICATIONS
- About 5% to 10% of patients are eventually disabled.
- Drugs used in treatment can cause adverse effects.
- Heart, lung, blood vessel, or eye problems.
- Anemia.

PROBABLE OUTCOME—The outcome varies. The disease course may be short and limited or progressive and severe. It is presently incurable. Pain relief, prevention of disability, and an active, normal life span are often possible.

HOW TO TREAT

GENERAL MEASURES
- Be sure to educate your-self about the disorder. Avoid arthritis treatment fads.
- Help the morning stiffness with a warm bath or shower, doing range-of-motion exercises, or a heating pad or cold pack (if it feels better).
- To learn more: Arthritis Foundation, P.O. Box 7669, Atlanta, GA 30357; (800) 283-7800; website: www.arthritis.org.

MEDICATION
- Nonsteroidal anti-inflammatory drugs, including aspirin and others will be prescribed.
- Disease-modifying drugs and biologic response modifiers are two classes of drugs that are often prescribed.

ACTIVITY
- Physical therapy will help maintain strength and joint mobility. Follow instructions for home exercising.
- Exercising in a heated pool is good for joints.
- Activity options include low impact aerobics, flexibility exercises, yoga, tai chi, or hydrotherapy.
- Mobility aids and splints may be helpful.

DIET—Eat a normal, well-balanced diet. Avoid arthritis diet fads, which are common. Lose weight if you are overweight. Being overweight stresses the joints.

CALL YOUR DOCTOR IF

- You or a family member has symptoms of rheumatoid arthritis.
- Symptoms appear in different joints or other symptoms get worse during treatment.

ASBESTOSIS

GENERAL INFORMATION

DEFINITION—Inflammation of the lung due to breathing asbestos particles. It is a chronic disorder, but is not contagious.

BODY PARTS INVOLVED—Lungs.

SEX OR AGE MOST AFFECTED—Men over age 40 who have been exposed to asbestos.

SIGNS & SYMPTOMS
* Shortness of breath.
* Cough that produces little or no sputum.
* General ill feeling.
* Fitful sleep.
* Appetite loss and weight loss.
* Chest pain.
* Hoarseness.
* Coughing up blood.
* Bluish nails.

CAUSES—Long-term exposure to small particles of asbestos at work or from other sources. The outer part of the lung becomes irritated by the asbestos fibers. This leads to inflammation and to a thickening and scarring of the lung tissue (pulmonary fibrosis). It may take up to 20 years or more between exposure to asbestos and the symptoms of the disease. This period may be shorter after intense exposure.

RISK INCREASES WITH
* Work that involves asbestos.
* Smoking.
* Excess alcohol use.

HOW TO PREVENT
* During exposure to asbestos, wear a protective mask or external-air-supplied hood.
* Follow recommended industrial safety procedures to suppress asbestos dust.
* For workers in asbestos industries, have regularly scheduled x-rays to detect any shadow on the lungs. If a problem develops, the person should stop working with asbestos, even if there are no symptoms.
* Don't smoke.

WHAT TO EXPECT

DIAGNOSTIC MEASURES
* Your own observation of symptoms.
* Your health care provider will do a physical exam and ask about your symptoms and past exposure to asbestos.
* Medical tests usually include a CT or x-rays of the lungs and lung function tests. A bronchoscopy may be done (an instrument with a lighted tip is used to view inside the lungs and remove tissue for a biopsy).

APPROPRIATE HEALTH CARE
* There is no specific treatment for asbestosis. Treatment can help relieve the symptoms and prevent complications.
* Obtain medical care for any respiratory infection, including the common cold.
* Chest physical therapy techniques will be provided by a respiratory therapist.
* Supplemental oxygen may be required.

POSSIBLE COMPLICATIONS
* Chronic obstructive pulmonary disease (COPD).
* Heart failure due to lung disease.
* It may lead to cancer of the lungs (the risk is greatly increased in cigarette smokers).
* Tuberculosis.

PROBABLE OUTCOME—There is no cure. In a few patients, it may remain unchanged, but in most, it is slowly progressive (even without further exposure to asbestos). Symptoms can usually be relieved or controlled.

HOW TO TREAT

GENERAL MEASURES
* Avoid any further contact with asbestos.
* Stop smoking. Find a way to quit that works for you.
* Learn and practice bronchial drainage.
* Use a cool-mist humidifier (if advised) to loosen bronchial secretions so they can be coughed up easily.
* Keep flu and pneumococcal vaccines current.
* Avoid crowds and persons with infections.
* To learn more: American Lung Association, 61 Broadway, 6th Floor, New York, NY 10006; (800) 586-4872; website: www.lungusa.org.

MEDICATION
* Bronchodilators (inhaled or oral) will help open up the bronchial tubes and allow passage of air. This is supervised at first by an inhalation therapist.
* For minor discomfort, use nonprescription drugs, such as acetaminophen or aspirin.

ACTIVITY—Regular exercise in whatever forms possible is important to preserve lung capacity.

DIET—No special diet.

CALL YOUR DOCTOR IF

* You or a family member has symptoms of asbestosis.
* New symptoms develop or other symptoms become worse, despite treatment.

ASTHMA

GENERAL INFORMATION

DEFINITION—Asthma involves blockage of normal airflow into and out of the lungs. The blockage develops when certain allergens or irritants are inhaled and cause a reaction in the airways. They become swollen (inflamed), produce excess mucus, and the airway muscles tighten. This leads to the wheezing and other symptoms.

BODY PARTS INVOLVED—Lungs; bronchi; bronchioles.

SEX OR AGE MOST AFFECTED—All ages, but 50% of the cases are in children under age 10. Boys with asthma outnumber girls. Women are more often affected in adult-onset asthma.

SIGNS & SYMPTOMS
* Chest tightness. Wheezes when breathes out.
* Coughing, especially at night, may have thick, clear or yellow sputum.
* Rapid, shallow breathing that is eased with sitting up.
* Breathing difficulty that gradually gets worse.
* Neck and chest may be sucked in with each breath.
* Severe symptoms of an asthma attack:
  - Cough that sounds tight and dry.
  - Rapid heart-beat and abnormal rapid rate of breathing that becomes more labored.
  - Unable to speak more than a few words without pausing for breath.
  - Sweating, and much anxiety and distress.

CAUSES—The exact cause of asthma remains unclear. It may be due to a combination of genetic factors, certain factors that may sensitize the airways (such as animal dander, and dust mites), and contributing factors (such as childhood respiratory infections).

RISK INCREASES WITH
* Other allergies, such as eczema or hay fever.
* Family history of asthma or allergies.
* Exposure to air pollutants.
* Exposure to allergens (such as pets).
* Smoking or exposure to second-hand smoke.
* For adults, exposure to occupational irritants (fumes, gases, latex products, metals, and others).

HOW TO PREVENT—No specific preventive measures for original disease. Avoiding risk factors where possible may help.

WHAT TO EXPECT

DIAGNOSTIC MEASURES
* Your own observation of symptoms.
* Your health care provider will do a physical exam and ask questions about your symptoms.

* Medical tests may include x-rays, pulmonary-function tests, an exercise tolerance test, and allergy tests (usually skin testing).

APPROPRIATE HEALTH CARE
* Treatment will depend on the severity of the symptoms. It may include daily drug therapy, drug therapy for attacks, avoiding triggers, lifestyle changes, self-care, and education. A written treatment plan is usually provided. It should be followed carefully.
* Counseling may help, if asthma is stress-related.
* Treatment (allergy shots) to desensitize the immune system to specific allergens may be recommended.
* Hospital care sometimes for severe attacks.

POSSIBLE COMPLICATIONS
* Missed workdays or school absenteeism.
* Pneumonia, pneumothorax, or respiratory failure.
* Status asthmaticus (a sustained attack that cannot be relieved).
* Poorly controlled asthma and chronic symptoms.

PROBABLE OUTCOME
* Symptoms can be controlled with treatment.
* Half the children will outgrow asthma.

HOW TO TREAT

GENERAL MEASURES
* Identify and avoid your triggering factors.
* A peak flow meter may be used at home. It is a small device that measures how well air flows into and out of the airways. You will be instructed on its use.
* To learn more: Asthma & Allergy Foundation of America, 1233 20th St., Suite 402, Washington, DC 20036; (800) 727-8462; website: www.aafa.org.

MEDICATION—Asthma drugs include:
* Quick relief. These drugs are prescribed for relief of asthma exacerbations and to prevent exercised-induced asthma (EIA) symptoms.
* Long-term control. These drugs are prescribed for use on a daily basis to prevent symptoms.

ACTIVITY—Stay active. Swimming is a good activity. Avoid sudden bursts of activity. If an attack follows exercise, sit, rest, sip warm water.

DIET—No special diet, but avoid foods to which you are sensitive. Drink plenty of fluids daily.

CALL YOUR DOCTOR IF

* You or a family member has asthma symptoms.
* Symptoms don't improve, despite treatment.
* Peak flow is in a zone that worries you.

ATELECTASIS

GENERAL INFORMATION

DEFINITION—Collapse of lung tissue affecting part or all of one lung. It prevents normal lung function.

BODY PARTS INVOLVED—Lungs.

SEX OR AGE MOST AFFECTED—Atelectasis can affect all ages, but is more common in children under age 10.

SIGNS & SYMPTOMS
Sudden, major collapse:
- Chest pain.
- Shortness of breath; rapid breathing.
- Shock (severe weakness, paleness of skin, rapid heartbeat).
- Dizziness.

Gradual collapse:
- Cough.
- Fever.
- Shortness of breath.
- Sometimes, no other symptoms.

CAUSES
- Obstructive atelectasis (most common type):
  - Thick mucous plugs from infection or other disease.
  - Inhaled objects, such as small toys or peanuts.
  - Surgery of the chest (thoracic) or abdomen.
- Nonobstructive atelectasis:
  - Pleural effusion (fluid in the lungs).
  - Pneumothorax (air in the area around the lung).
  - Tumors.
  - Lack of surfactant (a substance in the lungs).
  - Scarring of lung tissue (due to disease).
  - Trauma (injury) to the lung.
  - Enlarged lymph glands.

RISK INCREASES WITH
- Chronic obstructive pulmonary disease (COPD).
- Obesity.
- Congenital lung disease, such as cystic fibrosis.
- Neuromuscular disease.
- Smoking.
- Asthma.

HOW TO PREVENT
- Medical care to help prevent postsurgical problems.
- Keep small objects that might be inhaled away from young children (such as peanuts).

WHAT TO EXPECT

DIAGNOSTIC MEASURES
- Your own observation of symptoms.
- Your health care provider will do a physical exam.

- Medical tests may include blood studies to measure oxygen and carbon dioxide levels, x-rays, or CT of the chest.

APPROPRIATE HEALTH CARE
- Treatment depends on the cause. It may include drug therapy, chest physical therapy, bronchoscopy, and (rarely) surgery.
- Chest physical therapy may be done to help remove mucous from the lungs. It involves clapping, patting, and massaging the chest and back over the lungs. The lungs may be suctioned with a small plastic tube.
- Bronchoscopy (see Glossary) may be done to remove foreign objects or a mucous plug.
- Disabling, chronic atelectasis may have to be treated with surgery to remove the affected part of the lung.
- A tumor may require surgery or radiation therapy.

POSSIBLE COMPLICATIONS—Infection and chronic lung damage.

PROBABLE OUTCOME—Outcome is generally good. It usually resolves with treatment. Complications are rare, but will depend on any underlying cause.

HOW TO TREAT

GENERAL MEASURES
- Cooperate with requests to turn, cough and breathe deeply after surgery. Hold a pillow tightly against surgical incisions during the coughing exercises.
- Stop smoking.
- To learn more: American Lung Association, 61 Broadway, 6th Floor, New York, NY 10006; (800) 586-4872; website: www.lungusa.org.

MEDICATION
- Antibiotics for infection will be prescribed.
- Bronchodilators to assist breathing may be prescribed.
- Pain relievers may be prescribed.

ACTIVITY—Resume your normal activities as soon as symptoms improve. Take frequent showers. Try to avoid low-humidity environments.

DIET—No special diet, but drink plenty of fluids.

CALL YOUR DOCTOR IF

- You or a family member has symptoms of atelectasis.
- Symptoms return after treatment. Atelectasis can recur.

ATHEROSCLEROSIS
(Hardening of the Arteries)

 GENERAL INFORMATION

DEFINITION—A hardening or narrowing of the arteries. Arteries are blood vessels that carry blood and oxygen to the heart, brain, and other body parts. Atherosclerosis is an underlying medical problem that can lead to:
* Coronary artery disease.
* Stroke.
* Abdominal angina (pain).
* Bowel infarction (blood clot in the intestines).
* Atherosclerosis of the extremities. Legs get reduced blood flow, which leads to intermittent claudication (cramping with or without exercise).
* Other conditions, such as aortic aneurysm.

BODY PARTS INVOLVED—All arterial blood vessels in the body.

SEX OR AGE MOST AFFECTED—It can begin in childhood and progress slowly as people age. In some people, it progresses more rapidly. Up to age 45, it is more common in men. After menopause, women are equally affected.

SIGNS & SYMPTOMS
* Symptoms often are absent until atherosclerosis reaches advanced stages. Symptoms depend on what part of the body has a reduced blood flow and the extent of disease.
* Muscle cramps if it involves blood vessels in the legs.
* Angina pectoris (chest pain) or a heart attack if it involves blood vessels to the heart.
* Stroke or transient ischemic attack if it involves vessels to the neck and brain.
* Abdominal cramps or pain if blood vessels to the abdomen are involved.

CAUSES—Plaque (made up of cholesterol, muscle cells, fibrous tissue, and calcium) builds up on artery walls that have been damaged in some way. Plaque deposits can grow large enough to reduce blood flow and can also crack or break apart and form clots. Clots can block blood flow or travel to another part of the body and cause serious or fatal problems.

RISK INCREASES WITH
* High blood pressure or diabetes.
* High levels of LDL (the bad cholesterol).
* Low levels of HDL (the good cholesterol).
* Obesity.
* Sedentary lifestyle (lack of physical activity).
* Smoking.
* Family history of atherosclerosis.
* High fat diet.

HOW TO PREVENT
* Eat a healthy diet. Maintain a healthy weight. Exercise regularly. Don't smoke.
* Control diabetes and high blood pressure.
* Control cholesterol levels.

 WHAT TO EXPECT

DIAGNOSTIC MEASURES
* Your own observation of symptoms.
* Your health care provider may do a physical exam. Questions will be asked about your symptoms, smoking, alcohol use, drug use, exercise, and personal and family medical history. Blood pressure and pulse rate are checked. A stethoscope is used to listen for sounds of blood flow in the arteries.
* Blood studies are done for cholesterol, triglycerides, and blood sugar. Heart function tests (such as exercise stress tests and coronary calcium scores) and blood flow tests may be done.

APPROPRIATE HEALTH CARE—Treatment includes drug therapy and lifestyle changes. Treatment for organ damage caused by atherosclerosis depends on the organ involved.

POSSIBLE COMPLICATIONS
* Coronary artery disease, which is the number one cause of death in men and women.
* Other disorders as listed in Definition.

PROBABLE OUTCOME—There is no cure, but atherosclerosis can be slowed or stopped. If organ damage has developed due to reduced blood flow, the outcome will vary.

 HOW TO TREAT

GENERAL MEASURES
* Lifestyle changes include diet changes, losing weight, stopping smoking, and getting more exercise.
* To learn more: American Heart Association, local branch listed in telephone directory, or call (800) 242-8721; website: www.americanheart.org.

MEDICATION
* Drugs will be prescribed for any diagnosed disorders.
* Cholesterol-lowering drugs are usually prescribed.

ACTIVITY—Activity may depend on state of health. Try to get 20 to 30 minutes of aerobic exercise most days of the week.

DIET—Eat a low-fat, high-fiber diet, that includes fruits and vegetables. Begin a weight-loss diet, if overweight.

 CALL YOUR DOCTOR IF

You or a family member has symptoms of, or concerns about, atherosclerosis.

ATHLETE'S FOOT
(Tinea Pedis; Ringworm of the Feet)

GENERAL INFORMATION

DEFINITION—A common, contagious fungal (tinea) infection of the skin on the feet.

BODY PARTS INVOLVED—Feet, especially the soles and skin between toes (usually 4th and 5th toes).

SEX OR AGE MOST AFFECTED—It usually affects teens and adults (rare in young children).

SIGNS & SYMPTOMS
* Moist, soft, gray-white or red scales on feet, especially between toes.
* Dead skin between toes.
* Itching in inflamed areas.
* Damp, musty foot odor.
* Small blisters on the feet (sometimes).

CAUSES—Infection by a *Trichophyton* fungus. The germs can be spread by direct contact with an infected person, or by contact with the germs on shoes, socks, shower, or pool surfaces. Animals can also carry the germs and infect humans.

RISK INCREASES WITH
* Infrequent washing of the feet.
* Infrequent changes of shoes or socks.
* Use of locker rooms and public showers.
* Hot, humid weather.
* People who have immune system problems due to illness or medications.
* Persistent moisture around the feet.

HOW TO PREVENT
* Bathe feet daily. Dry completely between the toes and apply drying or dusting powder.
* Wear rubber thongs or wooden sandals in public showers.
* Go barefoot when possible.
* Change socks daily and wear socks made of cotton, wool, or other natural, absorbent fibers. Avoid synthetics.

WHAT TO EXPECT

DIAGNOSTIC MEASURES
* Your own observation of symptoms.
* See your health care provider if the symptoms are severe. Your health care provider can usually diagnose athlete's foot by looking at the affected skin area. Other skin tests may be done to rule out other skin disorders.

APPROPRIATE HEALTH CARE—Medical care is usually not needed for this disorder.

POSSIBLE COMPLICATIONS
* A bacterial infection may develop in the affected area.
* A skin rash can sometimes develop on the hands and face (rare).

PROBABLE OUTCOME—Usually curable in 3 weeks with treatment, but recurrence is common.

HOW TO TREAT

GENERAL MEASURES
* After soaking or bathing, carefully remove scales and material between the toes daily.
* Use a hair dryer to blow warm air on the feet to make sure they are completely dry.
* Keep affected areas cool and dry. Go barefoot or wear sandals during treatment. If socks are worn, keep them dry. If they get wet, change to dry ones.

MEDICATION
* Use nonprescription antifungal powders, creams, or ointments (such as terbinafine) after each bath.
* For severe cases, you may be prescribed oral, or stronger topical antifungal drugs.

ACTIVITY—No limits. Avoid activities that cause feet to sweat until healing is complete.

DIET—No special diet.

CALL YOUR DOCTOR IF

* You or a family member has symptoms of athlete's foot that persist, despite self-treatment.
* You develop a fever or the infection seems to be spreading.

ATRIAL FIBRILLATION

GENERAL INFORMATION

DEFINITION—An abnormal heart rhythm. Fibrillation pertains to a "quivering" of muscles. Atrial pertains to the atria, the upper chambers of the heart. The abnormal rhythm reduces the flow of blood through the heart to the brain and other body parts and can cause symptoms.

BODY PARTS INVOLVED—Heart muscles; the atrium (also called auricle), a chamber of the heart that connects to the left ventricle (main chamber); heart's electrical conduction system.

SEX OR AGE MOST AFFECTED—It usually affects older adults and men more than women.

SIGNS & SYMPTOMS
* There may be no symptoms.
* Irregular and often rapid beating of the heart.
* Weakness, dizziness, shortness of breath, chest pain, or faintness may occur.

CAUSES—The heart has an electrical system that controls the heart rate and the heart's contractions. The average heart beats at a rate of 60 to 100 times per minute. With atrial fibrillation, the electrical system does not function as it should. The atria quiver instead of contracting and heart rate increases (may reach 350 beats a minute). There are different risk factors that can lead to atrial fibrillation and sometimes no cause is found.

RISK INCREASES WITH
* Increased age.
* Coronary heart disease.
* High blood pressure.
* Abnormal heart muscle.
* Mitral valve disease.
* Hyperthyroidism.
* Lung disease (chronic obstructive pulmonary disease, emphysema).
* Pericarditis (heart lining inflammation).
* Pulmonary embolism.
* Congestive heart failure.
* Recent heart or lung surgery.
* Use of stimulant drugs (cocaine, decongestants).
* Excessive alcohol use.
* Congenital (present at birth) heart abnormality.
* Lone atrial fibrillation in young, healthy adults.

HOW TO PREVENT—No specific preventive measures. Avoid risk factors where possible.

WHAT TO EXPECT

DIAGNOSTIC MEASURES
* Your own observation of symptoms.
* Your health care provider will do a physical exam and ask questions about your symptoms. The rapid and irregular heart rate can be heard with a stethoscope (a device for listening to bodily sounds).
* Medical tests may include blood studies and heart function tests.

APPROPRIATE HEALTH CARE
* Treatment is aimed at treating the cause of the atrial fibrillation, slowing the heart rate, converting the abnormal rhythm to normal, preventing a recurrence, and preventing complications.
* Abnormal heart rhythm may be converted to normal rhythm with drug therapy or with electric shock (electrocardioversion). An electric shock stops the abnormal activity and allows the normal rhythm to take over.
* Recurring atrial fibrillation may be treated with a variety of procedures. These include a pacemaker or atrial defibrillator implantation, AV node ablation, Maze procedure (atrial surgery), and pulmonary vein isolation.
* Some patients may be left in atrial fibrillation long-term if the heart rate is under control.

POSSIBLE COMPLICATIONS
* Stroke.
* Arterial thrombosis or embolus (blood clots).
* Congestive heart failure.
* Other heartbeat irregularities can lead to cardiac arrest.

PROBABLE OUTCOME—It can often be controlled with treatment. Atrial fibrillation tends to become a chronic condition.

HOW TO TREAT

GENERAL MEASURES
* Don't smoke.
* Learn to check your own pulse for rate (beats per minute) and rhythm (regular or irregular).
* To learn more: American Heart Association, local branch listed in telephone directory, or call (800) 242-8721; website: www.americanheart.org.

MEDICATION—Drugs may be prescribed for the underlying risk factor, to slow the heart rate, and to prevent blood clots.

ACTIVITY—Aim for 20 to 30 minutes of aerobic exercise 3 or more days a week. Activity may depend on your health status.

DIET—Eat a low-fat, high-fiber diet that includes fruits and vegetables. Begin a weight loss diet, if overweight.

CALL YOUR DOCTOR IF

* You or a family member has symptoms of atrial fibrillation.
* Any change in heart rate or rhythm, chest pain, sweating, weakness, shortness of breath, or swollen feet and ankles occurs.

ATTENTION-DEFICIT HYPERACTIVITY DISORDER (ADHD)

GENERAL INFORMATION

DEFINITION—A consistent pattern of behavior that includes inattention, hyperactivity, and impulsivity. Attention deficit hyperactivity disorder (ADHD) is common and affects 3% to 5% of children.

SEX OR AGE MOST AFFECTED—Boys are affected 10 times more than girls. The symptoms may appear at ages 4 to 7 and peak between 8 and 10. It also affects adults.

SIGNS & SYMPTOMS
* Squirms in seat; fidgets with hands or feet.
* Unable to stay seated when required to do so.
* Easily distracted.
* Blurts out answers before a question is finished.
* Difficulty waiting turn in games and lines.
* Difficulty following instructions.
* Unable to sustain attention in work or play activities.
* Shifts from one uncompleted project to another.
* Difficulty playing quietly.
* Talks excessively.
* Interrupts or intrudes on others.
* Doesn't appear to listen.
* Loses items needed for tasks.
* Often engages in dangerous activities without considering consequences.

CAUSES—Unknown. Many theories have been proposed (but not yet proven). It is thought to have biologic origin. Recent studies suggest that TV watching by young children (age 3 and younger) may be a factor.

RISK INCREASES WITH—Family history of the disorder.

HOW TO PREVENT—No preventive measures known.

WHAT TO EXPECT

DIAGNOSTIC MEASURES
* The child's teacher may be the first to notice the behavior. A school psychologist, your child's doctor, or a special health care provider may diagnose the disorder.
* Several methods are used to help make the diagnosis. These include observing the child doing activities, mental, social, and intelligence tests, parent's and teacher's evaluation, and rating scales about behaviors.
* Adults are diagnosed based on their performance at work and at home. When possible, their parents rate how the person behaved as a child.

APPROPRIATE HEALTH CARE
* Treatment for children includes appropriate classroom setting, behavior therapy, drug therapy, and help for parents in managing the child's behavior. A combination of these techniques will have the best outcome.
* Adult patients may have drug therapy and counseling.
* Counseling can help, as can behavior and cognitive therapy. These help child and adult patients focus on ways to change the undesired behavior.
* Special education classes for all or part of the day may be needed for some children.

POSSIBLE COMPLICATIONS—Problems such as school failure, antisocial behavior, and later, (sometimes) criminal behavior.

PROBABLE OUTCOME—Most people don't outgrow ADHD, but do learn to adapt and live fulfilling lives.

HOW TO TREAT

GENERAL MEASURES
* Help your child at home by providing a structured environment, well-defined behavior limits, and consistent use of parenting techniques. Support groups or parenting skills training are helpful.
* Stay in close contact with the child's teacher. Arrange for extra lessons or tutoring if needed.
* To learn more: Attention Deficit Disorder Association, P.O. Box 543, Pottstown, PA 19464; (800) 487-2282; website: www.add.org.

MEDICATION
* Stimulant drugs (have a calming affect on persons with ADHD) or other drugs approved for ADHD may be prescribed. Some of these drugs have side effects, such as sleep problems, depression, headache, stomach ache, loss of appetite, and stunted growth.
* Antidepressants may be prescribed for adults.

ACTIVITY—Structure your child's activity to the extent possible.

DIET—Most medical research indicates that special diets benefit very few children. Many parents, however, report dramatic changes in behavior after this treatment. This change may result from the extra attention the child receives with preparation of special meals. Discuss any special diets with your child's doctor.

CALL YOUR DOCTOR IF

* You believe your child or a family member has symptoms of ADHD.
* New or worsening symptoms develop.

AUTISM

GENERAL INFORMATION

DEFINITION—Autism is a disorder that involves the way a child develops. Parents may notice that an infant or child is not behaving, talking, playing, or learning new skills as expected for their age group. Asperger's syndrome is like autism, but without the disabilities. It can range from mild to severe.

BODY PARTS INVOLVED—Total body.

SEX OR AGE MOST AFFECTED—It is usually discovered by the time a child is age 2 and a half, but could be later.

SIGNS & SYMPTOMS
* Does not talk or may talk using nonsense words. May use a sing-song voice and repeat what they hear. Unable to carry on a conversation.
* Does not respond to name and avoids eye contact.
* Is over active. Wants to play alone.
* Repeats the same movements over and over such as rocking and flapping or twisting hands.
* Has special routines and does not like change.
* Does not want to be touched, such as being cuddled.
* May injure self by head-banging or biting.
* Is bothered by noises.
* Overly interested in lights or moving objects.

CAUSES
* Unknown. Research continues in hopes of finding the cause. It is known that parents do not cause autism.
* There is no scientific proof to link childhood immunizations to autism.

RISK INCREASES WITH—Unknown. It does affect boys more than girls.

HOW TO PREVENT—None known. Autism cannot currently be detected at birth or through any prenatal tests.

WHAT TO EXPECT

DIAGNOSTIC MEASURES
* Your own observation of symptoms.
* Diagnosis is difficult, as the signs and symptoms may appear to be caused by another disorder or problem. There is no specific test for autism. Your health care provider (usually a mental health professional) will perform an exam of your child and ask you about your child's behavior and other signs or symptoms you may have observed.
* Tests for speech and other skills may be done to see how your child is developing compared to normal levels for his or her age group.

APPROPRIATE HEALTH CARE
* Treatment for autism should be started as soon as a child is diagnosed. Speech and behavior therapy and social skills training will help children with autism.
* There is no cure for autism. Treatments can help with many of the symptoms. The treatment plan for each child will depend on how mild or severe their symptoms are. Some children may be able to attend regular public schools. Others may require a special classroom.
* Counseling may help some parents cope with the stress involved with raising an autistic child.
* New treatments for autism are being studied and may be recommended for your child in the future. There are certain treatments that parents or others have tried and found to work for one or a few children. These treatments may or may not work for other autistic children. Always talk to your child's health care provider before you try any new type of treatment.

POSSIBLE COMPLICATIONS
* Parents of an autistic child have an increased risk of having another child with the disorder.
* Stress for the family raising an autistic child.
* The children have a higher seizure risk.

PROBABLE OUTCOME—The future is unknown for most autistic children. A child may be mentally retarded, have normal intelligence, or even have a genius-like ability. As they get older, their symptoms may improve, stay about the same, or worsen. Some children will need supervision for life. Some may be able to live independently.

HOW TO TREAT

GENERAL MEASURES
* The treatment steps take time and patience. Different treatment methods may need to be tried for a child.
* Join an autism family support group.
* To learn more: Autism Society of America, 7910 Woodmount Avenue, Suite 300, Bethesda, MD 20814-3015; (800) 328-8476; www.autism-society.org.

MEDICATION—Medicine is usually not needed for this disorder. A drug may be prescribed to help control symptoms that could be a danger to your child, such as self-injury.

ACTIVITY—Help your child to stay as physically active as possible.

DIET—Special diets will not improve the symptoms of autism.

CALL YOUR DOCTOR IF

Your child is not developing as expected for his or her age.

BACK PAIN, LOW
(Sciatica)

GENERAL INFORMATION

DEFINITION—Pain in the lower back usually caused by muscle strain. It may also include sciatica (pain that radiates from the back to the buttock and down into the leg). Onset of pain may be immediate or occur some hours after an activity or an injury. The symptoms occur in a cycle, starting with a muscle spasm, the spasm then causes pain, and the pain results in additional muscle spasm.

BODY PARTS INVOLVED—Lower back.

SEX OR AGE MOST AFFECTED—Adults of both sexes, usually between ages 20 and 40.

SIGNS & SYMPTOMS—Pain and stiffness. It may be ongoing, or only occur when you are in certain positions. The pain may get worse by coughing, sneezing, bending, or twisting.

CAUSES
• Strain or sprain. Muscles, tendons, ligaments of the low back become stretched or torn.
• Bone and joint conditions of the back. These include arthritis, osteoporosis, spinal nerve irritation or inflammation, disk problems, infections, weaker and thinner bones from aging, and others.
• Injury or a fracture.
• Congenital problem (something you were born with).
• Pregnancy, certain illnesses, or infections.

RISK INCREASES WITH
• Exertion or lifting; a severe blow, or a fall.
• Jobs that require a lot of sitting.
• Aging. After age 20, bones start to lose their strength.
• Gardening and other yard work.
• Sports and exercise activities.
• Driving for long periods of time.
• Overweight.
• Smoking.
• Poor body mechanics and poor posture.

HOW TO PREVENT
• Being in good physical condition.
• Exercises to strengthen lower back muscles.
• Learn how to lift heavy objects.
• Use good posture when sitting and standing.
• Lose weight, if overweight.

WHAT TO EXPECT

DIAGNOSTIC MEASURES
• Your own observation of symptoms.
• Your health care provider will do a physical exam and ask questions about your back pain symptoms.

• Tests may include blood studies, x-rays of the spine, and other imaging studies. These can help determine the specific cause of the pain.

APPROPRIATE HEALTH CARE
• Treatment will depend on the cause of the pain. Usually a combination of drugs and reduced activities for a short period of time is all that is needed.
• Physical therapy may be prescribed.
• Massage may help. Be sure that the person performing the massage is well-trained, or the massage may cause more harm than help.
• Other options are available depending on degree of injury, such as surgery for disk damage, electrical nerve stimulation, acupuncture, special shoes, and others.

POSSIBLE COMPLICATIONS—Chronic low back pain.

PROBABLE OUTCOME—Gradual recovery with time and treatment.

HOW TO TREAT

GENERAL MEASURES
• Ice pack or cold massage or heat applied to affected area with heating pad or hot water bottle.
• Wear a special back support device.
• Learn stress reduction techniques, if needed.
• Take breaks if you have to stand or sit for long periods.
• To learn more: National Institutes of Health, 800-352-9424; website: www.ninds.nih. gov/health_and_medical/pubs/back_pain.htm.

MEDICATION
• Use mild pain drugs such as aspirin, ibuprofen, or acetaminophen.
• Stronger pain drugs, muscle relaxants and drugs to reduce inflammation may be prescribed. Note: Drugs do not hasten healing. They only help to reduce symptoms.

ACTIVITY
• Try to continue with daily schedules to the extent possible.
• Avoid strenuous activity for 6 weeks.
• After healing, an exercise program will help prevent re-injury.

DIET—No special diet. A weight-reduction diet may help if overweight is a problem.

CALL YOUR DOCTOR IF

• You or a family member has mild, low back pain that persists for 3 or 4 days after self-care.
• Back pain is severe or recurrent.
• New or unexplained symptoms develop. Drugs used in treatment may cause side effects.

BALANITIS

 GENERAL INFORMATION

DEFINITION—Inflammation of the glans (head) of the penis and sometimes the foreskin as well. It is a common condition in males. It occurs more often in males who have a foreskin (have not been circumcised).

BODY PARTS INVOLVED—Penis and foreskin.

SEX OR AGE MOST AFFECTED—Males of all ages.

SIGNS & SYMPTOMS
- Tenderness, redness, itching, and swelling of the head of the penis.
- Inflammation of the foreskin.
- Unable to retract foreskin (phimosis).
- Impotence.
- Discharge from the penis.
- Burning during urination (rare).

CAUSES—The inflammation is a reaction to infection (most common cause), injury, or irritation of the penis. Sometimes the cause is unknown.

RISK INCREASES WITH
- Diabetes.
- Poor hygiene.
- Allergy to chemicals in clothing, contraceptive cream, or condom latex.
- Reaction to certain drugs.
- Trauma or minor injury to the foreskin and penis.
- Presence of foreskin.
- Sexual partner affected by vaginitis (rare).
- Being very obese.

HOW TO PREVENT
- Wash daily with soap and water and wash after sexual intercourse. Clean carefully under the foreskin.
- Control diabetes or other medical conditions.
- Weight loss for obese males.
- Use a latex condom during intercourse to help prevent some infections.

 WHAT TO EXPECT

DIAGNOSTIC MEASURES
- Your own observation of symptoms.
- Your health care provider can usually diagnose the disorder by an exam of the penis.
- A culture of the discharge from the penis may be done. Tests for other medical disorders such as diabetes may be done.

APPROPRIATE HEALTH CARE
- Treatment usually involves drugs applied to the penis and practicing good hygiene.
- A foreskin that cannot be retracted may be treated with topical steroid drugs, stretching techniques (done 2 to 3 weeks), or by a special slit made in the foreskin.
- Surgery may be recommended to circumcise the penis if balanitis recurs often or scar tissue develops.

POSSIBLE COMPLICATIONS—Chronic inflammation can cause:
- Scarring and narrowing of the opening of the penis (urethral stricture).
- Phimosis (difficult to retract the foreskin).
- Paraphimosis (unable to replace the foreskin to cover the head of the penis).

PROBABLE OUTCOME—Usually curable in 1 to 2 weeks with treatment.

 HOW TO TREAT

GENERAL MEASURES—Use warm-water soaks to relieve pain or discomfort.

MEDICATION
- Antibiotics to be applied to the penis are usually prescribed. Rarely, antibiotics to be taken by mouth may be prescribed.
- Steroid skin creams may be prescribed.
- Use acetaminophen or ibuprofen to relieve minor pain.

ACTIVITY
- Avoid sexual intercourse during treatment.
- Resume your normal activities when the infection is cured.

DIET—No special diet.

 CALL YOUR DOCTOR IF

- You or a family member has symptoms of balanitis.
- Symptoms don't improve in 3 days, despite treatment.

BALDNESS, PATTERN, MALE & FEMALE

GENERAL INFORMATION

DEFINITION—Gradual, painless hair loss that occurs in a certain pattern as a person ages. The medical term is androgenetic alopecia. The earlier the hair loss begins, the greater the eventual loss. Some persons have short periods of intense hair loss followed by long, stable periods.

BODY PARTS INVOLVED—Hair; scalp.

SEX OR AGE MOST AFFECTED—In men, hair loss appears as early as the teens; in women, it rarely appears before their 50's.

SIGNS & SYMPTOMS
* In men, hair thins on top of the head and recedes in the temple and front areas.
* In women, hair tends to thin on top of the head.
* Both sexes may have scattered hair loss.

CAUSES—It is probably due to a combination of hormonal and genetic factors. Male hormones (most often, androgens) are an important factor in balding. Estrogen (a female hormone) may be protective in women, because hair loss rarely begins before menopause. Hair loss that occurs after illness, pregnancy, or as an adverse reaction to drugs is a different form of baldness. Normal everyday stress is not a cause of pattern baldness.

RISK INCREASES WITH—Family history of pattern baldness.

HOW TO PREVENT—Some drug therapies have been shown to slow or reverse baldness to some degree in some men. Other medical treatments are undergoing study.

WHAT TO EXPECT

DIAGNOSTIC MEASURES
* Your own observation of symptoms.
* Medical history and physical exam by a health care provider, if diagnosis is in doubt.

APPROPRIATE HEALTH CARE—There is usually no need for medical care. If you do have concerns about the hair loss, see your health care provider. If it is not a typical hair loss, medical tests may be done to see if there is another cause.

POSSIBLE COMPLICATIONS
* There are no medical complications.
* Baldness can cause emotional distress, such as anxiety and a negative effect on self-image.

PROBABLE OUTCOME
* There is no cure. Balding can range from partial loss to complete baldness.
* In most cases, men let the process run its course. Use of a hairpiece or hair transplant is acceptable to some. Drug therapy may help others.

HOW TO TREAT

GENERAL MEASURES
* If you are not comfortable with the hair loss, there are options that you can consider.
   - Wear a hairpiece (toupee or a wig) or get a hair weave (synthetic hair is sewn into existing hair). Be sure to use care in keeping your scalp clean under the hairpiece.
   - Have a hair-transplantation procedure or scalp-reduction surgery. Be sure to seek information about the risks and benefits before undergoing these procedures.
   - Use drug therapy.
* Be cautious about buying and using hair products that claim to thicken or strengthen hair. They often use oils or waxes to give an effect of thickening.

MEDICATION
* A nonprescription topical drug, minoxidil, seems to help hair growth in some patients. Its effectiveness varies greatly. If it helps you, you need to continue its use indefinitely to sustain hair growth.
* A drug taken by mouth can be prescribed for hair loss in men. It is not approved for use in women as it may cause birth defects.

ACTIVITY—No limits.

DIET—No special diet.

CALL YOUR DOCTOR IF

You or a family member has concerns about hair loss.

ILLNESS & DISORDERS

BAROTITIS MEDIA
(Barotrauma)

 GENERAL INFORMATION

DEFINITION—Damage to the middle ear caused by pressure changes.

BODY PARTS INVOLVED—It affects the middle ear and the eustachian tube (a tube from the ear to the back of the nose and throat).

SEX OR AGE MOST AFFECTED—Both sexes; all ages.

SIGNS & SYMPTOMS
* Hearing loss (to varying degrees).
* A plugged feeling in the ear.
* Mild to severe pain in the ears, or over the cheekbones and forehead.
* Dizziness.
* Ringing noises in the ear.
* Crying in infants or young children.

CAUSES
* Damage caused by sudden, increased pressure in the air around you. This occurs in the rapid descent of an airplane or while scuba diving. In these activities, air moves from passages in the nose into the middle ear to maintain equal pressure on both sides of the eardrum. If the tube leading from the nose to the ear doesn't function properly, pressure in the middle ear is less than the outside pressure. The negative pressure in the middle ear sucks the eardrum inward. Blood and mucus may appear later in the middle ear. This damage is more likely if you have a nose or throat infection when scuba diving or traveling by air.
* Injury to external or middle ear (boxing, water skiing, accidents, etc.).

RISK INCREASES WITH
* Recent lung, nose, or throat infection.
* Airplane flight.
* Scuba diving.
* Sky diving.
* High-altitude mountain climbers.
* High-impact sports.

HOW TO PREVENT
* If possible, don't fly when you have a lung, nose, or throat infection. If you must fly anyway, use nonprescription decongestant tablets or sprays. Follow the package instructions.
* During air travel:
- While taking off or landing, suck on hard candy or chew gum to cause frequent swallowing.
- Take a moderate-size breath and hold your nose. Try to force air into the eustachian tube by gently puffing out the cheeks with the mouth closed. This is called the Valsalva maneuver.
- Give an infant a bottle of water or juice while taking off or landing during airplane travel.

 WHAT TO EXPECT

DIAGNOSTIC MEASURES
* Your own observation of symptoms.
* See your health care provider if symptoms continue. An ear exam usually confirms the diagnosis.

APPROPRIATE HEALTH CARE
* In most cases, no treatment is necessary and symptoms disappear in hours or days.
* Rarely, surgery may be required to open the eardrum and release fluid trapped in the middle ear. A plastic tube may be placed in the eardrum to keep it open. The tube falls out on its own in 9 to 12 months.

POSSIBLE COMPLICATIONS
* Permanent hearing loss.
* Ruptured eardrum.
* Middle ear infection.

PROBABLE OUTCOME—Most cases of barotitis media heal with self-care.

 HOW TO TREAT

GENERAL MEASURES—If fluid drains from the ear, place a small piece of cotton in the outer-ear canal to absorb it.

MEDICATION
* For minor pain, you may use nonprescription decongestants and pain relievers, such as acetaminophen.
* Your health care provider may prescribe stronger decongestant or anti-inflammatory nasal sprays or tablets.
* Antibiotics, if infection is present.

ACTIVITY—Resume your normal activities as soon as symptoms improve.

DIET—No special diet.

 CALL YOUR DOCTOR IF

* You or a family member has symptoms of barotitis media that do not heal on their own.
* The following occur during treatment: severe headache or other pain, fever and dizziness.

BED-WETTING
(Enuresis)

GENERAL INFORMATION

DEFINITION—Wetting the bed during sleep that occurs more often than once a month in girls over 5 and in boys over 6 years of age.

BODY PARTS INVOLVED—Urinary tract.

SEX OR AGE MOST AFFECTED—It is more common in boys than in girls. The occurrence of bed-wetting in children is 15% at age 5, 10% at age 6, 7% at age 8, 3% at age 12 and 1% at age 18.

SIGNS & SYMPTOMS—Bed-wetting at night (occasionally during the day). This is not usually a concern until a child is older than 6.

CAUSES—In most cases, the cause of bed-wetting is unknown. Most children who wet the bed are quite healthy. The following are other possible causes:
- Illness, such as diabetes or a urinary-tract infection.
- A small or weak bladder that cannot hold one night's urine production.
- Emotional problems caused by stress or separation from the mother.

RISK INCREASES WITH
- Diabetes.
- Urinary-tract infection.
- Family history of bed-wetting (44% chance if one parent was bed-wetter, 77% chance if both parents were bed-wetters).
- First-born child.

HOW TO PREVENT—No effective preventive methods known. Show your child love, support and understanding.

WHAT TO EXPECT

DIAGNOSTIC MEASURES
- Your own observation of symptoms.
- Talk to your child's health care provider about the bed-wetting problem. A physical exam will be done and questions asked about the symptoms.
- Medical tests are sometimes done to rule out infections and diabetes as causes.

APPROPRIATE HEALTH CARE—Medical care is usually not needed unless there is a health problem diagnosed or parents are interested in drug therapy as a treatment option.

POSSIBLE COMPLICATIONS
- Psychological and emotional scars that may affect the child's personality for years.
- Urinary-tract infection.

PROBABLE OUTCOME—Bed-wetting may continue for several years. If there are no medical or emotional problems, children normally outgrow the bed-wetting problem. Consider that your child's bed-wetting means a delay in maturing that will resolve with time.

HOW TO TREAT

GENERAL MEASURES
- Follow any medical advice. Basic ideas are listed here.
- Prepare the bed and the child:
  - Protect the mattress with a heavy plastic cover.
  - Stop using diapers or plastic pants by age 4. They may make it easy for the child to keep on wetting.
  - Have the child change the sheet on the bed and do the laundry, if he or she is old enough.
- Don't give any liquids to the child for 2 to 3 hours prior to bedtime.
- Have the child urinate at bedtime. You can also wake the child at night to urinate, but this is hard on parents.
- Reward the child for staying dry with praise and hugs. Use gold stars or happy faces to mark dry nights on a calendar.
- Respond gently to accidents. Don't blame, nag, restrict, or punish the child who has wet the bed. This can cause him to give up or lead to other problems.
- Try alarms that are triggered by wetting. These may be used in undergarments, pajamas, or mattresses. They have a high success rate.

MEDICATION—The drug vasopressin may be recommended if other methods fail and the family favors medical treatment.

ACTIVITY—No limits.

DIET—No special diet. Encourage your child to drink as much fluid as possible during the day. Limit or discontinue any fluid intake during the 2 to 3 hours before bedtime.

CALL YOUR DOCTOR IF

- You are concerned about your child's bed-wetting and your child is older than 6.
- The child dribbles urine, has a weak urinary stream, feels pain when urinating, or must strain to urinate.

BELL'S PALSY

GENERAL INFORMATION

DEFINITION—A paralysis or weakness on one side of the face. The onset may be sudden, or may come on over several days.

BODY PARTS INVOLVED—7th cranial nerve and the facial muscles that connect to the nerve.

SEX OR AGE MOST AFFECTED—All ages, but most common in adults.

SIGNS & SYMPTOMS
* Sudden paralysis on one side of the face, including muscles to the eyelid.
* Pain behind the ear on the affected side.
* Flat, expressionless features on one side of the face.
* Distorted smiles and frowns; drooling.
* Changes in taste, saliva, or tear formation.

CAUSES—Unknown. The paralysis is probably caused by swelling of the facial nerve. The swelling may be caused by a viral infection of the facial nerve as it passes through the temporal bone of the skull.

RISK INCREASES WITH
* Common cold, flu, other respiratory infection.
* Pregnancy.
* Diabetes.

HOW TO PREVENT—Cannot be prevented at present.

WHAT TO EXPECT

DIAGNOSTIC MEASURES
* Your own observation of symptoms.
* Your health care provider will do a physical exam of the affected area.
* Medical tests such as x-ray may be done to rule out other causes. A nerve study of the facial nerves may be done to determine the extent of nerve damage.

APPROPRIATE HEALTH CARE
* Treatment may include self-care measures, drug therapy if needed, and surgery.
* Surgery on the facial nerve may (rarely) be needed.
* Counseling may help for any emotional problems that develop.

POSSIBLE COMPLICATIONS
* Eye irritation or injury, because the eye does not close properly and is exposed to dust. If unprotected, the eye may develop ulcers on the cornea.
* Tooth decay and gum disease, due to reduced saliva and difficulty in chewing.
* Emotional and self-esteem problems.

PROBABLE OUTCOME
* Bell's palsy causes distress, but it is not dangerous. The amount of nerve damage determines the extent of recovery.
* Improvement is gradual. Recovery time varies, and sometimes requires many months.
* Patients with mild facial paralysis usually recover completely within several months. Those with more severe facial paralysis recover completely in 80% to 90% of cases.
* Surgery may help improve facial appearance and muscle function in patients who do not recover fully.

HOW TO TREAT

GENERAL MEASURES
* If you have pain, apply heat to the area twice a day. Use a moist, warm towel and apply for 15 minutes. Cover or close the eye during heat treatments.
* If you cannot wink or close your eye well, you should buy a pair of wrap-around, plastic sports goggles. Wear them to protect your eye from dirt, dust, and dryness.
* At night, apply an eye patch to shut the lid so that the eye stays moist and protected. Sometimes, a patch will be necessary during the daytime.
* As muscle strength returns, use facial massage and exercises. Massage muscles of the forehead, cheek, lips and eyes using cream or oil. Exercise the weak muscles in front of a mirror. Open and close the eye; wink, smile and bare your teeth. Perform the massage and exercises for 15 to 20 minutes several times a day.
* Brush and floss teeth regularly.

MEDICATION
* You may be prescribed eye drops for comfort and protection of the exposed eye.
* Cortisone drugs may be prescribed to reduce swelling and inflammation of the affected nerve.

ACTIVITY—Maintain your normal activities. Rest does not help Bell's palsy.

DIET—A soft diet may be necessary for a period of time.

CALL YOUR DOCTOR IF

* You or a family member has symptoms of Bell's palsy.
* Eye becomes red or irritated, despite treatment.
* Drooling or pain worsens or fever occurs.
* New, unexplained symptoms develop. Drugs used in treatment may produce side effects.

BENIGN PAROXYSMAL POSITIONAL VERTIGO (BPPV)

 GENERAL INFORMATION

DEFINITION—A common, inner ear disorder that causes dizziness or vertigo with certain movements of the head.
* Benign means "not very serious."
* Paroxysmal means "sudden and unpredictable in onset."
* Positional, because it comes about with a change in head position.
* Vertigo, causing a sense of the room-spinning or whirling.

BODY PARTS INVOLVED—Inner ear and the nervous system.

SEX OR AGE MOST AFFECTED—Both sexes; all ages. It is more common in people over age 40 and in women more than men.

SIGNS & SYMPTOMS
* A sensation of dizziness or vertigo (spinning). Vertigo begins 5 to 10 seconds after the head moves and lasts less than a minute. Feeling off balance may last longer.
* Most often, only one ear is affected, so symptoms occur when the head is turned that way. Symptoms are brought on when getting out of bed, rolling over in bed, or when looking up for an object on a high shelf.
* Falling, or a feeling of falling.
* Feeling lightheaded or woozy.
* Visual blurring.
* Nausea and vomiting (sometimes).
* Diarrhea, faintness, changes in heart rate and blood pressure, fear, anxiety, or (less often) panic.
* It does not cause hearing loss or noises in the ears (tinnitus).

CAUSES—It is thought to be caused by small crystals of calcium carbonate (also called "ear rocks", otoconia or otoliths) in the ear. Sometimes, these crystals get stuck and do not move normally with changes in position. This disrupts the balance centers in the inner ear and brings on the symptoms. The crystals usually return to normal within several weeks, and no longer cause symptoms.

RISK INCREASES WITH
* Head injury.
* Degeneration of the vestibular system of the inner ear (usually in older people).
* Ear infection or disorder.
* Surgery.
* Central nervous system disease.

HOW TO PREVENT—No specific preventive measures.

 WHAT TO EXPECT

DIAGNOSTIC MEASURES—A health care provider will do an exam of the ears and ask questions about your symptoms and activities. When BPPV occurs, there is an involuntary movement of the eyes, which is called nystagmus. To make the diagnosis, the patient's head is put into certain positions and the eye movements are observed.

APPROPRIATE HEALTH CARE
* Treatment may involve watchful waiting to see if the problem resolves on its own.
* An office procedure may be done for treatment. It is performed by placing the patient's head in various positions. This will cause the crystals to loosen and return to normal movement. The procedure takes about 5 to 10 minutes. Frequently, only one office procedure is needed. It is painless and has few side effects if any. There may be mild vertigo for a few days afterwards.
* Rarely, if other treatment is not effective, severe symptoms may require surgery.

POSSIBLE COMPLICATIONS—BPPV symptoms may come and go, recur after treatment, or become chronic.

PROBABLE OUTCOME—The condition heals on its own within several weeks. Treatment can hasten healing.

 HOW TO TREAT

GENERAL MEASURES
* Self-treatment exercises may be recommended. These can be done if symptoms recur, or office procedure was not effective. Instructions will be given on proper techniques for the head maneuvers. They are then done at home several times a day, usually for 2 weeks.
* To learn more: Vestibular Disorders Association, PO Box 4467, Portland, OR 97208-4467; (800) 837-8428; website: www.vestibular.org.

MEDICATION—Usually not needed for this disorder. Drugs may be prescribed for specific symptoms, such as nausea.

ACTIVITY—Instructions will be given if needed.

DIET—No special diet.

 CALL YOUR DOCTOR IF

* You or a family member has symptoms of benign paroxysmal positional vertigo.
* Symptoms recur after treatment.

BIPOLAR DISORDER
(Manic-Depressive Disorder)

 GENERAL INFORMATION

DEFINITION—A condition in which a person has episodes of mania, or cycles of mania and depression. There is usually no relationship between the moods and what is happening in the person's life. Periods of highs can alternate with periods of deep depression. The high periods are called mania. Periods of normal behavior occur in between the mania and the depression. The normal behavior period can last for a short time or for years.

SEX OR AGE MOST AFFECTED—Both sexes; all ages.

SIGNS & SYMPTOMS
Mania:
• Higher than normal energy levels. Person feels "high."
• Getting up earlier and earlier in the morning. Some people may not sleep at all for 3 to 4 days.
• Easily distracted and restless. Excited to start new projects, but then rarely finish.
• May go on spending sprees.
• May become sexually promiscuous.
• Often irritable. Often have attacks of rage.
• Speech becomes rapid. Speech may not make sense.
• May have very high opinion of one's abilities.
• May forget to eat. May lose weight. Can become exhausted.
• May have delusions of grandeur.
Depression:
• Becomes more and more withdrawn. Sleep may be disturbed. Late rising becomes a habit.
• May stay in one's room. May be afraid to face the world. Often lacks self-esteem.
• Self-neglect.
• Sex drive is lowered.
• Slow speech and movement.
• Imagined problems multiply.
• Worries about imagined illnesses.

CAUSES—There is no single cause. Genetics plays a part. Other factors may include changes in chemicals in the brain and environmental factors, such as stress.

RISK INCREASES WITH—Family history of bipolar disorder.

HOW TO PREVENT—No preventive measures.

 WHAT TO EXPECT

DIAGNOSTIC MEASURES
• Your health care provider will usually do a physical exam and ask questions about your symptoms and activities.

• Psychological testing may be done. Other medical tests are usually done to rule out infections or disorders that could be causing the symptoms.

APPROPRIATE HEALTH CARE
• Treatment will depend on the specific symptoms. Follow medical advice. Schedule regular office visits. Your health care provider will monitor the effectiveness of the treatment and watch for side effects.
• Hospital care may be required for severe symptoms. A stay at a mental health facility may be recommended.
• Electroconvulsive therapy (ECT) may be considered if other treatment steps do not help.

POSSIBLE COMPLICATIONS
• Relapse, especially if medicine is stopped.
• Problems at work, school, or home.
• Failure to get better.
• Alcohol or drug abuse.
• Suicide.

PROBABLE OUTCOME—Long-term therapy can help reduce how often the episodes occur and how severe the episodes are.

 HOW TO TREAT

GENERAL MEASURES
• Do not stop taking your medicine when you feel better. This may cause a relapse.
• Education and counseling can help you, and your family, cope with the condition. Family members should learn to recognize signs of a coming episode.
• Seek support groups. Call a suicide prevention hotline if needed.
• To learn more: Depression and Bipolar Support Alliance, 730 N. Franklin St., Suite 501, Chicago, IL 60610; (800) 826-3632; website: www.dbsalliance.org.

MEDICATION—Drugs will be prescribed to help relieve symptoms of the depression and the manic episodes. Other drugs may be prescribed to help prevent mood swings. Changes in drugs or dosages may be needed at various times to manage the illness more effectively.

ACTIVITY—Maintain daily activities. Exercise on a regular basis.

DIET—Eat a healthy diet.

 CALL YOUR DOCTOR IF

• You or a family member has symptoms of depression or mania.
• Symptoms don't improve despite treatment.
• You feel suicidal or hopeless. Call 911.

BLADDER INFECTION, FEMALE
(Cystitis in Women)

GENERAL INFORMATION

DEFINITION—Inflammation of the urinary bladder.

BODY PARTS INVOLVED—Urinary bladder.

SEX OR AGE MOST AFFECTED—Females of all ages.

SIGNS & SYMPTOMS
* Pressure, burning, or stinging during urination.
* Frequent urination, although the amount of urine may be small; increased urge to urinate.
* Sensation of incomplete bladder emptying.
* Pain in the abdomen over the bladder.
* Lower-back pain.
* Blood in the urine; bad-smelling urine.
* Low fever and, possibly, chills.
* Painful sexual intercourse.
* Lack of urinary control (sometimes).
* A need to urinate more often at night.

CAUSES—The inflammation is a reaction to infection (most commonly), injury, or irritation of the bladder lining. It can be brought on by a number of different factors. Sometimes the cause is unknown.

RISK INCREASES WITH
* Infection in other parts of the genitourinary system. Bacteria can reach the bladder from another part of the body through the bloodstream. Bacteria can enter the urinary tract from skin around the genital and anal area.
* Frequent or vigorous sexual activity.
* Pregnancy.
* Poor hygiene.
* Diabetes.
* Certain types of birth control. These can include a diaphragm that fits too-tightly, contraceptive foams or vaginal suppositories that irritate the urethra, or a condom that is not lubricated.
* Urinary tract problems (tumors, calculi, or strictures).
* Urethra (tube from the bladder to the outside) injury.
* Use of a urinary catheter to empty the bladder, such as during childbirth or surgery.
* Incomplete bladder emptying.

HOW TO PREVENT
* Urinate within 15 minutes after intercourse.
* Drink plenty of water every day.
* Get medical care for urinary-tract infections.
* Don't douche, use feminine hygiene sprays, or deodorants. Avoid bubble baths.
* Clean the anal area after bowel movements. Wipe from the front to the rear, not rear to front.
* Wear underwear that has a cotton crotch.
* Avoid postponing urination. Be sure to completely empty the bladder with urination.

* In women with frequent recurrence of infection, antibiotics may be prescribed for use before sexual intercourse.

WHAT TO EXPECT

DIAGNOSTIC MEASURES
* Your health care provider may do a physical exam.
* Medical tests will include a urine test.

APPROPRIATE HEALTH CARE—Treatment is usually with antibiotic drugs.

POSSIBLE COMPLICATIONS—Inadequate treatment can lead to chronic bladder infections, kidney infection, and (rarely) kidney failure.

PROBABLE OUTCOME—Curable in a few days to 2 weeks with treatment. Recurrence is common.

HOW TO TREAT

GENERAL MEASURES
* Warm baths may help relieve discomfort.
* Pour a cup of warm water over genital area while urinating. It will help to relieve burning and stinging.
* To learn more: National Kidney Foundation, 30 E. 33rd St., Suite 1100, New York, NY 10016; (800) 622-9010; website: www.kidney.org.

MEDICATION
* Antibiotics for bacterial infection will be prescribed. Antibiotics may reduce the effectiveness of some birth control pills. If you are using birth control pills, discuss this with your health care provider.
* Urinary analgesics may be prescribed for pain. If phenazopyridine (Pyridium) is taken, it will turn urine color to bright orange.

ACTIVITY—Avoid sexual intercourse until you have been free of symptoms for 2 weeks.

DIET
* Drink plenty of water daily to flush the bladder.
* Avoid caffeine and alcohol during treatment.
* Drink cranberry juice to acidify urine. Some antibiotic drugs have increased effectiveness when the urine is more acidic.

CALL YOUR DOCTOR IF

* You or a family member has symptoms of cystitis.
* Blood appears in the urine.
* Discomfort and other symptoms don't improve after you have taken the antibiotics for 48 hours or symptoms recur after treatment.

BLADDER INFECTION, MALE
(Cystitis in Men)

 GENERAL INFORMATION

DEFINITION—Inflammation of the urinary bladder.

BODY PARTS INVOLVED—Urinary bladder.

SEX OR AGE MOST AFFECTED—It can occur in males of any age. After age 50, men are affected more often (due to prostate problems).

SIGNS & SYMPTOMS
* Burning and stinging when you urinate.
* Urinating more often. The amount of urine may be small.
* Feeling like you need to go even when your bladder is empty.
* Pain in the pubic area.
* Discharge from the penis.
* Low back pain.
* Blood in the urine.
* Low fever.
* Urine that smells bad.
* Not being able to control urination.

CAUSES—Usually a bacterial infection. The infection may start in other parts of the genital or urinary system (such as the kidney or prostate). The bacteria may also enter the bladder from skin around the genitals and anus.

RISK INCREASES WITH
* Blockage in the urinary tract. This may be due to kidney stones or tumor.
* Enlarged prostate gland.
* Lack of circumcision (foreskin can harbor bacteria).
* Injury of the urethra (tube that carries urine from bladder).
* Use of a catheter to empty the bladder, such as following surgery.
* Defects in the urinary tract.
* Certain illnesses, such as diabetes.

HOW TO PREVENT
* Drink at least 8 glasses of fluid a day.
* Use a latex condom during sex. This can help prevent the spread of any infection.
* Avoid the use of catheters, if possible.
* Urinate when you feel the urge, empty the bladder completely, and keep the genital area clean.
* Get medical care for any prostate infection.

 WHAT TO EXPECT

DIAGNOSTIC MEASURES
* Your health care provider will usually do a physical exam and ask questions about your symptoms.
* Medical tests include urine studies. Additional tests may be done to rule out other disorders.

APPROPRIATE HEALTH CARE—Treatment is usually with drugs, or sometimes surgery if a physical defect is the cause.

POSSIBLE COMPLICATIONS
* Recurrent or chronic bladder infections.
* Kidney infection.

PROBABLE OUTCOME
* Usually curable with treatment.
* Complicated infections in males are sometimes more difficult to treat. The bacteria involved are often resistant to the commonly prescribed drugs.

 HOW TO TREAT

GENERAL MEASURES
* Warm baths may provide relief from symptoms.
* To learn more: National Kidney Foundation, 30 E. 33rd St., Suite 1100, New York, NY 10016; (800) 622-9010; website: www.kidney.org.

MEDICATION
* Drugs for bacterial infection are usually prescribed. To be sure of a cure, finish the entire prescribed dose even if symptoms improve. If infection recurs, drug therapy for 6 months to 2 years may be recommended.
* Drugs to relieve painful urination symptoms may be prescribed.

ACTIVITY
* Reduce activities as needed until symptoms improve.
* Avoid sexual intercourse until you have been free of symptoms for 2 weeks.

DIET
* Drink at least 8 glasses of fluid daily. Avoid citrus juice, caffeine, and alcohol. They can irritate the bladder.
* Drink cranberry juice if recommended by your health care provider.

 CALL YOUR DOCTOR IF

* You or a family member has symptoms of a bladder infection.
* Fever develops.
* Blood appears in the urine.
* Symptoms don't improve in one week.
* New, unexplained symptoms develop. Drugs used in treatment may produce side effects.
* Symptoms return after treatment.

BLADDER TUMOR

GENERAL INFORMATION

DEFINITION—An abnormal tissue growth in the bladder. It may be cancerous or noncancerous. If the tumor is cancerous, it may spread to lymph nodes, bones, liver and/or lungs.

BODY PARTS INVOLVED—Urinary bladder.

SEX OR AGE MOST AFFECTED—Adults over 50 of both sexes, but more common in men than women.

SIGNS & SYMPTOMS
- There are often no symptoms in the early stages.
- Blood in the urine.
- Pain or burning when urinating.
- Needing to urinate more frequently. There may be only small amounts of urine passed.
- Fever.
- Unexplained weight loss.

CAUSES—Unknown in some cases. Exposure to cancer-causing substances in the environment may be the cause in some cases.

RISK INCREASES WITH
- Smoking.
- Family history of bladder tumors.
- Exposure to certain dyes or to chemicals used in the manufacture of rubber.

HOW TO PREVENT
- Avoid exposure to chemical or environmental hazards. Improved methods of protecting workers from chemical hazards have lowered the number of bladder tumors. Regular screening of those who have been exposed in the past is also helpful.
- Don't smoke.

WHAT TO EXPECT

DIAGNOSTIC MEASURES
- Your own observation of symptoms.
- Your health care provider will do a physical exam and ask questions about your symptoms.
- Medical tests include urine studies. A lighted optical instrument (cystoscope) may be used to see inside the bladder. It can also be used to remove a small piece of tissue, or even a small tumor, for viewing under a microscope. X-ray, MRI, CT or other tests may be done to see if a cancerous tumor has spread (called staging).

APPROPRIATE HEALTH CARE
- Treatment may include surgery, radiation, chemotherapy (anticancer drugs) and biologic therapy.
- Small tumors may be removed by fulguration. This involves burning off the tumor by high frequency electrical current passed through the cystoscope.

- Larger tumors are removed surgically. This may require removal of part or all of the bladder (cystectomy) and other nearby body organs that may be involved. Various options are available for creation of a new bladder or to divert the urine flow to an external device (ostomy bag) on the outside of the body.
- Radiation and biologic therapy (the body's immune system is used to fight cancer) may be recommended.

POSSIBLE COMPLICATIONS
- Spread of cancer to other places in the body.
- Emotional stress about changes in body image.
- Side effects of treatments such as extreme fatigue.
- Treatment can lead to infertility for men and women.

PROBABLE OUTCOME—When diagnosed early, treatment can be successful. However, it is common for the tumors to return. Regular medical checkups are needed. If cancer has spread, the outcome will depend on many factors.

HOW TO TREAT

GENERAL MEASURES
- Counseling is helpful in learning to cope with the changes in your body.
- To learn more: American Cancer Society, (800) ACS-2345; website: www.cancer.org or National Cancer Institute at (800)4-CANCER; website: www.nci.nih.gov.

MEDICATION
- Anticancer drugs may be prescribed that are taken by mouth or given through a vein (IV).
- Drugs may be placed inside the bladder (biologic therapy); then a person waits 2 to 3 hours before urinating.

ACTIVITY—Resume your normal activities once your health care provider gives approval. This includes sexual relations.

DIET—No special diet.

CALL YOUR DOCTOR IF

- You or a family member has symptoms of a bladder tumor.
- Prescribed drugs produce unexpected side effects.

BLASTOMYCOSIS
(North American Blastomycosis; Gilchrist's Disease)

 GENERAL INFORMATION

DEFINITION—An infectious fungal disease that starts in the lungs. It can occasionally spread through the bloodstream to other body parts, especially the skin. Blastomycosis is not spread from person to person, but can be spread through bites from infected dogs. Higher rates of the disease are found in states bordering the Mississippi and Ohio rivers.

BODY PARTS INVOLVED—It can involve the lungs, mouth, skin (and tissue below the skin), and the prostate.

SEX OR AGE MOST AFFECTED—Both sexes, but most common in men from ages 20 to 40.

SIGNS & SYMPTOMS
* Symptoms may begin slowly or infection may be sudden.
* Cough, either wet or dry.
* Chest pain.
* Chills, fever, and sweats.
* Shortness of breath.
* Fatigue, loss of appetite.
* May have bumps or sores on the skin.

CAUSES—Infection with a fungus found in wood and soil. Skin lesions occur most commonly in gardeners or farmers, but the natural source of this fungus is not known.

RISK INCREASES WITH
* Gardening and farming, especially in southeastern states and the Mississippi River valley of the United States.
* Diabetes.
* Use of drugs that suppress the immune system.

HOW TO PREVENT—Cannot be prevented at present.

 WHAT TO EXPECT

DIAGNOSTIC MEASURES
* Your own observation of symptoms.
* Your health care provider will do a physical exam and ask questions about your symptoms.
* Medical tests may include blood tests; culture of the skin lesions, pus, saliva, or lung secretions; x-ray; and biopsy. Biopsy is when a small amount of tissue is removed for viewing under a microscope.

APPROPRIATE HEALTH CARE
* Treatment is with drugs and other supportive care.
* A hospital stay is usually needed at start of treatment.

POSSIBLE COMPLICATIONS—Spread to other body parts, with serious illness and death. If the infection spreads, the following may appear:
* Pain in long bones.
* Skin lesions that begin as small, raised bumps or small, white blisters with pus. They spread slowly. When fully developed, the lesions become open sores with sloping, reddish-purple borders.
* Swelling and painful, tender lumps in the scrotum.

PROBABLE OUTCOME—This fungus can cause severe illness that may be fatal without treatment. With treatment, it is usually curable in several weeks.

 HOW TO TREAT

GENERAL MEASURES
* Heat may be helpful for joint pain.
* Weigh yourself daily and keep a weight chart. An unexplained weight loss might indicate that the infection has spread.
* Keep follow-up appointments with your health care provider. It is important to monitor the treatment and watch for side effects or reactions from the medications.

MEDICATION—Drugs will be prescribed to kill the underlying fungus.

ACTIVITY—Rest in bed during the worst stage. Resume activities slowly as your strength returns.

DIET—No special diet.

 CALL YOUR DOCTOR IF

* You or a family member has symptoms of blastomycosis.
* Any of the following occur during treatment:
  - Weight loss.
  - Fever.
  - Diarrhea that cannot be controlled with self-care.
  - Severe headache and stiff neck.
* New, unexplained symptoms develop. Drugs used in treatment may produce side effects.

BLEPHARITIS

GENERAL INFORMATION

DEFINITION—Inflammation (redness and soreness) of the eyelid edges.

BODY PARTS INVOLVED—Eyelids and eyelashes. It can also include the glands that lubricate the lid, and the white area of the eye.

SEX OR AGE MOST AFFECTED—Adults of both sexes.

SIGNS & SYMPTOMS
* Redness and greasy flakes on eyelid edges.
* Small sores on the eyelid. Crusts may form on the edges of the eyelid.
* Discharge from the lids during sleep. Lids may be stuck together in the morning.
* A feeling that something is in the eye. This can cause itching, burning, redness, and swelling of the lid. May also have tearing and be sensitive to bright light.
* Eye may become irritated if flakes from the lid fall into the eye.
* Eyelashes that fall out.

CAUSES
* Seborrheic blepharitis is caused by a skin condition called seborrhea. It is similar to dandruff.
* Bacterial infection of the eyelash follicles and the glands that lubricate the eye. The infection cannot be spread from one person to another.
* Plugged glands on the eyelid.
* Allergies or lice in the eyelashes.

RISK INCREASES WITH
* Dermatitis (skin infection) of the scalp and other body parts.
* Acne rosacea.
* Exposure to allergens (substances that cause allergic reactions).
* Exposure to chemical or environmental irritants, such as smoke or smog.
* Work that keeps the hands dirty for most of the day.
* Elderly.

HOW TO PREVENT
* Wash hands often.
* Keep face, eyelids, and scalp clean.
* Avoid places that have lots of dust or other irritating substances.
* Get treatment for any skin disorders.
* Control dandruff with dandruff shampoos.

WHAT TO EXPECT

DIAGNOSTIC MEASURES
* Your own observation of symptoms.
* Your health care provider can diagnose blepharitis by an exam of the affected eyelid.
* Other medical tests are not usually needed.

APPROPRIATE HEALTH CARE—Treatment will be prescribed for any problem that is causing the disorder or any complications.

POSSIBLE COMPLICATIONS
* Styes or chalazia (blocked oil gland on the eyelid).
* Conjunctivitis (eye inflammation).
* Loss of eyelashes.
* Ulceration of the cornea (the covering of the eye).
* Scarred eyelids.

PROBABLE OUTCOME—Symptoms can be improved with treatment. The condition is often chronic and the symptoms come and go. If treatment is stopped, it tends to recur. It is usually not a serious condition.

HOW TO TREAT

GENERAL MEASURES
* Use warm-water soaks to reduce discomfort and speed healing. Apply soaks for 20 minutes, then rest at least 1 hour. Repeat as often as needed.
* Wash the eyelid edge and eyelashes twice a day. Use a baby shampoo diluted with some water, or a commercial eyelid cleanser. Use a washcloth wrapped around the index finger or cotton swabs. Don't rub too hard as it can lead to irritation. Rinse with warm water and then dry the area.
* Avoid use of eye makeup until symptoms improve. When used, be sure to remove it each night at bedtime.
* Ask your health care provider about using contact lenses while you have the symptoms.

MEDICATION
* Eye drops or ointment may be prescribed for use after the eyelid area is cleaned.
* Drugs to be taken by mouth may be prescribed in more severe cases.

ACTIVITY—No limits.

DIET—No special diet.

CALL YOUR DOCTOR IF

* You or a family member has symptoms of blepharitis.
* You have pain in the eye(s).
* Your vision changes.
* Symptoms recur after treatment.

ILLNESS & DISORDERS

BLOOD POISONING
(Septicemia; Septic Shock; Bacteremia)

 GENERAL INFORMATION

DEFINITION—Bacterial infection (or toxins from bacteria) in the blood that invade the entire body via the bloodstream.

BODY PARTS INVOLVED—Total body.

SEX OR AGE MOST AFFECTED—Both sexes; all ages.

SIGNS & SYMPTOMS
* Shaking chills.
* High fever.
* Rapid, pounding heartbeat.
* Warm, flushed skin and sweating.
* Confusion and other symptoms of mental impairment.
* Drop in blood pressure.
* General ill feeling.
* Hyperventilation.

CAUSES—Infection in some other body part, such as: appendix, tooth, sinus, pelvis, gallbladder or urinary tract. The source may also be a burn, infected wound, or open abscess.

RISK INCREASES WITH
* Adults over 60.
* Newborns and infants.
* Weak immune system due to illness or drugs.
* Leukemia or other cancer.
* Intravenous drug abuse.
* Use of a catheter.
* Complicated labor or delivery.
* Certain surgical procedures.

HOW TO PREVENT
* It cannot always be prevented.
* Obtain medical treatment for any infection or wounds.
* If dental procedures have produced blood poisoning in the past or you have diseased heart valves, take antibiotics before any dental treatment—including simple prophylaxis by a dentist or dental hygienist.
* Influenza and pneumococcal vaccinations for high-risk patients.

 WHAT TO EXPECT

DIAGNOSTIC MEASURES
* Your own observation of symptoms.
* A health care provider will do a physical exam.
* Medical tests include culture of the blood to identify organisms responsible for the illness; urinalysis and blood count.

APPROPRIATE HEALTH CARE
* Hospital care with intensive care treatment for severe cases.
* Removal or drainage of source of infection.
* Mechanical ventilation for respiratory failure.
* Blood transfusions.

POSSIBLE COMPLICATIONS
* Shock, with very low blood pressure, overwhelming infection and death.
* Persistent infection of the heart valves.
* Adult respiratory distress syndrome.
* Multi-organ failure (heart, lungs, kidney, liver).

PROBABLE OUTCOME—Dependent on underlying conditions, patient's health, and any delay in treatment.

 HOW TO TREAT

GENERAL MEASURES—This can be a frightening time for the patient's family. Intensive care units are intimidating places. Try to keep your spirits up, stay in close communications with the doctors.

MEDICATION—Antibiotics to treat infections will be prescribed.

ACTIVITY—As advised.

DIET—May require tube or intravenous feedings.

 CALL YOUR DOCTOR IF

* You or a family member has symptoms of blood poisoning.
* The following occurs during treatment:
  - Fever.
  - Signs of infection (swelling, pain, redness) anywhere in your body.
* You plan elective surgery or a dental procedure after you have had an episode of blood poisoning.

BLOOD-TRANSFUSION REACTION

 GENERAL INFORMATION

DEFINITION—Symptoms triggered by a blood transfusion.

BODY PARTS INVOLVED—Blood; blood vessels; kidneys; heart; skin; central nervous system; lungs.

SEX OR AGE MOST AFFECTED—Both sexes. All ages.

SIGNS & SYMPTOMS
Less serious:
• Chills and fever.
• Backache or other aches and pains.
• Hives and itching.
More serious:
• Blood-cell destruction (hemolysis), causing shortness of breath, severe headache, chest or back pain and blood in the urine.

CAUSES—Transfusions of a different blood type than that of the patient. This may occur from errors in matching or from the use of incompletely matched blood in an emergency.

RISK INCREASES WITH
• Blood transfusions in emergency situations, when careful typing and matching of blood must be bypassed.
• Blood transfusions from donors who carry infections.
• Multiple blood transfusions.
• Rh negative mother.

HOW TO PREVENT
• Blood-bank and hospital personnel have safety procedures to prevent reactions except in situations that are uncontrollable (see Causes).
• Use of diphenhydramine (an antihistamine) and acetaminophen prior to transfusion may prevent minor reactions.
• Let health care providers know of any prior history of a response to transfusions.
• If surgery is planned at least 1 month in advance, your own blood may be drawn and stored for use during surgery, if necessary. Transfusion with your own blood is least likely to produce a reaction.

 WHAT TO EXPECT

DIAGNOSTIC MEASURES
• Your own observation of symptoms.
• A health care provider may do a physical exam.
• Blood tests to recheck compatibility and detect complications.

APPROPRIATE HEALTH CARE—Hospital care. Patients receiving transfusions are usually in a hospital or outpatient surgical facility, and reactions can be treated when they occur.

POSSIBLE COMPLICATIONS
• Acute kidney failure.
• Anaphylaxis (shock).
• Congestive heart failure from too rapid transfusion.

PROBABLE OUTCOME—Most reactions clear gradually after the transfusion is halted. A few reactions are fatal.

 HOW TO TREAT

GENERAL MEASURES—Stay awake and alert during a blood transfusion, if possible, so you can notify medical personnel immediately if symptoms occur.

MEDICATION:
• You may be prescribed antihistamines to decrease hives and itching and cortisone drugs to decrease the risk of acute kidney failure.
• Drugs to raise or lower blood pressure will be prescribed if needed.

ACTIVITY—Resume your normal activities as soon as symptoms improve after transfusion.

DIET—No special diet.

 CALL YOUR DOCTOR IF

You or a family member has symptoms of a blood-transfusion reaction during or after a transfusion. Call immediately. This is an emergency!

BOILS
(Furuncles; Carbuncles)

GENERAL INFORMATION

DEFINITION—A painful, deep, bacterial infection of a hair follicle. Boils are common and somewhat contagious. Carbuncles are clusters of boils that occur when the infection spreads through small tunnels underneath the skin.

BODY PARTS INVOLVED—They can occur anywhere on the skin, but most often appear on the neck, face, buttocks, and breasts.

SEX OR AGE MOST AFFECTED—Both sexes; all ages.

SIGNS & SYMPTOMS
* A domed nodule that is painful, tender, red, and has pus on the surface. Boils can appear suddenly and ripen in 24 hours.
* Fever (rarely).
* Swelling of the closest lymph glands.

CAUSES—Infection, usually from *Staphylococcus* bacteria, that begins in the hair follicle and gets into the skin's deeper layers.

RISK INCREASES WITH
* Poor general health.
* Diabetes.
* Other skin problems (such as acne or skin infection).
* Weak immune system due to illness or drugs.

HOW TO PREVENT
* Keep the skin clean.
* If someone in the household has a boil, don't share towels, washcloths, or clothing with that person.
* If you have a chronic disease (such as diabetes), be sure to follow your medical regimen.

WHAT TO EXPECT

DIAGNOSTIC MEASURES
* Your own observation of symptoms.
* Your health care provider can diagnose boils by looking at the affected skin area.
* A medical study may be made of the material from the boil.

APPROPRIATE HEALTH CARE
* Self-care.
* Your health care provider's treatment may include incision and drainage of the boil.

POSSIBLE COMPLICATIONS
* The infection may enter the bloodstream and spread to other body parts.
* Scarring.
* Boils may recur.
* Family members may need treatment.

PROBABLE OUTCOME—Without treatment, a boil will heal in 10 to 20 days. With treatment, the boil should heal in less time, symptoms will be less severe, and new boils should not appear. The pus that drains when a boil opens on its own may infect nearby skin, causing new boils.

HOW TO TREAT

GENERAL MEASURES
* Do not burst a boil as this may spread bacteria.
* Taking showers instead of baths reduces the chances of spreading infection.
* Relieve pain with gentle heat from warm-water soaks. Use 3 or 4 times daily for 20 minutes. Wash your hands carefully after touching the boil.
* Prevent the spread of boils by using clean towels only once or using paper towels and discarding them.

MEDICATION
* Antibiotics may be prescribed if infection is severe.
* Don't use nonprescription antibiotic creams or ointments on the boil's surface. They do not work for boils.

ACTIVITY—Decrease activity until the boil heals. Avoid sweating and avoid contact sports (such as wrestling) while lesions are present.

DIET—No special diet.

CALL YOUR DOCTOR IF

* You or a family member has a boil.
* The following occur during treatment:
  - Symptoms don't improve in 3 to 4 days, despite treatment.
  - New boils appear.
  - Fever.
  - Other family members develop boils.

BONE FRACTURE

GENERAL INFORMATION

DEFINITION—A break in a bone often caused by a fall. Different types of fractures can occur depending on the severity. A complete fracture means the bone is broken all the way through. An incomplete fracture means the bone is cracked. An open (or compound fracture) means the fractured bone sticks out through the skin.

BODY PARTS INVOLVED—Bones.

SEX OR AGE MOST AFFECTED—Both sexes; all ages.

SIGNS & SYMPTOMS
* Pain, swelling, or tenderness near the fracture site.
* Paleness and deformity (sometimes).
* Bleeding or bruising at the site.
* Weakness.
* Cannot bear weight.
* Numbness, tingling, or paralysis below the fracture (rare; this is an emergency).

CAUSES—Injury.

RISK INCREASES WITH
* Activities that carry the risk of injury.
* Reckless behavior that increases the chance of an accident.
* Age. Older adults have bones that are more fragile and also tend to have more falls.
* Osteoporosis and osteopenia.
* Tumors of the bone or bone marrow.

HOW TO PREVENT
* Don't drink alcohol or use mind-altering drugs and drive.
* Use your seat belt in cars.
* Wear protective gear for sports.
* If you have osteoporosis, adhere to your treatment program and avoid situations in which injury is likely.
* Maintain a safe home to prevent falls. No slippery rugs, slick floors, or loose stair railings. Provide mats in bathtubs.

WHAT TO EXPECT

DIAGNOSTIC MEASURES
* Your own observation of symptoms.
* Your health care provider will do a physical exam of the injured area.
* X-rays will be done to confirm the bone fracture. In some cases, other tests are needed.

APPROPRIATE HEALTH CARE
* Bone ends that have been displaced are maneuvered back into place (reduction).
* Most fractures require casts, splints, or a special brace for healing. Crutches or other aids may be used to walk.

* Hospital care may be needed for severe fractures.
* Surgery, if the fracture must be repaired with rods, plates, or screws. See fracture repair in Surgery Section.
* Physical therapy to help in restoring full function to the injured area.

POSSIBLE COMPLICATIONS
* Failure to heal (non-union).
* Shock from blood loss.
* Travel of a fat embolus (clump of fat cells) from the injury site to the lungs or brain.
* Obstruction of nearby arteries.

PROBABLE OUTCOME
* Usually curable with treatment.
* Healing time varies. Recovery is complete when there is no bone motion at the fracture site, and x-rays show complete healing.

HOW TO TREAT

GENERAL MEASURES—Give first aid treatment for bleeding, cover any open wounds, move patient as little as possible. Then transport to hospital or other emergency facility.

MEDICATION—Pain relievers and muscle relaxants, if needed.

ACTIVITY
* Immobility of a bone for a long period of time can cause loss of muscle mass, stiffness in nearby joints, and edema (excess fluid in the tissues). Begin to use the affected part as soon as is safely possible.
* Physical therapy may be prescribed to maintain flexibility of the joint and provide strength to the muscles.
* Resume normal activities as soon as symptoms improve and your health care provider advises you to.

DIET—No special diet. Take vitamin-C and zinc supplements to promote bone healing.

CALL YOUR DOCTOR IF

* You or a family member has symptoms of a bone fracture.
* The following occur after treatment:
  - Swelling above or below the fracture site.
  - Severe, persistent pain.
  - Blue or gray skin below fracture site (such as in the fingernails), or numbness or loss of feeling below the fracture site.

BOTULISM

GENERAL INFORMATION

DEFINITION
* Food-borne botulism is a serious form of food poisoning that is usually caused by eating food contaminated with a toxin. The toxin affects both the central nervous system and the muscular system. The symptoms usually appear suddenly 18 to 36 hours (but the range can be anywhere from 2 hours to 1 week) after eating contaminated food. The disorder can affect all ages.
* Infant botulism is a special type that occurs in children less than 12 months of age.
* Wound botulism occurs when the toxin in a wound spreads to other body parts.
* Adult intestinal colonization botulism occurs in older children and adults with colitis who have had recent bowel surgery or have other intestinal conditions.

BODY PARTS INVOLVED—Central nervous system; muscular system.

SEX OR AGE MOST AFFECTED—All ages, but most common in adults.

SIGNS & SYMPTOMS
* Blurred or double vision and drooping eyelids.
* Dry mouth.
* Slurred speech.
* Trouble swallowing.
* Vomiting and diarrhea.
* Weakness of the arms and legs. Paralysis.
* No fever.
* No change in mental abilities.

The following symptoms appear in infants:
* Severe constipation.
* Feeble cry.
* Unable to suck.

CAUSES
* A bacteria germ, *Clostridium botulinum* (other types may, rarely, be the cause). The germ may be found in contaminated or incompletely cooked foods. It can also be found in improperly canned foods. The germ generates a strong poison that is absorbed from the digestive tract. The poison spreads to the central nervous system.
* Foods likely to cause botulism: home-canned vegetables and fruits. Also, smoked meats, undercooked sausage, fish, and milk products.
* Honey and corn syrup may cause botulism in infants.
* The bacteria may also contaminate a wound and produce the toxin.

RISK INCREASES WITH
* Infants.
* Home-canned foods.

HOW TO PREVENT
* If a can of food is bulging, don't open it. If the contents of a can have a strange color or odor, don't taste the food. Throw it away (safely).
* Don't eat any foods that may not have been properly cooked or canned.
* Don't give infants under age 1 honey or corn syrup, not even a small taste.
* Get proper instructions about canning food.

WHAT TO EXPECT

DIAGNOSTIC MEASURES
* Your own observation of symptoms—especially if several persons eat the same food and become sick.
* Diagnosis and treatment involves emergency hospital care. Blood and stool studies can confirm the diagnosis.

APPROPRIATE HEALTH CARE
* Hospital care. For food-borne infection, vomiting may be induced, enemas given, or a washing out (lavage) of the stomach may be done to help rid the body of the toxin.
* Wound care for infected wounds.
* Breathing support with a machine (ventilator) may be needed, along with other supportive-care measures.
* Fluids may be given through a vein (IV) or through a tube placed in the nose (nasogastric).
* Health care providers will report the disease to state or federal health authorities. They will arrange to remove any contaminated food from stores.

POSSIBLE COMPLICATIONS
* Long-lasting weakness.
* Nervous system problems that can last up to a year.
* Lung infections, such as pneumonia.
* Respiratory failure caused by weak breathing muscles. It can lead to death.

PROBABLE OUTCOME—With prompt treatment, the outlook is good.

HOW TO TREAT

GENERAL MEASURES—If you suspect botulism, refrigerate some of the contaminated food for testing, if possible.

MEDICATION—A special drug (antitoxin) may be given by injection. It can prevent the symptoms from getting worse. It may be life-saving, but it has serious side effects.

ACTIVITY—Bed rest during treatment. Resume normal activities as your strength permits.

DIET—After treatment, no special diet is needed.

CALL YOUR DOCTOR IF

You or a family member has symptoms of botulism. Call for medical help immediately.

BRAIN OR EPIDURAL ABSCESS

GENERAL INFORMATION

DEFINITION—A collection of pus caused by a bacterial infection in the brain. The infection can also be in the membranes that cover the brain and spinal cord.

BODY PARTS INVOLVED—Brain; meninges (membranes that cover the brain); skull.

SEX OR AGE MOST AFFECTED—They can affect all ages and are more common in men than in women.

SIGNS AND SYMPTOMS—The following symptoms usually appear gradually over several hours. They resemble symptoms of a brain tumor or stroke:
• Headache, usually severe.
• Fever.
• Stiff neck.
• Confusion or delirium.
• Seizures (convulsions).
• Nausea and vomiting.
• Pain in the back. It may occur if the infection is in the covering of the spinal cord.
• One side of the body may feel numb or weak. The body may be paralyzed on one side.
• Unable to walk normally.
• Trouble speaking.

CAUSES
• An infection that spreads from another part of the head such as sinusitis or a middle ear infection.
• An infection due to a head injury or surgery.
• An infection that spreads through the blood from other infected organs. This includes the lungs, skin, heart valves, or dental infections.
• Infections such as fungal or protozoan, that occur in people with weak immune systems.

RISK INCREASES WITH
• Head injury.
• Chronic illness, such as diabetes.
• Recent infection (in the ears, nose, eyes, or face).
• Weak immune system due to illness or drugs.
• Drug abuse.
• Tongue piercing.

HOW TO PREVENT—None specific. To reduce risk factors:
• Seek medical care for infections.
• Wear protective headgear when you are involved in any activity that could lead to a head injury.

WHAT TO EXPECT

DIAGNOSTIC MEASURES
• Emergency hospital care is needed.
• Your health care provider will do a physical exam and ask questions about your symptoms and activities. Medical tests may include blood tests, CT, and MRI (see Glossary for both).

APPROPRIATE HEALTH CARE
• Medical or surgical treatment will depend on the location of the infection. Usually, surgery is needed to drain the infected area. Drugs will be given for the infection.
• Breathing support with a machine (ventilator) may be needed, along with other supportive-care measures. Fluids may be given through a vein (IV).

POSSIBLE COMPLICATIONS
• Seizures, coma, and death (without treatment).
• Rupture of the abscess.
• Brain hemorrhage.

PROBABLE OUTCOME—Usually curable with early diagnosis and treatment.

HOW TO TREAT

GENERAL MEASURES—The family should maintain an optimistic outlook, stay in close contact with the patient's doctor and help by making their visits with the patient brief and as supportive as possible.

MEDICATION
• Antibiotic drugs will be given for the infection. They may be continued for several weeks.
• Drugs to prevent seizures may be prescribed.
• Following surgery, you may be given drugs to reduce swelling.

ACTIVITY—While in the hospital, you will need bed rest. After a 2 to 3 week recovery, you should be as active as your strength and feeling of well-being allow.

DIET—While you are in the hospital, essential fluids may be given through a tube in a vein. Following treatment, eat a normal, well-balanced diet.

CALL YOUR DOCTOR IF

• You or a family member has any symptoms of a brain abscess.
• New, unexplained symptoms develop. Drugs used in treatment may produce side effects.

ILLNESS & DISORDERS

BRAIN TUMOR

GENERAL INFORMATION

DEFINITION—Abnormal cell growth in the brain. The growth may be benign (noncancerous) or malignant (cancerous). The symptoms can be caused by pressure, as the tumor gets larger, or can be caused by the location, size, and type of tumor.

BODY PARTS INVOLVED—Brain; central nervous system.

SEX OR AGE MOST AFFECTED—All ages, but most common in adults between ages 20 and 60.

SIGNS & SYMPTOMS
* Headache that is worse when lying down.
* Seizures (convulsions).
* Memory loss, confusion, and loss of concentration.
* Personality and behavior changes.
* Vomiting or nausea.
* Problems with vision. This includes double vision.
* Weakness on one side of the body.
* Lack of balance and dizziness.
* Loss of sense of smell and hearing.

CAUSES—Exact cause is unknown. There are genetic factors and environmental factors involved. Some tumors begin in the brain and are called primary. Other brain tumors are called secondary. They have spread (metastasize) from other cancers in the body. These includes cancers of the breast, lungs, colon, or skin (melanoma).

RISK INCREASES WITH
* Unknown for most brain tumors.
* Radiation to the head for other cancer treatment.
* Rarely, certain types of tumors run in families.

HOW TO PREVENT—No specific preventive measures are known.

WHAT TO EXPECT

DIAGNOSTIC MEASURES
* Your own observation of symptoms.
* Your health care provider will do a physical exam and ask questions about your symptoms and activities.
* A variety of medical tests will be done to diagnose the tumor and to see if it has spread to or from other places in the body (called staging).

APPROPRIATE HEALTH CARE
* The treatment plan will be determined by the stage, size, location and type of tumor, and your age and health status. Because there are over 120 different types of brain tumors, treatment needs to be specific for each person. Treatment can include surgery, radiation, chemotherapy (anticancer drugs) and biologic therapy.
* Surgery is often needed. It may involve removal of all or part of the tumor and nearby tissue.
* Radiation may be used for certain stages of the tumor. It is normally not used for children under age 3.
* Biologic therapy uses the body's immune system to help fight the cancer.
* Treatment may involve steps to relieve symptoms and make you comfortable, rather than treating the tumor.

POSSIBLE COMPLICATIONS
* Long-term physical and mental side effects. They may be due to the effect of the tumor or to treatment.
* Tumor may recur after treatment.
* Death.

PROBABLE OUTCOME—The outcome depends on several factors. These include type of tumor, its size, location, spread of tumor, other cancer in the body, age and health of the patient. and the patient's response to treatment.

HOW TO TREAT

GENERAL MEASURES
* The more you can learn and understand about a disease, the more you will be able to make informed decisions about where to go for your care, the treatments available, the risks involved, side effects of therapy and expected outcome.
* To learn more: American Brain Tumor Association, 2720 River Rd Ste 146, Des Plaines, IL 60018; (800) 886-2282; website: www.abta.org.

MEDICATION—Drugs may be prescribed:
* To reduce swelling of the brain tissue.
* To control seizures.
* For pain relief.
* For cancer treatment (chemotherapy).

ACTIVITY—Stay as active as your strength allows.

DIET—Eat a normal, well-balanced diet. You may need to take vitamins and minerals if you cannot eat normally.

CALL YOUR DOCTOR IF

* You or a family member has symptoms of a brain tumor.
* New, unexplained symptoms occur during treatment.

BREAST ABSCESS

GENERAL INFORMATION

DEFINITION—An infected area of breast tissue that becomes filled with pus when the body fights the infection.

BODY PARTS INVOLVED—It involves breast tissue, nipple(s), milk glands, and milk ducts.

SEX OR AGE MOST AFFECTED—They almost always occur in a breast-feeding woman.

SIGNS AND SYMPTOMS
* Breast pain.
* Breast is tender, red or hard.
* Fever and chills.
* Feeling ill.
* Tenderness in the area under the arm.

CAUSES—Bacteria that enter the breast through the nipple. This can happen if a nipple gets dry and cracked from breast-feeding.

RISK INCREASES WITH
* Breast infection, such as mastitis.
* Pelvic infection after delivery of a baby.
* Previous breast abscess.
* Diabetes.
* Rheumatoid arthritis.
* Use of steroid drugs.
* Heavy cigarette smoking. This is also a risk factor for women who are not breast-feeding.
* Lumpectomy with radiation.
* Some breast implants.

HOW TO PREVENT
* Clean the nipples and breasts carefully, before and after nursing.
* Lubricate the nipples after nursing. Use vitamin A & D ointment or an other topical drug if recommended.
* Avoid clothing that irritates the breasts.
* Don't allow a nursing infant to chew nipples.

WHAT TO EXPECT

DIAGNOSTIC MEASURES
* Your health care provider will do a physical exam of the affected area. This is often all that is needed for diagnosis.
* Medical tests such as a culture of the pus and ultrasound may be done.

APPROPRIATE HEALTH CARE—The abscess may need to be drained. Draining the abscess may be done with a needle inserted into the abscess or with a small incision. This will reduce the pain and help clear up the infection.

POSSIBLE COMPLICATIONS—An abnormal opening (fistula) may develop between the breast and the outside of the body.

PROBABLE OUTCOME
* Usually curable in 8 to 10 days with treatment. Draining the abscess is sometimes needed to speed healing.
* It is rarely required for a patient to stop breast-feeding, even with severe infection. Certain antibiotics and pain relievers will require that breast-feeding be stopped for a short period of time. It will then be necessary to pump the breasts.

HOW TO TREAT

GENERAL MEASURES
* You may or may not be able to keep breast-feeding with the affected breast. Your health care provider will help determine if this is possible. If you can't breast-feed, use a breast pump to remove milk from the infected breast until you can start nursing again on that side.
* Use a warm, moist compress on the breast to relieve pain, hasten healing, and help the flow of milk.

MEDICATION—Drugs for pain or antibiotics for infection may be prescribed.

ACTIVITY—After treatment, resume normal activity as soon as symptoms improve.

DIET—No special diet.

CALL YOUR DOCTOR IF

* You or a family member has symptoms of a breast abscess.
* Any of the following occur during treatment:
  - Fever.
  - Pain becomes more severe.
  - Infection seems to be spreading, despite treatment.
  - Symptoms don't improve in 72 hours.

BREAST CANCER

 GENERAL INFORMATION

DEFINITION—A malignant growth of the breast tissue. It is the most common form of cancer in women.

BODY PARTS INVOLVED—Nipple or tissue of the breast.

SEX OR AGE MOST AFFECTED—Breast cancer is rare before age 30, and is most common after the age of 50. Men can develop breast cancer also.

SIGNS & SYMPTOMS
• No symptoms in early stages. It may be detected by a mammogram or by feeling a breast lump.
• Swelling or lump in the breast.
• Vague discomfort in the breast without true pain.
• Inversion of the nipple.
• Distorted breast contour.
• Dimpled or pitted skin in the breast.
• Enlarged nodes under the arm (late stages).
• Bloody discharge from the nipple (rare).

CAUSES—Unknown.

RISK INCREASES WITH
• Women over 50.
• Women who have not had children or who conceived in the late fertile years.
• Family history of breast cancer (especially mother or sister).
• Benign tumors of the breast (fibrocystic disease).
• Early menstruation, late menopause, or first pregnancy after age 30.
• Previous breast cancer in one breast.
• Radiation exposure.
• Patients with endometrial or ovarian cancer.
• Studies of estrogen therapy are not conclusive about their role in increased breast cancer risk.

HOW TO PREVENT
• None specific. Avoid risk factors where possible and follow early detection steps.
• Monthly self-exam of breasts for cancer signs.
• Get medical breast exams as recommended.
• Mammograms every 1 to 2 years starting at age 40 (or as recommended).
• Eat a well-balanced diet that is low in fat. Studies are unclear about a high-fat diet and breast cancer risk.
• Exercise regularly to lower breast cancer risk.
• Breast-feeding for at least 6 months (a year is better for mother and baby) will reduce breast cancer risk.
• A drug, such as tamoxifen, may be prescribed for women at high risk for breast cancer.
• A woman with very high risk may choose to have the breasts removed as a preventive step.

 WHAT TO EXPECT

DIAGNOSTIC MEASURES
• Your own observation of symptoms.
• Your health care provider will do a breast exam and ask questions about your symptoms.
• A number of medical tests will be done. The tests first help diagnose the cancer and then determine if it has spread (staging).

APPROPRIATE HEALTH CARE
• Treatment depends on location and size of the tumor, any spread of the cancer, your health, age, and preferences. Treatment may include chemotherapy (anticancer drugs) and/or radiation therapy, surgery, and biologic therapy.
• Chemotherapy uses drugs and radiation therapy uses radiation to attack the cancer cells. Biologic therapy uses the body's immune system to fight cancer.
• Surgery may be recommended to remove the lump, breast, lymph glands, lymphatic channels, or muscles under the breast.
• Counseling may help you cope with cancer.

POSSIBLE COMPLICATIONS
• Spread to vital organs if not treated early.
• Complications may occur from treatments.

PROBABLE OUTCOME—It can be curable with early diagnosis and treatment.

 HOW TO TREAT

GENERAL MEASURES
• The decision for treatment is very complex and often confusing. Learn about your options and understand the risks and benefits of each.
• To learn more: National Cancer Institute, (800) 422-6347; website: www.nci.nih.gov or Y-Me National Breast Cancer Organization hotline (800) 221-2141; website: www.y-me.org or American Cancer Society, (800) 227-2345; website: www.cancer.org.

MEDICATION
• For minor discomfort, use nonprescription drugs such as acetaminophen or ibuprofen.
• Anticancer drugs, hormones, drugs for biologic therapy, or cortisone drugs may be prescribed.

ACTIVITY
• Physical therapy after surgery in some cases.
• Exercise after recovery. It improves survival.

DIET—Eat a well-balanced diet.

☎ **CALL YOUR DOCTOR IF**

• You or a family member has breast changes.
• New, unexpected symptoms occur during or after treatment

BRONCHIECTASIS

GENERAL INFORMATION

DEFINITION—A rare lung disease, in which the bronchial tubes become enlarged and distended (stretched). Pockets form where infections may develop.

BODY PARTS INVOLVED—Lungs; bronchial tubes.

SEX OR AGE MOST AFFECTED—All ages, but most common in adults.

SIGNS & SYMPTOMS
* Frequent coughing. There may be foul-smelling mucus. The mucus may be green or yellow. The mucus may be flecked with blood.
* Chest pain and wheezing.
* Repeated lung infections.
* Shortness of breath.
* Feeling tired and weak.
* Weight loss.

CAUSES—The bronchial walls become damaged and weak usually as a result of infections. This damage may develop over years. The cilia (small hairs) that help keep the bronchial tubes clean are destroyed. This allows dust, bacteria and mucus to accumulate.

RISK INCREASES WITH
* Repeated lung infections such as pneumonia.
* Chronic bronchitis.
* Inhaling a foreign object (such as a peanut).
* Tuberculosis, lung cancer, or lung abscess.
* Cystic fibrosis.
* Family history of lung disease.
* Cigarette smoking.
* Weak immune system due to illness or drugs.

HOW TO PREVENT—None specific. Avoid risk factors where possible:
* Don't smoke.
* Obtain medical care for lung infections.
* Prompt removal of any foreign body that has entered the lungs.
* Get vaccines for flu and pneumonia.

WHAT TO EXPECT

DIAGNOSTIC MEASURES
* Your own observation of symptoms.
* Your health care provider will do a physical exam and ask questions about your symptoms.
* Medical tests may include blood or sputum (material coughed up from the lung) tests, CT, x-ray, bronchoscopy (looking in the airways with a lighted tube), and pulmonary function tests.

APPROPRIATE HEALTH CARE
* Treatment includes postural drainage to remove lung secretions, drugs (as needed), treatment for underlying disorder (such as cystic fibrosis), and lifestyle changes.
* Postural drainage involves ridding the lungs of the secretions. You will be taught the proper technique. It is usually done by lying on a bed and hanging your head over the side with the affected lung uppermost. Clapping the chest can help mucus drain. A family member can do this by hand or a mechanical device can be used. This routine is done 1 to 3 times a day.
* Surgery to remove areas of damaged lung tissue may be recommended if other treatments are not effective.

POSSIBLE COMPLICATIONS
* Chronic obstructive pulmonary disease.
* Repeated pneumonia or other infections.
* Cor pulmonale (heart disorder due to lung disease).
* Hospital care and breathing support may be needed for complications.

PROBABLE OUTCOME—With treatment, many patients can lead nearly normal lives without major problems.

HOW TO TREAT

GENERAL MEASURES
* Don't smoke. Find a way to quit.
* To learn more: American Lung Association, 61 Broadway, 6th Floor, New York, NY 10006, (800) 586-4872; website: www.lungusa.org.

MEDICATION—You may be prescribed:
* Antibiotic drugs for infections.
* Inhaled beta-agonists to assist breathing.
* Drugs, such as guaifenesin, to loosen mucus in the lungs.
* Drugs to treat any underlying disorder.

ACTIVITY—Remain as active as possible.

DIET—You may be advised to increase fluid intake.

CALL YOUR DOCTOR IF

* You or a family member has signs of bronchiectasis.
* Symptoms of lung infection develop or fever occurs.
* Sputum contains blood, changes color, or thickens.
* Chest pain increases or you become short of breath.

BRONCHIOLITIS

GENERAL INFORMATION

DEFINITION—Inflammation and infection of the smallest airways (bronchioles) of the respiratory tract. These airways normally carry air from the large bronchial tubes to tiny air sacs in the lungs.

BODY PARTS INVOLVED—Bronchioles.

SEX OR AGE MOST AFFECTED—Bronchiolitis mainly affects infants and young children. Boys are affected more often than girls.

SIGNS & SYMPTOMS
* Often there is a mild common cold and cough before symptoms of bronchiolitis appear.
* Sudden trouble with breathing and wheezing.
* Rapid, shallow breathing.
* Chest and stomach are pulled in and out in seesaw movements with breathing.
* Fever may occur.
* Dehydration.
* Blue skin or nails in severe cases.

CAUSES—Usually a viral infection. Respiratory syncytial virus (RSV) is the most common infection. Other viral infections may sometimes be the cause. Germs are spread by sneezing, coughing, or by contact of hands to nose, mouth, or eyes. Symptoms start 2 to 5 days after the exposure.

RISK INCREASES WITH
* Young children (usually under age 2).
* Winter and early spring seasons.
* Daycare centers.
* Crowded living conditions.
* Exposure to cigarette smoke.
* Children who were born premature, had low birth weight, were born with health problems (neurologic, heart, or lung), or have developed a lung disorder.

HOW TO PREVENT
* No specific preventive measures.
* Wash hands carefully to prevent spread of any germs.
* Avoid exposure to infected persons.
* Don't allow any smoking around a baby or child.
* Children at risk for complications of RSV infections may be given therapy to prevent the infection.

WHAT TO EXPECT

DIAGNOSTIC MEASURES
* Your own observation of symptoms.
* Your health care provider will do a physical exam and ask questions about the symptoms and activities.
* Medical tests are usually not needed, but may be done to confirm the diagnosis.

APPROPRIATE HEALTH CARE
* Home care.
* There is no specific treatment for this disorder. Mild cases may be treated at home. Extra rest and drinking plenty of fluids is usually all that is needed.
* If the symptoms are more severe, hospital care may be required. Oxygen may be provided through a facemask. Some patients require breathing support with a ventilator (a device to help the lungs). Treatment to help remove lung secretions may be needed.

POSSIBLE COMPLICATIONS
* Respiratory failure.
* Chronic lung disease.
* Heart disorders.
* Bronchiolitis obliterans (collapse of part of the lung).
* Other infections.

PROBABLE OUTCOME—The disorder usually heals on its own. Mild cases may last for one or two days. Other cases may take 5 to 12 days for recovery. A few children who have other health problems are more at risk for complications.

HOW TO TREAT

GENERAL MEASURES
* Use an ultrasonic, cool-mist humidifier if recommended by your health care provider. Clean the humidifier daily.
* A blocked-up nose may be suctioned with a rubber suction device.

MEDICATION—Hospital care may include drugs to help relieve breathing problems, treat infections, and to prevent complications.

ACTIVITY—Rest until symptoms have improved for 48 hours. Then gradually return to normal activities.

DIET—Offer the child clear fluids often. These include water, tea, or carbonated drinks. Also, lemonade, weak bouillon, fruit juice, or gelatin.

CALL YOUR DOCTOR IF

* You or a family member has symptoms of bronchiolitis.
* Cold symptoms become worse.
* Temperature rises to 101°F (38.3°C) or higher.
* Breathing becomes more difficult.
* A cough begins that produces colored mucus.
* The skin, lips, or nails turn bluish in color.
* The child becomes drowsy and lacks energy.

BRONCHITIS, ACUTE

GENERAL INFORMATION

DEFINITION—Inflammation (swelling) of the mucous lining of the bronchi (main air passages) to the lungs. Symptoms of acute bronchitis may start suddenly and last just a few days. Chronic bronchitis persists over a long period of time.

BODY PARTS INVOLVED—Trachea; bronchi; bronchioles.

SEX OR AGE MOST AFFECTED—It is a common disorder affecting all age groups.

SIGNS & SYMPTOMS
* A common cold or sore throat may occur prior to bronchitis.
* Cough that produces little or no mucus at first. Later, mucus may be produced.
* Low fever (usually less than 101°F/38.3°C).
* Burning feeling in chest. Feeling of pressure behind the breastbone.
* Wheezing. There may also be trouble breathing.
* Feeling tired.

CAUSES
* Viral infection usually. Most cases begin with a cold virus in the nose and throat. The virus then spreads to the lungs. A bacterial infection may also cause bronchitis. Infection causes the mucous membranes to become inflamed and produce thick, sticky mucus. This narrows the airways and causes the symptoms.
* Irritative bronchitis is caused by allergies, chemicals, and other irritants in the environment.

RISK INCREASES WITH
* Chronic lung disease or chronic sinusitis.
* Smoking or second hand smoke.
* Poor nutrition.
* Allergies.
* Areas with polluted air.
* Elderly and very young age groups.

HOW TO PREVENT
* Avoid close contact with people who have a cold or the flu. Wash hands often to avoid germs.
* Don't smoke.
* If you work around chemicals, dust or other lung irritants, wear a special facemask.

WHAT TO EXPECT

DIAGNOSTIC MEASURES
* Your own observation of symptoms.
* Your health care provider will do a physical exam and use a stethoscope to listen to your lungs.
* Medical tests are usually not done. A chest x-ray may be done if symptoms are more severe.

APPROPRIATE HEALTH CARE
* Self-care, if you are in good overall health.
* Treatment is directed toward relieving the symptoms. Get extra rest and increase fluid intake.

POSSIBLE COMPLICATIONS
* Pneumonia.
* Chronic bronchitis.
* Bronchiectasis (bronchial tubes become blocked).
* Pleurisy (swelling of the lining of the lungs).

PROBABLE OUTCOME—Usually curable in 1 week. Cases with complications are usually curable in 2 weeks, with drug therapy. In some people, the cough may continue for several weeks, even after the infection is gone.

HOW TO TREAT

GENERAL MEASURES
* If you are a smoker, don't smoke during your illness. This delays recovery and makes complications more likely.
* Increase air moisture. Take frequent hot showers. Use a cool-mist, ultrasonic humidifier by your bed. Clean humidifier daily.
* To learn more: American Lung Association, 61 Broadway, 6th Floor, New York, NY 10006, (800) 586-4872; website: www.lungusa.org.

MEDICATION
* Use acetaminophen for fever and minor pain.
* Nonprescription cough suppressants (to ease coughing) or expectorants (to thin mucus) may be used to relieve symptoms. The mucus should be coughed up, so use cough suppressants with caution.
* Antibiotics may be prescribed for bacterial infection. They will not help a viral infection.
* Drugs may be prescribed for specific symptoms.

ACTIVITY—Get extra rest until symptoms improve. Then return to normal activities, as you feel better.

DIET—No special diet. Drink extra fluids if advised.

CALL YOUR DOCTOR IF

* You or a family member has symptoms of acute bronchitis.
* You develop a high fever and chills.
* You have chest pain.
* You cough up mucus that is thick, colored, or has blood in it.
* You feel short of breath, even when resting.

BRONCHITIS, CHRONIC

GENERAL INFORMATION

DEFINITION—Inflammation (swelling) of the mucous lining of the bronchi (main air passages) to the lungs. It often occurs along with emphysema (damaged air sacs in the lungs).

BODY PARTS INVOLVED—Bronchial tubes (bronchi).

SEX OR AGE MOST AFFECTED—All ages, but most common in adults, usually men.

SIGNS & SYMPTOMS—Symptoms don't start suddenly. They develop over time. They include: presence of a mucus-producing cough most days of the month, 3 months of the year for 2 consecutive years.

CAUSES—Repeated irritation or infection in the bronchial tubes. The tubes begin to thicken and become more narrow. They begin to lose their elasticity. The main cause is smoking.

RISK INCREASES WITH
• Smoking.
• History of lung disorders.
• Family history of lung disease.
• Exposure to air pollutants or cigarette smoke.
• Work that involves exposure to high levels of dust and irritating fumes.

HOW TO PREVENT
• Don't smoke. This is the best prevention.
• Avoid fumes in the environment.
• Get prompt medical care for lung infections.

WHAT TO EXPECT

DIAGNOSTIC MEASURES
• Your own observation of symptoms.
• Your health care provider will do a physical exam and ask questions about your symptoms, smoking habits and exposure to pollutants or irritants. Many lung and heart disorders cause symptoms identical to those of chronic bronchitis.
• Medical tests will be used to make a diagnosis.

APPROPRIATE HEALTH CARE
• Treatment can help relieve symptoms and help prevent complications. A treatment plan will be developed based on your individual needs.
• Your health care provider can teach you exercises to help improve your breathing.
• Lung transplantation may be recommended for advanced cases.

POSSIBLE COMPLICATIONS
• Pneumonia.
• Chronic obstructive pulmonary disease (COPD).
• Cor pulmonale (heart disorder).

PROBABLE OUTCOME—There is no cure for this disorder. Treatment can help relieve the symptoms and slow the progress of the disease. Smokers must stop smoking.

HOW TO TREAT

GENERAL MEASURES
• Stop smoking. Find a way to quit that works for you.
• Avoid areas with air pollution, dust, or fumes. Consider changing jobs if you need to.
• Install air-conditioning with a filter and humidity control in your home.
• Avoid shouting, laughing loudly, and crying if these make you cough.
• Get a pneumococcal vaccine and annual flu vaccine.
• To learn more: American Lung Association, 61 Broadway, 6th Floor, New York, NY 10006, (800) 586-4872; website: www.lungusa.org.

MEDICATION
• Don't take drugs to lessen your cough. They can make this condition worse.
• Antibiotics for infection may be prescribed.
• Oral or inhaled bronchodilator drugs may be prescribed to relax and open the airways in the lungs.
• Oral or inhaled steroids may be prescribed to reduce inflammation.
• Drugs to thin the mucous may be prescribed.

ACTIVITY
• Regular exercise is important. Long periods of being inactive can add to your disability.
• Avoid sudden temperature changes. Avoid cold, wet weather.
• Be careful when exercising or working. Work at a pace that does not make you cough.

DIET—No special diet. Drink plenty of fluids.

CALL YOUR DOCTOR IF

• You or a family member has symptoms of chronic bronchitis.
• You have a fever or vomiting.
• Mucus gets thicker or has blood in it.
• Your chest pain gets worse.
• You feel short of breath even when you are resting or not coughing.

BRUCELLOSIS
(Undulant Fever; Bang's Disease)

GENERAL INFORMATION

DEFINITION—A rare infection passed to humans from infected cows, pigs, sheep, or goats. It cannot be passed from person to person. It affects the bone marrow, lymph glands, liver, and spleen. The infection may be acute (short lasting) or chronic (persisting over months or years).

BODY PARTS INVOLVED—Blood-producing organs, including bone marrow, lymph glands, liver and spleen.

SEX OR AGE MOST AFFECTED—Both sexes and all ages, but most common in men between ages 20 and 60.

SIGNS & SYMPTOMS
• Sweating, chills, and fever (may come and go).
• Tiredness.
• Upset stomach.
• Tenderness along the spine.
• Headache.
• Muscle and joint aches.
• Constipation.
• Weight loss.
• Depression.
• In later stages of the infection, mental problems and seizures may occur.

CAUSES—Infection from a bacterium, which is passed to humans by ingesting infected food products, direct contact with an infected animal, or breathing in germs in the air. After a person is exposed, symptoms may develop in 1 to 8 weeks.

RISK INCREASES WITH
• Persons who work with animals. This includes farmers, ranchers, meat processors, and veterinarians.
• Travel to some foreign countries.
• Biological warfare.

HOW TO PREVENT
• Don't drink milk from any source that has not been pasteurized.
• Protect yourself when working around animals. Use safety protection (gloves and mask) as needed.
• Farm animals should be immunized.

WHAT TO EXPECT

DIAGNOSTIC MEASURES
• Your own observation of symptoms.
• Your health care provider will do a physical exam and ask questions about your symptoms and activities. Be sure to discuss any contact with animals you have had in the last few months.
• Medical tests may include studies of blood, urine, and spinal fluid. X-ray, CT, heart tests, and others may be done depending on the symptoms.

APPROPRIATE HEALTH CARE
• Treatment usually consists of drugs for infection and getting extra rest.
• If symptoms are more severe, hospital care may be needed.

POSSIBLE COMPLICATIONS
• Endocarditis (heart inflammation).
• The infection may recur.

PROBABLE OUTCOME—Can usually be cured in 3 to 4 weeks with treatment. Some muscle aches may continue for a period of time.

HOW TO TREAT

GENERAL MEASURES
• It usually is not necessary to keep the ill person away from others.
• Avoid contact with animals that may be the source of the infection.
• Family members who may have been exposed to the same infected food products should see their health care provider.

MEDICATION
• Antibiotic drugs will be prescribed for the infection. You usually need to take them for several weeks.
• Drugs to reduce swelling in severe cases and for relief of muscle pain may be prescribed.

ACTIVITY—Get extra rest until fever and other symptoms improve. Return to your normal activities slowly.

DIET—No special diet.

CALL YOUR DOCTOR IF

• You or a family member has symptoms of brucellosis.
• Fever or other symptoms return after treatment.
• New, unexplained symptoms develop. Drugs used in treatment may produce side effects.

BUERGER'S DISEASE
(Thromboangiitis Obliterans)

GENERAL INFORMATION

DEFINITION—Blockage of small and medium arteries due to inflammation of blood vessels. The symptoms come on gradually over a period of time.

BODY PARTS INVOLVED—Arteries (and sometimes veins) in the extremities.

SEX OR AGE MOST AFFECTED—The disease is most common in men between ages 20 and 40 who are heavy cigarette smokers. However, it is now being diagnosed more in women and in people of both sexes over age 50.

SIGNS & SYMPTOMS
* Numbness and tingling in the legs, feet, arms, and fingers.
* Pain in the feet and legs while walking or during exercise. This pain occurs less often in the hands and fingers. Pain comes from not having enough blood flow to these areas of the body. Pain becomes persistent as disease progresses.
* Raynaud phenomenon. A condition where the hands, fingers, feet, and toes turn white, blue, or red when exposed to cold.
* Painful sores (ulcers) and gangrene (dead tissue) on the toes and fingertips.

CAUSES—Unknown. The disease is probably triggered by smoking combined with an immune reaction in the body. Most patients are heavy smokers, but some are moderate smokers, and some use smokeless tobacco.

RISK INCREASES WITH—Smoking or using smokeless tobacco.

HOW TO PREVENT—There are no specific preventive measures, except never to smoke.

WHAT TO EXPECT

DIAGNOSTIC MEASURES
* Your own observation of symptoms.
* Your health care provider will do a physical exam and ask questions about your symptoms and smoking history. This is often enough to make the diagnosis.
* Medical tests may be done to confirm the diagnosis and check for complications.

APPROPRIATE HEALTH CARE
* There is no specific medical treatment for the disorder. Lifestyle changes are the main form of treatment. Drug therapy may be prescribed for certain symptoms.
* Counseling may be recommended to help with lifestyle changes required to cope with the disease.

POSSIBLE COMPLICATIONS
* Blood clots in the legs.
* Finger and toe ulcers, gangrene, and amputation.
* Life expectancy is shorter.

PROBABLE OUTCOME—This condition is currently considered incurable. Stopping smoking is the only effective treatment to stop the progress of the disease.

HOW TO TREAT

GENERAL MEASURES
* The disease will get worse if smoking continues, so stop smoking. Join a program to help you stop.
* Avoid exposure to the cold if possible. Cold causes blood vessels to constrict. This deprives your body of a normal blood supply. If you are going out in cold weather, wear warm footwear and gloves.
* Clip nails carefully to avoid injuring the skin.
* Wear shoes that fit well. Wear cotton or wool socks.
* Insert soft pads in your shoes to protect your feet.
* Don't go barefoot outdoors.
* Get treatment for any infection or injury that occurs.

MEDICATION—Drugs that open the blood vessels may be prescribed. These drugs will not help if you continue smoking.

ACTIVITY—Stay as active as you can. Begin an exercise program to become as physically fit as possible.

DIET—No special diet.

CALL YOUR DOCTOR IF

* You or a family member has symptoms of Buerger's disease.
* You have pain that cannot be controlled.
* Sores develop on your fingers or toes.
* New, unexplained symptoms develop. Drugs used in treatment may produce side effects.

BULIMIA

GENERAL INFORMATION

DEFINITION—An eating disorder. It involves bingeing (uncontrolled overeating) and purging (getting rid of unwanted food in the body).

BODY PARTS INVOLVED—Brain and central nervous system; kidneys; liver; endocrine system; gastrointestinal tract.

SEX OR AGE MOST AFFECTED—Bulimia affects both sexes (women much more than men). It often starts in the teen years.

SIGNS & SYMPTOMS—Recurrent episodes of binge eating. This is rapid eating of a large amount of food in a short time (usually less than 2 hours), plus at least 3 of the following:
• Preference for high-calorie, convenience foods during a binge.
• Secretive eating during a binge. Patients are aware that the eating pattern is abnormal, and they fear being unable to stop eating.
• Following the eating binge with purging measures, such as laxative use or self-induced vomiting.
• Depression and guilt following an eating binge.
• Repeated attempts to lose weight with severely restrictive diets, self-induced vomiting, and use of laxatives or diuretics.
• Frequent weight changes greater than 10 pounds from first fasting and then extreme overeating.
• There is no underlying physical disorder.

CAUSES—Unknown (thought to be largely emotional).

RISK INCREASES WITH
• Strict, compulsive, perfectionistic family.
• Anorexia nervosa (another eating disorder).
• Depression.
• Stress, including lifestyle changes, such as moving or starting at a new school or job.
• Personality disorders.
• Concerned with being physically attractive.
• Certain occupations (such as ballet dancer, model, or actor).
• Certain activities (such as cheerleading).
• Athletes (such as gymnasts, runners, cyclists, weight-lifters, and wrestlers).

HOW TO PREVENT—No specific preventive measures. Early treatment may help keep it from progressing.

WHAT TO EXPECT

DIAGNOSTIC MEASURES
• Your own observation of symptoms. Many patients are secretive, and parents may be unaware of this condition.
• Your health care provider can usually diagnose bulimia with a physical exam and by asking questions about your symptoms, eating habits, and weight concerns.
• There is no one test to diagnose bulimia. Medical tests may be done to check for underlying disorder or complications.

APPROPRIATE HEALTH CARE
• The goal of treatment is to establish healthy eating patterns and to maintain normal weight.
• Treatment may include counseling for the patient and the family, nutrition counseling, and drug therapy if needed. Hospital care or care in an eating disorder facility may be required.
• A dental exam is usually recommended.
• Counseling focuses on the misconceptions that patients have of themselves (physically, mentally, emotionally). Support groups may help some patients.

POSSIBLE COMPLICATIONS
• Fluid/electrolyte imbalance, dental disease, stomach and esophagus problems, constipation, and dry skin.
• Not enough nutrients for body's needs (that could lead to death).
• Relapse after treatment.

PROBABLE OUTCOME—Outcome is variable. Patients, if they desire to change, can often be helped with therapy. For some patients, it may continue long-term. Others just have episodes of bulimia that occur with life events and crisis.

HOW TO TREAT

GENERAL MEASURES
• Denial of the severity or even the existence of the problem is common in patients. Most patients resist treatment and behavior changes at first. Some want a quick and easy solution and that is not possible.
• To learn more: National Eating Disorders Association, 603 Stewart St., Suite 803, Seattle WA 98101; (800) 931-2237; website: www.nationaleatingdisorders.org.

MEDICATION
• Antidepressants are often prescribed.
• Vitamin and mineral supplements if needed.

ACTIVITY—May be limited at first. Then exercise for enjoyment and fitness and not to lose weight.

DIET—A dietitian will help plan healthy meals that are not rigid, but provide food choices.

CALL YOUR DOCTOR IF

• You have symptoms of bulimia or you suspect your a family member has bulimia.
• Treatment does not improve bulimia behavior.

BUNION
(Hallux Valgus)

GENERAL INFORMATION

DEFINITION—A bony swelling or bump that occurs along the side of the big toe joint.

BODY PARTS INVOLVED—Great (big) toe.

SEX OR AGE MOST AFFECTED—Bunions may start in the teenage years, but usually occur in the 20 to 30 age group. Three times as many women as men have bunions.

SIGNS & SYMPTOMS
* A big toe that points in, toward the other toes. This is called hallux valgus.
* Thickened skin over the bony bump at the base of the big toe.
* Fluid may build up under the thickened skin.
* Foot pain and stiffness.
* The symptoms progress slowly over a period of years.

CAUSES—The big toe has been forced into an incorrect position. This causes the joint to stick out. The big toe may overlap one or more of the other toes.

RISK INCREASES WITH
* Family history of foot problems (inherited weakness in the toe joints).
* Flat feet.
* Arthritis.
* Shoes that have high heels and narrow toes that push the toes together.

HOW TO PREVENT
* Exercise daily to keep muscles of the feet and legs in good condition.
* Wear shoes that have wide toes and fit well. Don't wear high heels or shoes without room for toes in their normal position.

WHAT TO EXPECT

DIAGNOSTIC MEASURES
* Your own observation of symptoms.
* Your health care provider can diagnose a bunion by its appearance.
* An x-ray of the toe joint may be done.

APPROPRIATE HEALTH CARE
* Use self-care in the early stages. This may prevent a bunion from worsening.
* Custom-made orthotics (shoe inserts) may be prescribed.
* Surgery (bunionectomy) may be recommended when bunion makes walking painful. The bunion is removed and the toe may be straightened. Specific instructions will be provided for self-care after surgery (see Bunion Removal in Surgery section).

POSSIBLE COMPLICATIONS
* Infection of the bunion, especially in persons with diabetes.
* Inflammation and arthritis in other joints caused by difficulty in walking. Arthritis can result from abnormal stress on the foot, hip, and spine.
* Bunion may grow back after surgery.

PROBABLE OUTCOME—A bunion is permanent unless surgery is performed to remove it. Self-care can help improve the symptoms.

HOW TO TREAT

GENERAL MEASURES
* Wear comfortable shoes that fit well.
* If there is swelling, redness, and pain, keep pressure off the affected toe.
* At bedtime, separate the first toe from the others with a foam-rubber pad. Leave it there while you sleep.
* Wear a thick, ring-shaped pad around and over the bunion. Use arch supports to relieve pressure on the bunion. These are available in drugstores or shoe-repair shops.

MEDICATION—Use nonprescription drugs such as aspirin or ibuprofen for pain, swelling, and soreness.

ACTIVITY—If you have surgery, resume your normal activities slowly after surgery. Recovery may take 2 months or more.

DIET—No special diet.

CALL YOUR DOCTOR IF

* You or a family member has a bunion that is interfering with normal activities.
* You develop signs of infection after treatment or surgery. Signs of infection include fever, tenderness, or pain.

BURNS

GENERAL INFORMATION

DEFINITION—Injury to the skin from contact with heat, radiation, electricity, sunlight, or chemicals. Sometimes internal organs may also be injured.

BODY PARTS INVOLVED—Skin; underlying tissue and respiratory system (sometimes).

SEX OR AGE MOST AFFECTED—Both sexes; all ages. The risk of damage is greatest with infants and young children.

SIGNS & SYMPTOMS
* Thin or superficial burns (1st-degree burns) are limited to the upper skin layer. They cause redness, tenderness, pain, and swelling.
* Partial thickness burns (2nd-degree burns) affect deeper skin layers. Symptoms are more severe and usually include blisters.
* Full thickness burns (3rd-degree burns) involve all skin layers. Skin is white and appears cooked. There may be no pain at first.

CAUSES
* Rise in skin temperature from heat sources such as fire, steam, or electricity. Open flame and hot liquid are the most common causes.
* Tissue injury caused by chemicals or radiation, including sunlight.
* Lightning strikes can cause internal burns with few external signs.

RISK INCREASES WITH
* Stress, carelessness, smoking in bed, or excess alcohol use. All of these make accidents more likely.
* Job involving exposure to heat or radiation (e.g., firefighting, police work, or factory work).
* Faulty electrical wiring.
* Hot water heaters set too high.

HOW TO PREVENT
* Fireproof your home. Install smoke alarms. Plan emergency exits and do regular fire drills.
* Wear protective gear around heat or radiation.
* Don't touch uncovered electric wires.
* Teach children safety rules for matches, fires, electrical outlets, cords, and stoves.
* Use extension cords only when necessary.
* If you have small children, put safety covers on outlets. Get rid of frayed cords.
* Buy flame-resistant sleepwear for children.

WHAT TO EXPECT

DIAGNOSTIC MEASURES
* Your own observation of symptoms.
* For extensive burns call 911 for emergency help. Emergency care and a hospital stay are usually needed for treatment. Complications, such as lung damage from smoke, may also need treatment.

APPROPRIATE HEALTH CARE
* Self-care for most 1st-degree burns.
* See your health care provider for burns that are more severe or cause concern. The burn area will be examined and treatment given depending on the type of burn and size of the area affected.
* Special dressings and skin-care products may be prescribed.
* Surgery may be needed to graft skin, and rehabilitation may be needed after burns start healing (see Skin Graft in Surgery section).

POSSIBLE COMPLICATIONS
* Infection.
* Shock, due to loss of fluids from the body.
* Severe burns can cause serious health problems that can lead to death.

PROBABLE OUTCOME—Most persons recover if the burns affect less than 50% of the body's surface. With less severe burns, skin usually heals in 1 to 3 weeks.

HOW TO TREAT

GENERAL MEASURES—For minor burns treated at home:
* Place the burned area in cold water, hold it under running water, or use wet compresses on it for 15 minutes (longer for chemical burns). This will reduce pain and swelling. Don't use ice on a burn.
* Use an aloe vera cream or antibiotic ointment. Wrap the area loosely with sterile gauze dressing. This helps protect the area. Change the dressing each day.
* Don't break blisters. This can cause infection.
* Keep the burned area higher than the rest of the body, if possible.

MEDICATION
* You may take acetaminophen or ibuprofen for pain.
* Hospital care may include drugs to treat the burns, for pain, and to prevent infection. A tetanus booster is needed if it is not up to date.

ACTIVITY—Resume normal activity as soon as possible. This will help speed recovery.

DIET—No special diet for minor burns. Severe burns may require use of a feeding tube until symptoms improve.

CALL YOUR DOCTOR IF

* You or a family member has a less severe burn that does not heal in 5 to 6 days.
* Child under age 2 has a burn, even if it seems minor.
* You develop chills, fever; increased pain, redness, swelling, or pus in the burn area.

BURSITIS

GENERAL INFORMATION

DEFINITION—Inflammation (swelling and pain) of a bursa. A bursa is a soft, fluid-filled sac that serves as a cushion between tendons and bones.

BODY PARTS INVOLVED—Bursae, especially near the shoulders, elbows, knees, pelvis, hips or Achilles tendons.

SEX OR AGE MOST AFFECTED—Both sexes; usually in adults.

SIGNS & SYMPTOMS
* Pain, swelling, tenderness, and limited movement in the affected joint. Pain may spread into nearby areas of the body.
* A feeling of warmth over the affected joint.

CAUSES—Inflammation can be caused by overuse, injury, disease, or infection. Sometimes no cause is found.

RISK INCREASES WITH
* Injury to a joint.
* Overuse of a joint.
* Exercising more than usual.
* Calcium deposits in shoulder tendons.
* Infection.
* Arthritis.
* Gout.
* People who suddenly increase their activity levels ("weekend warriors").
* Not stretching properly or over-stretching.

HOW TO PREVENT
* Avoid injuries when possible. Don't overuse muscles. Wear protective gear for contact sports.
* Warm-up before exercise. Cool-down after exercise.
* Stay physically fit.

WHAT TO EXPECT

DIAGNOSTIC MEASURES
* Your own observation of symptoms.
* See your health care provider if self-care does not help or symptoms are severe. Bursitis can be diagnosed by a physical exam.
* Medical tests are usually not needed.

APPROPRIATE HEALTH CARE
* Your health care provider may sometimes drain fluid from the joint with a needle. Surgery is rarely needed.
* Physical therapy may be needed to maintain flexibility, mobility, and strength of the joint.

POSSIBLE COMPLICATIONS
* Prolonged healing time if activity is resumed too soon.
* Chronic bursitis may occur due to repeated injuries or recurrent attacks of bursitis.

PROBABLE OUTCOME—This is a common, but not serious problem. Symptoms usually improve in 7-14 days with treatment.

HOW TO TREAT

GENERAL MEASURES—Self-care may be all that is needed.
* Use RICE therapy (rest, ice, compression, and elevation). Rest the affected joint. Use an ice pack to massage the area several times a day. Use compression by wearing an elastic bandage. Elevate the affected joint by resting it on a pillow.
* You may use heat also. Apply a hot, wet towel or use a heating pad. A deep-heating ointment may help in some cases.

MEDICATION
* Use nonprescription acetaminophen or ibuprofen for mild pain.
* Your health care provider may prescribe:
  - Nonsteroidal anti-inflammatory drugs or creams.
  - Antibiotics (if the bursa is infected).
  - Prescription pain relievers for severe pain.
  - Injection with a local anesthetic mixed with a corticosteroid drug.

ACTIVITY
* Rest the affected joint as much as possible. It may help to wear a sling or a brace, or to use crutches until the pain becomes easier to bear. Begin normal, slow joint movement as soon as pain permits.
* Follow directions for any recommended home exercise routines.

DIET—No special diet.

CALL YOUR DOCTOR IF

* You or a family member has symptoms of bursitis that is severe or self-care methods do not help.
* New symptoms develop after treatment.

CALCIUM IMBALANCE
(Hypercalcemia; Hypocalcemia)

 GENERAL INFORMATION

DEFINITION—Calcium is a mineral that helps regulate the heartbeat, transmit nerve impulses, and contract muscles. It also helps form bone and teeth. Too much calcium (hypercalcemia) or too little calcium (hypocalcemia) can cause serious medical problems. The problems may be life-threatening. Most calcium is stored in the bones, but it is also found in the blood and cells.

BODY PARTS INVOLVED—Membranes of all body cells; muscles; bones; parathyroid glands and parathyroid hormones (these regulate calcium absorption and utilization).

SEX OR AGE MOST AFFECTED—Both sexes; all ages.

SIGNS & SYMPTOMS
Too little calcium:
* Muscle spasms, twitching, or cramping.
* Arms, hands, legs, and feet may tingle or feel numb.
* Seizures (convulsion).
* Heart-beat is irregular.
* High blood pressure.
Too much calcium (often produces no symptoms):
* Feeling tired and sluggish.
* Loss of appetite.
* Vomiting, diarrhea, dehydration, and thirst.
* Heart-beat is irregular.
* Low blood pressure.
* Depression or mental changes (confused or delirious).
* Seizures or coma (in severe cases).

CAUSES
Too little calcium:
* Parathyroid glands that are underactive. This can be caused by disease or damage to the parathyroid.
* Not getting enough calcium and vitamin D.
* The body does not absorb calcium from the stomach.
* Severe burns or infections.
* Problems with the pancreas.
* Kidney failure.
* Low levels of certain minerals in your blood.
Too much calcium:
* Parathyroid gland that is overactive.
* Broken bones and long periods of bed rest.
* Cancer of the bone marrow.
* Tumors that destroy bone.

RISK INCREASES WITH
Too little calcium:
* Use of certain drugs such as diuretics.
* Injury, cancer, or surgery of the thyroid or parathyroid glands.
* Excess alcohol use.
* Poor nutrition.

Too much calcium:
* Diet that is too high in dairy products or excess use of antacids that contain calcium.
* Kidney disease.
* Being inactive or confined to bed for long time.

HOW TO PREVENT
* Eat a normal, well-balanced diet.
* Avoid alcohol, or limit it to 1 to 2 drinks a day.
* Avoid regular use of nonprescription antacids.

 WHAT TO EXPECT

DIAGNOSTIC MEASURES
* Your own observation of symptoms.
* Your health care provider may do a physical exam. Medical tests can include blood studies of calcium levels, x-rays of bones and echocardiogram (a heart study).

APPROPRIATE HEALTH CARE—Treatment involves correcting the problem or treating the disorder causing the imbalance. This may be all that is required. In other cases, treatment may be needed to remove excess calcium or replace low calcium levels.

POSSIBLE COMPLICATIONS
* Heart attack.
* Bones may become weak and break easily.
* Kidney stones from high calcium.
* Ulcer from high calcium.

PROBABLE OUTCOME—Most cases can be cured with treatment in 1 week.

 HOW TO TREAT

GENERAL MEASURES—None specific.

MEDICATION
* Drugs may be prescribed to raise or lower your calcium levels, depending on the need. Drugs may be given by mouth or through a needle placed in your vein (IV).
* Drugs may be prescribed to treat a disorder that is the cause of the calcium imbalance.

ACTIVITY—After treatment, return to your normal activities slowly as symptoms improve.

DIET
* For mild, low calcium level, calcium pills and vitamin D may be recommended. Get more protein, milk, and milk products in your diet.
* For a mild, high-calcium level, reduce dairy products and antacids that contain calcium.

 CALL YOUR DOCTOR IF

* You or a family member has symptoms of calcium imbalance.
* Symptoms get worse or they don't improve.

CANDIDIASIS OF SKIN
(Moniliasis)

 GENERAL INFORMATION

DEFINITION—A yeast infection in skin folds, or in areas of skin that touch other areas of skin.

BODY PARTS INVOLVED—It can affect the skin of the scrotum, vagina and vaginal lips; underarm area; spaces between fingers and toes; inner thighs; under the breasts; and over the base of the spine (sacrum).

SEX OR AGE MOST AFFECTED—Both sexes; all ages.

SIGNS & SYMPTOMS
* Plaques (patches or flat areas) on skin.
* Bright-red patches with poorly defined borders. They are often 2.5 to 5 inches across, but may be larger.
* Patches may weep or ooze.
* Skin appears moist and crusted.
* Itching is usually severe.
* Smaller patches may surround larger patches. They sometimes form small white blisters with pus inside.

CAUSES—Yeast infection of the skin is caused by *Candida*, a type of fungus. *Candida* fungi actually live on the skin and normally cause no harm. If skin is damaged or there is excess moisture and warmth, the fungus germs can grow and cause infection. The infection can be spread from one person to another by direct contact, and less often, by sexual contact. Germs are also spread by sharing damp towels or washcloths.

RISK INCREASES WITH
* Use of oral antibiotics.
* Use of any type of steroids.
* Diabetes.
* The elderly or infants (it causes diaper rash).
* Pregnant women or use of birth control pills.
* Use of plastic pants in infants or pantyhose in women.
* Obesity.
* Existing skin infection or skin disorder.
* Weak immune system due to illness or drugs.
* Work that involves skin being wet continuously.

HOW TO PREVENT
* Take antibiotics only when prescribed.
* Keep skin cool and dry.
* Avoid risk factors where possible.

 WHAT TO EXPECT

DIAGNOSTIC MEASURES
* Your own observation of symptoms.
* Your health care provider can diagnose the infection by an exam of the affected skin area.
* Medical tests may include a study of a skin scraping or pus.

APPROPRIATE HEALTH CARE
* Treatment involves drugs and self-care measures.
* Any skin condition that may have lead to the candidiasis infection should be treated also.

POSSIBLE COMPLICATIONS
* Nail infection, causing them to thicken or crumble.
* Bacterial infection, in addition to the fungal infection.
* Infection spreading to the whole body (in those with weak immune systems).

PROBABLE OUTCOME
* Usually curable in 2 weeks with treatment. Without treatment, healing may be slow.
* It is common for these fungal infections to recur.

 HOW TO TREAT

GENERAL MEASURES
* Keep skin cool and dry. Expose affected skin areas to air as much as possible.
* Wear loose cotton clothing. Avoid synthetic or wool fabrics. Change socks often if feet are affected.
* To avoid spreading germs, don't go barefoot on wet floors where other people may walk. Don't share towels. Clean the bathtub or shower after you use it.
* Protect skin from injury, but don't bandage the affected skin.

MEDICATION—Antifungal drugs to be applied to the skin are usually prescribed. Gently massage a small amount into the affected area as directed. Use only enough to cover the affected area. Larger amounts don't help. In more severe cases, an antifungal drug taken by mouth may be prescribed.

ACTIVITY—No restrictions, except to avoid heat and sweating.

DIET—No special diet. Eating yogurt may or may not help prevent yeast infections (research is unclear).

 CALL YOUR DOCTOR IF

* You or a family member has symptoms of candidiasis.
* The following occur during treatment:
  - Infection continues to spread despite treatment.
  - Signs of bacterial infection develop (pain, tenderness, redness, warmth, and oozing).
* New unexplained symptoms develop. Drugs used in treatment may produce side effects.

CANKER SORES
(Aphthous Ulcers)

GENERAL INFORMATION

DEFINITION—Painful ulcers (sores) that occur in the lining of the mouth. They cannot be spread from one person to another. They may be confused with herpes infections.

BODY PARTS INVOLVED—Mouth and adjacent areas.

SEX OR AGE MOST AFFECTED—Both sexes, but more common in women.

SIGNS & SYMPTOMS
* Ulcers are small, very painful, shallow, and covered by a gray membrane. Borders are surrounded by an intense red halo.
* Ulcers appear on lips, gums, inner cheeks, tongue, palate, and throat. Usually, 2 or 3 ulcers appear during an attack. As many as 10 to 15 ulcers is not uncommon.
* Ulcers may be so painful during first 2 or 3 days that they interfere with eating or speaking.
* Sometimes there is tingling or burning for 24 hours before the ulcer appears.

CAUSES—Exact cause is unknown.

RISK INCREASES WITH
* Emotional or physical stress; anxiety or premenstrual tension.
* Injury to the mouth lining caused by rough dentures, hot food, toothbrushing, or dental work.
* Irritation from foods, such as chocolate, citrus, acidic foods (e.g., vinegar, pickles), salted nuts, or potato chips.
* Changes in the body's immune system.
* Family history of canker sores.

HOW TO PREVENT
* Brush teeth at least twice a day. Floss regularly to keep the mouth clean and healthy.
* Avoid risk factors where possible.
* Pay attention to your diet and when canker sores develop. Don't eat foods that seem to trigger the sores.

WHAT TO EXPECT

DIAGNOSTIC MEASURES
* Your own observation of symptoms.
* If you are concerned about the sores, see your health care provider. Canker sores can normally be diagnosed by an exam of the mouth.
* A culture of the sores may be done to rule out herpes infection.

APPROPRIATE HEALTH CARE
* Medical care is usually not needed.
* If a canker sore is caused by a rough tooth, braces, or dentures, consult your dentist. The sore won't heal until the cause is treated.

POSSIBLE COMPLICATIONS—Rarely, dehydration may occur if eating and drinking are limited by the pain of the canker sores.

PROBABLE OUTCOME—Most will heal on their own in 2 weeks. It is common for them to recur. Recurrence can vary from a single canker sore 2 or 3 times a year, to frequent episodes of many sores.

HOW TO TREAT

GENERAL MEASURES—Rinse the mouth 3 or more times a day with a salt solution (1/2 teaspoon salt to 8 oz. water) if this isn't painful.

MEDICATION
* A dental paste that contains steroids may be used. If applied as soon as the ulcer begins, it helps reduce pain.
* Aphthasol (amlexanox), a paste used only for canker sores may be prescribed. It helps with pain and hastens healing. Follow instructions on the label on how to use.
* Special mouthwashes may be prescribed.

ACTIVITY—No limits.

DIET
* Avoid foods that irritate the sores. Drink lots of fluids. If possible, eat a well-balanced diet while healing.
* To avoid pain, sip liquids through straws. Foods that cause the least pain are milk, liquid gelatin, yogurt, ice cream, and custard.

CALL YOUR DOCTOR IF

* You or a family member has canker sores that don't improve in 2 weeks.
* Other symptoms occur at the same time as canker sores.
* New, unexplained symptoms develop. Drugs used in treatment may produce side effects.

ILLNESS & DISORDERS

CARBON MONOXIDE POISONING

 GENERAL INFORMATION

DEFINITION—Breathing in carbon monoxide (CO), a poison gas that has no color or smell. CO is produced when gas or wood is burned. Common sources include smoke from fires, motor vehicle or boat exhaust, space heaters, furnaces, charcoal grills, and gas burning appliances.

BODY PARTS INVOLVED—Total body.

SEX OR AGE MOST AFFECTED—Both sexes; all ages.

SIGNS & SYMPTOMS
* The first symptoms may be mild and flu-like.
* Headache, feeling dizzy and tired.
* Nausea and vomiting; stomach pain.
* Feeling like you might faint, trouble with walking.
* Difficulty breathing, chest pain, and changes in heartbeat.
* Seizure.
* Vision changes.
* Confusion, depression, and other behavior changes.
* Coma (loss of consciousness).

CAUSES—Carbon monoxide is breathed into the lungs. It gets into the blood system and prevents the flow of oxygen that the body needs for survival. It is the most common form of accidental poisoning in the United States.

RISK INCREASES WITH
* Furnaces or space-heating devices that do not work properly; a fireplace with a clogged chimney.
* Riding in the back of a pickup truck under a closed cover of some type.
* Poor venting (exhaust fumes escape into buildings or homes).
* Use of charcoal grill in enclosed place, such as a tent.
* Faulty motor vehicle exhaust system, or leaving a car running in a garage attached to a house.
* Winter months when heaters are in use and houses are more closed up.

HOW TO PREVENT
* Avoid the risk factors where you are able.
* Install a carbon monoxide alarm in your home. If it goes off, leave the house right away and call 911.
* Make sure the furnace, fireplaces, gas appliances, and heaters in your home work properly. Call your gas company if you think there may be a gas leak.
* Use products that will help prevent fires in your home (such as smoke alarms, fire extinguishers).

 WHAT TO EXPECT

DIAGNOSTIC MEASURES
* Your own observation of symptoms.
* Your health care provider will do a physical exam and test your blood for carbon monoxide.
* Other medical tests may be done for more severe symptoms.

APPROPRIATE HEALTH CARE
* For mild cases, the symptoms usually disappear after you breathe in pure oxygen through a mask for a few hours.
* Some patients with more severe symptoms will require the use of breathing support in a hospital.
* Rarely, a patient is placed in a sealed chamber where high-pressure oxygen is used for treatment.

POSSIBLE COMPLICATIONS
* Poisoning can result in damage to the brain, heart, or lungs; and death. Children, the elderly, and those with lung disease are at high risk for adverse effects.
* Pregnant women may suffer miscarriage, early labor, fetal death, or a child with cerebral palsy.

PROBABLE OUTCOME
* In milder cases with quick treatment, recovery is complete and without complications.
* Some patients have delayed symptoms weeks later. They may feel extra tired, have memory problems, feel confused, or have mood and behavior changes.

 HOW TO TREAT

GENERAL MEASURES
* This type of poisoning can not be treated at home. Medical care is needed.
* To learn more: Consumer Product Safety Commission, (800) 638-2772, or Medline Plus website: www.nlm.nih.gov/medlineplus/carbonmonoxide poisoning.html.

MEDICATION—Usually not needed. Drugs may be used for seizures if they occur.

ACTIVITY—Depends on severity of symptoms.

DIET—No special diet.

 CALL YOUR DOCTOR IF

* You or a family member has symptoms of carbon monoxide poisoning.
* Symptoms get worse, recur, or new symptoms occur after recovery.

CARCINOID SYNDROME

 GENERAL INFORMATION

DEFINITION—A group of symptoms caused by tumors (carcinoids). Carcinoids secrete hormones and chemicals that cause the symptoms to develop.

BODY PARTS INVOLVED—The tumors can occur in the small intestine, appendix, rectum, colon, stomach, pancreas, liver, lungs, and (rarely) other organs.

SEX OR AGE MOST AFFECTED—Adults (of both sexes) usually ages 50 to 70.

SIGNS & SYMPTOMS
* Carcinoids grow slowly and can be benign or malignant (cancerous). Many persons have no symptoms.
* The primary tumor may cause intestinal obstruction (painful cramps in the middle of the abdomen, vomiting, swelling, and weight loss).
* In a few cases, carcinoid cells spread to other body parts and produce secondary, hormone-producing (serotonin) tumors. Heavy exercise, alcohol use, or eating bananas, tomatoes, plums, avocados, pineapple, or walnuts may trigger symptoms of these secondary tumors. These symptoms include:
- Flushed skin on the head and neck.
- Watery eyes.
- Diarrhea with abdominal cramps.
- Respiratory symptoms similar to asthma.
- Irregular heartbeat.
- Nausea and vomiting.
- Low blood pressure.
- Unexplained weight loss.

CAUSES—Unknown.

RISK INCREASES WITH
* Older adults.
* Smoking.
* Family history of multiple endocrine neoplasia, type 1 (a hereditary disorder).

HOW TO PREVENT—Cannot be prevented at present.

 WHAT TO EXPECT

DIAGNOSTIC MEASURES
* Carcinoids may be discovered during a diagnostic test or surgery for some other disorder.
* Your health care provider will do a physical exam and ask questions about your symptoms.
* A number of medical tests will be done. The tests help diagnose any cancer and then determine if it has spread (staging).

APPROPRIATE HEALTH CARE
* Treatment varies and depends on the location and size of the tumor, any spread of a cancer, your health, age, and preferences.

* Treatment may include surgery, anticancer drugs (chemotherapy), or other drugs.
* Surgery to remove the carcinoid tumor depends on the location. In some cases, surgery can bring about a cure. The entire tumor may be removed, or a portion of the tumor (as large a as possible) will be removed. This relieves symptoms because less of the harmful hormones are produced.

POSSIBLE COMPLICATIONS
* Cancer may spread to other body parts.
* Low blood pressure.
* Risk for stroke, blood clots, and similar disorders.
* Bowel obstruction.
* Heart failure.
* Angioedema (hives).
* Renal failure.

PROBABLE OUTCOME—The outcome will vary. In some, it can be cured with surgery. In others, the problem may progress, recur, or relapse.

 HOW TO TREAT

GENERAL MEASURES
* The more you can learn and understand about a disease, the more you will be able to make informed decisions about where to go for your care, the treatments available, the risks involved, side effects of therapy and expected outcome.
* To learn more: The American Cancer Society, (800) ACS-2345; website: www.cancer.org or National Cancer Institute, (800)4-CANCER; website: www.nci.nih.gov.

MEDICATION—The following may be prescribed:
* Antidiarrheal drugs.
* Anticancer drugs (they do not cure these tumors, but may help symptoms).
* Drugs to prevent serotonin production.
* Drugs to prevent flushed skin.
* Cortisone drugs to reduce inflammation
* Multivitamins and niacin supplements.

ACTIVITY—Resume your normal activities once symptoms improve. Avoid strenuous exercise.

DIET
* Include at least 2 servings of protein a day (or as advised).
* Avoid foods that trigger symptoms.
* Don't drink alcohol.

 CALL YOUR DOCTOR IF

* You or a family member has symptoms of carcinoid syndrome.
* Symptoms become worse, despite treatment.
* New, unexplained symptoms develop. Drugs used in treatment may produce side effects.

CARDIAC ARREST

 GENERAL INFORMATION

DEFINITION—Total loss of heart-pumping action. Delay of treatment for only 3 to 5 minutes may cause death or permanent brain damage.

BODY PARTS INVOLVED—Heart.

SEX OR AGE MOST AFFECTED— Up to age 45, it is more common in men. After age 45, the incidence is equal in men and women.

SIGNS & SYMPTOMS
• Brief dizziness, followed by fainting and unconsciousness.
• No pulse. Usually breathing also stops.
• Skin color becomes bluish-white. The pupils of the eye may get bigger.
• Seizures.
• Loss of bowel and bladder control (sometimes). Simple fainting may seem like a cardiac arrest, but heartbeat and breathing continue.

CAUSES—Heart stops beating suddenly. This may be due to a heart that is beating too fast, too slow, or that has an irregular heartbeat. Other causes include electrical shock, drowning, choking, trauma, or respiratory arrest (lungs stop working).

RISK INCREASES WITH
• Heart attack or heart disease.
• Lack of blood circulation and profound shock caused by uncontrolled bleeding or overwhelming infection.
• Loss of oxygen from drowning, choking, or during surgery from the anesthesia.
• Potassium or fluid imbalance in the blood.
• Diabetes.
• Use of certain heart medicines.
• Use of medicines that help with fluid retention. These can cause low potassium in the blood.
• Use of any drug that raises blood pressure in a heart patient. This can include cold capsules, decongestant tablets, and nasal sprays.
• Using drugs of abuse, such as cocaine and intravenous drugs.

HOW TO PREVENT
• Live a healthy lifestyle. Get regular exercise, eat a healthy diet, maintain ideal weight for height, and don't smoke.
• If you have heart disease or other risk factors, follow your treatment instructions carefully.
• Have family members and close friends learn CPR (cardiopulmonary resuscitation).
• Automated external defibrillators (AEDs) are being placed in public places (such as airports). They can be used by anyone to help a person who is having cardiac arrest.

 WHAT TO EXPECT

DIAGNOSTIC MEASURES—Your observation of symptoms. Once the patient is in the hospital, medical tests will confirm the diagnosis.

APPROPRIATE HEALTH CARE
• People who know how to recognize cardiac arrest and can perform CPR can often get the heart beating again. Someone may mistake fainting or other causes of unconsciousness for cardiac arrest. Check for a neck pulse before starting CPR.
• The victim must be taken to the nearest emergency facility as soon as the heartbeat is restored. Cardiac arrest may recur.
• Emergency medical care may involve shocking the heart back into a normal heartbeat. This process is called defibrillation.

POSSIBLE COMPLICATIONS
• Death or permanent brain damage if heart action cannot be resumed in 3 to 5 minutes.
• Mistaking a faint or other causes of unconsciousness for cardiac arrest. Check for a neck pulse before starting cardiopulmonary resuscitation (CPR).

PROBABLE OUTCOME—The final outcome, depends on the underlying cause of the cardiac arrest.

 HOW TO TREAT

GENERAL MEASURES
• Ensure that you and your family members learn CPR. Call your local Red Cross or hospital for information. You may save a life.
• If you have heart disease or have risk factors, wear a medical alert identification (a bracelet or neck tag).

MEDICATION—Drugs may be prescribed to treat the cause of cardiac arrest once the crisis is over.

ACTIVITY—After recovery, activities should be resumed gradually. Follow your health care provider's instructions.

DIET—Don't give fluids or foods to anyone with signs of cardiac arrest. He or she could choke.

 CALL YOUR DOCTOR IF

If the victim is not conscious and not breathing:
• Call 911 (emergency) for an ambulance or medical help.
• Yell for help. Don't leave the victim.
• Begin mouth-to-mouth breathing immediately.
• If there is no heartbeat, give CPR.
• Don't stop CPR until help arrives.

CARDIOMYOPATHY

 GENERAL INFORMATION

DEFINITION—An inflammatory disorder of the heart muscle. Damage to the heart muscle causes the heart to weaken and not be able to pump enough blood to the body. In addition, blood moves more slowly through an enlarged heart, allowing blood clots to easily form. Cardiomyopathy can lead to heart failure.

BODY PARTS INVOLVED—Heart muscle. Decreasing heart function eventually affects the lungs, liver and circulatory system.

SEX OR AGE MOST AFFECTED—Adults of any age and is more common in males.

SIGNS & SYMPTOMS—If the condition is severe enough to cause heart failure, the following symptoms may occur:
- Rapid and abnormal heartbeat.
- Shortness of breath (may be worse when lying down or being physically active).
- Swollen legs, feet, and ankles.
- Feeling tired and weak.
- Chest pain.
- Loss of appetite (weight gain may still occur).
- Dizziness or fainting.
- Cough.

CAUSES—There are different types of cardiomyopathy. They can be caused by a variety of heath problems. Sometimes, no cause is found.

RISK INCREASES WITH
- Viral infection of the heart muscle.
- Severe coronary artery disease.
- High blood pressure and high levels of fats in the blood.
- Alcoholism.
- Heart surgery.
- Family history of heart disease.
- Congenital (being born with) heart disease.
- Certain infections (amyloidosis and sarcoidosis).
- Postpartum (after pregnancy and delivery).
- Smoking.
- Diabetes.
- Stress.
- Being physically inactive (sedentary lifestyle).
- Obesity.

HOW TO PREVENT—No specific preventive measures. Avoid risk factors, where possible.

 WHAT TO EXPECT

DIAGNOSTIC MEASURES
- Your own observation of symptoms.
- Your health care provider will do a physical exam and ask questions about your symptoms and activities.

- Medical tests may include chest x-ray, heart function studies, and blood tests. A tube-like instrument may be inserted into the heart and a biopsy (removal of a sample of heart tissue for testing) may be done.

APPROPRIATE HEALTH CARE
- The goals of treatment are to improve symptoms and to prevent complications. Treatment steps may involve lifestyle changes, drug therapy, and/or surgery.
- Lifestyle changes can include stopping the use of alcohol and cigarette smoking, diet changes, weight loss, and limiting physical activity.
- Surgery may include implanting a pacemaker to change the heart rate and pattern. Surgery to remove part of the thickened heart wall or replace heart valves may be needed.
- A heart transplant may be recommended if other treatments are not successful. A long wait for a transplant is normal. A mechanical device may be used to temporarily help the heart.

POSSIBLE COMPLICATIONS—Congestive heart failure (which can be life-threatening).

PROBABLE OUTCOME—Sometimes, the heart damage cannot be reversed. Improvement can occur. Treatment may help relieve symptoms and prevent further damage. Some patients may be considered for a heart transplant.

 HOW TO TREAT

GENERAL MEASURES
- Stop smoking, Find a way to quit that works.
- Get regular medical and dental checkups.

MEDICATION—Drugs may be prescribed to improve heart function, to slow and regulate the heart rate, get rid of extra fluid, lower blood pressure, relax blood vessels, and suppress the immune system.

ACTIVITY—Follow medical advice about physical activity limits and when it is safe to resume sexual relations.

DIET
- If advised, eat a diet that is low in salt and fat. Avoid alcohol.
- Begin a weight-loss diet if you weigh more than is healthy for your body type.

 CALL YOUR DOCTOR IF

- You or a family member has symptoms of cardiomyopathy.
- Symptoms return after treatment.
- You have chest pain.
- New, unexplained symptoms develop. Drugs used in treatment may produce side effects.

CARPAL-TUNNEL SYNDROME

GENERAL INFORMATION

DEFINITION—A nerve disorder that causes pain, loss of feeling, and loss of strength in the hands.

BODY PARTS INVOLVED—It usually affects the thumb and first three fingers. In some cases, it may affect the 4th and 5th fingers only.

SEX OR AGE MOST AFFECTED—Both sexes, but most common in women between ages 29 and 62.

SIGNS & SYMPTOMS
* Tingling or numbness in part of the hand.
* Sharp pains that shoot from the wrist up the arm, especially at night.
* Burning sensations in the fingers.
* Morning stiffness or cramping of hands.
* Thumb weakness.
* Inability to make a fist.

CAUSES—It appears to result from either repetitive hand and wrist movement (repeating the same motion over and over) or an injury. The tendons or ligaments of the wrist become stretched and swollen. This puts pressure on the nerve that goes into the hand and fingers.

RISK INCREASES WITH
* Work that requires repetitive hand or wrist action. This includes factory assembly or packaging work, cashiering, janitors, or cleaning jobs, dental hygienists, butchers and meat cutters, or using a computer mouse.
* Certain medical or physical conditions may increase the risk. These include arthritis, diabetes, untreated hypothyroidism, obesity, menopause, and pregnancy.
* Sports activities, such as racquetball or handball.
* People who smoke, use alcohol, or have high levels of stress may be more at risk.

HOW TO PREVENT
* Take a break at least once an hour if doing repetitive work involving the hands. Stand up, stretch, and/or walk around.
* Learn to use a computer mouse safely. Don't squeeze or grip it too tightly. Use your arm to move it around, not just your wrist in a side-to-side movement.
* Don't wear tight watch bands or bracelets, or clothing that fits tightly at the wrists.
* Ask your health care provider if wrist splints will help you in the work that you do.

WHAT TO EXPECT

DIAGNOSTIC MEASURES
* Your own observation of symptoms. For a simple test, place the backs of your hands together with your fingers pointing straight down and your elbows pointing straight out to the side (wrists are at a 90° angle). If symptoms are brought on by you holding this position for one minute, you may have carpal-tunnel syndrome.
* Your health care provider will examine your hand and wrist and ask questions about your symptoms and activities.
* Medical tests may be done to study nerve conduction.

APPROPRIATE HEALTH CARE
* Conservative therapy is often tried first. Follow medical advice about how to treat. Consider techniques listed in General Measures.
* Surgery to free the pinched nerve may be needed. The procedure may be done as an outpatient. Allow 2 weeks for healing. Physical therapy will then help rebuild wrist strength.

POSSIBLE COMPLICATIONS—If untreated or treated too late, permanent numbness and a weak thumb or fingers in the affected hand may occur.

PROBABLE OUTCOME—Symptoms usually improve with treatment.

HOW TO TREAT

GENERAL MEASURES
* If you awaken at night with hand pain, hang it over the side of the bed, rub it, or shake it.
* Use ice or warm and cold soaks if they help with symptoms.
* Wearing a splint on the affected wrist may be recommended.
* For work at a computer terminal, be sure that the desk, keyboard, and chair are at the proper height. Take a break once an hour.

MEDICATION
* You may try aspirin or ibuprofen to reduce pain and inflammation.
* Anti-inflammatory drugs, cortisone injections at the wrist to reduce inflammation, and vitamin B6 injections or tablets may be prescribed.

ACTIVITY—Once symptoms get better, begin a routine of both aerobic and weight-training exercise to improve fitness.

DIET—Eat a normal, well-balanced diet.

CALL YOUR DOCTOR IF

* You or a family member has symptoms of carpal tunnel syndrome.
* Symptoms of carpal tunnel syndrome don't lessen in 2 weeks after treatment.
* New, unexplained symptoms develop. Drugs used in treatment may produce side effects.

CAT-SCRATCH DISEASE

GENERAL INFORMATION

DEFINITION—A mild, infectious disease caused by a small bacteria resulting from a scratch by a cat (most often a kitten). It is not contagious from person to person. More than one family member can be infected at one time.

BODY PARTS INVOLVED—Skin and the lymph nodes.

SEX OR AGE MOST AFFECTED—Both sexes; all ages.

SIGNS & SYMPTOMS
• A lump, with or without pus or fluid, which starts on the scratched skin 3 to 10 days after the cat scratch.
• Swollen lymph nodes near the affected area.
• Fever of 99°F to 101°F (37.2°C to 38.3°C).
• Fatigue.
• Headache.
• Loss of appetite.
• AIDS patients or patients on immune-suppression drugs may have more severe symptoms.

CAUSES—A bacterium (*Bartonella henselae*) carried on cat's claws. The infection spreads to lymph glands near the scratch by way of lymphatic vessels. Most of the animals involved are healthy.

RISK INCREASES WITH—Owning or handling cats.

HOW TO PREVENT
• Teach children to avoid rough play with a cat or kitten.
• Don't pick up strange cats.

WHAT TO EXPECT

DIAGNOSTIC MEASURES
• Your own observation of symptoms.
• Your health care provider can usually diagnose the disorder by an exam of the affected skin, feeling the swollen lymph nodes, and knowing about the exposure to a cat.
• Medical tests may include skin or blood tests to rule out other disorders that can cause swollen lymph nodes.

APPROPRIATE HEALTH CARE
• Medical care is usually not needed. An antibiotic drug may be prescribed.
• Needle aspiration to drain the lymph gland is rarely needed.

POSSIBLE COMPLICATIONS—Unlikely to occur in otherwise healthy persons. People with weak immune systems may develop central nervous system problems.

PROBABLE OUTCOME—The condition normally heals on its own. The skin symptoms usually clear up in 1 to 3 weeks. Swollen lymph nodes may take 2 to 4 months (and sometimes longer) to heal.

HOW TO TREAT

GENERAL MEASURES
• Apply heat to affected areas; use warm soaks or use heating pad.
• It is not necessary to isolate the ill person because the disease is not transmitted from person to person.
• Consult your veterinarian about the cat or kitten that caused the infection.

MEDICATION
• Antibiotics may be prescribed.
• To ease discomfort or soreness, use nonprescription acetaminophen or ibuprofen.

ACTIVITY—Get extra rest if you feel tired. Avoid activities that might cause injuries to swollen lymph nodes.

DIET—No special diet.

CALL YOUR DOCTOR IF

• You or a family member has symptoms of cat-scratch disease that cause concern.
• A swollen lymph gland becomes painful and red.

ILLNESS & DISORDERS

CATARACT

GENERAL INFORMATION

DEFINITION—A clouding of the lens of the eye. The lens is a clear, flexible structure near the front of the eyeball. It helps to keep vision in focus and screens and refracts light. Cataracts may form in one or both eyes. If they form in both eyes, their growth rate may be very different. They can take several months or several years to develop. They do not spread from one eye to the other.

BODY PARTS INVOLVED—Lens of the eye(s).

SEX OR AGE MOST AFFECTED
• Adults over 60.
• Newborns (congenital form only).

SIGNS & SYMPTOMS
• Blurred vision. It may be worse in bright light. The blurring may first become apparent while driving at night, when lights seem to scatter or have halos.
• Difficulty reading.
• Faded colors.
• Poor night vision.
• Double or multiple vision.
• Opaque, milky-white pupil (advanced stages only).
• Frequent changes in prescription for eyeglasses.

CAUSES
• The lens of the eye is made up of water and protein. The protein is arranged in a certain way that keeps the lens clear and lets light pass through it. A cataract forms when some of the protein clumps together and begin to cloud a small area of the lens. Over time, it grows larger and affects vision.
• Congenital (present at birth) cataracts can occur.

RISK INCREASES WITH
• Natural aging.
• Illnesses with high blood sugar, such as diabetes.
• Prolonged exposure to sunlight.
• Chronic eye disease.
• Exposure to some types of radiation.
• Family history of cataracts.
• Smoking.
• Use of steroid drugs.
• Surgery for other eye problems.
• Injury to the eye (cataract can occur years later).

HOW TO PREVENT— No specific preventive measures. Getting medical care for eye disorders, wearing sunglasses (that filter UV light) outside during the day, and not smoking may help reduce the risk or delay cataract development.

WHAT TO EXPECT

DIAGNOSTIC MEASURES
• Your own observation of symptoms.
• Cataracts are usually diagnosed with an exam done by an eye doctor (ophthalmologist).

APPROPRIATE HEALTH CARE
• Treatment depends on amount of vision problems.
• Surgery to remove cataracts is recommended if vision loss interferes with daily activities, such as reading, watching television, or driving.
• Surgery may be done on an inpatient or outpatient basis. Usually one eye is operated on at a time (if cataracts are in both eyes). The eye lens is usually removed and replaced with an artificial lens. Different types of surgery are available. Your options will be explained to you. After surgery, you will be given instructions for home care. (See Cataract Removal with Intraocular Lens Replacement in Surgery section.)

POSSIBLE COMPLICATIONS
• Loss of vision.
• After surgery complications. These include inflammation, infections, bleeding, loss of vision, and light flashes. These can usually be treated successfully.

PROBABLE OUTCOME—Some cataracts never impair vision enough to require surgery. During the time cataracts are forming, frequent eyeglass changes may help vision. Cataracts that cause vision problems can be cured with surgery.

HOW TO TREAT

GENERAL MEASURES—Wear eyeglasses that provide maximum benefit, if vision is not too badly affected.

MEDICATION—Eye drops or drugs taken by mouth may be prescribed after your surgery.

ACTIVITY—No limits. Don't drive at night if your vision is poor.

DIET—No special diet.

CALL YOUR DOCTOR IF

(Or call your eye care provider).
• You or a family member has symptoms of cataracts.
• Any eye symptoms develop after cataract surgery.

CELIAC DISEASE
(Gluten Enteropathy; Nontropical Sprue)

 GENERAL INFORMATION

DEFINITION—An allergic condition in the small intestine, triggered by gluten. Gluten is a protein found in most grains. It prevents the intestine from absorbing nutrients. Most forms of celiac disease are inherited.

BODY PARTS INVOLVED—Digestive system.

SEX OR AGE MOST AFFECTED—It usually begins during infancy or early childhood (2 weeks to 1 year). Symptoms may appear when the child first begins eating food with gluten. In adults, symptoms may develop gradually over months or even years.

SIGNS & SYMPTOMS
* Weight loss or slowed weight gain in an infant following the introduction of cereal to the diet.
* Poor appetite.
* Loose, pale, bulky, bad-smelling stools; frequent gas.
* Swollen abdomen; stomach pain.
* Mouth ulcers.
* Anemia or vitamin deficiency, with fatigue, pale skin, skin rash, or bone pain.
* Mildly bowed legs in children.
* Vague tiredness and weakness.
* Swollen legs.

CAUSES—Celiac disease is a congenital (present at birth) disorder. It is caused by an intolerance for gluten, a protein present in most grains.

RISK INCREASES WITH
* Family history of celiac disease.
* Pregnancy.
* Other allergies.

HOW TO PREVENT—Cannot be prevented at present.

 WHAT TO EXPECT

DIAGNOSTIC MEASURES
* Your own observation of symptoms.
* Your health care provider may do a physical exam and ask questions about your symptoms.
* Medical tests may include blood, urine, and stool studies. A biopsy may be done (a small sample of tissue is taken from the small intestine for viewing under a microscope). Sometimes, diagnosis is based on a person going on a gluten-free diet to see if the symptoms stop.

APPROPRIATE HEALTH CARE—The only treatment is a gluten-free diet.

POSSIBLE COMPLICATIONS—In rare cases, gluten withdrawal does not bring immediate improvement.

PROBABLE OUTCOME—With a strict, gluten-free diet, most persons with celiac disease can expect a normal life. Improvement begins in 2 to 3 weeks.

 HOW TO TREAT

GENERAL MEASURES
* Pay careful attention to the dietary instructions provided by your doctor or dietitian.
* To learn more: Celiac Sprue Association, P.O. Box 31700, Omaha. NE 68131; (877) 272-4272; website: www.csaceliacs.org or Celiac Disease Foundation, 13251 Ventura Blvd., Studio City, CA 91604; (818) 990-2354 (not toll free); website www.celiac.org.

MEDICATION
* Iron and folic acid for anemia may be prescribed.
* Calcium and multiple-vitamin supplements for deficiencies may be recommended.
* Cortisone drugs to reduce the body's inflammatory response may be prescribed.

ACTIVITY—No limits.

DIET—Gluten-free diet. Gluten is found in wheat, rye, barley, and possibly oats. It is difficult to exclude gluten from the diet completely. Be patient while becoming familiar with the diet. A dietitian can help you with a diet plan.

 CALL YOUR DOCTOR IF

* You or your child has symptoms of celiac disease.
* Symptoms don't decrease after 3 weeks of eating a gluten-free diet.
* The child fails to regain lost weight or grow and develop as expected.
* Fever develops.

ILLNESS & DISORDERS

CELLULITIS
(Erysipelas)

GENERAL INFORMATION

DEFINITION—An inflammation of the skin and the tissues just below the skin (subcutaneous).

BODY PARTS INVOLVED—Skin anywhere on the body, but most likely on the face or lower legs. Erysipelas is the name of a severe cellulitis of the face.

SEX OR AGE MOST AFFECTED—Both sexes; all ages.

SIGNS & SYMPTOMS
* Tenderness, warmth, swelling, and redness in an area of the skin. A thin red line may extend from the area toward the heart. Fluid or pus may leak out.
* Fever, chills, sweating, and a general ill feeling.
* Lymph glands nearest the area may be swollen.

CAUSES—Infection with bacteria, or, rarely, a fungal infection. It can begin with a minor injury to the skin that is invaded by the bacteria. The infection leads to inflammation, which is the body's response to infection. Cellulitis cannot be passed from one person to another.

RISK INCREASES WITH
* Chronic illness, such as diabetes.
* Weak immune system due to illness or drugs.
* Any injury that breaks the skin.
* Use of drugs by injection.
* Burns.
* Surgical wound infection.
* Skin disorders (eczema or psoriasis) or infections that cause skin symptoms, such as chickenpox.
* Poor blood circulation.

HOW TO PREVENT
* Keep the skin clean.
* Avoid skin damage. Use protective clothing or proper gear for work or sports where injuries may occur.
* Wear shoes that fit well. Avoid going barefoot in areas where there may be risk of injury.
* If the skin is injured, wash the area with soap and water. Check the injured skin for the next few days to make sure it is healing. If not, seek medical care.
* Avoid swimming if you have any skin sores.

WHAT TO EXPECT

DIAGNOSTIC MEASURES
* Your own observation of symptoms.
* Your health care provider can usually diagnose the disorder by a physical exam of the affected area.

* Medical tests may include blood tests and study of a sample of fluid removed from the affected skin.

APPROPRIATE HEALTH CARE
* Treatment is with drugs for the infection, rest, and hospital care, if needed.
* If too much fluid is lost from the skin, you may need hospital care. Replacement fluids will be given through a tube into a vein under the skin.

POSSIBLE COMPLICATIONS
* Blood poisoning, if bacteria enter the bloodstream.
* Brain infection, if the condition occurs on the central part of the face.
* Infection of the bone, muscle, and tissue beneath the affected areas.
* Vein or lymph gland inflammation.

PROBABLE OUTCOME—With treatment, symptoms will begin to improve in 2 to 3 days, and complete recovery occurs in 7 to 10 days. Complications are rare, but may develop in those with chronic disease or weak immune systems.

HOW TO TREAT

GENERAL MEASURES
* Soak the area in warm water to help it heal. This may also reduce pain and swelling.
* Elevate the affected area. Rest the arm or leg on a pillow. Don't move that area of your body unless you have to. This can help reduce swelling.

MEDICATION
* Antibiotics will be prescribed for infection. They may be taken by mouth or injection. Complete the entire dose prescribed, even if symptoms disappear quickly.
* Use acetaminophen or ibuprofen for minor pain and fever.

ACTIVITY—Get extra rest until symptoms improve. Then return to your normal level of activity.

DIET—No special diet.

CALL YOUR DOCTOR IF

* You or a family member has symptoms of cellulitis.
* The following occur during treatment:
  - High fever and chills.
  - Pain, redness, or swelling increases.
  - Red streaks continue to extend, despite treatment.
  - Vomiting.
* New, unexplained symptoms develop.

CEREBRAL PALSY (CP)

 GENERAL INFORMATION

DEFINITION—A group of chronic disorders that affect muscle movement and body coordination. Cerebral refers to the brain and palsy refers to a disorder of movement.

BODY PARTS INVOLVED—Central nervous system; muscular system.

SEX OR AGE MOST AFFECTED—It is often diagnosed in the first 1 to 2 years of life.

SIGNS & SYMPTOMS
* The number and severity of the following symptoms vary widely among children with cerebral palsy.
* Early sucking difficulty with the breast or bottle.
* Lack of normal muscle tone (early).
* Slow development (walking, talking).
* Unusual body postures.
* Stiffness and muscle spasms (later).
* Uncontrolled body movements.
* Poor coordination or balance.
* Crossed eyes.
* Impaired hearing, vision, or speech.
* Convulsions.
* Normal or above normal intelligence or degrees of mental retardation.

CAUSES—Damage to motor areas of the brain that disrupts its ability to adequately control movement and posture. The reason is often unknown. In most cases, the damage occurs before, during, or shortly after birth, or during infancy. Cerebral palsy is not inherited.

RISK INCREASES WITH
* Birth injury, including severe oxygen shortage.
* Congenital malformation of the nervous system.
* Jaundice in an infant.
* Rh incompatibility (a blood disorder).
* Stroke in a fetus or newborn, or seizures in newborn.
* Low Apgar score (a rating scale done on newborns).
* An infection in the mother during pregnancy, such as rubella (German measles) or toxoplasmosis.
* Prematurity and low birthweight.
* Breech birth, complicated labor and delivery, or maternal bleeding late in pregnancy.
* Mothers that have hyperthyroidism, mental retardation, or seizure disorder.
* Brain disease (meningitis or encephalitis).
* Head injuries during infancy or childhood.

HOW TO PREVENT—Get treatment for, or avoid, preventable risk factors. Get good medical care during pregnancy and don't smoke, use alcohol, or abuse drugs. Protect infants from accidents or injuries.

 WHAT TO EXPECT

DIAGNOSTIC MEASURES
* Your child's health care provider will do a physical exam.
* Medical tests include testing motor skills and reflexes. Tests are also done to rule out other disorders.

APPROPRIATE HEALTH CARE
* You and your child's health care team will decide on a treatment program based on your child's special needs. The program will change over time as the child matures and the needs change.
* The program can include drug therapy, physical therapy, occupational and speech therapy, behavior therapy, and emotional help. Braces, casts, mechanical aids, hearing aids, and surgery help some specific problems.

POSSIBLE COMPLICATIONS—Joint deformities; problems with nutrition, speech, vision, or hearing; mental retardation; or seizures.

PROBABLE OUTCOME—It is not progressive and children will vary widely in the severity of the condition. A child with CP may have high intelligence despite major muscular disability. Those with less-severe impairment can lead relatively normal, productive lives. Children with severe impairments may require special care.

 HOW TO TREAT

GENERAL MEASURES
* Parents may join a support group to seek help from other parents whose children have CP.
* To learn more: United Cerebral Palsy Foundation, 1660 L St. NW, Suite 700, Washington, DC 20036; (800) 872-5827; website: www.ucp.org.

MEDICATION
* Drugs may be prescribed for seizures, to control spasticity, or to reduce abnormal movements. Alcohol "washes" or injections into muscles may be done to reduce spasticity.
* Stool softeners can be used for constipation.

ACTIVITY—Limits or abilities will depend on degree of impairment.

DIET—Eating and swallowing may be difficult. Special diets and feeding techniques may be needed.

 CALL YOUR DOCTOR IF

* You are concerned about your child's development or suspect cerebral palsy.
* After diagnosis, you have any concerns.

CERVICAL CANCER

GENERAL INFORMATION

DEFINITION—Cancer of the cervix. The cervix is part of the female reproductive system.

BODY PARTS INVOLVED—Cervix (the lower third of the uterus, which opens into the vagina).

SEX OR AGE MOST AFFECTED—While the average age of women at diagnosis is about 45, this cancer can affect women of all ages.

SIGNS & SYMPTOMS
* The early stages usually have no symptoms.
* Pelvic pain. Pain may occur in the hip and thigh.
* Heavy menstrual periods.
* Spotting or bleeding between menstrual periods.
* Vaginal discharge.
* Pain and bleeding after intercourse.
* Abdominal pain.
* Leaking of feces and urine through vagina.
* Appetite and weight loss.
* Anemia.
* Weakness.

CAUSES—Unknown. It is probably related to viral infections, specifically human papillomavirus (genital warts).

RISK INCREASES WITH
* Early age of first intercourse (before age 18).
* Multiple sex partners.
* Multiple pregnancies.
* Human papillomavirus infection (genital warts).
* History of abnormal Pap smears.
* Recurrent vaginal infections.
* Smoking.
* Weak immune system due to illness or drugs.
* Sexually transmitted diseases.
* Daughters of mothers who took DES (diethylstilbestrol) to prevent miscarriage between 1938 and 1971.

HOW TO PREVENT
* Avoid the risks listed above if possible.
* Use latex condoms each time you have sexual intercourse. This is important if you or your partner has had multiple previous partners.
* Get regular pelvic exams and Pap smears. It is a test done to detect cancer of the cervix in an early and treatable stage.

WHAT TO EXPECT

DIAGNOSTIC MEASURES
* Your health care provider will do a pelvic exam.
* Medical tests will be done, first to diagnose the cancer, and then others to see if it has spread (called staging).

APPROPRIATE HEALTH CARE
* Surgery is usually done to remove the cancerous area.
  - During early cancer stages, this may involve only a small area of the cervix. This will still allow childbearing. The surgery is usually done as an outpatient.
  - The cancer cells may be frozen (cryotherapy), cut out with an electrical loop, burned away by laser, or removed in a cone biopsy. Your health care provider will explain these options and any risk factors involved.
  - More advanced stages may require removal of the reproductive organs and other affected tissue (radical hysterectomy).
* Chemotherapy and radiation therapy (internal, external, or both) are other treatments for advanced cancer.

POSSIBLE COMPLICATIONS
* If cervical cancer is not treated early, cancer cells can spread in the body which may be fatal.
* Complications often occur from treatments.

PROBABLE OUTCOME—Usually curable with early diagnosis and treatment.

HOW TO TREAT

GENERAL MEASURES
* The more you can learn and understand about cervical cancer, the more you will be able to make informed decisions about where to go for your care, the treatments available, the risks involved, side effects of therapy, and expected outcome.
* To learn more: The American Cancer Society, (800) ACS-2345; website: www.cancer.org or National Cancer Institute, (800)4-CANCER; website: www.nci.nih.gov.

MEDICATION—Anticancer drugs (chemotherapy) may be prescribed.

ACTIVITY
* Usually no limits.
* Avoid tampons following surgery.
* You will be advised when you can resume sexual activity.

DIET—Eat a well-balanced diet. Nutritional supplements may be needed if regular food cannot be tolerated.

CALL YOUR DOCTOR IF

* You or a family member has persistent vaginal bleeding or other symptoms of cervical cancer.
* You have not had a pelvic exam or Pap smear in the past year.
* New symptoms develop after treatment.

CERVICAL DYSPLASIA

 GENERAL INFORMATION

DEFINITION—Cervical dysplasia is the growth of abnormal cells on the lining of the cervix. It may be mild, moderate, or severe, depending on the spread and type of the abnormal cells. Dysplasia is not cancer, but can become cancerous.

BODY PARTS INVOLVED—Cervix (the lower third of the uterus, which opens into the vagina).

SEX OR AGE MOST AFFECTED—It occurs in females age 15 and over, and most often in those age 25 to 35.

SIGNS & SYMPTOMS—Usually no signs or symptoms occur. The diagnosis results from a routine Pap smear test.

CAUSES—It is believed to be due to human papillomavirus (genital warts) or similar viruses. The human papillomavirus (HPV) is acquired from sexual intercourse, and can, in rare instances, be acquired from skin-to-skin contact.

RISK INCREASES WITH
- History of infection with the human papillomavirus (HPV), which causes genital warts.
- Having a sexually transmitted disease.
- Smoking.
- Weak immune system due to illness or drugs.
- Multiple sexual partners or having sex with a man who has had multiple sexual partners.
- Pregnancy.
- Daughters of mothers who took DES (diethylstilbestrol) to prevent miscarriage between 1938 and 1971.
- Early age of first sexual intercourse (before age 18).
- Lack of folic acid in the diet may play a role.

HOW TO PREVENT
- Sexual monogamy of both partners.
- Yearly Pap smears (will not prevent dysplasia, but will aid in early diagnosis).
- Don't smoke. Avoid second-hand smoke.
- Use of a diaphragm by the female or a condom by the male for sexual intercourse.
- Eat a healthy diet.

 WHAT TO EXPECT

DIAGNOSTIC MEASURES
- Your health care provider will do a pelvic exam.
- Medical tests include a Pap smear. A swab of cervical cells may be taken for exam to check for HPV. A colposcopy (exam of the cervix with an instrument with a lighted tip) may be done. It can be combined with a biopsy. A biopsy involves removal of any tissue that appears abnormal for viewing with a microscope. Other tests may be done if further diagnosis is needed. The results of these tests help classify the dysplasia.

APPROPRIATE HEALTH CARE
- Treatment will vary depending on the degree and extent of the cervical dysplasia. No treatment may be recommended in some cases. Follow up visits will be needed to be sure the dysplasia clears up on its own.
- The abnormal cells may be frozen (cryotherapy), cut out with an electrical loop, burned away by laser, or removed in a cone biopsy. Your health care provider will explain your options and any risk factors involved.

POSSIBLE COMPLICATIONS
- Some moderate or severe dysplasia may progress to cancer of the cervix. It can take years for this to happen.
- Dysplasia may recur after treatment. If a woman has completed childbearing, recurrent dysplasia can be treated with a hysterectomy.
- Rarely, treatment may cause bleeding or infection.

PROBABLE OUTCOME—Most dysplasia is the mild form. Many of these cases resolve without treatment. Moderate to severe dysplasia can usually be cured with treatment.

 HOW TO TREAT

GENERAL MEASURES
- Follow-up care will depend on the treatment method.
- Follow-up Pap smears every 3 to 6 months, for 1 to 2 years, are usually recommended. This will verify the success of treatment and detect any recurrence. Be sure to schedule annual Pap smears after that time.

MEDICATION
- You may use nonprescription drugs, such as acetaminophen, for minor pain.
- Prescription pain drugs may be prescribed depending on the treatment procedure.

ACTIVITY
- After treatment, resume daily activities, including work, as soon as you are able.
- Delay sexual relations until a follow-up medical exam shows that healing is complete.

DIET—No special diet.

 CALL YOUR DOCTOR IF

- You or a family member needs to schedule a visit for pelvic exam and Pap test.
- After dysplasia treatment, any new symptoms occur.

CERVICAL EROSION

GENERAL INFORMATION

DEFINITION—A condition in which the lining of the uterus spreads to cover the tip of the cervix. This abnormally placed tissue is more likely to become inflamed or infected. It is not cancerous.

BODY PARTS INVOLVED—Cervix; uterus lining.

SEX OR AGE MOST AFFECTED—Adolescent and adult females.

SIGNS & SYMPTOMS
* No symptoms (usually).
* Increased mucus discharge from the vagina (sometimes).
* Unexplained vaginal bleeding (sometimes).

CAUSES—Often unknown. It may be due to:
* Trauma (injury) from intercourse, use of tampons, or insertion of a foreign object.
* Infections, such as herpes, tampons that were not removed, or a vaginal infection that is more severe.
* Chemicals, such as used in spermaticides, douches, creams or foam products.

RISK INCREASES WITH
* Multiple sexual partners.
* Using vaginal douches or other vaginal products.

HOW TO PREVENT—Cannot always be prevented at present. Practice safe sex behaviors and do not use douches.

WHAT TO EXPECT

DIAGNOSTIC MEASURES
* Your health care provider will do a pelvic exam.
* Medical tests may include a Pap smear and a colposcopy (an optical magnifying instrument is used to view the cervix). A culture of vaginal discharge and a cervical biopsy may also be done to rule out other disorders.

APPROPRIATE HEALTH CARE
* Treatment depends on the cause. Sometimes, no treatment is recommended (such as with trauma). The cervix will heal on its own in time.
* Treatment, if needed, may involve drugs, cauterization, cryosurgery (see both in Surgery section), diathermy or laser treatment.

POSSIBLE COMPLICATIONS—Rarely, erosion may be an early sign of cervical cancer.

PROBABLE OUTCOME—The disorder may clear up on its own. Treatment, if needed, will bring about a cure.

HOW TO TREAT

GENERAL MEASURES
* Don't douche unless instructed to by your health care provider.
* Obtain medical treatment for any vaginal infection you may have.

MEDICATION
* Antibiotics taken by mouth or topical antibiotics to apply to the cervix may be prescribed for infection.
* Estrogen vaginal cream may be prescribed.

ACTIVITY—No limits unless advised by your health care provider.

DIET—No special diet.

CALL YOUR DOCTOR IF

* You or a family member has symptoms of cervical erosion.
* The following occurs after treatment:
  - Increased discharge.
  - Pain with intercourse or bleeding afterward.
  - Vaginal bleeding between periods.

CERVICAL POLYPS

GENERAL INFORMATION

DEFINITION—A common disorder that involves a small growth on the cervix. The cervix is the long neck at the end of the uterus where it meets the vagina. Polyps vary in size and look like a bulb on a thin stem. There may be one (usually) or groups of polyps. A polyp can't be seen or felt by a woman.

BODY PARTS INVOLVED—Endometrium (thin membrane lining the uterus); cervix (lower third of the uterus).

SEX OR AGE MOST AFFECTED—Women of all ages. They occur most often in women over age 20 who have had at least one child.

SIGNS & SYMPTOMS
* No symptoms usually. They are often found on a routine pelvic exam.
* Bleeding between monthly menstrual periods.
* Heavier bleeding during periods.
* Spotting of blood after sexual intercourse.
* Vaginal discharge.

CAUSES—Exact cause is unknown. Inflammation of the cervix may be involved. This can be from infection, erosion, or other problems. The majority of polyps are benign (not cancerous). In very rare cases, they represent early cancer of the cervix. They are not contagious.

RISK INCREASES WITH
* Women over age 20 who have had one child.
* Recurrent vaginitis or cervicitis (inflammation or infection of the cervix).

HOW TO PREVENT
* No specific preventive measures.
* Get regular pelvic exams and Pap tests. This is the best way to identify cervical polyps.

WHAT TO EXPECT

DIAGNOSTIC MEASURES
* Your health care provider can diagnose the polyps during a pelvic exam.
* Medical tests are usually not needed, but may be done to rule out other disorders.

APPROPRIATE HEALTH CARE
* Treatment involves surgery to remove the polyps. This can usually be done in a simple office procedure. All tissue removed is examined in a laboratory for any sign of cancer.
* Polyps are usually removed by gently twisting the stem with forceps to break it off.
* A dilation and curettage (D & C) may be done. This involves a scraping procedure. You may feel brief, mild pain during the procedure. Mild to moderate cramps may occur for several hours. Spotting of blood may last for a few days.
* If the polyp is large or has a thick stalk, it may require surgery that is more extensive. This may be done in a hospital.

POSSIBLE COMPLICATIONS
* Infection can develop following surgery.
* In very rare cases, cancer may first appear as a polyp.
* After treatment, polyps may grow again on another area of the cervix.

PROBABLE OUTCOME—Polyps are easily treated and seldom grow back.

HOW TO TREAT

GENERAL MEASURES
* Don't douche unless you are advised to by your health care provider.
* Use small sanitary pads to protect your clothing from creams or suppositories.

MEDICATION
* Use acetaminophen or ibuprofen for minor pain.
* Antibiotics may be prescribed if signs of an infection are present. Antibiotics can interfere with the effectiveness of some birth control pills. If you are currently taking birth control pills, discuss this with your health care provider.

ACTIVITY—No limits on regular physical activities. Delay sexual relations until a follow-up pelvic exam confirms that healing is complete.

DIET—No special diet.

CALL YOUR DOCTOR IF

* You or a family member has symptoms of cervical polyps.
* The following occur after treatment:
  - Discomfort persists longer than 1 week.
  - Unexplained vaginal bleeding or swelling develops.

CERVICAL SPONDYLOSIS

GENERAL INFORMATION

DEFINITION—Changes to the spine, at the back of the neck, that occur with aging. These changes can cause problems when they put pressure on the nerves and blood vessels.

BODY PARTS INVOLVED
* 7 bones of the neck.
* Disks between the bones.
* Blood vessels to the head.
* Bladder and lower legs (advanced stages).

SEX OR AGE MOST AFFECTED—The
disorder is more common in people over age 50, and affects males more often than females.

SIGNS & SYMPTOMS
* Stiffness and pain in the neck that extends to the shoulder blades, top of the shoulders, upper arms, hands, or back of the head.
* Crunching sounds with movement of the neck or shoulder muscles.
* Numbness and tingling in the arms, hands, and fingers. There is some loss of feeling in the hands, as well as slowing of reflexes.
* Muscle weakness or muscle spasms.
* Headache.
* Dizziness; unsteady walk.
* Feeling extra tired and having disturbed sleep.

CAUSES—With aging, there is wear and tear on the vertebrae (bones of the spine) and the disks between these vertebrae. Bony growths called osteophytes (or spurs) can develop on the vertebrae. Because of these changes, there can be pressure on nerves and blood vessels.

RISK INCREASES WITH
* Adults over age 50.
* Arthritis (inflammation of a joint).
* Previous injuries such as automobile accidents with "whiplash" injury, athletic injuries, or falls.
* Osteoarthritis (wear and tear on joints that comes with aging).
* Smoking may be a risk factor.

HOW TO PREVENT
* There are no specific preventive measures for cervical spondylosis. It comes with aging.
* You can prevent some neck injuries, which might help prevent the risk. Wear protective headgear for contact sports. Use seat belts in vehicles and keep headrests at proper height.

WHAT TO EXPECT

DIAGNOSTIC MEASURES
* Your health care provider will do a physical exam and ask questions about your symptoms.
* X-rays or MRI (see Glossary) scans may be obtained to confirm the diagnosis.

APPROPRIATE HEALTH CARE
* Self-care for mild symptoms.
* Ultrasonic treatments may be recommended.
* Surgery (sometimes) to fuse neck bones, remove a damaged disk, or enlarge the spinal-cord space.

POSSIBLE COMPLICATIONS
* Reduced neck flexibility.
* Chronic neck pain.
* Unable to control bowel or urine functions.

PROBABLE OUTCOME—Treatment does not
cure the disorder, but does help improve the symptoms and prevent further problems.

HOW TO TREAT

GENERAL MEASURES
* Follow any instructions from your health care provider or try the treatment steps listed.
* Wear a cervical collar (neck brace) to prevent unexpected neck-muscle strain.
* Apply moist heat. Take warm showers twice a day and let the water beat on neck and shoulders. Between showers, apply warm soaks to neck. Soak towel or cloth in hot water, wring out, and apply.
* Gentle massage will often help.
* Improve your posture. Pull in the chin and abdomen when sitting or standing. Use a firm chair and sit with buttocks against the back.
* Sleep without a pillow. Instead, use a cervical pillow, wear a soft fabric collar, or put a small rolled towel under the neck.
* If numbness or pain affects the hands or arms, buy or rent a cervical-traction device. To set it up, follow the directions that come with the device.

MEDICATION
* For minor pain, you may use aspirin or ibuprofen.
* For serious discomfort, stronger pain medicine, muscle relaxants, or antidepressants may be prescribed.

ACTIVITY—Decrease activity or rest in bed for 2 to
3 days. Increase activity as symptoms improve. Swimming and walking are good ways to exercise.

DIET—No special diet.

CALL YOUR DOCTOR IF

* You or a family member has symptoms of cervical spondylosis.
* Symptoms persist or worsen despite, treatment.

CERVICITIS

GENERAL INFORMATION

DEFINITION—Inflammation of the cervix. The cervix is the long neck at the end of the uterus where it meets the vagina.

BODY PARTS INVOLVED—Cervix and mucous membranes covering the cervix.

SEX OR AGE MOST AFFECTED—Females of all ages, but it occurs more often in women under age 25.

SIGNS & SYMPTOMS
• Often no symptoms occur.
• Vaginal discharge. It may be thick and creamy, foamy and greenish-white, white and curd-like, or thin and grey.
• There may be bleeding after sexual intercourse.

CAUSES
• Infection. Cervicitis is most often caused by an infection (usually a sexually transmitted disease). Bacteria infections, *Neisseria gonorrhoeae* or *Chlamydia trachomatis,* are the most common. Herpes simplex or human papillomavirus (HPV) can also be the cause.
• Allergic reaction (such as to latex).
• Injury or irritation.

RISK INCREASES WITH
• Multiple sexual partners.
• Women who begin having sex at an early age.
• History of sexually transmitted diseases.
• Acute or recurrent vaginitis (vaginal inflammation).

HOW TO PREVENT
• Avoid sexually transmitted diseases. Do not have sexual intercourse with an infected partner. If unsure, have your sexual partner wear a condom during sexual activity.
• Have regular pelvic exams and Pap smear. This is important if you are sexually active.
• Get treatment for any vaginal infections before they spread to the cervix.
• Avoid irritants to the cervix, such as douches or sprays.

WHAT TO EXPECT

DIAGNOSTIC MEASURES
• Your own observation of symptoms.
• Your health care provider will do a pelvic exam.
• Medical tests usually include a culture of the vaginal discharge and blood studies and a Pap smear.

APPROPRIATE HEALTH CARE
• Treatment is with drug therapy to cure any infection. If a sexually transmitted disease caused the cervicitis, your sexual partner must also be treated.
• Repeated or prolonged cervicitis may require other treatment, such as surgery to destroy the infected cervix tissue.

POSSIBLE COMPLICATIONS
• Pelvic inflammatory disease (PID). The infection spreads to other parts of the reproductive system. PID does not cause symptoms and can lead to infertility.
• Salpingitis (inflammation of the fallopian tubes).
• Endometritis (inflammation of the uterus).
• Cervicitis may recur. This happens more often with an untreated sexual partner.

PROBABLE OUTCOME—Cervicitis can be cured with treatment.

HOW TO TREAT

GENERAL MEASURES
• Use sanitary pads instead of tampons during treatment.
• Don't douche unless it is recommended by your health care provider.

MEDICATION
• Oral (or sometimes injected) antibiotics will be prescribed for bacterial infection. Antibiotics may interfere with the effectiveness of some birth control pills.
• Antiviral drugs may be prescribed for viral infection.

ACTIVITY
• Avoid sexual relations until the treatment is complete and the symptoms have gone away— for at least 7 days.
• Do not have sexual relations until your partner is treated.

DIET—No special diet.

CALL YOUR DOCTOR IF

• You or a family member has symptoms of cervicitis.
• During treatment, discomfort lasts longer than one week or symptoms worsen.
• Vaginal bleeding or swelling develops during or after treatment.

CHALAZION

GENERAL INFORMATION

DEFINITION—A lump (also called a cyst) on the eyelid resulting from chronic inflammation of a gland that lubricates the edges of the eyelid. A chalazion is not a stye.

BODY PARTS INVOLVED—Eyelid.

SEX OR AGE MOST AFFECTED—Adults of both sexes.

SIGNS & SYMPTOMS—A painless swelling on the eyelid. At first, it may seem like a stye. The eyelid may swell, and the eye may feel irritated. After a few days, these early symptoms go away. There is then a painless, slow-growing, firm lump in the eyelid. Skin over the lump can be moved loosely. The upper eyelid is the one usually affected.

CAUSES—Blockage of a type of sweat gland in the eyelid. The blockage may be due to infection.

RISK INCREASES WITH—Skin conditions such as acne or dermatitis.

HOW TO PREVENT—There are no specific measures to prevent chalazions.

WHAT TO EXPECT

DIAGNOSTIC MEASURES
• Your own observation of symptoms.
• See your health care provider if you are concerned about the problem. An exam will be made of the affected eyelid area.
• Medical tests are not required.

APPROPRIATE HEALTH CARE
• Self-care.
• Treatment may involve drugs to be applied to the eyelid, drugs injected into the chalazion, or surgery to remove it.
• Surgery to remove the chalazion may be recommended. This is usually done in a medical office. The area will be numbed before the lump is removed. See Chalazion Removal in Surgery section.

POSSIBLE COMPLICATIONS—Some people are prone to chalazions. Once you have one chalazion, you are more likely to get another one.

PROBABLE OUTCOME—A chalazion may heal by itself. If not, it can be treated.

HOW TO TREAT

GENERAL MEASURES
• Self-care is often all that is needed.
• Use warm-water soaks to reduce irritation and swelling. The soaks may also make the area heal faster. Apply soaks for 20 minutes, then rest at least 1 hour. Gently massage the area several times a day. Do not squeeze or try to pop the chalazion.
• If you have a tendency to get chalazions, wash your eyelid area every day. Wash with water and baby shampoo that is diluted with water. There is also a commercial product available to clean eyelids. Apply either solution with a cotton swab and rinse with warm water.
• When you first notice that your eyes are getting irritated, use warm compresses and massage the area several times a day. Repeat as often as needed.

MEDICATION
• Ointments, drops, or creams that are put on the eye may be prescribed. These drugs help to kill bacteria. Follow instructions provided with the prescription.
• Injection of a drug into the chalazion may be recommended.

ACTIVITY—No limits.

DIET—No special diet.

CALL YOUR DOCTOR IF

• You or a family member has symptoms of a chalazion that is not better after 3 to 4 days of self-care.
• Fever, headache, vision changes, eye pain, eye discharge, or swollen eyes occur.

CHICKENPOX (Varicella)

GENERAL INFORMATION

DEFINITION—A very contagious disease caused by the herpes zoster virus. Symptoms are usually mild in children and may be more severe in adults.

BODY PARTS INVOLVED—Skin and mucous membranes.

SEX OR AGE MOST AFFECTED—All ages, but most common in children.

SIGNS & SYMPTOMS
* Fever.
* Abdominal pain or a general ill feeling that lasts 1 to 2 days.
* Skin eruptions that appear almost anywhere on the body, including the scalp, penis, and inside the mouth, nose, throat, or vagina. They may be scattered over large areas, and they occur least on the arms and legs. Blisters collapse within 24 hours and form scabs. New crops of blisters erupt every 3 to 4 days.
* Adults have other symptoms that resemble influenza.

CAUSES
* Infection with the herpes zoster virus. It is spread from person to person by airborne droplets or contact with a skin eruption on an infected person. Symptoms may appear 7 to 21 days after exposure.
* A newborn is protected for several months from chickenpox if the mother had the disease before or during pregnancy. The immunity diminishes in 4 to 12 months.

RISK INCREASES WITH
* Children who are not vaccinated.
* Weak immune system due to illness or drugs.

HOW TO PREVENT
* Varicella vaccine for healthy children 12 months or older. It may not completely prevent an infection, but symptoms are milder.
* An immune globulin may be used for high-risk persons, such as those who take anticancer or immunosuppressive drugs if they become exposed to the virus.

WHAT TO EXPECT

DIAGNOSTIC MEASURES
* Your own observation of symptoms.
* Your health care provider can diagnose chickenpox by the appearance of the skin eruptions.
* Medical tests are usually not needed.

APPROPRIATE HEALTH CARE—Medical care is usually not needed. Drug therapy may be prescribed for some patients.

POSSIBLE COMPLICATIONS
* Bacterial infection of chickenpox blisters. Scarring, if blisters become infected (rare).
* Pneumonia.
* Central nervous system complications (rare).
* Shingles (can occur years later in adulthood).

PROBABLE OUTCOME
* Children usually recover in 7 to 10 days. Adults may take longer. Adults and persons with weak immune systems are more at risk for complications.
* After recovery, a person has lifelong immunity against a recurrence of chickenpox.
* After chickenpox runs its course, the virus sometimes remains dormant in the body (probably in the roots of nerves near the spinal cord). The same virus may cause shingles many years later.

HOW TO TREAT

GENERAL MEASURES
* Use cool-water soaks or cool-water compresses to reduce itching.
* Keep the patient as quiet and cool as possible. Heat and sweat trigger itching.
* Keep the nails short to discourage scratching, which can lead to secondary infection.

MEDICATION
* To decrease itching: Topical anesthetics and topical antihistamines provide quick, short-term relief. Preparations containing lidocaine and pramoxine are least likely to cause allergic skin reactions. Lotions that contain phenol, menthol, and camphor (such as calamine lotion) may be recommended. Follow package instructions.
* To reduce fever, use acetaminophen or ibuprofen. Don't give children aspirin, as it may contribute to the development of Reye's syndrome (a form of encephalitis) when given to children during a viral illness.
* An antiviral drug may be prescribed for some.

ACTIVITY
* Bed rest is not needed. Allow quiet activity indoors or outdoors (during nice weather).
* Keep an ill child away from others, and from school, until all blisters have crusted and no new ones occur.

DIET—Blisters in the mouth may make eating and drinking painful. Fluid intake is needed to prevent dehydration. Try Popsicles, cool drinks, and bland foods.

CALL YOUR DOCTOR IF

* You or your child has symptoms of chickenpox.
* Cough, headache, or sensitivity to bright light develop, fever rises or blisters appear infected.

CHILD ABUSE

 GENERAL INFORMATION

DEFINITION—The major types of child abuse (or maltreatment) are:
* *Physical abuse* is physical injury (from minor injury to broken bones, or death). A child may be hit, bitten, shaken, punched, kicked, beaten, burned, or harmed in other ways.
* *Sexual abuse* includes touching a child's genitals, intercourse, forcing a child to watch sexual acts, having a child touch or look at an adult's genitals, watch or be in pornographic films, and any other sexual act.
* *Emotional abuse* harms a child's emotional growth or can destroy a child's confidence. Constant yelling and screaming, name-calling, threats, and not giving love and affection are forms of this abuse.
* *Child neglect* is when the child's basic needs are not met. This can include lack of proper food, clothes, school, hygiene, medical care, or leaving a child alone.

BODY PARTS INVOLVED—All.

SEX OR AGE MOST AFFECTED—All children.

SIGNS & SYMPTOMS
* All types of abuse will cause both physical and behavioral signs. Parents or other adults who know the child are unlikely to suspect child abuse. A child's injuries or behavior changes can result from other problems also.
* Physical signs. Any type of injury (mild or serious), pain when they urinate, genital bleeding, weight loss or no weight gain (in infants), stomach pain, headaches, or infections. Pregnancy in young adolescents.
* Behavioral signs. Avoiding family and friends, a change in eating habits, sleeping problems, emotional upsets, and poor school performance. Outgrown habits such as bed-wetting or thumb-sucking may recur. There may be inappropriate sexual behavior.
* Older children may abuse drugs or alcohol, talk about suicide, or behave in a reckless and destructive manner.

CAUSES—Abusers are more likely to be someone the child knows, rather than a stranger. Abusers may be parents, relatives, neighbor, babysitters, or other caregivers.

RISK INCREASES WITH
Children:
* A child of any age, sex, race, religion, rich or poor can be a victim of abuse.
* Infants under age one (high risk for injury).
* Females (more likely to suffer sexual abuse).
Adult abusers:
* Parents lacking parenting skills, and those with financial, relationship, mental, emotional, or stress problems.
* Adults who were victims of child abuse.

HOW TO PREVENT
* For children, age-appropriate education about abuse.
* If you suspect child abuse, report it now.

 WHAT TO EXPECT

DIAGNOSTIC MEASURES
* Children are often afraid to tell anyone about abuse. They feel they are at fault and no one will believe them.
* If your child tells you about abuse, stay calm and let the child know that he or she is believed. Take steps to protect the child. Take action to report the abuse. You may want to call the local Child Protective Service. If you are unsure what to do, ask someone you trust.
* Call your child's health care provider if you think your child has been abused. Treatment will be given for any injuries. The child may need hospital care. Health care providers must report any suspected or known cases of child abuse to the proper authorities.

APPROPRIATE HEALTH CARE
* Medical treatment as needed for any physical problems.
* Other therapy and counseling will be needed depending on each individual situation.

POSSIBLE COMPLICATIONS
* Physical injuries that could be fatal.
* Serious emotional and mental problems.
* Risk for many types of problems later in life.

PROBABLE OUTCOME—The best hope for the child is early discovery of the problem, and prompt action and treatment.

 HOW TO TREAT

GENERAL MEASURES
* To learn more: Childhelp USA, 15757 N. 78 Ave., Scottsdale, AZ 85260; (480) 922-8212 (not toll free); website: www.childhelpusa.org.
* To report child abuse, call the Local Child Protective Services or the national hotline (800) 422-4453.
* If you have abused a child or think you might, seek help. Call your health care provider or a local help line.

MEDICATION—Drugs may be needed to treat or prevent a sexually transmitted disease (STD), or to prevent a pregnancy.

ACTIVITY—No limits usually.

DIET—No special diet.

 CALL YOUR DOCTOR IF

An abused child needs medical or emotional help. You suspect someone is abusing a child.

CHILDHOOD OBESITY

 GENERAL INFORMATION

DEFINITION—Obesity (or being overweight) means having too much body fat. In children or adolescents, it means they weigh more than normal for their age, height, and sex.

BODY PARTS INVOLVED—All.

SEX OR AGE MOST AFFECTED—Children and adolescents of all ages and both sexes.

SIGNS & SYMPTOMS—A health care provider will usually diagnose an overweight child, but a parent may notice that a child:
• Appears heavier than other children of the same age.
• Eats a lot of food, but is always hungry.
• Often feels tired and is not active physically.

CAUSES
• Usually it is a combination of too little physical activity, being sedentary (sitting for long periods), and poor eating habits (eating too many high-calorie foods).
• A child's genes can play a small part. Genes are what determine a person's height; hair, eye, and skin color.
• A few children may have a hormone problem.

RISK INCREASES WITH
• Not being physically active. Watching television or sitting at a computer for several hours a day.
• Poor eating habits. Eating while watching television. Eating when not hungry. Eating foods high in fat and sugar or many fast-food meals.
• A child who has obese parents.

HOW TO PREVENT
• Children learn from their parents. If parents practice healthy eating and physical activity habits themselves, their children are more likely to make the right choices.
• Parents not using food as a reward system.
• More healthful food served in school meals.

 WHAT TO EXPECT

DIAGNOSTIC MEASURES
• Your own observations of your child.
• Health care providers use growth charts as one tool to track children's growth and development. These charts list ideal weights and normal BMI (body mass index) scores for the child's age, height and sex.
 - A BMI score is computed using a child's age, height, and weight. During well-child exams, your child's weight and height are compared to these charts.
 - The results may show the child is overweight. If the child's excess weight is a health concern, a proper eating program that involves the entire family can be started.

APPROPRIATE HEALTH CARE—Follow advice from your child's health care provider. A plan of action specific for your child will be discussed. It may involve goals for pounds to lose, new eating habits, more physical activity, behavior changes, and family involvement.

POSSIBLE COMPLICATIONS
• Emotional problems (being teased by other kids, low self-esteem, depression, and anxiety).
• Health risks while still a child and later as an adult. These include type 2 diabetes, problems that can lead to heart disease, orthopedic (bone and muscle) problems, liver disease, asthma, and overweight as an adult.

PROBABLE OUTCOME—Concerned and involved parents can help a child learn to eat properly and increase physical activity levels. It will take time and effort and is a long-term goal.

 HOW TO TREAT

GENERAL MEASURES—Some suggestions:
• Any goals for weight loss and physical activity should start low. Your child can see results and not feel stressed.
• Have child keep a food and activity diary. Write down information about what they eat and do. It helps to see where there is success or a possible problem.
• Reward a child (but not with food) when a behavior change or certain goal or is achieved.
• To learn more: American Obesity Association, 1250 24th St., NW, Suite 300, Washington, DC 20037; (800) 98-obese; website: www.obesity.org. To calculate a child's BMI: www.obesityhelp.com/kidscalc.php. The Centers for Disease Control and Prevention (CDC) has a website to answer children's questions: www.bam.gov.

MEDICATION—Drugs used for adult obesity are not used for children.

ACTIVITY
• Set limits on TV watching and computer time.
• Your child should spend 30 to 60 minutes daily being physically active. This can be sports, exercise, active games, and doing chores. Get the whole family to walk, skate, or bike together.

DIET
• Plan healthy meals for the whole family that you sit down and eat together. This way your child won't feel alone in changing eating habits.
• Don't buy foods high in calories, sugar or fat.
• Limit number of fast-food meals each week.
• Drink fat-free milk (if the child is over 2).
• Avoid juices and drinks high in sugar.

 CALL YOUR DOCTOR IF

You have concerns about your child's weight.

CHLAMYDIA INFECTION

 GENERAL INFORMATION

DEFINITION—Infection and inflammation caused by a bacterium. It is a common sexually transmitted disease in the United States. It can affect anyone who is sexually active. Chlamydial infection may also be transmitted to the eyes or lungs of a newborn infant.

BODY PARTS INVOLVED—The urethra (the tube that allows urine from the bladder to pass outside the body), vagina, cervix, uterus, fallopian tubes, ovaries, penis, and anus.

SEX OR AGE MOST AFFECTED—Both sexes, age 12 and older.

SIGNS & SYMPTOMS
* Sometimes there are no symptoms during the early stages.
* Women commonly have more symptoms than men.
* Vaginal discharge.
* Urethral discharge (males).
* Anal swelling, pain, or discharge.
* Vagina or tip of the penis becomes reddened.
* Stomach pain.
* Fever.
* Pain when urinating.
* Genital discomfort or pain.

CAUSES—*Chlamydia trachomatis* bacteria. Symptoms may appear 1 to 3 weeks after exposure. It is spread by:
* Vaginal sexual intercourse.
* Anal sexual intercourse.
* Oral-genital contact.
* Vaginal infection during delivery of a newborn, which may infect the baby.

RISK INCREASES WITH
* Sexually active persons.
* Unprotected sexual activity, especially in young females.
* Having other sexually transmitted diseases.
* Multiple sex partners.
* Diabetes.
* General poor health.

HOW TO PREVENT—Practice safe sex. Do not have sexual intercourse with an infected partner. If unsure, have your sexual partner wear a condom for sexual activity.

 WHAT TO EXPECT

DIAGNOSTIC MEASURES
* Your own observation of symptoms.
* Your health care provider will do an exam of the genital area.
* Medical tests may include vaginal smear, rectal smear, and urethral smear for analysis.
* Testing for other sexually transmitted diseases is usually recommended.

APPROPRIATE HEALTH CARE
* Treatment is with antibiotic drugs. All sexual partners must be treated.
* Home care after diagnosis.
* A follow-up medical exam may be needed after completing the prescribed treatment.

POSSIBLE COMPLICATIONS
* Infertility and/or sterility in female.
* Infecting one's sexual partner.
* Infections in pelvic organs, genitals, or rectum.
* Ectopic pregnancy.
* Liver infection (perihepatitis).
* Reiter's syndrome (a type of arthritis).

PROBABLE OUTCOME—Complete cure with adequate antibiotic treatment.

 HOW TO TREAT

GENERAL MEASURES
* Keep the genital area clean. Take showers rather than baths. Use plain unscented soap.
* Women should wear cotton underpants and pantyhose with a cotton crotch. Avoid materials that are non-ventilating, such as nylon.
* After urination or bowel movements, cleanse by wiping or washing from front to back (vagina to anus).
* Avoid douches.
* If urinating causes burning, urinate through a tubular device, such as a toilet-paper roll or plastic cup with the bottom cut out, or pour a cup of warm water over the genital area while urinating.

MEDICATION—Oral antibiotics are usually prescribed. Antibiotics may interfere with the effectiveness of some birth control pills. If you are currently taking birth control pills, discuss this with your health care provider.

ACTIVITY—Avoid sexual relations until treatment is completed and symptoms are cleared up.

DIET—No special diet.

 CALL YOUR DOCTOR IF

* You or a family member has symptoms of chlamydial infection.
* Symptoms last longer than one week or get worse.
* Unusual vaginal bleeding or swelling develops.
* New, unexplained symptoms develop. Drugs used in treatment may produce side effects.

CHOLECYSTITIS OR CHOLANGITIS

GENERAL INFORMATION

DEFINITION—Cholecystitis is inflammation of the gallbladder. Cholangitis is inflammation of the ducts (tubes) that drain bile from the gallbladder to the small intestine. In both conditions, a bacterial infection may develop.

BODY PARTS INVOLVED—Gallbladder (located under the liver, in the upper right abdomen); bile ducts in the liver, leading to the gallbladder.

SEX OR AGE MOST AFFECTED—The conditions usually occur in older adults (women more than men). They may rarely occur in children or teens.

SIGNS & SYMPTOMS
* Cramping pain in the upper right of the abdomen. Pain may also occur in the chest (imitating a heart attack), in the upper back, or the right shoulder. These symptoms frequently follow a meal rich in fats.
* Tenderness in the upper abdomen.
* Nausea and vomiting.
* Belching.
* Slight fever (higher fever and chills if infected).
* Jaundice (yellow skin and eyes) may occur.
* Pale stools (sometimes).
* Skin itching (sometimes).

CAUSES
* Cholecystitis usually results when a gallstone blocks the outlet of the gallbladder and bile builds up. Chronic cholecystitis results from recurrent inflammation.
* Acalculous cholecystitis is inflammation not caused by gallstones. It may be due to severe illness, surgery, burns, or injury.
* Cholangitis occurs when one or more gallstones pass from the gallbladder into the main bile duct and become lodged. Bile builds up behind the blockage.

RISK INCREASES WITH
* Gallstones.
* Injury or trauma.
* Heart surgery.
* Pregnancy.
* Rapid weight loss or lost weight is regained.
* Parasite infection.

HOW TO PREVENT—Avoid risk factors.

WHAT TO EXPECT

DIAGNOSTIC MEASURES
* Your own observation of symptoms.
* Your health care provider will do a physical exam and ask questions about your symptoms.
* Medical tests may include blood studies, ultrasound, x-rays, CT, HIDA scans (special type of x-rays), and gallbladder ejection fraction.

APPROPRIATE HEALTH CARE
* Specific treatment will depend on degree of severity, infection, size of stones, and your general health.
* Hospital care with emergency treatment may be required for complications.
* In some patients, a tube may be placed through the skin to drain the gallbladder.
* Surgical treatment is usually a cholecystectomy (gallbladder removal) done by laparoscopic technique. (See Surgery section.)
* Nonsurgical treatment methods for gallstones are less often used. They include drugs to dissolve the stones or extracorporeal shock wave lithotripsy to shatter stones.

POSSIBLE COMPLICATIONS
* Gallbladder perforation and peritonitis (inflammation of the lining of the abdomen).
* Blood infection (sepsis).
* Hepatitis (liver inflammation).
* Gallstones may cause intestinal blockage.
* Choledocholithiasis (gallstone in common bile duct).

PROBABLE OUTCOME
* Some mild, uncomplicated symptoms heal on their own in 1 to 4 days. Most episodes will require treatment.
* Recurrences are common. Symptoms will stop after surgery to remove the gallbladder.

HOW TO TREAT

GENERAL MEASURES—To learn more: National Digestive Diseases Information Clearinghouse, 2 Information Way, Bethesda, MD 20892; (800) 891-5389; website: www.niddk.nih.gov.

MEDICATION
* Drugs for pain and vomiting may be prescribed.
* A drug to dissolve gallstones may rarely be recommended. It will take about 2 years, works in 50% of patients, and is taken indefinitely.
* Antibiotics may be prescribed for infection.

ACTIVITY
* Rest as needed until symptoms disappear or recovery from surgery is complete.
* Other limits on activity depend on treatment.

DIET—Because of nausea and vomiting, intravenous fluids are usually needed during attacks. Begin taking clear liquids or a soft diet as soon as you can tolerate solid foods.

CALL YOUR DOCTOR IF

* You or a family member has symptoms of cholecystitis or cholangitis. If symptoms are severe, call immediately!
* Symptoms recur after diagnosis or treatment.

CHOLESTEROL, HIGH
(Hypercholesterolemia)

 GENERAL INFORMATION

DEFINITION—A total cholesterol level that is higher than the healthy range. The medical term is hypercholesterolemia. Cholesterol is a lipid (similar to fat) carried in the blood. It has several important functions in the body, but too much of it can cause problems. The liver makes all the cholesterol the body needs. More cholesterol comes from foods, such as meat, dairy products, and eggs.

BODY PARTS INVOLVED—Blood vessels.

SEX OR AGE MOST AFFECTED—Adults of both sexes, but more common in men.

SIGNS & SYMPTOMS—High cholesterol in itself does not produce symptoms.

CAUSES—Total cholesterol is made up of low-density (LDL) cholesterol and high-density (HDL) cholesterol. A high level of LDL causes a fatty buildup in the walls of the arteries (blood vessels). That means less blood and oxygen get to the heart. This can lead to heart disease or stroke. LDL is called the "bad" cholesterol. HDL, the "good" cholesterol, seems to have a protective effect against heart disease. Triglycerides are another form of fat in the blood. High levels of triglycerides may increase the risk of disease.

RISK INCREASES WITH
• Diet high in saturated fat and cholesterol.
• Being overweight.
• Not being physically active.
• Heredity. High cholesterol can run in families.
• Age. Cholesterol levels rise with aging. LDL levels in women tend to rise after menopause.

HOW TO PREVENT
• Eat a low-fat, healthy diet.
• Exercise on a routine basis.
• Maintain the proper body weight.

 WHAT TO EXPECT

DIAGNOSTIC MEASURES
• Your blood will be tested for cholesterol levels. The blood test will check for levels of total cholesterol, LDL, HDL, and triglycerides.
• Test results are looked at on an individual basis, and take into account your other risk factors for heart disease. Cholesterol levels are measured in milligrams per deciliter (mg/dL).
  - Desired level for total cholesterol is less than 200; 200 to 239 is borderline high risk; over 240 is high risk.
  - LDL below 130 is the recommended level; below 100 is ideal; over 160 is high risk.

  - HDL of 60 and above is good; under 40 is high risk.
  - Triglyceride level of 150 is borderline high; 200 is high.

APPROPRIATE HEALTH CARE—You and your health care provider can decide on an action plan to reduce your risks of heart disease and stroke. This may include changes in diet, more exercise, weight loss, quitting smoking, and drug therapy.

POSSIBLE COMPLICATIONS
• Heart disease and stroke. Other factors that can increase their risk include:
  - Smoking.
  - Stress.
  - Medical problems, such as diabetes.
  - Use of some drugs.
  - High blood pressure.
  - Age (men over 45, women over 55).
  - Family history of early heart disease.
• Atherosclerosis (hardening of the arteries).
• May be some decrease of kidney function.
• Poor circulation.

PROBABLE OUTCOME—High cholesterol can be lowered to desired levels with changes in diet, lifestyle, and/or drugs, if needed.

 HOW TO TREAT

GENERAL MEASURES
• Diet and lifestyle changes do not mean you have to give up all the good things you enjoy.
• To learn more: American Heart Association, 7272 Greenville Ave., Dallas, TX 75231; (800) 242-8721; website: www.americanheart.org.

MEDICATION—Cholesterol-lowering drugs may be prescribed if diet and exercise changes are not effective, or if you are at high risk for heart disease.

ACTIVITY—Increase physical activity. Try to get at least 30 minutes of aerobic exercise (such as walking) every day.

DIET
• Limit foods that contain saturated fats and high amounts of cholesterol. Read food labels carefully.
• Eat a diet that is high in fiber with lots of fruits and vegetables.
• Begin a weight-reduction diet if you are overweight.

 CALL YOUR DOCTOR IF

You or a family member wants to find out about cholesterol levels or wants help with diet and exercise planning.

CHRONIC FATIGUE SYNDROME

GENERAL INFORMATION

DEFINITION—Chronic fatigue syndrome (CFS) is a disorder that involves profound fatigue. There is usually an abrupt onset of symptoms that come and go for at least six months. It is unknown whether it represents one or many disorders. It is difficult to diagnose because there is no specific medical test, or a defined set of signs and symptoms.

BODY PARTS INVOLVED—Endocrine system, muscles, gastrointestinal system, central nervous system.

SEX OR AGE MOST AFFECTED— It is seen most often in young adults between 20 and 40. Women outnumber the men about two to one.

SIGNS & SYMPTOMS
* Fatigue.
* Sore throat.
* Mild fever.
* Lymph node pain.
* Muscle weakness, stiffness, and discomfort.
* Headache.
* Sleep disturbances.
* Mood swings; irritability; depression.
* Confusion; forgetfulness.
* Inability to concentrate.
* Vision changes; sensitivity to light.
* Dry eyes, mouth.
* Diarrhea.
* Loss of appetite.

CAUSES—Unknown. An abnormal immune system response may be involved. Many theories center on an infectious agent, but no such agent has been identified. Epstein-Barr (a virus that causes mononucleosis) and others have been implicated.

RISK INCREASES WITH—Unknown.

HOW TO PREVENT—Unknown.

WHAT TO EXPECT

DIAGNOSTIC MEASURES
* Your health care provider will do a physical exam and ask questions about your symptoms. There is no one test to identify CFS. Medical disorders that could be causing the fatigue and symptoms will be ruled out first.
* The guidelines used to help define cases are:
 - Persistence of relapsing fatigue that does not resolve with bed rest and is severe enough to reduce average daily activity by at least 50% for at least 6 months.
 - Other chronic clinical conditions have been satisfactorily excluded, including preexisting psychiatric disease.

APPROPRIATE HEALTH CARE
* Steps in therapy may include a combination of lifestyle changes, starting a gradual exercise program, counseling, behavior therapy, and drug therapy.
* Counseling and/or behavior therapy may be helpful for coping with the emotional aspects of the disorder and learning how to reduce stress.

POSSIBLE COMPLICATIONS—None specific to the disorder. Symptoms are usually most severe during the first 6 months.

POSSIBLE OUTCOME—Symptoms will usually come and go over a period of time. Generally, there is very slow improvement over months or years.

HOW TO TREAT

GENERAL MEASURES
* Lifestyle changes may include finding ways to cut back on work or other activities. This may help reduce physical and emotional stress. Stop smoking (find a way to quit that works for you).
* Joining a CFS support group is helpful for some patients.
* Learn more: Chronic Fatigue & Immune Dysfunction Syndrome Association, P.O. Box 220398, Charlotte, NC 28222; (800) 442-3437; website: www.cfids.org.

MEDICATION
* There is no specific drug to treat CFS. Drugs may be prescribed for depression, pain, low blood pressure, allergy-like symptoms, insomnia, or other specific symptoms.
* Other drugs are being studied and may prove to be helpful in treatment. Talk to your health care provider before taking herbal remedies or dietary supplements.

ACTIVITY
* Strenuous exercise should be avoided. Some exercise, however, is important. Begin a gradual program that may be just 3 to 5 minutes a day to start with. Increase the activity by about 20% every 2 to 3 weeks. Setbacks will sometimes occur, so don't be discouraged.
* Get enough sleep at night. Limit daytime napping.

DIET—Eat a healthy diet and drink plenty of fluids. Limit caffeine and avoid alcohol.

CALL YOUR DOCTOR IF

* You or a family member has symptoms of chronic fatigue syndrome.
* Symptoms worsen after treatment is started.

CHRONIC OBSTRUCTIVE PULMONARY DISEASE (COPD; Emphysema)

GENERAL INFORMATION

DEFINITION—A term used to describe two related disorders (chronic bronchitis and emphysema) that involve impaired airflow in and out of the lungs.

BODY PARTS INVOLVED—Lungs.

SEX OR AGE MOST AFFECTED—Women are more often affected by chronic bronchitis, while men are more often affected by emphysema.

SIGNS & SYMPTOMS
Chronic bronchitis:
• Frequent cough or coughing spasm. Mucus is usually present. It is thick and difficult to cough up. The mucus color and thickness may change according to whether infection is present.
• Shortness of breath.
Emphysema:
• Often, no symptoms in the early stages.
• Shortness of breath. It becomes worse over several years.
• Lung infections.
• Weight loss.
• Some wheezing or coughing.
• Little mucus is produced.

CAUSES—Bronchitis is caused by production of excess mucus in the lungs. Emphysema causes tiny air sacs in the lungs to become permanently enlarged. Patients with COPD have features of both conditions.

RISK INCREASES WITH
• Cigarette smoking or secondhand smoke.
• An inherited form of emphysema.
• Chronic exposure to dust, ozone, chemicals, smoke, traffic exhaust fumes, sulfur, and others.
• Frequent lung infections in childhood. They can lead to scarring of lung tissue.
• Aging.
• Personal history of allergies or lung disorders.

HOW TO PREVENT—The most important measure is to avoid smoking. Also, avoid breathing smoke from other people's cigarettes. Secondhand smoke can lead to this condition.

WHAT TO EXPECT

DIAGNOSTIC MEASURES
• Your own observation of symptoms.
• Your health care provider will do a physical exam and ask questions about your symptoms and activities.
• Medical tests may include blood studies, lung function testing and x-rays.

APPROPRIATE HEALTH CARE
• Goals of treatment are to relieve symptoms, slow progression of the disorder, and prevent complications.

• Treatment may include drug therapy, lifestyle changes, supplemental oxygen, special exercises, and sometimes, surgery. You and your health care provider will discuss a treatment plan depending on your individual needs. Educate yourself about this disorder.
• Usually, you can be treated at home. Hospital care may be needed for infections or if symptoms get worse.
• Lung surgery or a lung transplant may be an option for a few patients.

POSSIBLE COMPLICATIONS
• Frequent infections, anxiety, and depression.
• Other lung diseases, heart failure, and death.

PROBABLE OUTCOME—Lung function will continue to worsen over time. More and more effort is needed to get air in and out of the lungs. Treatment can help relieve symptoms and help prevent infections. Treatment may help you to lead a more active and productive life. Survival times are very different from person to person.

HOW TO TREAT

GENERAL MEASURES
• If you smoke, stop immediately. This is the most important thing you can do. Avoid secondhand smoke and other lung irritants (air pollution, fumes, dust).
• Get pneumonia vaccine and annual flu shot.
• Avoid excessive heat, cold, and very high altitudes. Talk to your health care provider about airplane travel you are planning.

MEDICATION
• Drugs may be prescribed to improve the symptoms. They can help open narrowed airways, reduce inflammation, treat or prevent infections, and reduce the amount of mucus in your lungs.
• Drugs may be prescribed for depression or anxiety.

ACTIVITY
• Not being active for long periods of time can make your disability worse. Try to maintain a regular exercise program. Walking is usually a good way to exercise.
• Your health care provider may prescribe physical therapy or special breathing exercises.

DIET—Eat a well-balanced diet.

CALL YOUR DOCTOR IF

• You or a family member has symptoms of COPD.
• Any signs of infection develop (such as fever).
• Symptoms get worse despite treatment.

CHRONIC PELVIC PAIN

GENERAL INFORMATION

DEFINITION—Chronic pelvic pain is any pain in the pelvic area that has lasted for at least 6 months. Pelvic pain is a common problem in women and the pain symptoms will vary for each woman.

BODY PARTS INVOLVED—Pelvic area, genitals, back and abdomen area.

SEX OR AGE MOST AFFECTED—Females, usually ages 18-50.

SIGNS & SYMPTOMS
• The main symptom is pain in the pelvic and lower stomach and back area. Other terms women use to describe the problem include discomfort, pressure, aches, tenderness, or a heavy feeling.
• The pain may be mild or severe. It may come and go, or it may be there all the time.
• The pain may occur before or during menstrual periods. Some women may have the pain when they have sex or when they exercise.
• Urination and bowel symptoms may occur, such as diarrhea or constipation.

CAUSES—There are many possible causes for this type of pain and sometimes the exact cause is not found. It may involve health problems that are both physical (such as with menstrual periods) and mental (such as stress).

RISK INCREASES WITH
• Prior health problem such as a pelvic infection or pelvic surgery.
• History of abuse as a child or adult.
• Having family members with chronic pelvic pain.

HOW TO PREVENT—Since there are many causes, there is no sure way to prevent it.

WHAT TO EXPECT

DIAGNOSTIC MEASURES
• Diagnosis begins with a physical exam plus a pelvic exam by your health care provider. You will be asked questions about the pain symptoms you are having.
• Different tests may be ordered to help find the cause of your pain. These include blood and urine studies, a pregnancy test, and a Pap smear (to check the cells in your cervix). X-rays may be needed.
• Minor surgery using a laparoscope may be necessary. This is an instrument with a thin, lighted tube that is inserted into the body through a small incision. It can help diagnose and sometimes treat chronic pelvic pain at the same time.

APPROPRIATE HEALTH CARE
• Treatment will depend on any health problems diagnosed.
• Your health care provider will talk to you about the treatment options for chronic pain and what may work best for you. Options may include drugs (oral and injections), physical therapy, and possibly surgery. It may be helpful to consult a behavior counselor and learn how to relax and control stress in your life.
• If the cause for the pain is unclear, you may be asked to keep a pain diary for 2 or more months. This can help you and your health care provider see how the pain symptoms relate to what is going on in your life day to day.

POSSIBLE COMPLICATIONS
• Depression, sleep problems, poor appetite, and weight loss occur along with the pain.
• Pain limits your normal activities and lifestyle.

POSSIBLE OUTCOME—Pain symptoms can usually be helped with one or more types of treatment.

HOW TO TREAT

GENERAL MEASURES
• For self-care, apply a heating pad to the painful area or soak in a warm bath.
• To learn more: National Women's Health Information Center (800) 994-9662; website: www.4woman.gov or the OBGYN.net: The Universe of Women's Health website: www.obgyn.net.

MEDICATION
• You may use nonprescription pain relievers such as ibuprofen or naproxen.
• Drugs to treat any medical problems diagnosed or to help control severe pain symptoms will be prescribed if needed.
• Drugs may be prescribed to stop your menstrual periods for 2 months to see if this helps stop pain.

ACTIVITY—Try to maintain a regular exercise program. It can help with the pain. It will also help you build strength and be more flexible.

DIET—No special diet is usually needed.

CALL YOUR DOCTOR IF

• You or a family member has symptoms of chronic pelvic pain.
• Your pelvic pain continues despite treatment.

CIRRHOSIS OF THE LIVER

GENERAL INFORMATION

DEFINITION—Damage to the liver that develops gradually over months to years. This can lead to serious health problems because the body depends on the liver for a number of vital functions.

BODY PARTS INVOLVED—Liver and its major blood vessels.

SEX OR AGE MOST AFFECTED—It usually occurs in people ages 40 to 60. It is more common in men than women.

SIGNS & SYMPTOMS
Early stages:
- There may be no symptoms.
- Feeling tired and weak. Some have nausea.
- Loss of appetite and weight loss.
- Pinhead-sized red spots on the skin.

Later stages:
- Yellow skin and eyes (jaundice).
- Palms may be reddish and blotchy.
- Urine may be dark yellow or brown.
- Loss of body hair and itchy skin.
- Excess fluid in the stomach (ascites) and legs.
- In men, testicles may shrink; breasts may be swollen.
- Stool may be black or bloody.
- Bleeding and bruising.
- Mental/personality changes.

CAUSES—Liver damage is due to scar tissue that replaces healthy tissue. This blocks the flow of blood through the liver and decreases liver function. A number of disorders can lead to the liver damage.

RISK INCREASES WITH
- Alcoholism. People are all affected differently by alcohol. An amount that causes cirrhosis in one person may not be a problem for another. Nutrition may be a factor.
- Chronic hepatitis B, C, and D.
- Chronic autoimmune hepatitis.
- Blood vessel disease or chronic heart failure.
- Certain inherited disorders.
- Nonalcoholic steatohepatitis (NASH)—fat in the liver.
- Blocked bile ducts.
- Certain drugs, toxin exposure, and some infections.

HOW TO PREVENT
- Limit alcohol use, or avoid it entirely.
- Avoid other risk factors, where possible.

WHAT TO EXPECT

DIAGNOSTIC MEASURES
- Your health care provider will do a physical exam and ask questions about your symptoms, activities and use of alcohol.
- Medical tests may include blood and urine tests, liver function studies, CT, and ultrasound. A biopsy of your liver may be done. This involves removing a sample of liver tissue for viewing under a microscope.

APPROPRIATE HEALTH CARE
- Treatment may include drugs, diet and lifestyle changes, prevention or treatment of complications, and liver transplant. Your health care provider will devise a treatment plan based on your individual needs.
- Bleeding (hemorrhage) or excess fluid (ascites) may be treated with drugs or medical procedures.
- Liver transplant may be an option for severe disease. (See Liver Transplantation in Surgery section.)
- Counseling or a support group may help.

POSSIBLE COMPLICATIONS
- Continued alcohol use will lead to more liver damage.
- Cirrhosis can cause serious, sometimes fatal problems in any organ system in the body.

PROBABLE OUTCOME—It will vary due to the many causes and possible complications. Stopping alcohol use and treatment of the disorder that lead to cirrhosis may slow or stop the progress of the disease.

HOW TO TREAT

GENERAL MEASURES
- If the condition is caused by alcoholism, stop drinking. Ask for help from family, friends, or support group. Contact Alcoholics Anonymous.
- To learn more: American Liver Foundation, 75 Maiden Lane, Suite 603, New York, NY 10038; (800) 465-4837; website: www.liverfoundation.org.

MEDICATION—You may be prescribed:
- Drugs for the underlying disorder, or to decrease excess fluid in the body, and to prevent bleeding.
- Supplements, such as vitamins.
- Drugs to help remove toxins from the body.
- Drugs for complications, such as infection.

ACTIVITY—Stay as active as possible. Rest when you feel tired.

DIET—Eat a well-balanced diet. You will be advised about any limits for fat, salt, or protein.

CALL YOUR DOCTOR IF

- You or a family member has symptoms of cirrhosis.
- Unusual bleeding, bloody vomit, fluid build-up, sudden weight gain, jaundice, mental changes, fever, pain, or breathing problem develops.

CLAUDICATION

 GENERAL INFORMATION

DEFINITION—A feeling of muscle fatigue or cramp-like pain, usually in one or both legs. The discomfort occurs after minimal exercise, such as a short walk, and is normally relieved by resting.

BODY PARTS INVOLVED—The calf is more frequently affected, but it can occur in the thighs, buttocks, hips or feet.

SEX OR AGE MOST AFFECTED—It is more common in men than women, particularly men over age 55.

SIGNS & SYMPTOMS
* Pain, tension, weakness, or cramping in the limb.
* Pain occurs while walking, and pain stops when resting.
* Unable to walk distances.
* Loss of the hair on the toes or lower legs.
* Lameness or limping.

CAUSES
* Blockage or narrowing of the arteries of the legs due to atherosclerosis.
* Rarer cause is spinal stenosis (pressure on nerve roots that pass into either leg).

RISK INCREASES WITH
* Males, females after menopause, and ages over 60.
* Smoking.
* Diabetes.
* Being sedentary (getting little or no exercise).
* High blood pressure.
* Overweight.
* Heart disease.
* High blood cholesterol.

HOW TO PREVENT
* Stop smoking.
* Weight loss, if overweight.
* Routine exercise program.
* Reduce saturated fats in the diet.

 WHAT TO EXPECT

DIAGNOSTIC MEASURES
* Your health care provider will do a physical exam and ask questions about your symptoms.
* A variety of medical tests, including an ultrasound (sometimes done with exercise), may be ordered. These will help confirm the diagnosis and rule out other disorders that have similar symptoms.

APPROPRIATE HEALTH CARE
* You will be given exercises to do at home, and/or supervised exercises that are done on a treadmill.
* High blood pressure and high cholesterol may be treated with drugs.
* Various surgical procedures, depending on the site of the disease and the health of the patient, are available for more severe cases.

POSSIBLE COMPLICATIONS
* Pain while resting, as well as when walking.
* Increased risk of falls, due to being unsteady.
* People with diabetes are at highest risk for problems.
* Blood clots, tissue loss, gangrene, and amputation (rare).

POSSIBLE OUTCOME—Gradual improvement in ability to walk distances without pain. Improvement may take 6 to 12 months. It is important to follow an exercise program.

 HOW TO TREAT

GENERAL MEASURES—Quit smoking. Find a way to stop that works for you.

MEDICATION
* Low doses of aspirin may be prescribed.
* Drugs to lower blood pressure and reduce cholesterol levels, and special drugs to increase blood flow may be prescribed.
* Taking vitamins C, E, and B has helped some people. Ask your health care provider about taking them.

ACTIVITY
* Begin an exercise program. Walking or riding an exercise bike is recommended. Stop and rest if the pain becomes more severe. Try for 30 to 60 minutes of exercise 3 to 5 days a week.
* Strength training for the arms and legs also helps to improve symptoms.

DIET—Eat a healthy diet (include fruits, vegetables, and fiber). Consider a weight-loss diet, if overweight is a problem.

 CALL YOUR DOCTOR IF

* You or a family member has symptoms of claudication.
* You experience chest pain, shortness of breath, or rapid heart-beat during exercise.
* Drugs used for treatment cause unexpected side effects.

COCCIDIOIDOMYCOSIS
(Valley Fever; San Joaquin Valley Fever)

 GENERAL INFORMATION

DEFINITION—A lung infection caused by a fungus that lives in soil. Coccidioidomycosis cannot be spread from person to person.

BODY PARTS INVOLVED—Lungs (most commonly), but the kidneys, lymph system, brain, and spleen can be affected.

SEX OR AGE MOST AFFECTED—Both sexes, all ages.

SIGNS & SYMPTOMS
The infection is usually so mild that it produces no symptoms. People may think they have a mild case of flu. In a few cases the symptoms may include one or more of the following:
* Cough.
* Fatigue.
* Sore throat.
* Chills and fever.
* Chest pain.
* Headache.
* Muscle and joint aches.
* Skin rash.
* General ill feeling.
* Sweating at night.
* Weight loss.
* Stiff neck (sometimes).

CAUSES—Infection by the fungus, *Coccidioides immitis*, which thrives in soil, especially soil that lines rodent burrows. A person becomes infected when they breathe the dust from such soil, and the fungi lodge in the lungs. Symptoms may begin 1 to 4 weeks after exposure.

RISK INCREASES WITH
* Geographic location. The disease is most common in the Southwest: California's San Joaquin Valley, some regions in southern and central Arizona, and southwest Texas.
* Work or environmental exposure to dust, such as farmers, construction workers, landscaping work, an archeology site, dirt biking, and others.
* Risk increases on windy days when the soil is dry and when the soil is disturbed, as with excavation. Outbreaks occur following dust storms or earthquakes. Cases increase during and after rainy seasons.

HOW TO PREVENT—Cannot be prevented at present.

 WHAT TO EXPECT

DIAGNOSTIC MEASURES
* Your health care provider may do a physical exam and ask about your symptoms and activities.

* Medical tests may include a skin test, blood studies, sputum cultures, chest x-ray and others.

APPROPRIATE HEALTH CARE
* Treatment usually involves care at home. Get extra rest if needed.
* Hospital care is required only for severe cases. Very rarely is surgery needed.

POSSIBLE COMPLICATIONS
* Spread of infection to other parts of the body, which can cause serious complications and could be fatal.
* Pneumonia.
* The disorder may become chronic.
* People with weak immune systems, pregnant women, African Americans, and Filipinos are more at risk for complications.

PROBABLE OUTCOME—Infected persons recover on their own in 3 to 6 weeks. Patients may continue to feel ill for 3 to 6 weeks after signs of infection disappear. Antifungal drugs may be used for persons with severe, widespread infection.

 HOW TO TREAT

GENERAL MEASURES
* Keep follow-up appointments with your health care provider to be sure there are no complications and the infection is healed.
* To learn more: Valley Fever Center for Excellence, Mail Stop 1-111INF, 3601 S. 6th Ave., Tucson, AZ 85732; (520) 629-4777 (not toll free); website: www.vfce.arizona.edu.

MEDICATION
* Drugs are usually not needed for treatment. You may use nonprescription nonsteroidal anti-inflammatory drugs for pain, and antitussives for cough if needed.
* For infection that spreads outside the lungs and for certain patients (infants, patients with pneumonia, or immune system problems, diabetes, or pregnancy), antifungal drugs may be prescribed.

ACTIVITY—Stay as active as your strength allows.

DIET—No special diet.

 CALL YOUR DOCTOR IF

* You or a family member has symptoms of coccidioidomycosis.
* Continued weight-loss, fever, diarrhea that cannot be controlled, stiff neck with headache develop.

COLD, COMMON

GENERAL INFORMATION

DEFINITION—A contagious viral infection of the upper-respiratory tract. Colds are the most common disease in the world.

BODY PARTS INVOLVED—Nose, throat, sinuses; ears, eustachian tubes, trachea, larynx, and bronchial tubes.

SEX OR AGE MOST AFFECTED—Both sexes; all ages.

SIGNS & SYMPTOMS
* Stuffy or runny nose. Nasal discharge may be watery at first, becoming thick and yellow.
* Throat feels scratchy or sore.
* Coughing and sneezing.
* Loss of voice.
* Mild headache.
* Fatigue.
* Low-grade fever.
* Watering eyes.
* Cold symptoms start slowly. Flu symptoms are more sudden and may include higher fever, chills, major aches, sweats, weakness, severe sore throat, chest discomfort, and cough.

CAUSES—Any of at least 100 viruses. Virus particles spread through the air or from person-to-person contact. Colds are often spread with hand-shaking.

RISK INCREASES WITH
* Winter (colds are more likely in cold weather).
* Children attending school or daycare.
* Household member who has a cold.
* Crowded or unclean living conditions.
* Stress, fatigue, and allergies.

HOW TO PREVENT
* To prevent spreading a cold to others, avoid contact if possible during the contagious phase (first 2 to 4 days).
* Wash hands often, especially after blowing your nose or before handling food.
* Avoid crowded places when possible, especially during the winter.
* Eat a well-balanced, healthy diet. Include plenty of citrus fruits and other sources of vitamin C.

WHAT TO EXPECT

DIAGNOSTIC MEASURES
* Your own observation of symptoms.
* Diagnosis by a health care provider.

APPROPRIATE HEALTH CARE
* Self-care at home.
* Medical treatment (for complications only).

POSSIBLE COMPLICATIONS—Bacterial infections of the ears, throat, sinuses, or lungs.

PROBABLE OUTCOME—Recovery in 7 to 14 days.

HOW TO TREAT

GENERAL MEASURES
* Self-care and time is usually all that is needed for a cold. There is no cure for a cold. There are many remedies for cold symptoms. They include nonprescription cold preparations, getting extra rest, drinking plenty of fluids, and others that may be suggested by friends and family members. One or more of these may help you feel better until the body's defenses fight off the germs.
* To help relieve nasal congestion, use salt-water drops (1/2 teaspoon of salt to 1 cup of warm water). Put 2 or 3 drops of salt solution into each nostril.
* Don't smoke. It can further irritate the nasal passages.
* For a baby too young to blow his or her nose, use an infant nasal aspirator. If mucus is thick and sticky, loosen it by putting 2 or 3 drops of salt solution (see above) into each nostril. Don't insert cotton swabs into a child's nostrils.

MEDICATION—No drugs, including antibiotics, can cure the common cold. To help relieve symptoms, you may use nonprescription drugs, such as acetaminophen, decongestants, nose drops or sprays, cough remedies, and throat lozenges. It is best to get a product that works for one symptom, such as a runny nose, rather than a multi-symptom product. If you take other drugs, talk to your health care provider or pharmacist about possible drug interactions.

ACTIVITY—Bed rest is not needed. Do reduce activity and exercise.

DIET—Regular diet. Drink extra fluids, including water, fruit juice, tea, and carbonated drinks.

CALL YOUR DOCTOR IF

* You have increased throat pain, or white or yellow spots on the tonsils or other parts of the throat.
* You have long coughing episodes. Your cough produces thick, yellow-green or gray sputum. You have a cough that lasts longer than 10 days.
* A fever lasts several days, or is over 101°F (38.3°C).
* You have chills, chest pain, or shortness of breath.
* You develop a painful earache or severe headache.
* You develop a skin rash or bruised skin.
* You feel pain in the teeth or over the sinuses.
* You develop enlarged, tender glands in the neck.
* Infant with a cold is unable to bottle-feed or breast-feed.

COLIC IN INFANTS

 GENERAL INFORMATION

DEFINITION—Repeated episodes of excessive crying that cannot be explained. The baby is healthy and does not have a specific disorder, such as an ear infection. Colic is different in each baby, but is sometimes defined as crying for 3 hours a day at least 3 days a week for 3 consecutive weeks.

BODY PARTS INVOLVED—Possibly the lower intestinal tract.

SEX OR AGE MOST AFFECTED—Colic affects infants up to 5 months old and is more common in a first child and boys.

SIGNS & SYMPTOMS
* Crying ranges from being fussy to a high-pitched, loud cry. Crying periods usually occur in late afternoon or evening.
* Colic usually begins at 2 to 4 weeks and can last through 3 or 4 months.
* The infant's stomach may rumble, face may be flushed (red), and the child may draw up the legs as if in pain. There may be passing of gas.
* Colic can cause loss of sleep and feeding problems in infants. In parents, it causes distress, depression, sleep loss, marital problems, and feeling a lack of parenting ability.

CAUSES—Unknown. Some possible, but not proven, causes include an immature nervous or digestive system, food allergy or food intolerance, or the baby is extra sensitive to things going on in the home.

RISK INCREASES WITH—None known.

HOW TO PREVENT—None specific.

 WHAT TO EXPECT

DIAGNOSTIC MEASURES
* Your own observation of symptoms.
* See your baby's health care provider if you are concerned about colic symptoms. A physical exam can be done to make sure there are no health problems.
* Medical tests are usually not required.

APPROPRIATE HEALTH CARE
* Home care.
* Medical treatment (rarely).

POSSIBLE COMPLICATIONS—None expected.

PROBABLE OUTCOME—All babies cry, and many have fussy periods. Crying is an important activity and is a way for babies to communicate. Colic is a distressing, but not dangerous, condition. The symptoms can sometimes be relieved. Colic will usually stop after the 3rd or 4th month.

 HOW TO TREAT

GENERAL MEASURES
* Be patient and tolerant. Colic is not the parent's fault, so do not blame yourselves.
* Don't feed the baby every time he or she cries. Look for a reason, such as a gas bubble, cramped position, too much heat or cold. Check for a soiled diaper, open diaper pin, or a desire to be cuddled.
* There are many options to try and help soothe the baby. These include:
  - Walking. Carry the baby or put baby in a stroller.
  - Rocking in a rocking chair or swinging in an automatic baby swing.
  - Take baby for a car ride.
  - Massage. Lay baby down on his/her stomach and gently rub the baby's back.
  - Swaddle the baby tightly in a baby blanket.
  - Use noise to help soothe. Run a vacuum or shower. Play soothing music (this may help baby and parents).
  - Vibration. Put the baby in a car seat and place seat on top of a dryer. Watch the baby carefully.
  - Lower lights and reduce noise in the home.
  - Some overtired infants may need to cry themselves to sleep. Once you know your baby is not hungry, not soiled, has no fever, no open pins, and you have done all you can, put your baby down for sleep.
  - Colic is distressing, but not harmful.
* Ask someone to take care of the baby in order to give you a break as often as possible. Parents need to get rest and try to avoid becoming too stressed.

MEDICATION—Drugs are usually not helpful for colic. Don't use any herbs or other supplements without medical approval.

ACTIVITY—No limits.

DIET
* Interrupt bottle feedings after every ounce and burp the baby. Interrupt breast-feedings every 5 minutes.
* Allow at least 20 minutes to feed the baby. Hold the baby in an upright position for 20 minutes after feeding.
* Breast-feeding mothers may try and adjust their diet. Try to avoid dairy, caffeine, foods that cause gas (beans, cabbage, and others) and spicy foods.
* A change in baby formula may be prescribed.

 CALL YOUR DOCTOR IF

* Your baby has colic that causes you concern.
* You fear that you are about to lose emotional control.

COLITIS, ULCERATIVE (Granulomatous Colitis)

GENERAL INFORMATION

DEFINITION—A serious, chronic, inflammatory disease of the colon (large intestine). The inflammation causes small sores or ulcers.

BODY PARTS INVOLVED—It usually affects the rectum (the lower end of the colon), but may affect the entire colon. Rarely, a portion of the small intestine is involved.

SEX OR AGE MOST AFFECTED—Both sexes and all ages (more common in young women).

SIGNS & SYMPTOMS
* Symptoms may be mild, moderate, or severe.
* Pain in the left side of the abdomen. It may improve after bowel movements.
* Episodes of bloody diarrhea with mucus, alternating with symptom-free intervals.
* Severe cramps and pain around the rectum.
* Appetite and weight loss.
* Sweating and nausea.
* Bloated abdomen.
* Fever.
* Symptoms may occur outside the abdomen.

CAUSES—Unknown. Genetic, infectious, immunologic, and psychological factors have all been suggested.

RISK INCREASES WITH—Family history of ulcerative colitis.

HOW TO PREVENT—No specific measures.

WHAT TO EXPECT

DIAGNOSTIC MEASURES
* Your health care provider will do a physical exam and ask questions about your symptoms.
* Medical tests may include stool and blood studies and x-ray of the colon (barium enema). A sigmoidoscopy or colonoscopy may be done. In these procedures, a thin tube with a lighted tip is used to view inside the colon and rectum. At the same time, a small piece of tissue can be removed for biopsy.

APPROPRIATE HEALTH CARE
* Treatment will depend on the severity and extent of the inflammation. Treatment steps may include drug therapy, surgery and, sometimes, diet changes.
* Hospital care may be needed if bleeding or dehydration develops. Fluids may be given through a vein (IV).
* Surgery to remove part of or the entire colon may be needed. This is done for severe symptoms (such as bleeding), rupture of the colon, cancer risk, failure of other treatments, or side effects of steroid drugs. The options for surgery and stool elimination will be explained to you.

* Counseling may help with emotional aspects of the disease or the surgery. Learn relaxation techniques.

POSSIBLE COMPLICATIONS
* Life-threatening blood loss, ulceration through the intestinal wall or peritonitis.
* Malnutrition (lack of nutrients).
* Inflammation of joints, eyes, and skin.
* Risk of colon cancer.
* Life-threatening blood poisoning.

PROBABLE OUTCOME— Symptoms tend to come and go throughout life. Treatment can help. It is curable with surgery.

HOW TO TREAT

GENERAL MEASURES
* To reduce cramps, apply a hot-water bottle, warm moist towels or heating pad to the abdomen or try taking a warm bath.
* To learn more: Crohn's and Colitis Foundation of America, 386 Park Ave. South, 17th Floor, New York, NY 10016; (800) 932-2423; website: www.ccfa.org.

MEDICATION
* Antidiarrheal drugs may be prescribed for diarrhea.
* Sulfa drugs, such as sulfasalazine may be prescribed to help control inflammation.
* Cortisone drugs may be prescribed for more severe symptoms. They may be taken by mouth, injected, given through an enema, or as a suppository.
* Drugs called immunomodulators may be prescribed.
* Antibiotics will be prescribed for infection.
* Vitamin and mineral supplements may be prescribed.
* Iron replacement may be needed.

ACTIVITY—Bed rest may be needed during acute attacks. Resume normal activity as soon as symptoms improve.

DIET
* Eat a healthy diet. Some foods aggravate symptoms in different people. Keep a food diary to learn which foods cause you symptoms so you can avoid them.
* Avoid milk products if you have a lactose intolerance.

CALL YOUR DOCTOR IF

* You or a family member has symptoms of ulcerative colitis.
* After diagnosis and treatment, fever and chills develop, the frequency of bowel movements or bleeding increases, jaundice (yellow eyes and skin with dark urine) develops, vomiting begins, or pain increases.

CONGESTIVE HEART FAILURE

GENERAL INFORMATION

DEFINITION—The heart has lost some of its ability to pump blood. The weak pumping causes fluid (congestion) to build up in the lungs and body tissues.

BODY PARTS INVOLVED—Heart; blood vessels; lungs; liver; extremities.

SEX OR AGE MOST AFFECTED—It is more common in older adults, and affects men more than women.

SIGNS & SYMPTOMS
- Feeling short of breath with activity or after lying down for a while.
- Feeling tired and weak.
- Coughing or wheezing.
- Sleep apnea (disturbed breathing at night).
- Swollen legs, ankles, and stomach.
- Appetite loss. A weight gain is due to retained water.
- Muscle wasting (loss of muscle mass).
- Swollen or protruding neck veins.
- Less urine, and a need to urinate at night.
- Less mentally alert, or unable to concentrate.
- Having to sleep propped up or in a recliner.

CAUSES—Over time, various disorders cause the muscles, valves, and blood vessels of the heart to become damaged and weak. The heart is not able to pump enough blood, oxygen, and nutrients to other organs in the body that they need in order for them to function properly.

RISK INCREASES WITH
- Uncontrolled high blood pressure.
- Disease of the heart valves.
- Damage following a heart attack.
- Coronary artery disease.
- Cardiomyopathy (enlarged heart).
- Congenital (being born with) heart disease.
- Abnormal rhythm or irregular heartbeat.
- Risk factors for heart disease that can lead to heart failure include: Smoking, obesity, high levels of fats in the blood, use of certain drugs, diet high in fat or salt, diabetes, alcohol abuse, and lack of physical activity.

HOW TO PREVENT—If you have a condition that can lead to congestive heart failure, get medical care. Follow the treatment plan. Eat a diet high in fiber, and low in fat and salt. Don't abuse alcohol and don't smoke. Exercise on a regular basis.

WHAT TO EXPECT

DIAGNOSTIC MEASURES
- Your own observation of symptoms.
- Your health care provider will do a physical exam and ask questions about your symptoms and activities.

- Medical tests may include blood studies and x-rays. Studies may be done of heart activity, function, and size. They help see if there has been a heart attack and the extent of any heart damage.

APPROPRIATE HEALTH CARE
- The goal of treatment is to improve the heart's pumping function. This may include drugs, lifestyle changes, and surgery. Your health care provider will devise a treatment plan based on your individual needs.
- Hospital care may be needed for severe cases. Supplemental oxygen may be used to help breathing.
- Surgery may be required for heart valve problems.
- A heart transplant may be recommended for severe cases that do not respond to other treatment. A mechanical device may be used temporarily to help the heart's pumping function.

POSSIBLE COMPLICATIONS—Heart attack, cardiac arrest, severe heart rhythm problems, pulmonary edema (fluid in the lungs), side effects of drugs, total heart failure, and death.

PROBABLE OUTCOME—Symptoms may be relieved with treatment. Long-term outcome depends on each individual patient and the severity of heart failure.

HOW TO TREAT

GENERAL MEASURES
- Don't smoke. Find a way to quit.
- Wear or carry identification that says you have this disorder. Be sure it lists the drugs you take.
- To learn more: American Heart Association, local branch listed in telephone directory, or call (800) 242-8721; website: www.americanheart.org.

MEDICATION—Drugs may be prescribed to improve heart function, to slow and regulate the heart rate, remove extra fluid, lower blood pressure, relax blood vessels, suppress the immune system, and to treat any underlying disorder.

ACTIVITY—Follow medical advice about physical activity limits and when it is safe to resume driving and sexual relations.

DIET
- Eat a diet that is low in salt and fat. Avoid alcohol.
- Go on a weight loss diet if you are overweight.

CALL YOUR DOCTOR IF

- You or a family member has symptoms of congestive heart failure.
- After diagnosis, any new symptoms occur or other symptoms become worse.

CONJUNCTIVITIS
(Pink Eye)

GENERAL INFORMATION

DEFINITION—An inflammation (redness and soreness) of the conjunctiva.

BODY PARTS INVOLVED—The conjunctiva is a clear membrane that covers the white part of the eye and the inside of the eyelids.

SEX OR AGE MOST AFFECTED—Both sexes and all ages, but more common in children.

SIGNS & SYMPTOMS
* Symptoms vary depending on the cause.
* One or both eyes may be affected.
* Eye discomfort or pain.
* Gritty feeling in the eye (like there is a piece of sand in the eye).
* Redness of the eye (leading to the term "pinkeye").
* Clear, green, or yellow discharge from the eye.
* After sleeping, crusts on lashes that cause eyelids to stick together.
* Swollen eyelids.
* Sensitivity to bright light.
* Intense itching (allergic type only).

CAUSES
* Bacterial or viral infection. Conjunctivitis may occur with colds or childhood diseases such as measles. These infections can be spread from one eye to the other. They can also be spread from one person to another.
* Chemical irritation or dust, smoke, chlorine, and other types of air pollution, or home chemicals.
* Allergies caused by cosmetics, pollen, animal dander, or other allergens. (Both eyes are usually affected.)
* A blocked tear duct.

RISK INCREASES WITH
* Children and the elderly.
* Contact lens wearers.
* Contact with an infected person.
* Newborns of mothers who are carriers of gonorrhea or chlamydia.

HOW TO PREVENT
* Wash hands often to avoid spreading germs.
* Avoid exposure to eye irritants.
* Newborns in hospital deliveries are routinely given antibiotic eye drops.
* Do not share eye makeup. Discard mascara after 4 to 6 months.

WHAT TO EXPECT

DIAGNOSTIC MEASURES
* Your own observation of symptoms.

* See your health care provider if you have any concerns about the symptoms. An exam of the affected eye will confirm the diagnosis.

APPROPRIATE HEALTH CARE—Medical care is usually not needed unless there are complications.

POSSIBLE COMPLICATIONS—Complications are rare, but may include other eye infections or problems of the cornea.

PROBABLE OUTCOME
* Most forms will heal on their own in 1 to 2 weeks with no serious harm.
* Allergic conjunctivitis can be cured if the allergen is removed. However, it is likely to recur.

HOW TO TREAT

GENERAL MEASURES
* Wash hands often with antiseptic soap, and use paper towels to dry. Don't touch the eyes. Gently wipe the discharge from the eye using disposable tissues.
* For infectious conjunctivitis, use warm-water compresses on the eye to reduce discomfort. Cool compresses feel better with allergic conjunctivitis. Apply for 5 to 10 minutes several times a day.
* Do not use eye makeup while symptoms are present.
* Do not wear contact lenses until symptoms are gone.

MEDICATION
* You may use nonprescription artificial tears in the eyes to help relieve symptoms.
* Antibiotic eye drops or ointments may be prescribed. Antibiotics taken by mouth may be prescribed for more severe cases.
* Steroid eye drops or ointments may be prescribed. Follow instructions carefully as these products can cause other, more severe eye problems.
* For allergic conjunctivitis, you may use nonprescription anti-allergy eye drops.

ACTIVITY—Return to work or school once symptoms improve.

DIET—No special diet.

CALL YOUR DOCTOR IF

* You or a family member has signs of conjunctivitis that does not improve in 48 hours.
* Fever occurs or pain increases.
* There are vision changes.

CONSTIPATION

GENERAL INFORMATION

DEFINITION—Having fewer bowel movements than usual and difficulty in passing stools. In most people, constipation is harmless. In some, it can be a sign that something else is wrong with the body. People may think they are constipated when their bowel movements are actually regular. There is no right number of daily or weekly bowel movements. Everyone has different bowel patterns.

BODY PARTS INVOLVED—Colon.

SEX OR AGE MOST AFFECTED—Both sexes; all ages.

SIGNS & SYMPTOMS
* Hard, dry, or lumpy stools.
* Having to strain to have a bowel movement.
* Fewer than three bowel movements a week.
* Pain or bleeding with bowel movements.
* Feeling bloated or sluggish.
* Feeling like you still need to go after having a bowel movement.

CAUSES—The slow movement of feces (stool) through the large intestine. This results in a dry, hard stool.

RISK INCREASES WITH
* Constipation can be a symptom or a complication of many different medical disorders.
* Emotional factors such as depression or anxiety.
* Not getting enough fluids.
* Not enough fiber in the diet.
* Being inactive.
* Taking certain drugs.
* Problems with the rectum.
* Laxative abuse.
* Travel-related constipation.
* Advancing age.

HOW TO PREVENT
* Eat a well-balanced diet. Include lots of fiber.
* Exercise regularly.
* Drink at least 8 glasses of fluid a day.

WHAT TO EXPECT

DIAGNOSTIC MEASURES
* Your own observation of symptoms.
* If you have any concerns about constipation, see your health care provider. A physical exam may be done and questions asked about your symptoms and activities.
* Medical tests may be done depending on the severity of the symptoms.

APPROPRIATE HEALTH CARE
* Self-care may be all that is needed for treatment.
* Other treatment may be prescribed for any specific cause that is diagnosed.

POSSIBLE COMPLICATIONS
* Hemorrhoids.
* Becoming dependent on laxatives.
* Uterine or rectal problems.
* Colon problems; blocked bowel.
* Chronic constipation.

PROBABLE OUTCOME—Usually curable with time, diet changes, drinking enough fluids, and getting more exercise.

HOW TO TREAT

GENERAL MEASURES
* In most cases, constipation can be helped with changes in diet and lifestyle (such as more exercise). Laxatives are usually not needed for mild constipation.
* Have a regular time each day for bowel movements. The best time is often within 1 hour after breakfast. Don't try to hurry. Sit at least 10 minutes, even if a bowel movement doesn't occur.

MEDICATION
* For occasional constipation, you may use stool softeners, mild nonprescription laxatives, or enemas. Don't use laxatives or enemas regularly, because you can become dependent on them. Avoid harsh laxatives. Ask your pharmacist or health care provider which laxatives are best to use.
* A person dependent on laxatives should slowly stop using them. Normal bowel function will begin again.

ACTIVITY—Get regular exercise and stay physically fit. This helps stimulate the bowel and helps maintain healthy bowels.

DIET
* Drinking hot water, tea, or coffee may make you feel the need to have a bowel movement.
* Drink at least 8 glasses of fluid each day.
* Include foods such as bran and raw fruits and vegetables in your diet.

CALL YOUR DOCTOR IF

* Constipation persists despite self-care, especially if the constipation is a change in your normal bowel patterns. Changes in bowel patterns may be a sign of cancer.
* You have a fever or severe stomach pain.

COR PULMONALE
(Pulmonary Hypertension)

 GENERAL INFORMATION

DEFINITION—An enlarged heart due to chronic lung disease or lung dysfunction. Cor pulmonale is usually chronic (ongoing), but may be acute (short term).

BODY PARTS INVOLVED—Lungs; heart; blood vessels.

SEX OR AGE MOST AFFECTED—Both sexes and all ages, but more common in adults over 50, and occurs in men more than women.

SIGNS & SYMPTOMS
Early stages:
* No symptoms (usually).
Later stages:
* Shortness of breath with physical activity.
* Feeling weak and tired.
* Chest pain.
* Fainting or near fainting.
* Rapid heartbeat.
* Cough or wheezing.
* Swelling of the ankles, feet.
* Swelling of the stomach (ascites).
* Bluish color of the skin.
* Neck veins swollen (distended).

CAUSES—Lung disease or lung dysfunction leads to pulmonary hypertension (high blood pressure in the lungs). This slows or blocks blood flow in the lungs. This in turn causes an extra load on the right side of the heart as it tries to pump enough blood through the lungs. The heart muscle becomes overdeveloped (enlarged) and the load on the heart becomes too great leading to heart failure.

RISK INCREASES WITH
* Chronic lung disease, such as emphysema, chronic bronchitis, silicosis, cystic fibrosis, and others.
* Pulmonary embolism (blood clot in the lungs).
* Major loss of lung tissue due to surgery or injury.

HOW TO PREVENT
* Avoid risk factors for lung disease, such as smoking.
* Obtain medical care for any heart or lung disorder.

 WHAT TO EXPECT

DIAGNOSTIC MEASURES
* Your own observation of symptoms.
* Your health care provider will do a physical exam and ask questions about your symptoms and activities.
* Medical tests may include blood studies, x-ray, lung scan, lung function tests, and echocardiogram (heart study).

APPROPRIATE HEALTH CARE
* Treatment steps usually include drug therapy, supplemental oxygen, and surgery (if needed).
* Hospital care may be required, especially if a blood clot is diagnosed.
* Supplemental oxygen is usually needed on a continuous basis. An oxygen therapist can arrange for the type of oxygen that allows you to be up and about.
* Surgery may be needed to correct heart defects.
* Lung transplant or heart-lung transplant may be recommended in some cases.

POSSIBLE COMPLICATIONS—Serious, sometimes fatal, heart failure.

PROBABLE OUTCOME—The outcome will depend on the underlying lung disorder. Symptoms can often be relieved or controlled with treatment.

 HOW TO TREAT

GENERAL MEASURES
* Avoid contact with people with infections.
* Avoid air irritants (e.g., smoke).
* To learn more: American Heart Association, 7272 Greenville Ave., Dallas, TX 75231; (800) 242-8721; website: www.americanheart.org.

MEDICATION—Drugs may be prescribed to improve heart function, to slow and regulate the heart rate, get rid of extra fluid, lower blood pressure, thin the blood, relax blood vessels, and to treat any underlying disorder.

ACTIVITY—Be as active as your condition allows, but don't overexert. Rest between activities.

DIET—You may be advised to follow a low-salt diet and limit your fluid intake.

 CALL YOUR DOCTOR IF

* You or a family member has symptoms of cor pulmonale.
* The following occur during treatment:
  - Temperature of 101°F (38.3°C) or higher.
  - Weight gain of 3 to 4 pounds in 1 or 2 days.
  - Increased shortness of breath.
  - Increased swelling of the ankles or stomach.
  - Cough with mucus that is discolored or bloody.

CORN OR CALLUS

GENERAL INFORMATION

DEFINITION
* A corn is a thickening (bump) of the outer skin layer, usually over bony areas such as the joints of the toes.
* A callus is a painless thickening of skin caused by repeated pressure or irritation.

BODY PARTS INVOLVED
* Corn: toe joints and skin between toes.
* Callus: any part of the body, especially hands, feet or knees, that endures repeated pressure or irritation.

SEX OR AGE MOST AFFECTED—Both sexes and all ages except infants.

SIGNS & SYMPTOMS
* Corn: A small, tender and painful raised bump on the side or over the joint of a toe. Corns are usually 3 mm to 10 mm in diameter and have a hard center.
* Callus: A rough, thickened area of skin that appears after repeated pressure or irritation.

CAUSES—Corns and calluses form to protect a skin area from injury caused by repeated rubbing or squeezing. Pressure causes cells in the irritated area to grow at a faster rate, leading to overgrowth.

RISK INCREASES WITH
* Shoes that fit poorly. Socks that bunch up.
* Persons with jobs that involve pressure on the hands or knees, such as carpenters, writers, guitar players, or tile layers.
* Foot deformity.
* Athletic activities that put stress on hands or feet.

HOW TO PREVENT
* Don't wear shoes or socks that fit poorly.
* Avoid activities that create constant pressure on specific skin areas.
* When possible, wear protective gear, such as gloves or knee-pads.
* Keep skin moisturized.

WHAT TO EXPECT

DIAGNOSTIC MEASURES
* Your own observation of symptoms.
* See your health care provider or a foot care provider if self-care is not effective. Diagnosis is done by an exam of the affected area.
* Medical tests are usually not needed, but an x-ray may be done.

APPROPRIATE HEALTH CARE—Medical care may involve shaving or cutting off the hardened area of skin, removing the corn or callus with a medicine used on the skin, and (rarely) surgery. Surgery does not remove the cause, and scarring from surgery is painful and may complicate healing.

POSSIBLE COMPLICATIONS—Back, hip, knee, or ankle pain caused by a change in the way you walk due to pain in your foot.

PROBABLE OUTCOME—Usually curable if the problem that caused it can be removed. Allow 3 weeks for recovery. Corns and calluses are likely to recur, even with treatment, if the cause is not removed.

HOW TO TREAT

GENERAL MEASURES
* Remove the source of pressure, if possible. Get rid of shoes that do not fit well.
* Use corn and callus pads to reduce pressure on the irritated areas.
* Peel or rub the thickened area with a pumice stone to remove it. Don't cut it with a razor. Soak the area in warm water to soften it before peeling.

MEDICATION
* Peel the upper layers of the corn once or twice a day, and then apply a nonprescription 5% or 10% salicylic ointment. Cover with adhesive tape.
* A health care provider may sometimes inject a corn or callus with a cortisone drug to reduce swelling or pain.
* An antibiotic may be prescribed for skin infection.

ACTIVITY—Resume your normal activities as soon as symptoms improve.

DIET—No special diet.

CALL YOUR DOCTOR IF

* You or a family member has corns or calluses that do not heal, despite self-treatment.
* You develop signs of infection around a corn or callus. Signs of infection include redness, swelling, pain, heat, or tenderness.

CORNEAL ABRASION AND ULCER

GENERAL INFORMATION

DEFINITION—An abrasion is a worn-off, scratched, or scraped area of the cornea. An ulcer is an open sore of the cornea.

BODY PARTS INVOLVED—Cornea (covering); conjunctiva (white of the eye); iris (colored part of the eye); and aqueous humor (fluid in the eyeball).

SEX OR AGE MOST AFFECTED—Both sexes; all ages.

SIGNS & SYMPTOMS
* Eye pain that may be severe.
* Eyes are sensitive to bright light.
* Feeling as if a foreign body is in the eye.
* Watering of the eye.
* Blurred vision.
* Redness in the white of the eye.
* Discharge from the eye.
* Clouding of the cornea.

CAUSES
* Corneal abrasion usually occurs from some type of injury to the eye. It may be a direct injury by a pencil, staple, pin, fingernail, or other object. It may be due to particles flying in the air, such as sand, dust, or from woodworking.
* Corneal ulcer usually occurs when the cornea has been injured and germs enter the injured area and cause an infection. The germs may be viral, bacterial, fungal, or may be a parasitic infection.

RISK INCREASES WITH
* Contact lens wear.
* Recent eye infection or injury, or general infection.
* Very dry eyes (lack of tearing).
* Small children playing with pointed objects.
* Athletes playing sports without using eye protection.
* Work or hobbies that use pointed tools or produce dust, and construction or farm workers.
* Weak immune system, such as with HIV.
* Severe allergies.
* Eyelids that do not close completely.

HOW TO PREVENT
* Avoid eye injury. Wear safety goggles or protective eye gear when using power tools or when participating in certain sports activities.
* Don't touch your eyes if you have cold sores.
* Handle contact lenses properly.
* Wash hands often to prevent spread of any germs.

WHAT TO EXPECT

DIAGNOSTIC MEASURES
* Your own observation of symptoms.
* Usually, an eye doctor (ophthalmologist) will examine the eye using a slit lamp (an eye microscope). A yellow dye may be used in the eye to make it easier to see the affected area.
* Medical tests may include a vision test and a culture study of corneal scraping.

APPROPRIATE HEALTH CARE
* Treatment will depend on the underlying cause. This may involve removing any foreign object in the eye and drug treatment for the eye.
* Rarely, hospital care may be needed for severe ulcers.
* If corneal ulcers cause scarring that affects vision, a corneal transplant may be needed.

POSSIBLE COMPLICATIONS—Scarring of the cornea, which can cause permanent partial or complete blindness.

PROBABLE OUTCOME—Abrasions are usually mild and heal on their own in a few days. Corneal ulcers are a more serious eye problem, but should heal in 2 to 3 weeks with treatment.

HOW TO TREAT

GENERAL MEASURES
* An eye patch may be used for a short term with an abrasion.
* Apply cool-water compresses to the eye as often as they feel good.
* Wear sunglasses. They may help relieve pain.

MEDICATION
* Eye drops or ointments for an eye infection will be prescribed.
* For minor pain, you may use a nonprescription drug such as acetaminophen. Stronger pain drugs may be prescribed if needed.
* A tetanus shot may be needed if it is not up to date.

ACTIVITY—Resting your eyes will help with healing. Limit your reading. Don't drive until you have medical approval.

DIET—No special diet.

CALL YOUR DOCTOR IF

* You or a family member has symptoms of a corneal abrasion or corneal ulcer. Seek medical care right away.
* After diagnosis, eye pain becomes more severe, vision changes (blurring or loss of vision), or eye becomes red.

CORONARY ARTERY DISEASE
(Coronary Atherosclerosis; Ischemic Heart Disease)

GENERAL INFORMATION

DEFINITION—Heart disease that is due to hardening and narrowing of the coronary arteries that provide the blood supply to the heart. There are three main coronary arteries. When any or all become narrowed, they can no longer provide adequate oxygen for heart cells.

BODY PARTS INVOLVED—Blood vessels to the heart.

SEX OR AGE MOST AFFECTED—Adults of both sexes over age 40. Coronary artery disease is uncommon in premenopausal women.

SIGNS & SYMPTOMS
* Usually no symptoms occur in the early stages.
* Angina pectoris (burning, squeezing, heaviness, or tightness in the chest that may extend to the left arm, neck, jaw, or shoulder blade).
* Irregular heart rate.
* Heart attack.

CAUSES—Usually results from atherosclerosis. This is a build-up of plaque on the artery walls.

RISK INCREASES WITH
* Smoking.
* Hypertension (high blood pressure).
* Family history of coronary artery disease, diabetes, high blood pressure, or atherosclerosis.
* Poor nutrition, especially high fat diet.
* Previous heart attack or stroke.
* Lack of exercise.
* Hostile or impatient personality type.
* Elevated cholesterol or LDL (low density lipoprotein) and/or low level of HDL (high-density lipoprotein).
* Overweight.

HOW TO PREVENT
* Don't smoke.
* Eat a low-fat, low-salt, high-fiber diet.
* Exercise regularly.
* One aspirin a day (if medically advised).
* Reduce stress level when possible.
* If you have diabetes or hypertension, adhere to the treatment plan, including diet limits.
* Maintain ideal body weight.

WHAT TO EXPECT

DIAGNOSTIC MEASURES
* Your health care provider will do a physical exam.
* Medical tests may include electrocardiogram (measures electrical activity of the heart), echocardiogram (measures sound waves), exercise-tolerance test, coronary calcium scoring, radionuclide stress test, blood studies, x-rays of the chest, and coronary angiogram (cardiac catheterization).

APPROPRIATE HEALTH CARE
* Treatment may include drug therapy, lifestyle changes, and surgery.
* Lifestyle changes include diet changes, losing weight, exercising, stopping smoking, and stress control.
* Counseling for stress problems may be helpful.
* Surgical treatment is available in some high-risk patients. Balloon angioplasty can open narrowed vessels. Vein graft bypass can help restore blood to the heart. Endarterectomy can remove large arterial obstructions. Entire segments of diseased vessels can be replaced by woven plastic tube grafts.
* End-stage coronary artery disease can still be cured with a heart transplant (in rare cases).

POSSIBLE COMPLICATIONS
* Heart attack or stroke.
* Kidney disease.
* Congestive heart failure.
* Heartbeat irregularity problems.
* Sudden death.

PROBABLE OUTCOME—Symptoms can usually be controlled with treatment and help prolong life and improve quality of life.

HOW TO TREAT

GENERAL MEASURES
* Stop smoking. Find a way to quit that works.
* To learn more: American Heart Association, local branch listed in telephone directory, or call (800) 242-8721; website: www.americanheart.org.

MEDICATION
* Nitroglycerin, anticoagulants, drugs for angina pectoris and blood-vessel spasms, and drugs to increase the blood supply to the heart may be prescribed.
* Drugs to lower cholesterol may be prescribed.
* Vitamin supplements may be recommended.

ACTIVITY—Get 20 to 30 minutes of aerobic exercise each day (if able).

DIET—Eat a low-fat, high-fiber diet that includes fruits and vegetables. Begin a weight loss diet, if overweight.

CALL YOUR DOCTOR IF

* You or a family member has symptoms of coronary artery disease
* After diagnosis, new or unexplained symptoms occur.

COSTOCHONDRITIS
(Tietze's Syndrome)

 GENERAL INFORMATION

DEFINITION—An inflammation of the cartilage of one or more ribs, most commonly the second or third ribs. The pain that results is often increased by movements that change the position of the ribs, such as lying down, bending over, coughing, or sneezing. Pain may mimic that of heart disease or digestive disorders. The term Tietze syndrome is often used for costochondritis.

BODY PARTS INVOLVED—Cartilage of one or more ribs.

SEX OR AGE MOST AFFECTED—More common in young adults, but can occur in any age group.

SIGNS & SYMPTOMS
• Pain in the chest wall, usually sharp in nature.
• Pain worsens with movement.
• Pain may occur in more than one location and may radiate into the arm.
• Tightness in the chest.
• Affected area is sensitive to the touch.

CAUSES—Inflammation (soreness and swelling) of the cartilage where the ribs attach to the sternum. The cause of the inflammation is often unknown.

RISK INCREASES WITH
• Trauma, such as a severe blow to the chest.
• Unusual physical activity.
• Upper respiratory infection.

HOW TO PREVENT—Avoid activities that may strain or cause trauma to the rib cage.

 WHAT TO EXPECT

DIAGNOSTIC MEASURES
• Your own observation of symptoms.
• Your health care provider will do a physical exam and ask questions about your symptoms.
• There is no specific test that can diagnose costochondritis. An x-ray or bone scan may be done to rule out other disorders.

APPROPRIATE HEALTH CARE—Self-care is usually all that is needed. Medical care may include drug therapy.

POSSIBLE COMPLICATIONS—None likely.

PROBABLE OUTCOME—Complete healing. The disorder is benign and the course is usually of a short duration.

 HOW TO TREAT

GENERAL MEASURES
• Use a heating pad or ice massage on the affected area. Use the one that feels better.
• Avoid sudden movements that will intensify the pain.
• Gently stretching the chest muscles several times a day may be helpful.

MEDICATION
• Mild pain drugs, such as aspirin or ibuprofen, may help relieve discomfort.
• Stronger pain drugs or steroid injections may be prescribed, but these are rarely needed.

ACTIVITY—Activities may need to be limited until symptoms improve. Get extra rest when you are able to.

DIET—No special diet.

 CALL YOUR DOCTOR IF

• You or a family member has symptoms of costochondritis.
• Pain continues or gets worse after treatment.

ILLNESS & DISORDERS

CROHN'S DISEASE
(Regional Ileitis; Granulomatous Ileitis or Ileocolitis)

GENERAL INFORMATION

DEFINITION—An inflammation (painful swelling) of the digestive tract. It can affect any part of the tract from the mouth to the anus, but most often affects the ileum. The ileum is the lower part of the small intestine. Crohn's is a type of inflammatory bowel disease (IBD). Symptoms can come and go. Periods between flare-ups vary from every few months to every few years. Sometimes, symptoms appear only once or twice, and then the disease disappears.

BODY PARTS INVOLVED—Ileum, colon and other parts of the gastrointestinal tract; regional lymph nodes; the mesentery (outside covering of the intestines).

SEX OR AGE MOST AFFECTED— It often starts between ages 15 to 35, and affects men and women equally.

SIGNS & SYMPTOMS
• Cramps and pain in the abdomen (stomach area). The pain is often in the lower-right part of the abdomen.
• Diarrhea.
• Loss of appetite and weight loss.
• Stools may be bloody or contain mucus.
• General ill feeling with fatigue.
• Fever may occur.
• Children with this condition may not grow at a normal rate, and have delayed puberty.

CAUSES—Unknown. Inflammation may result from the body's immune system overreacting to an infection. Genetic and environmental factors (such as your diet) may play a role.

RISK INCREASES WITH
• Family history of Crohn's or other bowel disease.
• Smoking.
• History of allergies.
• People of Jewish and European ancestry.
• A diet high in fat or refined foods may be a risk factor.

HOW TO PREVENT—Cannot be prevented at present.

WHAT TO EXPECT

DIAGNOSTIC MEASURES
• Your own observation of symptoms.
• Your health care provider will do a physical exam and ask questions about your symptoms and activities.
• Medical tests may include blood and stool studies, special x-rays, CT, MRI, or ultrasound (see Glossary for all). A colonoscopy (a colon exam using a thin, lighted tube) may be done.

APPROPRIATE HEALTH CARE
• Treatment steps can include drugs, diet changes, and surgery. Hospital care may be needed for severe symptoms.
• Surgery may be required. It may improve the symptoms and delay progress of the disease.

POSSIBLE COMPLICATIONS
• Intestines may become blocked (bowel obstruction).
• An abnormal opening (fistula) may develop between the bowel and nearby areas.
• Abscess (pus-filled sore).
• The bowel may burst or begin to leak.
• Higher risk of colon cancer.
• The body may not be able to absorb nutrients.
• Bleeding (can lead to low iron levels in blood).

PROBABLE OUTCOME—There is no cure for the disease, but patients can have a reasonable quality of life. Treatment can help relieve symptoms. Over time, the treatment usually becomes less effective, and many patients develop complications that require surgery.

HOW TO TREAT

GENERAL MEASURES
• Use heat to relieve pain. Apply a heating pad or take warm-water baths. Check stool daily for signs of bleeding.
• To learn more: Crohn's and Colitis Foundation of America, 386 Park Ave. South, 17th floor, New York, NY 10016; (800) 932-2423; website: www.ccfa.org.

MEDICATION—Your health care provider may prescribe one or more of the following:
• Anti-inflammatories or steroids.
• Anti-TNF (tumor necrosis factor) drugs.
• Drugs to relieve pain.
• Antidiarrheals to control diarrhea.
• Vitamin supplements.
• Drugs that suppress the immune system.
• Antibiotics for infection.

ACTIVITY—Remain as active as you can.

DIET
• Avoid foods that aggravate the condition. This may include alcohol, milk products, fatty foods, fiber, popcorn, nuts, and spices. Keep a food diary to help find what foods you cannot eat.
• Eat small, frequent meals. Take small bites and chew food completely. Drink fluids with meals. Drink liquid nutrient formulas if it is difficult to eat regular food.

CALL YOUR DOCTOR IF

• You or a family member has symptoms of Crohn's disease.
• Symptoms get worse or new ones develop.

CROUP
(Laryngotracheobronchitis)

GENERAL INFORMATION

DEFINITION—Infection, redness, and swelling of the larynx (vocal cords). It may extend into other parts of the throat or into the lungs.

BODY PARTS INVOLVED—Larynx; throat; trachea (windpipe) and bronchi (airways in the lungs).

SEX OR AGE MOST AFFECTED—Children under age 5 are most often affected.

SIGNS & SYMPTOMS
* The infection can start gradually with a cold, cough, and low fever. Frequently, symptoms come on suddenly in the middle of the night.
* Barking cough. It may be worse when child cries.
* Trouble breathing, especially at night.
* Noisy breathing or wheezing (called stridor).
* Hoarseness.
* Throat discomfort with difficulty in swallowing.
* More severe symptoms include fast breathing, ribs that seem to pull in when breathing, paleness, and bluish skin around the mouth.

CAUSES—A contagious, viral infection is the usual cause. Croup often occurs in outbreaks in the winter and early spring months. Symptoms may begin 3 to 5 days after exposure, but time will vary depending on the type of virus.

RISK INCREASES WITH
* Repeated colds and lung infections or lung disease.
* Previous croup.
* Allergies.

HOW TO PREVENT—No specific preventive measures. Wash your hands often to prevent the spread of any germs.

WHAT TO EXPECT

DIAGNOSTIC MEASURES
* Your own observation of symptoms.
* If symptoms are more severe or you are concerned about the symptoms, see your child's health care provider. A physical exam is usually all that is needed for diagnosis.

APPROPRIATE HEALTH CARE
* Most children can be treated at home using supportive care. There are no specific drugs to treat croup.
* A child who has severe breathing problems may need hospital care. Oxygen may be given to help breathing.

POSSIBLE COMPLICATIONS
* Recurrence of croup.
* Ear infection.
* Pneumonia.
* Lymph node inflammation.

PROBABLE OUTCOME—Croup can be frightening, because attacks usually happen at night and the child has trouble breathing. In almost all cases, croup is not serious and clears up in about a week or less. Complications are rare, but they may occur in children born prematurely or children with lung disease such as asthma.

HOW TO TREAT

GENERAL MEASURES
* Turn on the hot water in the bathroom shower and let the room fill with steam. Hold the child in your arms in the bathroom filled with steam for 10 to 15 minutes. Repeat this procedure if another attack occurs.
* Wrapping the child in a blanket and walking around outdoors may help. It is better if outdoor air is cool.
* Keep the child comfortable in a semi-seated position. Use TV, radio, or a story to distract the child so he or she can relax. Crying can aggravate symptoms.
* Use a cool-mist humidifier or vaporizer near the child's bed for several nights during and after an attack even if the child appears well. Simple croup can recur. Clean the humidifier daily.

MEDICATION
* Since the cause is usually viral, antibiotics do not help. Cough medicines are also not helpful.
* Acetaminophen may be given to lower fever.
* Injected drugs may be given to a child in the hospital.
* Steroids and/or bronchodilators (to help open the airways) may be prescribed.

ACTIVITY—Rest until symptoms improve.

DIET—Usually, a child with croup is not as hungry as normal. It is important to drink plenty of fluids. Offer frequent small amounts of clear fluids or Popsicles.

CALL YOUR DOCTOR IF

* Your child is having trouble breathing and cannot swallow saliva or water. This is an emergency! Call 911 or take the child to the nearest emergency room.
* Nails or lips become bluish.
* Mild croup symptoms don't improve with home care.

ILLNESS & DISORDERS

CRYPTOCOCCOSIS
(Torulosis)

GENERAL INFORMATION

DEFINITION—A fungal disease that usually affects the lungs, but may spread to other body parts. It is much more serious when there are underlying illnesses or risk factors. This condition has become more common since the emergence of AIDS.

BODY PARTS INVOLVED—Lung; central nervous system; kidney; bone; skin.

SEX OR AGE MOST AFFECTED—Both sexes and all ages. It is most common in men between ages 40 and 60.

SIGNS & SYMPTOMS
* Some people may have no symptoms or symptoms are mild and go unnoticed.
* Fever.
* Cough, sometimes with mucus.
* Headache, sometimes severe.
* Shortness of breath.
* Weight loss.
* Tiredness.
* Personality or mental changes if the infection affects the nervous system. This can include confusion or depression or being agitated.
* If the skin is infected, sores or ulcers may occur.
* The infection may cause symptoms in bones, the prostate, and the eyes.

CAUSES—Infection with *Cryptococcus neoformans*. A person gets the infection by breathing in air that contains the germs. The germs are found throughout the world, often in pigeon droppings. The infection is not passed from one person to another. Animals may also get the infection, but do not spread it to humans.

RISK INCREASES WITH
* Persons who have AIDS.
* Organ transplant patients.
* Drugs that suppress the immune system.
* Cancer (Hodgkin's disease, leukemia, myeloma, lung cancer, and others).
* Chronic lung disease, diabetes, cirrhosis, rheumatoid arthritis, lupus, and splenectomy (spleen removal).

HOW TO PREVENT—Avoid being in areas that have pigeon droppings.

WHAT TO EXPECT

DIAGNOSTIC MEASURES
* Your own observation of symptoms.
* Your health care provider will usually do a physical exam and ask questions about your symptoms and activities.
* Medical tests may include blood, urine, and spinal fluid studies. A brain CT or MRI may be done (see Glossary for both).

APPROPRIATE HEALTH CARE
* Some patients require no treatment. Those with underlying disorders are usually treated with drugs.
* Hospital care may be needed for severe symptoms.

POSSIBLE COMPLICATIONS
* Infection or inflammation of the brain (encephalitis) or the membranes that surround the brain (meningitis).
* Permanent brain damage, vision loss, and death.

PROBABLE OUTCOME—In those with normal immune systems, the infection usually heals on its own or with treatment. In those with weak immune systems, treatment may control the disease, but not cure it. Lifelong drug therapy may be needed to prevent a relapse.

HOW TO TREAT

GENERAL MEASURES
* It is usually not necessary to isolate ill persons.
* Weigh daily and keep a weight chart. An unexplained weight loss might indicate that infection has spread.

MEDICATION—Antifungal drugs are often prescribed. One drug is usually given by injection at first, followed by another drug that is taken by mouth. People with HIV or AIDS will usually need to take an antifungal drug for life.

ACTIVITY—Get extra rest until the symptoms improve.

DIET—No special diet.

CALL YOUR DOCTOR IF

* You or a family member has symptoms of cryptococcosis, especially if you have a severe headache.
* Symptoms recur after treatment.
* New, unexplained symptoms develop. Drugs used in treatment may produce side effects.

CUSHING'S SYNDROME

GENERAL INFORMATION

DEFINITION—A disorder due to excess levels of cortisol, a hormone. Cortisol helps the body respond to stress and change. The adrenal gland and pituitary gland are involved in the production of cortisol.

BODY PARTS INVOLVED—Adrenal gland (located over the kidney); pituitary gland (at the base of the brain).

SEX OR AGE MOST AFFECTED—Both sexes and all ages. It is most common in adults ages 20 to 50 and in women more than men.

SIGNS & SYMPTOMS
* Round (moon-like) face and puffy eyes.
* Thin, fragile skin; easy bruising.
* Weakness.
* Weight gain. Fat areas, such as around the torso.
* Growth of facial hair in women.
* Stretch marks (red/blue streaks on the skin).
* Mental, mood, and emotional changes.
* Menstrual changes (increase, irregular, or no period).
* More likely to get infections.
* Sexual and fertility problems.
* High blood pressure.
* Children may have growth retardation, acne, or very early or very late puberty.

CAUSES
* It may result from an overproduction of cortisol by the adrenal glands due to a variety of medical disorders.
* It may result from long-term use of cortisol-like drugs (steroid hormones) to treat medical disorders (such as asthma, arthritis, and inflammatory bowel disease).

RISK INCREASES WITH
* An abnormal growth in the pituitary gland. This causes production of excessive ACTH (adrenocorticotropic hormone). This in turn stimulates the adrenal glands to secrete hormones. This is called Cushing's disease.
* Adrenal gland tumor (benign or cancerous).
* Tumors in other places in the body produce hormones that in turn cause the adrenal glands to produce excess cortisol.
* Prolonged use of steroid hormone drugs.

HOW TO PREVENT—If steroid hormone drugs are prescribed, take the lowest dose possible for the shortest time.

WHAT TO EXPECT

DIAGNOSTIC MEASURES
* Your health care provider will do a physical exam and ask questions about your symptoms and about the drugs you take.

* Medical tests may include studies of blood and urine to measure hormone levels, pituitary gland and adrenal gland function tests, and CT, MRI, or x-rays (see Glossary for these tests).

APPROPRIATE HEALTH CARE
* Treatment will depend on the cause.
* If it is due to steroid hormone use, the dosage may be slowly reduced (depending on the disease being treated). If the steroid hormone needs to be continued, other drugs may be taken to control the side effects.
* Pituitary gland tumors may be treated with surgery or radiation. If the pituitary gland is removed, life-long hormone therapy is needed.
* Adrenal gland adenoma tumors are removed with surgery. The other adrenal gland is left in place and will take over hormone production.
* Adrenal gland cancerous tumors can be cured if diagnosed early. Often, they are not diagnosed until they have spread beyond the adrenal gland. When this happens, they are not curable. Drugs can treat symptoms.
* Tumors in other places in the body may be treated with surgery, chemotherapy or radiation. This may improve Cushing's syndrome.

POSSIBLE COMPLICATIONS
* Osteoporosis and bone fractures.
* Side effects of steroid hormones.
* Diabetes, high blood pressure, infections, kidney stones, or spread of cancerous tumors.

PROBABLE OUTCOME—it will depend on the cause, the degree of excess cortisol, the length of the disease, and the person's basic health. If the cause is treatable, the symptoms may resolve in 2 to 18 months.

HOW TO TREAT

GENERAL MEASURES—Wear a medical alert type bracelet or pendant indicating your medical problem and the drugs you take.

MEDICATION
* Drugs to suppress adrenal gland function, cortisone drugs (if adrenal gland removed), or drugs to replace pituitary hormones may be prescribed.
* Drugs to lower blood pressure, to prevent bone loss, and to reduce blood sugar may be prescribed.

ACTIVITY—As much as the condition allows.

DIET—No special diet, unless advised.

CALL YOUR DOCTOR IF

* You or a family member has symptoms of Cushing's syndrome.
* Signs of infection occur, other symptoms become worse or new symptoms develop.

CYSTIC FIBROSIS (CF)

GENERAL INFORMATION

DEFINITION—An inherited disease affecting the body's glands that produce secretions such as mucus, sweat, tears, saliva, and digestive juices. These secretions are normally thin and slippery and act as a lubricant. In cystic fibrosis (CF), the secretions are thick and sticky. This means the lungs, pancreas, intestines, and other organs are clogged up. One in 3,900 newborns is born with CF in the United States.

BODY PARTS INVOLVED—Pancreas; lungs; sweat glands of the skin; gastrointestinal tract.

SEX OR AGE MOST AFFECTED—Children of both sexes.

SIGNS & SYMPTOMS
* Symptoms will vary in different patients.
* Thick, sticky stools (meconium) in a newborn. They may cause intestinal obstruction.
* Delayed growth.
* Poor weight gain despite good appetite.
* Bad-smelling, large, fatty stools.
* Sometimes, because the air is chronically trapped in the chest, the child gets a barrel-chested appearance.
* Chronic cough or wheezing.
* Sticky, hard-to-cough-up sputum.
* Salty sweat.
* Polyps in the nose.
* Frequent chest and sinus infections.
* Rounding (clubbing) of the fingertips or toes.
* Rectal prolapse and intussusception (bowel disorder).

CAUSES—A defective gene. People can carry the gene for cystic fibrosis, but not develop it. If both parents are carriers of the defective gene, there is a 25% chance that a child will have the disease, a 50% chance the child will be a carrier, and 25% chance the child will not have the disease or be a carrier.

RISK INCREASES WITH—Family history of cystic fibrosis.

HOW TO PREVENT—If you have a family history of cystic fibrosis, seek genetic counseling before starting a family.

WHAT TO EXPECT

DIAGNOSTIC MEASURES
* Your child's health care provider will do a physical exam.
* Medical tests include a sweat test (repeated twice). CF is diagnosed if the sweat contains high amounts of salt. Very young infants may not produce enough sweat for this test, so genetic blood studies may be done to aid with diagnosis. Tests may be done for lung, pancreas, and liver functions.
* Testing of brothers and sisters of a child with CF is usually recommended even if they have no symptoms.

APPROPRIATE HEALTH CARE
* A medical team (for lung therapy, diet needs, and medical help) will provide for the child's care.
* Goals of therapy are to prevent and treat infections, keep lungs free of sputum, improve airflow, and provide adequate calories and nutrition.
* Transplants for lung, liver, and pancreas are possible (see Heart-Lung Transplantation in Surgery Section).

POSSIBLE COMPLICATIONS
* Repeated respiratory infections.
* CF can cause various other medical problems such as infertility, diabetes, osteoporosis, digestive system problems, and lung and heart disorders.

PROBABLE OUTCOME
* This condition is currently considered incurable and is often fatal in childhood. Careful long-term care by parents and a medical care team can help children lead reasonably comfortable lives. Children with milder forms are living to adulthood, especially if the disorder is detected early. Median survival age is 33.
* Medical research is ongoing to find a cure.

HOW TO TREAT

GENERAL MEASURES
* Learn as much as possible about CF. Parents may want to join a support group.
* You will be instructed on how to perform daily postural drainage to drain mucus from the lungs. This is done with clapping on the front and back of the chest. Mechanical aids and special vests are available to help.
* Keep your child's vaccines up-to-date.
* To learn more: Cystic Fibrosis Foundation, 6931 Arlington Road, Bethesda, MD 20814, (800) 344-4823; website: www.cff.org.

MEDICATION—Drug therapy may include digestive enzymes to help with digestion, antibiotics for infections, mucus-thinning drugs, and bronchodilators to help open airways.

ACTIVITY—As much as the condition permits.

DIET—High in calories, fat, and protein. Vitamin supplements and supplemental nutrition may be needed.

CALL YOUR DOCTOR IF

* You suspect your child has cystic fibrosis.
* After diagnosis, symptoms get worse at any time.

DECOMPRESSION SICKNESS (Bends)

 GENERAL INFORMATION

DEFINITION—A painful, sometimes life-threatening condition of blood gases that is caused by a sudden drop in environmental pressure.

BODY PARTS INVOLVED—Blood in all body parts.

SEX OR AGE MOST AFFECTED—Both sexes; all ages. Usually occurs in young males.

SIGNS & SYMPTOMS—The following may occur right away or up to 24 hours after the pressure change:
• Mild-to-severe joint pain, especially in the shoulders, elbows, hips, and knees.
• Chest pain, shortness of breath, and a burning sensation behind the breastbone.
• Chokes. This is severe breathing difficulty experienced by scuba divers and others who go from high to normal air pressure too rapidly. Bubbles of nitrogen develop in the blood stream and obstruct blood supply to vital organs, sometimes resulting in severe injury or death.
• Coughing.
• Weakness, loss of normal sensation, paralysis, unconsciousness, and coma (rare).
• Unable to speak, blindness, or deafness.
• Abdominal pain.
• Difficult urination.

CAUSES—Formation of nitrogen bubbles in the blood. Nitrogen is a normal blood component. If the pressure around the body drops rapidly, as in surfacing too quickly while scuba diving, or climbing too rapidly in a non-pressurized aircraft, the nitrogen collects in bubbles in the blood vessels. This blocks normal blood flow and deprives the body of blood and oxygen.

RISK INCREASES WITH
• Commercial diving or recreational scuba diving. Repeated dives in one day increase risk.
• Some kinds of high-performance aircraft.
• Working in compression chambers.

HOW TO PREVENT
• Get certified instruction before scuba diving.
• Don't dive if you are not in good general health. You are at risk if you are obese or have a medical history of:
- Lung conditions, such as asthma.
- Pneumothorax.
- Heart disease.
- Chronic sinusitis.
- Alcoholism.
• Allow for a slow, gradual change to normal air pressure when scuba diving. (The U.S. Navy has tested and set up guidelines.)
• Avoid air travel for 24 hours after diving.

 WHAT TO EXPECT

DIAGNOSTIC MEASURES
• Your own or a diving partner's observation of symptoms.
• Physical exam and medical tests by a health care provider.

APPROPRIATE HEALTH CARE
• Self-care is impossible for this condition. If you observe someone with symptoms of decompression sickness, get emergency medical care immediately.
• Treatment involves time in a decompression chamber to force nitrogen bubbles to dissolve into the blood.
• Treatment is best when it is done early. However, some patients may benefit even at 6 to 9 days after the incident. Medical care is critical even if symptoms resolve because 25% of patients will relapse.
• For assistance in locating the nearest treatment chamber in your area, call the emergency Divers Alert Network (DAN) at any hour (919) 684-8111. For nonemergency information, call (919) 684-2948; website: www.diversalertnetwork.org.

POSSIBLE COMPLICATIONS
• Permanent brain damage.
• Permanent bone destruction due to blockage of blood supply.

PROBABLE OUTCOME—Usually good for patients who receive early treatment. In others, it depends on duration and severity of symptoms prior to treatment.

 HOW TO TREAT

GENERAL MEASURES—None specific.

MEDICATION—Drugs are usually not needed for this disorder. Don't take pain relievers. These may further decrease normal breathing function.

ACTIVITY—Resume your normal activities as soon as symptoms improve after treatment.

DIET—No special diet.

 CALL YOUR DOCTOR IF

You develop any symptoms of decompression sickness within 24 hours after scuba diving or rapid ascent without pressurization.

DEHYDRATION

GENERAL INFORMATION

DEFINITION—The body is not able to function properly due to excess fluid loss, or not enough fluid intake. Dehydration is most dangerous in newborns, infants, and persons over 60. The dehydration may be mild, moderate, or severe depending on the percent of body weight lost.

BODY PARTS INVOLVED—Blood; gastrointestinal tract; kidneys.

SEX OR AGE MOST AFFECTED—Both sexes; all ages.

SIGNS & SYMPTOMS
* Dry mouth and swollen tongue. Severe thirst.
* Decreased or no urination; urine color may be deep yellow. In infants, there may be no wet diapers.
* Sunken eyes and wrinkled skin.
* Inability to sweat.
* Infants may have no tears when crying.
* Fatigue.
* Low blood pressure.
* Increase in heart rate and breathing.
* Dizziness, confusion, coma.

CAUSES
* Severe vomiting or diarrhea from any cause.
* Heavy sweating.
* Too much urine output.
* Not taking in a sufficient amount of food or water.

RISK INCREASES WITH
* Newborns, infants, and adults over 60.
* Illness with high fever.
* Not eating or drinking due to illness or mouth sores.
* Use of drugs, such as diuretics ("water pills").
* Excess exposure to sun or heat.
* Diabetes or kidney disease.
* Injuries to the skin, such as burns, can cause fluid loss through the damaged skin.

HOW TO PREVENT
* If you are vomiting or have diarrhea, take small sips of a fluid replacement product. This is important during an illness with a fever. Children need to be observed for any symptoms of dehydration.
* If you use diuretics, weigh yourself daily.
* Carry water with you to outdoor activities. Drink plenty of water while exercising. Avoid exercising outdoors in very hot weather.
* Avoid drinking alcohol in hot weather.

WHAT TO EXPECT

DIAGNOSTIC MEASURES
* Your own observation of symptoms.
* Your health care provider will do a physical exam and ask questions about your symptoms.
* Blood tests may be done to check electrolyte levels (these include sodium, potassium, bicarbonate, and others). Electrolytes are vital for the body to function normally. Other tests may be needed to find the specific cause of the dehydration.

APPROPRIATE HEALTH CARE
* Treatment will be aimed at restoring body fluids and treating any illness that is diagnosed.
* If the dehydration is severe, a hospital stay may be needed for fluid replacement.

POSSIBLE COMPLICATIONS
* Depends on any medical problems. Usually with mild to moderate symptoms, no complications are expected.
* Severe dehydration or electrolyte imbalance may lead to seizures, heart problems, brain damage, or death.

PROBABLE OUTCOME—Curable with control of the underlying cause and replacement of necessary fluids.

HOW TO TREAT

GENERAL MEASURES
* For mild dehydration, drink frequent small amounts of clear liquids. Large amounts may bring on vomiting.
* Drink electrolyte solutions. For adults, dilute solutions such as Gatorade or Recharge with an equal amount of water. For children, use special products (such as Pedialyte or Ricelyte). Instructions are on the labels.

MEDICATION—Usually not needed for dehydration.

ACTIVITY—Avoid any unnecessary activity until you recover.

DIET—A special diet is usually not needed. Resume a normal diet after the diarrhea and vomiting decreases or stops. Avoid alcohol and highly seasoned foods for several more days.

CALL YOUR DOCTOR IF

You or a family member has symptoms of dehydration.

DELAYED ONSET MUSCLE SORENESS (DOMS)

GENERAL INFORMATION

DEFINITION—Delayed onset muscle soreness (DOMS) occurs hours after an exercise is over. DOMS is not an injury as such, but can be painful. Nearly every healthy adult has had DOMS no matter what the person's fitness level is. The symptoms of DOMS are a normal response, and are part of the process that leads to improved strength once the muscles recover. You can expect a certain amount of DOMS when getting in shape.

BODY PARTS INVOLVED—Muscles.

SEX OR AGE MOST AFFECTED—Both sexes; all ages.

SIGNS & SYMPTOMS
• Symptoms start about 8 to 24 hours after the activity and end within 3 to 7 days. They may be worse the second day than they are the first day.
• Muscle pain, aches, soreness, stiffness, and swelling.
• The muscles may be less flexible.
• Muscle areas feel tender when touched.

CAUSES—Exact cause is not clear and there may be several factors involved including the buildup of lactic acid. DOMS results from doing any new or changed exercise or activity.

RISK INCREASES WITH
• Too much exercise, or a change in activity from non-impact, such as biking, to high-impact (such as running).
• New or heavy strength exercises. Even if you exercise on a regular basis, any new type of activity may cause delayed soreness.

HOW TO PREVENT
• There are no sure ways to prevent DOMS. Some ways to help reduce the amount of soreness are listed here.
• Most reports show that stretching prevents DOMS. If you do stretch before or after exercising, do so slowly, and only to the point at which you feel slight discomfort. Hold the stretch for anywhere between 10 and 30 seconds.
• Warm-up before you start an activity. Do a few minutes of slow walking or biking.
• Give your muscles time to adjust to an activity. Make changes slowly (over several weeks if needed) to a new exercise program or new or different sports activity.
• Cool down after a workout.
• If you start a new weightlifting program, begin with weights you can lift easily, and then add weight slowly.
• Drink plenty of fluids to help clear lactic acid from the tissues.

WHAT TO EXPECT

DIAGNOSTIC MEASURES—Your own observation of symptoms.

APPROPRIATE HEALTH CARE—Self-care is often all that is needed. If pain is severe, see your health care provider.

POSSIBLE COMPLICATIONS—None expected. There is no long-term damage or change in function of the muscles involved.

PROBABLE OUTCOME—The soreness is usually gone within 3 to 7 days. Your muscles will not get sore again if you keep doing the exercise or activity on a regular basis.

HOW TO TREAT

GENERAL MEASURES
• Use ice massage. Fill a Styrofoam cup with water and freeze it. Tear a small amount of foam from the top so ice sticks out. Rub the ice gently over the painful area in a circle about the size of a softball. Do this for 15 minutes at a time, 3 or 4 times a day, and before workouts.
• After 72 hours, if muscle is still sore, apply heat, such as hot soaks, instead of ice if it feels better.
• Use your hands to massage the muscle gently and often. Massage will provide comfort and reduce swelling, but it won't speed the recovery.

MEDICATION
• For minor pain and inflammation, you may try aspirin (not for children) or ibuprofen, but they do not always work for DOMS.
• Some people find that vitamin C supplements help.
• Nonprescription topical products may be used to soothe sore muscles.
• Drugs will not help to prevent DOMS.

ACTIVITY
• Keep on with some exercising. Perform low-impact aerobic exercise to increase blood flow to the muscles.
• If muscle soreness or pain increases after you begin exercising, stop and use ice on the muscles.

DIET—No special diet.

CALL YOUR DOCTOR IF

You or a family member has delayed onset muscle soreness that is severe or has lasted more than a week.

ILLNESS & DISORDERS

DEMENTIA
(Senility)

 GENERAL INFORMATION

DEFINITION—Dementia is a disease that attacks the brain. It is not a normal part of aging. Dementia results in problems with memory, thinking, and behavior. It can interfere with a person's ability to function and take care of everyday tasks. There are many types of dementia. Common types are Alzheimer's disease, multi-infarct, and vascular dementia.

BODY PARTS INVOLVED—Brain.

SEX OR AGE MOST AFFECTED—Adults over age 65.

SIGNS & SYMPTOMS
• Memory problems. Forgetfulness, such as about recent events or ordinary information such as birth date and address; not able to recognize family and friends.
• Confusion and poor judgment.
• Loss of interest in normal activities.
• Trouble speaking well.
• Disorientation, especially at night.
• Poor personal hygiene and appearance.
• Sleep problems.
• Personality changes.
• Anxiety, depression, being suspicious, agitation, wandering, verbal abuse, or being assaultive.
• Incontinence, hallucinations, delusions (later stage).

CAUSES—Nerve cells in the brain become damaged and die. Once the cells die, they cannot be replaced. The brain shrinks and brain function deteriorates. Most dementias are progressive (get worse with time) and cannot be cured. There are a few causes of dementia that may be potentially reversible, such as with a brain tumor.

RISK INCREASES WITH
• Inadequate blood supply to the brain. It may be due to blood clots, strokes, tumor, high blood pressure, or hardening of the arteries (atherosclerosis).
• Severe, or repeated, head injury (such as in boxing).
• Infections, such as AIDS or syphilis.
• Down syndrome, Parkinson's disease, Huntington's chorea, and some hereditary disorders.
• Metabolic disorders, such as thyroid disease.
• Certain nutritional deficiencies.
• Toxic causes (alcoholism, drugs, heavy metals).

HOW TO PREVENT—Most dementias are not preventable. Reducing risk factors may help. Maintain a healthy lifestyle, protect yourself from head injuries, and control chronic illnesses.

 WHAT TO EXPECT

DIAGNOSTIC MEASURES
• Family members may notice early behavior changes and seek medical care. The health care provider will do a physical exam and ask questions about the symptoms.
• There is no specific test to diagnose dementia. Medical tests may include cognitive tests (answering questions), blood, urine, and spinal fluid studies, heart studies, CT, MRI, PET scans (see Glossary for these 3), or others. Testing rules out other disorders or helps find a cause of dementia that can be treated.

APPROPRIATE HEALTH CARE
• Treatment will depend on the severity of the symptoms. Drugs are available that help slow the progress of some dementias.
• Drugs to treat the behavior symptoms can help the patient and make their care easier.

POSSIBLE COMPLICATIONS—Each type of dementia has its own complications. Most have a downward course that leads to death.

PROBABLE OUTCOME—Most dementias progress at varying rates. A few stay the same. A few may reverse with treatment of a cause.

 HOW TO TREAT

GENERAL MEASURES
• A diagnosis of dementia is overwhelming, both for the patient and the family. Educate yourselves as much as possible about what to expect and how to plan for it. In early diagnosis, the patient can take part in making decisions.
• Caring for a family member with dementia is a difficult task. Caregivers need to take care of themselves. Joining a support group can help.
• To learn more: Alzheimer's Association, 225 N. Michigan Ave., Fl 17, Chicago. IL 60601; (800) 272-3900; website: www.alz.org.

MEDICATION
• Drugs may be prescribed to help control behavior symptoms (insomnia, agitation, wandering, depression, anxiety, and others).
• Drugs that slow the progress of dementia or to treat causes of dementia may be prescribed.

ACTIVITY—Patient activity eventually requires supervision at all times.

DIET—Feeding help will eventually be needed.

 CALL YOUR DOCTOR IF

You observe symptoms of dementia in a family member or have concerns after a diagnosis.

DEPRESSION

 GENERAL INFORMATION

DEFINITION—Depression is a mood disorder. The symptoms that occur (emotional and physical) interfere with everyday life for an extended period of time. Symptoms may be mild, moderate, or severe. Depression is common and affects children and adults.

BODY PARTS INVOLVED—Nervous system.

SEX OR AGE MOST AFFECTED—Both sexes, but is more common in women; all ages.

SIGNS & SYMPTOMS
* Loss of interest in life, feeling bored and listless.
* Fatigue and lack of energy.
* Insomnia, excess sleep, or sleeping problems.
* Lack of pleasure, or withdrawal, from usual activities.
* Change in appetite that leads to weight gain or loss.
* Loss of sex drive.
* Difficulty making decisions; concentration difficulty.
* Unexplained crying bouts.
* Inappropriate guilt feelings, self-hate, lack of self-esteem, and feeling unworthy.
* Irritability, anger, and agitation.
* Headache or other aches and pains.

CAUSES—It is not fully known what causes depression. It appears to be a combination of factors. Chemical imbalances in the brain may cause or contribute to depression. Other factors may include biologic, genetic, psychological, environmental, and developmental events.

RISK INCREASES WITH
* Women are more at risk than men.
* Previous episode of depression.
* Family history of depression.
* Advanced age.
* Compulsive, rigid, perfectionistic, or highly dependent personality.
* Other emotional or personality disorder.
* Substance abuse, such as alcoholism or drugs.
* Failure in job, marriage, or a personal relationship.
* Death or loss of a loved one.
* Recent, stressful life experience.
* Living alone, social isolation.
* Surgery, major illness, or disability.
* Passing from one life stage to another (e.g., retiring).
* Use of some drugs, not taking prescribed drugs, or side effect of drugs.
* Some chronic diseases.

HOW TO PREVENT—Depression is often not preventable. Reduce your risks where possible. If you have recurring depression, drugs may be prescribed for prevention.

 WHAT TO EXPECT

DIAGNOSTIC MEASURES
* Your health care provider will do a physical exam and ask questions about your symptoms.
* Screening tests for depression are helpful in diagnosis. Medical tests may be done to rule out other disorders.

APPROPRIATE HEALTH CARE
* Therapy consists of treating acute symptoms, avoiding a relapse, and preventing recurrence.
* Psychotherapy or counseling along with drug treatment appears to obtain the best results.
* Types of psychotherapy include cognitive therapy, behavioral therapy, and interpersonal therapy. Therapy will take weeks to months.
* Severe depression may require hospital care or inpatient care at a special treatment center.

POSSIBLE COMPLICATIONS
* Alcohol or substance abuse.
* Problems with physical health.
* Failure to improve with treatment.
* Suicide.

PROBABLE OUTCOME—Treatment helps most patients. Depression may sometimes recur or it may be a one-time episode.

 HOW TO TREAT

GENERAL MEASURES
* If symptoms appear mild to moderate, try some self-care ideas: talk to friends and family; stay active and exercise regularly; eat a balanced diet; avoid alcohol; maintain normal routines (if over-scheduling is a problem, try to slow down); see fun movies; learn and practice relaxation techniques; take a vacation if you can; write down your feelings in a journal/diary; try to resolve interpersonal problems (it's best however, not to make major decisions now).
* Try a support group. Contact social agencies for help. Call your local suicide-prevention hot line if you feel suicidal.

MEDICATION
* Antidepressant drugs will usually be prescribed. More than one type of drug is needed in some cases. It will take 2 to 4 weeks or longer for improvement.
* Drugs for other symptoms may be prescribed.

ACTIVITY—Regular exercise helps depression.

DIET—Eat a normal, well-balanced diet.

 CALL YOUR DOCTOR IF

You or a family member has symptoms of depression or symptoms don't improve with treatment or time.

DERMATITIS, ATOPIC
(Eczema)

GENERAL INFORMATION

DEFINITION—A common, chronic skin disorder. *Dermatitis* means skin inflammation (redness and soreness). *Atopic* refers to hereditary disorders. It is not contagious.

BODY PARTS INVOLVED—Skin.

SEX OR AGE MOST AFFECTED—It affects males and females equally, but symptoms may be worse in females. Children are most commonly affected.

SIGNS & SYMPTOMS
* Itchy, dry skin. Scaling, redness, swelling, weeping, cracking, and crusting of the skin may occur. It often affects the skin creases of elbows, knees, neck, face, hands, feet, groin, genitals, and around the anus. It may also affect the skin around the eyes.
* Itching is worse during sleep.
* An itch-scratch cycle develops. The itch causes a person to scratch, which in turn worsens the itch.
* An infant may be irritable and restless.

CAUSES—Unknown. It may be a combination of environmental factors and genetic (hereditary) factors.

RISK INCREASES WITH
* Hay fever or asthma or food allergy.
* Family history of atopic dermatitis or other allergic disorders.
* Weak immune system due to illness or drugs.
* People living in dry climates.

HOW TO PREVENT
* No preventive measures for the first outbreak.
* Identify and then avoid the factors that may trigger an outbreak in an individual. These can include:
  - Emotional factors (stress and anger).
  - Irritants (wool, perfumes, fabric softeners, smoke, some soaps, etc.).
  - Allergens (substances that inflame the skin) such as pollen, or cat and dog dander.
  - Temperature or climate.
  - Skin infections.

WHAT TO EXPECT

DIAGNOSTIC MEASURES
* Your own observation of symptoms.
* Your health care provider will perform a skin exam and ask questions about your symptoms and medical history.
* There is no test to diagnose atopic dermatitis. Skin tests may be done to rule out other skin problems.

APPROPRIATE HEALTH CARE—Treatment steps involve healing the skin, preventing flare-ups, and treating symptoms when they occur.

POSSIBLE COMPLICATIONS
* Skin infections.
* Skin may become thick and leathery or scarred from scratching.
* Eye problems (blepharitis, cataracts, conjunctivitis).
* Herpes simplex infections are more severe in people with atopic dermatitis.

PROBABLE OUTCOME—The disorder can come and go throughout life. Symptoms may decrease with age. Treatment and self-care will help relieve symptoms in most people.

HOW TO TREAT

GENERAL MEASURES
* Lubricate the skin often, especially after bathing. Use petroleum, or alpha-hydroxy containing lanolin-based ointments.
* Bathe in cool to warm water (not hot) with products other than soap. Use cool-water soaks for crusting, oozing skin. These decrease itching and remove crusts.
* Wear loose fitting, cotton clothing. Avoid fabric softeners and anti-static laundry products.
* Reduce any emotional problems in your life, if possible. The itching often increases during stressful periods.
* To learn more: National Eczema Association, 4460 Redwood Hwy, Suite 16-D, San Rapheal, CA 94903; (800) 818-7546; website: www.nationaleczema.org.

MEDICATION
* To relieve minor itching, use nonprescription topical steroids or coal-tar preparations.
* You may be prescribed stronger topical steroids, oral or injected steroid drugs (for short periods only), antihistamines, antibiotics for infections, drugs to suppress the immune system, or other, newer drugs.
* A treatment called PUVA may be helpful. It combines a special light used with a cream applied to the skin.

ACTIVITY—No limits.

DIET—If food allergy is suspected, ask your health care provider if a diet change will help.

CALL YOUR DOCTOR IF

* You or a family member has symptoms of atopic dermatitis.
* A fever or other signs of infection develop, or uncontrolled itching occurs during a flare up.

DERMATITIS, CONTACT

GENERAL INFORMATION

DEFINITION—A common skin disorder caused by substances that irritate the skin or cause an allergic skin reaction. When an irritant causes the dermatitis, the symptoms usually begin right after exposure. With an allergen-caused dermatitis, the symptoms may take several hours or more to develop. Contact dermatitis can not be spread from one person to another.

BODY PARTS INVOLVED—Skin, especially of the hands, feet and groin.

SEX OR AGE MOST AFFECTED—All ages and both sexes, but most common in women.

SIGNS & SYMPTOMS
- Itching and swelling of the skin.
- Slight redness in milder cases.
- Bright red weeping areas in some cases.
- Blisters that break open and ooze, crust, or scale.
- Swelling of face, eyes, genital area (severe allergy).

CAUSES
- There are many causes of contact dermatitis. It may take time and effort to find the exact cause for each person, and sometimes, the cause is not found. Sometimes the causes may be from a mix of allergens and irritants, especially dermatitis on the hands.
- Irritants include soaps, detergents, bleaches, cleaners; bromine or chlorine used in swimming pools. Also, some oils, tars, a variety of plants including poinsettia, and numerous other items.
- Allergic reaction may come from nickel (found in earrings, rings, and watches); glues; household cleansers; leather; paints; latex (in balloons, rubber bands, elastic waist bands); chemicals (in hair dyes, perfumes, deodorants, and cosmetics); plants such as poison ivy, oak, or sumac; and numerous other possibilities.
- Reaction to topical drugs such as antibiotics or anesthetics.

RISK INCREASES WITH
- Ongoing use of hot water, detergents, or any irritant that changes the skin's moisture content.
- Jobs or hobbies that bring you in contact with substances that irritate or cause an allergic reaction.

HOW TO PREVENT
- Avoid contact with any irritant or allergen that has caused dermatitis in the past.
- Wear appropriate protective clothing.
- Protect skin from sunburn and other burns.
- Use bath oil or glycerin soap for bathing.
- Reduce water temperature to lukewarm for bathing or other uses.
- Minimize the use of solvents, and wear heavy-duty, cotton-lined vinyl gloves to prevent contact with irritating substances. Dry the insides of gloves after use.
- Wear leather or heavy-duty fabric gloves for housework or gardening.
- Use a dishwasher (if available).

WHAT TO EXPECT

DIAGNOSTIC MEASURES
- Your own observation of symptoms.
- See your health care provider if self-help steps are not working. A skin exam is usually all that is needed for diagnosis. Questions will be asked about any contact with possible irritating and allergic substances to help find the cause.
- Skin allergy testing may be done.

APPROPRIATE HEALTH CARE—Self-care usually. Medical care for severe symptoms.

POSSIBLE COMPLICATIONS
- Recurrence is common.
- Bacterial infection or other skin problems.

PROBABLE OUTCOME—Symptoms can usually be controlled with treatment and avoiding the irritant or allergen in the future.

HOW TO TREAT

GENERAL MEASURES
- Once the cause is known, avoid contact with that substance. Wear protective gloves for wet work. Use petroleum jelly to protect the hands.
- Treatment most often involves products applied to the skin to relieve the itching, redness, and soreness.

MEDICATION
- Use a nonprescription cream, ointment or lotion product to help relieve symptoms. These can add moisture to the skin, have an anti-itching effect, and may include a mild topical anesthetic. Use these skin care products for mild cases. For more severe cases, use 0.5% or 1% hydrocortisone product.
- Oral antihistamines may help relieve itching.
- You may be prescribed:
  - Other topical skin care products, such as stronger steroid drugs (to reduce redness and soreness) or lubricants (to preserve moisture).
  - Oral steroids for severe cases.
  - Topical or oral antibiotic for bacterial infection.

ACTIVITY—No limits.

DIET—No special diet.

CALL YOUR DOCTOR IF

- You or a family member has contact dermatitis and self-care is not working.
- Signs of infection occur the site of irritation.

DERMATITIS, HERPETIFORMIS

GENERAL INFORMATION

DEFINITION—A chronic skin inflammation that involves clusters of small itching blisters. The disorder is hereditary, but not contagious or cancerous. It is often associated with gluten sensitivity (which usually does not have symptoms). Gluten is a protein present in wheat, barley, rye, but not in rice.

BODY PARTS INVOLVED—Skin of the elbows, knees, shoulders, arms, legs and over the bottom of the spine (sacrum).

SEX OR AGE MOST AFFECTED—Adults and adolescents of both sexes.

SIGNS & SYMPTOMS
- Small clusters of 5 to 20 blisters.
- Clusters appear at the same time on both sides of the body in the same places.
- They itch, but are not usually painful (if there are no complications).
- May feel a burning or stinging sensation.
- Symptoms of gluten sensitivity may include bloating and diarrhea.

CAUSES—It is thought to be an autoimmune disorder.

RISK INCREASES WITH
- Gluten sensitivity.
- Family history of dermatitis herpetiformis.

HOW TO PREVENT—Cannot be prevented at present. To help prevent a recurrence of symptoms, continue drug therapy and diet changes as directed and prevent injury to normal skin.

WHAT TO EXPECT

DIAGNOSTIC MEASURES
- Your own observation of symptoms.
- Your health care provider will do a physical exam of the affected skin area.
- Biopsy of the skin may be done. This involves removal of a small amount of tissue or fluid for viewing under a microscope for diagnosis.

APPROPRIATE HEALTH CARE—Treatment usually includes drug therapy and diet changes.

POSSIBLE COMPLICATIONS
- Symptoms of gluten sensitivity (such as bloating, diarrhea, and poor absorption of needed nutrients).
- Certain cancers of the intestine.
- Thyroid disease.

PROBABLE OUTCOME—This is a chronic disease. Treatment can control symptoms (including itching) but it will not cure the disease.

HOW TO TREAT

GENERAL MEASURES—Soak in cool water or use cool-water compresses to reduce itching.

MEDICATION
- To control symptoms, usually one of two oral drugs, dapsone or sulfapyridine, is prescribed.
- For itching, you may use nonprescription drugs such as a low-dose steroid lotion, ointment, or cream. They reduce inflammation and itching in 24 to 48 hours.
- Topical anesthetics and topical antihistamines. These provide quick, short-term relief. Many cause skin sensitivity, but lidocaine and pramoxine usually do not.
- Lotions containing phenol, menthol, and camphor (such as calamine lotion). These are soothing, but use with care. Large amounts may be absorbed through the skin into the bloodstream; they can be toxic.
- To learn more: Celiac Sprue Association, P.O. Box 31700. Omaha, NE 68131; (877) 272-4272); website www.csaceliacs.org.

ACTIVITY—Avoiding overheating and moisture may help reduce itching symptoms.

DIET—Gluten-free diet. Get medical advice about restricting gluten in your diet. This will help improve the symptoms and often can reduce the amount of drug therapy you need.

CALL YOUR DOCTOR IF

- You or a family member has symptoms of dermatitis herpetiformis.
- New, unexplained symptoms develop. Drugs used in treatment may produce side effects.

DERMATITIS, SEBORRHEIC

GENERAL INFORMATION

DEFINITION—A skin condition with greasy, or dry, white scales. Dandruff and cradle cap are both forms of seborrheic dermatitis. It can not be spread from person to person.

BODY PARTS INVOLVED—Skin of the scalp, eyebrows, forehead, face, folds around the nose, behind ears, external ear canal or skin of the trunk, especially over the breastbone (sternum) or in skin folds.

SEX OR AGE MOST AFFECTED—Both sexes; all ages.

SIGNS & SYMPTOMS—Flaking, white scales over reddish patches on the skin. Scales stick to hair shafts. They may itch, but they are usually painless unless complicated by infection.

CAUSES—Unknown. Causes may be different in infants and adults.

RISK INCREASES WITH
* Hot, humid weather, or cold, dry weather.
* Oily skin.
* Other skin disorders, such as acne rosacea, acne, or psoriasis.
* Family history of seborrheic dermatitis.
* Obesity.
* Parkinson's disease, stroke, or head injury.
* Use of drying lotions that contain alcohol.
* People with immune disorders.

HOW TO PREVENT—Cannot be prevented. To reduce severity or frequency of flare-ups:
* Shampoo often.
* Dry skin completely after bathing or showering.
* Wear loose, ventilating clothing.

WHAT TO EXPECT

DIAGNOSTIC MEASURES
* Your own observation of symptoms.
* See your health care provider if self-help steps are not working. A skin exam is usually all that is needed for diagnosis.

APPROPRIATE HEALTH CARE—Self-care is usually all that is needed. Medical care may include drug therapy.

POSSIBLE COMPLICATIONS
* Embarrassment and social discomfort.
* Bacterial skin infection in affected areas.

PROBABLE OUTCOME—This is a chronic condition, but it is often characterized by long periods of inactivity. During active phases, symptoms can be controlled with treatment. It does not cause hair loss.

HOW TO TREAT

GENERAL MEASURES
* Shampoo hair once a day. Loosen scales with your fingernails while shampooing. Leave the shampoo on for about 5 minutes and then rinse.
* For infants, use mild baby shampoo to wash the hair and rinse completely. Brush the hair gently with a soft brush after shampooing and other times during the day.

MEDICATION
* For minor dandruff, you may use nonprescription dandruff shampoos. They may contain different types of ingredients, and all are effective.
* For seborrheic skin infections in teens and adults, a nonprescription steroid lotion may be used.
* For more severe problems, shampoos that contain coal tar, or scalp creams that contain cortisone may be prescribed. Follow instructions that are provided with each product on how to apply to hair or skin.

ACTIVITY—No limits.

DIET—No special diet.

CALL YOUR DOCTOR IF

* You or a family member has symptoms of seborrheic dermatitis that don't respond to self-care.
* Patches of seborrheic dermatitis ooze, form crusts, or drain pus.

ILLNESS & DISORDERS

DIABETES FEET & SKIN PROBLEMS

 ## GENERAL INFORMATION

DEFINITION—Infections of the skin, often of the feet, are more common in people with diabetes than in nondiabetics. The feet of a diabetic person are more prone to all forms of trauma. The common response is infection.

BODY PARTS INVOLVED—Feet and skin.

SEX OR AGE MOST AFFECTED—Both sexes; all ages.

SIGNS & SYMPTOMS
* Often there is no pain associated with infection or injury to the foot.
* New sores or ulcers that take a long time to heal.
* Unusual, persistent warmth or coolness.
* Numbness or muscle weakness.

CAUSES—Infections and other foot problems result from blood circulation problems, nerve damage, and an impaired immune system in diabetic patients.

RISK INCREASES WITH
* Ingrown toenail.
* Plantar corn or callus; blisters.
* Poor-fitting shoes.

HOW TO PREVENT
* Wash feet daily with soap and warm (but not hot) water. Dry thoroughly and gently, especially between the toes. Powder the feet once a week with talcum.
* When the feet are thoroughly dry, apply a cream or lanolin lotion into the skin of the feet to keep skin soft, moist, and free from scales. Do not rub so hard that the feet become tender. Do not cut corns or calluses or try to remove them without medical advice.
* Prevent calluses under the balls of the feet by exercise: curl and stretch the toes 20 times a day; finish each step that you take on the toes (not on the balls of the feet).
* If toenails are brittle and dry, apply a cream or lanolin lotion under and around the nails for a few nights after soaking. Clean the nails carefully with clean orangewood sticks. Cut nails carefully and straight across. Do not cut on the sides of the nail or the cuticle. If you go to a foot health care provider (podiatrist, foot specialist, or chiropodist), be sure to tell them that you have diabetes.
* If your toes overlap or are pushed close together, separate them with lamb's wool.
* Remove shoes for short periods.
* Do not wear bedroom slippers when you should wear shoes. Slippers do not give proper support.
* Do not go outside with bare feet.
* Wear shoes of soft leather that fit, but are not tight. Break in new shoes slowly (1 hour a day).
* Use cotton bed socks if you need extra warmth for your feet when you are in bed to sleep, but do not use hot-water bottles or electric heating pads. Don't burn the feet! Electric blankets are satisfactory.
* Do not wear garters or sit with legs crossed. Either will decrease circulation to the feet. (The circulation may already be less than normal because of the effect diabetes may have on your blood vessels.)
* Wear thin socks of cotton (not wool) to prevent moisture, which stimulates germs that cause athlete's foot or other infections. Wear clean socks that you change at least daily. Do not wear loose socks with raised seams.
* Check your feet every day for any changes in the skin. Use a mirror to see the bottom of the feet or back of the heel.

 ## WHAT TO EXPECT

DIAGNOSTIC MEASURES
* Your own observation of symptoms.
* See your health care provider if new skin problems occur and don't improve in a day or two or they cause concern.

APPROPRIATE HEALTH CARE
* Self-care for preventive measures.
* Medical care may be needed if complications occur. This may include drug therapy, special wound care and dressings, surgery, use of aids for walking (such as crutches), and others,

POSSIBLE COMPLICATIONS—Without treatment, serious foot problems may develop including infections, ulcers, gangrene, and amputation.

PROBABLE OUTCOME—Using preventive measures and seeking early treatment of infections will help to avoid serious problems.

 ## HOW TO TREAT

GENERAL MEASURES—To learn more: Local or national office of the American Diabetes Association, Attention: National Call Center, 1701 Beauregard St., Alexandria, VA 22311; (800) 342-2383; website: www.diabetes.org.

MEDICATION—Drugs for infections may be prescribed.

ACTIVITY—Regular activities (unless foot problems interfere).

DIET—Follow prescribed diet.

 ## CALL YOUR DOCTOR IF

* Skin on the foot becomes red, itchy, swollen, or is painful.
* Foot problems occur despite taking preventive measures.

DIABETES HYPOGLYCEMIA

 GENERAL INFORMATION

DEFINITION—Hypoglycemia means low blood sugar. When blood sugar drops too far below normal, a group of symptoms develop. Signs and symptoms vary in different people. Get to know your signs and symptoms. Also, your daytime symptoms may vary from those that occur at night.

BODY PARTS INVOLVED—Endocrine and metabolic body systems.

SEX OR AGE MOST AFFECTED—Both sexes; all ages.

SIGNS & SYMPTOMS
Mild:
* Hunger.
* Weakness.
* Nervousness.
* Emotional ups and downs.
* Difficulty in concentrating.
* Sweating.
* Headache.

Moderately severe:
* Increased weakness.
* Excessive perspiration.
* Skin that is cold and clammy to touch.
* Numbness about the mouth, and sometimes, fingers.
* Pounding of heart.
* Loss of memory.
* Double vision.
* Staring expression.
* Difficulty walking.
* Unaware of surroundings.

Severe:
* Twitching of muscles.
* Unconsciousness.
* Convulsions.
* Unaware of passing urine.

CAUSES—Hypoglycemia occurs when there is too much insulin in the body and not enough intake of food. It is more frequent in insulin-dependent type diabetes.

RISK INCREASES WITH
* Eating meals at times other than regular time.
* Skipping meals or eating only parts of meals.
* Dosing with too much insulin or other diabetic drug.
* More exercise or activity than usual.
* Alcohol use.
* Other, rarer risk factors.

HOW TO PREVENT
* Maintaining a regular schedule of diet, medication and exercise.
* Regular blood-glucose testing.
* Learn to recognize the early symptoms of hypoglycemia and take prompt action.
* Be sure family and friends know about the symptoms so if you become disoriented or confused, they can give you something sweet.
* Always have access to a simple sugar.

 WHAT TO EXPECT

DIAGNOSTIC MEASURES
* Your own or other's observation of symptoms.
* Medical diagnosis if needed.

APPROPRIATE HEALTH CARE
* Self-care is usually all that is needed.
* Medical care for complications or if there is any doubt about the cause.

POSSIBLE COMPLICATIONS
* Diabetic shock or coma.
* Permanent brain damage or death.

PROBABLE OUTCOME—Full recovery is the usual outcome. It depends on quick diagnosis and treatment.

 HOW TO TREAT

GENERAL MEASURES
* If hypoglycemia symptoms begin, eat or drink something that has sugar in it. This includes hard candy, fruit juice, or glucose tablets that you can buy at a drug store. If there are 30 minutes or more to the next meal, some protein and starch foods should also be eaten. They can help prevent another reaction.
* If the patient passes out, glucagon needs to be injected. Patients and families should have glucagon at hand and know how to inject it.
* Check blood sugar about 15 to 20 minutes after treatment for hypoglycemia. Repeat treatment if needed.
* If no glucagon is at hand, get the patient to the nearest emergency center or telephone for emergency help.
* To learn more: Contact the local or national office of the American Diabetes Association, Attn: National Call Center, 1701 Beauregard St., Alexandria, VA 22311; (800) 342-2383; website: www.diabetes.org.

MEDICATION—Insulin dose may need to be adjusted if it is the cause of hypoglycemia.

ACTIVITY—Rest until symptoms resolve.

DIET—If eating habits cause the hypoglycemia. Changes may need to be made in your diet.

 CALL YOUR DOCTOR IF

* You or a family member has symptoms of hypoglycemia that are not helped by home care.
* Attacks are recurring.
* Changes need to be made in insulin dosages.
* Adjustments need to be made in insulin dosages.

DIABETES INSIPIDUS

GENERAL INFORMATION

DEFINITION—A rare disorder of the hormone system, centered in the pituitary gland. It disrupts normal fluid regulation in the body. This condition has nothing to do with blood sugar levels or other types of diabetes.

BODY PARTS INVOLVED—Pituitary gland; endocrine system.

SEX OR AGE MOST AFFECTED—It can affect all ages and occurs equally in men and women.

SIGNS & SYMPTOMS
• Excessive thirst that is difficult to satisfy.
• Passing large amounts of diluted, colorless urine (up to 15 quarts a day).
• Dry hands.
• Constipation.

CAUSES—The cause for diabetes insipidus may be known or unknown. Types include:
• In one type (neurogenic or central), the pituitary gland in the brain does not make enough of an antidiuretic hormone (called ADH) needed for the body to function.
• In another type (nephrogenic), there is enough ADH hormone produced, but the kidneys don't work with the hormone as they should.
• Two other types involve an abnormal thirst (dipsogenic) and pregnancy (gestagenic).

RISK INCREASES WITH
• Tumor of the pituitary gland or other brain tumor.
• Head injury, with damage to the pituitary gland.
• Brain infection, such as encephalitis or meningitis.
• Blockage of the arteries to the brain.
• Aneurysm or other blood vessel problems.
• Granulomas (chronic inflammation).
• Drugs, such as lithium.
• Kidney disorders.
• Family history of diabetes insipidus.

HOW TO PREVENT—No specific preventive measures.

WHAT TO EXPECT

DIAGNOSTIC MEASURES
• Your own observation of symptoms.
• Your health care provider will do a physical exam and ask questions about your symptoms.
• Medical studies may include water-deprivation tests to determine levels of ADH. Blood and urine studies are usually done. If diabetes insipidus is diagnosed, A CT or MRI (see Glossary for both) of the brain may be done to check for any problems.

APPROPRIATE HEALTH CARE—Treatment involves controlling fluid balance and preventing dehydration and identifying the cause of the diabetes insipidus.

POSSIBLE COMPLICATIONS
• Electrolyte imbalance, especially low levels of sodium or potassium. Either of these can cause heartbeat irregularity, fatigue, and congestive heart failure.
• Young children may have growth failure.

PROBABLE OUTCOME—The prognosis is generally good depending on the underlying disorder.

HOW TO TREAT

GENERAL MEASURES
• Check weight daily and maintain a record.
• Wear a medical identification bracelet or neck pendant that indicates your medical problem and the drugs you take.
• To learn more: Diabetes Insipidus Foundation, 5203 New Prospect Dr., Ellicott City, MD 21043; (706) 323-7576 (not toll free); website: www.diabetesinsipidus.org.

MEDICATION
• Desmopressin (DDAVP) may be prescribed. It is a synthetic ADH and may be used in nose drops, by mouth, or in an injection form.
• Drugs may be prescribed to help the body balance the amount of salt and water.

ACTIVITY—No limits, unless advised.

DIET
• Monitor fluid intake as advised by your health care provider.
• A low sodium diet may be prescribed.

CALL YOUR DOCTOR IF

• You or a family member has symptoms of diabetes insipidus.
• Symptoms don't improve, despite treatment.
• New, unexplained symptoms develop. Drugs used in treatment may produce side effects.

DIABETES TYPE 1

GENERAL INFORMATION

DEFINITION—Diabetes is a chronic condition in which the body is not able to control the amount of glucose (a form of sugar) in the blood. Glucose is needed by the body to produce energy, but too much glucose leads to serious problems. Glucose levels are normally controlled by the hormone, insulin, which is produced in the pancreas. With diabetes, there is either not enough insulin produced or the body is unable to use the insulin that is produced. There are two main types of diabetes, type 1 and type 2. Type 1 diabetes is also called insulin-dependent diabetes or juvenile diabetes. About 5% to 10% of people with diabetes have type 1.

BODY PARTS INVOLVED
• Islet cells of the pancreas that produce insulin.
• All body cells that need insulin to convert food into chemicals the body can use.

SEX OR AGE MOST AFFECTED—It can develop at any age, but often occurs in children, teenagers, or young adults of both sexes.

SIGNS & SYMPTOMS
• Fatigue and excess thirst.
• Increased appetite and weight loss.
• Frequent urination.
• Itching around the genitals.
• General ill feeling.
• Blurred vision.
• Increased risk of infections, such as urinary-tract infections and yeast infections of the skin, mouth, or vagina.

CAUSES—In type 1 diabetes, little or no insulin is made by the pancreas. It is one of a group of autoimmune disorders. In these disorders, the immune system mistakenly attacks the body itself. Why this occurs is unknown. Other possible factors include a viral infection or an injury to the pancreas.

RISK INCREASES WITH—Family history of diabetes. It occasionally skips one generation.

HOW TO PREVENT—Cannot be prevented.

WHAT TO EXPECT

DIAGNOSTIC MEASURES
• Your own observation of symptoms.
• Your health care provider will do a physical exam and ask questions about your symptoms.
• Medical tests include blood glucose and urine studies. A glucose tolerance test may be done. A hemoglobin A1C (HbA1c) may be done as a follow-up. This test measures average blood glucose levels for the past 2 to 3 months.

APPROPRIATE HEALTH CARE—Type 1 diabetes is treated with insulin, exercise, diet, and steps to prevent complications. A diabetes educator can teach you to manage diabetes.

POSSIBLE COMPLICATIONS
• Cardiovascular (heart and blood vessel) disease (stroke, atherosclerosis, and coronary-artery disease).
• Foot or leg amputation due to poor circulation.
• Kidney damage.
• Blindness.
• Nerve damage (neuropathy).
• Sexual impotence in men.
• Hypoglycemia (low blood sugar).
• Hyperglycemia (high blood sugar).
• Ketoacidosis (very high blood sugar).

PROBABLE OUTCOME—There is no cure. Adhering to a treatment plan can improve symptoms and delay progress of the disease. Long-term complications may occur.

HOW TO TREAT

GENERAL MEASURES
• Learn all you can about diabetes. Learn the techniques of self-monitoring of blood sugar and monitor regularly. Learn the signs and symptoms of high and low blood glucose levels and what to do. Keep glucose tablets handy for treating low blood sugar, if needed.
• Get regular foot care and routine eye exams.
• Stop smoking. Find a way to quit that works.
• Wear a medical alert type bracelet or pendant to indicate you have diabetes and take insulin.
• Get medical care for any infection.
• To learn more: American Diabetes Association, 1701 North Beauregard St., Alexandria, VA 22311, (800) 342-2383; website www.diabetes.org.

MEDICATION
• Insulin will be prescribed. Dosage will be based on your individual needs. It is self-injected, or in some cases, an infusion pump is used. Forms of insulin are classified by how fast they work or how long they last.
• Aspirin (for adults), cholesterol-lowering drugs, and drugs for high blood pressure may also be prescribed.

ACTIVITY—Exercise helps control diabetes. Follow medical advice about daily exercising.

DIET—A healthy diet is part of treatment. Don't skip meals. A dietitian can help with meal plans.

CALL YOUR DOCTOR IF

• You or a family member has symptoms of diabetes.
• After diagnosis, any symptoms cause you concern or problems occur with glucose control.

DIABETES TYPE 2

 GENERAL INFORMATION

DEFINITION—Diabetes is a chronic condition in which the body is not able to control the amount of glucose (a form of sugar) in the blood. Glucose is needed by the body to produce energy, but too much glucose leads to serious problems. Glucose levels are normally controlled by the hormone, insulin, which is produced in the pancreas. With diabetes, there is either not enough insulin produced or the body is unable to use the insulin that is produced. There are two main types of diabetes, type 1 and type 2 Type 2 is the most common type (about 90% to 95% of people with diabetes), and is also known as non-insulin dependent diabetes.

BODY PARTS INVOLVED
* Islet cells of the pancreas that produce insulin.
* All body cells that need insulin to convert food into chemicals the body can use.

SEX OR AGE MOST AFFECTED—Both sexes; usually adults.

SIGNS & SYMPTOMS
* Many people don't know they have diabetes. There may be no symptoms or symptoms develop gradually.
* Fatigue and excess thirst.
* General ill feeling, increased appetite, weight loss, and frequent urination.
* Slow healing of cuts and bruises.
* Blurred vision.
* Impotence (erectile dysfunction).
* Increased risk of infections.

CAUSES—The pancreas may produce enough insulin, but, for unknown reasons, the body is unable to use it effectively (insulin resistance). After several years, insulin production decreases and glucose builds up in the blood.

RISK INCREASES WITH
* Family history of diabetes.
* Gestational diabetes (diabetes in pregnancy).
* Overweight (more so if fat is in the abdomen).
* High blood pressure; high cholesterol or high triglycerides.
* Sedentary lifestyle (lack of physical activity).
* Metabolic syndrome (a set of conditions).
* African Americans, Native Americans, Hispanic Americans, Pacific Islanders, and Asian Americans.

HOW TO PREVENT—To help prevent or delay onset of type 2 diabetes:
* Control weight and lose weight if overweight.
* Exercise regularly.
* Eat a healthy diet.
* Get treatment to control high blood pressure and high cholesterol levels.

 WHAT TO EXPECT

DIAGNOSTIC MEASURES
* Your health care provider will do a physical exam and ask questions about your symptoms.
* Medical tests include blood glucose and urine studies. A glucose tolerance test may be done. A hemoglobin A1C (HbA1c) may be done as a follow-up. This test measures average blood glucose levels for the past 2 to 3 months.

APPROPRIATE HEALTH CARE—Type 2 diabetes is treated with lifestyle changes (exercise and diet) and drug therapy,

POSSIBLE COMPLICATIONS
* Type 1 diabetes (insulin-dependent diabetes).
* Heart and blood vessel disease.
* Kidney damage; blindness; or nerve damage.
* Hypoglycemia (low blood sugar), hyperglycemia (high blood sugar), or ketoacidosis (severe reaction).

PROBABLE OUTCOME—Good blood glucose control (with lifestyle changes and/or drugs) can help prevent or delay complications.

 HOW TO TREAT

GENERAL MEASURES
* Learn the techniques of self-monitoring of blood sugar and monitor regularly. Know the symptoms of high and low blood glucose levels and what to do. Keep glucose tablets handy.
* Get regular foot care and regular eye exams.
* Stop smoking. Find a way to quit that works.
* Wear a medical alert type bracelet or neck tag to show you have diabetes and drugs you take.
* Get medical care for any infection.
* To learn more: American Diabetes Association, 1701 North Beauregard St., Alexandria, VA 22311, (800) 342-2383; website www.diabetes.org.

MEDICATION
* One or more types of oral antidiabetic drugs may be prescribed. Your health care provider will discuss the options, the benefits, and the risks with you. Insulin may be prescribed if oral drugs are not effective.
* Aspirin (for adults), cholesterol-lowering drugs, and drugs for high blood pressure may also be prescribed.

ACTIVITY—Exercise helps control diabetes.

DIET—A healthy diet is part of treatment. Don't skip meals. A dietitian can help you plan meals.

 CALL YOUR DOCTOR IF

* You or a family member has symptoms of diabetes.
* After diagnosis, you have any concerns.

DIAPER RASH

GENERAL INFORMATION

DEFINITION—Skin irritation in infants. It involves the skin in the area covered by diapers. Diaper rash is very common.

BODY PARTS INVOLVED—Skin around the genitals, rectum and abdomen in the area covered by diapers.

SEX OR AGE MOST AFFECTED—Infants and young children who wear diapers.

SIGNS & SYMPTOMS
- Moist, painful, red, spotty, and sometimes itchy skin in the diaper area. The skin may be cracked and split.
- In male infants a red, raw and sometimes bloody area may appear around the opening at the tip of the penis.

CAUSES
- It is most often a form of contact dermatitis. Diaper rash results from the skin being irritated by moisture in the urine or stool.
- Less often, it may be an allergic reaction. This can be from disposable diapers or baby wipes, or soap used for washing cloth diapers.

RISK INCREASES WITH
- Not changing diapers often enough.
- Skin gets rubbed from rough diapers.
- Cloth diapers may not be washed properly.
- Family history of skin allergies.
- Hot, humid weather.

HOW TO PREVENT
- Change diapers often.
- Use diaper products that are breathable. These allow more air to circulate. Breathable disposable diapers, cloth diapers, and diaper covers are available.
- Avoid using plastic pants.
- Leave diaper off for 10 to 30 minutes between diaper changes for air exposure.

WHAT TO EXPECT

DIAGNOSTIC MEASURES
- Your own observation of symptoms.
- See your child's health care provider if you are concerned about the rash.

APPROPRIATE HEALTH CARE
- Home care is all that is usually needed.
- Medical care if home treatment fails to cure the rash.

POSSIBLE COMPLICATIONS—Skin infection in the rash area.

PROBABLE OUTCOME—Curable with treatment. The rash is rarely serious. Recurrence is common.

HOW TO TREAT

GENERAL MEASURES
- Leave off the diaper and expose the affected skin area to air when possible.
- Change diapers often, even at night, if the rash is more severe.
- Clean the skin under the diaper with warm water and mild soap that is not perfumed. Baby wipes may also be used, but they might irritate skin in some babies.
- Don't use talcum powder or cornstarch.
- Apply small amounts of petroleum jelly, lanolin ointment, or zinc oxide ointment to the skin at the first sign of diaper rash, and thereafter 2 or 3 times a day.
- After you launder cloth diapers, put them in boiling water for 15 minutes. This will remove any leftover soap and kill any germs.

MEDICATION—Your child's health care provider may recommend medicated ointments or creams to be applied to the skin to help clear up the rash.

ACTIVITY—No limits.

DIET—No special diet. Avoid baby foods that cause diarrhea.

CALL YOUR DOCTOR IF

- Home treatment doesn't cure the rash in 1 week.
- The following occur during treatment:
  - Fever.
  - Sores develop in the rash area.

DIARRHEA, ACUTE

GENERAL INFORMATION

DEFINITION—An abnormal increase in the liquidity and frequency of stools. This is a symptom, not a disease.

BODY PARTS INVOLVED—Colon; small intestine.

SEX OR AGE MOST AFFECTED—Both sexes; simple diarrhea is common among all age groups.

SIGNS & SYMPTOMS
* Cramping abdominal pain.
* Loose, watery or unformed bowel movements.
* Lack of bowel control (sometimes).
* Fever (sometimes).

CAUSES—Either the intestines produce too much fluid or not enough fluid is absorbed from the intestines. There are many causes, including infections.

RISK INCREASES WITH
* Viral gastroenteritis (stomach "flu").
* Food intolerance or lactose intolerance.
* Emotional upsets or stress.
* Food poisoning.
* Eating foods, such as prunes or beans.
* Children in daycare.
* Food allergy.
* Malabsorption syndromes.
* Disease or tumor of the pancreas.
* Diverticulitis, appendicitis, or fecal impaction.
* Excess alcohol use.
* Use of drugs, such as laxatives, antacids, antibiotics, quinine, or anticancer drugs.
* Radiation treatments for cancer.
* Recent illness.
* Irritable bowel syndrome.
* Inflammatory bowel disease.
* Crowded or unsanitary living conditions.
* Weak immune system due to illness or drugs.
* Travel to foreign country.
* Drinking contaminated water.

HOW TO PREVENT
* Wash hands often to prevent spread of germs, especially after using the bathroom.
* Avoid undercooked or raw seafood, buffet or picnic foods left out for several hours, and food served by street vendors.

WHAT TO EXPECT

DIAGNOSTIC MEASURES
* Your own observation of symptoms.
* See your health care provider if symptoms are more severe or they cause you any concern. A physical exam may be done.
* Medical tests may include studies of blood and stool.

APPROPRIATE HEALTH CARE
* In most cases, this disorder will be self-treated at home.
* Medical care (if symptoms persist longer than 2 to 3 days).
* Hospital care may be needed, if dehydration is severe.

POSSIBLE COMPLICATIONS—Dehydration if diarrhea is prolonged, especially in infants.

PROBABLE OUTCOME—It goes away by itself and leaves no lasting effects. Most cases of diarrhea last a short time (24 to 48 hours) and a search for the cause may be unnecessary.

HOW TO TREAT

GENERAL MEASURES
* Treatment usually involves drinking plenty of fluids and rest as needed. There is no specific drug therapy.
* It is not necessary to keep persons with diarrhea away from others in the family or household. Try to avoid close contact if possible. Wash hands often.

MEDICATION
* Drugs are usually not needed for treatment. If symptoms are severe or prolonged, you may use drugs for nausea or diarrhea such as loperamide or Pepto-Bismol.
* Some infections may require specific drug treatment.
* If a drug you take is the cause of the problem, you may be advised to change drugs or stop taking the drug.

ACTIVITY—Get extra rest if needed. Be sure to have access to a toilet or bedpan.

DIET
* Suck ice chips or drink small amounts of clear fluids often. Replace lost fluids and electrolytes with products such as Pedialyte or Ricelyte for infants and children, and diluted rehydration fluids (Gatorade) for adults.
* Once the symptoms improve, try a diet of complex carbohydrates (rice, wheat, potatoes, bread, cereal, and lean meat such as chicken). Milk and dairy products usually do not need to be limited.
* Avoid high sugar foods or fatty foods for a few days.

CALL YOUR DOCTOR IF

* Diarrhea lasts more than 48 hours.
* Mucus, blood, or worms appear in the stool, or fever or severe pain develops.
* Dehydration develops. Signs include dry mouth, wrinkled skin, excess thirst, and little or no urination.

DIARRHEA, CHRONIC, NONSPECIFIC OF CHILDHOOD

 GENERAL INFORMATION

DEFINITION—Diarrhea is called chronic when it lasts more than three weeks. Most cases of diarrhea in children are acute and last less than 10 days.

BODY PARTS INVOLVED—Colon.

SEX OR AGE MOST AFFECTED—Young children (1-1/2 to 3-1/2 years).

SIGNS & SYMPTOMS
• Loose stools, sometimes watery.
• Stools are sometimes normal.
• Stools are more frequent than usual.
• Pain in the stomach area.
• Occasional soreness of the anal area caused by many bowel movements.

CAUSES—Nonspecific means no cause has been found such as infection or food intolerance. It may have to do with some aspect of the diet. Sometimes, the children affected drink excessive amounts of fluid or juices (such as apple juice).

RISK INCREASES WITH—No specific risk factors.

HOW TO PREVENT—Cannot be prevented at present.

 WHAT TO EXPECT

DIAGNOSTIC MEASURES
• Your own observation of symptoms.
• Your child's health care provider will do a physical exam and ask questions about the symptoms. Information about your child's activities, and eating and drinking habits will help with the diagnosis.
• Medical tests may be done to rule out any specific cause.

APPROPRIATE HEALTH CARE—Treatment may include diet changes for your child or lifestyle changes such as being more active.

POSSIBLE COMPLICATIONS—Usually no complications. Emotional problems such as anxiety may occur with parents and children.

PROBABLE OUTCOME—Despite the chronic diarrhea, affected children grow and develop normally. Diet changes can help resolve the diarrhea symptoms in some children. In others, bowel movements often become normal at about age 4.

 HOW TO TREAT

GENERAL MEASURES—Don't blame or criticize your child for this problem. Don't expect toilet training to be successful as soon as with some other children. Treat your child as normal and try to ignore the problem. Avoid tension. If the child becomes anxious about diarrhea, the problem may become worse or emotional problems may arise.

MEDICATION—Drugs are usually not needed for this disorder. Your child's health care provider may sometimes prescribe antidiarrheal drugs for a short period of time. Don't give your child herbal products or other dietary supplements without medical approval.

ACTIVITY—Your child should be physically active as appropriate for the age group.

DIET—Your child's health care provider will discuss diet changes with you. The goal is to achieve a healthy diet with regard to fat, fiber, fluids, and fruit juices. High-fiber foods such as beans, fruit, breads, and cereals are important in the diet.

 CALL YOUR DOCTOR IF

• Your child has diarrhea that lasts over 3 weeks.
• There is blood in the stool.
• Fever occurs.
• Your child becomes listless, refuses to eat, or cries loudly and persistently, even when picked up.
• Your child begins to lose weight or is not growing as expected.

ILLNESS & DISORDERS

DIPHTHERIA

GENERAL INFORMATION

DEFINITION—An acute, highly contagious respiratory infection. Incubation period is from 2 to 5 days.

BODY PARTS INVOLVED—Throat; skin; heart; central nervous system.

SEX OR AGE MOST AFFECTED—Older children (5 years and up), adolescents and adults.

SIGNS & SYMPTOMS
Early stages:
* Sore throat.
* Low fever.
* Swollen neck glands.
Late stages:
* Airway obstruction and breathing difficulty.
* Shock (low blood pressure, rapid heartbeat, paleness, cold skin, sweating, and anxious appearance).

CAUSES—A bacterial germ, *Corynebacterium diphtheriae*, infects the throat and sometimes the skin. The germ produces poisons that spread to the heart, central nervous system, and other organs.

RISK INCREASES WITH
* Adults over 60 and children under 5.
* Poor nutrition.
* Outbreak in the community.
* Crowded or unclean living conditions.
* Lack of up-to-date immunizations.
* Alcoholism.

HOW TO PREVENT
* Immunization with diphtheria vaccine.
* Improved nutrition and standard of living.
* Notify the local health department of any case of diphtheria. Anyone having contact with the patient must be examined and treated.

WHAT TO EXPECT

DIAGNOSTIC MEASURES
* Your own observation of symptoms.
* Your health care provider will do a physical exam.
* Medical tests usually include a throat culture and blood studies.

APPROPRIATE HEALTH CARE—Hospital care and isolation of the patient are needed until fully recovered. Protect susceptible individuals (the non-immunized, very young, or elderly) from exposure. Patients may require mechanical assistance in breathing.

POSSIBLE COMPLICATIONS
* Heart inflammation and heart failure.
* Suffocation.
* Nerve inflammation.
* Misdiagnosis as a less-serious infection, resulting in dangerous delay of treatment.

PROBABLE OUTCOME—Usually curable in 1 week if treatment is begun promptly, followed by slow recovery for several weeks. A delay in treatment may result in death or long-term heart disease.

HOW TO TREAT

GENERAL MEASURES
* Dispose of all secretions (nose and mouth) and excretions (urine and feces) in an acceptable manner. Call the local health department for instructions.
* People who have been in close contact with the patient and who have not been immunized should have throat cultures and be immunized. They should be watched closely for possible symptoms. A booster vaccine may be given for people who have been immunized.

MEDICATION
* Diphtheria antitoxin to neutralize the diphtheria toxin will be given during hospital care.
* Antibiotics to fight remaining diphtheria germs will be prescribed.

ACTIVITY—Prolonged bed rest (2 to 3 months or until fully recovered), especially if the heart is involved.

DIET—Liquid to soft diet as tolerated.

CALL YOUR DOCTOR IF

* You or a family member has symptoms of diphtheria or you observe them in someone else.
* Anyone in your family is exposed to diphtheria.
* Your immunizations are not current.
* The following occur during treatment:
  - Temperature rises to 102°F (38.9°C).
  - Increasing difficulty breathing.
  - Increasing shortness of breath.
  - Confusion.

DISK, RUPTURED
(Herniated Disk; Slipped Disk)

 GENERAL INFORMATION

DEFINITION—A ruptured disk is one that has moved or slipped out of its normal position.

BODY PARTS INVOLVED—Disks are part of the backbone and normally help the back to flex and bend. Disks are pads that are soft and gel-like in children and get harder as a person ages. Disks act as a cushion between each of the hard bones (vertebrae) of the spine.

SEX OR AGE MOST AFFECTED—Adults of both sexes.

SIGNS & SYMPTOMS
• Sharp or shooting pain in the lower back. Pain goes from the buttock down the back of one or both legs (sciatica). Movement can make it worse.
• Unable to bend or straighten the back.
• Back pain may develop over time in some cases. It may be more apparent when getting out of bed or when coughing.
• Numbness or tingling in an arm or leg. There may be some loss of strength in one or both legs.

CAUSES—A disk ruptures due to wear and tear or excess strain. The ruptured, bulging disk can be painless. It becomes painful when it puts pressure on nearby ligaments or nerves. Most disk injuries occur in the lower back. The disks in the upper back are less often affected.

RISK INCREASES WITH
• Heavy lifting.
• Poor physical condition.
• Twisting violently or jumping hard.
• Obesity.
• Elderly.
• Degenerative disk disease (changes that occur in disks as person ages).

HOW TO PREVENT
• Use proper posture when lifting.
• Exercise regularly to maintain good muscle tone and flexibility.

 WHAT TO EXPECT

DIAGNOSTIC MEASURES
• Your own observation of symptoms.
• Your health care provider will do a physical exam and ask questions about your symptoms and recent activities.
• To confirm diagnosis, tests may include x-rays of the neck or lower spine.

APPROPRIATE HEALTH CARE
• For most patients, treatment with simple measures is all that is needed. This starts with relief for pain and inflammation.
• Further measures include steps to restore back strength and a return to normal activity.
• In some cases, electrical stimulation, or a neck collar, or a back brace may be prescribed.
• Other treatment options include chiropractic care, acupuncture, or massage therapy.
• Surgery is needed if the disk is causing any loss of body function (such as bowel function) or nerve damage. Different procedures are available depending on the individual problem.
• Physical therapy is often needed after surgery to restore full function to the back.

POSSIBLE COMPLICATIONS
• Loss of bladder and bowel function.
• Muscle loss and weakness.

PROBABLE OUTCOME—Recovery usually takes about 6 weeks and is helped with simple treatment measures. If needed, surgery can relieve serious symptoms.

 HOW TO TREAT

GENERAL MEASURES
• Use ice packs to the painful area during the first 72 hours. After that, try using heat. Take warm showers or baths. Use warm compresses or a heating pad.
• Be patient about your recovery. It will take time and energy.

MEDICATION
• For minor pain, you may use nonprescription drugs such as acetaminophen or ibuprofen.
• Other drugs may be prescribed:
 - Pain relievers.
 - Muscle relaxants.
 - Drugs to reduce swelling around the rupture.
 - Laxatives or stool softeners for constipation.

ACTIVITY
• A long bed rest does not help. Rest for only 1 to 2 days, then start resuming normal activities.
• Take short walks. Don't sit for long periods. Follow any exercise routine prescribed by your health care provider or physical therapist.

DIET—No special diet.

 CALL YOUR DOCTOR IF

• You or a family member has symptoms of a ruptured disk.
• The following occur during treatment: Increased pain or weakness in back or legs, problems with bladder or bowel control, fever, or stomach pain.

DISLOCATION OR SUBLUXATION

GENERAL INFORMATION

DEFINITION—A dislocation is a joint injury in which the ends of the bones are forced from their normal position. They are no longer connected. If the bones still have some contact, it is called a subluxation. An injury may also affect the joint capsule, ligaments, and nerves.

BODY PARTS INVOLVED—Bones in joints, especially the jaw, shoulder, knee and spine. Some infants are born with a hip dislocation.

SEX OR AGE MOST AFFECTED—Both sexes; all ages.

SIGNS & SYMPTOMS
• Sudden joint pain, swelling, or an out-of-place joint after an injury. The shoulder is most often affected, but it may happen to any joint including the elbow, finger, knee, ankle, toe, hip, or jaw.
• Limited or no movement around a joint.

CAUSES—Injury (fall or hit) that puts too much pressure on a joint. Less often, a dislocation may occur as a result of disease that affects the structure of the joint. A joint is where two or more bones come together in the body. Ligaments connect bones to bones.

RISK INCREASES WITH
• Contact sports.
• Sports or activities that require quick motion, twisting, or pivoting.
• Hypermobile (loose) joints that move beyond their normal range with little effort.
• Previous dislocation or subluxation of the joint.

HOW TO PREVENT
• For sports or recreational activities (such as skating), wear proper equipment to protect the joints.
• Use safety measures in the home to prevent falls or other accidents.
• Do weight training to strengthen muscles and joints.

WHAT TO EXPECT

DIAGNOSTIC MEASURES
• Your own observation of symptoms.
• Your health care provider will do an exam of the injured joint and ask questions about the activity that caused the injury.
• Medical tests usually include x-rays of the joint and nearby bones to check for fractures.

APPROPRIATE HEALTH CARE
• Treatment to realign the bones after a dislocation or subluxation is called reduction. It may include maneuvers to put the bones back into the normal position. In some cases, surgery may be needed.

• After reduction treatment, the joint may be put into a splint or cast. This allows it to heal.
• Crutches may be needed while the injury heals.
• Frequent dislocations in the same joint may need surgery to correct or replace the joint.

POSSIBLE COMPLICATIONS
• Damage to nearby nerves or major blood vessels.
• Soreness and swelling may persist for many months.
• Repeated injuries in the joint may lead to arthritis.

PROBABLE OUTCOME—Usually curable with prompt treatment. After the dislocation has been treated, the joint may require a cast or sling for 2 to 8 weeks. Full recovery after surgery may take up to 6 months.

HOW TO TREAT

GENERAL MEASURES
• Right after an injury:
  - An untrained person should not try to move the joint back into position. It could cause further injury.
  - Apply ice packs to the involved joint. Elevate it (prop it up) if possible to ease pain and prevent swelling.
  - If needed, use a splint or sling to prevent movement while taking the injured person to a medical facility.
• After treatment, elevate the injured area on a pillow when you are resting.

MEDICATION
• Anesthesia or muscle-relaxing drugs may be used to make the joint realignment possible.
• Use acetaminophen or ibuprofen for mild pain.
• Stronger pain relievers may be prescribed.

ACTIVITY
• Physical therapy may be prescribed to restore normal strength and range of motion to the joint.
• Your health care provider will advise you about returning to sports and other physical activities.

DIET—Do not eat any food before treatment in case a general anesthetic is needed.

CALL YOUR DOCTOR IF

• You or a family member has symptoms of a dislocation or subluxation.
• Difficulty moving a joint develops after injury.
• Any joint area becomes numb, pale or cold, after injury. This is an emergency!
• Dislocations occur repeatedly that you can "pop" back into normal position.

DISSEMINATED INTRAVASCULAR COAGULATION (DIC)

GENERAL INFORMATION

DEFINITION—A serious, life-threatening disorder that involves blood clotting factors. This disorder is a complication of a variety of other diseases.

BODY PARTS INVOLVED—Blood vessels and blood in all parts of the body.

SEX OR AGE MOST AFFECTED—Both sexes; all ages.

SIGNS & SYMPTOMS
- Bleeding from any or several body parts, such as the nose or gums. Bleeding may be heavy. Common signs of bleeding include:
  - Vomiting up blood or material that looks like coffee grounds.
  - Red or black stools.
  - Vaginal bleeding.
  - Red or cloudy urine.
  - Bruising, pinpoint red spots on the skin, or bleeding under the skin (purpura).
- Severe stomach or back pain caused by bleeding into body organs.
- Cough, shortness of breath, fever, and confusion.

CAUSES—A decrease in blood-clotting factors which leads to severe bleeding (hemorrhaging).

RISK INCREASES WITH
- Widespread or major infection.
- Cancer.
- Certain types of surgery.
- Diseases such as arthritis, ulcerative colitis, Crohn's disease, sarcoidosis, Raynaud disease, and others.
- Burns or injuries.
- Pregnancy complications such as placental abruption, eclampsia, or retained dead fetus.
- Poisonous snakebite.
- Transfusion or blood disorders.
- Heart attack.
- Prosthetic devices, shunts, or heart assist devices.

HOW TO PREVENT—Obtain prompt medical care for any of the risk factors listed.

WHAT TO EXPECT

DIAGNOSTIC MEASURES
- Your own observation of symptoms.
- Patients with this condition are often very ill. Hospital care is needed for diagnosis and treatment.

APPROPRIATE HEALTH CARE
- Treatment will be provided for the DIC symptoms such as bleeding, and for any underlying disorder.
- Oxygen may be provided through a face-mask. Some patients require breathing support with a ventilator (a device to help the lungs).
- Surgery for the underlying disorder (sometimes).

POSSIBLE COMPLICATIONS
- Kidney failure.
- Shock.
- Gangrene and amputation.
- Blood clots and hemorrhage (excess bleeding).
- Hemothorax (blood in the lungs).
- Death.

PROBABLE OUTCOME—Outcome depends on the underlying cause, severity of the DIC, age, and health status.

HOW TO TREAT

GENERAL MEASURES—Patients with this condition are often desperately ill and require intensive hospital care. Family members can help by maintaining a positive, hopeful attitude.

MEDICATION
- Blood transfusions or replacement of blood products may be needed.
- Drugs to prevent blood clots and to help control hemorrhage are usually prescribed.
- Drugs as needed to treat the underlying disorder or medical problem.

ACTIVITY—Bed rest.

DIET—Whatever type of diet is tolerated depending on patient's condition.

CALL YOUR DOCTOR IF

- You or a family member has symptoms of DIC. This is an emergency.
- Symptoms recur after treatment.

DIVERTICULAR DISEASE
(Diverticulosis; Diverticulitis)

 GENERAL INFORMATION

DEFINITION
• Diverticulosis is the presence of small, shallow, sac-like depressions (diverticula) in the wall of the colon. These diverticula may be present without any symptoms.
• Diverticulitis occurs when diverticula become infected or inflamed. It can be a serious and dangerous disorder.

BODY PARTS INVOLVED—Left side of the large intestine.

SEX OR AGE MOST AFFECTED—Adults.
Diverticula are present in 30% to 40% of persons over age 50. They increase with each decade of life.

SIGNS & SYMPTOMS
Diverticulosis symptoms:
• No symptoms (usually).
• Mild cramping that comes and goes. Bloating or tenderness in the abdomen. Passing gas or bowel movements may relieve these symptoms.
• Constipation or diarrhea.
Diverticulitis symptoms:
• Pain in the abdomen that becomes constant. Pain may be disabling from the start or may not become disabling for several days.
• Areas of the abdomen are tender to the touch.
• Fever, chills, nausea, and vomiting.
• Blood in the stool.

CAUSES—Exact cause is unknown. A low-fiber diet is thought to be the main factor in developing diverticula. Why they become infected or inflamed is also unknown. It is possible that stool or bacteria are caught in the diverticula.

RISK INCREASES WITH
• Diet that does not have enough fiber.
• Constipation.
• Age over 50.
• Smoking. It is a risk factor for complications.

HOW TO PREVENT—None specific. To reduce risk, eat a high-fiber diet, exercise daily, avoid constipation, and don't smoke.

 WHAT TO EXPECT

DIAGNOSTIC MEASURES
• Your own observation of symptoms.
• Your health care provider may do a physical exam and a digital rectal exam (a gloved, lubricated finger is inserted into the rectum). Questions will be asked about your symptoms and bowel habits.
• Medical tests may include blood and stool studies, x-ray or CT.

APPROPRIATE HEALTH CARE
• If no symptoms, no treatment may be needed. For mild symptoms, treatment may include a change in diet and the use of stool softeners. For more severe symptoms, bed rest, drugs, hospital care, and surgery may be needed.
• Surgery may be done for complications. These include abscess, fistula, intestinal obstruction, perforation, or peritonitis. A part of the affected colon may be removed (resection) and the remaining sections rejoined. A colostomy involves creating a temporary hole (stoma) in the abdomen to remove stool. (See Sigmoid-Colon Removal in Surgery section.)

POSSIBLE COMPLICATIONS
• Intestinal bleeding or infections.
• Perforation, tear, or blockage of the intestines.
• Abscess (pus-filled, infected area).
• Peritonitis (inflammation of the abdominal cavity lining).
• Recurrent attacks of diverticulitis.
• Fistula (abnormal opening in the body).

PROBABLE OUTCOME—Most cases are mild, respond well to treatment, and have no recurrence. If complications occur, they can usually be treated successfully.

 HOW TO TREAT

GENERAL MEASURES—For self-care:
• Try to have a bowel movement at the same time each day. Allow about 10 minutes, and don't strain.
• Check your stool for bleeding. Ask your health care provider if a sample is to be taken to the medical office.
• To relieve mild pain, use a heating pad.
• To learn more: National Digestive Diseases Information Clearinghouse, 2 Information Way, Bethesda, MD 20892; (800) 891-5389; website: www.digestive.niddk.nih.gov.

MEDICATION
• Antibiotics will be prescribed for infections.
• Stool softeners may be recommended.
• Avoid laxatives, unless they are prescribed.

ACTIVITY—If you have fever or severe pain, stay in bed. Resume normal activity as soon as symptoms improve.

DIET—Eat a diet that is high in fiber. Drink plenty of fluids.

 CALL YOUR DOCTOR IF

• You or a family member has symptoms of diverticular disease.
• Symptoms don't improve or they become worse.

DOMESTIC VIOLENCE
(Battering; Spousal Abuse)

 GENERAL INFORMATION

DEFINITION—Any violence between current or former partners in an intimate relationship. It may include physical, sexual, emotional, or financial abuse. The victim is usually a woman (95% of abuse cases). Because of shame and guilt, the victim may not report the abuse to police, medical care givers, or talk about it with family or friends. Abuse is common. It may occur in any race, age group, economic or educational level, or nationality.

BODY PARTS INVOLVED—May affect all.

SEX OR AGE MOST AFFECTED—Both sexes, all ages, but most common in females.

SIGNS & SYMPTOMS
In female victims:
• Physical or sexual abuse injuries. These include broken bones, bruises, burns, choking, bites, rape and others. Most injuries are to the head, neck, chest, abdomen and breasts. Arm injuries may result from self defense.
• Other symptoms may include chronic pelvic pain, sexual dysfunction, anxiety, sleep disorders, depression, post-traumatic stress disorder (PTSD), eating disorders, psychological problems, and thoughts of suicide.
In male abusers:
• Angry, suspicious, tense and/or moody behaviors. Sometimes they can be very charming. They go from periods of abuse to periods of affection.
• May display extreme jealousy and be very possessive. May not allow partner's friends/family to visit or call.
• Makes threats of violence or legal threats (such as custody of the children). May play with guns or knives.
• Limits access to money or other basic needs.

CAUSES—The abuser's goal is to control the victim by the use of fear and force. It is unclear why some men are abusers and other men with similar risk factors are not.

RISK INCREASES WITH
• A history of abuse in a family. Many male abusers and, often, female victims, witnessed abuse or were victims.
• Male abusers tend to use alcohol or drugs, are often unemployed, and may be less educated. However, many educated, professional men are abusers.
• Males dependent on women, have money worries, feelings of inadequacy, and have traditional (or archaic) attitudes (such as about sex).
• Females lacking self-esteem and females who feel dependent and useless.
• Pregnant females.

HOW TO PREVENT—Victims should seek help at the first sign of abuse. Don't assume the abuser will change or stop the abuse.

 WHAT TO EXPECT

DIAGNOSTIC MEASURES—Exam by a health care provider and medical tests as needed.

APPROPRIATE HEALTH CARE
• Treatment steps for a victim:
- Get medical care for any injuries.
- Counseling is important. Treatment will help a woman learn to cope, regain self-confidence and her ability to function.
• Treatment for the abuser:
- Treatment is often resisted by an abuser. Educational and treatment groups have had some success.
- Abusers must be confronted with the results of the behavior; that they can go to jail if they don't change.

POSSIBLE COMPLICATIONS
• Years of emotional and physical abuse.
• Alcohol and drug abuse by a female victim.
• Murder or suicide.

PROBABLE OUTCOME
• For victims, help is available, if they choose to seek it.
• Abusers are unlikely to change their behavior.

 HOW TO TREAT

GENERAL MEASURES—If you are abused:
• Protect yourself, especially the head and abdomen. Get away from the abuser and get help. Document the abuse with pictures, telling someone, or calling 911.
• Have a personal safety plan set up. Have a place to stay, a way to get there, transportation, and survival funds. Have clothing and personal essentials packed.
• Seek legal help. Police departments are improving in responding to the problems of domestic violence.
• Numerous agencies and shelters for helping abused women and children are available. Call a local crisis line.

MEDICATION—Drugs may be prescribed for anxiety or depression.

ACTIVITY—No limits.

DIET—No special diet.

 CALL YOUR DOCTOR IF

You or a family member is a victim of domestic violence.

DOWN SYNDROME
(Trisomy 21)

GENERAL INFORMATION

DEFINITION—A chromosome abnormality that usually results in abnormal physical appearance, mental retardation and other health conditions. It is the single most common cause of birth defects.

BODY PARTS INVOLVED—Central nervous system; heart; skeletal system.

SEX OR AGE MOST AFFECTED—Newborns.

SIGNS & SYMPTOMS
Appearance: (some may have only a few of the recognizable traits, while others may have many).
* Lack of normal muscle tone; child seems "floppy."
* Head that is not shaped normally, including a small or odd-shaped skull.
* Facial features may include small, flattened nose, small mouth, and large tongue.
* Slanting, almond-shaped eyes. The inner corner of the eyes may have a rounded fold of skin (epicanthal fold). Iris may be abnormal.
* Ears that are not of normal shape.
* Broad hands with large, unusual palm creases. The little finger curves inward (sometimes).
Other conditions:
* Heart and gastrointestinal defects may be diagnosed.
* Slow growth and development. The child never reaches full height.
* Mental retardation.

CAUSES—Genetic. An extra chromosome creates abnormalities. Studies have shown that something goes wrong with the egg itself. It is not yet known why this occurs.

RISK INCREASES WITH—Many risk factors have been studied to see if they increase the risk of having a baby with Down syndrome. The only one that has been proven is the increasing age of the woman.

HOW TO PREVENT
* If you or your partner has a family history of Down syndrome, get genetic counseling prior to starting a family.
* If you are pregnant and over age 40, or you or your partner have a family history of Down syndrome, get a test that can detect if the fetus has Down syndrome.

WHAT TO EXPECT

DIAGNOSTIC MEASURES—Down syndrome is usually diagnosed at birth by the appearance of the baby. It is an extremely difficult time for new parents, and counseling may be helpful.

Some parents blame themselves and need help to cope with feelings of guilt.

APPROPRIATE HEALTH CARE
* Home care.
* Medical care is important. Children with Down syndrome are more likely to get infections and other illnesses. Surgery may be needed to correct heart or intestinal disorders.

POSSIBLE COMPLICATIONS
* Risk of infections, leukemia, and thyroid disease.
* Heart failure caused by heart defects.
* Alzheimer's disease (25% of those over 35).
* Death often occurs before age 40, but advances in care are helping patients lead longer lives.

PROBABLE OUTCOME—With help, those with Down syndrome can reach their full potential and lead happy, loving, and useful lives.

HOW TO TREAT

GENERAL MEASURES
* Raising the child to his or her full potential should be the goal for parents of a child with Down syndrome.
* Learn all you can about programs in your city to help children with Down syndrome. Join a support group.
* Learning programs for these children begin in infancy and continue all through their lives. Some children can be taught in regular classrooms (with extra help), while others may need special education. They can take part in, and enjoy, sports, music, art, and other activities.
* As adults, they can hold jobs, live in group-homes, have social lives, and some may marry.
* To learn more: National Down Syndrome Society, 666 Broadway, New York, NY 10012; (800) 221-4602; website: www.ndss.org or National Down Syndrome Congress, 1370 Center Dr, Suite 102, Atlanta, GA 30338; (800) 232-NDSC; website: www.ndscenter.org.

MEDICATION—Drugs are usually not needed unless an illness occurs.

ACTIVITY—Encourage the child to be as active as possible in a protected environment.

DIET—No special diet. Feeding an infant with Down syndrome may be a problem. Some have difficulty sucking or are not eager to eat.

CALL YOUR DOCTOR IF

* Your infant seems "floppy" or does not seem to be developing normally.
* A child with Down syndrome develops symptoms of infection or other medical problem.

DROWNING, NEAR

GENERAL INFORMATION

DEFINITION—Almost drowning. It results from being submerged in water or other fluid.

BODY PARTS INVOLVED—Lungs; blood; heart.

SEX OR AGE MOST AFFECTED—Both sexes; all ages. Children under age 4 and young adults (ages 15 to 24) are often the victims.

SIGNS & SYMPTOMS
* Difficulty breathing or shortness of breath.
* Fast or slow heartbeat.
* May be unconscious.
* Anxious appearance.
* Skin may be bluish-white, cold, and pale.
* Coughing or vomiting.
* May have breathed foreign material into lungs.

CAUSES—Submersion in water results in the larynx (the tube from the throat to the lungs) relaxing and letting water enter the lungs. Water in the lungs means the lungs can't function properly and transfer oxygen to the blood. The body's organs can become damaged from lack of oxygen.

RISK INCREASES WITH
* Not able to swim or overestimating swimming ability.
* Alcohol or drug use combined with water activity.
* Accidents from diving, surfing, or water skiing.
* Seizure, stroke, or heart problem while swimming.
* Unsupervised children in or near water. This includes bathtubs or pails of water (such as used for mopping).
* Unfenced swimming pools.
* Boating or scuba diving.

HOW TO PREVENT
* Learn cardiopulmonary resuscitation (CPR).
* Have all family members learn to swim.
* Adult supervision of children near water.
* Install a fence around a home swimming pool. Always be sure that pool gates are locked.
* Never swim alone.
* Don't drink alcohol or abuse drugs and swim.
* Wear life jackets in boats.
* Scuba divers should be fully trained and use proper caution when diving. Avoid risky dives.

WHAT TO EXPECT

DIAGNOSTIC MEASURES—Emergency care usually includes supplemental oxygen, body temperature control, maintenance of the body's electrolytes and blood sugar levels, and prevention of complications. Treatment for any injuries will be provided.

APPROPRIATE HEALTH CARE
* Immediate cardiopulmonary resuscitation (CPR).
* Hospitalization for observation for delayed, serious reactions.

POSSIBLE COMPLICATIONS
* Pulmonary edema (fluid in the lungs).
* Lung infection.
* Permanent brain damage.
* Heart problems, including cardiac arrest and death.

PROBABLE OUTCOME
* With mild symptoms, patients are usually sent home after 6 to 8 hours in the emergency room/hospital. Complications are unlikely.
* More severe symptoms require extended time for treatment and could result in complications.

HOW TO TREAT

GENERAL MEASURES
* If the victim is unconscious and not breathing, yell for help. Have someone call 911 (emergency) for an ambulance or medical help. Don't leave the victim.
* Try to warm the person with whatever means are at hand (blankets, towels, jackets).
* Begin mouth-to-mouth breathing.
* If there is no pulse, give external cardiac massage.
* Don't stop rescue effort until medical help arrives.
* The near-drowning victim should be taken to the nearest hospital for intensive care even if the victim has become conscious.
Complications may occur several hours after the near drowning.

MEDICATION—Drugs used for treatment may include:
* Cortisone drugs, to prevent or treat inflammation of the lungs.
* Antibiotics, to prevent lung infection.
* Bronchodilators, to enable oxygen to enter the lungs.
* Anticonvulsants, to prevent seizures.

ACTIVITY—Complete bed rest for at least the first 24 hours.

DIET—Nutrition may be provided through a vein (IV) while in the hospital. After recovery, no special diet is needed.

CALL YOUR DOCTOR IF

* Someone appears to have drowned. Call for emergency help immediately!
* Cough, shortness of breath, or fever develop after treatment.

DRUG HYPERSENSITIVITY

 GENERAL INFORMATION

DEFINITION—Allergic reaction caused by drugs. The reaction may happen immediately after using the drug or days to weeks later.

BODY PARTS INVOLVED—Skin; blood vessels; lungs.

SEX OR AGE MOST AFFECTED—Both sexes; all ages. Females are more often affected than males.

SIGNS & SYMPTOMS
- Rash (most common), hives (urticaria), itching skin.
- Wheezing.
- Swelling (lips, tongue, and/or face).
- Anaphylaxis (a life-threatening reaction). Symptoms can include difficult breathing, wheezing, hives, swelling, fainting, lightheadedness, dizziness, confusion, rapid pulse, fast heart rate, diarrhea, nausea or vomiting, and stomach pain or cramping.
- Serum sickness (a delayed type of reaction that occurs a week or more after exposure). It can occur with the first time use of a drug. Symptoms include fever, rash, joint pain, and nerve damage.

CAUSES—Hypersensitivity of the immune system in certain people. It leads to a misdirected response against a substance that does not cause a response in most people. The body becomes sensitized by the first exposure to the drug. The second or subsequent exposure causes an immune response (production of antibodies and release of histamine). Injected drugs are more of a risk than those taken by mouth or applied to the skin.

RISK INCREASES WITH
- Use of almost any drug. The following are more likely:
  - Penicillin and cephalosporin antibiotics.
  - Sulfa drugs.
  - Animal serums.
  - Vaccines.
  - Anesthetics applied to the skin.
  - Allergy extracts.
  - Iodine-containing compounds (used in some x-rays).
- Injected drugs, especially in high doses.
- Personal or family history of other allergies, such as hay fever, asthma, or eczema.
- Serious illness.
- Weak immune system due to illness or drugs.

HOW TO PREVENT
- Tell any health care provider you consult about the drug reactions you have had.
- Learn the name of any drug you are given. If it causes a reaction, avoid it in the future.

 WHAT TO EXPECT

DIAGNOSTIC MEASURES
- Your own observation of symptoms.
- Your health care provider may do a physical exam. Questions will be asked about your symptoms and the drugs you take (including nonprescription, herbals, or other supplements). Usually, a diagnosis can be made based on the type of reaction, the timing of the reaction, and that a drug you took is known to cause reactions.
- Sometimes, skin tests or blood tests are done.

APPROPRIATE HEALTH CARE
- The first step of treatment is to stop using the drug that caused a reaction. Usually, another drug can be safely substituted. Symptoms of the drug reaction may be treated with other drugs.
- If there is no substitute drug that can be used, other treatment steps may be taken. There are methods (called desensitizing) that gradually introduce a drug into the body in small doses.

POSSIBLE COMPLICATIONS
- Asthma.
- Anaphylaxis (can be life-threatening if not treated).

PROBABLE OUTCOME—In many cases, stopping the drug is all that is needed. In other cases, symptoms can be relieved with treatment. Most symptoms should resolve in about 2 weeks.

 HOW TO TREAT

GENERAL MEASURES
- Wear a medical alert type pendant or bracelet if you have drug hypersensitivity.
- Keep an anaphylaxis kit at home, on your person, nearby at work, and in your car for emergency use if anyone in the family has had a severe drug reaction.

MEDICATION
- Cortisone drugs to decrease inflammation, antihistamines for itching symptoms, and bronchodilators for wheezing may be prescribed.
- Epinephrine may be injected to treat anaphylaxis.

ACTIVITY—No limits once symptoms improve.

DIET—No special diet.

☎ **CALL YOUR DOCTOR IF**

- You have symptoms of drug hypersensitivity or observe them in someone else.
- You or a family member has anaphylaxis symptoms. This is an emergency! Call 911. Get help immediately!

DUMPING SYNDROME

 GENERAL INFORMATION

DEFINITION—A group of symptoms that are usually a complication of stomach surgery. Most patients experience the problem to a minor degree for 1 to 6 months after surgery. The symptoms are of 2 types: early dumping syndrome and late dumping syndrome. Symptoms of the first begin a few minutes to 45 minutes after every meal. Symptoms of the second begin 2 to 3 hours after eating. Most persons experience late dumping syndrome, and a person cannot have both forms. People with a rare disorder called Zollinger-Ellison syndrome may also have dumping syndrome.

BODY PARTS INVOLVED—Gastrointestinal system; cardiovascular system.

SEX OR AGE MOST AFFECTED—Both sexes of adults following surgery on the stomach.

SIGNS & SYMPTOMS
Early dumping syndrome:
- Weakness and fainting.
- Sweating.
- Irregular or rapid heartbeat.
- Decreased blood pressure.
- Skin gets flushed (reddens).
- Dizziness.
- May become hard to breathe.
- Vomiting.
- Explosive diarrhea and stomach cramps.

Late dumping syndrome:
- Sweating, anxiety, and tremors.
- Exhaustion and faintness.
- Decreased blood pressure.
- Headache.

CAUSES
- Early dumping syndrome: Rapid entry of food and fluids directly into the small intestine, producing decreased blood pressure and increased blood flow to the intestines.
- Late dumping syndrome: Low blood sugar caused by too much insulin being made by the body in response to sudden dumping of food and fluids into the intestine.

RISK INCREASES WITH—The larger the amount of stomach removed, the more severe the dumping syndrome.

HOW TO PREVENT—Cannot be prevented. Recurrence and severity can be reduced with changes in the diet.

 WHAT TO EXPECT

DIAGNOSTIC MEASURES
- Your own observation of symptoms.
- Your health care provider will do a physical exam and ask questions about your symptoms.
- Medical tests may be done to confirm the diagnosis.

APPROPRIATE HEALTH CARE
- Treatment includes diet changes and sometimes drugs.
- In ongoing severe cases of dumping syndrome, surgery may be considered.

POSSIBLE COMPLICATIONS
- Poor nutrition and weight loss.
- Anxiety.

PROBABLE OUTCOME—The problem clears up on its own for most patients. Early dumping syndrome usually lasts 3 to 4 months. Late dumping syndrome usually lasts 1 year, but it may persist for many years.

 HOW TO TREAT

GENERAL MEASURES
- Lie down as soon as you finish any meal. This helps reduce the symptoms.
- To learn more: National Digestive Diseases Information Clearinghouse, 2 Information Way, Bethesda, MD 20892, (800) 891-5389; website: www.niddk.nih.gov.

MEDICATION
- You may be prescribed drugs to help with digestion or lower blood sugar.
- Vitamin and mineral supplements to compensate for poor absorption.

ACTIVITY
- Between symptoms: no restrictions.
- With symptoms: rest until they pass.

DIET—Diet control is the most important treatment. Eat a diet low in sugar and other simple carbohydrates. Increase fat and protein food items. Avoid milk and milk products. Avoid foods that are very hot or very cold. Eat 6 small, evenly spaced meals a day. Take meals dry without water or beverages and drink fluids only between meals.

 CALL YOUR DOCTOR IF

- You or a family member has symptoms of dumping syndrome not relieved by diet changes.
- You vomit blood, have black, tarry stools, or other signs of internal bleeding.
- New, unexplained symptoms develop. Drugs used in treatment may produce side effects.

DYSENTERY, BACILLARY
(Shigellosis)

GENERAL INFORMATION

DEFINITION—A bacterial infection of the intestinal tract that is spread by close person-to-person contact. It often happens in epidemics (affects a large number of people at the same time).

BODY PARTS INVOLVED—Lower small intestine (ileum); large intestine (colon).

SEX OR AGE MOST AFFECTED—Both sexes; all ages. It occurs most often in young children.

SIGNS & SYMPTOMS
* Stomach cramps.
* Fever.
* Diarrhea (up to 20 or 30 watery bowel movements in one day). There may be small amounts of blood, mucus, or pus in the stool.
* Nausea or vomiting.
* Muscle aches or pain.

CAUSES—Bacteria called *Shigella* bacillus that attack the lining of the colon. It spreads from person to person, usually from germs on the hands. The infection is also spread from germs on objects such as toys, in food, or in drinking water (in areas with poor sanitation). Symptoms start 1 to 7 days after being exposed to germs.

RISK INCREASES WITH
* Travel to foreign countries.
* Crowded or unclean living conditions.
* Poor health.

HOW TO PREVENT
* Wash hands after bowel movements and before handling food. Children need to be reminded often.
* Avoid contact with an infected person.
* Put soiled clothes and bedclothes in covered buckets of soap and water until they can be washed.

WHAT TO EXPECT

DIAGNOSTIC MEASURES
* Your own observation of symptoms.
* Your health care provider will do a physical exam and ask questions about the symptoms.
* Tests and culture of a stool sample may be done to confirm the diagnosis.

APPROPRIATE HEALTH CARE
* Home care.
* Treatment usually includes fluids (to replace those lost from diarrhea), a bland diet, and drug therapy.
* A hospital stay may be needed if patient is severely ill. This may happen with small children with dehydration or severe rectal bleeding.

POSSIBLE COMPLICATIONS—Severe cases may occur in the very young or the elderly. Symptoms include convulsions, severe dehydration, and disorders that cause kidney failure and a type of arthritis.

PROBABLE OUTCOME—The infection resolves on its own or with treatment in about 5 to 7 days. Most *Shigella* infections are mild.

HOW TO TREAT

GENERAL MEASURES
* Watch for signs of dehydration. These include severe thirst, dry mouth and tongue, tiredness, sunken eyes, dry skin, being irritable and less urination.
* Keep the patient away from others if possible.
* Use warm compresses on the stomach to help relieve pain.

MEDICATION
* Antibiotics are usually prescribed. They help speed recovery and reduce risk of spreading germs. Be sure to take them for as long as prescribed.
* Don't use antidiarrhea drugs, unless they are prescribed. These may extend the illness.

ACTIVITY—Keep the ill person at home and away from others when possible. Return to daycare, school, or work is permitted after taking antibiotics for five days.

DIET—Be sure to drink plenty of liquids. A soft or liquid diet may be recommended. Use special drinks (or popsicles) that replace body fluids quickly.

CALL YOUR DOCTOR IF

* You or your child has symptoms of the infection.
* The following occur during treatment:
  - Rectal bleeding or bloody stools.
  - Signs of dehydration appear.
  - Symptoms get worse despite treatment.

DYSHIDROTIC ECZEMA
(Dyshidrosis; Pompholyx)

 GENERAL INFORMATION

DEFINITION—A skin condition, with small blisters on the hands or feet. It is a type of eczema (dermatitis).

BODY PARTS INVOLVED—Tips and sides of the fingers, toes, palms and soles.

SEX OR AGE MOST AFFECTED—Both sexes and all ages, but most common in women between ages 20 and 40.

SIGNS & SYMPTOMS
* Burning and itching in the hands and feet before the skin breaks out. Small blisters appear. They may be on the tips and sides of fingers, toes, palms, and soles of the feet.
* Blisters are nontransparent and deep; they are either even with the skin, or slightly raised. They don't break easily. Eventually, small blisters come together and form large blisters.
* Hands and feet may be wet with perspiration.
* Blisters may worsen after contact with soap, water, or irritating substances.

CAUSES—Unknown. Excessive sweating is not a cause of this problem, but is often linked to it.

RISK INCREASES WITH
* Females (affected more often than males).
* Periods of anxiety, stress, anger, and frustration seem to play a role.
* Other risk factors are being studied.

HOW TO PREVENT—No specific preventive measures are known.

 WHAT TO EXPECT

DIAGNOSTIC MEASURES
* Your own observation of symptoms.
* Your health care provider can diagnose the condition by an exam of the affected skin area.
* Medical tests are usually not needed.

APPROPRIATE HEALTH CARE.—Treatment involves drug therapy and self-care measures.

POSSIBLE COMPLICATIONS
* Continued peeling and cracking of the involved skin.
* Bacterial skin infection may occur.

PROBABLE OUTCOME—Outcome varies for different patients. Some recover completely with or without treatment. Others may continue to have symptoms even with treatment.

 HOW TO TREAT

GENERAL MEASURES
* Keep heat and moisture away from the affected areas whenever possible.
* Wear cotton socks and leather-soled shoes. Don't wear tennis shoes or other footwear made of man-made materials.
* Remove shoes and socks frequently to allow sweat to dry.
* Wear heavy-duty, cotton-lined vinyl gloves when in contact with water, soap, detergent, and other chemicals. Dry insides of gloves after use. Throw away gloves if they develop a hole.
* Wear gloves when you peel or squeeze acid fruits and vegetables.
* Wear leather or heavy-duty fabric gloves for housework or gardening.
* Avoid contact with irritating chemicals, such as paint; paint thinner; and polish for cars, floors, shoes, furniture, and metal.
* Use cool, moist compresses to help soothe the affected skin.
* Use lukewarm water and very little mild soap to shower or bathe.
* If emotional stress is a problem, try to identify the cause and find ways to control it. Counseling or learning stress management techniques may help.

MEDICATION
* Steroid creams or ointments are usually prescribed.
* If symptoms worsen, steroids or other drugs taken by mouth may be prescribed.

ACTIVITY—Avoid activities or environments that lead to stress or excessive sweating. Sweating does not cause the disorder, but may aggravate it.

DIET—No special diet.

 CALL YOUR DOCTOR IF

* You or a family member has symptoms of dyshidrotic eczema.
* Signs of infection (swelling, redness, tenderness, or warmth) appear around blisters.
* Symptoms don't improve after 1 week, even with treatment.
* Symptoms recur after treatment.

DYSMENORRHEA
(Menstrual Cramps)

 GENERAL INFORMATION

DEFINITION—Painful menstrual cramps. Primary dysmenorrhea often begins within a year or two of the first menstrual period (puberty). Secondary dysmenorrhea usually occurs after a woman has had normal periods for some time.

BODY PARTS INVOLVED—Female reproductive system, especially the uterus.

SEX OR AGE MOST AFFECTED—Women of childbearing age.

SIGNS & SYMPTOMS
* Severity of symptoms varies from woman to woman, and from one time to the next in the same woman.
* Cramping and, sometimes, sharp pains in the lower abdomen, lower back, and thighs. The pain usually begins with your period and lasts for hours to days. For some women, the pain may begin a week or more before her period and last for a few days after it stops.
* Other symptoms that may occur:
 - Nausea, vomiting, diarrhea, headache, and sweating.
 - Lack of energy.
 - Fainting.
 - Feeling irritable, anxious, or depressed.

CAUSES—Menstrual pain is a result of strong contractions of the muscles of the uterus. In primary dysmenorrhea, this is due to excess prostaglandin (a hormone-like substance) production. In secondary dysmenorrhea, this is due to an abnormality or disease of the uterus, fallopian tubes, or ovaries.

RISK INCREASES WITH
* Pelvic infections.
* Sexually transmitted diseases.
* Endometriosis or endometritis (uterine lining disorders).
* Adenomyosis (benign growth in uterine lining).
* Fibroids or other conditions of the uterus.
* Congenital (being born with) uterine or vaginal abnormalities.
* Use of an intrauterine device (IUD).
* Smoking or alcohol use.
* Not having given birth.
* Family history of dysmenorrhea.
* Obesity.

HOW TO PREVENT
* Take female hormones that prevent ovulation, such as oral contraceptives.
* Treatment of the underlying cause.

 WHAT TO EXPECT

DIAGNOSTIC MEASURES
* Your health care provider will do a physical exam and a pelvic exam. Questions will be asked about your menstrual history.
* Medical tests may include blood and urine studies, and an ultrasound.

APPROPRIATE HEALTH CARE
* Initial treatment aims are to relieve pain. Long term treatment goals may involve treating the cause with drugs, counseling, or surgery.
* Transcutaneous electrical nerve stimulator (TENS) treatment may help relieve pain.
* Counseling may help, if stress is a problem.
* Hypnosis therapy may help some women.
* Surgery may be recommended for women whose pain is not controlled by other methods.

POSSIBLE COMPLICATIONS
* Severe pain that interferes with a normal life.
* Infertility from underlying cause.

PROBABLE OUTCOME
* Symptoms can be helped with treatment.
* Symptoms improve with age or with childbirth. Symptoms are rare in postmenopausal women.

 HOW TO TREAT

GENERAL MEASURES
* Heat helps relieve pain. Use a heating pad on the abdomen or back. Take warm baths.
* Try to stop smoking and reduce alcohol use.

MEDICATION
* For minor discomfort, use nonsteroidal anti-inflammatory drugs (NSAIDs) such as ibuprofen, naproxen or aspirin (if over age 18).
* Antiprostaglandins (for painful menstrual periods) and oral contraceptives, which prohibit ovulation, may be prescribed.
* In severe cases, hormones (e.g., gonadotropin-releasing hormone [Gn-RH]) can stop ovary function to relieve pain.
* You may be prescribed vitamin B or vitamin E supplements. They may help relieve symptoms.

ACTIVITY—Exercise may help reduce the discomfort of menstrual cramps.

DIET
* Avoid drinking caffeine-containing beverages.
* Herbal teas may help reduce symptoms.

 CALL YOUR DOCTOR IF

* You or a family member has symptoms of dyspareunia.
* Pain worsens or recurs, despite treatment.

DYSPAREUNIA

GENERAL INFORMATION

DEFINITION—Pain that occurs with sexual intercourse. Dyspareunia and vaginismus (spasm of the pubic muscles of the lower vagina) may occur together in a woman.

BODY PARTS INVOLVED—Genital area, vaginal muscles, uterus (sometimes), brain.

SEX OR AGE MOST AFFECTED—Sexually active females of all ages. Dyspareunia also occurs in men, but less often.

SIGNS & SYMPTOMS
- Pain in the genital area during sexual activity. It can occur before, during, or after sexual intercourse.
- Women may have pain on entry or during intercourse (with deep thrusts of partner's penis).
- Men may have pain in the penis or testes.
- Pain may be mild or severe, and vary with different intercourse positions.

CAUSES
- Physical and medical problems.
- Emotional, interpersonal, and environmental problems (often referred to as psychosocial problems).
- It may be a combination of factors. Sometimes no cause is found.

RISK INCREASES WITH
Physical:
- Infection, inflammation, or injury of the genitals or the urinary tract.
- A lack of vaginal lubrication. This can be due to illness, drugs, or lack of estrogen (such as at menopause).
- Vaginal scarring from operations or radiation.
- Episiotomy scar (from repair after childbirth).
- Intact hymen (covering of the vaginal opening).
- Allergy to diaphragms, condoms, or contraceptive foams and jellies.
- Endometriosis or pelvic inflammatory disease.
- Muscle spasms of the vagina (vaginismus).
- Vulvodynia (chronic vulva pain).
- Tilted or enlarged uterus.

Emotional (psychosocial)
- Lack of sexual arousal or sexual foreplay, being unhappy with a sexual partner, fatigue, or anxiety.
- Lack of sexual experience or information.
- Past sexual abuse (such as rape) or emotional trauma.
- Fear of pregnancy.

HOW TO PREVENT
- Get medical care for genital infections.
- Don't use perfumed soaps or bubble baths. Don't douche.
- Get medical care for depression, anxiety, or stress problems.

WHAT TO EXPECT

DIAGNOSTIC MEASURES
- Your health care provider will do a physical exam and a genital exam. You will be asked about your symptoms and sexual history.
- Medical studies, such as a Pap smear and culture of vaginal discharge may be done to diagnose medical problems that can be treated.

APPROPRIATE HEALTH CARE
- Treatment will be directed to any physical or emotional cause that is diagnosed.
- In cases of scarring, problems with the hymen, or others, a minor surgical procedure may relieve symptoms.
- Instructions may be given for exercises or techniques to dilate (widen) the vagina. They involve use of fingers or dilators to condition the body and mind to the sensation of something being inserted into the vagina.
- Treatments for emotional causes will vary. They can involve education, counseling, sensate focus exercises, and teaching of appropriate foreplay techniques.

POSSIBLE COMPLICATIONS—Treatment may be long-term and may not always help. An intimate relationship with partner may suffer.

PROBABLE OUTCOME—Physical causes are often curable with treatment. Psychosocial causes may be helped with treatment.

HOW TO TREAT

GENERAL MEASURES
- Sitz baths relieve tenderness. Sit in a tub of warm water for 15 minutes, 3 or 4 times a day.
- Use a nonprescription lubricant, such as K-Y Lubricating Jelly, during sexual intercourse.
- Try different positions for sexual intercourse that reduce the depth of penile penetration.
- Discuss the lack of sexual arousal with your partner, including ways to improve foreplay.
- To learn more: American College of Obstetricians and Gynecologists, website: www.acog.org.

MEDICATION—Drugs may be prescribed for infection or inflammation. Steroid creams or estrogen creams may be prescribed.

ACTIVITY—A regular exercise program, while not a treatment for dyspareunia, is helpful for general well-being.

DIET—No special diet.

☎ CALL YOUR DOCTOR IF

- You or a family member has symptoms of dyspareunia.
- Symptoms do not improve with treatment.

DYSPHAGIA

 GENERAL INFORMATION

DEFINITION—Difficulty or pain in swallowing. It may involve solid foods, liquids or both. It is a common symptom with a wide variety of causes that can be benign or malignant. Chances of a serious disorder are slight.

BODY PARTS INVOLVED—Pharynx; esophagus.

SEX OR AGE MOST AFFECTED—Both sexes; all ages. It occurs more often in older adults.

SIGNS & SYMPTOMS
• Pain that occurs with swallowing. Pain and swallowing difficulty may progress over several weeks.
• Sore throat.
• The feeling that food "gets stuck" on the way down.
• Coughing or choking with eating or drinking. Food may come back out through the nose.
• Drooling, belching, and bad breath.
• Pressure sensation in mid-chest.

CAUSES—The swallowing difficulty may involve the mouth, the throat, and the esophagus. There are numerous risk factors that may be the cause.

RISK INCREASES WITH
• Gastroesophageal reflux disease (GERD) or acid reflux.
• Tumors (benign or cancer).
• Stricture (narrowing of the passage).
• Inflammation (esophagitis).
• Infections.
• Recent head, neck, or throat surgery.
• Laryngitis, pharyngitis, or tonsillitis.
• Foreign object lodging at the back of the throat.
• Scratch in the throat lining caused by a foreign object.
• Insufficient production of saliva.
• Esophageal spasm (loss of normal muscle movement).
• In children, it may be caused by delayed maturation, malformation, cerebral palsy, or muscular dystrophy.
• Hernia of part of the esophagus through a weak area in the surrounding muscle.
• Nervous system disorder (stroke, Alzheimer's disease, myasthenia gravis, Parkinson's disease, and others).
• Pressure on the esophagus (a goiter or aortic aneurysm).
• Emotional disorders (anxiety, fear, and others).
• Anemia.
• Smoking.

HOW TO PREVENT—No specific preventive measures. Avoid risk factors where possible.

 WHAT TO EXPECT

DIAGNOSTIC MEASURES
• Your health care provider will do an exam of the mouth, throat, head, and neck. You may be asked to chew and swallow so the action can be observed.
• Medical tests may be done to find the cause. These may include blood tests, swallowing studies (endoscopy, esophageal manometry, barium x-ray exam), ultrasound, or CT scan.

APPROPRIATE HEALTH CARE
• Treatment will be provided for the cause of the dysphagia. Specific treatment for the swallowing difficulty may include diet changes and swallowing therapy.
• Hospital care may be if problem is severe.
• Devices to dilate (widen) the esophagus or surgery may be needed for some disorders.

POSSIBLE COMPLICATIONS
• Dehydration or malnutrition due to not eating or drinking enough to meet the body's needs.
• Aspiration. It is the passage of food or liquid through the vocal folds ("going down the wrong way"). Food, fluid, or vomit may enter the lungs.

PROBABLE OUTCOME—Many causes are minor and easily treated. Other outcomes will vary depending on the cause.

 HOW TO TREAT

GENERAL MEASURES
• Brush teeth twice a day.
• For dry mouth, suck lozenges or chew gum.

MEDICATION—Drugs will be prescribed as needed for the cause.

ACTIVITY
• Swallowing therapy may be prescribed. It can include exercises to strengthen the swallowing muscles or exercises that are done while swallowing.
• Posture changes may help swallowing: tilting or turning the head to one side, tucking the chin in, using a head-back position, or lying on one's side or back. You will be given instructions about using these positions.

DIET
• May start with pureed foods, progress to soft food and semi-solids, and then to a regular diet.
• Hospital care may involve intravenous (IV) feeding, or feeding with nasal or stomach tube.

 CALL YOUR DOCTOR IF

You or a family member develops swallowing difficulty.

DYSPLASTIC NEVI

GENERAL INFORMATION

DEFINITION—Nevi is another word for moles. Dysplastic nevi are moles that are atypical. This means they do not have the appearance of common moles, and that they are a risk for melanoma. Melanoma is a serious type of skin cancer. A large number of dysplastic nevi increase the melanoma risk. The melanoma risk is even higher for a person with dysplastic nevi along with a family history of melanoma. This is called familial atypical mole/ melanoma (FAMM). It is also known as dysplastic nevus syndrome.

BODY PARTS INVOLVED—Skin.

SEX OR AGE MOST AFFECTED—Both sexes; late teens and adults.

SIGNS & SYMPTOMS—Dysplastic nevi may have the following appearance:
* Borders are irregular and ill defined.
* Have both flat and elevated areas.
* Are larger than common moles.
* Color may range from tan to dark brown or have other various shades of color within them.
* They can appear anywhere on the body, but most often are found on the back, chest, buttocks, breast, and scalp. They are found in sun-exposed as well as sun-protected areas.
* A person may have one (nevus), or a few, or more than 100 dysplastic nevi. (An average person with common moles has 15 to 20.)

CAUSES—Dysplastic nevi are acquired. A person is not born with them. The exact cause is unknown. Sunlight damage may play a part, but is not always a factor. Dysplastic nevi can appear on the buttocks and female breasts, which are generally covered. The tendency to develop dysplastic nevi does run in families.

RISK INCREASES WITH—Family history of dysplastic nevi or melanoma.

HOW TO PREVENT
* There are no specific preventive measures.
* Routine use of sunscreens may help reduce risks. Use one with an SPF of 15 or higher and that protects against both ultraviolet A and ultraviolet B radiation.
* If you have a family history of dysplastic nevi or skin cancer, get regular medical skin exams to detect any new moles or changes in existing ones. Exams may be as often as every 3 months for high-risk persons.
* Perform routine skin self-exams to check for any changes in skin appearance. Have a family member help check the areas of your body that you cannot see.

WHAT TO EXPECT

DIAGNOSTIC MEASURES
* Your own observation of symptoms.
* Your health care provider will do a physical exam of the skin.
* A biopsy may be done of a nevus (single mole) if skin cancer is suspected. Biopsy involves removing all or a portion of a nevus for viewing under a microscope. If the biopsy shows cancer, the whole nevus is removed.

APPROPRIATE HEALTH CARE
* Other dysplastic nevi may be removed or watched over time to see if they change. Most dysplastic nevi will not develop into melanoma; removing all of them is unnecessary. If the nevi look like melanoma, have changed over time, or are new and look abnormal, then removal may be the recommended treatment.
* In some cases, nevi may be removed because of bleeding, irritation, or they are a cosmetic concern.
* Removal usually involves excision (cutting out) of the nevi. The procedure is done in a medical office while the patients is under a local anesthetic. Sometimes stitches are required. A small scar may remain. If there are numerous nevi to be removed, it may be done over several office visits. Plastic surgery may be needed if the skin area involved is extensive.
* Color photographs may be taken of your body, so that on future office visits any changes can be verified.

POSSIBLE COMPLICATIONS—Melanoma.

PROBABLE OUTCOME—Prompt diagnosis and treatment, if needed, can help reduce the risk of melanoma.

HOW TO TREAT

GENERAL MEASURES—Follow medical instructions for post-treatment care.

MEDICATION—No drugs are needed for this disorder.

ACTIVITY—Be sure to use sunscreens and protective clothing for any exposure to the sun. Avoid sun exposure between 10 a.m. and 3 p.m., if possible.

DIET—No special diet.

CALL YOUR DOCTOR IF

* You or a family member has nevi (moles) that have changed in appearance or new ones developed and cause concern.
* New nevi appear after treatment.

ILLNESS & DISORDERS

DYSTHYMIA
(Low-Grade Depression)

 GENERAL INFORMATION

DEFINITION—A chronic, mild type of depression. The start of dysthymia often goes unnoticed. Many people are not aware of the change in their lives.

BODY PARTS INVOLVED—Nervous system.

SEX OR AGE MOST AFFECTED—Both sexes; late teens, young to middle-age adults. Symptoms may begin in childhood or in adolescence and go on for years.

SIGNS & SYMPTOMS
- The depressed mood has occurred for most of each day, for most days, for two years or more (one year for children/teens). There has been no more than two months without some of the symptoms listed.
- Poor appetite or overeating.
- Sleeping too much or too little.
- Lack of energy; feeling tired all the time.
- Feelings of hopelessness.
- Low self-esteem.
- Trouble with concentration and making decisions.

CAUSES—Probably a combination of genetic, developmental, and social factors (such as job loss or divorce).

RISK INCREASES WITH
- Family history of depressive illnesses.
- Loss of a caregiver in childhood.

HOW TO PREVENT—No specific preventive measures. A healthy lifestyle with good nutrition and exercise, having friends, and a job you enjoy may help reduce the risk.

 WHAT TO EXPECT

DIAGNOSTIC MEASURES
- Your own observation of symptoms.
- Your health care provider may do a physical exam, and will ask questions about your symptoms and activities.
- There is no medical test to diagnose dysthymia. Medical tests may be done to rule out other disorders.

APPROPRIATE HEALTH CARE
- Treatment may include some form of counseling along with drug therapy.
- Cognitive-behavioral therapy is often recommended. The cognitive part teaches people how to change thoughts, behaviors or attitudes. The behavior part teaches people ways to reduce anxiety, such as with deep breathing and muscle relaxation.
- Interpersonal therapy can help a patient identify personal relationship problems and how to correct them.
- Job counseling may be recommended for some patients to be sure their work suits their temperament.

POSSIBLE COMPLICATIONS
- Dysthymia recurs after treatment.
- Major depression develops.
- Alcohol abuse.

PROBABLE OUTCOME—Most people are helped by treatment. It may take several months before symptoms improve. Sometimes it isn't until a patient has been treated and is feeling better that they realize how depressed they have been.

 HOW TO TREAT

GENERAL MEASURES
- Join a support group. They help many people with sharing their problems.
- Avoid alcohol. If you need help stopping, ask your health care provider, or contact an Alcoholics Anonymous group in your area.
- Try to reduce emotional stress in your life. Learn techniques to cope with stress.
- To Learn More: National Institute of Mental Health (NIMH), 9000 Rockville Pike, Bethesda, MD 20892, (800) 232-3472; website: www.nimh.nih.gov.

MEDICATION
- An antidepressant may be prescribed. The drug may be needed for several months or several years. If one antidepressant doesn't work, another type may help.
- Thyroid supplements may be prescribed.

ACTIVITY—No limits. A daily exercise program is recommended. It can help improve well-being.

DIET—Eat a normal well-balanced diet.

 CALL YOUR DOCTOR IF

- You or a family member has symptoms of dysthymia.
- Symptoms worsen or don't improve despite treatment.

EAR INFECTION, MIDDLE
(Otitis Media)

 GENERAL INFORMATION

DEFINITION—Infection and inflammation (redness and soreness) in the middle ear. The medical term is acute otitis media (AOM). Otitis media with effusion (OME) is fluid in the middle ear, but without the symptoms of infection. It often follows AOM.

BODY PARTS INVOLVED—Middle-ear space where nerves and small bones connect to the eardrum on one side and the eustachian tube on the other side.

SEX OR AGE MOST AFFECTED—Both sexes and all ages, but most common in infants and children ages 3 months to 3 years.

SIGNS & SYMPTOMS
* Earache.
* Feeling of fullness in the ear.
* Hearing may be reduced.
* Child is fussy or irritable.
* Fever.
* Dizziness.
* Discharge or leakage from the ear.
* Diarrhea or vomiting (sometimes).
* Pulling at the ear (small children).

CAUSES—The ear infection is usually caused by bacteria, and less often by a virus. The infection creates a build up of fluid or pus in the middle ear. Middle ear infections often occur after a cold or other illness of the nose or throat.

RISK INCREASES WITH
* Recent illness, such as a cold or sore throat.
* Having asthma, allergies, or previous ear infections.
* Family history of ear infections.
* Being in daycare.
* Winter and spring seasons.
* Being bottle-fed while lying down, and (possibly) use of a pacifier.
* Smoking in the household.
* Use of antibiotic drugs in the past 1 to 3 months.
* Genetic factors. American Indians and Eskimos seem to get more ear infections than is usual.

HOW TO PREVENT
* Bottle-feed or breast-feed infants in a sitting position with head up, never lying down. Breast-feeding reduces chances of child having ear infections.
* No smoking in household.
* Wash hands often to prevent spread of germs that can cause colds, sore throats, or other infections.
* Possibly, a pneumococcal vaccine.

 WHAT TO EXPECT

DIAGNOSTIC MEASURES
* Your own observation of symptoms.
* Your health care provider can diagnose a middle ear infection by an exam of the ear.
* Other medical tests are normally not needed.

APPROPRIATE HEALTH CARE
* Treatment may include drugs and other steps to relieve pain. Not all infections need antibiotic treatment.
* Sometimes surgery is done to put in plastic tubes through the eardrum to drain pus or fluid from the middle ear. Surgery may be done to remove the adenoids.
* If the eardrum is bulging, a small cut may be made in it to relieve pressure and pain.

POSSIBLE COMPLICATIONS
* Middle ear infections often recur.
* Chronic otitis media (infection lasts over 6 weeks).
* Rarely, more serious ear problems, hearing loss, brain infection, and other complications may occur.

PROBABLE OUTCOME—The outcome is good in almost all cases.

 HOW TO TREAT

GENERAL MEASURES
* Apply heat to the area around the ear to relieve pain. Use a warm washcloth.
* Avoid swimming until the infection clears up.

MEDICATION
* An oral antibiotic may be prescribed for 7 to 10 days. Take the full dose even if symptoms get better. In severe cases, antibiotic injections may be given.
* Ear drops may be prescribed for pain.
* You may use acetaminophen to reduce pain and fever. Do not give aspirin to children.
* Don't use cold remedies, decongestants, or antihistamines. They won't help an ear infection.

ACTIVITY—Rest in bed or reduce activity until symptoms get better.

DIET—No special diet.

 CALL YOUR DOCTOR IF

* You or your child has symptoms of a middle ear infection.
* The following occur during or after treatment: fever, severe headache, earache that persists longer than 2 days despite treatment, swelling around the ear, twitching of the face muscles, or dizziness.

EAR INFECTION, OUTER
(Otitis Externa; Swimmer's Ear)

 GENERAL INFORMATION

DEFINITION—Inflammation (redness and soreness), infection or irritation of the ear canal that extends from the eardrum to the outside. The medical term is otitis externa.

BODY PARTS INVOLVED—Skin of the ear canal.

SEX OR AGE MOST AFFECTED—Both sexes; all ages.

SIGNS & SYMPTOMS
* Ear pain that worsens when the earlobe is pulled.
* Itching in the ear.
* Slight fever (sometimes).
* Discharge of pus from the ear.
* Temporary loss of hearing on the affected side.
* A small, painful lump or boil in the ear canal.

CAUSES
* Bacterial (most common) or fungal infection of the delicate skin lining of the ear canal.
* Injury to the ear canal.

RISK INCREASES WITH
* Swimming in dirty or polluted water.
* Excess moisture in the ear from any cause.
* Irritation from cotton swabs or metal objects, such as bobby pins.
* Previous ear infections.
* Disorders like diabetes that affect the immune system.
* Use of hair spray or hair dye that may enter the ear canal.

HOW TO PREVENT
* Dry ears completely after they have become wet.
* Wear ear-plugs when swimming.
* Don't clean your ears with any object.
* If you have had otitis externa, ask your health care provider about keeping the prescribed ear-drops on hand. If the ear canals get wet for any reason, such as swimming or shampooing, put drops in both ears at bedtime.

 WHAT TO EXPECT

DIAGNOSTIC MEASURES
* Your own observation of symptoms.
* Your health care provider can diagnose an outer ear infection by an exam of the ear.
* Other medical tests are normally not needed.

APPROPRIATE HEALTH CARE
* Treatment may involve your health care provider cleaning and draining the ear, drug therapy, and other steps to relieve pain.
* Self-care after diagnosis.

POSSIBLE COMPLICATIONS
* Chronic otitis externa. The infection persists or recurs often.
* Spread of infection to bones or cartilage. This is a rare, yet serious complication.

PROBABLE OUTCOME—Usually curable with treatment in 7 to 10 days.

 HOW TO TREAT

GENERAL MEASURES
* Apply heat to the area around the ear to relieve pain. Use a warm washcloth.
* Avoid swimming until the infection clears up.
* Gentle cleaning of the ear canal; remember that a small amount of ear-wax helps protect against infection.
* Keep the infected ear dry. Wear ear-plugs or shower cap for showering.

MEDICATION
* You may use acetaminophen or ibuprofen for minor pain. Don't give aspirin to children.
* Your health care provider may prescribe:
  - Eardrops for bacterial infections and cortisone drugs to help other symptoms. An ear wick may be used that allows the drug to reach the end of the ear canal.
  - Oral antibiotics for severe infection.

ACTIVITY—Resume your normal activities as soon as symptoms improve. Avoid getting water in the ears if possible. If you do, dry ears carefully.

DIET—No special diet.

 CALL YOUR DOCTOR IF

* You or a family member has symptoms of outer ear infection.
* Pain persists, despite treatment.

EARDRUM, RUPTURED
(Tympanic Membrane Perforation)

GENERAL INFORMATION

DEFINITION—A hole or tear in the eardrum. The eardrum is involved in hearing.

BODY PARTS INVOLVED—The eardrum which is a thin membrane (called the tympanic membrane) that separates the inner ear from the outer ear.

SEX OR AGE MOST AFFECTED—Both sexes; all ages.

SIGNS & SYMPTOMS
* Sudden pain in the ear.
* Some loss of hearing.
* Bleeding or discharge from the ear (sometimes).
* Ringing in the ear.
* Dizziness.

CAUSES
* An infection of the middle ear. Fluid or pus builds up behind the eardrum and causes it to burst.
* Injury or trauma to the eardrum.

RISK INCREASES WITH
* Using a sharp object to clean the ear or relieve an itch. This can be a cotton swab, hairpin, or paperclip.
* Changes in air pressure due to scuba diving or during an airplane flight.
* A loud noise such as a nearby explosion.
* Injury to the head, such as a skull fracture.
* A blow or hit directly to the ear.
* Middle-ear infection (otitis media).

HOW TO PREVENT
* Don't put any object into the ear canal.
* Get prompt medical treatment for ear infections.

WHAT TO EXPECT

DIAGNOSTIC MEASURES
* Your own observation of symptoms.
* Your health care provider can diagnose the problem by an exam of the ear.
* Fluid from the ear may be sent to the lab for a medical test.
* A hearing test may be performed.

APPROPRIATE HEALTH CARE
* Treatment may involve drugs to prevent infection and for pain.
* A patch may be used to repair the hole. In this procedure, a chemical is applied to the area to help the healing and a paper patch placed on the eardrum. This may need to be redone a few times until healing is complete.
* Surgery called tympanoplasty may be done to repair the hole if it doesn't heal within 2 months. This can be done in a medical office. Your health care provider will give you instructions for home care after surgery.

POSSIBLE COMPLICATIONS
* Ear infection, with fever, vomiting, and diarrhea.
* Mastoiditis. This is an infection of the mastoid (bony area just behind the ear).
* Permanent hearing loss (rare).

PROBABLE OUTCOME
* The eardrum will usually repair itself in 2 months. If it becomes infected, the infection is curable with treatment. Any hearing loss is usually short term.
* Surgery helps if the eardrum does not heal on its own.

HOW TO TREAT

GENERAL MEASURES
* Try to avoid blowing your nose. If you must, blow gently.
* Keep the ear as dry as possible. Don't swim. Take baths instead of showers. If you do shower, wear a plastic shower cap and be sure the ear is covered.

MEDICATION
* Antibiotics to prevent or treat infections may be prescribed.
* Pain relievers. For minor pain, you may use nonprescription drugs such as acetaminophen.

ACTIVITY—Resume your normal activities as soon as symptoms improve.

DIET—No special diet.

CALL YOUR DOCTOR IF

* You or a family member has symptoms of a ruptured eardrum.
* The following occur during treatment:
  - Fever.
  - Pain that persists, despite treatment.
  - Dizziness that continues longer than 12 to 24 hours.

EARWAX BLOCKAGE
(Cerumen Impaction)

 GENERAL INFORMATION

DEFINITION—Overproduction of earwax (cerumen), causing blockage of the external ear canal. Wax is produced by glands in the ear to protect the canal leading from the eardrum to the outside. The amount of wax produced varies from person to person. Some produce so little wax that it never accumulates. Others produce enough to block the canal every few months.

BODY PARTS INVOLVED—External ear canal on one or both sides.

SEX OR AGE MOST AFFECTED—Both sexes; all ages.

SIGNS & SYMPTOMS
* Decreased hearing.
* Ear pain.
* Plugged feeling in the ear.
* Ringing in the ear.

CAUSES—Overproduction of wax by glands in the external ear canal.

RISK INCREASES WITH
* Exposure to dust or debris.
* Family history of overproduction of earwax.
* Water in the ear, which can cause the wax to swell.
* Use of cotton swabs in an attempt to clean the ear canal.

HOW TO PREVENT
* Avoid areas where the air is dusty or filled with debris. This stimulates overproduction of earwax. Consider wearing earplugs if you must be in this type of environment.
* Monthly use of 1 to 2 drops of glycerin in the ear may soften the wax and prevent recurrent blockage.

 WHAT TO EXPECT

DIAGNOSTIC MEASURES
* Your own observation of symptoms.
* If concerned, see your health care provider. An ear exam can confirm the diagnosis.

APPROPRIATE HEALTH CARE
* Self-care. Sometimes wax can be removed easily at home with ear drops and irrigation of the ear canal.
* Medical care if the wax is difficult to remove.

POSSIBLE COMPLICATIONS
* Ear infection.
* Eardrum damage.

PROBABLE OUTCOME—Earwax can be removed, but stubborn cases require patience.

 HOW TO TREAT

GENERAL MEASURES—To remove earwax at home:
* Buy wax-softening ear-drops at a drug store.
* Lie down with the affected ear toward the ceiling.
* Pull the top of the ear gently up and back toward the back of the head.
* Instill the ear-drops as directed by the instructions on the package.
* Leave the drops in the ear for 20 minutes or as directed. Continue to lie down, if possible. Plug the ear with cotton.
* Sit up, leaning a little toward the affected side.
* Use a soft, rubber bulb syringe to irrigate the ear canal gently with plain warm water.
* Repeat irrigations until the ear feels clear. If the ear doesn't clear, see a health care provider so that wax can be removed using other methods.
* Don't try to remove wax with a stick or cotton swab. You may damage the eardrum or cause infection in the ear canal. Caution: If you have a perforated eardrum, don't try to remove wax; call a health care provider.

MEDICATION—For minor pain, you may use nonprescription drugs such as acetaminophen.

ACTIVITY—No limits.

DIET—No special diet.

 CALL YOUR DOCTOR IF

* You or a family member has symptoms of an earwax blockage that does not clear, despite treatment described above.
* A child younger than 4 has an earwax blockage.
* Fever and ear pain accompany an earwax blockage. Do not irrigate the ear in this case.

ECTOPIC PREGNANCY

GENERAL INFORMATION

DEFINITION—An ectopic pregnancy is one that develops outside the uterus. The most common site is in one of the narrow fallopian tubes that connect each ovary to the uterus. Other sites include the ovary or outside the reproductive organs in the abdominal cavity or the cervix. About 1 in 100 pregnancies is ectopic.

BODY PARTS INVOLVED—Female reproductive system; abdominal cavity.

SEX OR AGE MOST AFFECTED—Females of childbearing age.

SIGNS & SYMPTOMS
Early stages:
* Missed or late menstrual period.
* Vaginal spotting or bleeding.
* Pain and cramps in the lower abdomen.
* Pain in the shoulder (rare).
Late stages:
* Sudden, sharp, severe pain in the abdomen.
* Dizziness, fainting, and shock (paleness, rapid heartbeat, drop in blood pressure and cold sweats). These may occur before or along with the pain.

CAUSES—An egg from the ovary is fertilized and becomes implanted outside the uterus. This usually occurs in a fallopian tube that has been damaged (resulting in blockage or narrowing). As the fertilized egg enlarges, the fallopian tube may stretch and rupture. This leads to life-threatening internal bleeding.

RISK INCREASES WITH
* Prior abdominal or pelvic infection.
* Pelvic inflammatory disease (PID).
* Pregnancy after a tubal ligation.
* Assisted reproduction techniques, such as in vitro fertilization.
* Adhesions (scar tissue) from prior abdominal surgery.
* Previous ectopic pregnancy.
* Previous tubal or uterine surgery.
*History of endometritis (inflammation of the endometrium, which is the lining of the uterus).
* Endometriosis (disorder of the fallopian tube).
* Malformed (abnormal) uterus.
* Use of an intrauterine device (IUD) for contraception that results in a pelvic infection.
* Many women diagnosed with an ectopic pregnancy do not have a risk factor.

HOW TO PREVENT—It cannot be prevented.

WHAT TO EXPECT

DIAGNOSTIC MEASURES
* Your own observation of symptoms.

* Medical tests may include blood studies, pregnancy, ultrasound, and laparoscopy (a telescope-like tool is used to look inside the abdomen).
* Diagnosis and treatment may be done on an outpatient basis. Hospital care may be needed for surgery and supportive care. A blood transfusion may be required.

APPROPRIATE HEALTH CARE
* Before rupture of the tube, a diagnosed ectopic pregnancy may be treated using the laparoscope instrument, or with injected drug.
* Surgery may be needed to remove the developing embryo, placenta, and any damaged tissue. The fallopian tube is removed if it cannot be repaired. Future pregnancy is possible with one fallopian tube.
* Weekly blood tests may be recommended to be sure that treatment is successful. If persistent ectopic pregnancy is diagnosed, a drug may be prescribed for treatment.

POSSIBLE COMPLICATIONS
* Internal bleeding that can be life-threatening.
* Reduced fertility.
* Repeat ectopic pregnancy in the future.

PROBABLE OUTCOME—An ectopic pregnancy is always going to be lost. It may resolve on its own before a period is missed. Rupture of an ectopic pregnancy is an emergency. Full recovery is likely with early diagnosis and treatment.

HOW TO TREAT

GENERAL MEASURES
* At home, use heat to relieve pain. Apply a heating pad to the abdomen or back. Warm baths help. Sit in a tub of warm water for 10 to 15 minutes. Repeat as needed.
* To learn more: www.ectopicpregnancy.com.

MEDICATION
* In some ectopic pregnancies, methotrexate may be prescribed for treatment. Specific guidelines and close follow-up care are needed when this drug is used.
* After surgery, pain relievers may be prescribed.

ACTIVITY—Your obstetric provider will advise you when to resume normal activities, as well as sexual relations.

DIET—No special diet.

CALL YOUR DOCTOR IF

You or a family member has symptoms of ectopic pregnancy, especially a rupture (this is an emergency).

ECTROPION & ENTROPION

 GENERAL INFORMATION

DEFINITION—Ectropion is a disorder of the eyelid in which it turns outward (inside out). Entropion is a disorder of the eyelid (usually the lower) in which it curls inward toward the eye.

BODY PARTS INVOLVED—Eyelids.

SEX OR AGE MOST AFFECTED—Both sexes; all ages, but most often in adults over age 40.

SIGNS & SYMPTOMS
Ectropion:
* Turning out of the eyelid, usually the lower.
* Pain, redness, and swelling in the affected eyelid.
* Poor eye lubrication, caused when lubricating tears run down the cheek instead of into the eye.
Entropion:
* Swelling, redness, pain, and excessive tears of the eye. This is caused by the eyelid turning inward and the lashes rubbing against the cornea.

CAUSES
Ectropion:
* Weakening of the muscles and tissues that normally support the lid against the eye.
* Paralysis of the nerve that supplies the eyelid muscles.
* Shrinking of scar tissue from burns, wounds, or surgery near the eye.
Entropion:
* Relaxation of the eyelid's supporting tissue along with the inward pull of the eyelid muscles.
* Chronic eye inflammation (including allergy), creating scar tissue in the eyelid.

RISK INCREASES WITH—Older adults.

HOW TO PREVENT—Cannot be prevented at present.

 WHAT TO EXPECT

DIAGNOSTIC MEASURES–
* Your own observation of the symptoms.
* Your eye care provider can diagnose either disorder by an exam of the affected eye.

APPROPRIATE HEALTH CARE—Treatment involves minor surgery. See Ectropion Repair and Entropion Repair in Surgery Section.

POSSIBLE COMPLICATIONS
* Ectropion: Corneal damage caused by dryness.
* Entropion: Blister of the cornea from eyelash and eyelid irritation.

PROBABLE OUTCOME—Usually curable with surgery.

 HOW TO TREAT

GENERAL MEASURES
* Apply warm compresses to the eyelids several times a day for swelling and pain. To prepare compresses:
  - Pour warm water into a clean bowl. Soak a clean cloth in the water. Wring it out until it is almost dry.
  - Apply the warm, moist cloth to the closed eye for 10 to 15 minutes. Remoisten the cloth frequently.
* Wear protective glasses or goggles if you are exposed to wind or pollutants.

MEDICATION
* Artificial tears may be recommended until surgery can be performed.
* Antibiotics may be prescribed if infection is present.

ACTIVITY—No limits.

DIET—No special diet.

 CALL YOUR DOCTOR IF

* You or a family member has symptoms of ectropion or entropion.
* The following occur after surgery:
  - Eye pain, redness, or sensitivity to light.
  - Vision changes in any way.

ELECTRIC SHOCK

GENERAL INFORMATION

DEFINITION—Injury caused by electricity passing through the body.

BODY PARTS INVOLVED—Total body.

SEX OR AGE MOST AFFECTED—Both sexes; all ages.

SIGNS & SYMPTOMS—Depends on where the current enters the body and the kind of electrical current. Following are the most common:
* Burns at areas of contact. The burns are often deep.
* Heart damage, including cardiac arrest.
* Severe muscle spasms that may cause fractures.
* Breathing paralysis.

CAUSES—Contact with electricity from downed power lines, exposed appliance wires, faulty electrical equipment, lightning strikes or other electrical sources.

RISK INCREASES WITH
* Standing on wet ground or under a tree during an electrical storm.
* Mishandling of electrical equipment.
* Occupations that involve electrical machinery or lines.

HOW TO PREVENT
* Inspect your house, especially the kitchen, bathroom and workshop, for hazards. Use grounded plugs wherever possible.
* Don't use hair dryers, radios or other electrical products in the bathroom where they can fall into a tub or sink.
* Use safety plugs in empty electrical outlets to prevent children from inserting metal objects.
* Don't try to repair electrical equipment unless you know how.
* Wear protective gloves and clothing for work that involves exposure to electricity.
* Replace worn cords or wiring in your home.
* Use ground fault electrical interrupters when possible.
* Go indoors during electrical storms. Lightning may strike several miles away from actual rainfall.

WHAT TO EXPECT

DIAGNOSTIC MEASURES—Diagnosis is usually obvious from the circumstances. A physical exam and medical tests will be done as needed to check for complications.

APPROPRIATE HEALTH CARE
* Self-care after diagnosis (minor burns only).
* Emergency care with cardiopulmonary resuscitation (CPR) at the time of injury, if the victim is unconscious and not breathing.

* Hospital care (sometimes) for moderate to severe injuries. Care at a special burn center may be needed.
* Fluid replacement is often required to replace lost fluids and electrolytes.
* Severe burns may require surgery and skin grafts.
* Counseling may be recommended for patients with severe burns.

POSSIBLE COMPLICATIONS
* Pneumonia.
* Permanent brain damage.
* Severe burns of the skin and underlying muscle.
* Blood vessel damage that can lead to amputation or other problems.
* Death from heart damage.
* Other medical problems such as kidney failure, muscle damage, cataracts

PROBABLE OUTCOME—Depends on the extent of injury. Full recovery is likely if major brain or heart damage does not occur.

HOW TO TREAT

GENERAL MEASURES
* If the victim is touching live electrical wires, shut off the power or remove the wires with a nonmetal object (such as a wooden broomstick) before giving aid. Don't electrocute yourself trying to help someone else.
* If the victim is unconscious and not breathing:
  - Yell for help. Don't leave the victim.
  - Dial 911 (emergency) for an ambulance or medical help. Begin mouth-to-mouth breathing immediately.
  - If there is no heartbeat, give external cardiac massage.
  - Don't stop cardiopulmonary resuscitation (CPR) until help arrives.
* If multiple persons are struck, give CPR first to victims who are not moving (those moving are likely to recover).

MEDICATION—Antibiotics may be prescribed to prevent infections.

ACTIVITY—
* No limits, if the shock is mild.
* If the shock is severe, the victim may resume activities gradually as injuries heal.

DIET—Usually, no special diet.

CALL YOUR DOCTOR IF

* You or someone around you receives an electric shock severe enough to cause injury.
* The following occurs during recovery:
  - Irregular heartbeat.
  - Fever or cough with sputum.

ILLNESS & DISORDERS

EMPHYSEMA

GENERAL INFORMATION

DEFINITION—A chronic, progressive lung disease that causes decreased lung function. Emphysema and chronic bronchitis together are called chronic obstructive pulmonary disease (COPD).

BODY PARTS INVOLVED—Lungs, and eventually almost all body systems.

SEX OR AGE MOST AFFECTED—Both sexes (men more than women) and older adults.

SIGNS & SYMPTOMS
* In the early stages, there are often no symptoms.
* Trouble breathing that gets worse over several years.
* Breathing is more difficult after physical activity.
* Wheezing.
* Occasional repeated infections of the lungs or bronchial tubes.
* Blue skin and lips.
* Cough with sputum.
* Finger clubbing (fingertips become large).
* Barrel-chest.

CAUSES—Emphysema is caused by destroyed lung tissue, and inflammation and irritation of the airways in the lungs. Smoking is the main reason the lung damage occurs.

RISK INCREASES WITH
* Many years of cigarette smoking. About 15 to 20 percent of smokers get emphysema.
* Exposure to secondhand smoke.
* Family history of emphysema.
* Air pollution.
* Inherited alpha 1-antitrypsin deficiency. This is a disorder that can damage lungs as smoking does.
* Males (they are affected more than women).
* Older age.

HOW TO PREVENT
* Don't smoke. If you do smoke, quit now.
* Avoid places with polluted air.

WHAT TO EXPECT

DIAGNOSTIC MEASURES
* Your health care provider will do a physical exam and ask questions about your symptoms.
* Medical tests will be done to confirm the diagnosis and determine the extent of the disease. These may include blood tests, x-rays, and lung function tests.

APPROPRIATE HEALTH CARE
* Treatment is aimed at relieving symptoms, slowing the disease, and preventing complications.

* Get counseling for depression, anxiety, and other emotional problems.
* Pulmonary rehabilitation therapy.
* Surgery for lung reduction or lung transplant may be considered (rarely).

POSSIBLE COMPLICATIONS
* Lung infections, failure, or lung collapse.
* Anxiety, panic disorder, and depression.
* Congestive heart failure.

PROBABLE OUTCOME—Cannot be cured. Symptoms can be controlled to slow progress and severity of the disease. The disease shortens life expectancy, but patients live many years with it.

HOW TO TREAT

GENERAL MEASURES
* Don't smoke. Smoking will cause the disease to become worse, despite treatment.
* If you work in an area with severe air pollution, do all you can to reduce exposure. Change jobs, if necessary.
* Stay indoors during air pollution alerts.
* Install air-conditioning with a filter and humidity control in your home.
* Avoid sudden temperature or humidity changes, loud talking, laughing, crying, or exertion, if these trigger coughing episodes.
* Avoid higher altitudes where the air is thin.
* Raise foot of the bed with 4 or 5-inch blocks.
* Home oxygen use may be needed.
* To learn more: American Lung Association, 61 Broadway, 6th Floor, New York, NY 10006, (800) 586-4872; website: www.lungusa.org.

MEDICATION—You may be prescribed:
* Drugs to relax spasms of bronchial tubes.
* Steroids to reduce lung inflammation.
* Antibiotics to treat or prevent infections.
* Vaccines for influenza and pneumonia.
* Drugs for depression, anxiety, or panic disorder.

ACTIVITY—Physical exercises and breathing exercises are usually prescribed. Both are important in improving symptoms.

DIET—Drink plenty of nonalcoholic fluids each day. This thins lung secretions so they can be coughed up more easily.

CALL YOUR DOCTOR IF

* You or a family member has symptoms of emphysema.
* The following occur after diagnosis:
  - Signs of infection (fever, chills, or aches).
  - Increased trouble breathing or chest pain.
  - Sputum that increases, thickens, changes color, or is bloody.

EMPYEMA

GENERAL INFORMATION

DEFINITION—A collection of pus in a body cavity. It usually occurs in the space around the lungs (pleural cavity).

BODY PARTS INVOLVED—Lungs. It may rarely occur in the gall bladder or the pelvic cavity.

SEX OR AGE MOST AFFECTED—Both sexes; all ages.

SIGNS & SYMPTOMS
- Chest pain. Pain varies from slight discomfort to stabbing pain. It is often worse with coughing or breathing. Pain may extend to the lower chest wall or stomach.
- Rapid, shallow breathing.
- Chills.
- Fever.
- Extreme fatigue.
- Dry cough.
- Bad breath.
- Weight loss.

CAUSES—Usually a complication of pneumonia. Infection causes pus to build up in the pleural cavity. The pus, which can amount to a pint or more, puts pressure on the lungs and causes breathing problems.

RISK INCREASES WITH
- Lung or chest infections.
- Chest injury.
- Infection from elsewhere in the body that has spread to the lungs.
- Medical procedures that involve placement of a chest tube or inserting a needle into the chest to draw off fluid.

HOW TO PREVENT—No specific preventive measures.

WHAT TO EXPECT

DIAGNOSTIC MEASURES
- Your own observation of symptoms.
- Your health care provider will do a physical exam and ask questions about your symptoms.
- X-ray, CT, or ultrasound tests may be done of the chest. A sample of the pus may be taken for testing by using a needle inserted through the back into the affected area.

APPROPRIATE HEALTH CARE
- Treatment is done in a hospital and usually involves giving drugs to treat infection and a procedure to drain the pus (fluid).
- The fluid may be drained by using a chest tube or other type of surgery depending on the extent of the infection. The options will be explained to you by the surgeon.
- Treatment of empyema of the gall bladder involves drugs and surgical removal of the gall bladder.

POSSIBLE COMPLICATIONS—Complications are more likely in the elderly and very ill.

PROBABLE OUTCOME—Outcome will depend on several factors. The severity of the infection, the patient's health, any underlying disease, and how effective the treatment is. In otherwise healthy persons, the outcome is generally good.

HOW TO TREAT

GENERAL MEASURES—None specific.

MEDICATION—Antibiotics for infection are given through a vein (IV).

ACTIVITY—Gradually return to normal activity after treatment. Allow 2 months for recovery.

DIET—A special diet may be required while in the hospital. After treatment, resume a normal diet.

CALL YOUR DOCTOR IF

- You or a family member has symptoms of empyema.
- Following treatment, any signs of infection occur, such as fever, chills, aches, or pain.

ILLNESS & DISORDERS

ENCEPHALITIS, VIRAL

GENERAL INFORMATION

DEFINITION—Inflammation of the brain caused by a viral infection. It may occur in one part of the brain (focal), several parts of the brain (multi-focal), or throughout the brain (diffuse).

BODY PARTS INVOLVED—Brain; sometimes meninges (membranes that cover the brain).

SEX OR AGE MOST AFFECTED—It can occur at any age, but most often affects the very young or the elderly.

SIGNS & SYMPTOMS
* No symptoms (sometimes).
* Fever.
* Vomiting.
* In infants, a swelling or bulging of the soft spot of the skull.
* Headache.
* Stiff neck.
* Confusion.
* Seizures.
* Occasional weakness or paralysis of an arm or leg.
* Double vision.
* Trouble speaking.
* Hearing loss.
* Drowsiness.

CAUSES—Encephalitis can be caused by one of several types of viruses. These include arboviruses (which are transmitted by mosquitoes or ticks), viruses of the herpes virus family, and others, such as mumps or measles. In some cases, the viral infection may cause no problem until it enters the bloodstream and is carried to the brain cells. In other cases, the infection may first infect other body tissue and then spread to the brain.

RISK INCREASES WITH
* Newborns and infants.
* Adults over 60.
* Weak immune system due to illness or drugs.
* Living in areas with a large mosquito population.

HOW TO PREVENT
* Get medical care for viral infections.
* Take precautions to prevent mosquito bites.

WHAT TO EXPECT

DIAGNOSTIC MEASURES
* Your own observation of symptoms.
* Your health care provider will do a physical exam and ask questions about your symptoms and activities.

* Medical tests may include studies of blood and spinal fluid, CT, MRI (see Glossary for both), and electroencephalogram (which records brain waves). A brain biopsy (removal of a small amount of tissue for viewing under a microscope) may be done.

APPROPRIATE HEALTH CARE
* Hospital care is needed for severe symptoms. Supportive care will be provided for breathing or heart problems. Fluid and electrolyte levels will be monitored. Steps will be taken to prevent complications.
* If brain function is affected, physical therapy, speech therapy, and behavioral therapy may be recommended.

POSSIBLE COMPLICATIONS
* Bacterial infections may develop.
* A very small number of people suffer permanent brain damage that impairs mental or muscle functions.
* Coma and death (rare).
* Relapse (recurrence of the disease).

PROBABLE OUTCOME—Mild viral encephalitis may go unnoticed. In other cases, symptoms last 3 to 5 days. Complications from encephalitis are more likely in infants and the elderly. People in other age groups usually recover completely, but it may take several months.

HOW TO TREAT

GENERAL MEASURES
* Susceptible individuals should avoid contact with the patient.
* The illness can be frightening, both to the patient and to the family. Most hospitals have social workers who are there for your support.

MEDICATION—Your health care provider may prescribe:
* Pain relievers, for headache or fever.
* Antiviral drugs, for certain viral infections.
* Antibiotics drugs, for bacterial infection.
* Drugs to reduce inflammation.
* Drugs to control seizures if needed.

ACTIVITY—Reduce activity until the pain and fever are gone. Gradually return to normal activity. Allow 2 or more months for complete recovery.

DIET—No special diet. May require fluids given through a vein (IV) while in the hospital.

CALL YOUR DOCTOR IF

* You or a family member has symptoms of encephalitis.
* New, unexplained symptoms develop or symptoms recur after treatment.

ENCOPRESIS

GENERAL INFORMATION

DEFINITION—A condition in which a child over age four passes bowel movements (stools) on a regular basis into places other than a toilet.

BODY PARTS INVOLVED—Bowels.

SEX OR AGE MOST AFFECTED—Both sexes (boys more than girls) of children over age 4.

SIGNS & SYMPTOMS
* Bowel movements in underwear. Sometimes the bowel movements may be on the floor or other places.
* Not able to control bowel movements.
* Hard bowel movements.
* Secretive behavior about bowel movements.
* The child has a bad smell.
* The child may or may not have constipation.

CAUSES—There may be a physical or emotional factor, or both, involved. The child may be able to control the bowel movement, but chooses not to. The child may not be able to control the bowel movement. The child may have a more liquid bowel movement that leaks out.

RISK INCREASES WITH
* Boys are affected more often than girls.
* Constipation or diarrhea.
* A physical or emotional change in the child's life, such as the birth of a sibling or recent illness with diarrhea.
* Resistance to using the toilet because of too much pressure to do so.
* Painful bowel movements.
* Resistance to using toilet facilities at school, on camping trips, or outdoor toilets.
* Eating problems that cause constipation.
* Problems due to mental abilities or a medical illness that affects the colon.

HOW TO PREVENT
* Avoid undue emphasis on toilet training. Approach it calmly, with realistic expectations. Don't shame or blame the child for accidents.
* Be sensitive to stressful situations that your child faces. Talk together about the child's feelings.
* Maintain good diet and nutrition for your child.

WHAT TO EXPECT

DIAGNOSTIC MEASURES
* Your own observation of symptoms.
* Your child's health care provider will do a physical exam. Questions will be asked about the child's symptoms and other areas of the child's life.
* Medical tests may be done to check for illness or a physical problem.

APPROPRIATE HEALTH CARE—Treatment usually consists of diet changes, behavior training, and sometimes drugs, such as laxatives or stool softeners. Each child is different and will respond to different treatment steps. Follow any special instructions from your child's health care provider.

POSSIBLE COMPLICATIONS
* Child may suffer from embarrassment, shame, guilt, and low self-esteem.
* Skin rash in rectal area.
* Chronic constipation.
* Stool impaction (hard bowel movement remains in the colon).

PROBABLE OUTCOME—Usually curable. Parents need to be patient. It may take time for the problem to get better.

HOW TO TREAT

GENERAL MEASURES
* Respond gently to accidents. For children who are old enough, have them clean themselves and change into clean underwear. Don't blame, criticize, restrict, or punish the child for accidents. This may cause the child to give up, as well as lead to other emotional problems.
* After meals, have the child sit on the toilet for about 10 minutes. Praise the child for having bowel movements in the toilet. Give a reward for staying clean all day.
* Ask for the school's help. The child needs quick access to the bathroom at school, especially if shy or new at school.
* Don't make this problem the main focus of the child's or your family's life. Do try to identify stresses in the child's life and make every effort to ease them. Consider counseling for the child if needed.

MEDICATION—Lubricant laxatives or other types may be used. Enemas or suppositories may be needed for an impaction.

ACTIVITY—No limits.

DIET—Provide a diet high in fiber with plenty of fruits and vegetables. Use whole-grain products for cereals and breads. Be sure your child drinks enough fluids.

CALL YOUR DOCTOR IF

* Your child has encopresis, and it persists longer than 2 months, despite your efforts.
* Your child has a fever, diarrhea, hard or bloody bowel movements, or there is blood around the rectum.

ENDOCARDITIS
(Bacterial Endocarditis; Infective Endocarditis)

GENERAL INFORMATION

DEFINITION—An infection and inflammation involving the heart.

BODY PARTS INVOLVED—Heart muscle; heart valves; endocardium (lining of the heart chambers and valves).

SEX OR AGE MOST AFFECTED—Both sexes; all ages.

SIGNS & SYMPTOMS
* Fatigue and weakness.
* Recurrent fever, chills, and heavy sweating, especially at night.
* Loss of appetite and weight loss.
* Vague muscle aches and joint pains.
* Headache.
* Cough.
* Shortness of breath.
* Swelling of the feet, legs, and stomach.
* Fast or irregular heartbeat.
* Red spots on the skin.

CAUSES—An infection (usually bacterial, sometimes fungal) that enters the bloodstream and infects the heart valves. The infection may start with a skin disorder or injury, a medical or dental procedure, or a skin prick (as with an IV drug user).

RISK INCREASES WITH
* Rheumatic fever.
* History of endocarditis.
* Congenital (being born with) heart disease.
* IV (intravenous) drug abuse.
* Mitral valve prolapse with a heart murmur.
* Weak immune system due to illness or drugs.
* Artificial heart valves or other artificial devices in the heart, such as a pacemaker wire.

HOW TO PREVENT
* If you have heart-valve damage or a heart murmur, ask about antibiotic use before medical procedures that may bring bacteria into the blood. These include dental work, childbirth, and some surgeries.
* Once you have had endocarditis, follow your health care provider's advice about preventing a relapse.
* Don't abuse IV drugs.

WHAT TO EXPECT

DIAGNOSTIC MEASURES
* Your health care provider will do a physical exam and ask questions about your symptoms.
* Medical tests may include blood studies, echocardiogram and electrocardiogram (heart function tests), x-rays, and CT.

APPROPRIATE HEALTH CARE
* Treatment usually involves drugs for the infection, supportive care for symptoms, and steps to prevent complications.
* Hospital care is normally needed during acute phase. Once stable, some patients can continue with treatment at home.
* Surgery may be done to replace an infected heart valve in some patients.

POSSIBLE COMPLICATIONS
* Heart problems, including heart attack, congestive heart failure, arrhythmias, and others.
* Blood clots may break off and travel to other places in the body, such as the brain or kidneys.
* Kidney problems.

PROBABLE OUTCOME—Usually curable with early diagnosis and treatment. Recovery can take weeks. If untreated, or if treatment is delayed, heart function declines resulting in serious complications.

HOW TO TREAT

GENERAL MEASURES
* If you have damaged heart valves, tell any doctor or dentist who treats you.
* Ongoing dental hygiene is important to prevent infection.
* Wear a medical alert type bracelet or neck tag that indicates your medical problem. Carry a wallet card listing the antibiotic regimens needed for medical and dental procedures.

MEDICATION—Antibiotics (for a bacterial infection) will be prescribed. They are normally needed for 2 to 6 weeks. Antibiotic treatment is often given through a vein (IV), but in some cases may be taken orally.

ACTIVITY
* Rest in bed until fully recovered. While in bed, move your legs often to help prevent clots from forming in deep veins.
* Resume your normal activities, including sexual relations, when strength allows or upon medical advice.

DIET—No special diet.

CALL YOUR DOCTOR IF

* You or a family member has symptoms of endocarditis.
* The following occur during or after treatment:
  - Weight gain without diet changes.
  - Blood in the urine.
  - Chest pain or shortness of breath.
  - Sudden weakness or numbness in muscles of the face, trunk, or limbs.

ENDOMETRIAL HYPERPLASIA
(Adenomatous Hyperplasia of the Uterus)

 GENERAL INFORMATION

DEFINITION—Endometrial hyperplasia is an excess growth of tissue in the endometrium (inner lining of the uterus). It is not cancerous, but some hyperplasia is known to be precancerous (called atypia). Types of hyperplasia include:
* Simple or complex (adenomatous) hyperplasia without atypia.
* Simple or complex (adenomatous) hyperplasia with atypia.

BODY PARTS INVOLVED—Endometrium.

SEX OR AGE MOST AFFECTED—Women, usually over age 35.

SIGNS & SYMPTOMS
* Bleeding after menopause.
* Vaginal discharge, especially after menopause.
* Lower abdominal cramps (sometimes).
* Bleeding between normal menstrual periods.
* Heavy menstrual flow.

CAUSES—Excess estrogen (a female hormone) as compared with the amount of progesterone (another female hormone). This excess is caused internally, or from the use of hormone-containing drugs. Tamoxifen, a drug used for breast cancer, is a risk factor for hyperplasia.

RISK INCREASES WITH
* Estrogen replacement therapy without progesterone use.
* Diabetes.
* Obesity (25 or more pounds over normal weight).
* Women in the years around menopause.
* Polycystic ovary syndrome.
* Women who skip menstrual periods, or have none.

HOW TO PREVENT
* If taking estrogen, balance it with progesterone.
* Weight loss, if obesity is a problem.
* Birth control pills (oral contraceptives) contain estrogen, along with a form of progesterone. They may help protect against endometrial hyperplasia in women who do not have regular periods.

 WHAT TO EXPECT

DIAGNOSTIC MEASURES
* Your own observation of symptoms.
* Your health care provider will do a physical exam and a pelvic exam
* Medical tests may include blood tests of hormone levels and Pap smear. A vaginal

ultrasound, an endometrial biopsy, a D & C (dilatation and curettage) procedure, or a hysteroscopy (use of a telescopic instrument inserted through the vagina to look inside the uterus) may be done. They help to diagnose the type of hyperplasia and to rule out cancer.

APPROPRIATE HEALTH CARE
* Treatment will be based on findings from the medical tests, your age, and desires about future pregnancy.
* Drugs are normally the first step in treatment. They will cause the lining to shed and prevent it from building up again. This will show up as vaginal bleeding or a menstrual period.
* For some women, a hysterectomy (surgery to remove the uterus) is recommended. It may help when hormone therapy has failed and precancerous cells are discovered. (See Hysterectomy in Surgery section.)

POSSIBLE COMPLICATIONS
* Without treatment, women who have hyperplasia with atypia have a higher risk for endometrial cancer.
* Excessive, uncontrolled bleeding.

PROBABLE OUTCOME
* In most cases, treatment will reverse the hyperplasia caused by the excess estrogen.
* In other cases, it is often curable with surgery. If a woman chooses not to have surgery, hormone therapy usually controls symptoms.

 HOW TO TREAT

GENERAL MEASURES
* Long-term follow-up with your health care provider will be required to help avoid a recurrence. Periodic endometrial biopsies, and possibly other tests, will be used to watch for complications of this condition.
* Use heat to relieve pain. Place a heating pad on your abdomen or back. Take warm baths.

MEDICATION—Progesterone (progestin), a female hormone, may be prescribed. It may be taken by mouth or via a skin patch.

ACTIVITY—No limits unless you have surgery. Then resume your activities gradually. Resume sexual relations once medical approval is given.

DIET—Usually, no special diet is required. If you are overweight, losing weight might help decrease estrogen in the body.

 CALL YOUR DOCTOR IF

* You or a family member has symptoms of endometrial hyperplasia.
* Any unexpected symptoms occur with treatment.

ENDOMETRIOSIS

GENERAL INFORMATION

DEFINITION—The inner lining of the uterus (called the endometrium) is made up of endometrial tissue. This tissue normally builds up during the menstrual cycle. It is then shed each month during the normal menstrual period. Endometriosis occurs when this tissue grows outside the uterus in places such as the fallopian tubes or the ovaries. Rarely, the tissue may grow in other areas of the body.

BODY PARTS INVOLVED—Uterus; ovaries; fallopian tubes; outer layer of the intestines.

SEX OR AGE MOST AFFECTED—Females between puberty and menopause, but most common between ages 20 and 30.

SIGNS & SYMPTOMS
- Symptoms may begin suddenly or develop over years.
- Pelvic pain that may occur at anytime. It may increase during menstrual periods, especially the last days.
- Pain with sexual intercourse.
- Premenstrual spotting, blood in the urine, or blood in the stool (sometimes).
- Back pain.
- Infertility.

CAUSES—Unknown. One theory is that, during menstruation, some of the menstrual tissue backs up through the fallopian tubes into the abdomen, where it implants and grows. Another theory is that endometriosis may be genetic, or that certain families may have risk factors that lead to endometriosis. The body's immune system may also play a role in the cause.

RISK INCREASES WITH
- Women who don't become pregnant or who delay childbirth.
- Women with family history of endometriosis.
- Medical conditions that involve the cervix or vagina.

HOW TO PREVENT—There are no specific preventive steps.

WHAT TO EXPECT

DIAGNOSTIC MEASURES
- Your own observation of symptoms.
- Your health care provider will do a physical exam and a pelvic exam.
- Medical tests may include laparoscopy. A thin, lighted tube (called a laparoscope) is inserted through a small incision (cut) in the abdomen to view internal organs and to sometimes remove tissue. Open surgery (laparotomy) may be needed for diagnosis.

APPROPRIATE HEALTH CARE
- Treatment may include drug therapy, surgery, or both. Alternative treatments (such as acupuncture) may help. Treatment will vary depending on the severity of the disease and the patient's age and desire for pregnancy. A patient may desire pregnancy now, at a later time, or not at all.
- Different procedures are used for treatment. The options will be explained to you. A hysterectomy may be suggested for women who do not desire pregnancy.

POSSIBLE COMPLICATIONS
- Infertility.
- Severe pain that causes depression, stress, and problems with daily living activities.
- Adhesions (scar tissue) of pelvic organs.
- Endometriosis can recur after treatment.
- Cysts and pelvic masses (endometriomas).
- An increased risk of cancer is a possibility.

PROBABLE OUTCOME—It is an ongoing, long-term disorder that may get worse over time. Symptoms can often be relieved with treatment. Women with severe disease may have less success with treatment. The ability to become pregnant depends on factors such as severity of the disorder and success of therapy.

HOW TO TREAT

GENERAL MEASURES
- Use a heating pad or take warm baths to relieve pain. Cold therapy may help. Use ice packs on the abdomen.
- Put a pillow under your knees when you rest or sleep. When lying on your side, pull the knees up to the chest.
- To learn more: Endometriosis Association, 8585 N. 76th Place, Milwaukee, WI 53223, (800) 992-3636; website: www.endometriosisassn.org.

MEDICATION
- Use nonprescription nonsteroidal anti-inflammatory drugs to relieve minor pain.
- Stronger pain relievers may be prescribed.
- Hormonal drugs to stop ovulation may be prescribed.

ACTIVITY
- Exercise, such as walking, helps relieve pain.
- You may be taught to do Kegel exercises to help strengthen the pelvic floor muscles.

DIET—Avoid alcohol and caffeine. They can make the pain more severe in some women.

CALL YOUR DOCTOR IF

- You or a family member has symptoms of endometriosis.
- Severe pain occurs, or other symptoms recur.

EPIDIDYMITIS

GENERAL INFORMATION

DEFINITION—An inflammation and infection of the epididymis. These are thin-walled tubes at the top of a man's testicles. They carry sperm from the testicles to the vas deferens. The vas deferens is another tube that carries the sperm from the testicle to the prostate before ejaculation.

BODY PARTS INVOLVED—Epididymis.

SEX OR AGE MOST AFFECTED—Males (more often affects men ages 19 to 35).

SIGNS & SYMPTOMS
* Pain, heat, redness, and swelling at the back or top of one testicle (sometimes both).
* Fever and chills.
* Pain or burning with urination.
* Discharge from the penis (sometimes).

CAUSES
* Infection in the urinary tract or the prostate.
* Sexually transmitted diseases (STDs).
* Amiodarone (a heart drug).
* Intense exercise, such as heavy lifting, may be a cause.
* A whole body infection that spreads through the bloodstream to the epididymis.
* Sometimes, no cause is found.

RISK INCREASES WITH
* Recent urethral or urinary tract infection.
* Abnormalities or recent surgery involving the genitals or urinary tract.
* Unsafe sexual practices that lead to STDs.
* Catheter (use of a tube to carry urine from the body).
* Presence of a foreskin (being uncircumcised).

HOW TO PREVENT
* Practice safe sex or abstain from sexual activity.
* Avoid catheters if possible.
* Practice good hygiene, especially if uncircumcised.

WHAT TO EXPECT

DIAGNOSTIC MEASURES
* Your own observation of symptoms.
* Your health care provider will do an exam of the genitals.
* Medical tests usually include urine or discharge studies to check for bacteria or sexually transmitted diseases. Blood studies or ultrasound may also be done.

APPROPRIATE HEALTH CARE
* The goal of treatment is to cure the infection and reduce pain and swelling. Treatment can usually be done at home with rest, drug therapy, and self-care measures.
* Surgery may be recommended in cases of blockage or narrowing of the urethra, or for an abscess.

POSSIBLE COMPLICATIONS
* Abscess (pus-filled area).
* May become sterile (unable to father children) if untreated.
* The disorder may become chronic.
* Infection of the testicles or infection spreads into the bloodstream, or, rarely, a severe scrotal infection.

PROBABLE OUTCOME—Usually curable with treatment. Pain often goes away in 1 to 3 days. Complete healing may take several weeks.

HOW TO TREAT

GENERAL MEASURES
* Support the weight of the scrotum and tender testicles. Roll a soft bath towel and place it between the legs under the inflamed area.
* Apply an ice bag (wrapped in a cloth) to the inflamed parts to help reduce swelling and relieve pain. Do this for 10 to 15 minutes at a time several times a day. Don't use heat.
* Wear an athletic supporter or two pairs of athletic briefs when you return to normal activity.

MEDICATION
* Antibiotics will be prescribed for infection. They may be given by injection or taken orally.
* Use ibuprofen or naproxen for mild pain and inflammation. Stronger drugs may be prescribed for more severe pain.
* Stool softeners may be used to prevent constipation.

ACTIVITY—Rest in bed until fever, pain, and swelling improve. Don't engage in sexual intercourse. Wait at least 1 month (or as advised) after all symptoms disappear before resuming sexual relations.

DIET—Eat natural laxative foods, such as prunes, fresh fruit, whole-grain cereals, and nuts, to prevent constipation.

CALL YOUR DOCTOR IF

* You or a family member has symptoms of epididymitis.
* Pain is not relieved by treatment.
* You develop severe scrotal pain, urinary pain or a discharge, fever, chills, or you become constipated.

ILLNESS & DISORDERS

EPIGLOTTITIS

 GENERAL INFORMATION

DEFINITION—A life-threatening inflammation of the epiglottis. The epiglottis is a small flap of tissue in the back of the throat that keeps food from going into the windpipe (trachea). Immediate treatment is needed as swelling of the epiglottis may lead to complete blockage of the airway within 12 hours of onset.

BODY PARTS INVOLVED—Epiglottis and surrounding tissue.

SEX OR AGE MOST AFFECTED—It is more common in young children (ages 2 to 4) and boys more than girls. It can occur in adults as well.

SIGNS & SYMPTOMS
* Muffled voice or cry (with croup, it is more hoarse).
* Minimal cough (with croup, it is a barking cough).
* Sore throat.
* Fever.
* Hoarseness.
* Drooling caused by difficulty swallowing saliva.
* Increased breathing difficulty.
* Noisy, high-pitched, squeaky inhalations.
* Purple skin and nails.
* Odd head posture. The person tilts the neck back and leans forward with the tongue stuck out and the nostrils flared, trying to inhale more air.

CAUSES—Usually a bacterial infection. There may be other, more rare, causes.

RISK INCREASES WITH—Unknown.

HOW TO PREVENT—None specific. If your child has had epiglottitis previously, treat all respiratory infections early and with medical care. Immunize children against *Haemophilus influenza*.

 WHAT TO EXPECT

DIAGNOSTIC MEASURES
* Your own observation of symptoms.
* Hospital care is needed. Your health care provider will perform exams under special controls to prevent complications.

APPROPRIATE HEALTH CARE—Intensive care will be provided. A tube may be inserted in the throat to assist breathing (intubation). Surgery may be done to make an opening in the windpipe (trachea). Usually the tube is withdrawn or the opening is closed in 1 to 3 days.

POSSIBLE COMPLICATIONS
* Pneumonia, meningitis, septic arthritis, pericarditis, or cellulitis.
* Without treatment, complete airway obstruction and death can occur within hours.

PROBABLE OUTCOME—Full recovery with prompt diagnosis and treatment.

 HOW TO TREAT

GENERAL MEASURES
* Never attempt to look at the back of the child's throat if you suspect epiglottitis.
* Have the child sit up rather than lie down.
* Keep the child calm and still until reaching the hospital. Panic increases breathing difficulty.

MEDICATION
* Antibiotics will be prescribed for infection. Continue for a minimum of 10 days or as advised.
* Steroid drugs may be given to reduce inflammation.

ACTIVITY—Bed rest is needed until all symptoms disappear. Activities may then be resumed gradually.

DIET—Fluids only (usually through a vein) until the patient can swallow. Once the patient is home, return to a normal diet.

 CALL YOUR DOCTOR IF

* Your or a family member has symptoms of epiglottitis, especially signs of breathing difficulty. Or call 911. This is an emergency.
* Your child has had epiglottitis in the past, and symptoms of respiratory infection appear.

EPILEPSY
(Seizure Disorder)

 GENERAL INFORMATION

DEFINITION—Epilepsy is a brain disorder involving recurrent seizures of all types. Seizures are episodes of disturbed brain function that cause changes in attention and/or behavior. The two main categories of seizures are generalized seizures (the whole brain is involved) and partial seizures (a limited area of the brain is involved). Each category has different seizure types.

BODY PARTS INVOLVED—Nervous system.

SEX OR AGE MOST AFFECTED—Epilepsy affects both sexes and all ages. It often begins between ages 2 and 14.

SIGNS & SYMPTOMS
Generalized seizures types:
• Tonic-clonic (grand mal)—complete loss of consciousness, falling, jerking movements, urine incontinence.
• Absence (petit mal)—brief loss of consciousness.
• Myoclonic— brief jerking movements.
Partial seizures types:
• Simple partial—stays conscious, and weakness, numbness, unusual smells or tastes, muscle twitching, turning head to side, visual changes, or vertigo may occur.
• Complex partial—altered consciousness, automatic repetitive behavior, uncontrolled laughing, unusual thoughts, hallucinations, fears, or smells odd odors.

CAUSES—Abnormal changes in how the cells in the brain send signals to each other. The causes are often unknown.

RISK INCREASES WITH
• Family history of seizure disorders.
• Brain injury to the fetus during pregnancy.
• Birth injury (such as lack of oxygen).
• Poisoning from substance abuse or environmental toxins (such as lead poisoning).
• Infection of the brain (such as meningitis).
• Head injury (such as from accidents or shaken baby syndrome).
• Blood sugar problem (hypoglycemia).
• Metabolic illness (such as hypocalcemia).
• Brain tumor.
• Stroke.

HOW TO PREVENT—No specific preventive measures.

 WHAT TO EXPECT

DIAGNOSTIC MEASURES
• Your own observation of symptoms.
• Your health care provider will do a physical exam.

• Medical tests usually include blood studies; one or more types of brain scans; and electroencephalogram (EEG), a study of the brain's electrical activity.

APPROPRIATE HEALTH CARE
• Treatment for epilepsy usually involves drug therapy.
• Vagus nerve stimulation may be an option. A device implanted in the neck provides mild electrical stimulation to the vagus nerve to help control seizures.
• Surgery may be helpful in a few cases. An area of the brain causing seizures may be removed, or certain nerve pathways in the brain may be interrupted.

POSSIBLE COMPLICATIONS
• Seizures continue despite treatment.
• For some patients, epilepsy carries a stigma. It can lead to emotional problems, difficulty in social and family relationships, and problems in finding employment.
• Status epilepticus (a prolonged seizure state).
• Sudden, unexpected death.

PROBABLE OUTCOME—There is no cure. Treatment can prevent most seizures and allow a near-normal life.

 HOW TO TREAT

GENERAL MEASURES
• Seizures may result from too little sleep, stress, not taking your drugs, menstrual periods, or flashing lights.
• Wear a medical-alert type bracelet or pendant that shows you have epilepsy (in case you have a seizure).
• To learn more: Epilepsy Foundation of America, 4351 Garden City Dr., Landover, MD 20785; (800) 332-1000.

MEDICATION—Anticonvulsant drugs will usually be prescribed. Dosage changes are often needed. If a person is seizure-free for 2 or more years, drug withdrawal may be considered.

ACTIVITY—No limits usually. Most states allow persons with epilepsy to drive a vehicle after being seizure-free for 1 year.

DIET—No special diet. Don't drink alcohol.

 CALL YOUR DOCTOR IF

• You or a family member has symptoms of epilepsy.
• The pattern of seizure activity changes.
• Drugs used for treatment cause problems.
• Call 911 (emergency) if the seizure symptoms occur that require emergency care.

ERYTHEMA INFECTIOSUM
(Fifth Disease)

GENERAL INFORMATION

DEFINITION—An infectious, mild, viral illness that occurs in outbreaks (often during the winter and spring months). The word erythema means skin redness, and infectiosum means infectious. The name fifth disease comes from its place on a list made up many years ago of the five most common childhood infections.

BODY PARTS INVOLVED—Skin and body as a whole.

SEX OR AGE MOST AFFECTED—It most often affects children ages 5 to 14, and is rare in infants and adults.

SIGNS & SYMPTOMS
• The illness begins with a headache, stuffy or runny nose, and sometimes, a low-grade fever and feeling of fatigue. These symptoms may get better.
• From 3 to 10 days later, a rash appears. It is called "slapped cheeks appearance" because it starts as a rash on the cheeks. The rash spreads to the trunk, buttocks, and limbs. It has a lace-like pattern, and it may be itchy.
• Rarely, other symptoms may occur such as sore throat, red eyes, diarrhea, and swollen glands.
• In adults, there may be mild joint pain or swelling.
• About 20% of infected people will have no symptoms.

CAUSES—A virus called parvovirus B-19. The germs come from fluids in the nose, mouth, and throat of someone who has the infection. When an infected person coughs or sneezes, the germs are spread into the air. The period of time from exposure to the germs until symptoms begin is 4 to 28 days with an average of 16 to 17 days. Once the rash appears, the germs are no longer being spread.

RISK INCREASES WITH—Children in school and daycare centers.

HOW TO PREVENT
• No specific preventive measures. Outbreaks can last for months, so there is no need to keep a child out of school or daycare.
• A pregnant woman should avoid daycare centers and schools if there is an outbreak.
• Wash hands often to prevent spread of any germs.

WHAT TO EXPECT

DIAGNOSTIC MEASURES
• Your own observation of the symptoms. Call your health care provider if you have concerns

about the symptoms, or if you or a child has a chronic illness. Pregnant women should call their obstetric provider if they have been exposed or if they have any symptoms of the illness.
• Your health care provider will examine the appearance of the rash to diagnose the infection.
• In a few cases, a blood test is done to confirm the diagnosis.community.

APPROPRIATE HEALTH CARE—Home care is usually all that is needed for treatment.

POSSIBLE COMPLICATIONS
• None expected in most cases. In patients with disorders such as sickle-cell anemia or a weak immune (body's germ-fighting) system, the illness can cause a serious anemic reaction.
• In pregnant women there is a small risk of miscarriage if the infection occurs during the first 20 weeks of pregnancy. There is no evidence that it causes birth defects.

PROBABLE OUTCOME—Complete recovery. The rash usually clears in 10 days to 2 weeks. Once you have had the infection, you are immune (you cannot get it again).

HOW TO TREAT

GENERAL MEASURES
• For home care, use Aveeno (an oatmeal bath product) for a cool, soaking bath. This can help with the itching.
• The rash may become redder, or it may come back again after it seemed to clear up, after spending time in the sun, taking a warm bath, getting excited, or exercising. This is no cause for concern.

MEDICATION
• There are no drugs for treating the illness. You may use acetaminophen for fever. Don't give a child younger than 18 aspirin for fever.
• If the rash itches, use plain calamine lotion.
• Your health care provider may prescribe other drugs.

ACTIVITY—No limits needed. Get extra rest during the illness if you or your child feels tired.

DIET—No special diet. Drink plenty of fluids.

CALL YOUR DOCTOR IF

• If you or your child has symptoms of erythema infectiosum and you have concerns about the illness.
• Symptoms don't improve or worsen after home treatment.
• You are pregnant and have been exposed to erythema infectiosum.

ERYTHEMA MULTIFORME

GENERAL INFORMATION

DEFINITION—An inflammatory disorder of the skin and sometimes, the mucous membranes. The disorder is called erythema multiforme minor (80% of the cases) when only the skin is involved. It is called erythema multiforme major when the mucous membranes are also involved. More severe forms of the disorder are Stevens-Johnson syndrome and toxic epidermal necrolysis.

BODY PARTS INVOLVED—Skin and mucous membranes (thin, moist linings of body cavities).

SEX OR AGE MOST AFFECTED—Erythema multiforme affects children and teens, as well as adults of both sexes.

SIGNS & SYMPTOMS
• Rash spots that are red and evenly shaped. They often appear in rings like bull's-eyes.
• Rash usually appears on palms, soles, and other areas of arms and legs. It may spread to the face and the rest of the body.
• Rash is itchy, sometimes painful, or has a burning sensation.
• Rash develops into blisters, hives, or becomes ulcerated (open sores).
• With erythema multiforme major, the mucous membranes of the mouth, eyes, and genitals may become inflamed. Fever, headache, sore throat, or diarrhea may also occur.

CAUSES—It is thought to be an immune response. The most common cause is the herpes simplex virus (the same virus that causes cold sores). It is less often caused by drug reactions, cancer, radiation, other viruses, or bacteria. Sometimes, no cause is found.

RISK INCREASES WITH
• Previous history of erythema multiforme.
• Drugs such as sulfonamides, tetracyclines, barbiturates, metronidazole, nonsteroidal anti-inflammatories, oral contraceptives, pseudoephedrine, bupropion, and others. The reaction to the drug may not occur until days or weeks after first using it.
• Cancer.
• Radiation therapy.

HOW TO PREVENT—No specific prevention known except to avoid drugs that may be the cause. Drug therapy for herpes simplex virus outbreaks may be help prevent a recurrence.

WHAT TO EXPECT

DIAGNOSTIC MEASURES
• Your health care provider may diagnose the disorder by the appearance of the skin rash.
• A biopsy may be done (involves removing a small piece of the affected skin for viewing under a microscope). Blood tests may be done.

APPROPRIATE HEALTH CARE
• Self-care after diagnosis for mild cases.
• Treatment may involve drug therapy. In some cases, no treatment is needed. If a drug is the cause of the disorder, it will normally be discontinued.
• The more severe forms of the disorder may require hospital care.

POSSIBLE COMPLICATIONS
• May progress from the minor form to the major form of erythema multiforme.
• Recurrence of the disorder.

PROBABLE OUTCOME—Rash develops over 1 to 2 weeks. It usually clears up in 2 to 3 weeks, but it may take 5 to 6 weeks.

HOW TO TREAT

GENERAL MEASURES
• Wet dressings and soaks or lotions may help to soothe the skin. Bathing in lukewarm to cool water three times a day for 30 minutes is also helpful.
• If mouth sores are present, good oral hygiene is important to reduce risk of infection and to relieve discomfort.

MEDICATION
• Corticosteroids (topical or oral) may be prescribed to reduce inflammation and irritation.
• Antivirals may be prescribed to treat viral infection such as herpes simplex virus.
• Antibiotics will be prescribed for bacterial infection.
• If mouth sores are present, topical drugs or mouthwashes may be prescribed.
• If eyes are involved, eyewashes or other topical drugs may be prescribed.
• Pain remedies, sedatives, or antihistamines may be prescribed to help provide relief of symptoms.

ACTIVITY—As tolerated by your symptoms.

DIET
• Usually no special diet is needed.
• If mouth sores are present, a soft or liquid diet may be better tolerated.

CALL YOUR DOCTOR IF

• You or a family member has symptoms of erythema multiforme.
• Symptoms worsen during treatment.

ILLNESS & DISORDERS

ERYTHEMA NODOSUM

 GENERAL INFORMATION

DEFINITION—An inflammatory disorder of the skin and the tissue under the skin. It is not contagious. It usually affects the skin of the legs, especially areas over the large bone (shin bone) in the lower leg.

BODY PARTS INVOLVED—Skin of the legs, especially areas over the large bone in the lower leg. The disease occasionally involves the arms or other areas.

SEX OR AGE MOST AFFECTED—Both sexes and all ages, but more likely in females (ages 20 to 45).

SIGNS & SYMPTOMS
* An upper respiratory infection may precede the skin symptoms by 1 to 2 weeks. There may be a period of feeling generally unwell and fever. Joint aches may occur, especially of the knee.
* Red lumps (also called lesions or nodules) appear on the shins or about the knees or ankles. They vary in size from a cherry to a grapefruit. There may be 2 to 50 or more.
* The lumps are raised slightly above the skin. They are hot and painful. The color is bright red to start, then purple, and then fades to a bruise-like color.
* Other, smaller, red lumps may appear on the outer arms, face, and neck.
* Lumps continue to appear for about 10 days or more.
* Conjunctivitis (eye inflammation) may occur.Exact cause is unknown. Inflammation may be due to infection, use of certain drugs, or other factors.

RISK INCREASES WITH
* Drugs, such as birth-control pills (especially those high in estrogen), sulfonamides, iodides, and bromides.
* A preceding infection, including *Streptococcus* (most common), coccidioidomycosis, histoplasmosis, sarcoidosis, blastomycosis, tuberculosis, and *Yersinia* infections.
* Autoimmune disease.
* Chronic bowel inflammation.
* Dysproteinemia (involves protein in the blood).
* Eating foods with food dyes or preservatives.
* Cancer.
* Pregnancy.

HOW TO PREVENT—Remove or treat the cause if it can be identified.

 WHAT TO EXPECT

DIAGNOSTIC MEASURES
* Your health care provider can usually diagnose the disorder with an exam of the affected skin.
* Medical tests are not needed, but they may be done to diagnose an underlying disorder.

APPROPRIATE HEALTH CARE
* Erythema nodosum often heals on its own. Symptoms may be treated with drug therapy.
* Treatment may be provided for an underlying disorder. If a drug is the cause of the disorder, it will normally be discontinued.

POSSIBLE COMPLICATIONS
* None expected from erythema nodosum.
* Less than 20% of cases recur.
* Other complications can arise depending on the cause.

PROBABLE OUTCOME—Lumps diminish in size and tenderness and heal in about 3 to 6 weeks. Complete healing may take several months. It does not leave scars.

 HOW TO TREAT

GENERAL MEASURES—For self-care:
* Elevate the legs whenever possible.
* Use elastic wrap or support stockings.
* Soak the affected areas in water. Warm-water soaks are usually more soothing for pain or inflammation. Cool-water soaks feel better for itching.

MEDICATION
* For minor discomfort, use nonprescription drugs such as aspirin (not for children) or other nonsteroidal anti-inflammatory drugs.
* Potassium iodide may be prescribed.
* Corticosteroids may be prescribed in very severe cases.
* Topical drugs for the skin usually do not help.

ACTIVITY—Rest in bed as much as possible with the legs elevated. This may help prevent new lumps from developing. When symptoms improve, resume normal activity.

DIET—No special diet.

 CALL YOUR DOCTOR IF

* You or a family member has symptoms of erythema nodosum.
* Any new symptoms arise that you think may be due either to the disorder or the drugs prescribed.

ESOPHAGEAL STRICTURE

GENERAL INFORMATION

DEFINITION—Esophageal stricture is a narrowing of the tube (esophagus) that connects the throat to the stomach. The narrowing interferes with swallowing.

BODY PARTS INVOLVED—Esophagus.

SEX OR AGE MOST AFFECTED—Both sexes; all ages.

SIGNS & SYMPTOMS
* A gradual decrease in the ability to swallow. At first, it becomes difficult to swallow solid foods. Then it becomes difficult to swallow liquids.
* Uncomfortable feeling when swallowing.
* Food feels like it gets stuck in the throat.
* Stomach acid washing back into mouth.
* Vomiting (sometimes with mucus or blood).

CAUSES—Scarring of the lining of the esophagus. As the scar tissue builds up, it forms a ring that narrows the opening of the esophagus. The scarring most often results from excessive gastric acid in the stomach backing up (called reflux) into the esophagus. This causes repeated inflammation (esophagitis), which damages the lining of the esophagus. Other factors may also lead to scarring.

RISK INCREASES WITH
* Gastroesophageal reflux disease (GERD).
* Hiatal hernia (part of the stomach protrudes through the diaphragm).
* Prolonged use of feeding (nasogastric) tubes.
* Swallowing of corrosive (e.g., acid or lye) chemicals.
* Infections of the esophagus.
* Radiation injury to the esophagus.
* Injury from an endoscope (a tube-like device used to examine the internal organs).
* Cancer of the esophagus.

HOW TO PREVENT
* Get medical care for any problems that involve difficulty swallowing or acid reflux.
* Keep dangerous products out of child's reach.
* Don't swallow any substance that may harm the esophagus.

WHAT TO EXPECT

DIAGNOSTIC MEASURES
* Your own observation of symptoms.
* Your health care provider may do an endoscopy. This is a medical test using an instrument with a lighted tip (endoscope) that is inserted into the esophagus. A small amount of tissue may be removed for testing (biopsy) to make sure the stricture is benign. A special x-ray of the esophagus may be done.

APPROPRIATE HEALTH CARE
* Treatment will be provided for any underlying disorder, such as gastroesophageal reflux disease.
* Treatment for the stricture usually involves a medical procedure to widen (dilate) the esophagus. Different types of procedures are available. They are normally done with the patient sedated. Your health care provider will explain the options to you.
* Surgery to remove the stricture may be recommended, if other treatments fail.

POSSIBLE COMPLICATIONS
* Not able to eat and drink enough foods and fluids.
* Perforation (hole) in the damaged esophagus.
* Inflammation that may lead to internal bleeding.
* Stricture recurs after treatment.
* Aspiration, which is the passage of food or liquid through the vocal folds ("going down the wrong way"). The food, fluid, or vomit may enter the lungs.

PROBABLE OUTCOME—Treatment can help relieve the stricture, but treatment may need to be repeated.

HOW TO TREAT

GENERAL MEASURES
* Stop smoking. Smoking may make symptoms worse.
* See your dental care provider to be sure dentures and oral prostheses are fit well and are not loose.

MEDICATION—Drugs for reflux problems may be prescribed.

ACTIVITY—Usually no limits.

DIET
* Eat a soft or liquid diet after treatment, until normal swallowing is possible. Avoid spicy foods that irritate the esophagus.
* Don't drink alcohol.

CALL YOUR DOCTOR IF

* You or a family member has symptoms of esophageal stricture.
* The following occur during treatment:
  - Chest pain or fever.
  - Inability to speak.
  - Swallowing problems do not improve.

ESOPHAGUS CANCER

GENERAL INFORMATION

DEFINITION—A malignant (cancerous) tumor of the esophagus. This is the tube connecting the mouth to the stomach.

BODY PARTS INVOLVED—Esophagus.

SEX OR AGE MOST AFFECTED—This type of cancer usually affects adults over age 60 and both sexes, but is more common in men.

SIGNS & SYMPTOMS
* Early cancer does not usually cause symptoms.
* Swallowing difficulty that gradually gets worse.
* Pain when swallowing.
* Rapid weight loss.
* Chronic cough. May cough up blood
* Hoarseness.
* Feeling weak and tired.
* Vomiting.

CAUSES—Unknown. Risk factors for one type of cancer are due to smoking or alcohol use. Risk factors for a second type of cancer are due to esophageal conditions. Most esophagus cancers are primary (they begin there). Some are secondary (they spread from cancer elsewhere in the body).

RISK INCREASES WITH
* Ages over 60 and male.
* Smoking (including cigarettes, pipes, or cigars) or smokeless tobacco.
* Excess alcohol use.
* Barrett's esophagus (a precancerous condition).
* Previous esophagus, head, or neck cancer.
* Hiatal hernia.
* Esophageal stricture.
* Chronic gastric reflux (gastroesophageal reflux disease or GERD).

HOW TO PREVENT
* None specific. Try to reduce your risk factors.
* Don't smoke.
* Don't drink more than 1 or 2 alcoholic drinks, if any, a day.
* Obtain medical care for any gastrointestinal disorders.

WHAT TO EXPECT

DIAGNOSTIC MEASURES
* Your own observation of symptoms.
* Your health care provider will do a physical exam and ask questions about any symptoms.
* A number of medical tests will be done. The tests first help diagnose the cancer and then determine if it has spread (staging).

APPROPRIATE HEALTH CARE
* Treatment may include chemotherapy (anticancer drugs) and/or radiation therapy, surgery, and biologic therapy.
* Chemotherapy uses drugs and radiation therapy uses radiation to attack the cancer cells. Biologic therapy uses the body's immune system to fight cancer.
* Surgery may be performed to remove the tumor if the cancer has not spread in the body. Procedures may be done to allow passage of food and liquids.
* Treatment may involve steps to relieve symptoms and make you comfortable, rather than treating the cancer.
* Counseling may help you cope with having cancer.

POSSIBLE COMPLICATIONS—If treatment is delayed, esophagus cancer can spread rapidly to the lungs, liver, brain, and bones.

PROBABLE OUTCOME
* Recovery improves if diagnosed at an early stage. The diagnosis often comes too late for effective treatment. However, symptoms can be relieved or controlled.
* Research into causes and treatment continues. There is hope for improved treatment and cure.cure.

HOW TO TREAT

GENERAL MEASURES
* Stop smoking or the use of any tobacco product.
* To learn more: American Cancer Society, (800) ACS-2345; website: www.cancer.org; or National Cancer Institute, (800) 4-CANCER; website: www.nci.nih.gov.

MEDICATION—You may be prescribed:
* Pain relievers.
* Drugs to reduce anxiety.
* Chemotherapy (anticancer drugs).
* Anticholinergics or calcium-channel blockers for esophageal spasms.

ACTIVITY—Remain as active as possible.

DIET—Soft to liquid. Prior to surgery, special nutritional support may be required (such as a feeding tube).

CALL YOUR DOCTOR IF

* You or a family member has symptoms of cancer of the esophagus, especially difficulty swallowing.
* Pain or symptoms get worse despite treatment.

ESSENTIAL TREMOR

 GENERAL INFORMATION

DEFINITION—Essential tremor is one type of movement disorder. Movement disorders affect the ability to produce and control movement. Parkinson's disease is a different type of movement disorder.

BODY PARTS INVOLVED—Nervous system.

SEX OR AGE MOST AFFECTED—It is a common problem in people aged 60 and older. Men and women are affected equally.

SIGNS & SYMPTOMS
* The main symptom is tremor, which is a trembling or an up-and-down movement of the hands. The tremor may be noticed when doing simple tasks such as holding a glass of water. The tremor may occur in the arms, head, and voice. Rarely, it affects the trunk and legs.
* Walking in an unsteady manner.
* The symptoms start on a gradual basis, usually in mid-to-late life. In a few cases, symptoms begin in childhood, go away for many years, and then start up again.
* Being tired, feeling anxious, or being in hot climates can make the symptoms worse.
* Symptoms usually disappear when you sleep or rest.

CAUSES
* In about half of the cases, the cause is genetic. The genes were passed on by your parents. Familial tremor is the term used when it affects more than one person in a family.
* In the other half of the cases, the cause is unknown.

RISK INCREASES WITH
* Family history of essential tremor.
* Age. Most often, the disorder occurs in older people.

HOW TO PREVENT—None known.

 WHAT TO EXPECT

DIAGNOSTIC MEASURES
* Your own observation of symptoms.
* Your health care provider will do a physical exam, and ask questions about your symptoms and your activities.
* You may be asked to write, drink from a glass, or hold a piece of paper so that the tremor can be observed.
* There are a variety of medical problems that can involve similar symptoms. Medical tests on blood and urine are usually done to rule out other disorders.

APPROPRIATE HEALTH CARE
* Treatment may not be needed if the symptoms are mild and are not causing other problems.
* Treatment steps may include special exercises using weights for your hands and arms. These will be taught to you by a physical therapist. You can then continue doing them at home.
* Counseling may help if you are having emotional problems in coping with the changes in your life brought on by the symptoms.
* Surgery is rare, but may help if symptoms are severe.

POSSIBLE COMPLICATIONS
* The tremor makes it difficult to do everyday tasks in the home, perform hobbies, or other activities you may enjoy.
* Tremor may cause difficulty in performing your job.
* Feeling embarrassed about the tremor may lead to an avoidance of social activities.

PROBABLE OUTCOME
* In many people, the disorder may not get worse and the tremor may be mild throughout life.
* Others may have symptoms that get worse as they get older. There are treatments that can help relieve the symptoms.

 HOW TO TREAT

GENERAL MEASURES
* Joining a support group may help some people. Ask your health care provider about groups in your area.
* To learn more: We Move, 204 West 84th St., New York, NY, 10024; (800) 437-MOV2; website: www.wemove.org.

MEDICATION—There are several different classes of drugs that are used to treat tremors. Your health care provider will discuss the options with you and decide if they are appropriate.

ACTIVITY—Try to maintain an active lifestyle. Exercise each day to the extent possible.

DIET
* Avoid caffeine in coffee, tea, and soft drinks. It may make the symptoms worse.
* Avoid alcohol, or use it on a limited basis. It may help the tremors short term, but it is not wise to use it as a form of treatment.

 CALL YOUR DOCTOR IF

* You or a family member has symptoms of essential tremor.
* Symptoms get worse despite treatment.

EXOPHTHALMOS
(Proptosis)

GENERAL INFORMATION

DEFINITION—A protrusion or bulging of one or both eyes.

BODY PARTS INVOLVED—Eyes.

SEX OR AGE MOST AFFECTED—Both sexes; all ages. Females are more likely to have the type caused by thyroid problem.

SIGNS & SYMPTOMS
* Reduced eye movements causing double vision.
* Bulging eyes, which creates a staring or frightened look.
* Eyelids may not be able to close completely.
* Strabismus (crossed eyes).
* Gritty, dry feeling in the eye.

CAUSES—Inflammation of tissue (primarily the muscles) behind the eye. Inflammation can be caused by a variety of disorders that affect the eye and disorders that affect the body. In adults, an overactive thyroid gland is the most common cause. In children, it is often due to infection. A tumor or abnormal blood vessels behind the eye could push it forward also.

RISK INCREASES WITH
* Grave's disease (overactive thyroid gland).
* Bacterial infection (cellulitis).
* Tumor.
* Sinus disease.
* Aneurysm, blood clot or hemorrhage in the veins or arteries behind the eye.
* Vascular disease (such as Wegener's granulomatosis).
* Injury to the eye or face.

HOW TO PREVENT—There is no sure way to prevent the disorder. To reduce risk, get medical treatment for any possible underlying disorder and protect eyes from injury where appropriate.

WHAT TO EXPECT

DIAGNOSTIC MEASURES
* Your own observation of symptoms.
* Your eye care provider will do an exam of the eyes. A device called an exophthalmometer can be used to measure the protrusion.
* Medical tests may include thyroid function studies and other blood studies, and culture of nasal fluid. Imaging studies may include CT, MRI, or ultrasound (see Glossary for these tests).

APPROPRIATE HEALTH CARE
* Medical care will be directed at the cause of the disorder. This may involve drug therapy, surgery, and possibly, radiation therapy.
* Surgery may involve:
  - The thyroid gland.
  - Removing a tumor.
  - Returning the eyes to their normal position, if necessary, after the underlying cause is corrected.

POSSIBLE COMPLICATIONS—Effects on vision and appearance may be long term or permanent.

PROBABLE OUTCOME—Vision and appearance may return to normal with treatment of the underlying cause. In some cases, even with successful treatment of the cause, the bulging will remain.

HOW TO TREAT

GENERAL MEASURES
* If your vision is affected, don't drive or engage in dangerous activity.
* If eyelids don't blink properly, wear goggles to protect them from wind or dust.

MEDICATION
* Use nonprescription, lubricating eye drops or ointment to keep the eyes moistened.
* You may be prescribed drugs to treat the underlying cause, such as:
  - Antithyroid drugs for hyperthyroidism.
  - Antibiotics for infection.
  - Cortisone drugs to reduce inflammation.

ACTIVITY—No limits (unless vision is affected).

DIET—No special diet.

CALL YOUR DOCTOR IF

* You or a family member has symptoms of exophthalmos.
* Symptoms don't improve after treatment begins.

EXTRADURAL HEMORRHAGE
(Epidural Hemorrhage)

 GENERAL INFORMATION

DEFINITION—Bleeding between the skull and the outermost of 3 membranes that cover the brain (meninges). This disorder may be confused with meningitis. A hematoma (collection of clotted blood) forms and rapidly enlarges, increasing pressure within the skull and causing symptoms.

BODY PARTS INVOLVED—Skull; meninges; brain.

SEX OR AGE MOST AFFECTED—Both sexes, but more common in males and all ages, but rare in ages under two or over 60.

SIGNS & SYMPTOMS—These symptoms develop within 24 to 96 hours after a head injury:
* Headache that steadily worsens.
* Drowsiness or unconsciousness.
* Nausea or vomiting.
* Inability to move arms and legs.
* Seizures.
* Change in the size of eye pupils.
* Unable to control bladder or bowels.

CAUSES—Head injury.

RISK INCREASES WITH
* Use of anticoagulant drugs.
* Bleeding disorders, such as hemophilia, ITT or aplastic anemia.
* Injuries. These occur more often after excess alcohol consumption or use of mind-altering drugs.

HOW TO PREVENT—To reduce risk, avoid head injury:
* Use seat belts in motor vehicles.
* Wear protective head gear during contact sports or while riding a bicycle or motorcycle.
* Don't drink alcohol or use mind-altering drugs and drive.
* Seek medical advice for even a moderate blow to the head.

 WHAT TO EXPECT

DIAGNOSTIC MEASURES
* Your own observation of symptoms.
* Your health care provider will do a physical exam.
* Medical tests may include studies of blood and cerebrospinal fluid, x-rays of the head, arteriography, radioscopic scan, CT scan, and other tests as needed to check for complications.

APPROPRIATE HEALTH CARE
* Extradural hemorrhage is an emergency that requires rapid treatment to prevent permanent brain damage or death. Treatment will depend on the extent of the injury. Surgical treatment consists of drilling a hole in the skull, draining the blood clot and clipping the ruptured blood vessel.
* Home-care after surgery.

POSSIBLE COMPLICATIONS
* Brain damage or death.
* Seizures (may develop 1 to 3 months later).
* Postconcussion syndrome (headaches, dizziness, vertigo, fatigue, emotional problems, unable to concentrate, and restlessness).
* Ongoing nerve pain and incontinence.

PROBABLE OUTCOME—Outcome will depend on the extent of the injury, the quickness of treatment, and the age and health of the patient.

 HOW TO TREAT

GENERAL MEASURES—The family should maintain an optimistic outlook, stay in close contact with the patient's health care providers and help by making their visits with the patient as supportive as possible.

MEDICATION—You may be prescribed drugs to:
* Reduce swelling inside the skull.
* Treat the nausea and vomiting.
* Prevent seizures.
* Control fever.
* Prevent gastric ulcers.
* Treat bleeding problems and prevent blood clots.

ACTIVITY—Bed rest at first, then a gradual return to normal activity. You may need physical, occupational, or speech therapy.

DIET—Feeding through a vein (IV) may be needed while being treated.

 CALL YOUR DOCTOR IF

* You or a family member has had a head injury (even if it seems minor) and you develop any symptoms of extradural hemorrhage.
* The following occurs during treatment:
  - Fever.
  - Surgical wound becomes red, swollen or tender.
  - Headache worsens or other symptoms develop.

EYE CONTUSION OR LACERATION

GENERAL INFORMATION

DEFINITION—Eye injury, including blunt injury (contusion) or cut (laceration).

BODY PARTS INVOLVED—Eyeball; eyelid; bones around the eyeball (eye socket); muscles attached to the eyeball.

SEX OR AGE MOST AFFECTED—Both sexes; all ages.

SIGNS & SYMPTOMS
* Swelling, redness, tenderness, pain, bleeding, or bruising ("black eye") in or around the eye. A black eye may take 1 to 2 days to develop.
* Change in ability to see clearly.

CAUSES—A blunt or sharp blow or cut to the eye or the area around the eye.

RISK INCREASES WITH
* Doing work that may risk injury to the eyes. This includes bartending (opening bottles), carpentry, or construction work.
* Paintball, BB guns, rifles, or slingshot usage.
* Sports such as baseball, softball, basketball, soccer, football, or hockey.
* Using a rotary lawn mower.
* Fist fights. Eye injuries may occur in fights. Fights are more likely with alcohol use.

HOW TO PREVENT—When possible, wear appropriate eye protection for any activity that may lead to eye injury. This can include eye coverings or face shields.

WHAT TO EXPECT

DIAGNOSTIC MEASURES
* For most eye injuries, or if you are unsure if it is serious, see your health care provider. If you have any blurred vision, you must see a health care provider. Seek emergency care if the injury is severe.
* Your health care provider can diagnose the problem with an exam of the injured eye area.

APPROPRIATE HEALTH CARE—Treatment may involve stitches to repair cuts, or other surgical procedure.

POSSIBLE COMPLICATIONS
* Permanent vision loss.
* Infection.
* Cataract.

PROBABLE OUTCOME—Some injuries are mild and heal on their own. Others are usually curable with treatment. Allow at least 2 weeks for complete healing.

HOW TO TREAT

GENERAL MEASURES
* For a minor contusion (black eye) during the first 24 hours, use ice packs to reduce swelling. The next day, make a warm compress by folding a clean cloth in several layers. Dip in warm water, wring out slightly, and put on the eye. Dip the compress often to keep it moist. Apply compress for an hour, rest an hour, and repeat.
* For a minor cut or scrape around the eye, apply pressure to stop any bleeding. Use a clean cloth to clean the wound. Cover with a bandage if a cut or scrape is large.
* Sleep with the head raised with two pillows until symptoms get better.
* Protect eyes from bright light or sunlight by wearing dark glasses until healing is complete.

MEDICATION
* Antibiotic eye-drops to prevent infection may be prescribed.
* Use acetaminophen or ibuprofen for pain relief.
* Eye-drops, to dilate (enlarge) the eye pupil and rest the eye muscles, may be prescribed.

ACTIVITY—For minor injury, resume normal activities after healing. For other injuries, your health care provider will give you specific advice about sports and work activities.

DIET—No special diet.

CALL YOUR DOCTOR IF

* You have a cut or other eye injury. This may be an emergency.
* The following occur after eye injury: fever, vision changes, or eye pain that persists after treatment.

EYE, FOREIGN BODY IN

 GENERAL INFORMATION

DEFINITION—A small speck of metal, wood, stone, sand, paint, an eyelash, or other foreign material in the eye.

BODY PARTS INVOLVED—Eye, usually the conjunctiva (outer eye covering).

SEX OR AGE MOST AFFECTED—Both sexes; all ages.

SIGNS & SYMPTOMS
• Pain, irritation, watering, and redness in the eye.
• Eye is sensitive to light.
• Foreign body (object) that can be seen when the eye is examined. Sometimes the object is very small, trapped under the eyelid, and cannot be seen except with a medical exam.
• Scratchy feeling when blinking.

CAUSES—Accident.

RISK INCREASES WITH
• Windy weather.
• Jobs or activity, such as carpentry or grinding, in which fine pieces of wood or other materials fly loose in the air.

HOW TO PREVENT—Wear protective eye coverings if your job or hobby involves the risk of eye injury.

 WHAT TO EXPECT

DIAGNOSTIC MEASURES
• Your own observation of symptoms.
• Most eye injuries should be seen by your health care provider. Ask someone else to drive you to the medical office or emergency center. Don't try to drive yourself. Keep the eye closed, if possible, until the exam.
• Your health care provider will do an exam of the injured eye. It may include staining the eye with a harmless substance to outline the object, examining the eye through a magnifying lens, and/or use of a special ultraviolet light.

APPROPRIATE HEALTH CARE
• The procedure to remove the object will be determined by its size and location within the eye.
• An eye patch may be applied to keep the eye closed.
• A follow-up exam should be done in 1 to 2 days.

POSSIBLE COMPLICATIONS
• Infection, especially if the object is not removed completely.
• Permanent vision damage.

PROBABLE OUTCOME—Most objects can be removed simply with self-care, in a health care provider's office, or emergency room.

 HOW TO TREAT

GENERAL MEASURES
• For small foreign bodies, be sure not to rub the eye. Try to flush the eye using one of these options:
  - Gently pour warm (not hot) water from a pitcher over the eye. Keep eye open.
  - Stand at a sink with warm water running and cup your hands and put your face in the running water.
  - Use an eye dropper with warm water.
  - If outside, use a garden hose, but don't use high pressure. A water fountain may also be used to flush out the eye.
  - Check the eye often to see if the object is gone.
  - If flushing is not working, you may consider trying to remove the object with the tip of a tissue or cotton-tipped swab. Lift upper or lower eyelid (someone else may need to help you). Be extremely careful to not touch the eye itself with the swab. You could injure the cornea.
• If you removed the object, but it was large, or the patient is a child, then a health care provider should be seen for a follow-up check.
• Use moist compresses to relieve discomfort after removal of particle. Prepare by folding a clean cloth in several layers. Dip in warm water, wring out slightly and apply to the eye. Dip the compress often to keep it moist. Do this for 1 hour, rest 1 hour, and then repeat.

MEDICATION
• Antibiotic eye-drops may be prescribed to prevent infection.
• Pain relievers may be prescribed.

ACTIVITY—Resume your normal activities gradually after removal of the foreign body and the patch, if one is applied.

DIET—No special diet.

 CALL YOUR DOCTOR IF

• You or a family member has a foreign body in the eye that you are concerned about. If it is an emergency, call 911 to get emergency help right away.
• The following occur after removal:
  - Pain increases or does not disappear in 2 days.
  - Fever develops.
  - Vision changes.

FAILURE TO THRIVE

 GENERAL INFORMATION

DEFINITION—Failure of infants or young children to grow and develop normally. Failure to thrive is actually a group of symptoms, rather than a specific disorder. It has many possible causes.

BODY PARTS INVOLVED—All.

SEX OR AGE MOST AFFECTED—Children under 5, usually infants, ages 3-6 months.

SIGNS & SYMPTOMS
* Height and weight do not progress normally, as measured on standard growth charts.
* Physical skills may be slow to develop. This includes rolling over, sitting, crawling, standing, or walking.
* Mental and social skills may be delayed, such as talking, social interaction, or self-feeding.
* Child lacks energy, has small muscles, rash or other skin changes, swollen arms or legs, and changes in hair.
* Other symptoms (they may be due to a medical condition).

CAUSES—It may be due to medical conditions (sometimes called organic failure). It may involve psychosocial and environmental causes, such as family concerns or problems in the home (sometimes called nonorganic failure). It may also be a combination of the two.

RISK INCREASES WITH
* Pregnancy problems (such as alcohol use or intrauterine growth restriction) or premature infants or children with chromosomal abnormalities.
* Children who have trouble eating, are unable to suck, have vomiting or reflux problems, or have infections.
* Children who are unable to absorb nutrients or need extra nutrients, due to certain medical disorders.
* Children with chronic illness (cystic fibrosis, asthma).
* Child neglect, abuse, or lack of attention by parents.
* Child is not provided enough food or refuses to eat, or problems with weaning a child.
* Parents who lack parenting skills.
* Dysfunctional family, difficult parent-child interactions, or lack of support (family/friends).
* Depression, alcohol or drug abuse in a parent.
* Poverty of parents (can't provide needed foods).

HOW TO PREVENT
* Learn about proper nutrition for a new baby.
* Take your child regularly to "well-baby" checkups.
* Arrange for parenting classes if you are new parents.

 WHAT TO EXPECT

DIAGNOSTIC MEASURES
* Your own observation of symptoms.
* Your child's health care provider will do a physical exam. The child's height and weight will be compared to standard growth charts to determine if there is delayed growth.
* Medical tests may include blood and urine studies. To help pinpoint a cause for growth delay, questions may be asked about the pregnancy and birth, the child's behavior and eating habits, other family members, stress problems, and other concerns.

APPROPRIATE HEALTH CARE
* Treatment will depend on the cause. Organic causes may be treated medically. Nonorganic causes may be treated with counseling, education, and other help for the parents. The main goal of any treatment is to be sure your child has the proper nutrition.
* Hospital care may be needed in some cases.
* Home visits from a nurse may be prescribed.
* If child neglect or abuse is suspected, child protective services or other authorities may become involved.

POSSIBLE COMPLICATIONS—Ongoing mental, emotional, and physical delays.

PROBABLE OUTCOME—If the problem is short-term and the cause can be corrected, normal growth and development may resume. Recovery may take several months. In other cases, the outcome depends on the cause.

 HOW TO TREAT

GENERAL MEASURES—Community programs that help mothers and children are available. Other help can be provided to get financial aid (such as food stamps), medical benefits, parenting classes, or counseling for emotional problems.

MEDICATION—Drugs are not usually needed.

ACTIVITY—No limits.

DIET
* Diet changes may include special formulas for infants, high-calorie foods for older children, and high-energy shakes. Instructions will be provided. Be sure to follow them carefully.
* Tube feedings may be needed for severe cases. These can often be done at home.

 CALL YOUR DOCTOR IF

* You are concerned that your child is not developing properly or growing as expected.
* Symptoms continue despite treatment.

FAINTING
(Syncope)

GENERAL INFORMATION

DEFINITION—A sudden, temporary loss of consciousness due to a decrease in the supply of blood and oxygen to the brain. Fainting may be a symptom of a health problem or a one-time event. Syncope is the medical term for fainting.

BODY PARTS INVOLVED—Circulatory system (heart and blood vessels); brain.

SEX OR AGE MOST AFFECTED—Both sexes; all ages.

SIGNS & SYMPTOMS
- Paleness and sweating.
- Sudden light-headedness.
- General weakness, followed by a fall.
- Blurred vision (sometimes).
- Nausea (sometimes).
- Rapid heartbeat and rapid breathing.

CAUSES
- The heart can not pump enough blood for the body to function properly. This occurs with heart disease and blood vessel disorders.
- The blood volume (amount of blood) is low. This can be due to bleeding or dehydration.
- Stimulation of the vagus nerve (in the neck, chest, and intestine) may slow the heart. This can happen with pain, fear, distress, vomiting, a large bowel movement and even urinating.
- Blood flow back to the heart is reduced. This occurs with straining when coughing, passing a stool, or in older men when trying to urinate (called micturition).
- Standing up or sitting down too quickly causes a sudden change in blood pressure. This is called orthostatic hypotension. Standing for long periods on a hot day can cause a similar problem due to lack of leg muscle use.
- Very rapid breathing or hyperventilating due to anxiety. Too much carbon dioxide is exhaled which then causes blood vessels in the brain to narrow.
- Other causes may be due to stroke, anemia, low blood sugar, lung problems, and others.
- In some cases, the cause of fainting is unknown.

RISK INCREASES WITH
- Heart disease or other chronic disorders.
- Certain drugs, such as those that slow the heartbeat.
- Being elderly.

HOW TO PREVENT
- Often, fainting can not be prevented. If you feel faint, lie down with feet up or sit in a chair and bend over.
- Avoid the problems that can cause fainting if possible. Try not to get overly anxious. Get treatment for any medical disorder and avoid constipation. Men can urinate while sitting down if standing causes fainting. Avoid sudden changes in physical activity, such as when getting up from a chair or bed (move slowly).

WHAT TO EXPECT

DIAGNOSTIC MEASURES
- See your health care provider after any fainting event. A physical exam may be done and questions asked about your symptoms and activities.
- Medical tests may include an ECG (electrocardiogram). It measures the electrical activity of the heart. Other tests may be done depending on the results of the ECG, or if other health disorders are suspected.

APPROPRIATE HEALTH CARE
- Sometimes, no treatment is needed.
- In some cases, treatment may be prescribed for a diagnosed problem. Rarely, a patient may need hospital care during recovery.

POSSIBLE COMPLICATIONS
- Injury while fainting, such as from a fall.
- Complications caused by a disorder that lead to the fainting.
- Recurrent fainting can have a major impact on a person's lifestyle. It may prevent driving a motor vehicle.

PROBABLE OUTCOME—A person will recover from simple fainting in 1 or 2 minutes. There are normally no long-term effects.

HOW TO TREAT

GENERAL MEASURES—If you are subject to frequent fainting spells, avoid activities in which fainting may endanger your life or others. This includes climbing ladders, driving motor vehicles, or operating dangerous machinery. Take measures to make your home safe in case you fall during a fainting event.

MEDICATION—Drugs are usually not needed for fainting. They may be prescribed for a health problem that is diagnosed.

ACTIVITY—You can usually resume normal activities right away unless advised differently by your health care provider.

DIET—No special diet. Drink adequate fluids. Avoid alcohol.

CALL YOUR DOCTOR IF

You or a family member has a fainting event even if it seems mild. Fainting may be a symptom of a disorder that requires treatment.

FATTY LIVER
(Steatosis)

GENERAL INFORMATION

DEFINITION—The liver is one of the largest organs in the body and has many functions. Fatty liver is a build-up of fat in the liver cells. Alcohol-related fatty liver occurs in alcohol drinkers. Nonalcoholic fatty liver disease (NAFLD) occurs in people who seldom or never drink alcohol. Fat in the liver may cause no problems by itself. In some cases, it may be a sign of more serious problems.

BODY PARTS INVOLVED—Liver.

SEX OR AGE MOST AFFECTED—Both sexes; all ages.

SIGNS & SYMPTOMS
* Usually there are no symptoms. The fatty liver condition is often discovered during a routine physical exam, or when medical tests are done for other reasons.
* There may be some pain or tenderness in the upper-right abdomen, behind the ribs. This is where the liver is located.
* Feeling tired.
* Jaundice (yellow skin and eyes).

CAUSES—It is not known what causes fat to build-up in the liver. It is known that fat increases in the liver with a number of conditions or disorders. Eating fatty foods does not cause fatty liver.

RISK INCREASES WITH
* Heavy use of alcohol.
* Obesity.
* Diabetes.
* Use of certain drugs.
* Metabolic syndrome (a group of health problems).
* Malnutrition (poor diet).
* High triglycerides (high fat levels in the blood).
* Intestinal bypass surgery for obesity.
* Tuberculosis.
* Pregnancy. It is a rare complication.
* Other uncommon diseases and some poisons.

HOW TO PREVENT
* There are no specific preventive measures.
* Avoid alcohol.
* Eat a healthy diet. Maintain ideal body weight.
* Pregnant women get good prenatal care.

WHAT TO EXPECT

DIAGNOSTIC MEASURES
* Your health care provider will ask about alcohol and drug use, and do a physical exam. An enlarged liver can often be felt with fingertips during the exam.

* Blood tests are done to check liver function. Other tests, including a liver biopsy, can confirm fatty liver. In a biopsy, a long needle is used to remove a small bit of liver tissue for viewing with a microscope.

APPROPRIATE HEALTH CARE
* Simple fatty liver may require no treatment.
* Treatment of any medical condition and lifestyle changes will normally reverse fatty liver.
* Treatment of diabetes includes diet, drugs, or insulin.
* If a pregnancy is far enough along, the recommended treatment is delivery.

POSSIBLE COMPLICATIONS
* Inflammation of the liver. This is called alcoholic steatohepatitis or nonalcoholic steatohepatitis (NASH).
* Other types of liver problems.
* If untreated in a pregnant woman, it can be life-threatening for the mother and the fetus.

PROBABLE OUTCOME
* Fatty liver can be partially reversed when the underlying cause is treated or removed.
* In pregnancy, it usually resolves after delivery.

HOW TO TREAT

GENERAL MEASURES
* Stop drinking alcohol. For help, join a local support group such as Alcoholics Anonymous.
* To learn more: American Liver Foundation, 75 Maiden Lane, Suite 603, New York, NY 10038; (800) 443-7872; website: www.liverfoundation.com.

MEDICATION
* Drugs to treat fatty liver are being studied.
* Drugs may be prescribed for specific disorders.
* Certain drugs may be stopped if they are a risk factor.
* Weight loss drugs may be used for a short time.
* Vitamin and mineral supplements may be prescribed.

ACTIVITY—Start a daily exercise routine, such as walking.

DIET
* Eat a healthy diet (fruits, vegetables, and fiber), low in calories and low in cholesterol.
* Start a weight-loss diet if obesity is a problem.

CALL YOUR DOCTOR IF

* You or a family member has symptoms of fatty liver.
* You need information about diet or exercise.

FEBRILE SEIZURE

 GENERAL INFORMATION

DEFINITION—A febrile seizure is a convulsion that occurs with a fever in infants or small children. The fever may be from many causes, such as a cold or ear infection. Febrile seizures are common in young children. For many children, a febrile seizure occurs just one time. About one-third of the children will have recurrent febrile seizures. Few children have more than three.

BODY PARTS INVOLVED—Nervous system, circulatory system (heart and blood vessels), and musculoskeletal system.

SEX OR AGE MOST AFFECTED—Both sexes; infants and young children.

SIGNS & SYMPTOMS
- Repeated rhythmic jerking or stiffening of your child's arms and legs. The child may cry out initially.
- Eyes rolled back in the child's head.
- Lack of consciousness.
- Twitches in only a part of the body, such as an arm or a leg, or only on the right or left side.
- Usually occur on the first day of a fever. Parents may not even know the child is ill.
- Rectal temperature higher than 102°F (38.9°C).
- *Simple febrile seizure* stops by itself within a few seconds to 10 minutes. *Complex febrile seizure* lasts longer than 15 minutes, occurs in one part of the body, or recurs during the same illness.
- Confused or drowsy after a seizure.

CAUSES—Exact cause is unknown. The high fever, and possibly one that rises quickly, may trigger a brain disturbance.

RISK INCREASES WITH
- Children ages 6 months to 6 years.
- Slightly more common in boys than girls.
- Very high fever or a rapidly rising temperature.
- History of febrile seizures in other family members.
- Rarely, fever and seizure occurs after a vaccination.
- Risk factors for recurrent seizures include:
  - Young age (less than 15 months) for the first seizure.
  - Family members with a history of febrile seizures.
  - Fever was below 102°F (38.9°C) at time of first seizure.

HOW TO PREVENT
- None for a first febrile seizure. There is no way to know for sure if a child is at risk.
- Drugs to reduce fever may help reduce risk.
- Certain children with recurrent febrile seizures are sometimes given preventive drugs.

 WHAT TO EXPECT

DIAGNOSTIC MEASURES
- Medical care may include emergency room treatment or seeing your child's health care provider. Either way, your child will be examined and questions asked about the seizure symptoms.
- Medical tests may be done to be sure there is not a more serious illness causing the fever.

APPROPRIATE HEALTH CARE
- Sometimes, no treatment is needed.
- Reassurance to parents about the benign nature (not serious) of the seizure should help ease concerns.

POSSIBLE COMPLICATIONS
- Injury may result from bumping or falling into objects.
- There is a very small risk that certain children who have febrile seizures will develop epilepsy.

PROBABLE OUTCOME
- Outcome is usually excellent, with no lasting effects.
- Child will not be aware of having the seizure.
- Most children who have febrile seizures will outgrow them by four to five years of age.
- Febrile seizures do not cause brain damage.

 HOW TO TREAT

GENERAL MEASURES—If a febrile seizure recurs, follow these instructions:
- Stay calm!
- Do not put anything in your child's mouth.
- Place your child on his/her side to help drain saliva from the mouth. Don't try to hold your child still.
- Loosen clothing.
- Move objects away from child to avoid injury.
- Support child's head with a pillow or other soft object.

MEDICATION
- Drugs may be prescribed for any infection.
- In rare cases, drugs may be prescribed to help prevent future febrile seizures.
- Give acetaminophen or ibuprofen at the first sign of fever. Don't give aspirin to children under age 18.

ACTIVITY—Rest or sleep after a seizure.

DIET—No special diet.

 CALL YOUR DOCTOR IF

- Your child has another febrile seizure.
- A febrile seizure lasts more than 15 minutes.
- Your child has symptoms that cause concern.

FECAL IMPACTION

 GENERAL INFORMATION

DEFINITION—A large, firm amount of stool that cannot be passed voluntarily. In most cases, the impacted stool is in the rectum, which is the lowest end of the bowels. Sometimes, the impaction may extend further up into the bowels.

BODY PARTS INVOLVED—Lower colon; rectum.

SEX OR AGE MOST AFFECTED—Both sexes; all ages.

SIGNS & SYMPTOMS
* Lack of normal bowel movements.
* Sense of fullness in the rectum, but unable to pass stool.
* Pain or cramps in the stomach or abdomen area (often after meals).
* Thin, watery discharge from the rectum.
* Headache, nausea, vomiting, loss of appetite.
* General sick feeling.

CAUSES—Irregular bowel function causes dry, hardened feces to remain in the colon or rectum.

RISK INCREASES WITH
* Long term constipation.
* Rectal disorders that make normal bowel movements uncomfortable, such as painful hemorrhoids or fissures.
* Rectal or colon cancer.
* Swallowing substance for x-rays of the intestinal tract.
* Nerve problems in the colon or rectum, as with a spinal-cord injury, stroke, Parkinson's disease, or multiple sclerosis.
* Being elderly or bedridden (such as after surgery).
* Disorders such as hypothyroidism or hypercalcemia.
* Use of some drugs, such as narcotic pain remedies.

HOW TO PREVENT
* Increase the fiber in the diet. Drink adequate amounts of fluid each day. Begin a program of regular exercise.
* Set aside a regular time each day for bowel movement (within an hour after breakfast is best). Don't try to hurry. Sit at least 10 minutes.
* If mild constipation develops, use a stool softener or a suppository.

 WHAT TO EXPECT

DIAGNOSTIC MEASURES
* Your own observation of symptoms.
* Your health care provider will do an exam of the abdomen area and a digital rectal exam. The rectal exam is done with a gloved finger inserted into the rectum.
* Medical tests such as x-ray and others may be done to confirm the diagnosis and check for complications.

APPROPRIATE HEALTH CARE—The impacted mass may be removed partially by your health care provider. This is done as with the rectal exam. A gloved finger (sometimes two) is inserted into the rectum and the mass is broken up. The rest of the stool may be removed with the use of a suppository. In some cases, water irrigation with a special instrument inserted into the rectum is used.

POSSIBLE COMPLICATIONS
* Injury to the rectum.
* If the impaction is not removed, the problem can worsen and surgery may be required.

PROBABLE OUTCOME—Usually curable with treatment. Impaction may recur, unless the underlying cause is removed.

 HOW TO TREAT

GENERAL MEASURES—See Constipation (in Illness section) for suggestions to improve bowel habits.

MEDICATION—After treatment, stool softeners may be prescribed.

ACTIVITY—No limits. Be as active as your health permits. Good physical fitness improves bowel function.

DIET
* Eat a normal, well-balanced diet that is high in fiber.
* Drink plenty of fluids each day.

 CALL YOUR DOCTOR IF

* You or a family member has symptoms of a fecal impaction.
* Your normal bowel pattern changes.

FEMALE ATHLETE TRIAD

GENERAL INFORMATION

DEFINITION—Female athlete triad is a result of three related conditions. It can occur in females of any age, or athletic skill level. An athlete may have one, two, or all three of these conditions that make up the triad:
- Disordered eating (harmful eating behavior) combined with excessive exercise.
- Menstrual periods stop (amenorrhea).
- Loss of bone density (osteoporosis).

BODY PARTS INVOLVED—Reproductive system, musculoskeletal system, and gastrointestinal system.

SEX OR AGE MOST AFFECTED—Females, usually early teens to late 20s.

SIGNS & SYMPTOMS
- Weight loss
- Fatigue (sometimes).
- Not having monthly periods or periods that are not regular.
- Young females may not start their first period.
- Stress fractures (bones break for no apparent reason).
- Injuries to muscles.
- Eating only small amounts of food. Also, may overeat (binge) and then throw up or use laxatives (purge).

CAUSES—Not eating enough food for the energy being spent. Muscles and bones soon start wearing down. Estrogen hormone levels decrease, causing problems with menstrual periods and loss of bone density.

RISK INCREASES WITH
- Compulsive exercising. Workouts become the most important part of life.
- Overly concerned with reaching goals.
- Pushed by coach(es) or parents to lose weight for improved performance.
- Stress (emotional as well as physical).
- Activities where low body weights and thin body shape seem to be important. These include track and field, swimming, rowing, cycling, basketball, body-building, ballet, and gymnastics.

HOW TO PREVENT
- Eat a healthy, well-balanced diet. Don't skip meals.
- Maintain a healthy body weight for height.
- Keep track of your menstrual periods.
- Do not over exercise or over train.
- Education on good eating and exercise habits.

WHAT TO EXPECT

DIAGNOSTIC MEASURES
- Your health care provider will do a physical exam. It may include a pelvic exam. You will be asked about your diet and any weight changes, your exercise and physical activity routines, and menstrual-cycle history.
- Medical tests may include blood and urine studies and a bone density test.

APPROPRIATE HEALTH CARE
- Treatment involves an increase in the amount of food you eat, weight gain, and sometimes reducing physical activity. Small changes may be all that is needed.
- Parents, along with trainers and coaches should be involved in treatment plans. This is important with adolescent (early teens) patients.
- Physical therapy and other therapies.
- Some may benefit from seeing a mental health provider for any stress or emotional problems.

POSSIBLE COMPLICATIONS
- A decrease in athletic performance.
- Permanent bone loss and risk of bone fractures.
- Serious medical problems (can be life-threatening).

PROBABLE OUTCOME—Outcome will vary for each athlete. With prompt diagnosis and early treatment, menstrual periods can return to normal, and further bone loss can be halted.

HOW TO TREAT

GENERAL MEASURES—The treatment steps are not easy and will take time, but female athletes need to make the changes to improve their overall health now and in the future.

MEDICATION
- Hormones may be prescribed to stop bone loss.
- Calcium and vitamin D may be recommended to help prevent more bone loss.

ACTIVITY—Try for a balance in activity levels that will still allow you to train, compete, and achieve your goals while not harming your health. Ask your health care provider and coach to help you make specific plans.

DIET—It is important to get adequate calories, protein and calcium, and eat foods you enjoy. Proper nutrition can enhance athletic performance. Consult an expert in nutrition to help you in making the right choices.

CALL YOUR DOCTOR IF

- You or a family member has symptoms of any of the conditions that make up the female athlete triad.
- Symptoms don't improve after a few months of treatment.

FERTILITY PROBLEMS IN MEN

GENERAL INFORMATION

DEFINITION—Infertility is the inability to achieve pregnancy after 1 year of sexual activity without contraception. Infertility occurs in 10% to 15% of all couples. Fertility depends on the production of normal quantities of healthy sperm, ability to achieve an erection, and ejaculation of sperm into the vagina during sexual intercourse. About 30% of infertility causes can be linked to male partners.

BODY PARTS INVOLVED—Genitals; endocrine system; brain.

SEX OR AGE MOST AFFECTED—Males after puberty.

SIGNS & SYMPTOMS—Failure to impregnate a fertile woman.

CAUSES
* Certain physical problems of the penis or testicles, such as undescended testicles.
* Excess alcohol use.
* Urinary-tract infection.
* Hormone problems.
* Endocrine disorders.
* Severe chronic or metabolic disorders (such as uremia or cirrhosis).
* Mumps.
* Use of some drugs, such as antihypertensives, cytotoxic drugs, male hormones, and MAO inhibitors.
* Sexually transmitted disease, such as syphilis and nonspecific urethritis that causes scarring.
* Injury to the genitals.
* Varicose veins in the testicles (varicocele).
* Emotional reasons, such as fear of infertility.
* Overheating of the testicles caused by vigorous, repetitive exercise or underwear that is too tight and holds the testicles too close to the body.
* Intercourse problems (e.g., premature withdrawal, poor timing with menses, too infrequent).
* Ejaculatory dysfunction.
* Exposure to insecticides or industrial chemicals.

RISK INCREASES WITH
* Diabetes.
* Poor nutrition and poor general health.
* Smoking.

HOW TO PREVENT—Specific preventive measures depend on the cause.

WHAT TO EXPECT

DIAGNOSTIC MEASURES
* Your own observation of symptoms.
* Diagnosis begins with a detailed medical history and general physical exam.

* Further testing may include medical tests, such as blood studies of hormones and semen analysis (to determine quality, quantity, form, and motility). Surgical diagnostic procedures such as testicular biopsy and other special tests of sperm function and quality may be done.

APPROPRIATE HEALTH CARE—Results of the tests will determine the need for any special treatment such as drug therapy or surgery.

POSSIBLE COMPLICATIONS—Emotional stress caused by feelings of guilt, inadequacy, and loss of self-esteem.

PROBABLE OUTCOME—Some fertility problems are minor and reversible. Often, no clear cause for infertility is found. Each patient should approach treatment with optimism.

HOW TO TREAT

GENERAL MEASURES
* Some general suggestions include:
  - Counseling for sexual therapy techniques, marriage problems, or alcoholism may be helpful.
  - Heat may decrease sperm production in the testicles. To prevent this, don't wear tight underwear or athletic supporters that hold the testicles too close to the body. Don't take hot baths. Avoid long bicycle rides.
  - Advise your health care provider if you work with environmental chemicals or are exposed to radiation on a routine basis. These can be a risk factor for infertility.
  - Stop smoking. It can reduce sperm counts and impair sperm motility.
  - Avoid alcohol or any drugs of abuse.
  - Have sexual intercourse during the time your partner is ovulating. Don't ejaculate for 3 days prior to intercourse. Intercourse should occur about every 36 hours during fertile period.
* To learn more: American Infertility Association, 666 Fifth Ave., Suite 278, New York, NY 10103; (888) 917-3777; website: www.americaninfertility.org.

MEDICATION
* Drugs may be prescribed to treat a cause of infertility.
* Vitamin supplements may be recommended.

ACTIVITY—Usually no limits.

DIET—Eat a normal, well-balanced diet.

CALL YOUR DOCTOR IF

You or a family member has concerns about infertility.

FERTILITY PROBLEMS IN WOMEN

 GENERAL INFORMATION

DEFINITION—The inability to become pregnant after 1 year of sexual activity without contraception. Infertility occurs in 10% to 15% of all couples. Female fertility depends on normal functioning of the reproductive tract and the production of hormones needed for normal sexual development and functioning. About 30% of all infertility is attributed to the female, 30% to the male, and the rest is a combination or unknown.

BODY PARTS INVOLVED—Genitals; endocrine system; brain.

SEX OR AGE MOST AFFECTED—Females between puberty and menopause.

SIGNS & SYMPTOMS—Inability to conceive.

CAUSES—Infertility can be caused by a wide variety of factors, and sometimes the cause is unknown.

RISK INCREASES WITH
* Endometriosis (disorder of the uterine lining).
* Pelvic inflammatory disease.
* Ovulatory problem (unable to ovulate [release eggs]).
* Physical problems of the reproductive system.
* Repeated weight-gain/weight-loss cycles.
* Hormone problems (such as thyroid).
* Vaginitis (inflammation of the vagina).
* Disorders of the cervix, such as infection, laceration or tearing from previous childbirth, or narrowing of the cervical opening for any reason.
* Amenorrhea (no menstrual periods).
* Chemical changes in the cervical mucus.
* Ovarian cysts.
* Smoking.
* Tumors.
* Emotional stress.
* Use of some drugs.
* Intrauterine device (IUD) may be a possible cause.
* Diabetes.
* Compulsive or excessive exercising.
* Marriage problems and infrequent sexual intercourse.
* Age. Female fertility decreases with age.
* Drugs of abuse, such as heroin or cocaine.

HOW TO PREVENT—Obtain medical care for any treatable disorder that causes infertility. Avoid preventable causes of infertility.

 WHAT TO EXPECT

DIAGNOSTIC MEASURES
* The first diagnostic tests may include a health history, blood tests, and a pelvic exam.

* Further testing may then be done. Multiple tests are available to study specific aspects of reproduction. You may be referred to a fertility specialist. The causes of infertility can be complex.

APPROPRIATE HEALTH CARE—Treatment will be based on the findings. Drug therapy or surgery may be recommended.

POSSIBLE COMPLICATIONS
* Emotional stress, including feelings of guilt, inadequacy, and loss of self-esteem.
* Treatment costs are high and often not covered by insurance.
* Long-term effects of fertility drugs are unknown.

PROBABLE OUTCOME—Some fertility problems are minor and reversible. Other problems may be helped with treatment.

 HOW TO TREAT

GENERAL MEASURES
* General suggestions that may help you conceive:
  - Live a healthy lifestyle. Reduce stress. Eat a well-balanced diet. Exercise in moderation.
  - Avoid alcohol, drugs of abuse, and smoking.
  - Get counseling for depression or marital problems.
  - Keep a basal body-temperature chart to become familiar with your ovulation pattern. Have intercourse just before ovulation.
  - Don't use a lubricant during sexual intercourse.
  - Your partner should withdraw his penis quickly from your vagina after ejaculation.
  - After your partner's ejaculation, place pillows under your buttocks to provide easier access for the sperm.
  - Maintain a positive attitude.
* To learn more: American Infertility Association, 666 Fifth Ave., Suite 278, New York, NY 10103; (888) 917-3777; website: www.americaninfertility.org.

MEDICATION
* Drugs may be prescribed to treat a cause of infertility.
* Ovarian stimulating drugs may be prescribed.
* Begin taking folic acid. This will reduce the risk of birth defects once you become pregnant.

ACTIVITY—Too much exercising may contribute to infertility.

DIET—Eat a well-balanced diet. If overweight, try to lose weight. Avoid caffeine and alcohol.

 CALL YOUR DOCTOR IF

You or a family member is unable to become pregnant

FETAL ALCOHOL SYNDROME (FAS)

GENERAL INFORMATION

DEFINITION—A combination of irreversible birth abnormalities resulting from alcohol abuse by the mother during pregnancy. Fetal alcohol syndrome has been reported in babies of women who drank 2 mixed drinks or 2-3 bottles of beer or glasses of wine a day. Lesser degrees of alcohol abuse can result in less severe birth defects. There appears to be no safe level of alcohol during pregnancy.

SEX OR AGE MOST AFFECTED—Newborns.

SIGNS & SYMPTOMS
Newborn behaviors:
• Poor sucking ability; poor sleeping habits.
• Irritability; effects of alcohol withdrawal.
Possible physical abnormalities:
• Small head; small eyes; unusually short stature.
• Epicanthic folds (vertical folds of skin extending from upper eyelid to the side of nose).
• Small jaw; protruding forehead.
• Cleft palate.
• Small brain; heart defects.
• Hip dislocation; other joint deformities.
Later:
• Mental retardation; severe growth retardation.
• Poor coordination; learning disabilities.
• Speech and language difficulties; minimal brain dysfunction; hyperactivity; other behavioral problems.
Adolescence to adulthood:
• Maladaptive behaviors (social withdrawal, failure to consider consequence of actions, inappropriate emotional responses, excessive unhappiness, conduct problems).

CAUSES—Chronic (and probably binge-type) alcohol consumption during pregnancy. Alcohol intake can affect the unborn child during the first trimester by interfering with organ development, in the second trimester with mental retardation and the third trimester, retardation of fetal growth.

RISK INCREASES WITH
• The greater the alcohol consumption, the greater the risk for severe birth defects.
• Pregnant women not receiving prenatal health care.

HOW TO PREVENT
• Pregnant women (or those likely to become pregnant) should not drink any alcoholic drinks or abuse drugs. There is insufficient evidence that indicates an occasional glass of wine or beer is dangerous, but complete abstinence is recommended.
• If you are concerned about your alcohol consumption, seek help from your doctor, Alcoholics Anonymous or other support groups.
• Get early and continuing prenatal care.

WHAT TO EXPECT

DIAGNOSTIC MEASURES
• There is no diagnostic test that can determine an infant born with fetal alcohol syndrome. Some defects will be apparent at the time of birth; other defects will show up later.
• The diagnosis is difficult to confirm once the child is older. The mother may not remember if she drank during pregnancy or how much she drank. The child's academic performance may be blamed on behavior problems.

APPROPRIATE HEALTH CARE
• For the pregnant woman, get prenatal care.
• For the child, early diagnosis and recognition of a child at risk. A referral to medical professionals who can start immediately on special programs designed to enhance motor skills, improve communication skills and develop social interactions.

POSSIBLE COMPLICATIONS—The defects are generally irreversible. The complications may be mild or severe and include one or several of the problems listed in Signs and Symptoms.

PROBABLE OUTCOME—Since the effects of fetal alcohol syndrome can vary a great deal, the outcome is unpredictable.

HOW TO TREAT

GENERAL MEASURES
• If you are pregnant and continuing to drink alcohol, call your doctor and discuss.
• If you know a family member or friend who is pregnant and continues to drink alcohol, talk to her about your concern and the risk she is taking with her unborn child.
• If you are the parent of a child with fetal alcohol syndrome, get the appropriate help needed for the child's development. Get help for yourself if the alcohol problem is continuing or if you need other psychological support.

MEDICATION—Drugs are usually not needed for this disorder.

ACTIVITY—No limits.

DIET—No special diet.

CALL YOUR DOCTOR IF

• You are pregnant or think you might be pregnant and have not had a check-up.
• You are concerned about your newborn's behavior, physical development or appearance.

FEVER OF UNKNOWN ORIGIN

GENERAL INFORMATION

DEFINITION—Fever of unknown origin is a diagnosis given in cases where a person has had a fever (off and on) for at least 3 weeks, and no cause has been found after a basic medical evaluation.

BODY PARTS INVOLVED—Any body organs or system may be the source of a fever-producing condition.

SEX OR AGE MOST AFFECTED—Both sexes; all ages.

SIGNS & SYMPTOMS—Temperature above 101°F (38.3°C) on several occasions over a 3-week period.

CAUSES
In infants and children:
• Infections.
• Collagen or autoimmune diseases.
• Tumors and cancer, especially leukemia.
In adults:
• Infections.
• Collagen or autoimmune diseases.
• Tumors and cancer, especially kidney cancer and leukemia.
• Self-induced (in some emotionally unstable persons).
• Drugs can cause a fever as an adverse reaction.

RISK INCREASES WITH
• Weak immune system due to illness or drugs.
• Chemical or environmental exposure to polluted water or air.
• Travel in areas with unsanitary conditions.
• Exposure to others with infectious diseases.
• Elderly persons.
• Drug abuse.

HOW TO PREVENT—There are no specific preventive measures.

WHAT TO EXPECT

DIAGNOSTIC MEASURES
• Your own observation of symptoms.
• Your health care provider will do a physical exam and ask about your symptoms and activities.
• Because a fever may be the first evidence of a serious condition (in its early stages), careful medical testing may be done. This may include blood studies and a urine culture, x-rays of the chest, CT scan, an ultrasound, echocardiogram (heart function test), thyroid studies, liver function tests, an HIV antibody test, and others.

APPROPRIATE HEALTH CARE
• Treatment will depend on the underlying cause that is found.
• Hospital care may be recommended for elderly patients, patients with weak immune systems, and those with a serious chronic illness.

POSSIBLE COMPLICATIONS—Depends on the underlying condition causing the fever.

PROBABLE OUTCOME—Recovery without any treatment occurs in some cases. In other cases, the outcome depends on successful diagnosis and treatment of the underlying disorder.

HOW TO TREAT

GENERAL MEASURES—When at home, keep a daily temperature chart. Rectal temperatures are most accurate.

MEDICATION
• Acetaminophen or ibuprofen may be prescribed, to lower the fever. Don't give children under age 18 aspirin for fever.
• Until the cause is found, other prescription drugs may be withheld to avoid masking symptoms of the underlying disorder.
• In certain patients, antibiotics, steroids, or other drugs may be prescribed prior to a specific diagnosis.

ACTIVITY—Get extra rest while you have a fever.

DIET—No special diet. Drink extra fluids while you have a fever.

CALL YOUR DOCTOR IF

• You or a family member has an unexplained fever that lasts longer than 24 hours.
• New symptoms develop. They may provide a clue about the underlying cause of the fever.

ILLNESS & DISORDERS

FIBROCYSTIC BREAST CHANGES

GENERAL INFORMATION

DEFINITION—Fibrocystic changes are the most common cause of breast lumps in women. Over 50% of women have these changes at some point in their lives. The changes are not cancerous and are not a threat to health.

BODY PARTS INVOLVED—Breasts.

SEX OR AGE MOST AFFECTED—They can affect females from puberty to around age 50.

SIGNS & SYMPTOMS
* The changes may affect one or both breasts. Single lumps may occur, but multiple lumps are common.
* Lumps may offer resistance when pressed with fingertips and they may feel tender. They often enlarge before menstrual periods and shrink afterward.
* Breasts may be swollen and engorged.
* Mild to severe breast pain. It may be constant, on or off, irregular, or occur just before menstrual periods.
* Some women develop cysts, which are fluid-filled sacs that feel smooth and firm.
* Lumps come in different sizes. When the lumps are relatively large and near the surface, they can be moved freely within the breast.

CAUSES—The cause is not clear. Ovarian hormones appear to play a role. Fibrocystic changes may be caused by abnormal hormone levels or by an increased response of breast tissue to normal hormone levels.

RISK INCREASES WITH—Women who have not had children, have irregular menstrual cycles, or have a family history of fibrocystic breast changes or breast cancer. Studies on caffeine use, high-fat diet, and smoking as risk factors are inconclusive.

HOW TO PREVENT—Specific preventive measures are unknown. It may help to eat a low-fat diet, avoid smoking, and avoid caffeine.

WHAT TO EXPECT

DIAGNOSTIC MEASURES
* Your own observation of symptoms.
* Your health care provider will do a breast exam and examine the underarm area.
* Medical tests may include mammogram, ultrasound, and surgical diagnostic procedures, such as cyst aspiration.

APPROPRIATE HEALTH CARE
* Some cysts can be aspirated (removing the fluid). This is done in a health care provider's office. Removing the fluid should cause the lump to disappear. If the lump does not disappear, further diagnostic testing is done.

* The breast changes may get better without treatment. If symptoms continue, diet changes may help and drug therapy may be an option. Keep a pain diary for 2 to 3 months to determine the pattern of the pain.
* Surgery may be done to remove a lump.

POSSIBLE COMPLICATIONS—Only about 5% of fibrocystic breast changes have atypical cells that are a risk factor for developing cancer.

PROBABLE OUTCOME—Women with fibrocystic breast changes continue to have breast lumps that appear and dissolve. Some remain permanently. Treatment may help relieve symptoms. The condition often disappears after menopause (unless estrogen-replacement therapy is used).

HOW TO TREAT

GENERAL MEASURES
* Applying heat to the breasts may help discomfort.
* Wear a well-fitting bra (day and night).
* Stop smoking. Find a way to quit that works.
* Examine your breasts carefully each month. Report new lumps or any changes in lumps that have been diagnosed previously.
* Get routine mammogram studies as advised.
* Visit your health care provider at least every year for a breast exam. If you have a family history of cancer, more frequent follow-up visits may be recommended.

MEDICATION
* A mild diuretic may be prescribed.
* Birth control pills may be prescribed to help control hormone levels. For more severe symptoms, danazol or bromocriptine may be prescribed.
* Use nonprescription pain remedies for pain.
* Some women take vitamin A, vitamin B-6, vitamin E, or evening primrose oil to relieve symptoms. Ask your health care provider about these supplements.

ACTIVITY—No limits. A regular exercise program is usually recommended. Avoid activities that cause breast discomfort.

DIET
* Avoiding beverages that contain caffeine (coffee, tea, and some soft drinks) may help relieve symptoms.
* Eat a low-fat diet. Reducing salt and sugar may help.

CALL YOUR DOCTOR IF

* You or a family member has undiagnosed lumps in the breast.
* Lumps change, or new lumps appear.

FIBROMYALGIA
(Fibrositis)

 GENERAL INFORMATION

DEFINITION—Fibromyalgia is a painful condition that involves muscles, tendons, and joints. It may affect the muscle areas of the low back, neck, shoulder, chest, arms, hips, and thighs. It is a chronic problem that can come and go for years. Symptoms may be brought on by a change in the weather, being in cold or damp places, stress, hormone changes, or in response to activity. It is a common condition.

BODY PARTS INVOLVED—Muscular areas of the low back, neck, shoulder, chest, arms, hips and thighs.

SEX OR AGE MOST AFFECTED—It occurs in both men and women in all age groups, including children. It most often affects women ages 20 to 50.

SIGNS & SYMPTOMS
* Pain and aches in the muscles, often described as "hurting all over all the time."
* Fatigue and sleep problems.
* Areas of the body are tender to the touch (tender points). Common tender points are the front of the knees, the elbows, the hip joints, and around the neck.
* Feeling stiffness in mornings; having swollen joints, and the hands and feet may be numb and tingly.
* Headache, anxiety, and depression.
* Other symptoms may also occur, such as digestion, bowel, and urinary problems; vision changes; emotional or mental changes; allergies; dry eyes and mouth; and painful menstrual periods.

CAUSES—The cause is unknown and there are many theories. Research is ongoing into finding possible causes.

RISK INCREASES WITH
* Females ages 20 to 50.
* Having a relative with the condition. It appears to run in families.

HOW TO PREVENT—There are no steps that will prevent fibromyalgia.

 WHAT TO EXPECT

DIAGNOSTIC MEASURES
* Your own observation of symptoms.
* There is no special test to diagnose fibromyalgia. Your health care provider will do a physical exam, check the tender points in your body, and ask about all the symptoms you have. These same symptoms occur in other health problems. Tests such as blood work and x-rays may be done to be sure of the diagnosis.

APPROPRIATE HEALTH CARE
* There is no cure for fibromyalgia. Taking steps to reduce the symptoms is the main goal.
* Treatment steps vary. They may include prescribed drugs and injections, exercise, physical therapy, acupuncture, chiropractic care, or massage therapy. Counseling can help reduce stress and anxiety and promote well-being.

POSSIBLE COMPLICATIONS—Stress or other problems may cause the pain symptoms to worsen or flare up, usually only for a short time.

PROBABLE OUTCOME—The symptoms vary and may improve on their own or can be helped with treatment. The condition does not lead to more serious illness, nor is it life-threatening.

 HOW TO TREAT

GENERAL MEASURES
* Make changes in your life that may be needed to help you cope day-to-day. Maintain your social life and contact with friends.
* Join a local support group so you can talk with others about self-help ideas that work.
* Keep your activity levels about the same each day.
* Get as much sleep as you need.
* Don't smoke. Find a way to quit that works.
* To learn more: National Fibromyalgia Association, 2200 N. Glassell St., Suite A, Orange, CA 92865, (714) 921-0150 (not toll-free); website: www.fmaware.org.

MEDICATION
* For minor pain, use nonprescription drugs such as acetaminophen or ibuprofen.
* Drugs may be prescribed for symptoms of pain, depression, anxiety, and sleep problems. They will take a few weeks to work and side effects are common.

ACTIVITY—A daily exercise program is important. It will improve your fitness level, help reduce muscle pain, and let you sleep better. Talk to your health care provider about an exercise routine that will suit your needs.

DIET
* Avoid caffeine and alcohol.
* Eat a healthy diet. Your health care provider or a dietician can help you plan a diet.

 CALL YOUR DOCTOR IF

* You or a family member has some of the symptoms of fibromyalgia.
* Symptoms continue or worsen despite treatment.
* New symptoms develop.

FLUID & ELECTROLYTE DISORDERS

GENERAL INFORMATION

DEFINITION—An imbalance of the fluids and electrolytes in the body. Electrolytes are minerals found in the body that maintain many important body functions. The major electrolytes are sodium, calcium, potassium, magnesium, bicarbonate, phosphate, and chloride. An imbalance problem can affect any age group.

BODY PARTS INVOLVED—All.

SEX OR AGE MOST AFFECTED—Both sexes; all ages.

SIGNS & SYMPTOMS
* Dry mouth and wrinkled skin.
* Increased, decreased, or no urination.
* Fatigue.
* Muscle weakness, cramping, or twitching.
* Puffy legs, hands, face, or stomach.
* Lung congestion. Problems with breathing.
* Changes in mental status, depression, irritability.
* Fast or slow heartbeat.
* Constipation, nausea, and vomiting.
* Seizures or coma.

CAUSES—A variety of diseases and medical problems can lead to an imbalance. When the body loses fluids (such as with diarrhea) or retains fluids (such as with heart failure), the electrolyte balance is affected. Electrolytes may be too low (hypo-) or too high (hyper-).

RISK INCREASES WITH
* Diarrhea and/or vomiting.
* Heavy sweating.
* Serious burns, wounds, or other injuries.
* Heart or kidney disorders.
* Excess fluid intake.
* Use of diuretics (water pills).
* Laxative abuse.
* Certain types of prescription drugs.
* Diabetes.
* Endocrine diseases.
* Bone disorders.
* Milk-alkali syndrome (excess calcium intake).
* Fever.
* Unusual or extreme diets, or eating disorders.
* Alcoholism.
* Infants, young children, and people over 60. These people lose fluids very quickly when sick.

HOW TO PREVENT
* Avoid risk factors, where possible.
* Get medical care for chronic medical disorder.

WHAT TO EXPECT

DIAGNOSTIC MEASURES
* Your health care provider may do a physical exam and ask questions about your symptoms and activities.

* Medical tests include blood studies of electrolyte levels.

APPROPRIATE HEALTH CARE
* Treatment will depend on the underlying cause. This may include changes in diet or fluid intake, changes in drugs that may have caused the problem, prescribing new drugs, or other therapies as needed.
* Treatment steps include correcting the fluid and electrolyte imbalance. Electrolytes that are too low will be replaced. Electrolytes that are too high will be reduced. Hospital care may be needed for some patients to provide IV (intravenous) treatment. Patients with milder symptoms may be cared for at home.
* Dialysis (use of a machine to filter wastes) may be needed for some patients with kidney disorders.

POSSIBLE COMPLICATIONS—Severe imbalances can cause serious and fatal disorders.

PROBABLE OUTCOME—Treatment of electrolyte imbalance is usually effective. A long-term outlook depends on the underlying cause.

HOW TO TREAT

GENERAL MEASURES—None specific.

MEDICATION
* Electrolyte replacements may be prescribed. They may be given through a vein (IV) or taken orally.
* Drugs to reduce high electrolyte levels may be prescribed.
* Drugs to treat an underlying disorder may be prescribed.

ACTIVITY—Rest in bed until treatment is complete. Resume normal activities gradually.

DIET
* For a severe imbalance, solid food may be withheld until fluids and electrolytes return to normal.
* Diet changes may be recommended by your health care provider to help prevent problems in the future.

CALL YOUR DOCTOR IF

* You or a family member has symptoms of a fluid and electrolyte imbalance or dehydration.
* Your weight increases or decreases several pounds in one day.

FOLLICULITIS

GENERAL INFORMATION

DEFINITION—An inflammation of the hair follicles. Follicles are where the roots of body hair grow. Folliculitis can involve the hair on the skin anywhere on the body. It usually affects the face (such as the beard area in men), scalp, legs, armpits, and groin area. A stye is folliculitis on an eyelid.

BODY PARTS INVOLVED—Skin anywhere on the body, but usually the exposed areas of arms, legs and beard area of the face.

SEX OR AGE MOST AFFECTED—Both sexes; all ages.

SIGNS & SYMPTOMS
* Small groups of bumps (called papules or pustules) develop, usually with a hair in the middle of each bump. The bumps are small, and yellow-white in color, with a red area around them.
* Pain, redness, and swelling of the skin may occur.

CAUSES—Most often it is an infection of the hair follicles with *Staphylococcus or Pseudomonas* bacteria. It may also be caused by a fungal infection or irritation. Folliculitis may be superficial (on the surface of the skin) or deep in the hair follicle.

RISK INCREASES WITH
* Recent illness such as a nasal infection.
* Diabetes.
* Weak immune system due to illness or drugs.
* Excess sweating (hyperhidrosis).
* Eczema or dermatitis.
* Skin injuries, abrasions, surgical wounds, or draining abscess.
* Shaving, waxing, or plucking hairs.
* Tight clothing.
* Poor hygiene.
* Obesity.
* Use of hot tubs or saunas.
* Use of certain skin care products or overuse of topical steroids.

HOW TO PREVENT
* Wash hands often to prevent spread of any germs.
* Frequent bathing. Keep fingernails short and clean.
* Wash towels and linens often to prevent spread of germs.
* Avoid risk factors where possible.

WHAT TO EXPECT

DIAGNOSTIC MEASURES
* See your health care provider if you have concerns about the disorder. A health care provider can diagnose folliculitis by an exam of the affected area.
* A culture of fluid from the pustule or other tests may be done.

APPROPRIATE HEALTH CARE—Treatment involves supportive care of the skin and drug therapy if needed.

POSSIBLE COMPLICATIONS
* May progress to other types of skin problems.
* Scarring may occur.
* Folliculitis may recur or become chronic.

PROBABLE OUTCOME—Most cases clear up within 2 weeks. Some may take longer.

HOW TO TREAT

GENERAL MEASURES
* Don't scratch the affected area. The germs can be transferred from under the fingernails to other parts of the body.
* Use warm-water soaks to relieve itching and help healing.
* Clean area with antibacterial soap. Shampoo daily if the scalp is involved.
* Avoid using oils or greasy-type ointments on the skin.
* If you shave, change razor blades daily or use an electric razor.
* If folliculitis recurs or becomes chronic, shaving may need to be discontinued for a period of time.

MEDICATION
* If there are only a few bumps, you may use nonprescription, topical antibiotics (such as mupirocin). Apply as directed.
* Oral antibiotics may be prescribed.
* A topical antibiotic drug applied into the front of the nose may be prescribed. The nostrils are a source of bacteria that can be spread to other parts of the body.
* Other drugs may be prescribed if a cause other than bacteria is diagnosed.

ACTIVITY—No limits.

DIET—No special diet. A weight-loss diet may be recommended for obese patients.

CALL YOUR DOCTOR IF

* You or a family member has symptoms of folliculitis.
* You develop a boil or signs of spreading infection or folliculitis recurs after treatment.

FOOD ALLERGY

GENERAL INFORMATION

DEFINITION—Food allergy is a reaction of the body's immune system to some foods. Many people think they have a food allergy when it is food intolerance. Intolerance is caused by digestion problems, such as lactose or milk intolerance. A food allergy can cause severe symptoms. Food intolerance symptoms are rarely serious. It is important to know which one you have. Your health care provider can help you with the diagnosis.

BODY PARTS INVOLVED—Skin, lungs, gastrointestinal, central nervous system.

SEX OR AGE MOST AFFECTED—Males more often than females; all ages; food allergies are more common in children.

SIGNS & SYMPTOMS
* Diarrhea, stomach pains, nausea, or vomiting.
* Skin hives, rash (called eczema), itching, redness, and swelling of hands, feet, face, and lips.
* Cough, wheezing, or sneezing; runny nose.
* Infants may have blood in the stool or colic.

CAUSES
* The immune system reacts to certain proteins found in foods. It treats them as harmful to the body and tries to fight them off by releasing chemicals and histamines. This is what starts the allergic symptoms. Why it occurs in some people is unknown.
* Just about any food can cause an allergic reaction. Most common are milk, eggs, wheat, soy, peanut, tree nuts (walnuts and pecans), fish, and shellfish. Chocolate is not a common cause.

RISK INCREASES WITH
* People who have other allergy problems.
* Having family members who have a food allergy.
* Young children. Food allergy is more common.

HOW TO PREVENT
* Food allergy cannot be prevented. Reactions can be prevented if food causing it is known.
* It has not been proven that breast-feeding an infant prevents food allergies later in life. It does help delay the baby's exposure to foods that can cause allergies. Start solid foods at about age six months.

WHAT TO EXPECT

DIAGNOSTIC MEASURES
* Your own observation of symptoms.
* For diagnosis, your health care provider will ask questions about your symptoms and your diet, and may include a physical exam. Testing might involve skin and blood allergy tests, a food challenge test, or an elimination diet that you do at home.

APPROPRIATE HEALTH CARE—Once you know for sure that you have a food allergy, the treatment is to avoid the food or foods involved.

POSSIBLE COMPLICATIONS—None expected as long as the foods are avoided. Rarely, anaphylaxis (a severe, life-threatening reaction) occurs. Symptoms come on very quickly. They can include the symptoms listed plus troubled breathing, fast heart rate, and loss of consciousness. Get emergency help.

PROBABLE OUTCOME
* Infants often outgrow food allergy by 2 to 4 years.
* Adults with food allergy (particularly to milk, fish, shellfish, or nuts) are more likely to have their allergy for many years.
* Research is ongoing so new methods for treatment and prevention may be available.

HOW TO TREAT

GENERAL MEASURES
* Often, the food allergy is in a young child. Parents will need to discuss the allergy with any persons who will be caring for, teaching, or working with the child. They need to know what foods are involved and how to handle a severe reaction if one occurs. Once a child is older, parents can begin to teach the child how to take control of the allergy.
* To learn more: Food Allergy & Anaphylaxis Network, 10400 Eaton Place, Suite 107, Fairfax, VA 22030; (800) 929-4040; website: www.foodallergy.org.

MEDICATION
* Drugs will not cure a food allergy. Drugs may be prescribed to relieve some of the symptoms such as an antihistamine for itching or rash.
* If your food allergy is severe, you should carry a kit with a self-injecting device that contains the drug epinephrine. It can be used if the food is eaten by mistake and a reaction occurs. Know how to use the device. In addition, your family or others need to know how to give the injection if you are unable to do so.

ACTIVITY—No limits.

DIET
* Read labels carefully on food products.
* Use a food allergy cookbook to plan meals.
* Ask waiters in restaurants for details about foods and other items on the menu.

CALL YOUR DOCTOR IF

You or a family member has symptoms of food allergy.

FOOD POISONING

GENERAL INFORMATION

DEFINITION—A term used to describe illnesses suspected of being caused by contaminated food (or beverages). Food poisoning can affect all ages. Outbreaks can affect several members of a household, customers who dined at the same restaurant, nursing home patients, cruise ship passengers, university students, children in daycare, or shoppers who bought contaminated food in a store.

BODY PARTS INVOLVED—Gastrointestinal.

SEX OR AGE MOST AFFECTED—Both sexes; all ages.

SIGNS & SYMPTOMS
* Symptoms can begin within hours to days after eating the food. It depends on the cause of the contamination and how much food was ingested (eaten).
* Nausea, vomiting, stomach cramps or pain, diarrhea and/or bloody stools.
* Fever, chills, headache, and weakness may occur. In severe cases, shock and collapse.

CAUSES
* Certain bacteria such as *Campylobacter, Escherichia coli, Salmonella,* and others. Botulism is a rare, life-threatening food poisoning.
* Virus infection such as Norwalk virus (a common contaminant of shellfish), adenovirus, and rotavirus.
* Chemical causes such as contamination with insecticide or food served in lead-glazed pottery.
* Eating plants or animals that contain a naturally occurring poison, such as mushrooms or toadstools. Shellfish may contain a toxin that is not destroyed by cooking.

RISK INCREASES WITH
* Eating food that is improperly prepared.
* Lack of good hygiene when preparing food.
* Drinking water or eating raw foods when traveling in a foreign country.

HOW TO PREVENT
* Avoid raw seafood or meat.
* Avoid unpasteurized food products.
* Properly cook and store foods.
* Keep food preparation areas and utensils clean.
* Throw food items away that are old, have an "off" smell, or those in bulging tin cans.
* Always wash hands before preparing food.

WHAT TO EXPECT

DIAGNOSTIC MEASURES
* Your own observation of symptoms.

* See a health care provider if symptoms are other than mild. A health care provider may do a physical exam. Questions will be asked about your symptoms and recent foods you have eaten, and if others have eaten the same foods.
* Cultures may be made from a stool sample. If some of the food that made you sick is available, you may be asked to bring it in for testing.

APPROPRIATE HEALTH CARE
* In mild cases, self-care measures may be all that is needed.
* Hospital care may be required if symptoms are severe. Fluids may be given through a vein.
* If several persons are affected, contact the local health department. They can interview patients and food handlers and take samples of suspected contaminated food.

POSSIBLE COMPLICATIONS—Dehydration is the most common complication. More serious complications are rare but can be life-threatening, especially in very young or elderly patients or persons with weak immune systems.

PROBABLE OUTCOME—Most cases are mild and clear up within a few days.

HOW TO TREAT

GENERAL MEASURES—The main treatment is to replace fluid and electrolytes (salts and minerals) lost through vomiting or diarrhea.

MEDICATION
* Drugs are not needed to treat food poisoning. They may be prescribed for certain symptoms.
* Antibiotics may be prescribed.
* Don't take drugs for diarrhea unless they are prescribed. They may prolong the symptoms.

ACTIVITY—Get extra rest until diarrhea, vomiting, and fever are improved.

DIET
* Suck ice chips or drink small amounts of clear fluids often. Replace lost fluids and electrolytes with products such as Pedialyte or Ricelyte for infants and children, and diluted rehydration fluids (Gatorade) for adults.
* Once the symptoms improve, try a diet of complex carbohydrates (rice, wheat, potatoes, bread, cereal, and lean meat such as chicken). Milk and dairy products usually do not need to be limited.
* Avoid high-sugar foods or fatty foods for a few days.

CALL YOUR DOCTOR IF

You or a family member has signs or symptoms of food poisoning that cause concern or are not improving.

FROSTBITE

GENERAL INFORMATION

DEFINITION
• Frostbite is the destruction of body tissue from exposure to temperatures or wind chill below freezing. Arms, legs, fingers, toes, face, nose, and ears are areas of the body that are usually affected.
• Nonfreezing cold injuries include frostnip, chilblains, and immersion foot (cold and wet exposure).

BODY PARTS INVOLVED—Arms and legs (especially fingers and toes); face (especially nose and ears).

SEX OR AGE MOST AFFECTED—Both sexes; all ages (more common in males ages 30 to 49).

SIGNS & SYMPTOMS
• In milder cases, there may be burning, numbness, tingling, itching, or coldness in the affected area. Skin may be white and frozen in appearance, and may have some resistance when pressed.
• In more severe cases of frostbite, there may be no sensations in the affected area. Swelling and blood-filled blisters may appear. Skin may be white or yellow, look waxy, and turn purple as it is rewarmed. The area is hard when it is pressed. The affected area can look blackened and dead.
• Hypothermia (low body temperature) can cause uncontrolled shivering, weakness, and confusion.

CAUSES—Frostbite occurs when ice crystals form in skin and blood vessels, which leads to destruction of the cells. Further damage can occur upon rewarming when blood flow resumes into the damaged blood vessels.

RISK INCREASES WITH
• Car accidents or car breakdowns in bad weather (especially in remote areas).
• Drinking too much alcohol or abusing drugs.
• Elderly persons.
• Diabetes, blood-vessel diseases, or smoking.
• Persons with mental disorders.
• Homeless persons.
• High-altitude travel or activities.
• Poor conditioning, inadequate clothing, clothing that is wet and tight, dehydration, malnutrition, and fatigue.

HOW TO PREVENT
• Dress for the cold weather.
• Avoid smoking and alcohol.
• Travel with someone, in case help is needed.

WHAT TO EXPECT

DIAGNOSTIC MEASURES
• An exam by a health care provider is done to check for life-threatening problems and to diagnose frostbite or other types of cold injury, such as frostnip.

APPROPRIATE HEALTH CARE
• Rewarming for frostbite is usually done in a warm bath until the thaw is complete. It can be a painful process. Fluids are often given through a vein (IV). Supplemental oxygen may be needed.
• Hospital care may be required to treat skin damage, assess the extent of injury, and to prevent infection. Whirlpool bath therapy may be done to remove dead tissue. The affected area may be elevated and splinted.
• It may take months to see if the affected tissue will be healthy or permanently damaged. Surgery may be done to remove damaged tissue, including amputation.

POSSIBLE COMPLICATIONS
• Minor complications, such as pain, changes in sensitivity of the affected area, and skin color changes.
• Major complications, such as amputation.

PROBABLE OUTCOME—For milder cold injuries, complete recovery is expected. More severe frostbite may have complications. Full recovery can take months.

HOW TO TREAT

GENERAL MEASURES—Emergency care for frostbite:
• Call for help. Arrange transport to a hospital.
• Move patient to a warm area. Keep the affected area elevated. Keep the person warm to prevent hypothermia. Remove tight clothing or jewelry (they may block blood flow).
• Don't rewarm the affected area if there is a chance it may freeze again. Don't rewarm it using an open fire or dry heat. Put the affected area in warm (not hot) water.
• Give warm fluids to drink (no alcohol or caffeine).
• Never massage (rub) the affected areas.
• Cover the area with soft, cloth bandages. Place cloth or cotton between toes/fingers to prevent rubbing.

MEDICATION—You may be prescribed drugs for pain relief, antibiotics to prevent infection, and/or a tetanus booster.

ACTIVITY—Will depend on extent of damage. Physical therapy may be needed.

DIET—Warm fluids to start with, as tolerated thereafter.

CALL YOUR DOCTOR IF

You or a family member has symptoms of frostbite or cold injury, or you observe them in someone else.

GALLSTONES
(Cholelithiasis)

GENERAL INFORMATION

DEFINITION—Stones in the gallbladder. The gallbladder is an organ in the body that stores bile.

BODY PARTS INVOLVED—Gallbladder; bile ducts.

SEX OR AGE MOST AFFECTED—They can affect young people and adults of both sexes, and are more common in women.

SIGNS & SYMPTOMS
* No symptoms in about 40% of cases.
* Sharp pain in the upper-right stomach area or between the shoulder blades.
* Nausea and vomiting.
* Bloating or belching.
* Fatty foods cause indigestion.
* Jaundice, which causes yellow skin and eyes.

CAUSES—Bile is a liquid made by the liver and stored in the gallbladder. Its use in the body is to help with digestion. Gallstones form when substances in the bile liquid harden. This may be due to too much cholesterol or bilirubin, or not enough bile salts, or the gallbladder not emptying as it should. Stones may be small like a grain of sand or as large as a golf ball. There may be one or hundreds of tiny stones.

RISK INCREASES WITH
* People over age 60.
* Women get gallstones twice as often as men.
* Disorders such as cirrhosis of the liver, blood disorders, Crohn's disease, cystic fibrosis, sickle-cell anemia, or biliary tract infection.
* Stomach reduction surgery.
* Genetic factors. Some ethnic groups are more likely to have gallstones.
* Overweight.
* Diabetes.
* Too much estrogen in the body. It may be from pregnancy, birth control pills, or hormone replacement.
* Rapid weight loss or fasting.
* Drugs that lower cholesterol can actually increase the cholesterol in the bile, which can lead to gallstones.

HOW TO PREVENT—There are no specific preventive measures.

WHAT TO EXPECT

DIAGNOSTIC MEASURES
* Your own observation of symptoms.
* Your health care provider will do a physical exam and ask questions about your symptoms.
* Medical tests may include blood tests and an ultrasound, which can detect the stones by sound waves. Other tests may be done to confirm the diagnosis or check for complications.

APPROPRIATE HEALTH CARE
* There are several ways to treat gallstones that are causing symptoms. They include surgery, shockwave treatment, drugs, and sometimes diet changes.
* Surgery to remove the gallbladder. For most people, this will relieve the symptoms. Surgery options include:
  - Laparoscopic procedure. This procedure uses tiny incisions through the skin and a special instrument to remove the gallbladder.
  - Open surgery. A more serious procedure that requires a longer incision to remove the gallbladder.
* Shockwave (lithotripsy) treatment to break up (shatter) the stones may be an option for some patients.

POSSIBLE COMPLICATIONS
* A stone becomes lodged in a duct. Ducts are tubes that carry bile to and from the gallbladder. A lodged stone can cause serious problems with the gallbladder, pancreas, or liver.
* Gallstones may recur if treatment does not include removing the gallbladder.

PROBABLE OUTCOME—Gallstones that cause no symptoms can safely be left alone. They are unlikely to cause problems. For those who do have symptoms, treatment is available.

HOW TO TREAT

GENERAL MEASURES
* Some people try diet changes and drugs to help symptoms. This may work for a while, but not permanently.
* To learn more: National Digestive Diseases Information Clearinghouse, 2 Information Way, Bethesda, MD 20892; (800) 891-5389; website: www.digestive.niddk.nih.gov.

MEDICATION—Drugs can be taken by mouth to dissolve stones. This treatment is used for certain types of stones and can require up to 2 years to be effective.

ACTIVITY—You will be advised of limits depending on the type of treatment. Get extra rest while you recover.

DIET—No special diet unless advised.

CALL YOUR DOCTOR IF

* You or a family member has symptoms of gallstones.
* Fever rises to 101°F (38.3°C).
* Pain occurs that lasts for more than 3 hours.

ILLNESS & DISORDERS

GANGRENE

GENERAL INFORMATION

DEFINITION—Gangrene is dead tissue. It forms when a wound becomes infected or body tissue is destroyed by an accident. It can affect any body part, including internal organs.

BODY PARTS INVOLVED—Any body part, but the most common sites are toes, feet, legs, fingers, hands and arms.

SEX OR AGE MOST AFFECTED—Both sexes; all ages.

SIGNS & SYMPTOMS
* Skin may be pale at first, then turn red or bronze, and finally, a purple or blue-black color.
* Crackling of the skin. This feels like pressing on air bubbles under the skin.
* Swelling of the skin tissue.
* Pain or loss of sensation in affected area.
* Bad-smelling discharge from the dead tissues.
* Fever, sweating, and fast heartbeat.

CAUSES—Gangrene occurs when blood flow to a section of the body is blocked or reduced. There are two types. Dry gangrene is when there is no infection and is often caused by a blood clot or frostbite. Wet (gas) gangrene occurs when a wound becomes infected with bacteria.

RISK INCREASES WITH
* Infection with bacteria.
* Body injury caused by accidents, surgery, or deep puncture wounds.
* Crush injury that cuts off blood supply.
* Blood clot in an artery.
* Hardening of the arteries.
* Prolonged frostbite.
* Diabetes.
* Smoking.
* Excess alcohol use.
* Poor blood circulation.
* Old age.

HOW TO PREVENT
* Avoid any risk factors where possible.
* If you have diabetes, check your feet often for signs of unhealthy tissue.
* Seek medical advice for signs of infection (warmth, swelling, redness, pain, or tenderness) in a skin injury.

WHAT TO EXPECT

DIAGNOSTIC MEASURES
* Your health care provider will do an exam of the affected area.
* Medical tests will be done to determine the extent of the problem. These may include blood studies and a culture of the fluid from the wound. Imaging tests such as x-ray, CT, or MRI (see Glossary for these tests) may help with diagnosing complications.

APPROPRIATE HEALTH CARE
* Hospital care is needed for treatment.
* Treatment for gangrene will involve drugs and surgery to remove dead tissue. Removal of the dead tissue may need to be repeated over several days.
* Treatment will be given for any medical problem that is causing the gangrene, and to help restore blood flow to the affected area.
* You may need oxygen supplied through a mask or into the nose to help you breathe.
* You may be placed in a sealed chamber (hyperbaric) where high-pressure oxygen is used for treatment.
* Amputation of an infected body part may be needed to keep the infection from spreading. This often involves part of an arm or leg. Instructions will be provided for ongoing home care and physical therapy following surgery.

POSSIBLE COMPLICATIONS
* Liver damage, kidney failure, shock, and coma.
* Limb removal (amputation).
* Gangrene can be fatal, even with treatment.

PROBABLE OUTCOME—Can be cured in the early stages with drugs and treatment to remove dead tissue.

HOW TO TREAT

GENERAL MEASURES—The family should maintain an optimistic outlook, stay in close contact with the patient's doctor and help by making their visits with the patient as supportive as possible.

MEDICATION—In the hospital, you will be given antibiotics, pain relievers, and usually blood thinners to prevent blood clotting. Additional drugs may be needed to treat other disorders diagnosed.

ACTIVITY
* Rest in bed until healing begins. Your health care provider will advise you of any limits to your activities.
* Physical therapy may be needed after an amputation.

DIET—Eat a high-protein, high-calorie diet while your body is repairing damaged tissue. Take vitamin and mineral supplements if advised.

CALL YOUR DOCTOR IF

* You or a family member has symptoms of gangrene.
* Pain continues, despite drugs and treatment.
* Fever or infection develops during recovery.

GASTRIC EROSION

GENERAL INFORMATION

DEFINITION—A sore or raw area on the inner lining (mucosa) of the stomach. Gastric erosions can affect all ages. They are more common in men than in women.

BODY PARTS INVOLVED—Stomach.

SEX OR AGE MOST AFFECTED—All ages and both sexes, but most common in men.

SIGNS & SYMPTOMS
* Vomiting blood. Blood may be bright red or look like black coffee grounds.
* Blood in the stool. Blood will appear black or "tarry."
* Often there are no symptoms. A person may be unaware of the bleeding.

CAUSES—The stomach's lining is delicate and can easily be damaged by too much stomach acid or other irritants. The damage can result in erosions or ulcers that may cause bleeding. Erosions can be shallow or deep and are often in the shape of a circle.

RISK INCREASES WITH
* Drugs that irritate the stomach lining. These include aspirin and other nonsteroidal anti-inflammatory drugs.
* Tobacco use. It increases stomach acid.
* Excess alcohol intake. It irritates the stomach lining.
* Bacteria infection.
* Physical stress such as from burns or surgery.
* Rarely, in children, a swallowed coin that contains zinc can cause erosion.
* Emotional stress was once considered the main risk factor. Medical experts are now unsure of its role and research is ongoing.
* No specific food (or diet) has been identified as a risk factor. A person should avoid any foods that cause an upset stomach.

HOW TO PREVENT
* If possible, take pills that have a protective coating.
* Don't smoke or drink alcohol.

WHAT TO EXPECT

DIAGNOSTIC MEASURES
* Your own observation of symptoms.
* Your health care provider will do a physical exam and ask questions about your symptoms.
* Medical tests may include studies of the stool and blood, and x-rays of the stomach.

APPROPRIATE HEALTH CARE—Treatment usually involves taking drugs to reduce stomach acid. This helps relieve symptoms and promote healing.

POSSIBLE COMPLICATIONS
* Perforation, in which the erosion opens a hole through the stomach wall. Surgery is sometimes needed to correct the problem.
* Anemia due to blood loss.

PROBABLE OUTCOME—Usually curable in 2 weeks.

HOW TO TREAT

GENERAL MEASURES
* Your health care provider may have you check your stool daily for any signs of bleeding. You will be given instructions on how to do this.
* Stop smoking. Find a way to quit.

MEDICATION
* Drugs to reduce stomach acid may be recommended. These may be prescription drugs or others that are nonprescription.
* An antibiotic may be prescribed for bacteria infection.
* If a drug you are currently taking is a cause of erosion, a change in dosage or a different drug may be prescribed.
* For minor pain, you may use acetaminophen.

ACTIVITY—Resume normal activities as soon as symptoms improve.

DIET—Eat small, frequent meals for 1 to 2 weeks. No specific foods need to be avoided. Don't drink alcohol.

CALL YOUR DOCTOR IF

* You or a family member has signs of bleeding described in Frequent Signs and Symptoms.
* You develop diarrhea. This may represent a reaction to drugs used in treatment.
* You have severe pain that is not helped by treatment.
* You are unusually weak, pale, or lightheaded.
* Symptoms of gastric erosion recur after treatment.

ILLNESS & DISORDERS

GASTRITIS

GENERAL INFORMATION

DEFINITION—Inflammation of the stomach lining. Inflammation causes pain, swelling, redness, and heat. Gastritis may start as a sudden attack, or develop slowly over a period of time.

BODY PARTS INVOLVED—Stomach.

SEX OR AGE MOST AFFECTED—Both sexes; all ages.

SIGNS & SYMPTOMS
* Stomach pain and cramps.
* Black stool or bloody vomit due to stomach bleeding.
* Appetite loss.
* Fever.
* Weakness.
* Swollen stomach.
* Sharp, dull, or annoying pain in the chest.
* Acid taste in the mouth.
* Mild nausea and diarrhea (rare).
* Belching or gas.

CAUSES—The inflammation is a reaction to injury, infection, or irritation of the stomach lining. It can be brought on by a number of different factors. Sometimes the cause is unknown.

RISK INCREASES WITH
* Drinking too much alcohol.
* Use of nonsteroidal anti-inflammatory drugs such as aspirin or ibuprofen.
* Illness that has weakened the body.
* Surgery and being in the hospital for other problems.
* Serious injury or severe burns.
* Smoking.
* The presence of a bacteria in the stomach.
* Pernicious anemia, immune problems, and chronic bile reflux.

HOW TO PREVENT
* Eat and drink moderately.
* Don't skip meals or eat irregularly.
* Avoid foods you find hard to digest.
* Don't smoke.
* Avoid drugs that irritate your stomach, if possible.

WHAT TO EXPECT

DIAGNOSTIC MEASURES
* Your own observation of symptoms.
* Your health care provider will do a physical exam and ask questions about your symptoms.
* Diagnosis is made by examining the stomach through a tube passed down the throat to the stomach. A small amount of tissue may be removed for a test. Samples of blood and stool may be tested.

APPROPRIATE HEALTH CARE
* Goals of treatment are to relieve the symptoms and get rid of the gastric irritant or other cause. Drug therapy can help.
* A hospital stay may be necessary if extreme bleeding occurs.

POSSIBLE COMPLICATIONS—Bleeding is an uncommon but dangerous complication, especially in the elderly.

PROBABLE OUTCOME—Usually can be cured in several days with treatment, and if the cause is taken away.

HOW TO TREAT

GENERAL MEASURES
* Consider lifestyle changes if they are contributing to symptoms.
* Smoking and alcohol drinking should be stopped.

MEDICATION
* Drugs are usually prescribed to reduce stomach acid. Acid irritates the stomach lining.
* Take acetaminophen for minor pain. Don't use aspirin.
* Other drugs, such as antibiotics for infection, may be prescribed.
* A drug you take may be causing the problem. Your health care provider may stop the drug, change the dose, or prescribe a new drug.

ACTIVITY—Resume normal activities as soon as symptoms improve.

DIET—Don't eat solid food on the first day of the attack. Drink liquids often, preferably milk or water. Resume a normal diet slowly. Avoid hot and spicy foods, coffee, and acidic foods until symptoms are gone.

CALL YOUR DOCTOR IF

* You or a family member has symptoms of gastritis.
* You vomit blood.
* Bowel movements become black or tarry.
* Pain becomes severe.
* Signs of dehydration develop.

GASTROENTERITIS (Stomach Flu)

GENERAL INFORMATION

DEFINITION—Irritation and inflammation of the stomach and intestines. Gastroenteritis is a general term and is often used when there is a nonspecific, uncertain, or unknown cause. The disorder is most severe in young children. Adults usually have mild cases, sometimes with no symptoms.

BODY PARTS INVOLVED—Stomach; small intestine; colon.

SEX OR AGE MOST AFFECTED—All ages, both sexes.

SIGNS & SYMPTOMS
* Diarrhea is the main symptom, and sometimes, the only one. Diarrhea may range from 2 or 3 loose stools to many watery stools.
* Nausea and vomiting.
* Stomach cramps, pain, or tenderness.
* Fever or chills.
* Appetite loss.
* Weakness.
* Dehydration.

CAUSES
* Viral infections are the most common cause. They are spread by contact with an infected person or by touching an object that has germs on it. Contaminated food or water is another source for infection.
* Other causes are bacterial or parasitic infections, food-borne toxins, shellfish and marine animal poisoning, food intolerance, drug-caused diarrhea, and colitis.

RISK INCREASES WITH
* Children in daycare centers.
* Crowded living or working conditions.
* Older adults in nursing homes.
* Schools, dormitories, camps, or cruise ships
* Weak immune system due to illness or drugs.
* Drugs, such as antibiotics, laxatives, or antacids.
* Contaminated food or water.
* Travel to foreign countries.

HOW TO PREVENT
* No specific preventive measures.
* Wash hands often to stop spread of germs.
* Don't share eating utensils or towels.
* Store and cook foods in a safe manner.
* When traveling in foreign countries, take care to eat food and drink water that is safe.

WHAT TO EXPECT

DIAGNOSTIC MEASURES
* Call your health care provider if symptoms are severe or if they cause you any concern.

* Your health care provider may do a physical exam. Medical tests may include studies of blood and stool.

APPROPRIATE HEALTH CARE
* Care at home is usually all that is needed.
* Hospital care may be needed, if dehydration is severe.

POSSIBLE COMPLICATIONS—Serious dehydration that requires special treatment. Other complications are rare.

PROBABLE OUTCOME—The prognosis is excellent. Diarrhea and other symptoms usually clear up in 2 to 5 days. Adults may feel somewhat weak and fatigued for about a week.

HOW TO TREAT

GENERAL MEASURES
* Treatment usually involves rest and fluids. There is no specific drug for viral infections.
* It is not necessary to keep persons with gastroenteritis away from others in the family or household. Try to avoid close contact if possible.

MEDICATION
* Drugs are usually not needed for treatment. If symptoms are severe or prolonged, you may take antinausea and antidiarrhea drugs such as Pepto-Bismol or loperamide.
* Some infections may require specific drug treatment.
* If a drug you take is the cause of the problem, you may be advised to change drugs, reduce the dosage, or stop taking the drug.

ACTIVITY—Get extra rest until diarrhea, nausea, vomiting, and fever are improved. Be sure to have access to a toilet or bedpan.

DIET
* Suck ice chips or drink small amounts of clear fluids often. Replace lost fluids and electrolytes with products such as Pedialyte or Ricelyte for infants and children, and diluted rehydration fluids (Gatorade) for adults.
* Once the symptoms improve, try a diet of complex carbohydrates (rice, wheat, potatoes, bread, cereal, and lean meat such as chicken). Milk and dairy products usually do not need to be limited.
* Avoid high-sugar foods or fatty foods for a few days.

CALL YOUR DOCTOR IF

* Symptoms of gastroenteritis last longer than 2 days.
* Symptoms continue or worsen after treatment.
* Blood or mucus appears in the stool.

GASTROESOPHAGEAL REFLUX DISEASE (GERD)

GENERAL INFORMATION

DEFINITION—A condition that occurs when acids from the stomach move backward (reflux) into the esophagus (the food pipe that carries food from the mouth to the stomach).

BODY PARTS INVOLVED—Gastrointestinal.

SEX OR AGE MOST AFFECTED—All ages, but most common in adults over 60.

SIGNS & SYMPTOMS
* Persistent heartburn (stomach acid touches the lining of the esophagus and causes a burning sensation in the chest). You can have GERD without having heartburn.
* Regurgitation (acid can be tasted in the back of the mouth).
* Hoarseness in the morning.
* Difficulty swallowing.
* Feels like you have food stuck in your throat, like you are choking, or your throat is tight.
* Dry cough and bad breath.
* Excessive clearing of the throat.
* Burning in the mouth.
* Infants and children may have repeated vomiting, coughing, and other respiratory (lung) problems. Most babies grow out of GERD by their first birthday.

CAUSES—The problem occurs when the lower esophageal sphincter (LES) does not close properly. This allows stomach contents to leak back, or reflux, into the esophagus. The LES is a ring of muscle at the bottom of the esophagus. It acts like a valve between the esophagus and stomach. It is unknown why people get GERD.

RISK INCREASES WITH
* Hiatal hernia may contribute. It occurs when part of the stomach protrudes into the diaphragm (the muscle wall that separates the stomach from the chest).
* Alcohol use.
* Overweight.
* Pregnancy.
* Smoking.
* Certain foods can trigger symptoms (chocolate, caffeine, fatty and fried foods, garlic, onions, mint, spicy foods, spaghetti, chili, pizza, and citrus fruits).

HOW TO PREVENT—Follow steps listed in General Measures.

WHAT TO EXPECT

DIAGNOSTIC MEASURES
* Your health care provider will do a physical exam and ask questions about your symptoms, diet, and activities.

* Medical tests may be done at this time or after simple treatment measures are tried.

APPROPRIATE HEALTH CARE
* Treatment will depend on how severe your GERD is. It may involve lifestyle changes, drugs, further medical testing, or surgery.
* If lifestyle changes and drugs don't help, medical tests may be done to check for other problems:
    - Barium swallow (a type of x-ray).
    - Endoscopy (a thin, flexible plastic tube with a tiny camera is used to view the esophagus).
    - A device may be inserted into the esophagus that measures acid reflux. The device remains for 24 or 48 hours while you go about your regular activities.
* Surgery is a treatment option when drugs and lifestyle changes do not work. Surgery may also be a reasonable alternative to a lifetime of drugs and discomfort.

POSSIBLE COMPLICATIONS
* Inflammation of the esophagus (esophagitis).
* Ulcers.
* Scars from tissue damage narrow the esophagus.
* Barrett's esophagus (can lead to cancer).
* Erosion or weakening of the teeth.
* Asthma, chronic cough, or pulmonary fibrosis may be aggravated or even caused by GERD.

PROBABLE OUTCOME—Symptoms can be improved with treatment. GERD may come and go for weeks or months, or it may persist.

HOW TO TREAT

GENERAL MEASURES—Lifestyle changes:
* If you smoke, stop. Find a way to quit.
* Make changes in your diet.
* Wear loose-fitting clothes.
* Avoid lying down for 3 hours after a meal.
* Raise the head of your bed 6 to 8 inches by putting blocks of wood under the bedposts.

MEDICATION—Antacids, or drugs that stop acid production or help the muscles that empty your stomach may be prescribed. Combinations of these drugs can help control symptoms.

ACTIVITY—No limits.

DIET—Do not drink alcohol. Lose weight, if needed. Eat small meals. Avoid the foods that trigger symptoms.

CALL YOUR DOCTOR IF

* You or a family member has symptoms of GERD.
* Symptoms continue despite treatment.

GESTATIONAL DIABETES
(GDM; Gestational Carbohydrate Intolerance)

 GENERAL INFORMATION

DEFINITION—A type of diabetes that occurs only in pregnant women. Gestational diabetes mellitus (GDM) affects 2% to 5% of all pregnancies.

BODY PARTS INVOLVED—Pancreas.

SEX OR AGE MOST AFFECTED—Females of childbearing age.

SIGNS & SYMPTOMS
• Usually no symptoms are apparent. A prenatal exam may find that the fetus is larger than normal for the stage of pregnancy.
• Diagnosis is based on glucose testing done during the 24th to 28th week of pregnancy for nondiabetic mothers. Earlier testing is often done for patients diagnosed with GDM in a previous pregnancy, a birth weight over 9 pounds in a previous infant, or for other risk factors.

CAUSES—Your body isn't able to use the sugar (glucose) in your blood as well as it should, so the level of sugar in your blood becomes higher than normal.

RISK INCREASES WITH
• Previous pregnancy with GDM.
• Obesity (especially if excess fat is around the waist).
• Mother over age 30.
• Polycystic ovarian syndrome (PCOS).
• Family history of diabetes.
• Excess weight gain in pregnancy.
• Previous birth of an infant weighing over 9 pounds.
• Four or more previous pregnancies.
• History of an unexplained fetal death or stillbirth.
• Some population groups, such as Native Americans, Mexican-Americans, Asians, and East Indians.

HOW TO PREVENT—There are no specific preventive measures. Weight loss in overweight women prior to pregnancy may help. Careful attention to diet and exercise in pregnant women with risk factors may help.

 WHAT TO EXPECT

DIAGNOSTIC MEASURES—Your obstetric provider will do a glucose test.

APPROPRIATE HEALTH CARE
• Treatment will include diet changes, moderate exercise program, and drug therapy, if needed.
• You will learn how to monitor your glucose levels. At first, glucose checks may need to be done up to 4-6 times daily. Once glucose levels are in the desired range and diet changes are made, glucose checks may be reduced with your obstetric provider's approval.

POSSIBLE COMPLICATIONS
• Excess amniotic fluid (polyhydramnios).
• Premature labor.
• May need to have labor induced.
• Preeclampsia.
• Miscarriage (rare).
• Risk for mother of diabetes in the future.

PROBABLE OUTCOME
• Successful treatment and a healthy baby often depend on the mother's motivation and ability to change her lifestyle. For some, dietary control is sufficient. Others may require drug therapy.
• In most cases, labor occurs naturally, and the birth is usually vaginal. Cesarean section may be required if the fetus is considered too large for vaginal birth.
• Gestational diabetes usually clears up with delivery of the baby.

 HOW TO TREAT

GENERAL MEASURES—To learn more: Contact the local or national office of the American Diabetes Association, Attention: National Call Center, 1701 Beauregard St., Alexandria, VA 22311; (800) 342-2383; website: www.diabetes.org.

MEDICATION
• Drugs are usually not needed if glucose control is achieved with diet and exercise.
• Insulin injections or oral antidiabetic drugs may be prescribed for some patients.

ACTIVITY—A program of moderate, non–weight-bearing exercise is usually recommended. Exercising for even small time periods can have major benefits. Follow any prescribed exercise program carefully.

DIET
• Diet changes are an important part of the treatment. Specific diet instructions will be provided. Following this diet will decrease the risks to the mother and her unborn child.
• The diet changes will involve increased fiber intake, fat limits, avoiding sweets, and monitoring caloric intake to prevent excess weight gain.

 CALL YOUR DOCTOR IF

• You are 24 to 28 weeks pregnant and have not had a screening test for gestational diabetes.
• After diagnosis, you develop any new signs or symptoms that cause you concern.

GENITOURINARY INJURY
(Bladder Injury; Kidney Injury; Urethra Injury; Ureter Injury; Penis or Testis Injury)

GENERAL INFORMATION

DEFINITION—Injury to a part of the genitourinary tract that may result from a variety of causes.

BODY PARTS INVOLVED—Kidney (organ that filters the blood and excretes waste products); bladder (the organ that stores urine); ureter (two tubes that carry urine from the kidneys to the bladder); urethra (the tube through which urine travels from the bladder to the outside); penis; scrotum.

SEX OR AGE MOST AFFECTED—Both sexes; all ages.

SIGNS & SYMPTOMS
* Severe abdominal pain.
* Shock (sweating; faintness; nausea; panting; rapid pulse; pale, cold, moist skin).
* Painful urination or inability to urinate.
* Pain or tenderness in the back, just below the ribs on the injured side.
* Fever (sometimes).
* Blood in the urine.
If you have severe pain with large amounts of blood in your urine, one or both kidneys may be seriously injured.

CAUSES—Forceful or penetrating blow or wound to lower abdomen (gunshot or stab wounds, pelvic surgery, pelvic fracture, straddle injuries, kicks, penis amputation).

RISK INCREASES WITH
* Excess alcohol consumption.
* Hazardous occupations.
* Motor vehicle accidents.
* Sexually abused children.
* Medical treatments including surgery, shock waves, laser therapy, instrument use, radiation.
* Physical combat or physical violence.
* Penile rings.
* Excessive trauma during intercourse or other sexual activity.

HOW TO PREVENT
* Protect yourself from injury whenever possible.
* Buckle your automobile seat belt to minimize internal injury in case of accident.
* Don't drink and drive.
* Avoid alcohol or limit amount you consume.

WHAT TO EXPECT

DIAGNOSTIC MEASURES
* Your own observation of symptoms.
* Your health care provider will do a physical exam.

* Medical tests may include urine studies.x-rays of the urinary tract,ultrasound, intravenous urography, and cystography (the last two special x-rays used to see inside the kidneys and bladder).

APPROPRIATE HEALTH CARE
* Emergency care and/or hospital care.
* Surgery may be needed to repair any wounds, control bleeding and repair damage to the organs involved. A temporary catheter may be necessary for urinary drainage while the body heals.
* Injury to external male genitalia may require skin grafts.
* An amputated penis may be re-implanted using microsurgical techniques.

POSSIBLE COMPLICATIONS
* Internal bleeding.
* Urine leakage into the abdomen, causing abdominal inflammation or infection.
* Recurrent infections from scars in the urethra that narrow the urinary passage.
* Scarring and narrowing of the injured ureter.
* Atrophy of testes following a rupture injury.

PROBABLE OUTCOME—A genitourinary tract injury usually requires emergency treatment. Most cases heal with bed rest, time, supportive treatment or surgery.

HOW TO TREAT

GENERAL MEASURES—No specific instructions except those under other headings.

MEDICATION—You may be prescribed:
* Antibiotics to prevent infection.
* Pain medicine as required.
* Anticholinergics for spasms.

ACTIVITY—Stay as active as your strength allows. Allow 1 month for recovery. Don't return to work or resume sexual relations until healing is complete.

DIET—No special diet.

CALL YOUR DOCTOR IF

* You or a family member has any symptoms of genitourinary injury.
* During or after treatment, you develop fever and chills.

GIARDIASIS

GENERAL INFORMATION

DEFINITION—An intestinal infection caused by a parasite. Giardiasis is a frequent cause of diarrhea. It may occur in clusters or outbreaks, affecting many persons at a time.

BODY PARTS INVOLVED—Gastrointestinal tract, especially the small bowel.

SEX OR AGE MOST AFFECTED—All ages, but most common in children.

SIGNS & SYMPTOMS
* Often, there are no symptoms.
* Symptoms can be mild and recurrent, persisting for months, or longer.
* Sudden diarrhea and stomach cramping. Some persons have only mild diarrhea and upset stomach.
* Stools may have a foul smell and be greasy.
* Nausea and vomiting.
* Slight fever (rare).

CAUSES—A parasite, *Giardia lamblia*. The germs may be spread in food or water contaminated by feces from infected animals or humans. Germs can be spread from one person to another due to poor hygiene. Symptoms begin in 1 to 3 weeks after being infected.

RISK INCREASES WITH
* Drinking from a water supply that is contaminated.
* Drinking unsafe water while camping or hiking.
* Swimmers who swallow contaminated water.
* Weak immune system due to illness or drugs.
* Children or workers at preschool or daycare center.
* Foreign travel.
* Oral or anal sex.

HOW TO PREVENT
* Don't drink unsafe water. Boil or treat it first.
* Avoid uncooked foods that may have been rinsed in contaminated water.
* Wash hands often to prevent spread of any germs.
* Keep children with diarrhea away from others.
* To avoid spreading the germs, don't swim if you have diarrhea.
* When traveling in foreign countries, take care to eat food and drink water that is known to be safe.

WHAT TO EXPECT

DIAGNOSTIC MEASURES
* Your health care provider may do a physical exam. Questions will be asked about your symptoms and activities. Health providers are often aware if there is an outbreak of giardiasis in the community.
* Medical tests may include stool studies to detect the parasites.

APPROPRIATE HEALTH CARE
* Giardiasis responds well to drugs. Treatment is usually done at home. Drug treatment for family members who are infected, but have no symptoms, may be recommended. Pregnant women may require special treatment.
* Hospital care to replace lost fluids may be required for patients with severe diarrhea and dehydration.

POSSIBLE COMPLICATIONS
* Dehydration.
* Chronic giardiasis.
* Malabsorption (unable to absorb nutrients from food) and weight loss.

PROBABLE OUTCOME—Complete recovery is expected within 1 to 2 weeks with treatment. Symptoms may go away even without treatment, but a person can carry the germs for weeks or months.

HOW TO TREAT

GENERAL MEASURES
* Prevention is the best treatment. Be cautious when away from normal drinking-water supplies.
* Practice careful personal hygiene if you, or others around you, have diarrhea.

MEDICATION—Antiparasitic drugs such as metronidazole (Flagyl) and others may be prescribed. Alcohol interacts with metronidazole to cause stomach cramps and nausea, so don't drink alcohol during this treatment.

ACTIVITY—No limits.

DIET
* Maintain an adequate fluid intake (at least 8 glasses of water or liquid a day).
* Some persons develop lactose intolerance. A lactose-free diet may be recommended.

CALL YOUR DOCTOR IF

* You or a family member has symptoms of giardiasis.
* New, unexplained symptoms develop. Drugs used in treatment may produce side effects.

ILLNESS & DISORDERS

GILBERT'S SYNDROME
(Hyperbilirubinemia)

 GENERAL INFORMATION

DEFINITION—A disorder that causes increased blood levels of bilirubin. Bilirubin is a yellow chemical that results from red-blood-cell breakdown. Gilbert's syndrome is usually a chance finding of routine testing.

BODY PARTS INVOLVED—Blood.

SEX OR AGE MOST AFFECTED—It affects both sexes, but is most common in men. It is present from birth, but symptoms may not appear until ages 20 to 40.

SIGNS & SYMPTOMS
* Usually there are no symptoms.
* Mild jaundice (yellow skin and eyes) may occur in some patients. It may come and go.
* Some patients have symptoms that are nonspecific. These include stomach cramps, tiredness, and general ill feeling. They may be related to anxiety in some cases.

CAUSES—A dysfunction of the liver in processing bile. This leaves above-normal levels of bilirubin in the blood. If blood levels are high enough, jaundice may appear.

RISK INCREASES WITH—None specific. The signs of jaundice may be brought on by dehydration, fasting, illness, menstrual periods, and stress (trauma or overexertion).

HOW TO PREVENT—No specific preventive measures.

 WHAT TO EXPECT

DIAGNOSTIC MEASURES
* Your own observation of symptoms (sometimes). The minor jaundice may be unnoticeable.
* Your health care provider will usually do a physical exam.
* Blood tests of bilirubin and liver function will be done to help confirm the diagnosis.

APPROPRIATE HEALTH CARE—No treatment is necessary. Your health care provider will explain that the syndrome is benign and will not cause health problems or affect lifestyle.

POSSIBLE COMPLICATIONS—No known complications.

PROBABLE OUTCOME—The condition is harmless.

 HOW TO TREAT

GENERAL MEASURES—If you or others notice a yellowing of your eyes or skin (it may seem like a good suntan) get a medical diagnosis. Some more serious conditions also begin with mild jaundice.

MEDICATION—Drugs are not necessary for this disorder.

ACTIVITY—No limits.

DIET—No special diet.

 CALL YOUR DOCTOR IF

You or a family member has symptoms of Gilbert's syndrome. This usually involves skin that looks a bit yellow.

GINGIVITIS

GENERAL INFORMATION

DEFINITION—Inflammation (redness, soreness, swelling) or infection of the gums. This is a mild form of gum disease, but it can lead to more serious problems.

BODY PARTS INVOLVED—Gum tissue around teeth.

SEX OR AGE MOST AFFECTED—All ages, but most common in adults.

SIGNS & SYMPTOMS
* Gums that have become swollen, tender, red, and soft around the teeth. Gums may bleed easily.
* Bad breath.
* No pain.
* Fever (rarely).

CAUSES—Plaque. It is a sticky substance made up of food particles, germs, and mucus that builds up on the teeth.

RISK INCREASES WITH
* Poor dental hygiene, other tooth problems, and mouth infections.
* Poor nutrition. This can include eating too much sugar or vitamin deficiencies.
* Adverse reactions to drugs, such as phenytoin and barbiturates.
* People with diabetes, gastroesophageal reflux disease (GERD), or osteoporosis.
* Disorders that affect the immune system such as arthritis, lupus, and AIDS.
* Smoking.
* Pregnancy.
* Female hormones can affect the gums.

HOW TO PREVENT
* Practice good oral hygiene to prevent plaque formation.
* Brush teeth and your tongue twice a day. Brush your teeth properly. A soft brush is less likely to damage teeth and gums than a hard brush. Scrub clear, sticky plaque off the teeth daily with a soft toothbrush. Place the brush at the gum line and gently rotate it, pointing bristles toward the gum. Brush one section of teeth at a time.
* Floss your teeth at least once a day. Use waxed or unwaxed dental floss. Wind most of it around the middle finger of each hand. Use index fingers as guides to force the floss between the teeth gently. Gently clean adjacent tooth surfaces with a back-and-forth, sawing motion at the gum line. Floss between all lower teeth. Loosen floss and place it on the tops of the thumbs. Floss between all upper teeth, using thumbs as guides.
* Make regular appointments with your dental health care provider for cleaning and treatment of cavities.

* Have regular dental checkups twice a year.
* Eat a well-balanced diet. Take vitamin supplements if you are unable to eat well-balanced meals.
* Quit smoking. Find a plan that works for you.

WHAT TO EXPECT

DIAGNOSTIC MEASURES
* Your own observation of symptoms.
* Your dental health care provider can diagnose gingivitis with an exam of your teeth and gums. A special tool is used to check the depth of pockets in the gums.
* X-rays of the teeth help reveal any bone loss.

APPROPRIATE HEALTH CARE
* Treatment usually includes cleaning the teeth by a dental hygienist or other dental health care provider. There are different techniques depending on the degree of plaque build-up.
* Other dental work may be needed. Teeth may need straightening, cavities filled, or missing teeth replaced.
* Surgery may be needed to remove infected gum tissue, if other treatment fails.

POSSIBLE COMPLICATIONS—Without treatment, gingivitis can lead to more serious gum disease, infections, and tooth loss.

HOW TO TREAT

GENERAL MEASURES—To learn more: American Dental Association, 211 E. Chicago Avenue, Chicago, IL 60611, (312) 440-2500 (not toll free); website: www.ada.org.

MEDICATION
* Antibiotics may be prescribed for infection. They may be taken by mouth (orally) or applied to the gums with special devices.
* Fluoride mouthwash may be recommended.

ACTIVITY—No limits.

DIET—No special diet. Avoid candy, sweet drinks, or sweet snacks. Sugar stimulates the production of acid, which attacks normal teeth.

CALL YOUR DOCTOR IF

OR CALL YOUR DENTIST
* You or a family member has symptoms of gingivitis.
* The following occur after treatment:
  - Bleeding increases or there is more pain.
  - Fever of 101°F (38.3°C) or higher.
  - Neck or face is swollen, or it is hard to swallow.

GLAUCOMA, ANGLE-CLOSURE

GENERAL INFORMATION

DEFINITION—Glaucoma is a progressive disease of the optic nerve that can lead to loss of vision. It is usually due to increased intraocular pressure (IOP), but it can be due to other causes. Angle-closure glaucoma is one of the two main types of glaucoma, and it is the less common type. Open-angle glaucoma is the more common type. The disease process, the treatment, and the prognosis are different for each type. Angle-closure glaucoma symptoms can occur suddenly (acute), or develop over time (chronic).

BODY PARTS INVOLVED—Eye.

SEX OR AGE MOST AFFECTED—Adults of both sexes. It occurs more often in people over 55 and in women more than in men.

SIGNS & SYMPTOMS
- Acute angle-closure glaucoma (symptoms are sudden, and often occur in a darkened room, such as a movie theater, or during periods of stress):
  - Severe, throbbing eye pain. Eye becomes red.
  - Blurred vision.
  - May see halos around lights.
  - Nausea, vomiting, and headache.
- Chronic angle-closure glaucoma (not acute):
  - There may be no symptoms.
  - Slightly blurred vision, mild eye pain, or seeing halos around lights. These symptoms may come and go.

CAUSES—Normal eye pressure is maintained by a balance of fluid (aqueous) that flows into the front of the eye and then drains out. The angle of the eye (where the iris and cornea meet) is where the drains (called trabecular meshwork) are located. With angle-closure glaucoma, the angle of the eye is not as wide (or open) as it should be. When the pupil dilates (gets larger), it pushes the iris forward and narrows the angle even more so that the drain is blocked or covered over. In acute cases, this happens suddenly. In chronic cases, it occurs over time. The blocked drain causes a buildup of fluid and pressure in the eye. The pressure can damage the optic nerve, sometimes within hours, and lead to vision loss.

RISK INCREASES WITH
- Adults over 55. Females more than males.
- Family history of glaucoma.
- Farsightedness.
- Asian or Eskimo descent.
- Use of certain drugs with cholinergic inhibition.

HOW TO PREVENT
- Regular eye exams:
  - Under age 45, have an exam every 4 years if there are no risk factors and every 2 years with risk factors.
- Over age 45, have an exam every 2 years if there are no risk factors and every year with risk factors.
- Get medical care for any changes in your vision.

WHAT TO EXPECT

DIAGNOSTIC MEASURES
- Your own observation of symptoms.
- An acute attack is an emergency situation. In the hospital, drugs are given to constrict the pupil and to reduce fluid production of the eye.
- A gonioscopy test may be done. This test is a way to view the trabecular meshwork in angle-closure glaucoma. (It is not visible in other types of eye tests.) The test involves placing a contact lens on the front of the eye. Topical anesthetic is used to prevent discomfort. The contact lens allows the person doing the exam to check the trabecular meshwork for signs of glaucoma.

APPROPRIATE HEALTH CARE—Surgery (iridectomy with a laser beam) to prevent further attacks is often performed. A small opening is made in the iris so that the aqueous humor (fluid in the eye) can drain. It is usually done in the other eye as a preventive measure.

POSSIBLE COMPLICATIONS—With acute glaucoma, blindness in the affected eye is possible, if treatment is delayed or unsuccessful.

PROBABLE OUTCOME—Symptoms can usually be controlled with treatment.

HOW TO TREAT

GENERAL MEASURES—To learn more: Glaucoma Foundation, 116 John St, Suite 1605, New York, NY 10038; (800) 452-8266; website: www.glaucomafoundation.org.

MEDICATION—Eye drops may be prescribed to lower pressure inside the eye. Follow the instructions and schedule carefully.

ACTIVITY—No limits after treatment, unless advised otherwise.

DIET—No special diet.

CALL YOUR DOCTOR IF

- You or a family member has symptoms of acute angle-closure glaucoma. This is an emergency!
- Other vision or eye problems develop.
- New, unexplained symptoms develop. Drugs used in treatment may produce side effects.

GLAUCOMA, OPEN-ANGLE

GENERAL INFORMATION

DEFINITION—Glaucoma is a progressive disease of the optic nerve that can lead to loss of vision. It is usually due to increased intraocular pressure (IOP), but it can be due to other causes. Open-angle glaucoma (or primary open-angle glaucoma [POAG]) is one of the two main types of glaucoma, and it is more common. The other type, angle-closure glaucoma, is less common. The disease process, the treatment, and the prognosis are different for each type.

BODY PARTS INVOLVED—Eye.

SEX OR AGE MOST AFFECTED—Adults of both sexes and all ages, but occurs more often in people over 40.

SIGNS & SYMPTOMS
• Usually, there are no warning symptoms.
• Later stages of the disease include loss of peripheral vision in small areas, blurred vision, halos around lights, blind spots, and poor night vision.

CAUSES
• Normal eye pressure is maintained by a balance of fluid (aqueous) that flows into the front of the eye and then drains out. The angle of the eye (where the iris and cornea meet) is where the drains (called trabecular meshwork) are located. For unknown reasons, the drains become clogged. The fluid builds up over time and eye pressure increases. This causes damage to the optic nerve, which leads to vision loss.
• Restricted blood supply to the optic nerve is another cause. People with normal eye pressure and open-angle glaucoma have what is called normal-tension glaucoma.

RISK INCREASES WITH
• Glaucoma suspect (IOP without optic nerve damage).
• Adults over 45.
• Family history of glaucoma.
• Diabetes.
• Myopia (nearsightedness).
• Previous eye injury.
• Regular, long-term steroid use.
• African Americans (have a greater tendency).
• Low blood pressure.

HOW TO PREVENT
• Regular eye exams:
 - Under age 45, have an exam every 4 years if there are no risk factors and every 2 years with risk factors.
 - Over age 45, have an exam every 2 years if there are no risk factors and every year with risk factors.
• Get medical care for any changes in your vision.

WHAT TO EXPECT

DIAGNOSTIC MEASURES
• An eye exam is usually done by an eye doctor (ophthalmologist). It includes a tonometry exam (measures pressure within the eyeball) and visual field test (to see how your vision is affected).
• An ophthalmoscope is used to see into the eye to view the optic nerve. A person has glaucoma if their eye exam shows changes to the optic nerve and blind spots.

APPROPRIATE HEALTH CARE
• There is no cure. The goal is to protect the optic nerve from future damage and possible loss of vision. Treatment may include drug therapy, laser surgery, eye operations, or a combination of methods.
• Laser surgery can help improve the draining of the excess fluid. Other eye surgery may be done to open up the draining area and relieve pressure.

POSSIBLE COMPLICATIONS—Optic nerve damage that cannot be reversed. A permanent vision loss can occur.

PROBABLE OUTCOME—The disorder can usually be controlled with treatment to prevent further vision loss.

HOW TO TREAT

GENERAL MEASURES—To learn more: Glaucoma Foundation, 116 John St, Suite 1605, New York, NY 10038; (800) 452-8266; website: www.glaucomafoundation.org.

MEDICATION—One or more types of eye drops to lower pressure inside the eye will be prescribed. Follow the instructions and schedule carefully, even if symptoms improve. If eye drops do not control the pressure, oral drugs (taken by mouth) will usually be prescribed.

ACTIVITY—No limits.

DIET—No special diet.

CALL YOUR DOCTOR IF

• You or a family member has symptoms of chronic glaucoma.
• Any sign of eye infection develops.
• Pain begins in the eye.
• Redness occurs in the eye.
• Vision changes suddenly.

ILLNESS & DISORDERS

GLOMERULONEPHRITIS

GENERAL INFORMATION

DEFINITION—A group of disorders that cause inflammation of the glomeruli. These are filtering units in the kidneys that help filter out waste products and water and salt from the blood. Over time, the inflammation can lead to loss of kidney function.

BODY PARTS INVOLVED—Kidneys.

SEX OR AGE MOST AFFECTED—It is more common in children 5 to 15 years old, and occurs in males more than females.

SIGNS & SYMPTOMS
* Mild inflammation produces no symptoms. Diagnosis is possible only with urine studies.
* Dark-colored urine (color of tea or cola drink).
* Reduced urine.
* Urine may be bloody.
* Puffy eyelids.
* Swelling of the face, hands, feet, and stomach.
* Side pain.
* Weakness.
* Headache, fever, nausea, or vomiting.
* High blood pressure. It causes no symptoms, but may be measured with home blood pressure monitors.
* Shortness of breath.
* Loss of appetite.

CAUSES
* Postinfectious type (more common). This type develops after a *streptococcus* (often referred to as strep) infection. It may be a strep infection such as a sore throat or a skin infection.
* Other types (less common). These may be caused by other types of infections, whole body (systemic) diseases, IV drug abuse, kidney (renal) disease, and other medical problems. Sometimes the cause is unknown.

RISK INCREASES WITH
* Strep infection, such as scarlet fever.
* Persons diagnosed with any of the possible causes.

HOW TO PREVENT—No specific preventive measures. Get treatment for any strep infection to help reduce risk.

WHAT TO EXPECT

DIAGNOSTIC MEASURES
* Your own observation of symptoms.
* Your health care provider will do a physical exam and ask questions about your symptoms and recent illnesses.
* Medical tests may include blood and urine studies, and x-rays. A kidney biopsy may be done. This involves removal of a small amount of kidney tissue for viewing under a microscope.

APPROPRIATE HEALTH CARE
* The goals of treatment are to relieve symptoms and to treat and prevent complications. Treatment may involve drugs, diet changes, and extra rest.
* Hospital care may be needed for severe symptoms.

POSSIBLE COMPLICATIONS
* Kidney failure. It may lead to dialysis (use of a machine to filter body waste) and a kidney transplant.
* Chronic glomerulonephritis.
* Complications may occur in patients who have other health problems such as severe high blood pressure.

PROBABLE OUTCOME
* Outlook is excellent for most post-streptococcal cases in children. Mild cases may recover on their own. Some may be helped with treatment. Symptoms usually improve in 2 weeks to several months.
* In those cases caused by other medical problems, the outcome will vary depending on the underlying cause.

HOW TO TREAT

GENERAL MEASURES
* None specific.
* To learn more: National Kidney Foundation, 30 E. 33rd St., Suite 1100, New York, NY 10016; (800) 622-9010; website: www.kidney.org.

MEDICATION—You may be prescribed:
* Antibiotics for strep infection.
* Drugs for high blood pressure.
* Diuretics, to help remove excess fluid.
* Steroids, to reduce inflammation.
* Drugs, to suppress the immune system.
* Drugs for other types of infection, or to treat an underlying disorder.

ACTIVITY—Stay in bed, except to go to the bathroom, until symptoms have improved. Bed rest ensures an adequate blood flow to the kidney. Blood flow is best when lying down. Resume normal activities gradually.

DIET—Diet changes may be recommended to help reduce the work of the kidneys. These may include eating less salt, potassium, and protein.

CALL YOUR DOCTOR IF

* You or a family member has symptoms of glomerulonephritis.
* Urine changes color or urine output is decreased.
* New symptoms occur during treatment.

GONORRHEA

GENERAL INFORMATION

DEFINITION—An infection caused by a sexually transmitted disease (STD). Gonorrhea can affect anyone (even young children) who has sexual contact with an infected person.

BODY PARTS INVOLVED
* In males, it usually involves the urethra (urine canal).
* In females, it usually involves the cervix and, sometimes, the urethra.
* In both sexes, the rectum, throat and other body parts may be involved.

SEX OR AGE MOST AFFECTED—Both sexes and all ages. It most often occurs in younger persons (ages 15 to 29), and in men more than in women.

SIGNS & SYMPTOMS
* Symptoms usually begin 2 to 5 days, or up to 30 days after being exposed. Females have few or no symptoms. Males usually have symptoms.
* Burning sensation when urinating.
* White to yellow-green discharge from the urethra.
* Rectal discomfort and discharge (sometimes).
* Sore throat (mild).
* Females may have abdominal cramps.
* Conjunctivitis (eye inflammation). This occurs when the person touches infected genitals and then the eyes.
* If the infection spreads to other body parts: joint pain, low fever, rash, headache, neck pain, and stiffness.

CAUSES—Infection from *Neisseria gonorrhoeae*, a bacteria. It grows easily on delicate, moist tissue. The bacteria is transmitted sexually (vaginal, anal, or oral sex). It can be spread from mother to child during birth.

RISK INCREASES WITH
* Any sexually active persons.
* Having sex with an infected person.
* Multiple sexual partners, whether heterosexual or homosexual.
* Child sexual abuse.
* Passage of newborn through the infected birth canal of the mother.

HOW TO PREVENT
* Abstain from sexual activity.
* Avoid sexual partners whose health practices and status are uncertain.
* Use a latex condom during sexual intercourse.

WHAT TO EXPECT

DIAGNOSTIC MEASURES
* Your health care provider will do a physical exam and a pelvic exam.

* Medical tests may include blood and urine studies and studies of the discharge from the vagina, urethra, rectum, throat, or eyes. Tests for other sexually transmitted diseases are usually done. Other tests may be done if complications are suspected.

APPROPRIATE HEALTH CARE
* Treatment is with antibiotic drugs. Follow-up tests may be done to confirm a cure.
* If the eyes are involved, an eye doctor (ophthalmologist) should be consulted.
* Hospital care may be needed in some cases.

POSSIBLE COMPLICATIONS
* Persons who have no symptoms are at risk for complications and can unknowingly spread the infection.
* Spread from mother to child during birth. This can cause complications in the newborn.
* Blood poisoning (gonococcal septicemia).
* Infectious arthritis.
* Pelvic inflammatory disease in females (PID), which can lead to infertility.
* Heart inflammation or infection around the liver.
* Epididymitis (which can lead to infertility), prostate problems, and urethral scarring in males.
* Risk of getting HIV is higher.

PROBABLE OUTCOME—Usually curable in 1 to 2 weeks with treatment.

HOW TO TREAT

GENERAL MEASURES
* Inform all sexual contacts so they can seek treatment.
* For self-care:
  - Use separate towels, washcloths, and disposable eating utensils during treatment.
  - Wash hands often.
  - Don't touch your eyes with your hands.
* To learn more: Centers for Disease Control & Prevention (CDC) National STD Hotline (800) 227-8922; website: www.cdc.gov/std.

MEDICATION
* Antibiotics will be prescribed.
* You may take nonprescription drugs, such as acetaminophen or aspirin (for adults), to reduce discomfort.

ACTIVITY—Don't resume sexual activity until treatment is complete.

DIET—No special diet.

CALL YOUR DOCTOR IF

* You or a family member has symptoms of gonorrhea.
* Symptoms don't improve with treatment.

GOUT

GENERAL INFORMATION

DEFINITION—Recurrent attacks of joint inflammation, especially the base of the big toe. Gout may also involve the foot, ankle, knee, elbow, hand, arm, or shoulder.

BODY PARTS INVOLVED—Joints: base of the big toe; may also involve the elbow, knee, hand, foot, ankle, arm or shoulder.

SEX OR AGE MOST AFFECTED—Adults of both sexes but it is more common in men than women, until after menopause.

SIGNS & SYMPTOMS
* Sudden onset of severe pain (usually at night) in the inflamed joint. This is often at the base of the big toe.
* Involved joints may be hot, swollen, and very tender. Skin over the joint is red and shiny.
* Fever, chills, or fatigue (sometimes).

CAUSES—A high level of uric acid in the blood. This may be due to increased production of uric acid or decreased elimination of uric acid by the kidneys.

RISK INCREASES WITH
* Men over 60.
* Family history of gout.
* Obesity.
* Excess alcohol use.
* Thyroid disorders.
* Use of certain drugs, such as diuretic drugs (water pills), high blood pressure drugs, aspirin, drugs that treat gout, and others.
* High blood pressure.
* Starvation or dehydration.
* Eating large amounts of foods that contain purines. These include anchovies, sardines, sweetbreads, kidney, liver, tongue, and large amounts of red meat, shellfish, peas, lentils, and beans.

HOW TO PREVENT—Avoid risk factors, where possible.

WHAT TO EXPECT

DIAGNOSTIC MEASURES
* Your own observation of symptoms.
* Your health care provider will do an exam of the joints.
* Medical tests may include blood and urine levels of uric acid and studies of fluid removed from the joint. X-ray or bone scan may be done.

APPROPRIATE HEALTH CARE
* Goals of treatment are to control the symptoms, prevent a recurrence, and to lower uric acid levels. Treatment usually involves drug therapy, lifestyle changes, and rarely, surgery.
* Lifestyle changes may include diet changes and weight loss (if overweight).

* Surgery is rare, but may be recommended if the disorder was untreated or treated late.

POSSIBLE COMPLICATIONS
* Crippled, deformed joints.
* Kidney stones.
* Continued gout attacks (if untreated).

PROBABLE OUTCOME—The first attack may last a few days. Recurrent attacks are common unless the uric acid level in the blood is reduced. Symptoms can be relieved with treatment.

HOW TO TREAT

GENERAL MEASURES—For home care:
* Use warm or cold compresses on painful joints.
* Keep the weight of bedclothes off any painful joint by making a frame that raises sheets off the feet.

MEDICATION
* Nonsteroidal anti-inflammatory drugs to control inflammation and pain are usually prescribed.
* Other drugs for an attack of gout may be prescribed.
* Lifelong treatment with drugs to decrease uric acid production or to increase the kidneys' excretion of uric acid may be needed. These drugs have side effects and adverse reactions. Obtain as much information as possible regarding their use.

ACTIVITY
* During an attack, rest and elevate the foot. Take care to avoid joint injury. Wear shoes that fit properly.
* When able, exercise daily.

DIET
* Limit foods that contain purines (see Risk Factors). Note: all protein foods contain purine, so no one should avoid all purines.
* Drink plenty of water and other liquids daily. Fluids keeps the urine diluted, which helps prevent kidney stones.
* Don't drink alcoholic beverages, especially beer or red wine. They can worsen or trigger an attack.
* If you are overweight, begin a medically approved weight-loss diet. Do not go on a crash diet, as rapid weight loss may bring on a gout attack.

CALL YOUR DOCTOR IF

* You or a family member has symptoms of gout.
* Pain gets worse, or fever and chills occur.
* New, unexplained symptoms develop.

GRANULOMA ANNULARE

 ## GENERAL INFORMATION

DEFINITION—A common benign skin disorder. It can involve the skin on the bottoms of feet and backs of fingers, hands, arms, elbows, legs, and knees.

BODY PARTS INVOLVED—Skin on the bottoms of feet and backs of fingers, hands, arms, elbows, legs and knees.

SEX OR AGE MOST AFFECTED—It can affect all ages but is more common in children and young adults. Females are more often affected than males.

SIGNS & SYMPTOMS
• Small, raised bumps (called papules) on the skin.
• Bumps have a domed or slightly flat shape. Their color may vary on different people. Bumps may be skin-colored, reddish, bluish, or yellowish.
• They don't hurt, and usually don't itch.
• The bumps cluster in a ring. Bumps around the ring border are close, but don't grow completely together. This gives the border a beaded appearance. The ring's center is often darker than the edge.
• The appearance may change in size and shape over a few weeks to 6 months.
• The area affected may be small (localized) or widespread (generalized) over the body.

CAUSES—Unknown.

RISK INCREASES WITH
• Diabetes.
• Damage to the skin such as from injury, sunburn, or insect bite.

HOW TO PREVENT—No specific preventive measures. Avoid injury to the skin. Protect skin from sunburn with sunscreen or clothing.

 ## WHAT TO EXPECT

DIAGNOSTIC MEASURES
• Your own observation of symptoms.
• Your health care provider can diagnose the disorder by an exam of the affected skin area.
• In some cases, other medical tests are done to confirm the diagnosis.

APPROPRIATE HEALTH CARE—Treatment is usually not needed, and currently, there is no effective drug treatment that works for everyone. Your health care provider will discuss options with you.

POSSIBLE COMPLICATIONS—No complications are expected.

PROBABLE OUTCOME—The disorder will heal on its own, but it usually takes months to years. The disorder may also recur with no apparent cause or timing.

 ## HOW TO TREAT

GENERAL MEASURES—You may use cosmetics or fake-tan products to help hide the affected skin areas.

MEDICATION
• Steroid creams or ointments to be applied to the skin may be prescribed.
• Your health care provider may inject steroids directly into the bumps.
• A treatment called PUVA may be recommended. It combines a special light, used with a cream applied to the skin.

ACTIVITY—No limits.

DIET—No special diet.

 ## CALL YOUR DOCTOR IF

• You or a family member has symptoms of granuloma annulare.
• The disorder recurs.

GRANULOMA INGUINALE
(Donovanosis)

GENERAL INFORMATION

DEFINITION—A sexually transmitted disease generally affecting people living in tropical climates. It is becoming more common in the U.S., especially in the south and southwest regions. Incubation period is 8 to 12 weeks.

BODY PARTS INVOLVED—Genitals.

SEX OR AGE MOST AFFECTED—Both sexes; all ages.

SIGNS & SYMPTOMS
* Formation of a nonpainful lesion (cyst, papule, or nodule) in the genital area that does not readily heal. This lesion ulcerates (becomes open and runny) and may spread so that it involves most of the vulva, and sometimes the buttocks and lower abdomen.
* Marked discomfort occurs if the ulceration spreads to the urethra or anal area. Walking, sitting and sexual intercourse become painful.
* Vaginal discharge that has an unpleasant odor.

CAUSES—An organism, *Calymmatobacterium granulomatis* (Donovan body), that is spread via sexual intercourse with an infected person.

RISK INCREASES WITH
* Multiple sexual partners.
* Unprotected intercourse.
* Infection with other sexually transmitted diseases.

HOW TO PREVENT
* Monogamous sexual relationship.
* Having the male partner use a latex condom.
* Cleansing of the genital area before and after sex. Douching is usually not effective.
* If there has been good possibility of exposure, seek medical care immediately. Early treatment may head off the infection.

WHAT TO EXPECT

DIAGNOSTIC MEASURES
* Diagnosis is confirmed with laboratory studies of scrapings or biopsies of the lesions.
* Testing (screening) for other sexually transmitted diseases is often recommended.

APPROPRIATE HEALTH CARE
* Treatment is with drug therapy.
* A follow-up medical examination after treatment is important to verify that healing is complete.

POSSIBLE COMPLICATIONS
* Secondary bacterial infection.
* Relapse may occur if treatment is stopped too soon.
* Scars may form where infection occurred.

PROBABLE OUTCOME—With treatment, healing should begin within a few days, but complete resolution will take up to 3 weeks.

HOW TO TREAT

GENERAL MEASURES
* Sitz baths frequently relieve soreness. Sit in a tub of hot water for 10 to 15 minutes. Repeat baths as often as 3 or 4 times a day.
* Sexual partners should be examined for infection.
* To learn more: Sexually Transmitted Diseases Hotline, (800) 227-8922.

MEDICATION—An antibiotic, such as trimethoprim-sulfamethoxazole, doxycycline, ciprofloxacin or erythromycin will be prescribed. If lesions do not respond within the first few days of therapy, another drug may be added to the treatment. Do not discontinue treatment until healing is complete or when advised to by your health care provider.

ACTIVITY—Avoid sexual intercourse during the active phase of the infection.

DIET—No special diet. If taking tetracycline, avoid dairy products within 3 hours of taking the medicine.

CALL YOUR DOCTOR IF

* You or a family member has symptoms of granuloma inguinale.
* Symptoms don't start improving within a few days after starting medication.
* Symptoms worsen despite treatment.
* New, unexplained symptoms develop. Drugs used in treatment may produce side effects.

GRANULOMA, PYOGENIC

GENERAL INFORMATION

DEFINITION—A fairly common skin growth. It is not contagious or cancerous. Pyogenic granuloma can involve skin anywhere on the body.

BODY PARTS INVOLVED—Skin anywhere on the body. It often affects the head, neck, upper trunk, and fingers. It can also affect the gums and other mucous membranes of the mouth.

SEX OR AGE MOST AFFECTED
- Children of both sexes (ages 5 to 15).
- Pregnant women.

SIGNS & SYMPTOMS
- Papule (small, raised bump on the skin). Usually, a single one is present, but in rare cases, there may be multiple papules.
- It first appears as pinhead-sized, but it grows rapidly over a period of a few weeks to about a half inch in size.
- The color is scarlet, brown, or blue-black.
- Will bleed easily when injured.
- They don't hurt or itch.
- May ulcerate (become an open sore) and form a crust.

CAUSES—Unknown. Pyogenic refers to an infectious process, but these lesions are misnamed. Because they frequently appear in late childhood or pregnancy, hormonal changes may be a factor in their development.

RISK INCREASES WITH
- Pregnancy.
- Recent injury (they may develop at the injured site).
- Use of certain drugs (such as oral contraceptives, retinoids, or protease inhibitors).

HOW TO PREVENT
- Cannot be prevented at present.
- Because pyogenic granuloma resembles melanoma (skin cancer), medical diagnosis can be important.

WHAT TO EXPECT

DIAGNOSTIC MEASURES
- Your own observation of symptoms.
- Your health care provider will do an exam of the affected skin area.
- Medical tests usually include a skin biopsy (removal of a small amount of tissue for viewing under a microscope).

APPROPRIATE HEALTH CARE
- The growths can be removed by several different methods.
- Often, they are scraped off with an instrument called a curette and then cauterized (using heat to heal tissue). This helps to decrease the chance that they will regrow.
- Laser surgery can be used to destroy the growth.
- In some cases, it may be treated with chemicals (such as silver nitrate).
- The growth may be removed by surgery excision and closed with stitches.
- If a drug is the cause of the pyogenic granuloma, stopping the drug often leads to healing.

POSSIBLE COMPLICATIONS—Recurrence is common.

PROBABLE OUTCOME—Some heal on their own (such as in pregnancy). Others can be successfully treated.

HOW TO TREAT

GENERAL MEASURES—Follow medical advice for self-care after any treatment procedure.

MEDICATION
- For minor pain, you may use nonprescription drugs such as acetaminophen or aspirin. Don't give aspirin to children under age 18.
- If the scab cracks or oozes, apply a nonprescription antibiotic ointment several times a day.

ACTIVITY—No limits, except to avoid injury to the area while it is healing.

DIET—No special diet.

CALL YOUR DOCTOR IF

- You or a family member has symptoms of pyogenic granuloma.
- The wound bleeds after surgery, and applying pressure for 10 minutes cannot stop it.
- The wound shows signs of infection, such as redness, swelling, pain, or increased tenderness.

GRIEF
(Bereavement)

GENERAL INFORMATION

DEFINITION—The emotional reaction following the death of a loved person, a divorce, loss of a body part or its function, loss of self-esteem (such as losing a job), or other significant loss. Grief is a normal, appropriate reaction to loss. It comes in many forms. Grieving people gradually adjust to their loss and begin to make positive plans for the future. There are no guidelines for the normal time for grieving. Sometimes, grief is serious or long-lasting enough that medical help is needed.

BODY PARTS INVOLVED—Sometimes all.

SEX OR AGE MOST AFFECTED—Both sexes; all ages.

SIGNS & SYMPTOMS
* Feelings of sadness, numbness, pain, anger, despair, or guilt. These feelings can come and go for months, and may be overwhelming at times.
* Sudden crying spells.
* Hallucinations (such as a sense of having seen or heard the dead person).
* Anxiety and depression.
* Being unwilling to accept the loss; for example, keeping the dead person's room or clothing as if he or she is expected to return.
* Unable to sleep.
* Nervousness and being overactive.
* Stomach problems.
* Tiredness, agitation, tearfulness.
* Increased use of alcohol and other drugs.

CAUSES—A normal reaction to a loss.

RISK INCREASES WITH—Existing emotional problems can affect how a person responds to loss. This includes depression, social aloneness, strong feelings of guilt, self-blame, or anger due to one's relationship with the dead person.

HOW TO PREVENT—Grieving should not be prevented or denied. It is a normal and expected response to a loss.

WHAT TO EXPECT

DIAGNOSTIC MEASURES
* Your own observation of symptoms.
* See your health care provider if the feelings of grief are severe, or continue interfering with your daily life and/or work. A physical exam may be done and questions asked about your symptoms and feelings.

APPROPRIATE HEALTH CARE—Grief counseling may be recommended. It can help bring about a healthy resolution of grief.

POSSIBLE COMPLICATIONS
* Difficulty maintaining relationships and jobs.
* Excess use of alcohol or other drugs.
* Chronic anxiety and depression.
* Symptoms that may need medical help include:
  - Severe depression, panic attacks, chronic anxiety.
  - Strong feelings of guilt, bitterness, or remorse.
  - Grief continues for 2 years or more. A person may build a life around the grief and never accept the loss.
  - Talk about or threats of suicide.

PROBABLE OUTCOME—With time, the grief lessens and adjustment begins. Your mind, body, and spirit will begin to heal. The feelings of grief may come and go, and will probably recur occasionally for years.

HOW TO TREAT

GENERAL MEASURES
* Express your feelings following the loss. Don't keep them "bottled up" inside. Look to family and friends for help and support.
* Religious or spiritual help may be of benefit to some people. Talk to your pastor or other religious professional about your feelings.
* Join a grief support group. They are available in most areas. People often find comfort in sharing their feelings with others who have had similar experiences.
* Slowly begin to rebuild your life. Interest yourself in things you have enjoyed in the past or try some new activities.
* Avoid the overuse of alcohol or drugs to suppress the emotions that you are feeling.
* Don't expect your feelings of grief to follow any pattern or a particular timetable.

MEDICATION—You may be prescribed drugs, such as sedatives or antidepressants, for a short time. In most cases, drugs are not needed.

ACTIVITY—Normally, no limits. Try to do some physical activity daily.

DIET—Eat a normal, well-balanced diet.

CALL YOUR DOCTOR IF

* You or a family member has symptoms of grief that are getting worse or not getting better with time.
* Any of the Possible Complications occur.

GUILLAIN-BARRé SYNDROME
(Infectious Polyneuropathy)

GENERAL INFORMATION

DEFINITION—A rare, inflammatory condition involving the peripheral nerves. These are nerves outside the brain and spinal column. It causes rapid weakness and loss of sensation.

BODY PARTS INVOLVED—Central nervous system.

SEX OR AGE MOST AFFECTED—Both sexes; all ages, but is more common in young adults and the elderly.

SIGNS & SYMPTOMS
- Muscle weakness starting in the lower limbs (feet and legs) and moving up to the abdomen and chest, and to the arms and hands. The weakness spreads over days to weeks.
- Facial weakness and drooping, double vision, difficulty in speaking, and in swallowing.
- Pain, often in the back and legs; muscle cramps and tenderness; numbness, tingling, or burning sensations.
- Irregular heart beat, high or low blood pressure.
- Shortness of breath.
- Complete paralysis (sometimes) for weeks or months.

CAUSES—Unknown. It may be an autoimmune disorder. It sometimes follows a bacterial or viral infection.

RISK INCREASES WITH—Recent illness, such as a respiratory infection or gastroenteritis (stomach flu).

HOW TO PREVENT—No preventive measures.

WHAT TO EXPECT

DIAGNOSTIC MEASURES
- Your own observation of symptoms.
- Your health care provider may be able to diagnose the disorder by the symptoms and with a physical exam.
- Medical tests may be done, such as lumbar puncture for spinal fluid analysis, electromyography (studying nerve and muscle disorders by recording electrical activity of muscles), and lung function tests.

APPROPRIATE HEALTH CARE
- Hospital care is needed in an intensive care unit so the condition can be closely monitored. There is no specific treatment for the disorder. Care involves supportive measures and methods to help speed recovery.
- A respirator (breathing machine) may be needed if muscles of respiration become greatly weakened. A tracheotomy (opening in the throat for breathing) may be required.

- Immunotherapy may be used to help shorten the duration and severity of the disease. It involves either plasmapheresis or IV immune globulin (injections).
- Plasmapheresis is a procedure where blood plasma is withdrawn from the patient, treated to remove antibodies, and then returned to the body by transfusion.
- Rehabilitation will begin as soon as it is feasible. It may involve physical therapy, occupational therapy (to promote self-care), speech therapy (to help with speaking and swallowing problems), and recreational therapy (helps the patient adjust to any disability).

POSSIBLE COMPLICATIONS
- A relapse may occur after initial improvement.
- Respiratory failure.
- Permanent muscle weakness or numbness.
- Permanent total or partial paralysis (rare).
- Pneumonia.
- Deep vein thrombosis.
- Contractures of joints.

PROBABLE OUTCOME
- Complete recovery without any lasting effects in many cases. Adults recover better than children. For some persons, symptoms clear in 15 to 20 days. Others require a year or more. Many mechanical devices can aid mobility until the person recovers.
- Some patients will have moderate lasting effects, and a few will have severe disabilities.

HOW TO TREAT

GENERAL MEASURES—To learn more: Guillain-Barré Foundation, P.O. Box 262, Wynnewood, PA 19096; (610) 667-0131 (not toll free); website: www.guillain-barre.com.

MEDICATION
- IVIG (IV immune globulin) may be prescribed.
- Drugs as needed for symptoms, such as pain.

ACTIVITY
- Remain as active as muscle strength permits. Have a family member or physical therapist passively move and stretch muscles.
- Ongoing physical therapy will be needed to rebuild strength.

DIET—A feeding tube may be needed for patient with severe swallowing problem.

CALL YOUR DOCTOR IF

- You or a family member has symptoms of Guillain-Barré syndrome.
- New symptoms occur after a patient returns home.

ILLNESS & DISORDERS

HAND, FOOT & MOUTH DISEASE

GENERAL INFORMATION

DEFINITION—A common childhood infection with symptoms that begin in the mouth and throat.

BODY PARTS INVOLVED—Throat; tonsils; skin; gastrointestinal tract; central nervous system.

SEX OR AGE MOST AFFECTED—It most often affects children under the age of 10. Adults may get the infection, but it is less common.

SIGNS & SYMPTOMS
* Sore throat with blisters and sores in the mouth and throat lining.
* Sudden fever that is usually mild.
* Rash with blisters on the hands, feet, and groin.
* Refusal to eat.
* Stomach pain or headache (sometimes).

CAUSES—Viral infection commonly caused by coxsackieviruses. The germs are spread from person to person or by touching an object (such as a toy) that has the germs on it. It takes about 3 to 6 days after exposure for the symptoms to start. Outbreaks may occur in nursery schools or child-care centers.

RISK INCREASES WITH—Summer and fall seasons.

HOW TO PREVENT
* No specific preventive measures.
* Try to prevent exposure of infants and young children to anyone with an infection. Wash hands often to prevent spread of germs.
* Pregnant women should consult their obstetric provider if they are exposed to an infected person.

WHAT TO EXPECT

DIAGNOSTIC MEASURES
* Your own observation of symptoms.
* See your health care provider if you are concerned about the symptoms. Diagnosing the infection can be done by an exam of the affected mouth and skin area.
* Other medical tests are normally not needed.

APPROPRIATE HEALTH CARE
* Home care is usually all that is required for this infection.
* There is no specific treatment for the infection, but treatment may help relieve pain and fever symptoms.

POSSIBLE COMPLICATIONS
* The infection may be more serious in some infants and dehydration can occur.
* Other complications are rare.

PROBABLE OUTCOME—The infection is usually mild and complete recovery occurs in about a week. It rarely recurs once someone has had the infection.

HOW TO TREAT

GENERAL MEASURES
* Rinse the mouth with salt water (1/2 teaspoon salt to 1 cup water) after eating, if the child is old enough to rinse without swallowing.
* Use separate dishes or disposable plates and cups to help avoid spreading the infection to other children in the family.

MEDICATION—To reduce high fever or for pain, you may use nonprescription drugs such as acetaminophen. Don't use aspirin in children under age 18. Antibiotics are not effective for this infection.

ACTIVITY—Have the child get extra rest at home until any fever is gone. Children may return to school or daycare while they still have the rash.

DIET—Encourage the child to increase their fluid and soft food intake. This may include milk, liquid gelatin, ice cream, custard, or special products that you can buy at grocery or drug stores.

CALL YOUR DOCTOR IF

* Your child has symptoms of hand, foot and mouth disease that cause you concern.
* Symptoms get worse or do not improve.

HANTAVIRUS
(Hantaviral Pulmonary Syndrome)

 GENERAL INFORMATION

DEFINITION—Hantavirus (named after a place in Korea) causes an illness called hantavirus pulmonary syndrome (HPS). Hantavirus has probably caused people to get sick for years in the United States, but it was not known about until recent years.

BODY PARTS INVOLVED—Respiratory system.

SEX OR AGE MOST AFFECTED—Both sexes; all ages.

SIGNS & SYMPTOMS
Early symptoms are flu-like:
• Chills.
• Fever.
• Muscle aches.
• Cough.
• General ill feeling.
• Feeling tired; lack of energy.
• Somewhat short of breath.
Later symptoms:
• Extreme difficulty in breathing.

CAUSES—Several types of mice can carry the hantavirus without getting ill. Where they nest, they leave the germs in their urine, feces (droppings), and saliva. If the nests are disturbed, the germs can get into the air as dust. When humans breathe in the air containing the germs, they can become infected. Infection may also come from a mouse bite, or from germs in food, water, or on something you touched. It may take a few days to 6 weeks for symptoms to appear once a person is exposed to the germs. The germs are not passed between humans.

RISK INCREASES WITH—No known specific risk factors.

HOW TO PREVENT
• Avoid exposure to rodent urine and feces.
• Use caution in cleaning areas where mice nests might be located.
• Keep a clean home. This includes clearing out potential nesting sites and maintaining a clean kitchen.

 WHAT TO EXPECT

DIAGNOSTIC MEASURES
• Your own observation of symptoms.
• The breathing problems progress very quickly and treatment must occur in the hospital. Usually this is in an intensive care unit. Your health care provider will do a physical exam and discuss the possible exposure to rodents.
• A number of medical tests will be done to confirm the diagnosis.

APPROPRIATE HEALTH CARE
• The main treatment is to help with any breathing problems.
• Supplemental oxygen is used to help the breathing. In severe cases, a machine may be needed to assist with the breathing.

POSSIBLE COMPLICATIONS—Hantavirus pulmonary syndrome is a serious infection, and is fatal in about one-third of cases.

PROBABLE OUTCOME—The outcome will vary for each patient. To date, there is no treatment to stop the infection once it sets in. But steps can be taken to help control the symptoms while your body fights off the infection.

 HOW TO TREAT

GENERAL MEASURES—The family should maintain an optimistic outlook, stay in close contact with the patient's doctor and help by making their visits with the patient brief and as supportive as possible.

MEDICATION—Drugs will be prescribed as needed to help control any bleeding and improve lung function.

ACTIVITY—Bed rest for acute illness; resume normal activities gradually.

DIET—May require feeding through a vein (IV) while in the hospital. Then return to a regular diet with recovery.

 CALL YOUR DOCTOR IF

You or a family member has symptoms of hantavirus pulmonary syndrome, especially if you live in an area, or have traveled to an area, where the virus is present.

ILLNESS & DISORDERS

HAY FEVER
(Allergic Rhinitis)

GENERAL INFORMATION

DEFINITION—An allergic response to an allergen in the air. Attacks occur in pollen season. The name is confusing as hay does not cause allergic an reaction and there is no fever.

BODY PARTS INVOLVED—Hay fever affects the eyes, nose, sinuses, throat, and bronchial tubes in the lungs.

SEX OR AGE MOST AFFECTED—Both sexes; all ages.

SIGNS & SYMPTOMS
* Itching, watery eyes.
* Frequent sneezing; stuffy nose with a clear discharge.
* Itching in the roof of the mouth.
* Wheezing (sometimes).
* Burning in the throat.

CAUSES
* The body's immune system produces antibodies that release a chemical called histamine. Histamine in turn produces swelling and irritation in the nose, sinuses, and eyes.
* Allergens in the air that cause an allergic sensitivity include: Pollen (from weeds, flowers, grasses, and trees), mold, dust, mites, tobacco smoke, and other air pollutants.

RISK INCREASES WITH
* Having other allergic reactions, such as eczema or asthma.
* Smoking.
* Spring and autumn. Most plants produce pollen during these seasons.
* Family history of allergies.
* Weak immune system due to drugs or illness.

HOW TO PREVENT—There is no way to prevent having allergies. You can take steps to help prevent having symptoms.

WHAT TO EXPECT

DIAGNOSTIC MEASURES
* Your own observation of symptoms.
* Your health care provider will do a physical exam and ask questions about your symptoms.
* Medical tests such as blood and allergy skin tests may be recommended, but are usually not required for diagnosis.

APPROPRIATE HEALTH CARE—Medical care may include drugs and desensitizing treatment.

POSSIBLE COMPLICATIONS
* Difficulty in sleeping and chronic fatigue.
* Increased risk for other infections.

PROBABLE OUTCOME—Symptoms can be helped with treatment. The condition persists over a lifetime. It is usually more troublesome than disabling.

HOW TO TREAT

GENERAL MEASURES
* Try to remove as many allergens from your home or the surrounding property area as able.
* Prepare your bedroom as follows:
  - Empty the room of furniture, rugs or carpet, and drapes or curtains. Clean the walls, woodwork, and floors with a damp mop. Wax the floor.
  - Cover box springs, mattress, and pillows with plastic covers. Use bedclothes that can be washed often.
  - Use throw rugs that can be washed easily.
  - Use wood or plastic chairs, not stuffed chairs.
  - Use window shade/blind, not drape/curtain.
  - Use vacuum cleaner, damp rags, and damp or oiled mop to clean bedroom every week.
* Other preventive measures:
  - Keep windows and doors closed if possible.
  - Don't handle objects that are very dusty, such as books or stored clothing.
  - No stuffed animals or toys in the house.
  - Remove all pets (except fish) from the house.
  - Wear a filter face-mask during exposure to allergens, including during housecleaning.
  - Install an air-purification unit in your home's heating and air-conditioning system, preferably a high-efficiency particulate (HEPA) filter.
  - Drive an air-conditioned car.
  - Have someone else mow the lawn.

MEDICATION—You may be prescribed:
* Antihistamines; decongestants; cortisone eyedrops or nasal spray; cortisone tablets (severe cases only); cromolyn nasal spray; or cromolyn nose drops. These drugs relieve symptoms, but they don't cure hay fever.
* Desensitization injections for known allergens for severe or year-round cases. Once allergens are known (through skin or blood tests), small amounts are injected over a period of time. This helps block the immune system from releasing the histamine. This process may take months or years for effective results.

ACTIVITY—No limits. Avoid areas with known allergens.

DIET—No special diet.

CALL YOUR DOCTOR IF

* You or a family member has symptoms of hay fever that are interfering with normal activities.
* Symptoms worsen or don't improve with treatment.

HEAD INJURY

GENERAL INFORMATION

DEFINITION—Injury to the head. Head injuries may be internal (penetrating) or external (closed). They can cause physical problems, cognitive (thinking) dysfunction, or emotional changes. Most head injuries are minor (such as a small bump or "goose egg" on the head), but some can be life-threatening or cause permanent brain damage.

BODY PARTS INVOLVED—It involves the scalp, skull, or brain.

SEX OR AGE MOST AFFECTED—Both sexes; all ages. Young children, teens, and the elderly are more often affected.

SIGNS & SYMPTOMS
- Head injury symptoms may occur right away, or hours or days later. Signs and symptoms can include one or more of the following effects.
- Swelling, bleeding at the site of the injury.
- Fracture of the skull.
- Loss of consciousness (short time or for long period).
- Abnormal breathing.
- Clear or bloody fluid from nose, mouth, or ear.
- Drowsiness, confusion, irritability, or loss of memory.
- Unable to feel or control muscle function.
- Black-and-blue color around the eyes.
- Vomiting and nausea.
- Changes in vision or speech.
- Pupils of different sizes.
- Dizziness.
- Pain, such as headache or stiff neck.
- Seizure.

CAUSES
- Accidents (motor vehicle, work-related, sports, falls, physical assault, outdoor activities, and in the home).
- Child abuse or shaken baby syndrome.

RISK INCREASES WITH
- Alcohol or substance abuse.
- Contact sports, such as football, soccer, or boxing.
- Prior head injury.
- Illnesses that affect balance or walking ability.
- Not using seat belts or not wearing helmets.

HOW TO PREVENT
- Don't drink or use drugs of abuse and drive.
- Use proper headgear if head injury is a risk.
- Use your auto seat belt always. Place young children in approved safety car seats.

WHAT TO EXPECT

DIAGNOSTIC MEASURES
- Your own observation of symptoms.
- Medical care starts with checking the person's ABCs (airway, breathing, and circulation). Any visible head injuries will be treated.
- Medical tests usually include testing the person's alertness. Other tests, such as x-ray, CT, or MRI (see Glossary for these tests) are often done to check for brain damage.

APPROPRIATE HEALTH CARE
- A person with a mild head injury can be sent home after initial medical care. Someone must stay with the person and watch for serious symptoms over the next 24 hours. Instructions may include waking the patient every 2 to 3 hours to check for alertness. Get medical help if you cannot awaken or arouse the person.
- In other head injuries, the treatment will depend on the severity. Hospital care may be needed for a period of time, and then rehabilitation care may be required.

POSSIBLE COMPLICATIONS—Permanent physical or mental disabilities, and social and economic problems (such as loss of job).

PROBABLE OUTCOME—The outcome will vary depending on a variety of factors (e.g., age, type of injury, severity of symptoms, and treatment). Many head injuries are mild and heal on their own with no lasting effects. Others can be treated successfully. Some may require extended hospital care and long-term rehabilitation.

HOW TO TREAT

GENERAL MEASURES
- Self-care is sometimes done for mild injuries. Get medical help right away if any of the symptoms listed occur or other head injury symptoms cause concern. Give first aid if needed. Call 911 for emergency help.
- To learn more: Brain Injury Association, 1776 Massachusetts Ave, NW, Washington, DC 20036; (800) 444-6443; website: www.biausa.org.

MEDICATION—For self-care, you may use acetaminophen for pain or discomfort. Avoid aspirin. It can increase bleeding risk.

ACTIVITY—After treatment, rest as needed. Follow your health care provider's instructions about resuming physical activity.

DIET—Food intake will depend on the extent of injury.

CALL YOUR DOCTOR IF

- You or a family member has symptoms of a head injury or observe them in someone else. Get emergency help if needed!
- After a head injury, you observe any new, changed, or worsening symptoms.

HEADACHE, CLUSTER

GENERAL INFORMATION

DEFINITION—A very severe headache that typically causes pain on one side of the head, behind the head, or around one eye. The headaches tend to recur at the same time each day for several days or weeks, separated by attack-free weeks or months.

BODY PARTS INVOLVED—Central nervous system.

SEX OR AGE MOST AFFECTED—About 90% of those affected are males. Onset is around age 30 in men, later in women.

SIGNS & SYMPTOMS
* Sudden onset of headache. It often occurs at night while sleeping.
* Headache reaches a peak within 15 minutes and lasts about 2 to 3 hours.
* Pain around the eye.
* Severe, piercing, or boring pain.
* Teary eyes.
* Swollen and droopy eyelid.
* Stuffy or runny nose.
* Slow heartbeat.
* Nausea.
* Sweating.

CAUSES—The cause is unknown. It may be a combination of factors, such as dilating blood vessels in the head, disturbance of the trigeminal nerve, or abnormal activity in part of the brain.

RISK INCREASES WITH
* Male, age over 30.
* Smoker.
* Previous head injury.
* Sleep apnea (periods of not breathing at night).
* Persons who are in stressful jobs, are self-employed, sociable, active, and responsible.
* Possibly a genetic factor (unproven as yet).

HOW TO PREVENT—Since the cause is unknown, no specific measures to prevent first episode.

WHAT TO EXPECT

DIAGNOSTIC MEASURES
* Your own observation of symptoms.
* Your health care provider can usually diagnose the disorder based on the history of the headache patterns and symptoms.
* Medical tests are normally not required.

APPROPRIATE HEALTH CARE
* Treatment goals are to treat the symptoms and prevent or abort future attacks. It may involve drug therapy, use of oxygen, and lifestyle changes.

* Surgical treatments may be considered when drug therapy is not helpful. Surgery has limited effectiveness.

POSSIBLE COMPLICATIONS—Cluster headaches do not cause complications or lead to other disorders. They are debilitating and can interfere with daily activities.

PROBABLE OUTCOME—The cluster headache attacks may come and go, or be ongoing. Many people are headache-free for a year or more, but then they may start up again. Various drug therapies are available that can help control attacks.

HOW TO TREAT

GENERAL MEASURES
* During cluster periods, avoid bright light or glare, alcohol, excessive anger, stressful activity, or excitement. These can trigger attacks. Keeping a headache diary may be useful to help identify other triggers.
* Don't smoke. It may interfere with drug therapy.
* Some patients also have sleep apnea. Treating the apnea (with a mechanical device) helps headaches also.
* To learn more: National Headache Foundation, 428 West St. James Pl., 2nd Flr., Chicago, IL 60614; (888) 643-5552; website: www.headaches.org.

MEDICATION—Your health care provider may prescribe one or more drugs to treat the headache and for prevention:
* Drugs called triptans (by mouth or by injection).
* Dihydroergotamine (Migranal) by injection.
* Ergotamine tartrate, in a tablet, suppository, aerosol, or injection form.
* Oxygen therapy for home use.
* Lidocaine nasal spray or nasal drops.
* Phenylephrine (can be used for nasal stuffiness).
* Other drugs as needed to help treat or prevent cluster headaches.

ACTIVITY—Vigorous physical activity at first symptoms may abort attack.

DIET—Avoid alcohol and foods containing nitrates (such as smoked meat).

CALL YOUR DOCTOR IF

* You or a family member has symptoms of cluster headache.
* Attacks continue after treatment is started.

HEADACHE, MIGRAINE

GENERAL INFORMATION

DEFINITION—A severe type of headache that involves more than just the headache pain. There are five stages that may occur with a migraine. Prodrome (warning signs), aura (beginning symptoms), headache itself, resolution (pain stops), and postdrome (tiredness and other symptoms).

BODY PARTS INVOLVED—Central nervous system.

SEX OR AGE MOST AFFECTED—Migraines may start occurring before age 20, affect both sexes, and are more common in females.

SIGNS & SYMPTOMS
• The nature of attacks varies between persons and from time to time in the same person.
• Prodrome (hours/days before attack). It can include changes in mood, behavior, energy, and appetite.
• Aura (minutes or an hour before attack). It affects vision, hearing, or smell.
 - The most common symptoms are the inability to see clearly and seeing bright spots and zig-zag patterns.
 - Visual disturbances may last several minutes or several hours and stop once the headache begins.
• Headache. Dull, boring pain in the temple that spreads to the entire side of the head.
 - Pain becomes worse and throbs. Nausea, vomiting, and/or sensitivity to light and sound.
 - Headaches can last from 4 to 72 hours.
• Postdrome (may occur after an attack and last for hours or days). It includes exhaustion, weakness, lethargy, and elation (in some cases).

CAUSES—Exact cause is unknown. It may be due to a central nervous system disturbance that sets off a chain of events in the body. Genetic factors are involved also.

RISK INCREASES WITH
• Females.
• Family history of migraines.
• Other disorders (such as asthma, allergies, *H. pylori* infection, epilepsy, fibromyalgia) and possibly, certain nasal cavity problems.

HOW TO PREVENT—No preventive steps for first attack. After diagnosis, take steps to help prevent future attacks. Try to avoid the triggers of migraines (such as some foods and drugs, bright lights, weather changes, high altitudes, and stress). Keep a diary to learn your own specific triggers.

WHAT TO EXPECT

DIAGNOSTIC MEASURES
• Your own observation of symptoms.

• Your health care provider can usually diagnose the disorder based on the history of the headache pattern and symptoms.
• Medical tests are normally not required.

APPROPRIATE HEALTH CARE
• Treatment is usually with drugs and self-care.
• Hospital care possibly for a severe attack.
• Counseling, behavior therapy, or stress reduction techniques may be recommended.
• Sinus surgery for nasal problem in rare cases.

POSSIBLE COMPLICATIONS
• Interferes with day-to-day life (work, family, or social).
• Status migraine (lasts over 72 hours) or stroke (rare).

PROBABLE OUTCOME—People with migraines tend to have them over many years. They can often be controlled with treatment. Migraines may end when a person gets older.

HOW TO TREAT

GENERAL MEASURES
• For self-care at the first sign of a migraine:
 - Apply a cold cloth to your head; lie down in a quiet, dark room; relax and sleep if possible.
 - Minimize noise, light, and odors (such as cooking odors and tobacco smoke). Don't read.
• To learn more: National Headache Foundation, 428 West St. James Pl., 2nd Flr., Chicago, IL 60614; (888) 643-5552; website: www.headaches.org.

MEDICATION—No single drug works best for everyone. A variety of drugs can be prescribed for symptoms and prevention:
• Triptans by subcutaneous (under the skin) self-injection, oral tablet, or nasal spray.
• Ergot preparations in a tablet, suppository, aerosol, or injection form.
• Use nonprescription drugs such as ibuprofen, or aspirin (if over age 18), or acetaminophen.
• Narcotics or butalbital.
• Antihistamines to expand blood vessels.
• Antiemetics to decrease nausea and vomiting.
• Vasoconstrictors to narrow blood vessels.
• Beta-adrenergic, calcium channel blockers, or antidepressants to prevent attacks.
• Note: Overuse of drugs can cause a "rebound" into another headache.

ACTIVITY—Exercise daily to maintain fitness.

DIET—Keep a diary to see if certain foods trigger migraines.

CALL YOUR DOCTOR IF

• You or a family member has migraine symptoms.
• Treatment is not helping the migraines.

ILLNESS & DISORDERS

HEADACHE, TENSION

GENERAL INFORMATION

DEFINITION—Tension headaches are the most common type of headache. These headaches may occur on 15 days out of a month (chronic) or less often (episodic).

BODY PARTS INVOLVED—Sensory nerves in the skin, scalp, blood vessels and muscles of the head.

SEX OR AGE MOST AFFECTED—Both sexes; all ages.

SIGNS & SYMPTOMS
- Dull, steady pain on both sides of the head. The pain may be mild to severe. It usually comes on gradually.
- Tight feeling or tenderness in the muscles of the head, neck or scalp. "Like a band around the head."
- Some people may clench their teeth.
- Tension headaches are different from migraines, which cause intense pain, usually on one side of the head. Migraines also cause nausea and light sensitivity.

CAUSES—The cause is not clearly understood. It now appears that it is caused by a problem of the central nervous system and changes in brain chemicals. It has been thought the cause was stress and tension that puts strain on the muscles of the neck, scalp, face, and jaw. There are other possible causes being studied also.

RISK INCREASES WITH
People who might get tension headaches:
- Women (more often affected than men).
- Those who are overworked on a continuous basis.
- Persons with chronic poor posture.
- Persons with sleep disorders.
- Those who suffer from depression, stress, or anxiety.
- Certain chronic medical problems.
- Abuse of alcohol or other substances.

Things that might bring on (trigger) a tension headaches include:
- A stressful event.
- Eating certain foods.
- Not eating on time; caffeine withdrawal.
- Intense physical exercise.
- Taking certain drugs.
- Hormone changes in women.
- Eyestrain.
- Fatigue.
- Having a cold or the flu.

HOW TO PREVENT—Avoid any of the risk factors when possible.

WHAT TO EXPECT

DIAGNOSTIC MEASURES
- Your own observation of symptoms.
- Your health care provider will do a physical exam, and ask questions about your symptoms and your lifestyle.
- Medical tests and blood studies may be done to be sure no other medical problem involved.

APPROPRIATE HEALTH CARE
- Chronic tension headaches may be treated with different methods for stress reduction and relaxation techniques, and prescribed drugs. Drugs that have been overused for headache pain may need to be withdrawn.
- There are more treatment options that you and your health care provider may discuss. These may include physical therapy, hypnosis, massage therapy, and others.

POSSIBLE COMPLICATIONS
- None expected for a simple headache.
- Chronic tension headaches may require trying several types of treatment. The headaches may continue if the risk factors are not changed or treated.

PROBABLE OUTCOME—Most tension headaches can be relieved with treatment, and do not disrupt home or work activities.

HOW TO TREAT

GENERAL MEASURES
- Self-care can include mild pain relievers. If possible, stop what you are doing and try to relax. Take a hot bath or shower. Lie down. Place a warm or cold cloth, whichever feels better, over the aching area.
- To learn more: National Headache Foundation, 820 N. Orleans, Suite 217, Chicago, IL 60610, (888) 643-5552; website: www.headache.org.

MEDICATION
- You may take nonprescription pain relievers such as ibuprofen, naproxen, aspirin (adults), or acetaminophen.
- Stronger drugs, for pain, and drugs to prevent chronic tension headaches may be prescribed.

ACTIVITY—Exercise on a regular basis and get enough sleep.

DIET—Eat a normal, healthy diet.

CALL YOUR DOCTOR IF

- You or a family member has tension headaches and self-care steps are not working.
- Headaches recur or get worse despite treatment or new drugs cause side effects.

HEARING IMPAIRMENT OR LOSS (Deafness)

GENERAL INFORMATION

DEFINITION—Hearing loss may be partial or total. It may develop gradually or suddenly. It may occur at any age. There are two types of hearing loss:
- Conductive loss. It is caused by anything that blocks the conduction of sound from the outer ear through to the inner ear.
- Sensorineural loss. It results from damage to the inner ear such as to the auditory nerve or hair cells of the cochlea. This type includes the gradual hearing loss that occurs with aging called presbycusis.
- A mixed loss is both types of hearing loss.

BODY PARTS INVOLVED—Middle-ear bones that conduct sound; branches of the 8th cranial nerve that transmit sound to the brain.

SEX OR AGE MOST AFFECTED—Both sexes; all ages.

SIGNS & SYMPTOMS
- In an infant, there is a lack of response to sounds.
- Trouble understanding speech. Misunderstanding others and responding inappropriately.
- Difficulty in hearing a phone ring, or problem hearing over the phone.
- Difficulty hearing in a group of people or when there is background noise.
- Avoiding social activities (may feel embarrassed).
- Turning up the volume of the radio or television.
- Asking others to repeat themselves.
- Ringing in the ears, dizziness, or pain.

CAUSES—Hearing loss occurs when any part of the hearing system is unable to function. A wide variety of conditions can cause hearing loss. Sometimes, no cause is found.

RISK INCREASES WITH
Conductive:
- Middle ear infection (otitis media).
- Collection of fluid in middle ear (glue ear).
- Blockage of the outer ear by wax.
- Damage to the eardrum from infection or injury.
- Otosclerosis (growth of spongy tissue in ears).
- Rheumatoid arthritis affects joints in ear (rare).
Sensorineural:
- Aging (hearing starts decreasing in the 30s and 40s).
- Noise exposure (repeated and continuous).
- Viral infection such as mumps.
- Ménière's disease.
- Certain drugs (aspirin, quinine, some antibiotics).
- Acoustic neuroma (benign tumor).
- Brain infection, inflammation or tumor.
- Multiple sclerosis.
- Stroke.
- Congenital (present at birth). A family history of hearing loss is also a risk factor.

HOW TO PREVENT—Avoid the risk factors where possible. Get medical care for any infections or any symptoms of hearing loss.

WHAT TO EXPECT

DIAGNOSTIC MEASURES
- Your health care provider will do an exam of the ears and ask about your symptoms.
- Hearing tests may include tests done with a tuning fork and an audiogram (to measure hearing levels). Other hearing studies and speech testing may be done. Tests help determine the extent of hearing loss and whether it is conductive or sensorineural.

APPROPRIATE HEALTH CARE
- Treatment will depend on the cause. It may involve simple procedures (like earwax removal), drug therapy, surgical treatments, and sound amplification (hearing aids). You may be asked to consult a health care provider who specializes in hearing problems.
- If the hearing loss is related to drugs, changes in dosage or stopping the drug may help.

POSSIBLE COMPLICATIONS
- Complete loss of hearing (deafness).
- Language delay or learning problems in a child.
- Emotional, social, and work-associated problems.

PROBABLE OUTCOME—The outcome depends on the cause. The hearing loss may be temporary, treatable, or manageable.

HOW TO TREAT

GENERAL MEASURES—To learn more: National Institute on Deafness and Other Communication Disorders, 31 Center Dr., MSC 2320, Bethesda, MD 20892, (800) 241-1044; website: www.nidcd.nih.gov/health/hearing.

MEDICATION—Drugs may be prescribed for any treatable disorder that is diagnosed.

ACTIVITY—No limits.

DIET—No special diet.

CALL YOUR DOCTOR IF

- You suspect you have a hearing loss, especially if you must ask others often to repeat themselves or family members frequently ask you if your hearing is all right.
- A family member shows signs of hearing loss.

HEART ATTACK
(Myocardial Infarction)

 GENERAL INFORMATION

DEFINITION—A sudden instance of abnormal heart function. A heart attack is a life-threatening event.

BODY PARTS INVOLVED—Coronary arteries; heart muscle; platelets and clotting factors circulating in the blood.

SEX OR AGE MOST AFFECTED—Adults over 40. This is more common in men, but the incidence is rising for women.

SIGNS & SYMPTOMS
* Chest pain or "heavy, squeezing, or crushing" feeling in the chest.
* Pain that radiates from the midchest over the breast bone to the jaw, neck, either arm, the area between the shoulder blades, or upper abdomen (sometimes).
* Feeling of impending doom.
* Shortness of breath.
* Nausea and vomiting.
* Sweating.
* Dizziness and/or weakness.
* Choking sensation.

CAUSES—A heart attack occurs when the supply of blood and oxygen to an area of heart muscle is blocked. This is usually due to a blood clot in a coronary artery. The blockage leads to an irregular heartbeat or rhythm that causes a severe decrease in heart function. When the heart actually stops, it is called cardiac arrest.

RISK INCREASES WITH
* Men over age 45 and women over age 55.
* Family history of early heart disease.
* Having coronary artery disease (CAD).
* Smoking.
* Obesity.
* High LDL cholesterol levels or low HDL cholesterol.
* High blood pressure.
* Diabetes.
* Sedentary lifestyle (lack of physical activity).

HOW TO PREVENT—Exercise daily. Maintain a healthy weight. Eat a healthy diet. Don't smoke. Get medical care for diabetes, high blood pressure, and high cholesterol. A daily, low-dose aspirin may be prescribed.

 WHAT TO EXPECT

DIAGNOSTIC MEASURES —Diagnosis and treatment of a heart attack begins when emergency medical personnel arrive after you call 911. In the emergency room, health care providers will work fast to find out if you are having or have had a heart attack and to give you treatment.

APPROPRIATE HEALTH CARE
* If you are having a heart attack, treatment is done to restore the blood flow to the heart, and to monitor your vital signs to detect and treat complications.
* Long-term treatment after a heart attack may include cardiac rehabilitation, checkups and tests, lifestyle changes (such as stopping smoking or weight loss), and drug therapy.

POSSIBLE COMPLICATIONS
* Irregular heart rhythms.
* Shock.
* Congestive heart failure.
* Pericarditis (heart lining inflammation).
* Blood clots in other parts of the body.

PROBABLE OUTCOME—The amount of damage from a heart attack depends on how much of the heart is affected, how soon treatment begins, and other factors. Survivors should allow 4 to 8 weeks for recovery. Repeat heart attacks are common.

 HOW TO TREAT

GENERAL MEASURES
* If you have symptoms of a heart attack, seek medical help right away. Don't drive yourself.
* If you suspect heart attack symptoms in someone, call 911 for help.
* To learn more: American Heart Association, 7272 Greenville Ave., Dallas, TX 75231; (800) 242-8721; website: www.americanheart.org.

MEDICATION
* Drugs to dissolve and/or prevent blood clots may be used for emergency care.
* After a heart attack, drugs may be prescribed to help the heart function better, treat high blood pressure, prevent blood clots, or to lower cholesterol levels.

ACTIVITY
* Resume your normal activities gradually during recovery. An exercise program will usually be recommended.
* You will be advised about when to return to work, resume sexual relations, or drive a car.

DIET
* After a heart attack, eat a low-fat, high-fiber diet.
* Maintain ideal weight. Start a reducing diet if overweight.

 CALL YOUR DOCTOR

* You or a family member has symptoms of a heart attack. This is a life-threatening emergency!
* New symptoms occur during recovery.

HEART BLOCK
(Atrioventricular Block)

 GENERAL INFORMATION

DEFINITION—A persistent disruption (either mild or major) in transmission of electrical signals between the heart's upper and lower chambers. Contractions of the atria (upper heart chambers) lose synchronization with those of the ventricles (lower heart chambers). The heartbeat is no longer regulated normally to quicken under exertion or stress and slow down at other times.

BODY PARTS INVOLVED—Heart's electrical-transmission system that coordinates contractions of heart-muscle cells. The heart's natural pacemaker initiates the electrical system.

SEX OR AGE MOST AFFECTED—All ages, but most common in men over 40 and women after menopause.

SIGNS & SYMPTOMS
* No symptoms (sometimes) for less-severe forms.
* Slow, irregular heartbeat.
* Sudden loss of consciousness.
* Convulsions (sometimes).
* Attacks of dizziness, weakness or confusion.

CAUSES
* Coronary artery disease, a result of atherosclerosis (hardening of the arteries).
* Congenital heart abnormalities.
* Excessive digitalis and some other medications.

RISK INCREASES WITH
* Adults over 60.
* Stress.
* Improper diet that is high in fat and salt.
* Obesity.
* Smoking.
* Diabetes.
* Heart disease, including atherosclerosis, congestive heart failure or heart-valve disease.
* High blood pressure.
* Previous electrolyte imbalance.
* Use of some drugs, such as digitalis, quinidine or beta-adrenergic blockers.

HOW TO PREVENT
* Obtain medical treatment for any underlying disease.
* Don't smoke.
* Exercise regularly.
* Eat a diet that is low in fat and low in salt and high in fiber.

 WHAT TO EXPECT

DIAGNOSTIC MEASURES
* Your own observation of symptoms.
* Your health care provider will do a physical exam.
* Medical tests may include electrocardiogram (ECG). The ECG provides information about the degree of heart block (1st, 2nd or 3rd) and will help decide what treatment, if any, is needed. Heart monitoring may be done while you go about your daily activities by wearing a special recording device (e.g., Holter monitor).

APPROPRIATE HEALTH CARE
* Some heart blocks require no treatment.
* Surgery is usually done to implant an artificial pacemaker. It provides a regular, mild electric stimulus that maintains a normal heartbeat.

POSSIBLE COMPLICATIONS—Uncontrolled slow, rapid or irregular heartbeat and cardiac arrest.

PROBABLE OUTCOME
* Heart blocks that do not bring on symptoms usually require no treatment.
* More serious heart blocks can be controlled with surgery to implant a pacemaker.

 HOW TO TREAT

GENERAL MEASURES
* Wear a medical alert bracelet or pendant showing the name of your condition.
* To learn more: American Heart Association, 7272 Greenville Ave., Dallas, TX 75231; (800) 242-8721; website: www.americanheart.org.

MEDICATION
* Atropine may be prescribed for a short term therapy.
* Don't take drugs to relieve allergy or nasal congestion without medical approval. They can worsen symptoms.

ACTIVITY—Don't think of yourself as an invalid. Mild exercise is helpful for most patients. Begin a regular exercise program (walking is ideal).

DIET
* Lose weight if you are overweight.
* Avoid excess use of alcoholic beverages. Alcohol depresses the heartbeat.

 CALL YOUR DOCTOR IF

* You or a family member has symptoms of heart block, especially an episode with loss of consciousness.
* After diagnosis, symptoms recur.

HEART MURMURS

 GENERAL INFORMATION

DEFINITION—Heart murmurs are not a disease or illness. They involve the sounds, as heard through a stethoscope, of blood flowing through the heart. With murmurs, there is an extra sound (sometimes described as "swishing") in addition to the normal sounds (described as "lub-dup") of the heartbeat. Most heart murmurs are harmless or "innocent" and are detected at a routine physical or well-baby examination. Murmurs are heard in many healthy people.

BODY PARTS INVOLVED—Heart.

SEX OR AGE MOST AFFECTED—All ages, both sexes; more often heard in children and teenagers.

SIGNS & SYMPTOMS—People with heart murmurs have no symptoms, unless associated with other disorders.

CAUSES—The stethoscope picks up sounds made when the ventricles of the heart contract and the 4 heart valves snap shut. Most extra sounds caused by turbulent blood flow are known as murmurs. What causes innocent type heart murmurs is unknown.

RISK INCREASES WITH
* Congenital heart defects.
* Rheumatic fever.
* Myocarditis.
* Children with anemia.
* Pregnancy.

HOW TO PREVENT—There are no preventive measures.

 WHAT TO EXPECT

DIAGNOSTIC MEASURES
* Heart murmurs are detected by a health care provider listening to the heart sounds through a stethoscope. By listening to these sounds, a trained person can judge by their quality, intensity, location and timing that the murmur is insignificant (most cases).
* In a few cases, the sounds that are heard may indicate a need for more testing in order to determine the cause. Chest x-ray, ECG and echocardiography may be done for further study.

APPROPRIATE HEALTH CARE—No medical treatment is necessary for an innocent heart murmur.

POSSIBLE COMPLICATIONS
* None expected with innocent heart murmurs.
* If there is any underlying organic heart problem, it can usually be corrected surgically.

PROBABLE OUTCOME—Most innocent heart murmurs detected (particularly in children) disappear or become undetectable over time. People with these murmurs live a completely normal life.

 HOW TO TREAT

GENERAL MEASURES—If your child has an innocent type heart murmur, treat him or her like any other healthy child. Parents sometimes become concerned about the idea of a heart murmur and become over-protective. This can cause problems for the child's emotional well-being.

MEDICATION—No drugs are needed.

ACTIVITY—Do not limit activity.

DIET—No special diet.

 CALL YOUR DOCTOR IF

You need further assurance about heart murmurs.

HEART RHYTHM IRREGULARITY
(Arrhythmia)

 GENERAL INFORMATION

DEFINITION—A change in the regular beat of the heart. Arrhythmias are common, and many are mild and require no treatment. Almost all adults have some amount of irregular heartbeats.

BODY PARTS INVOLVED—Heart; nerves that transmit impulses to coordinate heart muscle contractions. Most people have some irregular beats.

SEX OR AGE MOST AFFECTED—Both sexes; all ages, but most likely over age 65.

SIGNS & SYMPTOMS
- A fluttering in the chest; the heart seems to skip a beat, or beat irregularly, or beat very fast or slowly.
- Shortness of breath and/or mild chest pains.
- Faintness, dizziness, or weakness.
- Feeling anxious.
- No symptoms (frequently).

CAUSES—The heart has an electrical system that controls its rate and contractions. The average heart beats at a rate of 60 to 100 times per minute. With arrhythmias, the electrical system does not function as it should. There are different types of arrhythmias depending on what part of the heart is involved. They can be due to a number of causes. In some cases, no cause is found.

RISK INCREASES WITH
- Heart diseases. This includes rheumatic fever, congenital heart disease, cardiomyopathy, previous heart attack, or heart-muscle inflammation.
- Endocrine disorders, such as thyroid and adrenal gland diseases.
- Fluid and electrolyte imbalance, such as too little or too much potassium.
- Side effects of certain drugs, such as digitalis, beta-adrenergic blockers, stimulants, and diuretics.
- Use of certain drugs, such as caffeine, alcohol, amphetamines, and many nonprescription cough and cold remedies.
- Overdose of certain drugs, including antidepressants, marijuana, and cocaine.
- Postoperative effects following chest or heart surgery.
- Chronic kidney disease.
- High blood pressure.
- Smoking.
- Stress.
- Sleep deprivation (lack of sleep).

HOW TO PREVENT—Avoid risk factors where possible and get treatment for those that are treatable.

 WHAT TO EXPECT

DIAGNOSTIC MEASURES
- Your health care provider will do a physical exam and listen to the heart with a stethoscope.
- Medical tests usually include an electrocardiogram (ECG) or you may be asked to wear a Holter monitor (a portable ECG) for 1 to 5 days. These aid in diagnosing heart diseases by measuring the electrical activity of the heart. Other tests may be done to see if the cause is a heart disease.

APPROPRIATE HEALTH CARE
- Treatment, if needed, will depend on the cause.
- You may require cardioversion (brief electric shock to the heart) to restore normal rhythm.
- Surgery may be needed to correct some heart problems (coronary-artery bypass, to replace damaged heart valve, or insertion of a pacemaker or atrial defibrillator).
- Counseling may be helpful if stress is a major factor.

POSSIBLE COMPLICATIONS
- Complications may arise from the heart disease that is causing the arrhythmia.
- Some arrhythmias can lead to complications if they are untreated.

PROBABLE OUTCOME—Irregular heartbeats that occur only occasionally are typically harmless and require no treatment. Other arrhythmias can usually be controlled with treatment.

 HOW TO TREAT

GENERAL MEASURES
- Wear a medical alert bracelet or pendant showing the name of your condition.
- To learn more: American Heart Association, 7272 Greenville Ave., Dallas, TX 75231; (800) 242-8721; website: www.americanheart.org.

MEDICATION—Antiarrhythmic drugs may be prescribed. You may need to try several of them to find the most effective one. A few arrhythmias may also require anticoagulant drug therapy.

ACTIVITY—Your health care provider will advise you if there are any limits.

DIET—Avoid caffeine and alcohol (if advised).

 CALL YOUR DOCTOR IF

- You or a family member has symptoms of heart-rhythm irregularity.
- New, unexplained symptoms develop.

ILLNESS & DISORDERS

HEART VALVE DISEASE
(Valvular Heart Disease)

GENERAL INFORMATION

DEFINITION—A complication of diseases that distort or destroy valves of the heart. The heart has four valves. The mitral and tricuspid valves (main heart valves) control blood flow into the ventricles. The aortic and pulmonic valves control blood flow out of the heart. The proper functioning of the valves is vital to the heart as a pump.

BODY PARTS INVOLVED—Heart valves (aortic, mitral, tricuspid and pulmonic valves).

SEX OR AGE MOST AFFECTED—Both sexes; all ages.

SIGNS & SYMPTOMS
* No symptoms (sometimes).
* Fatigue and weakness.
* Dizziness or fainting.
* Chest pain.
* Shortness of breath, which may wake you out of a sleep.
* Lung congestion.
* Heart-rhythm problems.

CAUSES—Narrowed valves (stenosis) can obstruct blood flow. Widened or scarred valves allow blood to leak backward into the heart (insufficiency). The disorder may be inherited or caused by a variety of medical problems.

RISK INCREASES WITH
* Persons over 60.
* Family history of heart-valve disease.
* Pregnancy.
* Rheumatic fever.
* A complication of strep throat.
* Atherosclerosis.
* High blood pressure.
* Congenital (being born with) heart defects.
* Endocarditis (heart inflammation).
* Intravenous (IV) drug abuse.
* Syphilis (rare).
* Marfan's syndrome.

HOW TO PREVENT
* Obtain medical care for diseases that cause heart-valve damage, such as high blood pressure, endocarditis, and syphilis.
* Take antibiotics, if prescribed, for streptococcal infections to prevent rheumatic fever.
* If you have a family history of congenital heart disease, obtain genetic counseling before starting a family.

WHAT TO EXPECT

DIAGNOSTIC MEASURES
* Your health care provider will do a physical exam.
* Medical tests may include blood tests, electrocardiogram (which measures electrical activity of the heart), echocardiogram (uses sound waves to examine the heart), and x-rays of the heart, lungs, and blood flow (called angiography).

APPROPRIATE HEALTH CARE—Surgery may be recommended to repair a heart valve or to remove a diseased or damaged valve. It may be replaced by a mechanical valve, one made from human or bovine tissue, or a human valve from a donor.

POSSIBLE COMPLICATIONS
* Infection of the valves.
* Congestive heart failure.

PROBABLE OUTCOME—Depends on the underlying condition. Many complications of valvular disease can be controlled with treatment.

HOW TO TREAT

GENERAL MEASURES
* Tell any doctor, dentist, or anesthesiologist who treats you that you have heart-valve disease. Remind those involved, even if you think they know the details of your medical history.
* To learn more: American Heart Association, 7272 Greenville Ave., Dallas, TX 75231; (800) 242-8721; website: www.americanheart.org.

MEDICATION—You may be prescribed:
* Antibiotics to treat or prevent bacterial infection of abnormal heart valves.
* Antiarrhythmic or digitalis drugs for the heart.
* Anticoagulants (blood thinners) after surgery.

ACTIVITY—You will be advised about any limits. Sometimes, no limits are needed with certain forms of the disease.

DIET—You may be advised to eat a low-fat, low-salt diet.

CALL YOUR DOCTOR IF

* You or a family member has symptoms of heart-valve disease.
* Signs of infection develop, such as fever, chills, muscle aches, headache, fatigue, and a general ill feeling.

HEARTBEAT, RAPID
(Tachycardia; Paroxysmal Tachycardia)

 GENERAL INFORMATION

DEFINITION—A heart rate (or heartbeat) that is faster than normal. In adults, the resting heart rate is normally between 60 and 100 beats per minute. Tachycardia is the medical term for rapid heart rate. Bradycardia is the medical term for slow heart rate.

BODY PARTS INVOLVED—Heart muscle; electrical system of the heart.

SEX OR AGE MOST AFFECTED—Both sexes; all ages.

SIGNS & SYMPTOMS
* Some people may have no symptoms.
* Heart pounding or palpitations. The pulse at the wrist or neck will be 100 to 180 beats per minute, which is much faster than normal.
* Faintness; a feeling of doom or anxiety.
* Chest pain.
* Cough.
* Being short of breath.
* Dizziness.
* Heavy sweating.

CAUSES—An electrical system in the heart normally controls the heart rate so that it remains at 60 to 100 beats per minute. This allows the heart to provide the body with the blood and oxygen it needs to function. When something causes the heart to beat too fast, it may not be able to supply all the blood and oxygen needed by the body.

RISK INCREASES WITH
* Heart attack, heart disease, or surgery.
* Thyroid disease.
* Fever.
* Anemia.
* Stress, anxiety, fear, anger, or being nervous.
* Smoking.
* Dehydration.
* Infections.
* Sleep deprivation (not getting enough sleep).
* Too much caffeine.
* Use of some drugs, such as albuterol, cocaine, ephedrine, or others, and some herbal remedies.

HOW TO PREVENT
* Often, the problem cannot be prevented.
* Avoid the risk factors where possible.
* Regular exercise.

 WHAT TO EXPECT

DIAGNOSTIC MEASURES
* Your own observation of symptoms.
* Your health care provider will do a physical exam and ask questions about your symptoms and activities.

* Tests may be done to measure the heart's electrical activity. Other tests may be done to check for medical problems that could cause rapid heart rate.

APPROPRIATE HEALTH CARE
* A few patients may require immediate treatment, including electrical shock (cardioversion), to stop the rapid heart rate. In milder cases, no treatment may be required. Other treatment may depend on the cause.
* If the rapid heart rate occurs often, a small electrical device called implantable cardioverter-defibrillator (ICD) may be implanted under the skin. It can detect irregular heartbeats and shock the heart back into normal rhythm.
* Surgery may (rarely) be recommended.

POSSIBLE COMPLICATIONS—An ongoing rapid heartbeat can lead to life-threatening heart problems.

PROBABLE OUTCOME—Most heartbeat problems are temporary and harmless. If the rapid heartbeat is ongoing, it can usually be controlled with treatment.

 HOW TO TREAT

GENERAL MEASURES
* Ask your health care provider about ways to reduce stress in your life, and to stop smoking, if you smoke.
* The following steps sometimes slows the heartbeat:
  - Hold your breath briefly.
  - Pinch the skin on your arm enough to cause pain.
  - Bathe your face in cold water or put your head briefly in a sink of cool water.
  - Hold your nostrils closed and blow gently through the nose, making the eardrums pop.
* To learn more: American Heart Association, 7272 Greenville Ave., Dallas, TX 75231; (800) 242-8721; website: www.americanheart.org.

MEDICATION—For repeated attacks, one or more drugs to control heart rhythm may be prescribed.

ACTIVITY—Exercise regularly for 20 to 30 minutes a day (with medical approval). Being fit will improve heart health.

DIET—Avoid caffeine and alcohol (if advised).

 CALL YOUR DOCTOR IF

* You or a family member has an episode of rapid, irregular heartbeat that does not end in 4 or 5 minutes.
* Shortness of breath or chest pain develops.

HEARTBURN

GENERAL INFORMATION

DEFINITION—Heartburn (also known as acid indigestion) is a symptom, not a disease, and has nothing to do with the heart. The symptoms are sometimes mistaken for a heart attack. When heartburn occurs often or complications develop, the problem is known as GERD (gastroesophageal reflux disease).

BODY PARTS INVOLVED—Gastrointestinal system.

SEX OR AGE MOST AFFECTED—Both sexes; all ages. It is most common in adults over 60.

SIGNS & SYMPTOMS
* Belching or backward flow of stomach contents into the mouth and throat. This produces an acid taste.
* Heavy burning, discomfort, or pain in the chest.
* It may be difficult to swallow.
* Mild stomach pain or bloated feeling.

CAUSES—Heartburn is caused by a backflow of acid from the stomach into the esophagus. The esophagus is the tube that goes from the mouth to the stomach. The muscles that close off the upper stomach become lax (loose). This allows stomach juices to enter the esophagus and irritate its lining.

RISK INCREASES WITH
* Hiatal hernia (part of the stomach bulges into the chest).
* Ulcers (open sores) of the esophagus.
* Stress.
* Improper diet or overeating.
* Overweight.
* Smoking.
* Excess alcohol use.
* Use of certain drugs.
* Eating spicy or acidic (citrus, tomatoes) foods.
* Drinking carbonated beverages.
* Exercise, lying down, bending over, or straining too soon after a meal.
* Disorders of the gastrointestinal tract.

HOW TO PREVENT
* Avoid smoking.
* Don't overeat. Avoid excess use of alcohol.
* Reduce amount of fats, deep-fried foods, spices, coffee, and tomato products you eat.
* Don't bend over or lie down right after eating.
* Don't wear tight clothes that restrict your body.
* Raise head of bed 4 to 6 inches with blocks.
* Lose weight if you are overweight.

WHAT TO EXPECT

DIAGNOSTIC MEASURES
* Your own observation of symptoms.

* Your health care provider will do a physical exam and ask questions about your symptoms.
* Medical tests are usually not needed, but may be done to help diagnose any complications.

APPROPRIATE HEALTH CARE
* Treatment usually consists of self-care and drug therapy if needed.
* Rarely, surgery may be recommended when other treatment steps are not helping the symptoms.

POSSIBLE COMPLICATIONS—GERD (gastroesophageal reflux disease).

PROBABLE OUTCOME—Symptoms usually clear up on their own. In other cases, symptoms can be relieved with treatment.

HOW TO TREAT

GENERAL MEASURES
* Heartburn usually begins within about an hour after eating and may continue for several hours. Self-care involves taking preventive measures and heartburn drugs, if needed, to control the symptoms.
* If the problem gets worse or self-care is not working, see your health care provider.
* Stop smoking. Find a way that will works.
* To learn more: National Heartburn Alliance, 303 East Wacker Drive, Suite 440, Chicago, IL 60601; (877) 471-2081; website: www.heartburnalliance.org.

MEDICATION
* For minor discomfort, you may use any of the heartburn preventive drugs available without a prescription. Different ones work for different people. If one type does not work for you, a different type may help.
* A stronger type of heartburn drug may be prescribed.
* If a drug you take is causing heartburn, a change in dosage or a new drug may be prescribed.

ACTIVITY—Resume normal activities as soon as symptoms improve.

DIET
* Avoid foods and beverages that cause excess stomach acid, such as spicy dishes, coffee, acidic fruit juice, or alcohol. Avoid chocolate, and eat less high-fat foods.
* Eat small, frequent meals.

CALL YOUR DOCTOR IF

* If you or a family member has heartburn that continues or worsens despite self-care.
* If symptoms get worse or are severe, get medical help right away. They could mean a heart attack.

HEARTBURN DURING PREGNANCY

 GENERAL INFORMATION

DEFINITION—Heartburn is the term used to describe a burning pain in the chest and upper abdomen. It is common for pregnant women to have the symptoms of heartburn. It usually comes and goes until delivery. Although it can cause you some discomfort, heartburn will not hurt your baby.

BODY PARTS INVOLVED—Gastrointestinal system.

SEX OR AGE MOST AFFECTED—Pregnant women.

SIGNS & SYMPTOMS
* Burning pain in the center of the chest and upper abdomen. It is often causes an unpleasant taste in the mouth.
* Belching (burping).

CAUSES
* Heartburn is not a heart disorder. It is caused by a backflow of acid from the stomach into the esophagus. The esophagus is the tube that goes from the mouth to the stomach. The muscles that close off the upper stomach become lax (loose), allowing stomach juices to enter the esophagus and irritate its lining.
* Changes caused by pregnancy include an increase in the amount of stomach acid. It also takes longer for the stomach to empty.
* During late pregnancy, the enlarged womb presses on the stomach and may increase the symptoms.

RISK INCREASES WITH
* Overeating or eating and then lying down.
* Smoking.
* Excess use of alcohol.

HOW TO PREVENT—Avoid risk factors listed above.

 WHAT TO EXPECT

DIAGNOSTIC MEASURES—Heartburn is usually self-diagnosed. Your obstetric provider may make the diagnosis from the symptoms you describe, and rarely, may recommend other medical tests.

APPROPRIATE HEALTH CARE—Treatment usually consists of self-care

POSSIBLE COMPLICATIONS—Heartburn may affect your ability to eat a healthy diet. Low food and fluid intake might cause problems for the mother and the baby.

PROBABLE OUTCOME—The heartburn goes away after the baby is born unless the cause is not related to pregnancy. There are normally no complications.

 HOW TO TREAT

GENERAL MEASURES—General treatment suggestions:
* Avoid bending over or lying down right after eating.
* Don't wear tight underclothes or belts.
* Place books or blocks under the head of your bed to raise it about 4 inches, or sleep propped up with several pillows.
* Don't smoke.

MEDICATION
* While drugs are not usually needed for this disorder, in some cases they may be of benefit. Simple antacid mixtures or tablets, such as magnesium trisilicate, may be helpful. These drugs should be used only with your obstetric provider's approval. Other drugs may be prescribed if simple measures don't help the symptoms.
* Don't take any herbal remedies without asking your obstetric provider.
* If you can live with the symptoms, try to avoid use of drugs.

ACTIVITY—Stay active. Avoid exercises that require bending over.

DIET
* Eat small, frequent meals.
* Don't rush through your meals; eat slowly.
* Avoid drinking large quantities of fluids during meals.
* Don't eat before bedtime.
* Avoid highly seasoned food.
* Don't drink alcohol.
* Avoid very hot or very cold beverages.
* Avoid eating while lying down.
* Chewing gum may be helpful for some women.

 CALL YOUR DOCTOR IF

* You or a family member has symptoms of heartburn during pregnancy. This should be diagnosed.
* The following occur after diagnosis:
  - Simple measures don't bring relief.
  - You begin vomiting late in pregnancy.
  - You vomit material that has blood in it or looks like coffee grounds.
  - You have black or tarry stools.

HEATSTROKE OR HEAT EXHAUSTION
(Sunstroke)

 GENERAL INFORMATION

DEFINITION—Illness caused by excess exposure to heat, not enough fluid intake, or a failure of the body's ability to regulate its temperature.

BODY PARTS INVOLVED—Total body.

SEX OR AGE MOST AFFECTED—All ages, but most common in the elderly.

SIGNS & SYMPTOMS
Heat exhaustion:
- Dizziness, fatigue, faintness, headache.
- Skin that is pale and clammy.
- Pulse rapid and weak.
- Breathing is fast and shallow.
- Muscle cramps.
- Intense thirst.

Heatstroke:
- Often preceded by heat exhaustion and its symptoms.
- Skin that is hot, dry, and flushed.
- No sweating.
- High body temperature.
- Rapid heartbeat.
- Confusion.
- Loss of consciousness.

CAUSES
- Heat exhaustion is caused by a lack of fluid intake, a lack of salt intake, and a problem with the body's production of sweat. Sweat is what helps to cool the body.
- Heat stroke is caused by overexposure to extreme heat and a breakdown in the body's temperature regulation system. The body becomes overheated to a dangerous degree. The body's temperature can reach 107°F (41.7°C).

RISK INCREASES WITH
- Elderly persons.
- Excess alcohol use or drug abuse.
- Poor health or chronic illness, such as diabetes, high blood pressure, or heart disease.
- Exercise or work in a hot, humid location. This can be indoors or outdoors.
- Loss of body fluids, from sweating and failure to drink enough fluids.
- Heavy, tight clothing.
- High fever.

HOW TO PREVENT
- Wear light, loose-fitting clothing in hot weather.
- Drink fluids often; don't wait until you are thirsty. Drink extra water if you sweat a lot. If urine output decreases, increase water intake.
- If you become overheated, open a window or use a fan or air conditioner. This helps sweat dry up, which cools the skin.
- Take precautions when going outside in hot weather.

 WHAT TO EXPECT

DIAGNOSTIC MEASURES
- Your own observation of symptoms.
- Your health care provider will do a physical exam and ask questions about the symptoms and activities.
- Usually no medical tests are needed for diagnosis.

APPROPRIATE HEALTH CARE—Medical treatment will depend on how severe the symptoms are. Fluids may be given through a vein (IV).

POSSIBLE COMPLICATIONS
- Can involve any major organ system (heart, lungs, kidneys, brain).
- Related to duration and amount of heat and to speed of treatment.

PROBABLE OUTCOME—Fast treatment usually brings full recovery in 1 to 2 days.

 HOW TO TREAT

GENERAL MEASURES
- If someone with symptoms is very hot and not sweating: Cool the person rapidly. Remove their clothing, use a cold-water bath, or wrap in wet sheets. Get them to the nearest hospital. This is an emergency!
- If someone is faint but sweating: Lie the person down in a cool place. Give them cool water (not iced) to sip or a sports drink containing electrolytes. Get medical advice for proper care.

MEDICATION—Drugs are usually not needed for these disorders. Drugs may be needed for complications that develop.

ACTIVITY—Rest with legs elevated while symptoms are present. Normal activity may be resumed after symptoms improve.

DIET—No special diet.

 CALL YOUR DOCTOR IF

You or a family member has symptoms of heatstroke or heat exhaustion, or observe them in someone else. Call immediately! These conditions may be serious or fatal.

HEEL PAIN
(Heel Contusion; Heel Spur; Heel Bursitis)

 GENERAL INFORMATION

DEFINITION—Heel pain or discomfort caused by several conditions.
* Contusion or bruise of the heel bone. This causes inflammation of the tissue (periosteum) that covers the heel bone (calcaneus).
* Heel spur. A hard, bony sliver or needle that develops on the heel. It can cause inflammation and other problems in tendons and ligaments in the foot.
* Heel bursitis. This is inflammation of the connective tissue that surrounds a joint.

BODY PARTS INVOLVED—Heels.

SEX OR AGE MOST AFFECTED—Adults. The conditions are fairly common among runners and other athletes.

SIGNS & SYMPTOMS—Pain and tenderness in the heel and sole of the foot under the heel bone. Pain often occurs after resting or after rising in the morning. There may be no pain when sitting. One or both feet can be affected.

CAUSES—Heel pain is usually a result of putting too much stress on the heel bone and the soft connective tissues (called the fascia) that attach to it.

RISK INCREASES WITH
* Running, jogging, or fast walking.
* Previous, or recent, foot or leg injury.
* Poorly cushioned shoes; lack of arch support.
* Prolonged standing; sciatica (leg nerve pain).
* Overweight.

HOW TO PREVENT
* Avoid activities that put constant strain on the foot. Switch to swimming or cycling.
* Wear a shoe with inserts.
* Wear athletic shoes with good shock support in the heels, good flexibility, and good support to control side-to-side motion.
* No more than 1.5-inch heels on everyday shoes.

 WHAT TO EXPECT

DIAGNOSTIC MEASURES
* Your own observation of symptoms.
* Your health care provider will do a physical exam of the foot and ankle area. Questions will be asked about your symptoms and activities.

APPROPRIATE HEALTH CARE
* Most people try self-care first.
* Medical care may include physical therapy, casts, taping, night splints, injections, ultrasound, orthotics, or surgery. Treatment steps will depend on the symptoms.

POSSIBLE COMPLICATIONS—Soreness and arthritic changes in the heel that place extra stress on joints, such as those in the knee, hip, and spine.

PROBABLE OUTCOME—Usually curable with treatment. Different types of treatment work for different people.

 HOW TO TREAT

GENERAL MEASURES
* Use ice massage, or soak the heel in ice water. Do this for 15 minutes at a time, 3 or 4 times a day.
* Lightly massage the heel and calf before getting out of bed. Apply heat with a heating pad if it feels good.
* Taping helps some people. Apply athletic tape as directed on the product's instructions.
* Try heel cushions or lifts, arch supports, or medial wedge supports (available at sporting-goods stores and drug stores). Use products in both shoes so that other problems don't develop. Custom orthotics (inserts designed for an individual) may be helpful.
* Purchase shoes that fit well. Sandals help some people. Break in new shoes slowly by wearing them a few minutes per day to start.
* Stretching exercises will help.

MEDICATION
* To relieve minor pain, you may use ibuprofen or aspirin (adults only).
* Stronger anti-inflammatory drugs or injections of a steroid drug into the heel to reduce inflammation may be prescribed.

ACTIVITY—Stay off your feet as much as possible, especially at the beginning of treatment.

DIET—No special diet, unless you are overweight. If so, lose weight to reduce stress on the foot.

 CALL YOUR DOCTOR IF

You or a family member has heel pain that isn't helped by self-care.

ILLNESS & DISORDERS

HEMOPHILIA

GENERAL INFORMATION

DEFINITION—An inherited bleeding problem that causes dangerous bleeding. The two main types of hemophilia occur only in boys. Hemophilia is passed via a gene from mother to son. Most mothers who pass the gene on are carriers of hemophilia and have no symptoms of the condition.

BODY PARTS INVOLVED—All body parts.

SEX OR AGE MOST AFFECTED—It affects 1 in 10,000 males and appears early in childhood.

SIGNS & SYMPTOMS
• Symptoms often don't occur until the baby starts to crawl or walk. Sometimes, a circumcision procedure causes excess bleeding and is the first symptom.
• Painful, swollen joints or swelling in the leg or arm when bleeding occurs.
• Bruising. Bruises may be large and deep.
• Heavy bleeding from small cuts.
• Nosebleeds.
• Blood in the urine or stool.

CAUSES—Lack of a blood-clotting (coagulation) factor. Clotting is the process by which blood changes from a liquid to a solid substance in order to stop bleeding. There are 13 clotting factors in the body. Hemophilia occurs in three of them. Hemophilia A lacks enough clotting factor VIII. Hemophilia B lacks enough clotting factor IX. Hemophilia C (rare in the United States) lacks enough clotting factor XI.

RISK INCREASES WITH—Family history of the disorder.

HOW TO PREVENT
• Cannot be prevented at present. If your family has a history of this disorder, get genetic counseling before having children. If you are pregnant, talk to your obstetric provider about testing to see if the baby has inherited hemophilia.
• Testing for a female to check her hemophilia carrier status is done with a blood study. Blood studies of other family members are usually needed also.

WHAT TO EXPECT

DIAGNOSTIC MEASURES
• Your own observation of symptoms.
• Your child's health care provider will do a physical exam and ask questions about the symptoms and activities.
• Blood tests to diagnose blood-clotting problems.

APPROPRIATE HEALTH CARE
• Family education about the disorder is the first step. Parents need to learn how to recognize signs and symptoms of bleeding and how to provide therapy. They need to learn ways to keep a child safe and about appropriate physical activities. Vaccines need to be current.
• Bleeding episodes can usually be controlled with home care by self-administered replacement therapy.
• Hospital care to control bleeding may be needed when the bleeding is heavy or unusual.

POSSIBLE COMPLICATIONS
• Bleeding events needing emergency care.
• Joint damage and problems due to bleeding.
• Adverse reaction to clotting-factor treatment.
• Risk of getting other diseases through donated blood. Risk is less with genetically produced clotting products.

PROBABLE OUTCOME
• The disorder is not curable, but it is not fatal. With treatment, patients can have a near-normal life span.
• The disorder may be mild, moderate or severe. It depends on amount of the clotting factor produced.

HOW TO TREAT

GENERAL MEASURES
• Parents need to make sure anyone (sitters, relatives, teachers) taking care of a child with hemophilia knows what to do in an emergency.
• Use good dental hygiene to avoid problems that can cause bleeding, such as pulling a tooth.
• Wear a medical alert type of identification showing showing that they have hemophilia.
• To learn more: National Hemophilia Foundation, 116 West 32nd St., 11 Floor, New York, NY 10001, (800) 424-2634; website: www.hemophilia.org.

MEDICATION
• Bleeding can be controlled by injections of clotting factor. It can be taken as a preventive measure. Patients can be trained to give themselves the treatment.
• Desmopressin (DDAVP) may be injected into veins or given as a nasal drug to help stimulate a release of the body's own clotting factor.
• Drugs to reduce joint pain may be prescribed.
• Avoid aspirin and other nonsteroidal anti-inflammatory drugs. They increase bleeding.

ACTIVITY—Exercise daily. Avoid activities that can cause injury, such as contact sports. Swim, bicycle, or walk instead.

DIET—No special diet.

CALL YOUR DOCTOR IF

• A child has symptoms of hemophilia.
• Bleeding or other symptoms cause any concern.

HEMORRHOIDS

GENERAL INFORMATION

DEFINITION—Swollen veins of the rectum or anus. Hemorrhoids may be located inside of the anal canal, or at the anal opening. Hemorrhoids may be present for years, but go unnoticed until bleeding occurs.

BODY PARTS INVOLVED—Veins under the rectal or anal membrane.

SEX OR AGE MOST AFFECTED—Adults of both sexes.

SIGNS & SYMPTOMS
• Rectal bleeding. Bright-red blood may show as streaks on toilet paper or be a part of a bowel movement. Blood may be a slow trickle for a short while following bowel movements. It almost always colors the toilet water.
• Pain, itching, or discharge after bowel movements.
• A lump or swelling that can be felt in the anus.
• A feeling that the rectum has not emptied completely after a bowel movement.

CAUSES—Repeated pressure on the anal or rectal veins, which causes them to stretch.

RISK INCREASES WITH
• A diet that lacks fiber.
• Prolonged sitting or standing.
• Overweight people.
• Pregnancy.
• Chronic constipation or diarrhea.
• Loss of muscle tone in older adults.
• Rectal surgery or episiotomy.
• Liver disease.
• Anal sex.
• Colon cancer.

HOW TO PREVENT
• Don't try to hurry bowel movements, but do try to avoid straining and prolonged sitting on the toilet.
• Lose weight if you are overweight.
• Include plenty of fiber in your diet.
• Drink 8 to 10 glasses of fluid per day.
• Exercise regularly.

WHAT TO EXPECT

DIAGNOSTIC MEASURES
• Your own observation of symptoms.
• Your health care provider can diagnose hemorrhoids by a physical exam of the rectal area.
• Medical tests may be done to check for complications.

APPROPRIATE HEALTH CARE
• Treatment is aimed at easing the symptoms.
• Surgery may be recommended when simple treatment measures are not helping the symptoms.

POSSIBLE COMPLICATIONS
• Anemia, if there is a lot of blood loss.
• Severe pain caused by a blood clot in a hemorrhoid.
• Infection or inflammation of a hemorrhoid.

PROBABLE OUTCOME—Hemorrhoids usually clear up with proper care, but symptoms may come and go. Stubborn cases may require surgery.

HOW TO TREAT

GENERAL MEASURES
• Never strain to push your stool out.
• When sitting on the toilet, place feet on a low footstool to aid bowel movement.
• Clean the anal area gently with soft, moist paper after each bowel movement.
• To relieve pain, sit in 8 to 10 inches of warm water for 10 to 20 minutes several times a day.
• To reduce pain and swelling of a blood clot or swollen hemorrhoid, stay in bed for 1 day and apply ice packs to the anal area.

MEDICATION
• For minor pain, itching, or to reduce swelling, you may use drug products to relieve symptoms of hemorrhoids. If these symptoms occur during pregnancy, ask your obstetric provider which drugs are safe to use.
• Use a stool softener, if a laxative is needed.
• Other drugs may be prescribed for complications.

ACTIVITY—Get 30 minutes of exercise on a daily basis. Bowel function improves with good physical fitness.

DIET
• To prevent constipation, eat a well-balanced diet that contains many high-fiber foods.
• Drink 8 to 10 glasses of fluid daily.
• Go on a weight loss diet if you are overweight.

CALL YOUR DOCTOR IF

• You or a family member has symptoms of hemorrhoids
• Hemorrhoids continue to cause severe pain.
• A hard lump develops where a hemorrhoid has been.
• Rectal bleeding is heavy. Rectal bleeding can be an early sign of cancer.

ILLNESS & DISORDERS

HEPATITIS, VIRAL

GENERAL INFORMATION

DEFINITION—Inflammation of the liver caused by a virus infection. Viral hepatitis has several types. The most common are type A, type B, and type C. Other types are type D and type E.

BODY PARTS INVOLVED—Liver.

SEX OR AGE MOST AFFECTED—Both sexes; all ages.

SIGNS & SYMPTOMS
* After an infection occurs, there may be no symptoms, or symptoms may take weeks to months to appear. A person may first have flu-like symptoms, such as fever, fatigue, nausea, vomiting, diarrhea, and loss of appetite.
* Jaundice (yellow eyes and skin) caused by a buildup of bile in the blood.
* Dark urine and light, "clay-colored," or whitish stools.
* Pain in the upper-right abdomen.

CAUSES
* Types A and E: The virus usually enters the body through water or food (especially raw shellfish) that has been contaminated by sewage (fecal-oral contact).
* Type B: Usually sexually transmitted (contact with body fluids of an infected person), or by blood transfusions contaminated with the virus, or from injections with non-sterile needles or syringes. An infected mother can pass it to her newborn. Cause may be unknown.
* Type C: Usually spread through intravenous (IV) drug use, blood transfusions, and other exposures to contaminated blood or its products. Cause may be unknown.
* Type D: Occurs with hepatitis type B infection.

RISK INCREASES WITH
* Alcoholism, blood transfusions, kidney disease, blood-clotting disorders, organ transplants, having prior sexually transmitted diseases.
* Daycare centers (children and workers, especially those who change diapers).
* Infants born to mothers with hepatitis B or C.
* Health care workers.
* Work that involves contact with body fluids.
* Close contact with an infected person.
* Getting a tattoo or body piercing.
* People who engage in anal sex, and persons who have multiple sexual partners.
* IV drug abuse or intranasal cocaine use.
* Travel to countries where hepatitis is common.

HOW TO PREVENT
* Avoid the risk factors listed above if possible.
* If exposed to someone with hepatitis, seek medical advice about receiving gamma-globulin injections to prevent or decrease the risk of some types of hepatitis.
* Persons at risk for hepatitis should get hepatitis A and B vaccines (other vaccines are being studied) and immune globulin in addition to vaccine. Your health care provider can advise you if you are in a risk group.
* Routine hepatitis B vaccine for all newborns.

WHAT TO EXPECT

DIAGNOSTIC MEASURES
* Your health care provider will do a physical exam.
* Medical tests may include blood and urine studies and liver function tests. A liver biopsy may be done by using a needle to remove liver tissue for microscopic exam.

APPROPRIATE HEALTH CARE
* Acute (short term) hepatitis usually requires little or no treatment.
* Chronic hepatitis is treated with drugs.
* Hospital care for severe symptoms.

POSSIBLE COMPLICATIONS
* Liver disorders that could be fatal. This includes liver cancer.
* Chronic hepatitis. Some patients look and feel well and do not know they are infected. They can still pass the infection on to others. Some patients have symptoms that lead to liver damage (this can take 20 years).

PROBABLE OUTCOME—Most people recover fully in 1 to 4 months.

HOW TO TREAT

GENERAL MEASURES
* Most patients can be cared for at home. Keeping apart from others is not needed.
* If you have hepatitis or are caring for someone with it, wash your hands carefully.
* To learn more: Centers for Disease Control & Prevention (CDC) hotline: (888) 443-7232; website: www.cdc.gov/ncidod/diseases/hepatitis/index.htm.

MEDICATION—Interferon, steroids, or antivirals may be prescribed.

ACTIVITY
* Extra rest may be helpful.
* Avoid contact sports until tests show no virus.
* Food handlers may return to work when medically advised.

DIET—No special diet

CALL YOUR DOCTOR IF

* You or a family member has symptoms of hepatitis or has been exposed to hepatitis.
* After diagnosis, symptoms cause concern.

HEPATOMA
(Liver Cancer; Hepatocellular Carcinoma)

 GENERAL INFORMATION

DEFINITION—A malignant tumor that begins in the liver. This is a primary liver cancer. Cancers that develop elsewhere in the body (such as the breast) and spread to the liver are secondary liver cancers.

BODY PARTS INVOLVED—Liver.

SEX OR AGE MOST AFFECTED—Adults of both sexes (more common in men after age 40).

SIGNS & SYMPTOMS
• Hard lump in the right upper abdomen.
• Weight and appetite loss.
• Jaundice (yellow skin and eyes).
• Abdominal pain that feels like a pulled muscle.
• Low blood sugar (weakness, sweating, hunger, tremor, and headache).
• Fever.
• Fluid in the abdomen; enlarged spleen.
• Unusual bleeding.

CAUSES—Exact cause is unknown. There are certain known risk factors.

RISK INCREASES WITH
• Cirrhosis of the liver.
• Alcoholic liver disease.
• Hepatitis types B, C, D, and G infection.
• Family history of liver cancer.
• Alcoholism.
• Misuse of anabolic steroids.
• Geographic locations. This is especially common in South Africa and Southeast Asia.

HOW TO PREVENT
• No specific preventive measures. Steps can be taken to reduce a person's risk factors.
• Avoid alcohol or drink no more than 1 or 2 alcoholic drinks a day.
• Vaccine to prevent hepatitis B in high-risk persons.
• Screening tests for high-risk persons to diagnose and treat cancer at an early stage.

 WHAT TO EXPECT

DIAGNOSTIC MEASURES
• Your own observation of symptoms.
• Your health care provider will do a physical exam and ask questions about your symptoms.
• Medical tests may include blood studies and liver-function tests. Other tests are usually done to confirm the diagnosis and to determine if cancer has spread (called staging).

APPROPRIATE HEALTH CARE
• Treatment will depend on the stage of the cancer, your health, and your preferences. The treatments involve surgery, chemotherapy (anticancer drugs), and radiation (less often used). Since most hepatomas cannot be removed by surgery, alternate treatment forms are evolving. These include embolization, radiofrequency ablation, cryotherapy, and injections of alcohol. Your health care provider will discuss the options.
• Surgery is done only for cancer in an early stage. The cancer can still recur, because cancer cells may have spread before surgery.
• Liver transplants have been done in a few select patients.
• Counseling may help in coping with this disorder.

POSSIBLE COMPLICATIONS
• Liver failure.
• Internal bleeding.
• Spread to other organs, especially the lungs, adrenal glands, and bones.

PROBABLE OUTCOME
• This condition is considered incurable. Only a small number of patients survive 5 years after diagnosis. However, symptoms can sometimes be relieved.
• Research into causes and treatment continues, so there is hope for effective treatment.

 HOW TO TREAT

GENERAL MEASURES
• The more you can learn and understand about this disorder, the more you will be able to make informed decisions about where to go for your care, the treatments available, the risks involved, side effects of therapy and expected outcome.
• To learn more: American Cancer Society, (800) ACS-2345; website: www.cancer.org; or National Cancer Institute, (800) -4-CANCER; website: www.nci.nih.gov.

MEDICATION
• For minor discomfort, you may use nonprescription drugs such as acetaminophen. Stronger pain relievers will be prescribed as needed.
• Anticancer drugs may be prescribed.

ACTIVITY—Stay as active as your strength allows.

DIET—No special diet. Don't drink alcohol.

 CALL YOUR DOCTOR IF

• You or a family member has symptoms of hepatoma.
• Signs of bleeding develop, especially from the gastrointestinal tract. (bloody vomit or vomit that contains black material, blood in the stool, or black, tarry stools).

HERNIA

GENERAL INFORMATION

DEFINITION—A part of a body organ or tissue protrudes (pokes out) through the muscle wall that normally holds it in place. The most common types involve the lower torso (abdominal wall area). They include:
* Inguinal hernia and femoral hernia (both involve muscles in the groin).
* Incisional hernia (involves muscles at the site of a prior surgery).
* Umbilical hernia (in newborns, involves muscles around the navel).
* Epigastric hernia (occurs in the upper abdomen, between the breastbone and the navel).
* Periumbilical hernia (develops around the navel, more common in women).

BODY PARTS INVOLVED—Muscles.

SEX OR AGE MOST AFFECTED—Both sexes; all ages.

SIGNS & SYMPTOMS
* A swelling, lump, or bulge in the abdomen. It may be more apparent when standing or coughing. It may reduce in size when pushed back into the abdomen or when lying down.
* Heavy feeling, discomfort, or pain may occur in the abdomen, especially when bending over or lifting.
* Constipation.

CAUSES—Weakness in muscle wall or connective tissue (called fascia). The weakness may be present at birth or acquired later in life. Incisional hernias result from previous surgery.

RISK INCREASES WITH
* Premature infants.
* Adults over 60.
* Chronic cough or chronic lung disease.
* Obesity or overweight.
* Pregnancy.
* Straining, as with chronic constipation.
* Family history of hernias.
* Heavy lifting.

HOW TO PREVENT
* Most hernias cannot be avoided. Maintaining proper weight and regular exercise to keep muscles toned may help prevent some types of hernias.
* Seek medical help if constipation or a chronic cough are problems.

WHAT TO EXPECT

DIAGNOSTIC MEASURES
* Your own observation of symptoms.
* Your health care provider will usually diagnose the hernia by means of a physical exam.

* An x-ray or ultrasound may be done if any complications are suspected.

APPROPRIATE HEALTH CARE
* Surgery is usually advised to repair the hernia (called a herniorrhaphy). Many hernia repairs can now be done by laparoscopy. Surgery is usually done on an outpatient basis. In most cases, the surgery is elective (performed by choice), but there may be an emergency if the hernia is strangulated.
* If the hernia is causing only mild discomfort and can readily be pushed back, a supportive garment or truss may be used for treatment. This may be done if surgery is not possible or surgery needs to be delayed.

POSSIBLE COMPLICATIONS
* Strangulated hernia (loses its blood supply). It may cause serious complications, sometimes fatal.
* Hernia may recur after surgery.
* Surgery complications may develop.

PROBABLE OUTCOME—Umbilical hernias usually heal on their own by age 4 and rarely require surgery. Other hernias are usually curable with surgery.

HOW TO TREAT

GENERAL MEASURES
* For an explanation of surgery and post-operative care, see Hernia (in Surgery section).
* If surgery is not done, see your health care provider for periodic exams of the hernia.

MEDICATION—For minor discomfort, you may use nonprescription drugs such as acetaminophen or ibuprofen.

ACTIVITY
* Speed of recovery will depend on general heath and the type of hernia repaired. Work and regular activities can usually be resumed in a week (or as advised). Complete recovery can take 4 to 6 weeks. Avoid heavy lifting for about 3 months.
* Your health care provider will advise you about returning to sports or exercise activities.

DIET
* Eat a diet high in fiber to avoid constipation.
* Maintain ideal weight.

CALL YOUR DOCTOR IF

* You or a family member has symptoms of a hernia.
* If you have vomiting, fever, severe pain, or are unable to have a bowel movement. Call immediately! This can be an emergency.

HERPANGINA

GENERAL INFORMATION

DEFINITION—A virus of the mouth and throat. It may be mistaken for canker sores, strep throat, or herpes.

BODY PARTS INVOLVED—Soft palate (back of the mouth and tonsil area).

SEX OR AGE MOST AFFECTED—Young children (1 to 10 years).

SIGNS & SYMPTOMS
* Fever.
* Sudden sore throat, with redness, swelling, and painful swallowing.
* Tiny blisters in the affected areas. The blisters become small ulcers (open sores).
* General ill feeling.
* Vomiting and stomach pain (sometimes).

CAUSES—Infection from a virus (usually coxsackie) that is spread from person-to-person. Symptoms appear from 2 to 14 days (average time is 3 to 5 days) after being exposed. If blisters appear on the palms or soles, it is a different disorder called hand, foot and mouth disease.

RISK INCREASES WITH
* Summer and early fall seasons.
* Children in daycare or school where the infection is occurring.

HOW TO PREVENT
* Cannot be prevented at present.
* Wash hands carefully to prevent its spread.
* Avoid close personal contact with infected persons, such as kissing or sharing food.

WHAT TO EXPECT

DIAGNOSTIC MEASURES
* Your own observation of symptoms.
* Your health care provider usually diagnoses the disorder by an exam of the blisters in the mouth and throat.

APPROPRIATE HEALTH CARE—Home care. Usually no treatment is necessary other than simple pain relievers.

POSSIBLE COMPLICATIONS—There are usually no complications.

PROBABLE OUTCOME—Rapid recovery in a few days to a week.

HOW TO TREAT

GENERAL MEASURES—Careful handwashing and sanitary disposal of excretions is important.

MEDICATION
* You may use nonprescription drugs, such as acetaminophen or ibuprofen, to relieve pain and fever. Don't give aspirin to children under age 18.
* Antibiotics do not help a viral infection such as this.

ACTIVITY
* Extra rest until the fever and sore throat disappear.
* A child may be kept at home from daycare or school for a few days if symptoms are present.

DIET—No special diet. Drink extra fluids, such as water, fruit ices, ice chips, or cool-gelatin solutions. Avoid acidic fruit juices, which irritate inflamed tissues.

CALL YOUR DOCTOR IF

Your child has symptoms of herpangina.

ILLNESS & DISORDERS

HERPES, GENITAL

GENERAL INFORMATION

DEFINITION—An infection caused by one of two types of herpes simplex virus (HSV). Herpes type 2 virus (HSV-2) is the usual cause of genital herpes. Herpes type 1 virus (HSV-1) causes common cold sores around the mouth, but can also cause genital herpes.

BODY PARTS INVOLVED—Penis; vagina; cervix; thighs; buttocks (sometimes).

SEX OR AGE MOST AFFECTED—Both sexes and all ages of sexually active persons.

SIGNS & SYMPTOMS
- No symptoms may occur or they may not be noticed. A person may not realize they are infected.
- Early symptoms may include itching or burning in the genital or anal area. This may be followed by pain. Women may have vaginal discharge.
- Within a few days, sores appear in the vaginal area, on the penis, around the anal opening, on the buttocks, thighs, or the mouth. The sores start as red bumps, then turn into a cluster of blisters, that open and cause pain. They then crust over and heal. There is no scarring.
- First episode may include a general ill feeling, difficult and painful urination, swollen lymph glands, and fever.
- Symptoms can recur since the virus permanently remains in the body. Future outbreaks may be milder. They may occur several times a year in some, but others may have only one or two outbreaks in a lifetime.

CAUSES—Having sex (intercourse or oral sex) with someone who is having a herpes outbreak. An outbreak means that HSV is active and usually causes visible sores in the genital area. The sores shed the virus that can infect another person. In some cases, a person may have an outbreak with no visible sores. They can still shed the virus and infect the other person.

RISK INCREASES WITH—Anyone who is sexually active.

HOW TO PREVENT—Avoid sexual intercourse, oral or anal sex, or skin-to-skin contact if either partner has blisters or sores. Use a latex (rubber) condom during intercourse if either sex partner has inactive genital herpes.

WHAT TO EXPECT

DIAGNOSTIC MEASURES
- Your own observation of symptoms.
- Your health care provider usually diagnoses the disorder by an exam of the affected area.
- Medical tests may include blood studies or studies of fluid taken from the sores.

APPROPRIATE HEALTH CARE
- Treatment goals are to relieve the symptoms and prevent recurrences.
- Treatment steps may include drugs.
- Consider counseling for problems of emotional stress.
- If you are pregnant and have herpes, be sure to advise your obstetric provider so any safeguards can be taken.
- Women should have an annual pelvic exam and Pap smear.

POSSIBLE COMPLICATIONS—Complications are rare in otherwise healthy persons. A person with a weak immune system may have more severe and prolonged outbreaks.

PROBABLE OUTCOME—Genital herpes cannot be cured. During symptom-free periods, the virus returns to its dormant (inactive) state. Symptoms recur when the virus is reactivated. The symptoms vary from person to person and from time to time in the same person. Symptoms and recurrence can be relieved with treatment.

HOW TO TREAT

GENERAL MEASURES
- For self-care, keep the affected area clean and dry. Avoid touching the sores, but if you do, wash your hands right away. Warm baths with a tablespoon of salt added can ease some of the discomfort.
- Certain "triggers" can lead to outbreaks. They include skin friction, sex, stress, sunlight and sunburn, wind, fever, surgery, menstruation, infection, and some drugs. A person will begin to recognize their triggers and take steps to avoid them.
- To learn more: Herpes Resource Center, P.O. Box 13827, Research Triangle Park, NC 27709; hotline (919) 361-8488 (not toll-free); website: www.ashastd.org/hrc.

MEDICATION—Antiviral drugs in oral form are often prescribed for treatment and prevention of outbreaks. A topical form is available, but may not be as effective.

ACTIVITY
- No limits on daily activities.
- Avoid sexual relations until symptoms disappear.

DIET—No special diet.

CALL YOUR DOCTOR IF

- You or a family member has symptoms of genital herpes.
- Symptoms don't improve in 1 week, despite treatment.

HERPES SIMPLEX
(Cold Sores; Fever Blisters)

 GENERAL INFORMATION

DEFINITION—A common viral infection that affects the skin. In most cases, people become infected with the virus in childhood. The first time a person (usually a child) is infected, symptoms may include mouth sores, sore throat, fever, aching, tiredness, problems with eating, and swollen glands. The virus then stays inactive in the body (sometimes for months or years), until an active infection occurs and cold sores result.

BODY PARTS INVOLVED—Cold sores usually involve the lips. In some cases, they occur on nostrils, cheeks, or fingers.

SEX OR AGE MOST AFFECTED—Both sexes, all ages.

SIGNS & SYMPTOMS
• Prior to a cold sore, the skin area may feel itchy, tingly, or sensitive.
• A cluster of small, painful, fluid-filled blisters appear in the affected area. The blisters break and ooze. A yellow crust forms and sloughs off, leaving pink skin and no scarring.

CAUSES
• Herpes simplex virus type 1, or, less often, herpes simplex type 2 (the cause of genital herpes). The virus is spread from person to person by contact with fluid from a cold sore, saliva, contact with an item that has the germs on it, or sharing food or drinks with an infected person. The blisters and open sores can spread the virus until they heal.
• Risk factors (listed below) may trigger an outbreak of cold sores. Cold sores also recur for unknown reasons.

RISK INCREASES WITH
• Physical or emotional stress.
• Illness, including a cold, flu, or fever from any cause.
• Menstrual periods.
• Dental treatment that stretches the mouth.
• Weak immune system due to illness or drugs.
• Exposure to the sun.
• Certain foods or drugs.
• Eczema (a skin infection).
• In daycare settings, sharing toys that children put in their mouths.

HOW TO PREVENT
• Avoid contact (such as kissing or sharing food) with someone who has an active cold sore.
• Wash your hands often when you have a cold sore. This can help prevent spreading the virus.
• Use a sunscreen.

 WHAT TO EXPECT

DIAGNOSTIC MEASURES
• Your own observation of symptoms.
• See your health care provider if you are concerned about the symptoms. An exam of the infected area can confirm the diagnosis. Rarely, a medical test is be done of fluid from the sore.
• Medical care may include prescription drugs.

APPROPRIATE HEALTH CARE—Home care.

POSSIBLE COMPLICATIONS—Rarely, infection spreads to other places in the body, such as the eyes and brain. Prompt treatment is vital.

PROBABLE OUTCOME—Recovery takes a few days to a week. Recurrence will vary for different people. Cold sores may recur often or rarely. Complications are unlikely.

 HOW TO TREAT

GENERAL MEASURES
• Apply ice to the affected area, or use nonprescription products for cold sores, to ease discomfort.
• Don't squeeze or pick at the blisters. Avoid touching them except to apply cream or ointment. Then wash hands carefully. Be careful about touching other places in the body, especially the eyes and genital area, where the infection could spread.
• Don't share lip products, or cups and other utensils.

MEDICATION
• Use aspirin, acetaminophen, or ibuprofen to relieve minor pain. Don't give aspirin to children under 18.
• Nonprescription creams or ointments for treating cold sores may be used.
• Antiviral drugs may be prescribed. They can be taken by mouth or applied to the skin.

ACTIVITY—No limits on physical activity. Avoid close contact with others, especially newborns and persons who have weak immune systems.

DIET—No special diet.

 CALL YOUR DOCTOR IF

The following occur with a cold sore:
• The cold sore does not heal in a week.
• Signs of infection, such as fever or pus, instead of clear fluid in the blister. Sores form on the genitals, or the eyes get infected.
• You have a weak immune system due to illness or drugs.

ILLNESS & DISORDERS

HERPES ZOSTER
(Shingles)

 GENERAL INFORMATION

DEFINITION—A condition that causes pain, a rash, and blisters on the skin. You can get it only if you have had chickenpox in the past.

BODY PARTS INVOLVED—Sensory nerves of the skin on one side of the body.

SEX OR AGE MOST AFFECTED—Both sexes and all ages (most common in adults over 50).

SIGNS & SYMPTOMS
* Pain, tingling, or burning on the skin.
* A rash appears a few days after the first symptoms begin. It appears as a band of reddened skin on one side of the chest, neck, or face. The rash turns into fluid-filled blisters. These may itch or be very painful. The blisters then begin to dry out and crust over within several days.
* Mild chills and fever.
* General ill feeling.
* Mild nausea, stomach ache, cramps, or diarrhea.
* Chest pain, face pain, or burning pain in the skin of the stomach (depends on affected area).

CAUSES—Varicella-zoster virus, the same virus that causes chickenpox. After a chickenpox infection, the virus remains inactive in nerve cells in the body. In some people, the virus becomes active again and causes zoster. Why this happens is unknown.

RISK INCREASES WITH
* Anyone who has had chickenpox.
* Adults over 50.
* Cancer.
* High stress situations.
* People who have a weak immune system due to drugs or illness.

PREVENTIVE MEASURES—Cannot be prevented at present.

 WHAT TO EXPECT

DIAGNOSTIC MEASURES
* Your own observation of symptoms.
* Your health care provider can usually diagnose the disorder by a skin exam of the affected area and asking questions about your pain symptoms. If the rash has not appeared, it is more difficult to diagnose.
* Medical tests may be done to confirm the diagnosis.

APPROPRIATE MEDICAL CARE
* Goals of treatment are to relieve the itching and the pain as much as possible. This is usually done with topical and oral drugs.

* The nerve pain that remains after the skin clears up is the most difficult to treat.

POSSIBLE COMPLICATIONS
* Skin infection may occur in the blisters.
* Chronic pain, especially in the elderly. It lasts for months or years in the nerves where the blisters have been. This is called post-herpetic neuralgia.
* Spread of zoster over the body or to internal organs.
* If the face is affected, eye complications can occur.
* When blisters are present, herpes zoster patients can spread the virus and cause chickenpox in people who have never had it. Avoid physical contact with pregnant women, infants, and those with weak immune systems.

PROBABLE OUTCOME—The rash usually clears in 14 to 21 days. The nerve pain may last for a month or longer. One attack usually provides immunity against herpes zoster, but a few persons have had more than one attack.

 HOW TO TREAT

GENERAL MEASURES—For self-care:
* When bathing, wash blisters gently.
* Don't bandage the blistered area.
* Try applying cool, moist compresses to help decrease the pain.
* Soak in a tub of water to which cornstarch or an oatmeal product (such as Aveeno) has been added.

MEDICATION
* Use calamine lotion or capsaicin ointment for the blisters. For minor pain and discomfort, you may use drugs such as aspirin (not for children), acetaminophen, or ibuprofen.
* You may be prescribed one or more drugs to help treat the symptoms. Antiviral drugs can help if the disorder is diagnosed early. Injections of a nerve block may be recommended in severe cases.
* Other drugs for pain may be prescribed. Different ones may need to be tried, as they are not always effective for every person.

ACTIVITY—No limit, except those caused by the symptoms.

DIET—Maintain a healthy diet.

 CALL YOUR DOCTOR IF

* You or a family member has symptoms of herpes zoster.
* Pain gets worse, despite treatment.
* New symptoms develop. Drugs may have side effects.

HERPETIC WHITLOW

GENERAL INFORMATION

DEFINITION—An inflammation of skin folds around the fingernails caused by a contagious herpes virus.

BODY PARTS INVOLVED—Fingernail bed or toenail bed (less common).

SEX OR AGE MOST AFFECTED—Both sexes; all ages. It is more common in children.

SIGNS & SYMPTOMS
• The infected skin around a nail may have pain, tingling, itching, redness, swelling, and/or warmth.
• Groupings of tiny blisters that are barely visible around the nail. They may break open and crust over in a few days to a week.
• Swelling of the lymph glands nearby, such as in the elbow or armpit.
• In some cases, a fever or general ill feeling may occur before the skin symptoms.

CAUSES—Herpes simples virus, either type 1 (usually) or type 2. The herpes infection may be spread from one person to another. It may also start in the mouth as a cold sore and then is spread to the fingers through a break in the skin. In children this can occur when they suck their thumb or finger.

RISK INCREASES WITH
• Persons who have other types of herpes infections.
• Health care workers who are exposed to patients with herpes infections.
• Weak immune system due to illness or drugs.

HOW TO PREVENT
• If you have a herpes infection, do not touch the sores or blisters with bare fingers
• Health care workers should wear protective gloves, wash hands often, and follow proper procedures in disposing of fluids and waste.
• Antiviral drug may be prescribed to help abort a recurrence after the initial episode.

WHAT TO EXPECT

DIAGNOSTIC MEASURES
• Your own observation of symptoms.
• Your health care provider can diagnose the disorder by a skin exam.
• Medical tests may include a laboratory study of fluid removed from the blisters.

APPROPRIATE HEALTH CARE—Treatment involves self care and drugs if needed.

POSSIBLE COMPLICATIONS
• The disorder may be misdiagnosed at first as a bacterial infection.
• A bacterial skin infection may develop in the affected area.
• Rarely, scarring of the affected area.
• Spread of the herpes infection to other parts of the body or to other persons.

PROBABLE OUTCOME—The first episode is usually curable in a 3 to 4 weeks. Antiviral drugs may help shorten the duration of the infection. The disorder may recur.

HOW TO TREAT

GENERAL MEASURES
• Protect your hands to prevent further injury or spread of the infection to others. Wear the proper type of gloves to avoid contact with irritating substances, such as water, soap, detergent, metal scrubbing pads, scouring pads, scouring powder and other chemicals.
• Don't touch other persons until inflammation clears.

MEDICATION
• Topical or oral antiviral drug (usually acyclovir) may be prescribed to treat the symptoms. The oral antiviral drug may be prescribed to help abort future recurrences.
• Antibiotics may be prescribed if a bacterial infection develops.
• Use acetaminophen or ibuprofen for pain or fever.

ACTIVITY—No limits.

DIET—No special diet.

CALL YOUR DOCTOR IF

• You or a family member has symptoms of herpetic whitlow.
• Symptoms don't improve in a few days, despite treatment.
• Herpes infection breaks out elsewhere on the body.

ILLNESS & DISORDERS

HIATAL HERNIA

GENERAL INFORMATION

DEFINITION—A part of the stomach protrudes (pokes) through the diaphragm into the chest. The diaphragm is a thin muscle between the chest and the stomach. The esophagus (the tube from the mouth) connects to the stomach through an opening in the diaphragm called the hiatus. A hiatus may become weak and allow part of the stomach to push up through the weak area and into the chest. This becomes a hiatal hernia. It is a common problem.

BODY PARTS INVOLVED—Esophagus; stomach; diaphragm.

SEX OR AGE MOST AFFECTED—Both sexes; all ages, but most common in older adults.

SIGNS & SYMPTOMS—Hiatal hernias do not usually cause symptoms. A person with a hiatal hernia may be more likely to have reflux or it may make existing reflux worse. Reflux occurs when acid in the stomach backs up into the esophagus. This can lead to symptoms of heartburn such as burning in the chest after a meal.

CAUSES—A person may be born with a hiatal hernia or develop one as they get older. An injury or surgery may lead to the problem also.

RISK INCREASES WITH
* Muscle weakness and loss of elasticity (ability of muscles to stretch and regain shape) due to aging.
* Injury or surgery of the diaphragm.
* Obesity.
* Lifting or straining.
* Pregnancy (it increases pressure in the abdomen).
* Ascites (excess fluid in the abdomen).
* Smoking.

HOW TO PREVENT—No specific preventive measures.

WHAT TO EXPECT

DIAGNOSTIC MEASURES
* Your health care provider will usually do a physical exam and ask about your symptoms and eating habits.
* Medical tests may include x-rays of the esophagus and stomach. An endoscopy (the passing of a tube with a camera on the end into the esophagus) may be done.

APPROPRIATE HEALTH CARE
* The goals of treatment are to relieve any reflux symptoms and to manage and prevent complications.
* Self care and drug therapy are used in treatment. Rarely, surgery is recommended.

* Surgery to repair the hernia may be recommended for certain patients with complications of GERD or other health problems, such as chronic lung disease. Some repairs can now be done by laparoscopy.

POSSIBLE COMPLICATIONS
* Esophageal complications.
* Gastroesophageal reflux disease (GERD).

PROBABLE OUTCOME—Reflux and heartburn symptoms can usually be relieved with treatment.

HOW TO TREAT

GENERAL MEASURES
* Raise the head of your bed 4 to 6 inches. This allows gravity to keep stomach acid away from the hernia.
* Don't smoke. Find a way to stop that works.
* Don't wear tight pantyhose, undergarments, belts, or pants.
* Don't strain with bowel movements or urination.

MEDICATION
* Antacids in table or liquid form. These are most effective for some persons when they take them 1 hour before meals and at bedtime. Others find them more helpful 1 to 2 hours after meals and at bedtime. Try both ways to find the best schedule for you.
* Use stool softeners to prevent constipation.
* Nonprescription or prescription drugs called H2-receptor blockers or proton pump inhibitors are often prescribed for symptoms.
* Drugs that help the stomach empty more quickly may be prescribed.

ACTIVITY—No limits. Don't bend over or lie down immediately after a meal.

DIET
* Avoid large meals. Eat 6 small meals a day instead. Eat slowly. Don't eat anything 1 to 2 hours before bedtime.
* A diet with more fiber may help prevent constipation.
* Lose weight, if you are overweight.
* Avoid alcohol, caffeine-containing drinks (coffee, tea, cocoa, cola drinks), and any other food, juice, or spice that may cause symptoms.

CALL YOUR DOCTOR IF

* You or a family member has symptoms of heartburn.
* Call immediately if pain occurs along with shortness of breath, sweating, or nausea.
* You vomit blood or have recurrent vomiting.
* Fever occurs.
* Symptoms don't improve in 1 month with treatment.

HICCUP
(Hiccough; Singultus)

GENERAL INFORMATION

DEFINITION—Hiccups are a symptom, not a disease. Hiccups involve the diaphragm (the large, thin muscle that separates the chest from the abdomen) and the phrenic nerve (the nerve that connects the diaphragm to the brain).

BODY PARTS INVOLVED
• Diaphragm (big muscle which separates the chest from the abdomen).
• Phrenic nerve (nerve that connects the diaphragm to the brain).

SEX OR AGE MOST AFFECTED—Both sexes; all ages Almost everybody gets hiccups, even unborn babies.

SIGNS & SYMPTOMS—A sharp, quick sound produced from the mouth by a spasm of the diaphragm. The spasm closes muscles in the back of the throat.

CAUSES—Irritation of nerves that control breathing muscles, especially the diaphragm. The cause of short hiccup episodes is usually unknown. Prolonged or recurrent hiccup episodes may be caused by many different medical problems.

RISK INCREASES WITH
• Swallowing hot or irritating substances.
• Diseases of the pleura (thin membrane layers that cover the lung).
• Pneumonia.
• Uremia (a blood infection).
• Alcoholism.
• Disorders of the stomach, esophagus, bowel, or pancreas.
• Pregnancy.
• Bladder irritation.
• Hepatitis of the liver.
• Spread of cancer from another part of the body to the liver or part of the pleura.
• Recent surgery, especially abdominal surgery.
• Emotional causes.
• Use of drugs, such as those that irritate the stomach.
• Full stomach.
• Laughter or intense emotions.
• Changes in temperature.
• Alcohol use.
• Noxious fumes (bad smells in the air).

HOW TO PREVENT—Cannot be prevented at present.

WHAT TO EXPECT

DIAGNOSTIC MEASURES
• Your own observation of symptoms.

• See your health care provider if hiccups continue or recur often. A physical exam will be done and questions asked about your symptoms, eating habits, and activities.
• Medical tests are usually not needed, but may be done to check for a suspected medical problem.

APPROPRIATE HEALTH CARE
• Self-care almost always.
• In rare cases, drugs or nerve surgery may be needed for severe, persistent hiccups.

POSSIBLE COMPLICATIONS—None, unless hiccups are prolonged, which may indicate a medical problem.

PROBABLE OUTCOME—Short hiccup episodes usually don't indicate disease. They will go away on their own or with treatment. Continued hiccups can be a problem and require medical care to find and treat the cause.

HOW TO TREAT

GENERAL MEASURES—These instructions are for short hiccup episodes. Prolonged hiccups require medical care. Try one or more methods to see which works best for you.
• Hold your breath and count to 10.
• Breathe into a paper bag, and rebreathe air in the bag. Don't use a plastic bag because it may cling to nostrils.
• Insert your thumb between your teeth and upper lip; press the upper lip with your index finger just below the right nostril.
• Press a forefinger into each ear for about 20 seconds.
• Drink a glass of water rapidly.
• Swallow dry bread or crushed ice.
• Pull gently on the tongue.
• Close eyelids and apply gentle pressure to the eyeballs.
• Swallow a teaspoon of dry sugar.

MEDICATION—Usually no drugs are needed for this disorder. In some severe or prolonged cases, drugs may be prescribed to help control the hiccups.

ACTIVITY—No limits.

DIET—Avoid overeating or drinking carbonated drinks.

CALL YOUR DOCTOR IF

• Hiccups persist longer than 8 hours.
• You suspect a prescription drug may be the cause of hiccups.

HIDRADENITIS SUPPURATIVA

GENERAL INFORMATION

DEFINITION—Hidradenitis means inflammation of the sweat glands. Suppurative means there is pus.

BODY PARTS INVOLVED—The armpits are usually affected, but it can occur on the buttocks, groin, or under the breasts in females.

SEX OR AGE MOST AFFECTED—Both sexes; all ages, but more common in young females.

SIGNS & SYMPTOMS—Nodular lesions (sores) with the following features:
• They are firm, tender, and domed.
• Larger ones soften in the center and become painful.
• When pressed, they feel like an overfilled inner tube.
• They open, and often drain pus.
• Individual lesions (with or without drainage) heal slowly over 10 to 30 days.
• Scars are left on the skin after healing.
• Severity of the disorder varies from a few lesions per year to several lesions that form as old ones heal. They often show up at the same place on the skin.

CAUSES—Exact cause is unknown. The apocrine glands (a form of sweat glands) in the body seem to cause the problem. Substances in these glands enlarge the gland. The outlets become blocked, probably by heat, sweat, or incomplete gland development. The substances that are in the glands force sweat and bacteria into skin tissue, which then becomes infected.

RISK INCREASES WITH
• Exposure to heat and moisture.
• Family history. This disorder is most common in black females.
• Smoking may be a risk factor.
• Obesity does not cause the disorder, but may make it worse.

HOW TO PREVENT—No specific preventive measures.

WHAT TO EXPECT

DIAGNOSTIC MEASURES
• Your own observation of symptoms.
• Your health care provider can usually diagnose the disorder by an exam of the affected area.
• Medical tests may be done to check for infection or other problems.

APPROPRIATE HEALTH CARE
• Treatment involves self-care measures, drug therapy, and sometimes surgery.
• Surgery to open and drain abscesses or to remove involved skin may be recommended.

POSSIBLE COMPLICATIONS
• Extensive lesions that do not respond to treatment.
• Scarring may restrict movement of arm.
• Other medical problems due to infection or inflammation.

PROBABLE OUTCOME—This disorder may last many years, from puberty through the following 10 to 20 years. Symptoms can often be controlled with treatment. There is no cure for this disorder.

HOW TO TREAT

GENERAL MEASURES
• Avoid getting overheated and sweating.
• Avoid tight clothing or clothes that irritate the skin.
• Wash with antibacterial soap. A liquid form may be used for washing, and then applied as a lotion. It may help reduce odor.
• Don't shave the infected area.
• Avoid stress if you can. It may make symptoms worse.
• Use soaks to relieve itching and hasten healing. Warm-water soaks are usually more soothing for pain or inflammation. Cool-water soaks feel better for itching.

MEDICATION
• You may be prescribed:
  - Injection of cortisone drugs directly into the lesions.
  - Antibiotics to treat infection.
  - Hormones to help subdue inflammation.
  - Isotretinoin has been effective in some patients. This is a potent drug, and must be given under medical supervision.
• For minor discomfort, you may use drugs such as acetaminophen.

ACTIVITY—Restrict your activity in hot weather. Avoid working in the heat, if possible. Swimming is an excellent activity.

DIET—No special diet, unless you need to lose weight. Losing weight may help ease the symptoms.

CALL YOUR DOCTOR IF

• You or a family member has symptoms of hidradenitis suppurativa.
• Lesions don't improve after 5 days of treatment, or new symptoms develop.

HIP DISLOCATION, CONGENITAL

GENERAL INFORMATION

DEFINITION—A disorder in which the head of the thigh bone doesn't fit properly into, or is outside of, the hip socket. The condition is also called developmental dysplasia. Most often, the condition occurs after birth. The condition does not cause pain in the newborn.

BODY PARTS INVOLVED—One or both hip joints.

SEX OR AGE MOST AFFECTED—About 1 of every 60 newborns has a possible hip dislocation. About 85% are girls.

SIGNS & SYMPTOMS
• One limb may appear shorter than its mate. There may be less mobility or flexibility on one side.
• Skin folds of the buttocks will not be symmetrical; the side with the dislocated hip will have more creases than the other.
• When the child is old enough to walk, he or she may waddle, limp, or favor one side.

CAUSES—Unknown. Several risk factors have been identified. Hormonal changes in the mother during pregnancy may contribute to the development of the condition. High levels of the hormone, estrogen, relax ligaments in the mother and some babies may be more sensitive to the estrogen than others.

RISK INCREASES WITH
• Family history of hip dislocation.
• Females.
• First born.
• Twins or other multiple births.
• Breech birth.
• Little or no amniotic fluid.
• Swaddling an infant or using a cradle-board (as done in certain cultures) may increase the risk.
• It sometimes occurs along with congenital torticollis (the baby's head is bent or turned) and/or turned-in-feet.

HOW TO PREVENT—Cannot be entirely prevented at present. Ask your child's health care provider about swaddling or using a cradle-board for your baby.

WHAT TO EXPECT

DIAGNOSTIC MEASURES
• Your own observation of symptoms.
• Your child's health care provider may suspect the condition is present when doing a well baby physical exam.
• An ultrasound of the hip will aid in confirming the diagnosis. Other imaging tests may be done.

APPROPRIATE HEALTH CARE
• Treatment depends on the child's age and hip development. The goal is to hold the hips in place so they can continue their development.
• Splints or a harness, or, sometimes, a cast may be used to hold the hips in place. It will probably be used for 6 to 12 weeks.
• Closed (no incision is made) reduction may be needed. This is done under an anesthetic. A cast is placed for about 3 months. Leg traction may also be used for treatment.
• In some cases, open reduction surgery is done to correct the problem.

POSSIBLE COMPLICATIONS—Delayed diagnosis and treatment may lead to the need for more extensive surgery, possible treatment failure, long term hip damage, and osteoarthritis later in life.

PROBABLE OUTCOME—If congenital hip dislocation is detected early, it is normally curable. Surgery is used only when conservative treatment fails or the disorder has not been discovered until late in childhood.

HOW TO TREAT

GENERAL MEASURES
• Your child will develop normally during the treatment time. A child can still have some mobility depending on the type of treatment.
• You will be advised about home care during the treatment period, such as how to take care of a cast or if the harness is to be worn full time.

MEDICATION—Drugs are usually not needed for this disorder.

ACTIVITY—Will depend on the type of treatment prescribed. Your child's health care provider will advise you about specific activities allowed.

DIET—No special diet.

CALL YOUR DOCTOR IF

• Your child has signs of a congenital hip dislocation.
• Any symptoms develop during treatment that cause concern.

HIP FRACTURE (Femoral Neck Fracture)

GENERAL INFORMATION

DEFINITION—A complete or partial break (fracture) in the femur. The femur is the major bone in the hip joint.

BODY PARTS INVOLVED—Femur, including muscles and tendons that attach the head of the femur to the acetabulum (hip socket in the bony pelvis).

SEX OR AGE MOST AFFECTED
• Breaks from common injuries affect both sexes and all ages.
• Spontaneous (occurs without an injury) breaks, and breaks from minor injuries, affect mostly older people. Nine out of 10 hip fractures occur in persons over 65, and 3 out of 4 occur in women.

SIGNS & SYMPTOMS
• Severe pain when trying to walk.
• Pain may occur in the groin or thigh.
• Swelling, tenderness, and bruising in the hip area.
• Deformed hip appearance.

CAUSES—Hip fractures are usually caused by injuries (trauma) such as falls, other types of accidents, and sports injuries. Weakened bones are more at risk of a fracture.

RISK INCREASES WITH
• Female, over age 65, and Caucasian.
• Osteoporosis, especially in women after menopause.
• Decreased bone mineral density.
• Falls. Risk of falls increases with muscle weakness, problems with walking or balance, disorders such as Parkinson's and stroke, poor eyesight, foot problems, arthritis, previous falls, use of certain drugs, and home risks.
• Self-reported poor health.
• Family history of hip fracture.
• Sedentary (lack of physical activity) lifestyle.
• Previous fractures of any kind.
• Previous hyperthyroidism.
• Motor vehicle accidents and physical activities such as contact sports for younger hip fracture patients.

HOW TO PREVENT
• Protect against falls, especially in the home.
• Drug therapies to improve bone density.
• Daily exercise improves bone strength and maintains muscle strength and balance.

WHAT TO EXPECT

DIAGNOSTIC MEASURES
• Your own observation of symptoms.
• Your health care provider will do a physical exam.
• Medical tests include x-rays of the hip.

APPROPRIATE HEALTH CARE
• Hospital care with surgery is the main treatment. The surgeon reattaches fractured bone parts and secures them with surgical steel pins; the surgeon may replace body parts with a medical device (complete hip or parts of a hip) in people whose bones can no longer grow back together. Unlike most fractures, hip fractures usually don't require casts.
• After surgery, time is usually spent in a rehabilitation center for therapy to help regain mobility and functions of daily living.
• Ongoing physical therapy may be needed to rehabilitate the muscles, bones, and joints.

POSSIBLE COMPLICATIONS
• Surgical-wound infection, incomplete healing, and other surgery complications.
• Being immobile for a prolonged period can lead to blood clots, pulmonary embolism, pneumonia, and weakened muscles.
• Loss of mobility (may require wheelchair use), loss of independence, reduced quality of life, and depression.

PROBABLE OUTCOME—Outcome depends on the age and health of the patient and the location of the fracture. In older persons, there is often a loss of ability to function as they did before the fracture. The function loss may be mild to severe.

HOW TO TREAT

GENERAL MEASURES—See Hip Nailing for Hip Fracture in Surgery section.

MEDICATION
• Pain relievers as needed may be prescribed.
• Antibiotics for infection and blood thinners to prevent blood clots may be prescribed.
• Stool softeners to prevent constipation.
• Drugs to increase bone mass and to prevent bone loss may be prescribed.

ACTIVITY
• After surgery, move the unaffected leg often to decrease the risk of deep-vein blood clots. You will be urged to get up and move about.
• A physical therapist will help in rehabilitation, which can take several months. A walker or crutches will be used at first. Riding an exercise bike or swimming are good forms of therapy.
• Resume your normal activities to the extent possible as healing progresses.

DIET—Usually no special diet.

CALL YOUR DOCTOR IF

• You or a family member has symptoms of a hip fracture. Call right away if there is numbness or loss of feeling below the injury site.
• Any new symptoms develop after surgery.

HIRSUTISM

GENERAL INFORMATION

DEFINITION—Hirsutism is increased growth of hair on the face and body that occurs in women. It usually occurs gradually over an extended period of time. It may begin with puberty. Hirsutism is a benign condition and is mostly a cosmetic problem. When it occurs along with signs of masculinity (maleness), a more serious disorder may be involved.

BODY PARTS INVOLVED—Endocrine system.

SEX OR AGE MOST AFFECTED—Post-pubescent females.

SIGNS & SYMPTOMS
- Excessive growth of thick, dark hair in body areas of women where hair growth is normally absent or minimal. It grows in a male pattern (beard, moustache, chest, around the nipples, genitals, and other places).
- Hair growth may occur along with irregular or absent menstrual periods, acne, deepening of the voice, and infertility problems.

CAUSES—It may be due to genetic (hereditary) factors, hormonal dysfunction, certain drugs, and some medical disorders. In some cases, no cause is found.

RISK INCREASES WITH
- Family history of hirsutism.
- Dark-haired persons, especially those of Hispanic, African-American, Mediterranean, or Indian ancestry.
- Use of drugs such as testosterone, steroids, and others.
- Adrenal disorders.
- Adrenal or ovarian tumor.
- Polycystic ovarian syndrome.
- Anorexia, acromegaly, hypothyroidism, or porphyria.

HOW TO PREVENT—No specific preventive measures.

WHAT TO EXPECT

DIAGNOSTIC MEASURES
- Your health care provider will do a physical exam.
- A variety of medical tests may be done to help diagnose any disorder that could be the cause of the hair growth.

APPROPRIATE HEALTH CARE
- The treatment depends on the cause of the hirsutism. A mild case of hirsutism with no menstrual problems may not require treatment. For others, treatment sometimes depends on the patient's desire for pregnancy.
- Treatment may involve drugs, surgery, and hair removal techniques.
- Tumors may be treated with surgery.

- Permanent hair removal may be done with electrolysis or thermolysis. These use an electric current to remove hair. Multiple treatments are needed. It is time-consuming, can be costly, and cause some discomfort.
- Permanent hair removal may be done with a laser. Larger areas can be treated quickly and with minimal discomfort. Multiple treatments are needed. It is costly.
- Other forms of hair removal include pulsed light and photodynamic (use of a topical drug and special light).
- The various forms of hair removal can cause skin irritation, folliculitis (inflamed hair follicles), skin color changes, and, rarely, scarring.

POSSIBLE COMPLICATIONS
- Poor self-image. May feel unattractive, stressed, anxious, and find social activities with other people difficult.
- Complications may occur from underlying disorder.

PROBABLE OUTCOME—Diagnosis and treatment of the cause can often halt further hair growth. Treatment may take 6 to 12 months. Excess hair may be removed by various methods.

HOW TO TREAT

GENERAL MEASURES—Cosmetic treatments of hirsutism include covering up with makeup, bleaching, and removal with physical methods. These include rubbing, cutting, shaving, plucking, or waxing. Chemical depilatories are designed to use on specific body locations. Home hair-removal devices are available. All of these methods are temporary; their effects lasting from hours to days.

MEDICATION
- There are a variety of drugs used to treat the underlying cause of hirsutism. They may take 3 to 6 months for results. They can help decrease new hair growth. They will not change the amount of hair you already have.
- Eflornithine (Vaniqa), a topical drug, may be prescribed for reducing facial hair.
- If skin gets irritated, use nonprescription 1% hydrocortisone cream.
- If a drug is causing hirsutism, it is usually stopped.

ACTIVITY—Usually no limits.

DIET—No special diet. If overweight, losing weight may help.

CALL YOUR DOCTOR IF

- You or a family member has symptoms of hirsutism.
- New, unexplained symptoms develop.

HISTOPLASMOSIS

GENERAL INFORMATION

DEFINITION—A fungus infection that normally affects people who live in eastern and Midwestern parts of the United States. Most cases are minor and go undiagnosed.

BODY PARTS INVOLVED—Lungs; central nervous system; gastrointestinal system.

SEX OR AGE MOST AFFECTED—Both sexes; all ages.

SIGNS & SYMPTOMS
* Frequently, no symptoms are present.
* Persistent cough and other symptoms, similar to a cold.
* Loss of appetite, diarrhea, and weight loss.
* Fever; headache.
* Irritability.
* Paleness.
* Abdominal swelling.
* Breathing difficulty (rare).

CAUSES—Infection by the fungus, *Histoplasma capsulatum*. People become infected by breathing dust that contains fungus spores. The fungus is found in soil contaminated by feces of birds and bats that carry the fungus. This soil is most often found in pigeon lofts, barns, chicken houses, and in damp areas under bridges, along streams, and in caves.

RISK INCREASES WITH
* Geographic location. The disease is normally found in the western Appalachian slopes and the Mississippi, Missouri, and Ohio River valleys. Millions of people living in these areas have been infected, but never have symptoms or they are so mild that they go unnoticed.
* Working in construction-related activities that disturb contaminated soil (e.g., bulldozing or demolition).
* Spelunking (cave exploring).

HOW TO PREVENT—No specific preventive measures. Wear protective masks for work in areas that might be contaminated.

WHAT TO EXPECT

DIAGNOSTIC MEASURES
* Your own observation of symptoms.
* Your health care provider will do a physical exam and ask about your symptoms and activities.
* Medical tests may include sputum culture, blood studies, skin tests, and chest x-ray.

APPROPRIATE HEALTH CARE—Treatment is usually with drugs and supportive care.

POSSIBLE COMPLICATIONS
* People with weak immune systems or middle-aged smokers are more at risk for complications.
* Spread of infection to other organs. This is rare, but it can sometimes be fatal.
* Histoplasmosis often recurs in AIDS patients.
* Eye problems if infection spreads.

PROBABLE OUTCOME
* Mild cases usually resolve on their own. Most people only feel tired or "bad" for several weeks.
* Severe cases are treatable with antifungal drugs.

HOW TO TREAT

GENERAL MEASURES
* Isolation is not necessary. The disease is not transmitted from person to person.
* Don't smoke.
* Use warm compresses or a heating pad on the chest to relieve pain.

MEDICATION
* For mild cases, no drugs are usually needed.
* For more-severe cases, antifungal drugs will be prescribed. Some may be given intravenously (IV).
* For AIDS patients, chronic therapy with antifungal drugs will be necessary.
* You may use nonprescription drugs, such as acetaminophen or aspirin (not for children), to relieve pain.

ACTIVITY—Get extra rest until fever, pain, and shortness of breath disappear for at least 48 hours. Then resume your normal activities gradually. Many people are tired and weak after recovery. Don't expect too much too soon.

DIET—No special diet.

CALL YOUR DOCTOR IF

* You or a family member has symptoms of histoplasmosis.
* The following occur during treatment:
  - Weight loss continues.
  - Fever rises to 101°F (38.3°C) orally.
  - Diarrhea is severe.
  - Severe headache and stiff neck occur.

HIV & AIDS (Human Immunodeficiency Virus; Acquired Immunodeficiency Syndrome)

 GENERAL INFORMATION

DEFINITION—Human immunodeficiency virus (HIV) is a virus that gradually destroys the body's ability to fight infection and certain cancers. Acquired immunodeficiency syndrome (AIDS) is a secondary immunodeficiency syndrome resulting from HIV infection.

BODY PARTS INVOLVED—Lungs; central nervous system; gastrointestinal system.

SEX OR AGE MOST AFFECTED—Both sexes; all ages; most common in young males ages 25-44.

SIGNS & SYMPTOMS
- Initial infection with HIV may produce no symptoms.
- Fatigue and unexplained weight loss.
- Recurrent respiratory and skin infections and fever.
- Swollen lymph glands throughout the body.
- Genital changes.
- Diarrhea.
- Mouth sores.
- Night sweats.

CAUSES—HIV is a virus (retrovirus) that invades and destroys cells of the body's immune system.

RISK INCREASES WITH
- Sexual contact with infected persons. Homosexual men are at the greatest risk.
- Multiple sexual partners (particularly anal intercourse).
- Contaminated needles used by IV drug abusers.
- Transfusions of blood or blood products from a person with acquired immunodeficiency syndrome (rare).
- Children born to an HIV infected mother.
- Exposure of hospital workers and laboratory technicians to blood, feces, and urine of HIV-positive patients. Greatest risk is with an accidental needle injury.
- Note: Nonsexual contact does not transmit the disease. A person with HIV infection is not a risk to the general population.

HOW TO PREVENT
- Avoid sexual contact with HIV-affected person or known IV drug user. Limit sexual activity to partners whose sexual histories are known.
- Use condoms for intercourse (vaginal or anal). Their consistent use may reduce transmission.
- The risk of oral sex is not fully known. Ejaculation into the mouth should be avoided.
- Avoid IV drugs of abuse. Don't share unsterilized needles.
- Avoid unscreened blood products.
- Infected people or those in risk groups should not donate blood, sperm, organs, or tissue.

- Early diagnosis is helpful. If you are at risk, obtain a medical test even if you feel well.

 WHAT TO EXPECT

DIAGNOSTIC MEASURES
- Your health care provider will do a physical exam and ask questions about your sexual history.
- Medical tests may include blood studies and an HIV antibody test. It may not become positive for 6 months after exposure to HIV. Tests for other sexually transmitted diseases and infections are usually done.

APPROPRIATE HEALTH CARE
- Treatment incudes drug therapy and self-care. Hospital care may be needed for complications.
- Counseling helps you cope with having HIV.

POSSIBLE COMPLICATIONS—Serious infections, cancer, and once ill, survival averages vary.

PROBABLE OUTCOME—This condition is currently considered incurable. Symptoms can be relieved or controlled. AIDS may not develop for years following a positive HIV test.

 HOW TO TREAT

GENERAL MEASURES
- Advise past/present sexual partners to get HIV tests.
- Get regular medical and dental check-ups. Tell any health care provider you consult that you have HIV.
- Avoid exposure to people with infections.
- Join a support group.
- To learn more: National AIDS Hotline: (800) 342-2437; website: www.cdc.gov/hiv/dhap.htm.

MEDICATION—Drugs to treat HIV and AIDS, and drugs to treat infections or complications will be prescribed.

ACTIVITY—Fatigue or infections can limit some activities. Get the rest you need, but try to exercise to the extent possible.

DIET—Try to maintain good nutrition. Poor eating habits, changes in metabolism, and weight loss are common.

 CALL YOUR DOCTOR IF

- You or a family member has HIV.symptoms.
- Any infections occur after diagnosis. Symptoms include fever, cough, and diarrhea.
- Other new symptoms develop. Drugs used in treatment have many side effects.

HIVES
(Urticaria; Giant Urticaria)

GENERAL INFORMATION

DEFINITION—An allergic reaction that involves the skin. Hives may occur anywhere on the body, but the arms, legs, and trunk are most often affected. Urticaria is the medical name for hives. Hives are very common.

BODY PARTS INVOLVED—Skin anywhere, including the scalp, lips, palms and soles.

SEX OR AGE MOST AFFECTED—Both sexes; all ages.

SIGNS & SYMPTOMS
• Raised, red areas on the skin. They may be referred to as wheals or welts. They usually itch, but they may also burn or sting. The size may range from small spots to the size of a dinner plate. They can sometimes cause the whole lip or eyelid to swell.
• Wheals can join together quickly and form large, flat plaques. These are raised, skin-colored areas.
• Wheals and plaques change shape, go away, and come back in minutes or hours.

CAUSES—Release of histamines. These are chemicals in the cells of the human body that are released during an allergic reaction. They may be released due to a specific reaction or in some cases for unknown reasons.

RISK INCREASES WITH
• Drugs (many cause hives in some persons).
• Insect bites; viral infections; some chronic medical disorders.
• Exposure to cold, heat, water, or sunlight.
• Exposure to animals, especially cats.
• Eating eggs, fruits, nuts, and shellfish. Other foods may cause hives in infants but not adults.
• Food dyes and preservatives (possibly).
• Infection (bacterial, viral, fungal).
• Cancer, especially leukemia.
• Physical and emotional stress, other allergies, or family history of allergies.

HOW TO PREVENT
• There are no specific preventive measures to stop the first outbreak of hives. Once you have had hives and know the cause, you need to avoid it in the future.
• Your health care provider may advise you to keep an emergency injection kit handy if you have had severe reactions.

WHAT TO EXPECT

DIAGNOSTIC MEASURES
• Your own observation of symptoms.
• See your health care provider if the hives are more severe or cause concern. A diagnosis can

be made by a physical exam of the affected skin. Questions will be asked to help identify the cause.
• Medical tests are usually not needed.

APPROPRIATE HEALTH CARE
• Most persons will treat hives at home. Try to identify the cause of the hives.
• Treatment usually involves antihistamines, stopping the cause of the hives when known (such as a drug, cosmetic, or soap), and self-care measures. If the reaction is severe, hospital care may be needed.

POSSIBLE COMPLICATIONS—Other allergic reactions may occur with hives:
• Angioedema (face, throat, and tongue swelling).
• Anaphylaxis (severe reaction that causes shock and difficulty in breathing).

PROBABLE OUTCOME—Hives usually clear up within hours or days (even if the cause is unknown). They can be uncomfortable, but normally they cause no complications. A few cases become chronic and may last for weeks.

HOW TO TREAT

GENERAL MEASURES
• Don't wear tight clothing. Any skin irritation may trigger new outbreaks.
• Don't take hot baths or showers.
• Apply cold-water compresses or soaks.
• Try to relax and not become over-stressed.

MEDICATION
• Use nonprescription antihistamines for the itching.
• Prescription antihistamines, steroids, or other drugs to relieve itching and rash may be prescribed.
• Epinephrine by injection for severe symptoms.

ACTIVITY—Decrease activities until several days after hives disappear. Avoid getting hot, sweaty, or overly excited.

DIET
• If foods are suspected as a cause, keep a food diary to help identify the offending food.
• Avoid alcohol and coffee or other caffeine-containing beverages if they appear to trigger outbreaks.

CALL YOUR DOCTOR IF

• You or a family member has hives that aren't helped by self-care or last for more than 2 days.
• Any outbreak of hives leads to severe symptoms and breathing problems. This is an emergency!

HODGKIN'S DISEASE

GENERAL INFORMATION

DEFINITION—A cancer that involves the lymph glands. This is a form of lymphoma.

BODY PARTS INVOLVED
* Lymphocytes (white blood cells).
* Lymph glands (glands which help control infection and produce immune substances).
* Spleen (a large lymph gland).

SEX OR AGE MOST AFFECTED—All ages, but most common in young adults and older persons. Hodgkin's disease is rare in children under 10.

SIGNS & SYMPTOMS
* Swollen, non-tender, rubbery, distinct lymph glands anywhere in the body, but most commonly in the neck, armpit, or groin.
* Intermittent fever and night sweats.
* Itching all over the body.
* Weight loss.
* Jaundice (yellow skin and eyes).
* General ill feeling.
* Cough.

CAUSES—Unknown, but research suggests a viral infection may be a factor.

RISK INCREASES WITH—People with weak immune systems due to illness or drugs.

HOW TO PREVENT—No specific preventive measures.

WHAT TO EXPECT

DIAGNOSTIC MEASURES
* Your own observation of symptoms.
* Your health care provider will do a physical exam and ask questions about your symptoms and activities.
* Different medical tests are done to verify the diagnosis and to determine if the cancer has spread to other places in the body (called staging).

APPROPRIATE HEALTH CARE
* Treatment may be radiation alone, chemotherapy alone, or the two in combination. Treatment will depend on the stage of the disease, your health, and your preferences.
* Radiation therapy may consist of daily treatments, Monday through Friday, for about four weeks. Side effects that occur will stop once treatment is complete.
* Males receiving therapy may want to consider sperm-banking in case of sterility. Females may want to store fertilized eggs.
* Counseling may help a person to cope with having cancer.

POSSIBLE COMPLICATIONS
* Spread of cancer to other places in the body.
* Infertility in males and females.
* Heart or lung disorders, anemia, hypothyroidism, and infections.
* Cancer may return.

PROBABLE OUTCOME—Usually curable with radiation therapy and anticancer drugs, if diagnosed and treated early. With treatment, the 10-year survival rate is about 80%.

HOW TO TREAT

GENERAL MEASURES
* Try to remain optimistic about your treatment and chances for cure. A good mental attitude is a powerful ally.
* Good oral hygiene is important to prevent mouth sores, if receiving chemotherapy.
* To learn more: American Cancer Society, (800) ACS-2345; website: www.cancer.org or National Cancer Institute, (800) 4-CANCER; website: www.nci.nih.gov.

MEDICATION
* Anticancer drugs. These may cause side effects or adverse reactions in some people. They may be given as an outpatient or require a hospital stay.
* Steroid drugs may be prescribed for short periods.

ACTIVITY—Remain as active as your strength allows. Regular exercise can help both physical and emotional health.

DIET—No special diet.

CALL YOUR DOCTOR IF

* You or a family member has symptoms of Hodgkin's disease.
* Any new symptoms develop or other symptoms get worse during treatment.

HYPERALDOSTERONISM
(Aldosteronism)

 GENERAL INFORMATION

DEFINITION—An endocrine disease caused by too much aldosterone, a hormone made by the adrenal gland. Excess aldosterone causes the kidneys to take in too much sodium and water, and eliminate too much potassium.

BODY PARTS INVOLVED—Adrenal glands, which are attached at the upper part of the kidneys; kidneys; fluids and electrolytes in the bloodstream and body cells.

SEX OR AGE MOST AFFECTED
• Both sexes, but more common in females.
• All ages, but most common in adults between ages 30 and 50.

SIGNS & SYMPTOMS
• Fatigue and weakness.
• Temporary paralysis (sometimes).
• Tingling sensations in the arms, legs, hands, and feet.
• Urinary frequency, especially at night.
• Thirst.
• Severe muscle spasms.
• Vision problems.
The following may show up in medical tests:
• Low blood levels of potassium.
• High blood levels of sodium.
• High blood pressure.

CAUSES—It involves the adrenal glands, which are attached to the upper part of the kidneys. The increased adrenal secretion of aldosterone is caused by:
• A tumor of the adrenal gland.
• High blood pressure or kidney disease, causing increased production in the kidneys of a hormone (renin) that controls aldosterone levels.

RISK INCREASES WITH
• Kidney disease.
• Congestive heart failure.
• Cirrhosis of the liver.
• Use of oral contraceptives.
• Use of drugs that cause potassium loss.
• Pregnancy.

HOW TO PREVENT—If you have kidney disease or high blood pressure, remain under medical care, and adhere to your treatment program even if you have no symptoms.

 WHAT TO EXPECT

DIAGNOSTIC MEASURES
• Your own observation of symptoms.
• Your health care provider will do a physical exam and ask questions about your symptoms.
• Medical tests may include blood studies of electrolyte levels and CT or MRI scan (see Glossary for these tests) of the kidneys and adrenal glands.

APPROPRIATE HEALTH CARE
• Treatment usually involves drugs and a sodium-restricted diet.
• Surgery to remove adrenal gland in some patients.

POSSIBLE COMPLICATIONS
• Congestive heart failure.
• Atherosclerosis.
• Kidney failure.

PROBABLE OUTCOME—If the disorder is caused by an adrenal tumor, it is often curable with surgery. If it is caused by kidney disease or high blood pressure, medical treatment for these disorders will control the symptoms.

 HOW TO TREAT

GENERAL MEASURES
• Weigh daily and keep a record. Report a gain of 3 or more pounds in a 24-hour period.
• Wear a medical alert bracelet to identify your medical condition and any drugs that you take.

MEDICATION
• Drugs to decrease the aldosterone effect may be prescribed. This drug may cause breast enlargement and sexual impotence in men. Other drug options are available.
• Drugs for high blood pressure may be prescribed.

ACTIVITY—No limits usually.

DIET—Eat a diet that is low in sodium and high in potassium. Foods rich in potassium include dried apricots and peaches, raisins, citrus fruits, lentils, and whole-grain cereals.

 CALL YOUR DOCTOR IF

• You or a family member has symptoms of hyperaldosteronism.
• New, unexplained symptoms develop. Drugs used in treatment may produce side effects.

HYPEREMESIS GRAVIDARUM

GENERAL INFORMATION

DEFINITION—Severe nausea and vomiting in a pregnant woman. It is more serious than the typical morning sickness (milder nausea and vomiting) in pregnancy. Hyperemesis gravidarum usually occurs before the 20th week of pregnancy (often the 4th to 12th week).

BODY PARTS INVOLVED—Gastrointestinal tract; vomiting center in the brain.

SEX OR AGE MOST AFFECTED—Pregnant females.

SIGNS & SYMPTOMS
* Severe and frequent nausea and vomiting. Symptoms may increase over a few weeks or, sometimes, months.
* Dehydration (less urine, pale and dry skin).
* Failure to gain weight, or there is weight loss.
* Unable to eat and maintain proper nutrition.
* Some affected women may have a distinct odor to their breath (ketonic odor).
* Often unable to work, perform daily house-hold tasks and routines, or care for young children.
* Fast heartbeat (sometimes).
* Symptoms may come and go (wax and wane).

CAUSES—Unknown. The most common theories involve:
* Changes in hormones.
* Liver or stomach problems.
* Nutrition problems.
* Psychological factors, such as depression or a poor response to stress.
* Thyroid disorder or endocrine imbalance.
* *Helicobacter pylori* (a bacteria that can cause ulcers) may be a factor.

RISK INCREASES WITH
* Younger maternal age.
* First pregnancy.
* Being overweight.
* Multiple-pregnancy (more than one fetus).
* Single marital status.
* Diet high in fat.
* Women with eating disorders.
* Hyperemesis gravidarum in a previous pregnancy.
* Emotional stress.

HOW TO PREVENT—There is no known prevention. To reduce risk, maintain a healthy diet, get adequate sleep, and control stress.

WHAT TO EXPECT

DIAGNOSTIC MEASURES
* Your own observation of symptoms.
* Your obstetric provider will usually do a physical exam and ask questions about your symptoms.

* Medical tests may be done to check for other health problems.

APPROPRIATE HEALTH CARE
* Hospital care is often needed to replace lost fluids and electrolytes (substances needed for body function). Fluids are given through a vein (IV) to provide nutrition and relieve dehydration.
* If symptoms are not too severe, home care with diet instructions and rest may be recommended.
* Reduce stress whenever possible. Counseling is often helpful for emotional problems.
* You and your obstetric provider may discuss alternate treatments for nausea and vomiting. These include acupressure wristbands or nerve stimulation device (which have been used to help motion sickness) or hypnosis.

POSSIBLE COMPLICATIONS
* Emotional and physical complications may occur.
* May increase the risk of the baby having a lower than normal birth weight.

PROBABLE OUTCOME—Usually curable with time and treatment. Pregnancy can continue to the successful delivery of a healthy baby.

HOW TO TREAT

GENERAL MEASURES
* Weigh daily. Report unusual changes to your obstetric provider.
* To learn more: Hyperemesis Education and Research Organization, P.O. Box 452443, Garland TX, 75045; website: www.hyperemesis.org.

MEDICATION
* Intravenous (IV) fluid, vitamins, and electrolyte replacement may be required.
* Other drugs may be prescribed for nausea.
* Don't use any nonprescription drugs or herbal products to prevent vomiting without medical advice.

ACTIVITY—Increased rest is helpful.

DIET
* Avoid foods or smells that trigger symptoms.
* Drink fluids one half hour before or after meals.
* Eat dry toast or crackers before you get out of bed.
* Eat small, frequent meals. High-protein meals may help nausea. Sit upright for 45 minutes after eating.

CALL YOUR DOCTOR IF

* You or a family member has symptoms of hyperemesis gravidarum.
* You are unable to keep any food or fluids down for 24 hours.

HYPERHIDROSIS

GENERAL INFORMATION

DEFINITION—A condition of excessive sweating that may occur for no apparent reason.

BODY PARTS INVOLVED—Skin, especially of the underarms, palms and soles.

SEX OR AGE MOST AFFECTED—Both sexes and all ages, except young children.

SIGNS & SYMPTOMS
- Heavy sweat from underarm area, soles, palms, and other body parts.
- Sweating occurs without warning or cause.
- The amount of sweating, body parts involved, and when it occurs differs in different people.
- An odor, which is caused by bacteria in sweat.

CAUSES
- Primary hyperhidrosis is the term used when there is no physical cause for the excessive sweating. Sweating is normally regulated by the body's sympathetic nervous system. In some people, this system becomes overactive. Why this occurs is unknown.
- Secondary hyperhidrosis results from a specific factor such as diabetes.

RISK INCREASES WITH—Secondary hyperhidrosis may be caused by:
- Diabetes.
- Hyperthyroidism.
- Menopause.
- Some cancers.
- Some drugs, such as narcotics.
- Obesity.
- Certain psychiatric conditions.

HOW TO PREVENT—No specific measures to prevent hyperhidrosis. Steps may be taken to help control the sweating.

WHAT TO EXPECT

DIAGNOSTIC MEASURES
- Your own observation of symptoms.
- Your health care provider will do a physical exam and ask questions about your symptoms and activities.
- Medical tests may be done to identify any disorder that is causing the excessive sweating.

APPROPRIATE HEALTH CARE
- Treatment for an underlying condition will be provided.
- Counseling, if stress is a major factor.
- Drugs may be recommended.
- Electrical devices that temporarily reduce sweating of palms or feet may be recommended.
- Surgery to remove sweat glands or sever nerves to major sweat areas, in more serious cases.

POSSIBLE COMPLICATIONS
- Emotional distress caused by social embarrassment.
- Rashes from deodorants or antiperspirants.

PROBABLE OUTCOME—Secondary hyperhidrosis can often be controlled with treatment of the underlying condition. Primary hyperhidrosis can be helped using a variety of treatment options. No single treatment works for everyone.

HOW TO TREAT

GENERAL MEASURES
- Bathe often, using a deodorizing soap.
- Change clothes often.
- Wear loose-fitting clothes made of natural fibers, such as cotton.
- Use underarm sweat shields.
- Use antiperspirants and deodorants. Use an unscented product that contains aluminum chloride.
- Use drying powders.
- Wear cotton socks.
- Wear leather shoes or sandals. Don't wear shoes of man-made materials.
- Shave underarm hair.

MEDICATION
- Drugs to reduce activity of the central nervous system may be prescribed. Side effects can be a problem.
- Prescription antiperspirants may be prescribed.
- Botulinum toxin (Botox) injections may be prescribed. It helps reduce or stop the sweating for 3 to 6 months.
- Other drugs may be prescribed to be taken by mouth or applied to the skin.

ACTIVITY—No limits.

DIET—No special diet. Drink plenty of fluids each day.

CALL YOUR DOCTOR IF

- Excessive sweating is causing you problems at work or in social situations.
- Treatment for excessive sweating is not working.

HYPERLIPIDEMIA

GENERAL INFORMATION

DEFINITION—Hyperlipidemia is the medical term used to describe having high amounts of lipids in the blood. Lipids, such as cholesterol and triglycerides, are fat or fat-like substances that maintain important body functions. They travel in the bloodstream attached to proteins. The lipid-protein combinations are called lipoproteins. Lipoproteins help the lipids get absorbed by the body's cells. Hyperlipidemia is called primary if it is inherited and secondary if it is caused by illness or other health problem. Subcategories of hyperlipidemia include:
- Hypercholesterolemia (high levels of cholesterol).
- Hypertriglyceridemia (high levels of triglycerides).
- Hyperlipoproteinemia (high levels of lipoproteins).

BODY PARTS INVOLVED—Blood and arteries.

SEX OR AGE MOST AFFECTED—All ages, but most common in adults. Different types appear at different ages.

SIGNS & SYMPTOMS
- There are usually no symptoms. It may be discovered on routine blood studies.
- There may be pinkish-yellow deposits of fat in the skin beneath eyes, elbows, and knees.

CAUSES
- There are five types of lipoproteins—defined by size and density. Two types carry cholesterol and the other three types carry triglycerides.
- Cholesterol is carried through the blood by high-density lipoproteins (HDL) and low-density lipoproteins (LDL). High levels of LDL and/or low levels of HDL can increase the risk of heart disease and stroke.
- Triglycerides are carried by three lipoproteins. These are very low-density lipoprotein (VLDL), intermediate density lipoproteins (IDL), and chylomicrons. High triglyceride levels may increase the risk of heart disease and stroke.
- To reduce risks, HDL should be above 40, LDL should be below 130, and triglycerides should be below 150, for most people.

RISK INCREASES WITH
- Hereditary factors.
- A diet that is high in fat and cholesterol.
- Illness or medical problems, such as diabetes, hypothyroidism, nephrotic syndrome, alcoholism, or obstructive liver disease.
- Sedentary lifestyle (lack of physical activity).
- Age. Males over 40 and females over 55.

HOW TO PREVENT
- Exercise daily. Maintain a healthy weight. Eat a healthy diet.
- Don't smoke. Avoid or limit alcohol drinks.
- Get a medical test to check your blood levels of cholesterol and triglycerides.

WHAT TO EXPECT

DIAGNOSTIC MEASURES
- Your health care provider may do a physical exam and ask questions about any symptoms.
- For diagnosis, a blood study will be done to measure blood lipids.

APPROPRIATE HEALTH CARE
- Treatment will depend on the results of your blood studies, your health risks, and other medical problems.
- For some patients, an altered diet and lifestyle changes may be sufficient for treatment. Others may require drugs to reduce blood lipids.

POSSIBLE COMPLICATIONS—Fatty deposits on artery walls (atherosclerosis). This is a major cause of coronary heart disease and stroke.

PROBABLE OUTCOME—Usually treatable or controllable with diet and drugs.

HOW TO TREAT

GENERAL MEASURES
- Emotional stress can increase the risk of heart disease. Look for ways to reduce stress in your life. Learn relaxation methods.
- Quit smoking. Find a way to stop that works.

MEDICATION
- Many different drugs are now prescribed to control blood lipids. Your health care provider will discuss the options, and their risks and benefits with you.
- Drugs to treat diseases, such as high blood pressure, diabetes, or thyroid conditions may be prescribed.

ACTIVITY
Regular exercise is helpful for reducing weight, staying fit, and controlling stress. It might help in increasing the body's ability to clear fat from the blood after meals.

DIET
- Eat a diet that is low in fat (particularly saturated fat). Eat a high fiber diet with plenty of fruits and vegetables. Medical advice on a proper diet may be helpful.
- Lose weight, if you are overweight. The more overweight, the more lipids your body produces.
- Reduce alcohol intake.

CALL YOUR DOCTOR IF

- You or a family member has symptoms or a family history of hyperlipidemia.
- New, unexplained symptoms develop.

HYPERNEPHROMA
(Kidney Tumor; Renal Cell Carcinoma)

 GENERAL INFORMATION

DEFINITION—A form of kidney cancer with uncontrolled growth of malignant cells in the kidney.

BODY PARTS INVOLVED—Kidney.

SEX OR AGE MOST AFFECTED—Both sexes; (twice as common in men); usually affects adults between ages 40 and 60.

SIGNS & SYMPTOMS
* No symptoms may occur.
* Firm mass in an enlarged abdomen.
* Appetite and weight loss.
* Persistent low-grade fever.
* Night sweats.
* Mild abdominal pain.
* Red or smoky urine caused by bleeding from the tumor.
* General ill feeling.

If the tumor grows large enough to cause kidney failure, symptoms may include:
* Increasing fatigue and weakness.
* Headache
* Bad breath.
* Nausea, vomiting, or diarrhea.
* Shortness of breath.
* Chest pain.
* Itching skin.

CAUSES—Unknown. Certain risk factors are known.

RISK INCREASES WITH
* Smoking.
* Obesity (especially in women).
* Estrogen therapy without progestin
* High blood pressure and its treatment.
* Occupational exposure to certain toxins.
* Cystic kidney disease.
* Dialysis therapy.
* Kidney transplant.
* Tuberous sclerosis.
* von Hippel-Lindau syndrome

HOW TO PREVENT
* Cannot be prevented at present. If you are a woman of childbearing age with a family history of kidney tumors, seek genetic counseling before becoming pregnant.
* If kidney tumors run in your family, get medical advice about tests. Even if you feel well and don't have the disease, get regular checkups.

 WHAT TO EXPECT

DIAGNOSTIC MEASURES
* Your own observation of any symptoms.
* Your health care provider will do a physical exam and ask questions about your symptoms.

* Medical tests may include blood studies and liver-function tests. Other tests are usually done to confirm the diagnosis and to determine if cancer has spread (called staging).

APPROPRIATE HEALTH CARE
* Treatment may include chemotherapy, surgery, biologic therapy, hormone therapy, and/or radiation. Treatment will depend on the stage of the disease, your health, and your preferences.
* Chemotherapy uses drugs and radiation therapy uses radiation to attack the cancer cells. Biologic therapy uses the body's immune system to fight cancer. Surgery involves removal of the kidney.

POSSIBLE COMPLICATIONS
* Spread to other organs, especially the liver, lungs, brain and bones, before discovery of the primary tumor.
* Weakening of the bones (osteoporosis or osteomalacia).
* Increased risk urinary-tract infections.

PROBABLE OUTCOME—May be curable with treatment, if the tumor is detected before it spreads to other body parts. Other outcomes depend on the spread of the cancer and success of treatment.

 HOW TO TREAT

GENERAL MEASURES
* The more you can learn and understand about this disorder, the more you will be able to make informed decisions about where to go for your care, the treatments available, the risks involved, side effects of therapy and expected outcome.
* To learn more: American Cancer Society, (800) ACS-2345; website: www.cancer.org; or National Cancer Institute, (800) 4-CANCER; website: www.nci.nih.gov.

MEDICATION—Your health care provider may prescribe anticancer drugs (chemotherapy), drugs to stimulate the immune system (biologics), pain relievers, and others if needed.

ACTIVITY
* Follow medical advice about returning to normal activities after treatment.
* Stay as active as your strength allows.

DIET—Eat a low-fat, high-fiber diet.

 CALL YOUR DOCTOR IF

* You or a family member has symptoms of hypernephroma.
* New symptoms occur during or after treatment.

HYPERPARATHYROIDISM

GENERAL INFORMATION

DEFINITION—The parathyroids are four pea-sized glands located within the thyroid gland in the neck. They produce a hormone (PTH) that helps maintain the body's mineral levels. Hyperparathyroidism occurs when these glands become overactive and produce too much PTH. This triggers an imbalance of minerals (calcium and phosphorous) that affects the body's bones and muscles.

BODY PARTS INVOLVED—Parathyroid glands, teeth; blood, which affects all body tissues—especially the heart, blood vessels, bones, kidneys, gastrointestinal tract, central nervous system and skin.

SEX OR AGE MOST AFFECTED—Both sexes and all ages, but more common in women between ages 30 and 50.

SIGNS & SYMPTOMS
• There may be no symptoms, or the symptoms may be mild to severe. This disorder comes on over years, so symptoms may not get noticed at first. Many cases are first diagnosed on a routine blood test.
• Loss of appetite, thirst, frequent urination, weight loss, or constipation.
• Feeling tired, depressed, or anxious.
• Muscle weakness, bone and joint pain.
• Nausea, vomiting.
• Severe side (flank) pain caused by kidney stones.
• Easy bone fractures due to reduced calcium in the bones.
• High blood pressure.
• Pain in the upper abdomen caused by a peptic ulcer or pancreatitis (inflammation of the pancreas).

CAUSES
• Benign tumors (adenomas) that grow in one or two of the parathyroid glands. Why the tumors occur is unknown.
• Sometimes caused by an enlargement of the glands (hyperplasia); the cause for this is unknown.
• Very rarely is a cancer involved.

RISK INCREASES WITH—Females ages 30 to 50.

HOW TO PREVENT—No specific preventive measures.

WHAT TO EXPECT

DIAGNOSTIC MEASURES
• Your own observation of any symptoms.
• Your health care provider usually will do a physical exam and ask questions about your symptoms.

• Medical tests may include studies of blood and urine, x-rays of bones, and other tests to confirm the diagnosis.

APPROPRIATE HEALTH CARE
• Surgery is usually the best form of treatment. The parathyroid gland or glands that are producing the excess hormones are removed. There are different types of operations that are done. Your health care provider will explain them to you.
• In mild cases, or when there are no symptoms, watchful waiting may be an option. This means monitoring the patient for a time to see if the disorder shows signs of getting worse. A follow-up exam may be done every 6 months for 1 to 3 years, and then less often, if tests are normal.

POSSIBLE COMPLICATIONS
• Weak bones (osteopenia and osteoporosis).
• Kidney damage.
• Peptic ulcer.
• Pancreatitis.
• Nervous system problems.
• Hypoparathyroidism (too little PTH) caused by removal of too much parathyroid tissue during surgery.

PROBABLE OUTCOME—Outcome is favorable in almost all cases.

HOW TO TREAT

GENERAL MEASURES—None specific.

MEDICATION
• Don't take antacids that contain calcium without medical approval.
• Estrogen or bone-building drugs for postmenopausal females may be prescribed.

ACTIVITY
• Follow medical advice about returning to normal activities following surgery.
• Exercise daily to maintain good health.

DIET
• Drink extra water to help prevent complications.
• Your health care provider will discuss the amount of calcium intake that is recommended. This is usually about 1000 mg/day.

CALL YOUR DOCTOR IF

• You or a family member has symptoms of hyperparathyroidism.
• Any new symptoms occur after surgery.
• You did not have surgery and you need to schedule appointment for follow-up studies.

HYPERTENSION
(High Blood Pressure)

 GENERAL INFORMATION

DEFINITION—Blood pressure measures the force of blood as it flows through the arteries. Adult blood pressure is considered normal at 120/80. The first number is systolic pressure, which measures pressure as the heart contracts (pumps). The second number is diastolic, which measures pressure when the heart is relaxed (between beats). If blood pressure stays high over time (140/90 or above), it is called high blood pressure or hypertension. It is a common disorder. Prehypertension is when the blood pressure is between 120/80 and 140/90. The risk of stroke and heart attack begins to rise as the blood pressure goes above 115/75.

BODY PARTS INVOLVED—Heart; blood vessels; kidneys and eyes (advanced stages).

SEX OR AGE MOST AFFECTED—All ages, but most common in adults.

SIGNS & SYMPTOMS
• Usually no symptoms occur. It is often discovered when blood pressure is measured.
• Vague, mild symptoms such as headache, dizziness, blurred vision, or nausea may occur.

CAUSES—Mostly unknown (called primary hypertension). In some cases, it results from certain medical problems (called secondary hypertension).

RISK INCREASES WITH
• Aging and hardening of the arteries.
• Prehypertension.
• Chronic kidney disease or thyroid dysfunction.
• Narrowing of the aorta (major artery of the heart).
• Adrenal gland disorders.
• Alcoholism.
• Hormone problems of adrenals or pituitary glands.
• Overweight; smoking; stress.
• Sedentary (lack of physical activity) lifestyle.
• Sensitivity to sodium (salt).
• Genetic factors (it is common in African Americans).
• Family history of hypertension.
• Use of certain drugs. These include birth-control pills, steroids, diet pills, and decongestants.

HOW TO PREVENT—No specific preventive measures. Avoid risk factors where possible. Maintain a healthy weight, be physically active, eat a healthy diet (limit salt), drink little or no alcohol, and don't smoke. If you have a family history of hypertension, have frequent blood-pressure checks.

 WHAT TO EXPECT

DIAGNOSTIC MEASURES
• Your health care provider will do a physical exam, check your blood pressure, and ask questions about your medical history.
• Medical tests may include blood and urine studies. Other tests may be done to find a cause for the high blood pressure or to determine if there are any complications.

APPROPRIATE HEALTH CARE
• Treatment steps will depend on each individual. Steps may involve diet changes, weight loss, stopping smoking, increasing exercise, limiting alcohol use, reducing stress, and taking drugs.
• Counseling, meditation, biofeedback, relaxation techniques, or other therapies can help you reduce stress.

POSSIBLE COMPLICATIONS—Without treatment, high blood pressure can lead to heart attack, stroke, congestive heart failure, pulmonary edema, and kidney failure. High blood pressure is called the "silent killer".

PROBABLE OUTCOME—Outlook is good if blood pressure can be controlled.

 HOW TO TREAT

GENERAL MEASURES
• Take your blood pressure at home each day. Write down the results.
• Stop smoking. Find a way to quit that works.
• Get medical advice before trying alternate forms of treatment such as acupuncture, diet supplements, and others.

MEDICATION
• One or more antihypertensive drugs to reduce blood pressure may be prescribed. Do not stop taking them unless medically advised.
• Avoid nonprescription cold, allergy, and sinus decongestant drugs (may raise blood pressure).

ACTIVITY—Exercise moderately hard for 30 minutes, most, if not all, days of the week. It helps reduce stress, control body weight, and lowers blood pressure.

DIET—Eat a healthy diet, high in fiber, fruits and vegetables. Limit fat and salt use. If overweight, consider a weight loss diet.

 CALL YOUR DOCTOR IF

• You or a family member thinks they may have high blood pressure.
• After diagnosis, any symptoms cause concern.

HYPERTHYROIDISM (Thyrotoxicosis; Goiter; Graves' Disease; Overactive Thyroid)

 GENERAL INFORMATION

DEFINITION—Hyperthyroidism means the thyroid gland is overactive and produces too much thyroid hormone. The most common form of hyperthyroidism is called Graves' disease. The thyroid hormone is used by the body for metabolism (producing energy).

BODY PARTS INVOLVED—Thyroid gland and most other body organs, especially the endocrine system, which includes the pituitary gland, parathyroid glands, pancreas, adrenal glands, and ovaries or testicles.

SEX OR AGE MOST AFFECTED—Adults between ages 20 and 50, mostly women.

SIGNS & SYMPTOMS
- Anxiety, nervousness, and restlessness.
- Feeling warm or hot all the time.
- Sweating.
- Heart palpitations.
- Weight loss, even though appetite increases.
- Sleeplessness.
- Fatigue and weakness.
- Frequent bowel movements.
- Women may have less menstrual flow.
- Eyes appear to bulge out. There is swelling around the eyes. Vision changes may occur.
- Goiter (visibly enlarged thyroid) may occur.
- Hair loss.
- Tremor of the hands.

CAUSES—Graves' disease is an autoimmune disorder. In these disorders, the immune system by mistake attacks the body itself in different ways. In Graves' disease, abnormal antibodies from the immune system cause the thyroid to produce more hormone. Other causes of hyperthyroidism may be due to thyroid disorders.

RISK INCREASES WITH
- Thyroid nodules or tumors.
- Thyroiditis (inflammation of thyroid gland).
- Personal or family history of thyroid or autoimmune diseases.
- Radiation treatment.
- Females more than males.
- Excess iodine intake.
- Stress may be a contributing factor.

HOW TO PREVENT—No specific preventive measures.

 WHAT TO EXPECT

DIAGNOSTIC MEASURES
- Your health care provider will do a physical exam.
- Medical tests include blood studies for thyroid levels. Radioactive iodine studies may be done.

APPROPRIATE HEALTH CARE
- Treatment usually involves drugs to reduce thyroid hormone levels. Permanent treatment involves use of radioactive iodine or surgery. With these two treatments, thyroid hormone production is decreased. Sometimes, hypothyroidism (too little thyroid hormone) occurs, which will need to be treated.
- Radioactive iodine treatment is usually done as an outpatient. The iodine (taken by mouth) causes the thyroid gland to shrink over a period of months.
- Surgery to remove part of the thyroid (called a thyroidectomy) may be advised. It is usually done in a hospital with a general anesthetic.
- For eye symptoms, an exam and follow-up by an eye specialist (ophthalmologist).

POSSIBLE COMPLICATIONS
- Thyroid eye disease. This includes blurred and double vision, difficulty in seeing, tearing, and light sensitivity.
- Heart problems.
- Dermopathy (a skin disorder).
- Hypothyroidism (low thyroid hormone levels).
- Surgery complications (infection or bleeding).

PROBABLE OUTCOME—Treatment is effective in controlling the disorder. It may take 6 months for thyroid levels to return to normal.

 HOW TO TREAT

GENERAL MEASURES—It is important for your doctor to monitor the treatment. Be sure to keep follow-up appointments.

MEDICATION
- Antithyroid drugs to depress thyroid activity are usually prescribed. Follow-up blood tests are done to adjust the dosage until thyroid hormone levels are normal.
- Beta blockers to treat the heart and nervous system symptoms may be prescribed.
- Thyroid replacement drugs if the thyroid gland becomes underactive due to treatment.
- Avoid drugs or supplements containing iodide. Iodide may interfere with treatment drugs.

ACTIVITY—Usually no limits in otherwise healthy persons. In older persons or those with heart problems, decrease activity until thyroid levels are normal.

DIET—No special diet.

 CALL YOUR DOCTOR IF

- You or a family member has symptoms of hyperthyroidism.
- Symptoms worsen, or new, unexplained symptoms develop during treatment.

HYPOCHONDRIASIS

GENERAL INFORMATION

DEFINITION—A disorder that causes a person to feel that he or she has a serious or fatal disease, even though there is no medical evidence of this.

BODY PARTS INVOLVED—Brain.

SEX OR AGE MOST AFFECTED— It occurs equally in men and women. It may begin at any age, but is most common in early adulthood.

SIGNS & SYMPTOMS
• Preoccupied for over 6 months with the fear of having a serious disease. There may be constant thought about the possibility of heart disease or cancer.
• Anxiety and reports of symptoms involving any body part. Symptoms may be vague or specific.
• Symptoms may change, but the person's belief that a serious condition exists does not.

CAUSES—The cause is uncertain. It is based on misinterpreting normal body sensations. There are a number of risk factors that have been identified. A person with the disorder may be aware that the fear of having a serious disease is unfounded, excessive, or unreasonable.

RISK INCREASES WITH
• Other mental health problems, such as anxiety.
• Recent stressful event or major life change.
• Having a need for attention. (A person may be unaware of this.)
• Having personal relationship problems. (A person may be looking for care and concern.)
• Family history of hypochondriasis.
• People who had a serious illness or experience of adversity in childhood. Parents may have rewarded illness by giving a child special privileges and attention for being sick, or they may have neglected the child.

HOW TO PREVENT—No specific measures known. In childhood, don't reward illness by giving a child special privileges and undue attention for being sick. Provide adequate love and support during healthy periods.

WHAT TO EXPECT

DIAGNOSTIC MEASURES
• Your health care provider will do a physical exam and ask questions about your symptoms.
• Medical tests may include a blood study. A mental (emotional) health exam may be done.

APPROPRIATE HEALTH CARE
• Your health care provider will assure you that the diagnosis of the symptoms shows there is no threat to life or risk of disability. Regular

follow-up medical appointments may be scheduled for further assurance.
• Behavior therapy can help a patient understand what generates the symptoms and how to overcome worrisome thoughts.
• Interpersonal therapy can help a patient identify personal relationship problems and how to correct them.
• Group therapy may help some patients.
• Patients should depend on one health care provider for their treatment. Avoid going to different health care providers and having repeat medical tests.

POSSIBLE COMPLICATIONS
• It can affect all aspects of a person's life. This includes personal relationships, work, and social life.
• A real illness may be overlooked.
• Becoming dependent on pain relievers or sedatives.
• Patients tend to "doctor shop." They feel rejected if they aren't believed about the symptoms.
• Taking unnecessary medical tests that are dangerous or could result in complications.

PROBABLE OUTCOME—Patients may have periods of hypochondriasis for months and years, and then go months and years without hypochondriasis. Some patients recover from the disorder. For others, it may be a lifelong problem.

HOW TO TREAT

GENERAL MEASURES—Having the diagnosis of hypochondriasis is hard for anyone to accept. Feelings of anger, sadness, or frustration are normal. Education about the disorder for you and your family may help you cope. Your health care provider is the first source. Then learn what you can from books or an Internet search.

MEDICATION
• Antidepressants may be prescribed for anxiety or depressive symptoms.
• Other drugs may be prescribed for symptoms such as mood disorders or stress.

ACTIVITY—Exercise daily. This can improve physical fitness as well as having a positive affect on mental health. It helps improve mood, reduce tension, and improve sleep.

DIET—Eat three regular, healthy meals daily. Avoid alcohol or caffeine.

CALL YOUR DOCTOR IF

You or a family member has symptoms of this disorder and wants help with the problem.

HYPOGLYCEMIA, FUNCTIONAL

GENERAL INFORMATION

DEFINITION—A low level of blood sugar (glucose) in the body. Functional (or reactive) hypoglycemia is usually a reaction to eating. It is not a disease in itself and is not a common medical condition as many persons would believe. Symptoms vary greatly among people in frequency and severity.

BODY PARTS INVOLVED—Pancreas.

SEX OR AGE MOST AFFECTED—Both sexes; all ages.

SIGNS & SYMPTOMS
- Headache.
- Nervousness or anxiety.
- Sweating.
- Dizziness.
- Fast heartbeat.
- Weakness or faintness.
- Shaking muscles.
- Hunger.
- More severe symptoms are less likely. They may include being forgetful, poor concentration, confusion, poor coordination, or slurred speech.

CAUSES—The amount of sugar (glucose) in the blood normally increases for one to two hours after a meal, especially a high-carbohydrate meal (sugars and starches). In many people, instead of increasing, the glucose level may drop to a level that is lower than before the meal. It will then rise back again to normal levels. Most of these people do not have any symptoms from the drop in glucose levels. In a few, the symptoms of hypoglycemia occur.

RISK INCREASES WITH
- Improper diet.
- Obesity.
- Smoking, alcohol, stress, or other emotional or mental problems may contribute.

HOW TO PREVENT
- Follow instructions under Diet.
- Get treatment for emotional problems such as stress.
- Don't smoke.
- Don't drink alcohol.
- Recognize early symptoms and drink or eat something that contains sugar.

WHAT TO EXPECT

DIAGNOSTIC MEASURES
- Your health care provider may do a physical exam.
- Medical tests may include blood-sugar and glucose-tolerance studies to rule out other medical problems.

APPROPRIATE HEALTH CARE
- Long-term treatment usually involves diet changes.
- Short-term treatment during an episode can raise blood sugar more quickly.
- Counseling or other therapy may help you learn to cope with stress or emotional problems.

POSSIBLE COMPLICATIONS—None expected.

PROBABLE OUTCOME—The symptoms usually clear up on their own or with glucose in a very short period of time. A change in diet may help prevent symptoms from occurring in the future.

HOW TO TREAT

GENERAL MEASURES—Self care during an episode includes drinking juice or a soft drink or eating candy to raise the glucose level. Take a protein food, such as milk or cheese, at the same time. This helps the body slowly absorb the glucose and avoid a "seesaw" effect of glucose levels.

MEDICATION—Drugs are not usually needed for treatment.

ACTIVITY—Regular exercise may improve blood-sugar control. It can help to reduce stress and build self-esteem. It helps to control and maintain an ideal weight. It also helps improve heart and lung function, lower blood pressure, improve blood circulation, and lower cholesterol levels.

DIET
- Eat several smaller meals a day that are low in simple carbohydrates, moderate in fats, and high in protein.
- Don't skip meals.
- Between-meal snacks should include protein, such as chicken, eggs, cheese, nuts, or skim milk, rather than carbohydrates.
- Avoid sugar and foods containing sugar (especially on an empty stomach).
- Weight-loss diet will help if being overweight is a problem.
- Limit or avoid alcohol.
- Avoid caffeine (coffee, tea, or soft drinks).

CALL YOUR DOCTOR IF

- You or a family member has symptoms of functional hypoglycemia.
- Symptoms continue after treatment.

HYPOPARATHYROIDISM

GENERAL INFORMATION

DEFINITION—The parathyroid glands lie within the thyroid glands in the neck. They produce parathyroid hormones, which along with vitamin D and calcitonin (a hormone produced by the thyroid gland), regulates the calcium level in the body. With hypoparathyroidism, there is a decreased production of hormones by the parathyroid glands causing a low level of calcium in the blood. This disorder is rare.

BODY PARTS INVOLVED—Parathyroid glands (4 pea-sized glands located on the back and side of the thyroid gland); teeth; blood, which affects all body tissues, especially the heart, blood vessels, bones, kidneys, gastrointestinal tract, central nervous system and skin.

SEX OR AGE MOST AFFECTED—Both sexes; all ages. It affects children more than adults.

SIGNS & SYMPTOMS
Acute phase:
- Tetany (painful cramp-like spasms of the face, hands, arms, and sometimes feet).
- Tingling and numbness in feet or hands.
Chronic phase:
- Scaling skin.
- Splitting nails.
- Poor tooth development.
- Seizures.
- Mental retardation in children.
- Psychosis in adults.

CAUSES
- Complication of surgery on the parathyroid glands, the thyroid glands, or other neck tissues.
- Genetic autoimmune disorder (possibly).
- Radiation of the thyroid gland.
- Hemochromatosis (disease in which excessive iron accumulates in the liver).
- No apparent reason (sometimes).
- Occasionally the parathyroids are absent from birth.

RISK INCREASES WITH—Neck surgery or trauma.

HOW TO PREVENT—No specific preventive measures.

WHAT TO EXPECT

DIAGNOSTIC MEASURES
- Your own observation of symptoms.
- Your health care provider may do a physical exam.
- Medical tests may include blood and urine studies, ECG (electrocardiogram—method of diagnosing heart diseases by measuring electrical activity of the heart), CT, and x-rays of bones to detect increased bone density.

APPROPRIATE HEALTH CARE
- Treatment involves restoring the mineral balance in the body. This is done with supplements.
- If you are suffering an acute attack of tetany (see Symptoms), you may need hospital care for calcium injections to provide quick relief.

POSSIBLE COMPLICATIONS
- Cataracts.
- Brain damage.
- Heartbeat abnormalities and congestive heart failure.
- Difficulty breathing.
- Malformation of teeth.
- Seizures.

PROBABLE OUTCOME
- This condition is currently considered incurable. It requires lifelong replacement therapy to control symptoms. Without treatment, it is fatal.
- Scientific research into causes and treatment continues, so there is hope for increasingly effective treatments and a cure.

HOW TO TREAT

GENERAL MEASURES
- For self-care, if muscle cramps start, place a paper bag over your mouth. Blow into it and rebreathe your breath. This will raise carbon-dioxide levels in the blood and decrease muscle spasms.
- Apply lubricating creams or ointments to dry, scaling skin.
- Keep nails trimmed to prevent splitting.
- Get periodic medical tests to check calcium levels in your blood. It is important to remember to have these tests done on time.

MEDICATION
- Vitamin D and calcium supplements are normally prescribed. A lifelong course of these drugs is necessary.
- Intravenous (IV) calcium may be given for severe muscle spasms.
- Other drugs for treating muscle spasms may be prescribed.

ACTIVITY—No limits.

DIET—A high-calcium, low-phosphorus diet may be helpful. Your health care provider will advise you of special diet needs.

CALL YOUR DOCTOR IF

- You or a family member has unexplained muscle spasms of the hands, feet, or throat, or numbness, or tingling in the hands or feet.
- Muscle spasms do not decrease in 1 week, despite treatment.

HYPOTHERMIA

GENERAL INFORMATION

DEFINITION—A drop in body temperature to below normal usually due to exposure to cold. It can occur both indoors (such as lack of heat) and outside in cold weather, or from being in water. Hypothermia can take several hours or even several days to develop.

BODY PARTS INVOLVED—All major organ systems, including decreased blood flow through the kidneys and brain.

SEX OR AGE MOST AFFECTED—All ages, but most common in adults over 60.

SIGNS & SYMPTOMS
Early symptoms (they can start slowly):
• Poor muscle coordination.
• Mental confusion.
• Shivering.
• Low body temperature that is below 96°F (35.5°C). Normal body temperature is around 98.6°F (37°C).
• Slow pulse.
• Weakness, drowsiness.
Late symptoms:
• Rigid muscles.
• Temperature drops even lower.
• Purple fingers, toes, and nail beds.
• Loss of consciousness.

CAUSES—Cold starts affecting different functions of the body. The brain and nerves work more slowly. The heart rate becomes irregular. Muscles don't work normally. There are many risk factors besides being outdoors in cold weather that can lead to hypothermia.

RISK INCREASES WITH
• Adults over 60 or infants.
• Mentally impaired.
• Poorly heated homes.
• Outdoor work.
• Disease or injury (heart, lung, stroke, tumor, thyroid, burns, and others).
• Homeless persons.
• Indoor factors may include exposure to air conditioning or ice baths.
• Excess alcohol use.

HOW TO PREVENT
• Be sure the home is heated adequately. Prepare a winter survival kit for indoor safety (include water, blankets, first-aid kit, medicines, and nonperishable foods).
• In cold weather, wear windproof clothing in many loose layers, including a scarf, hat, and mittens. In the rain, change to dry clothing as soon as possible.
• Avoid alcohol use if you are going out into the cold.
• Don't skate or fish on ice unless you know that it's safe.

• If camping, walking, or hiking in a cold climate, carry emergency gear for use if stranded or injured. Travel with a partner.
• Persons who are unable to care for themselves fully, such as the elderly, the mentally impaired, or the alcoholic, should be visited or supervised during cold weather.

WHAT TO EXPECT

DIAGNOSTIC MEASURES—Diagnosis is done in the emergency care center. Medical tests are often needed to check for any complications.

APPROPRIATE HEALTH CARE—In the hospital or emergency center, the process of rewarming will be started. The patient will be treated until the temperature returns to normal.

POSSIBLE COMPLICATIONS—Many complications can occur depending on the patient's health, age, and the length of the exposure to cold.

PROBABLE OUTCOME—The outcome is usually good if the patient is otherwise healthy and treatment is started quickly. Some children have been revived despite being in ice water for an hour or more.

HOW TO TREAT

GENERAL MEASURES
• Urgent medical care is needed. Arrange transport to the nearest emergency center right away.
• The following may be helpful while waiting for emergency help: Dry the person if wet. Keep the person lying down and cover them with blankets. If the person is outdoors, move them inside. If unable to do so, cover with a blankets and protect them from the weather. Try to warm the main body area first, then the arms and legs. In wilderness conditions, if help is not near, undress the victim and yourself and establish skin-to-skin contact.

MEDICATION—Drugs will be provided as needed for any complications.

ACTIVITY—After treatment, normal activity should be resumed gradually.

DIET—Don't give alcohol to a person with hypothermia. Warm fluids may be given if the patient is able to swallow.

CALL YOUR DOCTOR IF

You or a family member has symptoms of hypothermia or you observe the symptoms in someone. This may be an emergency.

ILLNESS & DISORDERS

HYPOTHYROIDISM (Underactive Thyroid)

GENERAL INFORMATION

DEFINITION—Hypothyroidism means the thyroid gland is underactive and produces too little thyroid hormone. The thyroid is a small butterfly-shaped gland in the neck. Just about all chemical reactions in the body are affected by the thyroid hormone.

BODY PARTS INVOLVED—Thyroid gland and the endocrine system.

SEX OR AGE MOST AFFECTED—Both sexes of adults, but more common in women.

SIGNS & SYMPTOMS
- A person will have some, but not all of the symptoms listed.
- Feeling cold (especially hands and feet).
- Decrease in sweating.
- Dry, itchy skin; paleness.
- Loss of appetite, but a weight gain occurs.
- Constipation.
- Loss of energy, feeling tired or sluggish.
- Coarse, dry, brittle hair, or hair loss.
- Muscle aches.
- Blurred vision; hearing loss.
- Sleepiness or insomnia.
- Emotional or mental changes; mood swings.
- Puffy skin around the eyes.
- Decreased sex drive.
- Changes in menstrual cycle.
- Deepened or hoarse voice.

CAUSES—A variety of medical disorders or health problems can damage, inflame, enlarge, shrink or otherwise affect the thyroid gland and cause it to be underactive.

RISK INCREASES WITH
- Autoimmune disorder such as Hashimoto's thyroiditis. The body's immune system functions abnormally and attacks the thyroid gland.
- Hyperthyroidism treatment (e.g., surgery or iodine therapy).
- Drugs (e.g., lithium can cause thyroid dysfunction).
- Radiation or surgery of head, neck, or chest.
- Congenital (being born with hypothyroidism).
- Adults over 60. Women more than men.
- Personal or family history of thyroid disease.
- Disorders of the pituitary or hypothalamus.
- Too little iodine (rare in the United States).

HOW TO PREVENT—No known preventive measures. Screening tests for those at risk may help with early diagnosis.

WHAT TO EXPECT

DIAGNOSTIC MEASURES
- Your own observation of symptoms.
- Your health care provider will do a physical exam and ask questions about your symptoms.
- Blood tests will be done for thyroid hormone and TSH (thyroid-stimulating hormone) levels. Blood tests may result in a diagnosis of pronounced hypothyroidism or subclinical (mild) hypothyroidism.

APPROPRIATE HEALTH CARE
- Treatment for pronounced hypothyroidism involves restoring thyroid blood levels to normal with synthetic thyroid hormone. Follow-up is usually needed for several months to be sure of the correct dose of thyroid replacement. Then the follow-ups may be less frequent but still done on a regular basis.
- Treatment may be recommended for mild hypothyroidism, depending on symptoms and other factors.
- Rarely, hospital care may be needed if emergencies occur, such as myxedema coma.
- Pregnancy will require careful monitoring and additional thyroid replacement as the pregnancy advances.

POSSIBLE COMPLICATIONS
- Risk of infections, heart disease, and pituitary tumors.
- Infertility and risk of miscarriage in pregnant women.
- Myxedema coma (rare life-threatening complication).

PROBABLE OUTCOME—Normal thyroid levels can be achieved with treatment. Most people will need to take thyroid hormones for life.

HOW TO TREAT

GENERAL MEASURES
- Medical follow-up may be needed for several months to establish the correct dose of thyroid replacement.
- To learn more: American Thyroid Association, (800) 849-7643; website: www.thyroid.org.

MEDICATION—Thyroid hormone replacement is often prescribed. Dosage will depend on age, weight, capacity of thyroid function, other drugs you take, and intestinal function. Don't switch brand names of your thyroid drug without consulting your health care provider.

ACTIVITY—No limits.

DIET—No special diet for hypothyroidism. Avoid constipation by eating a high-fiber diet. A weight-loss diet is helpful if you are overweight.

CALL YOUR DOCTOR IF

- You or a family member has hypothyroidism symptoms.
- Symptoms don't improve with treatment, or new, unexplained symptoms develop.
- Coma or seizures occur. Get emergency help.

ID REACTION
(Autoeczematization; Autosensitization)

 GENERAL INFORMATION

DEFINITION—An allergic response to a skin condition that occurs somewhere else on the body.

BODY PARTS INVOLVED
• Parts with the original disorder: groin, ears, hands, feet.
• Parts with the allergic response: hands, feet, arms, legs or trunk.

SEX OR AGE MOST AFFECTED—Both sexes; all ages.

SIGNS & SYMPTOMS
• Itching (often severe).
• Vesicles (small, fluid-filled blisters) of varying size on the skin.
• It most often occurs on the sides of the fingers, but can be all over the body.

CAUSES—Unknown. An id reaction may be a disorder of the body's immune response to the original skin problem. It may occur with a fungal infection, such as athlete's feet, or other type of skin condition.

RISK INCREASES WITH
• Recent skin rash (such as diaper dermatitis, stasis dermatitis, external otitis, hand eczema, or foot eczema).
• History of allergies.
• Stress may play a role.

HOW TO PREVENT—Treat all skin infections until they are cured.

 WHAT TO EXPECT

DIAGNOSTIC MEASURES
• Your own observation of symptoms.
• Your health care provider will do a physical exam of the affected skin and ask questions about your symptoms.
• A medical test may be done to check for the type of infection that caused the original skin problem.

APPROPRIATE HEALTH CARE—Treatment of the first skin condition should also cure the id reaction.

POSSIBLE COMPLICATIONS—A bacterial infection may develop.

PROBABLE OUTCOME—Usually curable in 2 weeks. It may recur again if treatment is stopped before the id reaction and original condition are gone.

 HOW TO TREAT

GENERAL MEASURES
• Treat the original skin disorder until it heals completely to prevent a recurrence of the id reaction.
• Id reaction does not respond well to simple treatment measures such as soaks.

MEDICATION
• Topical or oral steroid drugs may be prescribed.
• An anti-itching cream for skin can help control the itching.
• Drugs (such as an antifungal) may be prescribed for other skin problems diagnosed.

ACTIVITY—No limits.

DIET—No special diet.

 CALL YOUR DOCTOR IF

• You or a family member has symptoms of an id reaction.
• The following occur during treatment:
  - Fever higher than 101°F (38.3°C).
  - Infection develops (heat, redness, pain, or tenderness in any of the lesions).

ILLNESS & DISORDERS

IDIOPATHIC HYPERTROPHIC SUBAORTIC STENOSIS (IHSS)

GENERAL INFORMATION

DEFINITION—A chronic heart condition that produces an enlarged heart muscle. This restricts the amount of blood the heart pumps. Cardiac output may be low, normal, or high depending on whether stenosis (a narrowing) is obstructive or nonobstructive. If output is normal, idiopathic hypertrophic subaortic stenosis (IHSS) could go undetected for years.

BODY PARTS INVOLVED—Heart.

SEX OR AGE MOST AFFECTED—Both sexes; all ages (young people usually have more severe symptoms).

SIGNS & SYMPTOMS
- Many patients have no symptoms.
- Chest pain (called angina pectoris).
- Strong, rapid heartbeat.
- Fainting from exertion.
- Shortness of breath.
- Swollen feet and ankles.
- Distended (sticking out) neck veins.
- Fatigue.

CAUSES—Thickening of the walls of the heart. This is caused by a defect in the genes and often runs in families. The thickened walls obstruct the flow of blood, and the heart may be unable to pump enough blood for the needs of the body.

RISK INCREASES WITH—Family history of IHSS.

HOW TO PREVENT—If you have a family history of IHSS, obtain genetic counseling before starting a family.

WHAT TO EXPECT

DIAGNOSTIC MEASURES
- Your health care provider will do a physical exam.
- Medical tests may include cardiac catheterization to measure blood flow through heart chambers, CT, MRI, and x-rays of the heart (see Glossary for these tests). An ECG (electrocardiogram) and echocardiogram, which are studies to check heart function, and other tests may be done.

APPROPRIATE HEALTH CARE
- Treatment may include drugs, lifestyle changes, pacemaker or defibrillator insertion, or surgery.
- Lifestyle changes involve reducing activity levels.
- An electronic cardiac pacemaker may be inserted. It helps relieve symptoms by changing the pattern of the heartbeat.

- An implantable-cardioverter defibrillator may be inserted. It can help prevent sudden death.
- A procedure that uses alcohol injected into an artery may be recommended. It can help to reduce obstruction and improve symptoms.
- Surgery may be recommended to reduce the obstruction, if other treatments do not control the problem.
- Counseling may be helpful in adjusting to emotional effects of chronic illness.

POSSIBLE COMPLICATIONS
- Abnormal heart rhythm.
- Sudden death.

PROBABLE OUTCOME—Symptoms can often be controlled with treatment. Life-style changes may be required.

HOW TO TREAT

GENERAL MEASURES
- Stay under close medical supervision.
- Wear a medical alert type bracelet or pendant to indicate you have this disorder.

MEDICATION—Beta-adrenergic blockers or calcium-channel blockers to prevent heartbeat irregularities will be prescribed.

ACTIVITY
- Instructions will be provided about how much physical activity is ideal. Your ability to increase activity is dependent on your response to therapy. Don't regard yourself as an invalid.
- Avoid strenuous activities and sports because of the high risk of sudden death.

DIET—Usually no special diet. A low-salt diet may be recommended if you have fluid buildup. This is a possible sign of congestive heart failure.

CALL YOUR DOCTOR IF

- You or a family member has symptoms of IHSS.
- Symptoms worsen during treatment.
- New, unexplained symptoms develop. Drugs used in treatment may produce side effects.

IMMUNODEFICIENCY DISEASE

GENERAL INFORMATION

DEFINITION
• Defects in the body's immune system, which means a person is more likely to develop infections and cancer. A healthy immune system protects the body against germs (bacteria, viruses, and fungi), cancer (partial protection), and any foreign material that enters the body.
• Primary immunodeficiency is inherited. Nearly 100 forms have been recognized. One form is common variable immunodeficiency (CVID). A rare form is severe combined immune deficiency (SCID).
• Secondary immunodeficiency is acquired. It occurs in persons who previously had a normal immune system. A form of this type (not discussed here) is the acquired immunodeficiency syndrome (AIDS).

BODY PARTS INVOLVED—Immune system (blood, bone marrow, lymph tissue, liver, spleen and thymus gland).

SEX OR AGE MOST AFFECTED—Both sexes; all ages.

SIGNS & SYMPTOMS
• Repeated, severe, and hard to cure infections, illnesses, and other health problems. Some are listed here.
• Ear infections (otitis media), and sinus or other respiratory infections, such as pneumonia. Yeast infections, such as candidiasis and eczema (a skin disorder).
• Cancer, especially leukemia and lymphoma.
• Bleeding disorders.
• Other immune disorders (anemia, arthritis).
• Meningitis or encephalitis (brain infections).
• Heart, digestive tract, or nervous system disorders.

CAUSES
• Primary: Being born with a faulty immune system. One or more or all of the essential parts of the immune system are missing due to a genetic defect.
• Secondary: Caused by diseases or other health problems that affect the immune system.

RISK INCREASES WITH
• Surgical removal of the spleen before age 2.
• Use of drugs to suppress the immune system.
• Radiation treatment or severe burns.
• Some cancers, such as leukemia.
• Viral infections, such as measles or influenza.
• Malnutrition (severe nutrient deficiency).
• Blood transfusion or IV drug use.
• Family history of immunodeficiency disease.

HOW TO PREVENT
• No preventive measures for primary type. If you have a family history, get genetic counseling before starting a family.
• Prevention of secondary type may or may not be possible. It depends on the cause.

WHAT TO EXPECT

DIAGNOSTIC MEASURES
• Your own observation of symptoms, especially repeated infections in children.
• Your health care provider will do a physical exam.
• Medical tests may include blood studies of antibodies, microscopic exams of blood and tissue cells, skin tests, chest x-rays of the thymus gland, and radioactive studies of immune function.

APPROPRIATE HEALTH CARE
• Specific treatment will depend on the type of immune deficiency. General treatment involves preventing and treating infections.
• Surgery to transplant bone marrow or the thymus gland may be recommended.
• Hospital care for treatment of serious infection may be required.

POSSIBLE COMPLICATIONS
• Infections and other diseases that may not respond to treatment.
• Complications can occur due to specific deficiency.

PROBABLE OUTCOME—Advances in treatment have improved outlook for many of the patients. Lifelong treatments may be needed.

HOW TO TREAT

GENERAL MEASURES
• Avoid exposure to persons with infections. Don't get any type of vaccine without medical advice. Wear a medical alert bracelet or neck tag to identify your medical condition.
• To learn more: Immune Deficiency Foundation, 40 W. Chesapeake Ave., Suite 308, Towson, MD 21204; (800) 296-4433; website: www.primaryimmune.org.

MEDICATION—Antibiotics for infection, transfusion of blood components, and gamma globulin injections may be prescribed.

ACTIVITY—Activity will depend on the type of deficiency. A risk of bleeding may limit activities.

DIET—No special diet.

CALL YOUR DOCTOR IF

• You or a family member has symptoms of immunodeficiency disease.
• After diagnosis, you have any signs of infection or illness or injury, or unexplained symptoms occur such as: chills; fever; muscle aches; headache; dizziness; and cough with thick, discolored or blood-streaked sputum.

ILLNESS & DISORDERS

IMPETIGO
(Pyoderma)

 GENERAL INFORMATION

DEFINITION—A common bacterial skin infection that affects the top layers of the skin.

BODY PARTS INVOLVED—Skin of the face, arms and legs.

SEX OR AGE MOST AFFECTED—All ages, but most common in infants and children.

SIGNS & SYMPTOMS
* A localized (not spreading) red rash with many small blisters. Some blisters contain pus, and yellow crusts form when they break. The blisters don't hurt, but they may itch.
* Slight fever (sometimes).

CAUSES—Staphylococcal or streptococcal (or both) bacteria growing in the upper skin layers. It is usually spread from person-to-person, or from germs on something an infected person has touched. The time from exposure to the germs and the start of symptoms is 1 to 3 days. A person is contagious when the rash is crusting or oozing pus.

RISK INCREASES WITH
* Contact with an infected person.
* Skin that is sensitive to sun and irritants, such as soap and makeup.
* Other skin problems, such as bites, burns, infections, sores, or injuries.
* Poor general health.
* Warm, moist weather.
* Children in daycare.
* Poor hygiene.

HOW TO PREVENT
* No specific preventive measures.
* Maintain good general health and good hygiene.

 WHAT TO EXPECT

DIAGNOSTIC MEASURES
* Your own observation of symptoms.
* Your health care provider can diagnose impetigo by an exam of the infected skin.
* Medical skin tests are usually not needed.

APPROPRIATE HEALTH CARE—Treatment is with drugs used for bacterial infection.

POSSIBLE COMPLICATIONS
* Can lead to other skin conditions and scarring (rare).
* Kidney disorder (rare).

PROBABLE OUTCOME—Curable in 7 to 10 days with treatment. It may recur in children.

 HOW TO TREAT

GENERAL MEASURES
* Keep fingernails short. Don't scratch the blisters.
* If there is an outbreak in the family, urge all members to use antibacterial soap. Wash hands carefully.
* Use separate towels for each family member, or substitute paper towels temporarily.
* Don't share razors with other people.
* Scrub sores with gauze and antiseptic soap. Break any pustules. Remove all crusts, and expose and cleanse all lesions. If crusts are difficult to remove, soak them in warm, soapy water and scrub gently.
* Cover impetigo sores with gauze and tape to keep hands away from them.
* Men should shave around sores on the face, not over them. Use an aerosol shaving cream and change razor blades each day. Don't use a shaving brush; it may have germs on it.

MEDICATION
* Antibiotic ointments may be prescribed.
* Oral antibiotics may be prescribed.

ACTIVITY—No limits.

DIET—No special diet.

 CALL YOUR DOCTOR IF

* You or your child has symptoms of impetigo.
* Fever occurs.
* The sores continue to spread or don't begin to heal in 3 days, despite treatment.

IMPOTENCE, MALE SEXUAL
(Erectile Dysfunction)

 GENERAL INFORMATION

DEFINITION—A consistent inability to sustain an erection as needed for sexual intercourse. Impotence can occur at any age. It is not a normal part of aging (though arousal may normally take longer). Impotence affects millions of men.

BODY PARTS INVOLVED—Male reproductive system; central nervous system.

SEX OR AGE MOST AFFECTED—Male adolescents and adults, but most common in men over 45.

SIGNS & SYMPTOMS
• Total inability to achieve an erection, an inconsistent ability to do so, or ability to achieve only brief erections.
• Sexual drive and the ability to have an orgasm may not be affected.

CAUSES—An erection requires a sequence of events. It starts with sexual stimulation in the brain, which sends nerve signals to the arteries and muscles of the penis. The penis fills with blood and grows firm and erect. After the stimulation ends, or ejaculation occurs, the blood leaves the penis, and it softens again. With erectile dysfunction, this sequence of events is disrupted. This can be due to physical (most often) or psychological (mental or emotional) factors.

RISK INCREASES WITH
Physical factors may include:
• Diabetes, endocrine disorder, liver or kidney disease.
• Atherosclerosis (hardening of arteries), high blood pressure, heart or blood vessel disease.
• Some drugs (e.g., high blood pressure drugs).
• Disorder or injury of central nervous system.
• Alcoholism, smoking, or drugs of abuse.
• Decreased penile blood flow from any cause.
• Surgery (such as for heart or blood vessels).
• Prostate cancer treatment.
• Hormone imbalance.
Psychological factors may include:
• Fear of sexual failure or performance anxiety, low self-esteem, or lack of interest in sex.
• Decreased sexuality in long-term relationship.
• Depression, anxiety, stress, anger, and guilt.
• Fear of disease (e.g., sexual) or heart attack.
• Other people around (such as mother-in-law).

HOW TO PREVENT
• None specific. General advice is listed.
• Maintain good health and proper weight.
• Avoid any of the risk factors where possible.
• Control any chronic medical conditions.
• Ask about side effects before taking new drug.
• Open communication with sexual partner.
• Avoid worries about sexual performance.

 WHAT TO EXPECT

DIAGNOSTIC MEASURES
• Your health care provider will do a physical exam and ask about your sexual history.
• Medical tests may be done to diagnose any underlying disorder.

APPROPRIATE HEALTH CARE
• Treatment steps may involve lifestyle changes, therapy for any illness diagnosed, erectile dysfunction drugs or devices, counseling, and surgery. A treatment plan will be based on your individual case.
• Lifestyle changes may include cutting back on alcohol, smoking, or drug abuse. Reducing stress, diet changes, and increased exercise may be recommended.
• Counseling can help. It may be for emotional problems (such as stress, anxiety, or guilt). Counseling may involve a sex therapist for you and your partner.
• Use of a vacuum inflation device is an option.
• Surgery for an inflatable or non-inflatable penile implant may help if other methods fail.
• Surgery to help blood flow to the penis may be advised if there are blood vessel problems.

POSSIBLE COMPLICATIONS
• Reduced quality of life for the man and his partner.
• Depression, anxiety, and low self-esteem.

PROBABLE OUTCOME—Impotence is treatable in all age groups. Near normal sexual activity can often be achieved with treatment.

 HOW TO TREAT

GENERAL MEASURES—To learn more: Erectile Dysfunction Institute, 10949 Bren Road East, Minnetonka, MN 55343; (866) 563-2432; website: www.erectile-dysfunction-impotence.org.

MEDICATION
• Drugs for erectile dysfunction (taken by mouth, self-injected, or by suppository) are often prescribed. Follow instructions carefully.
• If a drug you take is the cause of impotence, a change in drugs or a change in dosage amounts may be made.
• Drugs may be prescribed for other disorders.

ACTIVITY—No limits. Exercise daily for health.

DIET—Eat a well-balanced diet.

 CALL YOUR DOCTOR IF

• You or a family member has impotence.
• Impotence continues even with treatment.

INCONTINENCE, STRESS

 GENERAL INFORMATION

DEFINITION—An involuntary leaking of urine that occurs with sudden increased pressure in the abdomen.

BODY PARTS INVOLVED—Kidneys and urinary system.

SEX OR AGE MOST AFFECTED—Both sexes, but is more common in older women.

SIGNS & SYMPTOMS—Leaking of urine. This may happen with lifting, sneezing, singing, coughing, laughing, exercising, sports activity, crying, or straining to have a bowel movement. It may also occur with small movements such as rolling over in bed or standing up from a sitting position.

CAUSES—It is usually due to pelvic floor muscle or sphincter muscle problems. Pelvic floor muscles support the bladder. Sphincter muscles keep the opening of the bladder closed until it is time to urinate, and then they relax. When these muscles become weak or don't function properly, urine can leak out from the bladder.

RISK INCREASES WITH
* Repeated vaginal childbirth.
* Vaginal birth of large children.
* Adults over 60.
* Obesity.
* Surgery or radiation of the genitals or urinary tract.
* Chronic lung disease with a cough.

PREVENTIVE MEASURES
* Maintain good health.
* Get physical exams to detect early problems.
* Urinate regularly.
* Strengthen pelvic floor muscles with Kegel exercises.
  - First step is to identify pelvic floor muscles. When urinating, stop the flow by squeezing the pelvic floor muscles. Another way is to insert a finger into vagina (women) or rectum (men), then tighten the muscles around the finger. Repeat each method until you are sure you can feel which muscles are involved.
  - The exercises can be done any time and any place, lying down or sitting up. Start by emptying the bladder.
  - Tighten the pelvic floor muscles and hold for a count of 10.
  - Relax the muscles completely for a count of 10.
  - Perform 10 exercises, 3 times a day (morning, afternoon, and night). Don't do more than this.
  - It may take 6 weeks to 3 months for improvement.

 WHAT TO EXPECT

DIAGNOSTIC MEASURES
* Your health care provider will do a physical exam and ask questions about your symptoms.
* Medical tests of blood and urine may be done to check for other conditions. Additional tests may be done to help diagnose specific urinary-tract problems. You may be asked to keep a diary about your urination patterns.

APPROPRIATE HEALTH CARE
* Treatment may involve weight loss, stopping smoking, suppressing cough, Kegel exercises, drugs, pessary, other therapy, or surgery.
* Other therapies include biofeedback, electrical stimulation, bladder training, magnetic innervation, or special weights to strengthen pelvic muscles. These options will be explained.
* A pessary (support device) to fit inside the vagina to support the uterus is helpful for some women. Other types of devices include urethral plugging or stenting.
* If other methods fail, surgery to tighten relaxed or damaged muscles that support the bladder helps some. Even with surgery, some leakage may continue.

POSSIBLE COMPLICATIONS—Physical problems are rare. It can affect quality of life.

PROBABLE OUTCOME—Kegel exercises can be effective for mild symptoms. With more severe incontinence, other treatment steps may cure the problem or reduce symptoms.

 HOW TO TREAT

GENERAL MEASURES
* Learn and practice Kegel exercises. Try to use the squeezing technique just before any sneeze or a cough.
* Wear special underwear or incontinence pad.
* To learn more: National Association for Continence, (800) 252-3337; website: www.nafc.org or Simon Foundation for Continence, (800) 237-4666; website: www.simonfoundation.org.

MEDICATION
* Drugs to help sphincter muscles may be prescribed.
* Estrogen therapy may be prescribed.

ACTIVITY—No limits. Exercise daily for health.

DIET—Start a weight loss program if overweight. Decrease caffeine and alcohol.

 CALL YOUR DOCTOR IF

* You or a family member has symptoms of stress incontinence.
* Symptoms don't improve with treatment.

INCONTINENCE, URGE

GENERAL INFORMATION

DEFINITION—Feeling the need or urge to urinate and then being unable to control the bladder until you can get to a toilet.

BODY PARTS INVOLVED—Kidneys and urinary system.

SEX OR AGE MOST AFFECTED—Both sexes, but is more common in older women.

SIGNS & SYMPTOMS
- Loss of urine right after feeling an urge to urinate. It may be a few drops to complete bladder emptying.
- Symptoms may occur with sudden change in position or activity, hearing or touching running water, drinking a small amount of liquid, and during sleep.
- Key-in-lock syndrome may occur. This happens when you rush home, put a key in the door lock, and experience a sudden bladder contraction and urine leakage.

CAUSES—The usual cause is a spasm or contraction of the bladder muscle. It squeezes at the wrong time, earlier than it should, and causes the leakage. The spasm may result from bladder nerve damage, other nerve problems, or problems of the bladder muscles. The bladder may be described as spastic, overactive, or unstable.

RISK INCREASES WITH
- Repeated vaginal childbirth.
- Adults over 60. Women more than men.
- Hormonal changes after menopause.
- Obesity.
- Genitals or urinary tract surgery or radiation.
- Urinary-tract infection, stone, cancer, or obstruction.
- A neurological (nervous system) disorder.

PREVENTIVE MEASURES
- Maintain good health. Urinate regularly.
- Get physical exams to detect early problems.
- Do Kegel exercises for pelvic floor muscles.
 - The first step is to identify pelvic floor muscles. When urinating, stop the flow by squeezing the pelvic floor muscles. Another way is to insert a finger into vagina (women) or rectum (men), then tighten the muscles around the finger. Repeat each method until you are sure you can feel which muscles are involved.
 - The exercises can be done any time and any place, lying down or sitting up. Start by emptying the bladder.
 - Tighten pelvic floor muscles. Hold for a count of 10, then relax them for a count of 10.
 - Perform 10 exercises, 3 times a day (morning, afternoon, and night). Don't do more .
 - Improvement takes 6 weeks to 3 months.

WHAT TO EXPECT

DIAGNOSTIC MEASURES
- Your health care provider will do a physical exam and ask questions about your symptoms.
- Medical tests of blood and urine may be done to check for other conditions. Additional tests may be done to help diagnose specific urinary-tract problems. You may be asked to keep a diary about your urination patterns.

APPROPRIATE HEALTH CARE
- Treatment may involve drugs for bladder spasms or infection, weight loss, smoking cessation, Kegel exercises, pessary, other types of therapy, or surgery.
- Other therapies include biofeedback, electrical stimulation, bladder training, magnetic innervation, or special weights to strengthen pelvic muscles.
- A pessary (support device) fits inside vagina to support the uterus or other types of devices including urethral plugging or stenting may help.
- If other methods fail, surgery to tighten relaxed or damaged muscles that support the bladder helps some. Even with surgery, some leakage may continue.

POSSIBLE COMPLICATIONS—Physical problems are rare. It can affect quality of life.

PROBABLE OUTCOME—Treatment can help reduce symptoms.

HOW TO TREAT

GENERAL MEASURES
- Have quick access to a toilet. Urinate on schedule.
- Learn and practice Kegel exercises.
- Wear special underwear or incontinence pad.
- To learn more: National Association for Continence, (800) 252-3337; website: www.nafc.org or Simon Foundation for Continence, (800) 237-4666; website: www.simonfoundation.org.

MEDICATION
- Drugs to control bladder spasms may be prescribed.
- Women may be prescribed hormone therapy.
- Drugs may be prescribed for any infection.

ACTIVITY—No limits. Exercise daily for health.

DIET—Start a weight loss program if overweight. Decrease caffeine and alcohol.

☎ CALL YOUR DOCTOR IF

You or a family member has symptoms of urge incontinence and self-treatment isn't helping.

ILLNESS & DISORDERS

INDIGESTION
(Dyspepsia)

GENERAL INFORMATION

DEFINITION—Indigestion is the term used to describe chest or abdominal discomfort following meals. The medical term is dyspepsia. Almost everyone will experience indigestion at one time or another. Some people have it every day, others may have it occasionally.

BODY PARTS INVOLVED—Stomach; esophagus; small intestine.

SEX OR AGE MOST AFFECTED—Both sexes; all ages.

SIGNS & SYMPTOMS
- Mild nausea.
- Upset stomach.
- Upper abdominal discomfort.
- Gas or belching.
- Bloated or full feeling.
- Stomach feels full soon after starting a meal.
- Acid taste in the mouth.

CAUSES—There may be excess stomach acid produced, problems with motility (movement of food through the digestive system), irritation of the stomach lining, or an increase in gas. A bacterial infection with *Helicobacter pylori* may also be involved. A number of risk factors are known to lead to indigestion.

RISK INCREASES WITH
- Eating too much and eating too quickly.
- Eating food with a high fat content.
- Poor digestion of gas-forming foods (beans, cucumbers, cabbage, onions, and others).
- Smoking.
- Drinking too much alcohol.
- Lactose intolerance.
- Stress or anxiety.
- Some drugs can irritate the stomach lining. These include nonsteroidal anti-inflammatories (such as aspirin or ibuprofen), iron supplements, antibiotics, and others.
- Swallowing too much air when chewing.
- Exercising right after eating.
- Food allergy.
- Pregnancy.
- Overweight.

HOW TO PREVENT—Follow suggestions in General Measures. Avoid risk factors.

WHAT TO EXPECT

DIAGNOSTIC MEASURES
- If symptoms persist or cause concern, see your health care provider. A physical exam may be done and questions asked about symptoms.
- Medical tests may sometimes be needed to check for other disorders.

APPROPRIATE HEALTH CARE
- Most people will self-treat this disorder.
- Medical care may include drug therapy.

POSSIBLE COMPLICATIONS—Indigestion usually does not cause complications. It can occasionally be a symptom of another disorder that could be more serious.

PROBABLE OUTCOME—Indigestion is very common and is usually nothing to worry about. Symptoms can be controlled, but recurrence is likely.

HOW TO TREAT

GENERAL MEASURES—Treatment and prevention are similar. Follow the steps listed here to help relieve the symptoms.
- Eat slowly. Chew food carefully and completely.
- Don't smoke right before or during a meal.
- Relax after meals, but don't lie down.
- Avoid excitement or exercise right after a meal.
- Avoid situations that make you swallow air, such as chewing gum, or drinking carbonated drinks.
- Avoid tight clothing.
- Avoid foods you don't digest well.
- Avoid emotional problems during meals.
- Place blocks under the head of your bed to raise it a few inches.
- Avoid nonsteroidal anti-inflammatory drugs.

MEDICATION
- You may use nonprescription antacids to neutralize the stomach acid. Use H2 antagonists (such as cimetidine or ranitidine) or proton pump inhibitors (such as omeprazole) to reduce stomach acid.
- Stronger drugs may be prescribed if needed.

ACTIVITY—No limits. Daily exercise (such as 30 minute walk) helps promote good health. Don't exercise right after a meal.

DIET—Eat small meals. Don't eat near bedtime. Avoid foods that cause discomfort. Eat slowly; don't gulp food. Avoid alcohol or caffeine on an empty stomach. Lose weight, if you are overweight.

CALL YOUR DOCTOR IF

- You or a family member has symptoms of indigestion that persist, are severe, or cause concern.
- Other symptoms occur along with indigestion, such as chest pain, shortness of breath, or rapid weight loss.

INFLUENZA (Flu)

GENERAL INFORMATION

DEFINITION—A contagious infection caused by viruses that affect the nose, throat, and lungs. Influenza (flu) outbreaks occur in the late fall and winter with varying degrees of severity. The disease spreads through communities creating an epidemic.

BODY PARTS INVOLVED—Upper-respiratory system.

SEX OR AGE MOST AFFECTED—Both sexes; all ages except infants.

SIGNS & SYMPTOMS
- Chills and moderate-to-high fever.
- Headache.
- Muscle aches, including backache.
- Dry cough.
- Sore throat.
- Runny or stuffy nose.
- Fatigue.

CAUSES—The virus germs are spread when an infected person coughs, sneezes, or speaks. The germs get into the air, and nearby persons breathe in the germs. Flu can also be spread by touching a surface that has the germs on it and then touching your nose or mouth. Adults are contagious 1 day before symptoms and up to 7 days after getting sick. Children may be contagious for longer than 7 days. Symptoms start 1 to 5 days after exposure.

RISK INCREASES WITH
- Crowded places during an epidemic.
- Students in schools.
- Children and the elderly.
- Nursing homes or long-term care centers.
- Recent illness that has lowered resistance.
- Smokers.
- Chronic illness, such as chronic lung or heart disease.
- Weak immune system due to illness or drugs.

HOW TO PREVENT
- Have a yearly influenza vaccine injection or a nasal spray flu vaccine. A different vaccine is made every year because strains of the virus change from year to year. Sometimes, an unpredicted new strain appears and you may still get the flu, but it is usually a milder case. Talk to your health care provider if you have any questions.
- Some antiviral drugs may also help in preventing flu.
- Wash hands often to help avoid germs.

WHAT TO EXPECT

DIAGNOSTIC MEASURES
- See your health care provider if symptoms are more severe, cause any concern, or you are at risk for complications.
- Your health care provider may do a physical exam. A diagnosis of flu can usually be made based on the symptoms.
- Medical tests are not always needed, but may be done to verify the diagnosis or check for complications.

APPROPRIATE HEALTH CARE
- Most people who get the flu will use self-care methods at home.
- Treatment steps may include extra rest, drinking plenty of fluids, and using flu remedies or other drugs.

POSSIBLE COMPLICATIONS—Pneumonia, dehydration, or worsening of a chronic illness. Children may get sinus problems or ear infections.

PROBABLE OUTCOME—Most people who get the flu get better in a week. A cough or tired feeling may last a little longer. Elderly persons, children 6 months to 23 months, pregnant women, and people with chronic illnesses are more at risk for complications.

HOW TO TREAT

GENERAL MEASURES
- For nasal congestion, use salt-water drops in the nose. Mix one-quarter teaspoon of salt in four ounces of water).
- To help a sore throat, gargle often with warm or cold double-strength tea or salt water (mix one-half teaspoon of salt in one cup of water).
- Use a cool-mist humidifier (if advised) to increase air moisture. Clean humidifier daily.
- Avoid spreading germs. Wash hands often.
- Use a warm heating pad for aching muscles.

MEDICATION
- For minor discomfort, use nonprescription drugs, such as acetaminophen, aspirin, cough syrups, nasal sprays, or decongestants. Do not give aspirin to children under age 18.
- Antiviral drugs may be prescribed.

ACTIVITY—Get extra rest. Rest helps your body fight the virus.

DIET—You may just want liquids at first. Then progress to small meals of bland starchy foods (e.g., dry toast, rice, pudding, cooked cereal, baked potatoes).

CALL YOUR DOCTOR IF

- You or a family member has symptoms of influenza that seem severe or cause concern.
- Symptoms get worse, such as higher fever, shaking chills, chest pain with breathing, coughing that produces a yellow mucus, ear ache, sinus pain, neck pain or stiffness, nausea, or vomiting.

ILLNESS & DISORDERS

INSECT BITES & STINGS

GENERAL INFORMATION

DEFINITION—Skin eruptions and other symptoms caused by insect bites or stings from mosquitoes, fleas, chiggers, bedbugs, ants, spiders, bees, wasps, hornets, scorpions, and other insects. The victim often doesn't remember being bitten or stung.

BODY PARTS INVOLVED
• Skin on any part of the body.
• Lymph glands in the neck, armpit, groin or elbow.

SEX OR AGE MOST AFFECTED—Both sexes; all ages.

SIGNS & SYMPTOMS—Red lumps in the skin. The lumps usually appear within minutes after the bite or sting. Some don't appear for 6 to 12 hours. Skin reactions fall into 2 kinds:
• A toxic reaction with pain and sometimes fever, such as from bee stings.
• A toxic reaction with itching due to the body's release of histamine at the site of the bite, such as from mosquitoes.

CAUSES—The insect bite or sting causes an injection of venom into the skin. This starts a reaction from the body's immune system. The reaction may be mild to severe, depending on how sensitive a person is to the toxin.

RISK INCREASES WITH
• Areas with heavy insect infestations.
• Warm weather in spring and summer.
• Lack of protective measures.
• Perfumes, colognes.

HOW TO PREVENT
• If you cannot avoid exposure, use insect repellent with diethyltoluamide (DEET) on skin.
• Wear protective clothing. Apply permethrin to clothing to repel insects and ticks.

WHAT TO EXPECT

DIAGNOSTIC MEASURES
• Your own observation of symptoms.
• See your health care provider if any symptoms cause you concern.

APPROPRIATE HEALTH CARE
• For severe reactions to a bite or sting, get emergency help right away. They can be life-threatening.
• For most bites and stings, self-care is usually all that is needed.

POSSIBLE COMPLICATIONS
• A bacterial infection at the site of the bite.
• Anaphylaxis (life-threatening allergic reaction) for certain super-sensitive persons.
• Scarring on the skin.

• Disorders caused by certain insects. These include Lyme disease, Rocky Mountain spotted fever, West Nile virus, malaria, and others.

PROBABLE OUTCOME—Most of the symptoms are mild and go away in 2 to 3 days. Scratching may occur for several weeks. Treatment helps, but it doesn't cure quickly.

HOW TO TREAT

GENERAL MEASURES
• Remove stinger. Scrape it out. Don't use tweezers.
• For bee, wasp, yellow-jacket, or hornet stings, rub a paste of meat tenderizer and water into the site.
• For ant bites rub the bite with ammonia; repeat as often as necessary.
• For spider or scorpion bites, capture the insect, if possible, and seek medical help.
• For a tick, use a tweezer to remove it. Put it in a jar with alcohol to kill it. Save it in case more medical problems develop.
• Clean the wound. Apply an ice pack.
• Elevate and rest the affected body part.
• Warm-water soaks help soothe minor pain. Cool-water soaks feel better for itching.
• If you have had anaphylaxis (severe allergic reaction) following an insect bite, carry a special kit to treat it in the future.

MEDICATION
• For minor discomfort, you may use:
  - Nonprescription oral antihistamines to decrease itching.
  - Nonprescription topical steroid drugs to reduce redness and soreness and to decrease itching. For face and groin, use only low-potency steroid products without fluorine.
• For serious symptoms, you may be prescribed:
  - Stronger topical steroids or oral steroids if the reaction is severe.
  - Injection of drugs may be needed to prevent or reduce symptoms of anaphylaxis.
• A tetanus shot if needed for some patients.

ACTIVITY—No limits.

DIET—No special diet.

CALL YOUR DOCTOR IF

• You or a family member has an insect bite or sting and has a severe reaction. This is an emergency!
• Self-care does not relieve symptoms, or symptoms don't improve after 2 to 3 days of treatment.
• Fever occurs and bitten area becomes red, swollen, warm, and tender. This could mean an infection.

INSOMNIA

GENERAL INFORMATION

DEFINITION—Problems falling asleep, staying asleep, waking early, or a combination of these. Insomnia is often described by how long it has lasted. Transient is a few days, short-term is less than 3 weeks, and chronic is more than 3 weeks.

BODY PARTS INVOLVED—Nervous.

SEX OR AGE MOST AFFECTED—Both sexes; all ages. It is more common in the elderly.

SIGNS & SYMPTOMS
• Difficulty falling asleep.
• Wakefulness follows a brief period of sleep.
• Normal sleep until very early in the morning, then wakefulness (often with frightening thoughts).
• Daytime fatigue and tiredness.
• Lack of sleep causes problems with social, work, family, and other areas of one's life.

CAUSES—Insomnia is a symptom, not a disease. It can be caused by physical, mental, and environmental problems.

RISK INCREASES WITH
• Depression, anxiety, tension, or stress.
• Daytime napping.
• Noise (including a snoring partner).
• Allergies and early-morning wheezing.
• Heart or lung problems that cause shortness of breath when lying down.
• Painful disorders, such as arthritis.
• Frequent need to urinate at night.
• Night sweats, or disorders that cause excess itching.
• Sexual problems.
• Drinking caffeine drinks (coffee, tea, or cola).
• Use of some drugs.
• Odd work hours, such as swing shifts.
• A new environment or location.
• Jet lag after travel.
• Lack of exercise.
• Smoking, alcoholism, or drug abuse, including overuse of sleep-inducing drugs.
• Withdrawal from addictive substances.
• Sleep apnea.

HOW TO PREVENT
• Avoid lengthy daytime napping.
• Avoid risk factors, where possible.
• For general good health, eat a healthy diet, exercise daily, maintain weight for height, and don't smoke.

WHAT TO EXPECT

DIAGNOSTIC MEASURES
• See your health care provider if self-care doesn't help. A physical exam may be done and questions asked about your symptoms and activities.

• Medical tests may be done to check for any physical disorders. A special sleep study may be prescribed.

APPROPRIATE HEALTH CARE—Medical steps may include:
• Counseling for problems such as depression.
• Treatment for any medical order diagnosed.

POSSIBLE COMPLICATIONS—Insomnia can cause impaired thinking, and health and emotional problems that affect all aspects of life.

PROBABLE OUTCOME—Insomnia can usually be relieved by treating the cause, using self-care steps, or with other medical treatment.

HOW TO TREAT

GENERAL MEASURES—You may try these self-care steps:
• Try to reduce tension, stress, or anxiety in your life.
• Don't turn the bedroom into an office or den.
• Create a comfortable sleep setting.
• Relax in a warm bath before bedtime.
• After 15 to 20 minutes of trying to sleep, get up and do some relaxing activity. Don't watch television.
• Relax your mind. Focus on peaceful and relaxing thoughts. Play soft music or relaxation tapes.
• Set a strict sleep schedule and keep to it.
• Use ear plugs, eye shades, or an electric blanket.

MEDICATION
• Sleep-inducing drugs may be prescribed for a short time if: short-term insomnia is interfering with daily activities; you have a disorder that disturbs sleep; you need to establish regular sleep patterns.
• Long-term use of sleep inducers may be counter-productive or addictive. Don't use sleeping pills unless they are prescribed.

ACTIVITY
• Exercise daily to create healthy fatigue, but not within 2 hours of going to bed.
• Have sexual relations, if they are satisfying and fulfilling before going to sleep.

DIET—Avoid alcohol, caffeine, or a heavy meal within 3 hours of bedtime. Try a light snack with milk at bedtime.

CALL YOUR DOCTOR IF

• You or a family member has had insomnia for over 4 weeks or it is interfering with your ability to function.
• Medical care is not relieving insomnia.

ILLNESS & DISORDERS

INTERSTITIAL CYSTITIS

GENERAL INFORMATION

DEFINITION—Interstitial cystitis (IC) is a chronic bladder disorder. Symptoms are similar to cystitis (an infection of the urinary tract), but no infection is found. Hunner's ulcer is a rare, and more severe, form of IC.

BODY PARTS INVOLVED—Bladder.

SEX OR AGE MOST AFFECTED—The average age of onset is 40, but it affects all ages, women more commonly than men.

SIGNS & SYMPTOMS
- Symptoms vary greatly for each person.
- Pelvic pain and a feeling of pressure.
- Urgent need to urinate day and night (up to 40 times a day). This also causes sleep problems.
- Bladder does not feel like it empties completely when you urinate.
- Pain during sexual intercourse.
- Burning when urinating.
- Vaginal and rectal pain.

CAUSES—The lining (or wall) of the bladder breaks down. Urine stored in the bladder irritates the damaged lining and it becomes red and sore. Why the lining breaks down is not known. Medical tests find no bacteria or virus infection. There actually may be several causes, or there may be different disorders, rather than just one.

RISK INCREASES WITH
- Having allergies (such as to drugs or food).
- Hay fever or asthma.
- Rheumatoid arthritis, lupus (immune disorders).
- Certain bowel or urinary problems.

HOW TO PREVENT—No preventive measures.

WHAT TO EXPECT

DIAGNOSTIC MEASURES
- There are a number of medical problems that cause similar symptoms. They include kidney stones, urinary or vaginal infection, cancer, and others. Your health care provider will perform tests to rule out these other causes of the symptoms.
- A physical exam will be performed.
- Urine tests are needed to check for infection.
- A cystoscopy is usually done. In this test, a thin, tube-like device with a light is used to see inside the bladder. The test can be uncomfortable because the bladder is stretched. A drug (anesthetic) will be used to stop pain. A stretched bladder holds more urine so this test helps symptoms also.

APPROPRIATE HEALTH CARE
- There are a variety of treatment options. It is important to find out what works for you.

- Bladder instillation (a bladder wash or bath) is done at the medical office. It involves stretching the bladder by filling it with a solution for about 15 minutes.
- Bladder training involves teaching yourself to urinate at certain times.
- Counseling or behavior training. Learn how to relax and cope with stress, anxiety, or depression.
- A TENS (transcutaneous electrical nerve stimulation) device uses mild electric pulses to help block pain.
- Surgery is rarely needed. It may be done as a last resort when other methods have failed.

POSSIBLE COMPLICATIONS
- The symptoms may come and go over days, weeks, or months, sometimes years, even with treatment.
- Chronic symptoms can lead to problems with your work, friends, family, and sexual activity.

PROBABLE OUTCOME—Treatments can help control or relieve the symptoms, but they do not cure the disorder. It may take time to find the treatments that work best for you.

HOW TO TREAT

GENERAL MEASURES
- Don't smoke. Smoking worsens symptoms.
- Consider joining a support group.
- To learn more: The Interstitial Cystitis Association (ICA), 51 Monroe St, Suite 1402, Rockville, MD 20850; (800) 435-7422; website: www.ichelp.org.

MEDICATION
- You may use nonprescription pain relievers.
- Pentosan polysulfate, brand name Elmiron, may be prescribed. It is used for treating interstitial cystitis.
- Other drugs may be prescribed for depression, anxiety, sleep problems, and severe pain.

ACTIVITY
- No limits unless limited by the symptoms.
- Regular exercise may help patient feel better.

DIET—Diet changes help some patients. Avoid drinks with caffeine, alcohol, or artificial sweeteners; spicy foods, chocolate, soda/carbonated beverages, citrus fruits, and tomatoes.

CALL YOUR DOCTOR IF

- You or a family member has symptoms of interstitial cystitis.
- Treatment is not helping the pain or other symptoms.
- New symptoms occur. Drugs may cause side effects

INTESTINAL OBSTRUCTION

GENERAL INFORMATION

DEFINITION—Partial or complete blockage of the intestines. The material in the bowel cannot move pass the blockage. This causes the symptoms and also upsets the body's electrolyte balance. A mechanical obstruction occurs when the bowel is physically blocked. Nonmechanical obstruction (called ileus) occurs when peristalsis (wavelike motion of the intestine) stops.

BODY PARTS INVOLVED—Small and large bowel.

SEX OR AGE MOST AFFECTED—Both sexes; all ages.

SIGNS & SYMPTOMS
* Cramping abdominal pain.
* Nausea and vomiting. In the advanced stages, vomit resembles feces.
* Weakness, dizziness, or fainting.
* Little or no urine due to fluid loss.
* Failure to pass stools or gas.
* Audible noises from the abdomen in early stages; later, no sounds are audible.
* Abdominal bloating, swelling, and gas.
* Fever (sometimes).
* Diarrhea (partial obstruction only).
* Passing jelly-like mucus or bloody mucus.

CAUSES
Mechanical:
* Adhesions (constricting bands of fibrous tissue that result from previous surgery).
* Intestinal hernias.
* Intestinal inflammation or tumors (either benign or cancerous).
* Tumors in adjacent organs that cause pressure on the intestines.
* Inflammatory bowel disease.
* Foreign objects inside the intestines (gallstones, swallowed objects or parasites such as worms).
* Twisted bowel (volvulus).
* Fecal impaction.
* Bowel telescopes into itself (intussusception).
* In newborns or infants, it may be caused by a birth defect.
Nonmechanical:
* Certain drugs, such as narcotics.
* Decreased blood supply to intestines due to injury or other problem.
* Complication of abdominal surgery.
* Infection of the lining of the abdominal cavity.
* Kidney or thoracic (chest cavity) disease.
* Metabolic problems, such as decreased potassium.

RISK INCREASES WITH—Previous abdominal surgery.

HOW TO PREVENT
* There are no specific preventive measures. Suggestions listed may help in prevention.
* Eat a diet high in fiber and drink plenty of fluids each day to avoid constipation or fecal impaction.
* Obtain medical treatment for hernias.
* See your health care provider if your bowel habits change significantly for longer than 7 days. It may be an early sign of bowel cancer.

WHAT TO EXPECT

DIAGNOSTIC MEASURES
* Your own observation of symptoms.
* Your health care provider will do a physical exam and ask about your symptoms.
* Medical tests include blood and urine studies. Other tests may include a barium enema or air enema (either one may also resolve the problem by straightening the intestine). An x-ray, CT, and ultrasound may be done.

APPROPRIATE HEALTH CARE
* Emergency care is usually needed. A nasogastric tube is used to suction out the contents of the stomach and/or intestines above the blockage. Fluid and electrolyte replacement will be provided by an IV (intravenous).
* Surgery to remove the obstruction is necessary in some cases.

POSSIBLE COMPLICATIONS
* Obstruction may recur after treatment.
* Dehydration, shock, and sepsis.
* Bowel complications such as gangrene, perforation, abscess, or peritonitis. Without treatment, complications can be fatal.

PROBABLE OUTCOME—With proper diagnosis and treatment., the outcome is good.

HOW TO TREAT

GENERAL MEASURES—Intestinal obstruction usually develops rapidly into an emergency. Home remedies are of no value and some, such as enemas or laxatives, may be harmful.

MEDICATION—Antibiotics are often prescribed to prevent infection.

ACTIVITY—You will be advised about limits depending on the treatment.

DIET—Don't eat or drink anything until the obstruction is corrected. You will probably receive intravenous nourishment until then.

CALL YOUR DOCTOR IF

* You or a family member has symptoms of intestinal obstruction. This is an emergency!
* Your bowel habits change.

INTUSSUSCEPTION

GENERAL INFORMATION

DEFINITION—An intestinal obstruction in which the bowel telescopes (folds into itself), forming a tube within a tube.

BODY PARTS INVOLVED—Intestine, usually the large intestine.

SEX OR AGE MOST AFFECTED—All ages, but most common in infants and children between 2 months and 6 years. It is more common in boys.

SIGNS & SYMPTOMS
• Cramping pain in the abdomen. Infants cry out and bring the legs up to the abdomen. They become pale and sweaty during an attack. Pain attacks may occur 10 to 20 minutes apart.
• Vomiting.
• Rectal bleeding. This may be dark red material that resembles red current jelly.
• Weakness and lack of energy.
• Swollen abdomen.
• Mass in the abdomen that can be felt.
• Later symptoms: increased weakness, fever, shock (rapid heartbeat, weak pulse, rapid breathing).

CAUSES
• Unknown for infants. The disorder may be caused by a virus infection, but this is unproven.
• In older children (usually over age 3) or in adults, it may be due to an intestinal problem.

RISK INCREASES WITH
• Recent upper-respiratory infection.
• Recent diarrhea illness.
• Cystic fibrosis.
• Blunt injury to the abdomen.
• Lymph nodes that are enlarged; tumor or polyp in the intestine.
• Season of the year (for unknown reasons). It is most common in late spring, early summer, and midwinter.

HOW TO PREVENT—No specific preventive measures.

WHAT TO EXPECT

DIAGNOSTIC MEASURES
• Your child's health care provider will do a physical exam with careful attention to the abdomen. Medical tests may include blood studies, x-rays, and ultrasound.
• A barium or air enema may be done for diagnosis and treatment. In this procedure, a liquid containing barium is given with a tube into the rectum and special x-rays are taken. The barium helps show the intussusception on the x-ray. In many cases, the pressure of the barium unfolds the bowel and cures the problem. An air enema can work in the same way.

APPROPRIATE HEALTH CARE—Surgery to correct the problem may be needed. This is done if the child is too ill for the enema procedure or it was done and did not provide a cure. Surgery involves pushing out the telescoped portion of the intestine. In a few cases, a part of the bowel must be cut out.

POSSIBLE COMPLICATIONS
• Dehydration and shock.
• Intestinal perforation.
• Tissue damage that cannot be reversed.
• An infection may occur after surgery.
• The disorder may recur after barium treatment.
• Without treatment, complications are life-threatening.

PROBABLE OUTCOME—Outcome for most children is very good. With early diagnosis and treatment, complications are unlikely to develop.

HOW TO TREAT

GENERAL MEASURES—Observe your child carefully if symptoms develop. Prevent complications by seeking medical treatment during early stages.

MEDICATION
• Drugs are usually not needed for this disorder unless infection develops. Then antibiotics may be prescribed.
• Don't use home remedies or nonprescription drugs, such as laxatives, for this condition. They may be dangerous.

ACTIVITY—The child should rest in bed until the obstruction is cleared. Activities may then be resumed gradually.

DIET—Don't feed a child who has signs of intestinal obstruction. Intravenous (through a vein) fluids are given in the hospital until the child can eat again.

CALL YOUR DOCTOR IF

• Your child has signs or symptoms of intestinal obstruction. This condition changes quickly from a curable one to a life-threatening one.
• Any new symptoms develop after treatment.

IRITIS
(Uveitis; Eye Inflammation)

 GENERAL INFORMATION

DEFINITION—Redness and soreness (inflammation) of the iris. The iris is the colored part of the eye. Uveitis is a general term used to describe inflammation of the eye which includes iritis. Other eye inflammations are ciliary body (cyclitis), choroid (choroiditis) and retina (retinitis).

BODY PARTS INVOLVED—Eye.

SEX OR AGE MOST AFFECTED—Both sexes; all ages.

SIGNS & SYMPTOMS
May start suddenly:
• Severe eye pain.
• Photophobia (sensitivity to light).
• Eye redness.
• Smaller pupil in the affected eye (sometimes).
• Tears.
• Blurred vision.
Gradual onset:
• Eye pain.
• Photophobia.
• Floating spots in the field of vision.
• Blurred vision.

CAUSES—The cause is unknown for most people. It is sometimes one of the symptoms of a disease that affects other parts of the body, such as arthritis. Iritis may sometimes be confused with pink eye (conjunctivitis).

RISK INCREASES WITH
• Ankylosing spondylitis.
• Inflammatory bowel disease.
• Reiter's syndrome.
• Arthritis.
• Behçet syndrome.
• Herpes infections.
• Lyme disease.
• Injuries.
• Sarcoidosis.
• Candidal infection.
• Syphilis.
• Histoplasmosis.
• Toxoplasmosis.
• Tuberculosis.

HOW TO PREVENT—No specific preventive measures known.

 WHAT TO EXPECT

DIAGNOSTIC MEASURES
• Iritis can be diagnosed by your eye care provider using special equipment to look into the eye.
• Other medical tests may be needed to help diagnose any health problem that is associated with iritis.

APPROPRIATE HEALTH CARE
• Treatment goals are to reduce pain and redness, prevent complications, and treat other health problems that are diagnosed.
• Treatment usually involves drug therapy.

POSSIBLE COMPLICATIONS
• Glaucoma, cataracts, retinal detachment, cystoid macular edema, or other eye disorders.
• Permanent or partial vision loss.

PROBABLE OUTCOME—Vision can usually be preserved with prompt treatment. Recovery takes 6 to 8 weeks. It sometimes depends on the disorder that is associated with iritis.

 HOW TO TREAT

GENERAL MEASURES—Wear dark glasses, even indoors, until treatment is complete.

MEDICATION
• Eyedrops (mydriatics) that dilate the pupil and prevent scarring may be prescribed. You may need to use eyedrops for a long time.
• Oral cortisone drugs or cortisone eyedrops to reduce inflammation may be prescribed.
• Drugs for other medical problems may be prescribed.

ACTIVITY—No limits (unless advised).

DIET—Eat a normal well-balanced diet.

 CALL YOUR DOCTOR IF

• You or a family member has symptoms of iritis, either sudden or gradual. Call immediately.
• Vision changes in any way.
• New, unexplained symptoms develop. Drugs used in treatment may produce side effects.

ILLNESS & DISORDERS

IRRITABLE BOWEL SYNDROME
(Spastic Colon or Colitis; Mucous Colitis)

 GENERAL INFORMATION

DEFINITION—A functional disorder of the large intestine (bowel). It is not a disease. "Functional disorder" means the bowel doesn't work properly. Irritable bowel syndrome (IBS) can cause a variety of symptoms. Episodes may last for days, weeks, or months. It is not contagious, inherited, or cancerous. It is very common.

BODY PARTS INVOLVED—Small and large intestines.

SEX OR AGE MOST AFFECTED—Often begins in adolescents or young adults; twice as likely to affect women as men.

SIGNS & SYMPTOMS
- Cramp-like pain in the middle or to one side of the lower abdomen. Pain is usually relieved with bowel movements.
- Diarrhea or constipation; usually alternating.
- Swollen or bloated abdomen and gas.
- Mucus in the stools.
- Straining to have bowel movement.
- Urgency to have bowel movement.
- Feeling that the bowels still have to be emptied after having a bowel movement.

CAUSES—Exact cause is unknown. The nerves and muscles in the bowel seem to be extra-sensitive in people with IBS. Nerves can cause pain and discomfort if they become irritated. Muscles that contract to pass food through the intestines may contract too much and cause cramping and diarrhea. The bowel can overreact to food, stress, exercise, and hormones. Stress may trigger symptoms if you have IBS, but it doesn't cause IBS.

RISK INCREASES WITH
- Under age 35.
- Women more than with men.
- Family members with similar bowel problems.
- People who have panic disorder, or similar disorders.
- People who have had a history of sexual, physical, or emotional abuse.

HOW TO PREVENT—No specific measures to prevent IBS. After it is diagnosed, you can find ways to help prevent symptoms.

 WHAT TO EXPECT

DIAGNOSTIC MEASURES
- Your health care provider may do a physical exam and ask questions about your symptoms and activities.
- Medical tests may include blood and stool studies, as well as other tests to exclude more serious disorders. A mental health exam may be done also.

APPROPRIATE HEALTH CARE
- Treatment may involve a combination of diet changes, drugs if needed, and treating stress.
- Consider counseling for emotional or personal problems or stress.

POSSIBLE COMPLICATIONS
- IBS can affect all aspects of life. It can interfere with work schedules, limit physical activities, disrupt personal relationships, and cause a restricted social life.
- It won't cause physical damage to bowels, nor lead to bleeding, serious disease, or cancer.

PROBABLE OUTCOME—The condition is usually recurrent throughout life. Symptoms may be mild to severe and may come and go. Most people can be helped with treatment. No specific treatment works best for everybody. You may need to try more than one.

 HOW TO TREAT

GENERAL MEASURES
- Reduce stress in your life. Try various techniques that can help you relax. Meditation, self-hypnosis, or biofeedback may help. Keep a stress and symptom diary so you know who or what may trigger an episode.
- Quit smoking (nicotine may add to problem).
- Join a support group. This can be helpful.
- To learn more: National Digestive Diseases information Clearinghouse, 2 information Way, Bethesda, MD 20892, (800) 891-5389; website: www.niddk.nih.gov/health/digest.

MEDICATION
- Antispasmodics to relieve severe cramps and drugs to treat the constipation form of IBS may be prescribed.
- Drugs for depression or anxiety may be prescribed.
- Antidiarrheals or laxatives need to be used with caution. Get medical advice before using.

ACTIVITY—Daily exercise helps bowel function, keeps you fit, and reduces stress.

DIET
- Increase fiber in the diet to promote good bowel function. Add fiber to your diet slowly. Too much fiber can cause gas.
- Avoid foods or drinks that can worsen symptoms. These include fatty foods, milk products, chocolate, alcohol, caffeine, and carbonated drinks. Keep a food diary to help find the foods that cause you problems.
- Avoid large meals, but eat regularly.

 CALL YOUR DOCTOR IF

- You or a family member has IBS symptoms.
- Symptoms don't improve with treatment.

JET LAG

GENERAL INFORMATION

DEFINITION—Jet lag results from east-west travel between different time zones. (North-south travel does not cause jet lag.) The degree of severity depends on the number of time zones crossed and the direction traveled. Most people find traveling eastward and adapting to a shorter work day is more difficult than traveling westward and adapting to a longer work day.

SEX OR AGE MOST AFFECTED—Both sexes; all ages.

SIGNS & SYMPTOMS
* Extreme fatigue.
* Sleep disturbances.
* Loss of concentration.
* Malaise.
* Disorientation.
* Sluggishness.
* Stomach upset.
* Loss of appetite.
* Swollen feet.

CAUSES—Disturbance in the body's physiological processes that control not only sleep and wakefulness, but also alertness, hunger, digestion, urine production, temperature and hormone secretion.

RISK INCREASES WITH—Frequent travel in short periods of time.

HOW TO PREVENT
* Avoid alcohol.
* There are many jet lag prevention methods that have been proposed, written about, and discussed among travelers. There is no one method that works for everyone. You may want to try one or more prevention methods to see what might work for you. Check in bookstores, libraries, and the Internet for information.

WHAT TO EXPECT

DIAGNOSTIC MEASURES—Your own observation of symptoms.

APPROPRIATE HEALTH CARE—No medical care is necessary for typical cases of jet lag.

POSSIBLE COMPLICATIONS—Usually, no complications develop.

PROBABLE OUTCOME—Symptoms usually resolve themselves after a short period of time in the same geographic location.

HOW TO TREAT

GENERAL MEASURES
* Plan destination activities to accommodate for time differences.
* Spend some time every day in natural sunlight.
* Adjust your bed and mealtimes to the new timetable as soon as possible
* Set your watch to local time as soon as possible after takeoff.

MEDICATION
* Drugs for insomnia may be prescribed for a short period of time. You might try them before you leave to see how they effect you and if they cause any unwanted side effects.
* The hormone melatonin has been used for this condition, but long-term data are lacking.

ACTIVITY
* Continue with any regular exercise program once you arrive at your destination. Do not exercise close to bedtime.
* Don't operate motor vehicles or swim alone if you feel tired.

DIET
* Eat a normal well-balanced diet, even if you have no appetite.
* Drink plenty of liquids, but avoid alcoholic drinks.

CALL YOUR DOCTOR IF

You or a family member has symptoms of jet lag and they don't improve after one week.

ILLNESS & DISORDERS

KAPOSI'S SARCOMA

 ## GENERAL INFORMATION

DEFINITION—A form of skin cancer that is found most often in patients with advanced HIV (human immunodeficiency virus) infection. A second form of Kaposi's sarcoma is associated with some immunosuppressive drugs. A third form, referred to as classic, is found in elderly men of Mediterranean and Eastern European ancestry. A fourth form is found in young men in Africa.

BODY PARTS INVOLVED—Skin.

SEX OR AGE MOST AFFECTED—Usually adult males.

SIGNS & SYMPTOMS
* Skin lesions (sores) usually on the face, arms, and trunk. They may also be found in the mouth, lymph nodes, and other areas.
* The color may be brown, reddish-purple, or purple-black. They usually don't itch or cause pain.
* Lesions in the mouth may interfere with eating or swallowing.
* Lesions on the feet may interfere with walking.
* Swelling of the face, scrotum, and lower extremities if the lymph nodes are affected.
* May cause internal bleeding if the stomach is affected.
* May cause breathing problems if the lungs are affected.

CAUSES—The exact cause is unknown. Multiple causes are probably involved. It is known to be caused, in part, by a type of human herpesvirus called HHV-8.

RISK INCREASES WITH
* Weak immune system due to HIV-AIDS infection.
* Elderly men of Mediterranean and Eastern European descent.
* People with weak immune system, due to drugs taken for organ transplantation.

HOW TO PREVENT—If you have HIV or AIDS, using anti-HIV drugs can boost the immune system and help prevent Kaposi's sarcoma.

 ## WHAT TO EXPECT

DIAGNOSTIC MEASURES
* Your own observation of symptoms.
* Your health care provider will do an exam of the affected skin areas.
* Medical tests may be done to confirm the diagnosis and to see if the disorder has spread to other places in the body (staging).

APPROPRIATE HEALTH CARE
* Primary goals of treatment are to relieve symptoms and improve cosmetic appearance.
* If there are only a few skin lesions, they may be followed up for a period of time rather than being treated.
* More widespread skin lesions can be treated in several ways. They can be frozen (cryotherapy), treated with radiation, cut out surgically, or treated with drugs that are injected into the skin or used on the skin. Your health care provider will discuss your options.
* If lesions have spread to the inside (internal organs) of the body, drugs are used for treatment.

POSSIBLE COMPLICATIONS
* Lesions spread to other parts of the body.
* Other infections.
* Internal bleeding.
* Anemia.

PROBABLE OUTCOME
* There is no cure. It is a lifelong condition.
* For HIV-AIDS associated infection, the outcome depends on the extent and location of the lesions and the degree of immune system impairment. Treatment can help shrink the lesions, but they often recur.
* For Kaposi's due to an immune-suppressing drug, it often improves if drug is changed or dosage reduced.
* For classic type, patients may develop another form of cancer or die from other causes.

 ## HOW TO TREAT

GENERAL MEASURES—Cosmetic cover up products can be used on the skin to camouflage the lesions.

MEDICATION
* Drugs (antiretrovirals) for AIDS treatment are usually prescribed if they are not being taken already.
* Anticancer drugs may be given.
* Topical retinoic acid may be used for skin lesions.
* New drugs for treatment are being studied.

ACTIVITY—As tolerated.

DIET—You may need a special diet if the mouth is affected.

 ## CALL YOUR DOCTOR IF

* You or a household member has symptoms of Kaposi's sarcoma.
* New or unexplained symptoms develop. Drugs used in treatment may cause side effects.

KELOIDS

GENERAL INFORMATION

DEFINITION—An overgrowth of fibrous tissue (scar) on the skin.

BODY PARTS INVOLVED—Anywhere on the skin, but most commonly appear on the breastbone, upper back and shoulder.

SEX OR AGE MOST AFFECTED—Both sexes; all ages. Keloids are more frequent in black people than in white people and occur more often in young women.

SIGNS & SYMPTOMS
• Keloids begin as a small bump. The lump grows and turns into firm, raised, hard scars that are slightly pink.
• Scars may continue to grow over a period of time.
• May itch or cause burning sensation.
• They may become a cosmetic problem.
• Scars may become irritated from rubbing on clothing.

CAUSES—Keloids probably occur due to a defective healing process. An excess of collagen forms at the site of a healing scar. Keloids usually arise in an area of injury (such as after a burn or from severe acne), but sometimes arise from a very minor scratch. Why they occur in certain people is unknown.

RISK INCREASES WITH
• Family history of keloids.
• Dark skin pigment.
• Surgical wound.
• Acne.
• Burn injury.
• Ear piercing.
• Vaccination.
• Insect bite.
• Folliculitis barbae (inflammation of a hair follicle).

HOW TO PREVENT
• Avoid injuries to the skin, if possible.
• For patients with known tendency to keloid formation, elective surgery should be avoided. If a procedure is necessary, special precautions should be implemented.

WHAT TO EXPECT

DIAGNOSTIC MEASURES
• Your own observation of symptoms.
• Your health care provider can diagnose keloids by their appearance on the skin.
• Medical tests are usually not needed, but may be done to rule out any other skin problem.

APPROPRIATE HEALTH CARE
• There are a variety of treatment options. Your health care provider will discuss them with you.
• Treatment may include injections into the scars. This may be combined with surgery to help remove the scars.
• Surgery may also be done in combination with radiation therapy.
• Cryotherapy involves freezing the affected area with liquid nitrogen.
• Special gel sheeting can be used to flatten the scars. It is applied to the area and changed about every week or 10 days for as long as a year.
• Other new therapies are currently undergoing study.

POSSIBLE COMPLICATIONS—Recurrence, despite adequate treatment.

PROBABLE OUTCOME—Scars gradually diminish with treatment. Sometimes, keloids heal on their own. Keloids are generally considered harmless and noncancerous.

HOW TO TREAT

GENERAL MEASURES—There is no self-treatment for keloids. Follow medical instructions for follow-up measures after treatment.

MEDICATION—Injection of corticosteroid drugs directly into the keloid. May be repeated every 3 to 4 weeks until desired degree of flattening and softening has been achieved.

ACTIVITY—No limits.

DIET—No special diet.

CALL YOUR DOCTOR IF

• You or a family member has signs of keloids.
• Keloids recur after treatment.

ILLNESS & DISORDERS

KERATITIS

GENERAL INFORMATION

DEFINITION—A term used to describe a variety of conditions where there is inflammation, infection, or irritation of the cornea.

BODY PARTS INVOLVED—The cornea is the clear membrane on the front of the eye that covers the iris and the pupil.

SEX OR AGE MOST AFFECTED—Both sexes; all ages.

SIGNS & SYMPTOMS
* Symptoms may be mild to severe.
* Eye pain.
* Redness and itching of the eye.
* Feeling that there is something in the eye.
* Photophobia (sensitivity to light).
* Tearing or discharge of the eye.
* Blurry vision.

CAUSES—There are many causes and types of keratitis. In a lot of cases, an injury to the cornea has allowed an infection to occur. Prompt treatment is important.

RISK INCREASES WITH
* Viral, bacterial, or fungal infection. The most common is the same virus that causes cold sores.
* Drying of the eye, caused by an eyelid disorder or insufficient tear formation.
* Foreign object in the eye.
* Intense light, such as from welding arcs or the reflection of intense sunlight from snow or water. Symptoms may not appear for 24 hours after exposure.
* Vitamin A deficiency (rare in normal diet).
* Allergy or sensitivity to eye cosmetics, air pollution, airborne particles (pollen, dust, mold, or yeasts), and other allergens.

HOW TO PREVENT
* Wear protective glasses or goggles if work or sports activity involves eye hazards.
* Eat a well-balanced diet that contains sufficient vitamin A, or take a multiple-vitamin containing vitamin A.
* For dry-eyes, use eye drops recommended by your health care provider.
* Don't share eye makeup.
* Avoid rubbing the eyes when you have cold sores.
* Follow instructions provided with contact lenses for cleaning and length of wearing time.

WHAT TO EXPECT

DIAGNOSTIC MEASURES
* Your own observation of symptoms.
* A special eye exam can diagnose keratitis.
* A vision test and other medical tests may be done.
* You may be referred to an eye care provider (ophthalmologist).

APPROPRIATE HEALTH CARE
* Treatment usually involves eye medication.
* Surgery to replace the cornea (severe cases only).

POSSIBLE COMPLICATIONS
* Glaucoma.
* Ulceration of the cornea.
* Permanent scarring in the eye.
* Vision loss.

PROBABLE OUTCOME—Depends on the cause. With early treatment, most types of keratitis are curable. It may take several months.

HOW TO TREAT

GENERAL MEASURES—Cool compresses applied to the closed eye may help.

MEDICATION
* Antibiotic, antifungal, or antiviral eyedrops or ointments are prescribed depending on the infection.
* Steroid eyedrops may be prescribed.
* Don't treat any eye inflammation without medical advice. Don't use nonprescription eyedrops containing topical corticosteroids. These may worsen the condition or cause eyeball perforation.

ACTIVITY—No limits.

DIET—No special diet.

CALL YOUR DOCTOR IF

* You or a family member has symptoms of keratitis. Get treatment right away.
* Your vision changes in any way.

KERATOSES, SEBORRHEIC

 GENERAL INFORMATION

DEFINITION—Growths on the outer layer of the skin. They are not related to skin cancer.

BODY PARTS INVOLVED—They may involve the chest, back, face, and/or arms.

SEX OR AGE MOST AFFECTED—Adults of both sexes. By age 60, almost everyone has a few seborrheic keratoses.

SIGNS & SYMPTOMS
• Growths are raised, thick bumps. They are flat-topped with well-defined borders.
• Newer growths are relatively flat and light brown. Older ones are dark brown or black.
• Growths are wider than tall. They appear "stuck on."
• They may itch or bleed if they get irritated. They do not cause any pain.
• There may be only I or 2 growths, or there may be as many as 100.

CAUSES—Unknown. They are not caused by sunlight. They can not be spread from one person to another.

RISK INCREASES WITH
• Aging.
• Family history of the disorder.

HOW TO PREVENT—No specific preventive measures.

 WHAT TO EXPECT

DIAGNOSTIC MEASURES
• Your own observation of symptoms.
• If you are concerned, see your health care provider. The growths can be diagnosed with a skin exam.
• In some cases, a growth may be removed for viewing under a microscope to confirm the diagnosis

APPROPRIATE HEALTH CARE
• Usually, no treatment is needed.
• The growths can be removed if they are unsightly, are irritated by clothing, or cause problems with shaving. Removal methods include cryosurgery (freezing), chemocautery, light electrosurgery, or shave biopsy. Your health care provider will discuss the treatment options with you.
• Seborrheic keratoses on the eyelid borders may require special treatment.

POSSIBLE COMPLICATIONS—None expected.

PROBABLE OUTCOME—The number of growths usually increases with age. Each growth is permanent unless removed. Seborrheic keratoses are harmless and require no treatment. People may want them removed (especially if they are unsightly or irritated by clothing).

 HOW TO TREAT

GENERAL MEASURES—After removal, a blister (sometimes with blood) will develop at the treatment site. The top of the blister will come off spontaneously in about 2 weeks. You should have little or no scarring. Wash and use makeup or cosmetics as usual. If clothing irritates the blister, cover it with a small adhesive bandage.

MEDICATION—Drugs are usually not needed for this disorder.

ACTIVITY—No limits.

DIET—No special diet.

 CALL YOUR DOCTOR IF

• You or a family member has symptoms of seborrheic keratoses and are concerned.
• You want unsightly seborrheic keratoses removed.
• Treated areas become infected (sore, red, feels warm).

ILLNESS & DISORDERS

KERATOSIS, ACTINIC

GENERAL INFORMATION

DEFINITION—An area of sun-damaged skin. Actinic keratosis can be a problem for people who spend a lot of time in the sun. It is the most common sun-related skin growth. It is considered a precancerous condition.

BODY PARTS INVOLVED—Skin of exposed areas, especially the scalp, face, ears, lips, arms and hands.

SEX OR AGE MOST AFFECTED—Adults of both sexes.

SIGNS & SYMPTOMS
- Sharply outlined, scaly, or crusted areas on exposed areas of skin.
- There may be single or multiple areas (patches).
- May be red, brown, or skin colored; flat or elevated.
- The patches are usually painless, but may sometimes itch.

CAUSES
- Prolonged exposure to the sun's radiation is the most common cause. It may develop years after the person's most intense sun exposure.
- Exposure to tanning devices, or rarely, to x-rays or certain industrial chemicals may be a cause.

RISK INCREASES WITH
- Outdoor athletic activities and sports.
- Outdoor occupations, such as farming.
- Light (fair) complexion and blue, gray, or green eyes.
- Weak immune system due to illness or drugs.

HOW TO PREVENT
- Protect yourself against direct sun exposure. When outdoors, wear a hat and protective clothing. Use sunscreen lotions and creams with SPF ratings of 15 or more. Avoid sun between 10 AM and 4 PM if possible.
- Do skin self-exams on a regular basis (each month).

WHAT TO EXPECT

DIAGNOSTIC MEASURES
- Your own observation of symptoms.
- Your health care provider can diagnose the condition by an exam of the skin.
- Medical tests are usually not needed.

APPROPRIATE HEALTH CARE
- Several treatment options are available. Your health care provider will discuss which one will work best for you, depending on the extent of the condition, your health, and your age.
- Cryosurgery (the most common treatment) is the application of liquid nitrogen to the skin.
- Curettage is the scraping away of the lesions with a sharp instrument.
- Excisional (cutting) surgery removes the lesions.
- Laser surgery may be used to destroy the cells.
- Dermabrasion is a treatment where the top layers of the skin are ground away.
- Photodynamic therapy. Medicine is applied to the affected skin, and then it is exposed to a special light.
- Chemical peels may be used for facial lesions.

POSSIBLE COMPLICATIONS
- Skin damage.
- Some risk of skin cancer if untreated. This is usually squamous cell carcinoma, which is curable when treated early.

PROBABLE OUTCOME—There are several types of effective treatment, and outcome is usually excellent. New outbreaks do sometimes occur following treatment.

HOW TO TREAT

GENERAL MEASURES—After diagnosis:
- Minimize direct sun exposure.
- See your doctor for checkups every 6 months to ensure early detection and treatment of skin cancers.

MEDICATION
- Applications of 5-fluorouracil or masoprocol to the affected area may be used for a large affected area. These can cause irritation or an allergic reaction.
- Vitamin A and other drugs are being studied.

ACTIVITY—No limits.

DIET—No special diet.

CALL YOUR DOCTOR IF

You or a family member has signs of an actinic keratosis. Even though this causes no symptoms, it can be a risk for cancer.

KERATOSIS PILARIS

GENERAL INFORMATION

DEFINITION—A common skin disorder in which the openings of the hair follicles become filled with hard plugs.

BODY PARTS INVOLVED—Skin on the backs of upper arms, fronts of thighs or buttocks.

SEX OR AGE MOST AFFECTED—It may start in childhood, around age 2 or 3, affects many teenagers, and some adults.

SIGNS & SYMPTOMS
- Skin bumps that are small, firm, and skin-color or pink, or sometimes red. They have a dry "sandpaper" or "goosebumps" texture.
- They are located at the openings of hair follicles.
- The condition is usually worse in winter months when a person's skin is dryer.
- Bumps usually don't itch and they do not cause pain.

CAUSES—Unknown. It does run in families. It often occurs along with other skin disorders such as ichthyosis (an inherited dry skin condition). The condition cannot be spread from one person to another.

RISK INCREASES WITH
- Family history of keratosis pilaris.
- Ichthyosis (dry and scaly skin disorder).

HOW TO PREVENT—Cannot be prevented at present.

WHAT TO EXPECT

DIAGNOSTIC MEASURES
- Your own observation of symptoms.
- If you are concerned about the skin rash, see your health care provider. The condition can be diagnosed by an exam of the affected area.

APPROPRIATE HEALTH CARE—Usually, no treatment is needed, but self-care measures may help the appearance.

POSSIBLE COMPLICATIONS—Complications are unlikely. A skin infection may occur if the affected area is scratched or overly treated with abrasive methods.

PROBABLE OUTCOME—Keratosis pilaris is a chronic, harmless skin problem with no permanent cure. The bumps may come and go over a period of time. Many cases clear up on their own as a person gets older. Cosmetic appearance and rough skin texture are often bothersome to patients.

HOW TO TREAT

GENERAL MEASURES
- Use mild, unscented soap when bathing.
- Apply lubricating ointments or creams to the affected areas 2 or 3 times a day. The most useful time is immediately after bathing to help the skin retain moisture. There is no advantage to using expensive skin products or vitamin creams.
- Go over the affected skin area with a pumice stone, loofah sponge, or washcloth to gently loosen the plugs.

MEDICATION—Drugs are usually not needed for this condition. Your health care provider may prescribe a product to be applied to the skin if the condition is more severe.

ACTIVITY—No limits.

DIET—No special diet.

CALL YOUR DOCTOR IF

- You or a family member has signs of keratosis pilaris and are concerned about them.
- Appearance of the affected area changes. There may be a skin infection.

KIDNEY INFECTION, ACUTE
(Pyelonephritis, Acute)

GENERAL INFORMATION

DEFINITION—Infection and inflammation of one (sometimes both) kidneys. Kidneys filter waste matter from the blood and produce urine.

BODY PARTS INVOLVED—Kidneys; urinary tract.

SEX OR AGE MOST AFFECTED—Both sexes, but more common in females of all ages.

SIGNS & SYMPTOMS
* Symptoms often come on suddenly.
* Fever and shaking chills.
* Burning, frequent urination.
* Cloudy urine or blood in the urine.
* Aching (may be severe) in one or both sides of the lower back.
* Pain in the abdomen.
* Fatigue.
* Nausea and vomiting.

CAUSES—Most often, a bacteria called *Escherichia coli*. The infection begins in the bladder (cystitis) and the infected urine moves back up the tubes (ureters) that connect the bladder to the kidneys. This is called reflux.

RISK INCREASES WITH
* Sexual activity in women. Bacteria enters the urethra (tube from bladder to outside) and bladder.
* Blockage or abnormality of the urinary system. This can be caused by stones, obstructions, nerve diseases, tumors, or congenital (being born with) deformity.
* Prostatitis (prostate inflammation).
* Catheters, tubes, or certain surgical procedures.
* Diabetes.
* Chronic bladder infection or tumor.
* Spinal-cord injury or tumor.
* Pregnancy.
* Bubble bath use in young girls.

HOW TO PREVENT
* Women and girls should wipe from front to back (not back to front) after bathroom use.
* Avoid sitting around in wet clothing (such as wet swimsuits).
* Urinate within 15 minutes after sexual intercourse.
* Don't hold urine. If you have the urge to void, do so.
* Drink plenty of fluids every day.

WHAT TO EXPECT

DIAGNOSTIC MEASURES
* Your own observation of symptoms.

* Your health care provider will do a physical exam along with a pelvic exam in females and a rectal exam (for prostate problems) in males. Questions will be asked about your symptoms.
* Medical tests may include urinalysis, urine culture, and blood studies. Other tests may be done to diagnose kidney stones or obstructions.

APPROPRIATE HEALTH CARE
* Treatment usually involves antibiotic drugs, or, in some cases surgery or hospital care.
* Surgery may be needed for an obstruction or kidney stones, or for an abnormality diagnosed in a child.
* Hospital care (possibly) for severe symptoms or for people with other medical disorders.

POSSIBLE COMPLICATIONS
* Chronic kidney infection.
* Scarring of kidneys and permanent kidney damage.
* Blood infection.
* Hypertension (high blood pressure).

PROBABLE OUTCOME—With early diagnosis and treatment, an uncomplicated kidney infection is usually curable in 10 to 14 days.

HOW TO TREAT

GENERAL MEASURES
* Be sure to see your health care provider for follow-up tests to verify the infection is cured.
* To learn more: National Kidney & Urologic Diseases information Clearinghouse, 3 information Way, Bethesda, MD 20892, (800) 891-5390; website: www.kidney.niddk.nih.gov.

MEDICATION
* Oral antibiotics. Take all the antibiotics prescribed, even if symptoms clear up.
* Antibiotics intravenous or by injection, if oral antibiotics don't cure the infection.
* Take nonprescription drugs such as ibuprofen for pain symptoms.
* Urinary analgesics to relieve pain may be prescribed.

ACTIVITY—Extra rest. Resume sexual relations when advised by your health care provider.

DIET—No special diet. Drink plenty of fluids. Drinking cranberry juice may be recommended.

CALL YOUR DOCTOR IF

* You or a family member has symptoms of a kidney infection.
* Symptoms and fever persist after 48 hours of antibiotic treatment. A different antibiotic may be needed.
* Symptoms return after treatment is completed.

KIDNEY INFECTION, CHRONIC
(Pyelonephritis, Chronic)

GENERAL INFORMATION

DEFINITION—Infection and inflammation of the kidneys that develops slowly and lasts for months or years. It leads to scarring and eventual loss of kidney function. Kidneys filter waste material from the blood and produce urine.

BODY PARTS INVOLVED—Kidneys.

SEX OR AGE MOST AFFECTED—Adults of both sexes, but more common in women.

SIGNS & SYMPTOMS—Usually there are no signs or symptoms, unlike acute kidney infection. The following symptoms occur if chronic kidney failure develops:
- Anemia (paleness and fatigue).
- Weakness.
- Loss of appetite, nausea.
- High blood pressure and buildup of fluid in the body.
- Pain in one or both sides of the lower back.
- Blood in the urine.
- Numbness and tingling of the hands and feet.

CAUSES—The kidneys have been scarred or damaged by a variety of diseases. They begin to lose their ability to function as they normally would in removing waste products from the blood.

RISK INCREASES WITH
- Frequent, acute, bacterial kidney infections.
- Untreated lower urinary-tract infections.
- Diabetes.
- Urinary obstruction, such as stones or tumors.
- Long-term use of catheters.

HOW TO PREVENT—In many cases, there are no preventive measures. Controlling diabetes and getting treatment for urinary-tract infections can help reduce risks.

WHAT TO EXPECT

DIAGNOSTIC MEASURES
- Your health care provider will do a physical exam.
- Medical tests include urine studies and urine culture. X-ray, ultrasound, and cystoscopy (use of a tube with a camera on the end to see inside the urinary tract) may be done.

APPROPRIATE HEALTH CARE
- Treatment may include drugs, surgery, dialysis, and kidney transplant. Follow your treatment plan carefully. This may not be easy for an illness that causes few symptoms in the early stages.
- Surgery may be needed to relieve obstruction or correct any structural problem in the urinary tract.
- If chronic kidney failure develops, a kidney transplant or kidney dialysis can be lifesaving.

POSSIBLE COMPLICATIONS—Chronic kidney failure, which can be fatal.

PROBABLE OUTCOME—There is no cure. The disease progresses until dialysis or kidney transplant is required. If symptoms occur, they may be relieved with treatment.

HOW TO TREAT

GENERAL MEASURES
- Follow your treatment plan carefully. This may not be easy for an illness that causes few symptoms in the early stages.
- To learn more: National Kidney & Urologic Diseases information Clearinghouse, 3 information Way, Bethesda, MD 20892, (800) 891-5390; website: www.kidney.niddk.nih.gov.

MEDICATION
- Antibiotics may be prescribed. They are usually taken for months or years.
- Drugs to keep the urine slightly acidic may be prescribed.

ACTIVITY—No limits.

DIET—No special diet. Drink plenty of fluids each day. Drink cranberry juice to acidify the urine.

CALL YOUR DOCTOR IF

- You or a family member has symptoms of chronic kidney infection.
- You or a family member has symptoms of an acute kidney infection, such as urgent, frequent, or burning urination; fever and chills; fatigue; and cloudy urine.

KIDNEY, POLYCYSTIC

GENERAL INFORMATION

DEFINITION—An inherited kidney disorder in which cysts develop in the kidneys. The cysts replace normal kidney tissue and reduce kidney function. Most people show no symptoms until adulthood. Then symptoms progress slowly for up to 20 years. It is a common hereditary disease in the United States.

BODY PARTS INVOLVED—Kidneys.

SEX OR AGE MOST AFFECTED—Both sexes; all ages.

SIGNS & SYMPTOMS
Early stages:
• Blood in the urine that may be visible only by microscope exam.
• Repeated kidney infections.
• A mass in the abdomen.
• High blood pressure.
• No symptoms (often) until the cysts replace so much normal kidney structure that kidney failure occurs.
Symptoms of kidney failure:
• Pain in the lower back.
• Frequent urination.
• Increasing fatigue and weakness.
• Headache.
• Bad breath.
• Nausea, vomiting, or diarrhea.
• Fluid build-up (swelling around the ankles or eyes).
• Shortness of breath.
• Chest pain.
• Itching skin.
• Menstruation stops in women of childbearing age.

CAUSES—This disease is inherited; the cause is unknown.

RISK INCREASES WITH—Family history of polycystic kidney disease.

HOW TO PREVENT—Cannot be prevented at present. If polycystic kidney disease runs in your family, get medical advice about tests to discover if you have kidney cysts. Even if you feel well and don't have the disease, get regular checkups. If you have a family history of polycystic kidney, seek genetic counseling before starting a family.

WHAT TO EXPECT

DIAGNOSTIC MEASURES
• Your health care provider will do a physical exam and ask questions about your family medical history.
• Medical tests may include blood studies, CT scan, ultrasound, and others.

APPROPRIATE HEALTH CARE
• There is no specific treatment for the disorder. Treatment is aimed at preventing complications or treating them if they occur.
• Surgical procedures may be needed if kidney cysts rupture, large cysts cause pain, or if cysts in the liver cause problems.
• If kidney failure develops, dialysis or surgery to perform a kidney transplant may be recommended.

POSSIBLE COMPLICATIONS
• Kidney failure and end-stage renal disease (ESRD).
• High blood pressure.
• Aneurysms (ballooning of weak places in arteries).
• Infection or rupture of cysts.
• Cysts in the liver and other organs.

PROBABLE OUTCOME—There is no cure for polycystic kidney disease. Medical care may slow the progressive kidney damage by treating complications as they arise.

HOW TO TREAT

GENERAL MEASURES
• Check your blood pressure each day and keep a record.
• Prompt treatment of any infection is important.
• To learn more: National Kidney & Urologic Diseases information Clearinghouse, 3 information Way, Bethesda, MD 20892, (800) 891-5390; website: www.kidney.niddk.nih.gov.

MEDICATION
• Antibiotics for infection or antihypertensives to control high blood pressure may be prescribed.
• Most drugs are excreted by the kidney. If you have chronic kidney failure and take prescription drugs, the dose may need adjustment because of this disorder.
• Vitamins and supplements may be recommended.

ACTIVITY
• Take short, frequent rest periods during the day. Otherwise, stay as active as your strength allows.
• Avoid contact sports to reduce any risk of injury to the kidneys.

DIET—Usually, no special diet. A low-salt diet may be recommended if high blood pressure or kidney failure develops. Drink plenty of fluids.

CALL YOUR DOCTOR IF

• You or a family member has symptoms of polycystic kidney.
• You have symptoms of kidney failure, signs of infection, urination decreases, or blood appears in urine.

KIDNEY STONES
(Renal Calculi; Urinary Calculi)

 GENERAL INFORMATION

DEFINITION—Small, solid particles that form in one or both kidneys. They sometimes travel into the ureter (slender muscular tubes that carry urine from the kidneys to the urinary bladder). Stones vary from the size of a grain of sand to a golf ball, and there may be one or several.

BODY PARTS INVOLVED—Kidneys.

SEX OR AGE MOST AFFECTED—They usually affect adults of both sexes over age 30, but they occur more often in men.

SIGNS & SYMPTOMS
• Episodes of severe, off and on pain every few minutes. The pain usually appears first in the back, just below the ribs. Over several hours or days, the pain follows the stone's course through the ureter toward the groin. Pain stops when the stone passes.
• Frequent nausea.
• Cloudy or dark urine or blood in urine.

CAUSES—Stones are made up of crystals that form in the urine. Normally, the urine contains chemicals that stop crystals from forming. These chemicals do not seem to work for everyone, and some people form stones. Why this occurs is unknown. Kidney stones contain various chemicals. They may be made up of calcium (most common), struvite, uric acid, or cystine.

RISK INCREASES WITH
• Family history of kidney stones.
• Hyperparathyroidism (excess parathyroid hormone).
• Urinary-tract infections (UTI) or blockage.
• Gout (uric-acid stones).
• Kidney disorders.
• Certain inherited disorders.
• Excess vitamin C or D intake.
• Drugs such as diuretics (water pills), calcium-based antacids, or protease inhibitors (used for AIDS).
• Chronic bowel inflammation or bowel surgery.
• Bed rest for a long period of time.
• Too little fluid intake.

HOW TO PREVENT—No specific measures to prevent a first kidney stone. If you have had one kidney stone, you are more likely to have another and should take preventive measures. These will depend on the type of stone formed.

 WHAT TO EXPECT

DIAGNOSTIC MEASURES
• Your health care provider will do a physical exam and ask about your symptoms and activities.

• Medical tests may include urinalysis, urine culture, x-rays, and other tests to confirm the diagnosis.

APPROPRIATE HEALTH CARE
• Small stones may need no specific treatment. They usually pass within 72 hours. Strain all urine and save the stone for analysis of type of stone.
• Treatment may be done to remove larger stones if they don't pass on their own and are causing complications, infection, or severe pain. Options include chemical dissolution, endourologic stone extraction, percutaneous nephrolithotomy, extracorporeal shock wave lithotripsy, and rarely, open surgery. Other, new approaches are being studied. Your health care provider will discuss the options with you.
• Stones due to excess calcium in the body may require surgical removal of abnormal parathyroid tissue.

POSSIBLE COMPLICATIONS
• Urinary-tract infection.
• Kidney damage or scarring.
• Kidney function may be lost or reduced.

PROBABLE OUTCOME—Most kidney stones will pass out of the body on their own. Stones that cause symptoms or complications can be treated successfully. Stones often recur.

 HOW TO TREAT

GENERAL MEASURES—To learn more: National Kidney & Urologic Diseases information Clearinghouse, 3 information Way, Bethesda, MD 20892, (800) 891-5390; website: www.kidney.niddk.nih.gov.

MEDICATION
• Pain relievers may be prescribed.
• Antispasmodics to relax the ureter muscles and help the stone pass may be prescribed.
• Drugs may be prescribed that will stop the growth of new or existing stones.

ACTIVITY—During a kidney-stone episode, stay as active as possible. Activity may help the stone pass.

DIET—Drink lots of fluids (water is best). Eating less red meat may be helpful. You may be advised to make other diet changes to help prevent more stones.

 CALL YOUR DOCTOR IF

• You or a family member has symptoms of a kidney stone.
• Symptoms of a kidney infection develop (stinging, burning on urination, or a frequent urge to urinate).

LABYRINTHITIS

GENERAL INFORMATION

DEFINITION—Inflammation of the labyrinth (fluid-filled canals and sacs) in the inner ear. The labyrinth contains the vestibular system, which controls a person's balance and eye movement. It also contains the cochlea, which controls hearing. Labyrinthitis may affect one or both ears.

BODY PARTS INVOLVED—Ears.

SEX OR AGE MOST AFFECTED—It can affect both sexes and all ages, including children.

SIGNS & SYMPTOMS
- Vertigo. A sensation that you or your surroundings are spinning around. Head movements make it worse.
- Hearing loss (one or both ears; may be mild or severe).
- Involuntary eye movement.
- Nausea and vomiting.
- Loss of balance (may fall toward the affected side).
- Ringing in the ear (tinnitus).
- Feeling of fullness in the ears.

CAUSES—The exact cause of the inflammation is sometimes unknown or unclear. It may result from an infection or trauma. The whole inner ear is about the size of a dime, so inflammation often affects both hearing and balance.

RISK INCREASES WITH
- Bacterial infection in the middle ear.
- Upper respiratory viral infection.
- Cholesteatoma (a type of cyst in the middle ear).
- Head injury.
- Stress or fatigue.
- Allergies or family history of allergies.
- Smoking.
- Excess alcohol use.
- Use of some prescription or nonprescription drugs.
- Heart, brain, or blood-vessel disease.

HOW TO PREVENT
- Obtain prompt medical care for ear infections.
- Don't take drugs that have caused dizziness symptoms for you in the past.

WHAT TO EXPECT

DIAGNOSTIC MEASURES
- Your own observation of symptoms.
- Your health care provider will do an exam of the ears and your eye movements. Your head and body may be placed or moved in different positions to help determine what movements bring on the symptoms. You may be asked to walk so your balance can be checked.

- Medical tests may include hearing tests and others as needed to determine any underlying disorder.

APPROPRIATE HEALTH CARE
- Treatment includes steps to treat any underlying disorder, rest, and drugs for symptoms if needed.
- Surgical removal of cholesteatoma (an infected collection of debris in the middle ear) and drainage of infected areas may be needed.

POSSIBLE COMPLICATIONS
- Injuries from falls that occur due to vertigo.
- Permanent hearing loss on the affected side (rare).

PROBABLE OUTCOME—The disorder usually resolves on its own in 1 to 6 weeks. Treatment can help relieve symptoms. Some mild vertigo symptoms may continue for several months.

HOW TO TREAT

GENERAL MEASURES—This disorder can be frightening and debilitating but complete recovery is usual.

MEDICATION—Your health care provider may prescribe:
- Antinausea drugs (oral or suppositories).
- Tranquilizers to reduce dizziness.
- Diuretics to decrease excess fluid in the inner ear.
- Antibiotics for bacterial infection.
- Antivirals for virus infection.
- Antihistamines to relieve symptoms.

ACTIVITY—Keep the head as still as possible. Rest in bed until vertigo stops. Then resume your normal activities gradually. Avoid activities, such as driving, climbing, or working around dangerous machinery until symptoms clear up.

DIET—No special diet is needed. Nausea and vomiting symptoms may make eating difficult. Drink clear liquids and eat bland foods until symptoms improve.

CALL YOUR DOCTOR IF

- You or a family member has symptoms of labyrinthitis.
- The following occur during treatment:
  - Decreased hearing in either ear.
  - Persistent vomiting.
  - Convulsions or fainting.
  - Fever of 101°F (38.3°C) or higher.
- New, unexplained symptoms develop. Drugs used in treatment may produce side effects.

LACTOSE INTOLERANCE
(Milk Intolerance; Lactase Deficiency)

 GENERAL INFORMATION

DEFINITION—Difficulty digesting cow's milk. Lactose is the primary sugar in milk. Lactose intolerance occurs in 75% of the black population, 90% of Asians or American Indians, and less than 20% of Caucasians of northwest European origin.

BODY PARTS INVOLVED—Digestive system.

SEX OR AGE MOST AFFECTED—Both sexes; all ages.

SIGNS & SYMPTOMS
• Symptoms will vary depending on the amount of lactose each person can tolerate. Symptoms occur about 30 minutes to 2 hours after eating or drinking foods that contain lactose. They may be mild to more severe.
In children:
• Foamy diarrhea with diaper rash.
• Vomiting (sometimes).
• Slow weight gain, growth, and development.
In adults:
• Rumbling stomach sounds, stomach cramps, and diarrhea.
• Gas and bloating.
• Nausea.

CAUSES
• Deficiency or absence of the enzyme lactase. Lactase is needed to digest all milk except mother's milk. Without it, sugars in milk absorb fluid and cause diarrhea. Some infants are born with the disorder, but lactose intolerance usually develops in adulthood.
• Temporary lactose intolerance can occur in an infant after a severe case of gastroenteritis (stomach flu) that irritates the intestinal lining.

RISK INCREASES WITH—Family history of enzyme-lactase deficiency.

HOW TO PREVENT—Cannot be prevented at present. If you are pregnant and there is a history of lactose intolerance in your family, consider breast-feeding your baby. If not, you may need a non-milk formula.

 WHAT TO EXPECT

DIAGNOSTIC MEASURES
• Your own observation of symptoms.
• Your health care provider may do a physical exam. A trial period of no dairy products is usually recommended to see if symptoms stop.
• Medical tests may be done. For older children or adults, a hydrogen breath test or lactose absorption test indicate whether lactose is not being absorbed in the digestive tract. A stool acidity exam may be done. It can be used for infants or young children.

APPROPRIATE HEALTH CARE—Treatment involves diet changes. Using lactase enzymes is also an option.

POSSIBLE COMPLICATIONS—Calcium deficiency and weak bones (rare).

PROBABLE OUTCOME—There is no cure for this disorder, but it does not cause a threat to good health. Symptoms can be controlled with diet changes. Symptoms may worsen at times for unknown reasons.

 HOW TO TREAT

GENERAL MEASURES—To learn more: National Digestive Diseases Clearinghouse, 2 information Way, Bethesda, MD 20892; (800) 891-5389; website: www.digestive.nddic.nih.gov.

MEDICATION
• The enzyme lactase is available without a prescription. It can be taken as a tablet or as a liquid that is added to milk and milk products. It acts in much the same way as the naturally occurring enzyme does.
• Calcium supplements may be recommended.
• Some prescription and nonprescription drugs contain lactose as an ingredient. These include some birth-control pills and antacids. They may affect people who have severe lactose intolerance.

ACTIVITY—No limits.

DIET
• If the condition is present at birth, an infant formula that contains little or no lactose, such as a soybean-based formula, will be recommended.
• If the lactose intolerance is short-term and caused by gastroenteritis, a substitute formula is needed for a short time. Cow's milk can be introduced again later.
• Older persons with lactose intolerance should reduce or restrict milk and milk products, such as cheese and ice cream. Lactose-free milk is available.
• Yogurt and fermented products such as hard cheese are often tolerated better than milk.
• Read food labels with care. Avoid products that contain milk, lactose, milk sugar, whey, curds, milk by-products, dry milk solids, and nonfat dry milk powder.

 CALL YOUR DOCTOR IF

• You or your child has symptoms of lactose intolerance.
• Infant fails to gain weight or refuses food or formula.
• Vomiting or diarrhea occurs.
• A milk-free diet doesn't relieve symptoms.

LARGE-INTESTINE CANCER
(Colon Cancer; Colorectal Cancer)

GENERAL INFORMATION

DEFINITION—Growth of cancer cells in the rectum or colon (large intestine). It may involve the large intestine, including the cecum, ascending colon, transverse colon, descending colon and sigmoid colon, and rectum.

BODY PARTS INVOLVED—Large intestine, including the cecum, ascending colon, transverse colon, descending colon and sigmoid colon; rectum (50% of all colorectal cancers occur here).

SEX OR AGE MOST AFFECTED—Both sexes; often affects adults over age 50.

SIGNS & SYMPTOMS
- No symptoms in the early stages (frequently).
- Bloody or black, tarry stools or rectal bleeding.
- Cramping stomach pain; feeling of fullness.
- Change in bowel habits, such as diarrhea, constipation, or narrow stools.
- Unexplained weight loss.
- Anemia (pale skin and fatigue).
- Loss of bowel control (sometimes).
- Pain in the rectum (sometimes).

CAUSES—Exact cause is unknown. Genetic and environmental factors may contribute. There are known risk factors.

RISK INCREASES WITH
- Family history of colorectal cancer or colon polyps.
- Inherited genetic abnormality. Two types are familial adenomatous polyposis (FAP) including an attenuated form (AFAP), and hereditary nonpolyposis colorectal cancer (HNPCC).
- Inflammatory bowel disease (ulcerative colitis).
- Intestinal polyps (benign growths).
- Previous colorectal cancer.
- Age over 50.
- Diabetes.
- Diet high in fat and meat (both red and white).
- Obesity.
- Sedentary (not physically active) lifestyle.
- Smoking and alcohol use.

HOW TO PREVENT
- To reduce risk: Exercise daily; eat a low-fat, high-fiber diet; control weight; don't smoke; and limit alcohol.
- Colon cancer screening tests for adults over age 50 and adults over age 40 (or younger) with risk factors.
- Genetic tests for family members at risk.
- Precancerous conditions should be treated.
- Vitamins, calcium, folic acid, nonsteroidal anti-inflammatory drugs, or female hormones may be recommended for some patients as possible preventive therapies.

WHAT TO EXPECT

DIAGNOSTIC MEASURES
- Your health care provider will do a physical exam and ask questions about your symptoms.
- A number of medical tests will be done. The tests help diagnose the cancer and then determine if it has spread (staging).

APPROPRIATE HEALTH CARE
- Treatment varies and depends on location and size of tumor, any spread of the cancer, your health, age, and preferences. Treatment may include surgery, anticancer drugs (chemotherapy) and/or radiation therapy, and biologic therapy.
- Chemotherapy uses drugs and radiation therapy uses radiation to attack the cancer cells. Biologic therapy uses the body's immune system to fight cancer.
- The goal of surgery is to remove as much of the cancer as possible. Part, or all, of the colon, rectum, and nearby organs may be removed. A colostomy to collect stool or an urostomy to collect urine may be needed to help the body get rid of these wastes.
- Treatment may involve steps to relieve symptoms and make you comfortable, rather than treating the cancer.
- Counseling may help you cope.

POSSIBLE COMPLICATIONS
- Spread to other body parts. This can be fatal.
- Complications may occur due to treatments.

PROBABLE OUTCOME—Outlook varies. The earlier the cancer is diagnosed and treated, the greater the chances for recovery.

HOW TO TREAT

GENERAL MEASURES—To learn more: American Cancer Society, (800) ACS-2345; website: www.cancer.org; or National Cancer Institute, (800) 4-CANCER; website: www.nci.nih.gov.

MEDICATION—You may be prescribed anticancer drugs (chemotherapy), drugs to stimulate the immune system (biologics), and pain relievers.

ACTIVITY—You will be advised when to resume normal activities.

DIET— Eat a low-fat, high-fiber diet.

CALL YOUR DOCTOR IF

- You or a family member has symptoms of cancer of the large intestine.
- New symptoms occur during treatment.

LARGE-INTESTINE POLYP

GENERAL INFORMATION

DEFINITION—A growth that occurs on the lining of the colon or rectum. A polyp may grow with or without a stalk. Polyps occur singly or in groups. They are a health concern, because most colon cancers arise from polyps.

BODY PARTS INVOLVED—Large intestine, most often in the rectum and sigmoid colon.

SEX OR AGE MOST AFFECTED—Adults of both sexes. Polyps occur more often as people age.

SIGNS & SYMPTOMS
* No symptoms (usually).
* Rectal bleeding (sometimes).
* Mucous discharge from the rectum (sometimes).
* Cramps or stomach pain.

CAUSES—Unknown.

RISK INCREASES WITH
* Family history of intestinal polyps.
* Polyposis syndromes. These are genetic abnormalities that are passed down in families. Some syndromes may cause large numbers of polyps in the colon (such as familial adenomatous polyposis [FAP]).

HOW TO PREVENT
* No specific measures to prevent polyps.
* If you have had polyps in the past, you should have regular follow-up exams.
* Patients with a family history of polyps, colon cancer, or polyposis syndromes should have polyp screening tests starting at a young age, or as recommended.
* All adults starting at age 50 should have colon cancer screening tests.

WHAT TO EXPECT

DIAGNOSTIC MEASURES
* Your own observation of symptoms.
* Your health care provider will do a physical exam and a digital rectal exam (a gloved, lubricated finger is inserted into the rectum).
* Medical tests may include blood studies, stool studies, barium x-ray, or virtual colonoscopy (CT scan of the colon). A sigmoidoscopy (exam of rectum and lower end of the colon) or conventional colonoscopy (exam of entire length of colon) may be done. Both of these tests use a lighted tube with a camera on the end to see inside the body. A biopsy is done during a colonoscopy. This involves removal of a small amount of tissue for viewing under a microscope.

APPROPRIATE HEALTH CARE
* Treatment to remove polyps is usually recommended.
* Polyps can be removed during the colonoscopy procedure. Polyps are snipped off or destroyed by electric cauterization. If the removed polyp is diagnosed as cancer, this may be all the treatment that is needed.
* Surgery (laparotomy) is performed to remove some types of polyps. This is done through an incision made in the abdomen. Part of the colon may be removed and then the two cut ends are rejoined.

POSSIBLE COMPLICATIONS—Risk of colorectal cancer. It develops slowly over several years.

PROBABLE OUTCOME—Usually curable with treatment. Most polyps are benign (noncancerous). Polyps may recur after treatment.

HOW TO TREAT

GENERAL MEASURES—Follow medical instructions for self-care after any surgical procedure.

MEDICATION—Drugs are not usually needed for this disorder. Nonsteroidal anti-inflammatory drugs and others are being researched to see if they decrease the number and size of polyps.

ACTIVITY—No limits.

DIET—No special diet (unless advised otherwise).

CALL YOUR DOCTOR IF

* You or a family member has bleeding or mucous discharge from the rectum.
* Other members of your family have polyps or colorectal cancer. You should have regular exams.
* The following occur after surgery:
  - Increased rectal bleeding.
  - Fever, chills, or aches. This may indicate an infection.

LARVA MIGRANS, CUTANEOUS
(Creeping Eruptions)

 GENERAL INFORMATION

DEFINITION—A skin infection caused by hookworms. Hookworms are parasites that infest animals, particularly dogs and cats. Humans pick up the infection by coming in contact with sand or soil where an infected animal has passed feces. It is more common in warm, humid areas, such as the southeastern United States.

BODY PARTS INVOLVED—Skin areas that come in contact with the ground, usually feet, legs or buttocks.

SEX OR AGE MOST AFFECTED—Both sexes; all ages.

SIGNS & SYMPTOMS—First, there may be a tingling or prickling of the skin area. Then it begins to itch. This is followed by a rash or small blisters on the skin. They often form thin, raised tracks (or lines) on the skin leading from the parasite's entry point. The tracks can get longer each day. There are usually several tracks at the same time, each of different length and pattern.

CAUSES—An animal that has hookworms leaves feces on the ground that contains the hookworm eggs. The eggs hatch into larvae that infest the soil around the droppings. When a human comes in contact with the soil, the larvae are able to penetrate the skin and cause the symptoms. The infection cannot be spread from one person to another.

RISK INCREASES WITH
• Working or playing in warm, moist sand in which cats or dogs have defecated. They can be found in a child's sandbox.
• Walking barefoot in sand or dirt.
• Work that requires crawling in confined spaces and contact with infected soil (e.g., plumbers working under houses).

HOW TO PREVENT
• Handle cat litter carefully. Avoid touching soil.
• Don't work or play in soil used by cats and dogs for elimination.
• Have pets treated for worms.

 WHAT TO EXPECT

DIAGNOSTIC MEASURES
• Your own observation of symptoms.
• Your health care provider can usually diagnose the problem by an exam of the affected skin area.
• Other medical tests may be done to confirm the diagnosis.

APPROPRIATE HEALTH CARE
• Self-care is usually all that is needed.
• Medical care may involve drug therapy.

POSSIBLE COMPLICATIONS—If the blisters are scratched and opened, a bacterial infection may occur.

PROBABLE OUTCOME—The outcome is good. The infection may heal on its own over several weeks or months. Treatment with drugs can hasten the healing process.

 HOW TO TREAT

GENERAL MEASURES—Apply cool, moist compresses to the affected area to help relieve itching.

MEDICATION—Your health care provider may prescribe an anti-parasitic drug to be applied to the skin, or taken by mouth (if the infection is more severe).

ACTIVITY—No limits.

DIET—No special diet.

 CALL YOUR DOCTOR IF

• You or a family member has symptoms of larva migrans.
• Skin symptoms become worse or there are new symptoms.
• You take an oral anti-parasitic drug, and new, unexplained symptoms develop.

LARYNGITIS

GENERAL INFORMATION

DEFINITION—A minor inflammation of the larynx (voice box) and surrounding tissues. Inflammation causes swelling and pain and is a reaction to injury, infection or irritation. The disorder is common and occurs more often in late fall, winter, and early spring.

BODY PARTS INVOLVED—Larynx (voice box); the upper part of the neck, behind the Adam's apple.

SEX OR AGE MOST AFFECTED—Both sexes; all ages.

SIGNS & SYMPTOMS
* Hoarseness, weak voice, or loss of voice.
* Sore throat; tickling in the back of the throat.
* Feeling like you have a lump in your throat.
* Slight fever (sometimes).
* Swallowing difficulty (rare).

CAUSES—There are a variety of risk factors that can lead to the inflammation of the larynx. The most common is a viral infection.

RISK INCREASES WITH
* Viral infection from a recent cold or flu-like illness.
* Excessive use of the voice (such as singers, politicians, cheerleaders, or young children who cry or yell strenuously).
* Exposure to irritants such as mold, pollen and pollutants, or irritating chemicals.
* Allergies.
* Smoking or being around second-hand smoke.
* Gastroesophageal reflux disease (GERD).
* Rarely, it may be a bacterial infection, or be caused by disorders such as tuberculosis, syphilis, fungal infection, or tumor.

HOW TO PREVENT
* Most cases are caused by a virus. Taking steps to prevent viral infections such as hand washing may help.
* Take care to not overuse the voice.

WHAT TO EXPECT

DIAGNOSTIC MEASURES
* Your own observation of symptoms.
* If symptoms persist, are severe, or cause concern, see your health care provider. An exam of the throat, ears and nose, can usually confirm the diagnosis.
* Medical tests are normally not needed.

APPROPRIATE HEALTH CARE—Home care is the main form of treatment.

POSSIBLE COMPLICATIONS—Chronic hoarseness.

PROBABLE OUTCOME—Laryngitis usually clears up on its own in 10 to 14 days.

HOW TO TREAT

GENERAL MEASURES
* Avoid using your voice as much as possible. Don't whisper (it can irritate the throat). Write notes to communicate. For most cases, resting the voice for a few days is all that is needed.
* Suck on throat lozenges, cough drops, or hard candy.
* To help relieve minor pain, gargle often with double-strength tea or warm salt water (one-half teaspoon of salt to 8 oz. of water).
* Hot, steamy showers also help.
* Avoid smoking and second-hand cigarette smoke.

MEDICATION—For minor discomfort, you may use nonprescription drugs, such as acetaminophen or ibuprofen.

ACTIVITY—Usually no limits.

DIET—No special diet. Increased fluid intake may be helpful.

CALL YOUR DOCTOR IF

* You or a family member has hoarseness or other symptoms of laryngitis that last longer than 2 weeks.
* You feel very ill, are vomiting, have a high fever, or difficulty breathing. If these symptoms develop in a child, call immediately.

ILLNESS & DISORDERS

LARYNX CANCER
(Laryngeal Cancer)

 GENERAL INFORMATION

DEFINITION—Growth of malignant cells in the larynx (voice box). The larynx plays a role in helping a person breathe, swallow, and talk.

BODY PARTS INVOLVED—The larynx is about 2 inches long and 2 inches wide and located at the back of the throat.

SEX OR AGE MOST AFFECTED—Both sexes of adults over age 40 (more common in men).

SIGNS & SYMPTOMS
* Few or no symptoms in early stages.
* Hoarseness, scratchy, or weak voice.
* "Lump-in-the-throat" feeling.
* Painful or difficult swallowing.
* Trouble breathing.
* Hard, swollen lymph glands in the neck.
* Weight loss.
* Ear pain.
* Chronic cough.

CAUSES—Exact cause is unknown. Smoking or alcohol abuse are known major risk factors.

RISK INCREASES WITH
* Smoking.
* Excess alcohol use.
* Age over 55. Men more than women.
* African-Americans more than whites.
* Having had head or neck cancer.
* Exposure to certain chemicals, toxins, or asbestos.
* Gastroesophageal reflux disease (GERD).

HOW TO PREVENT
* Don't smoke. Don't drink more than 1 or 2 alcoholic drinks, if any, a day.
* Avoid exposure to known toxins.

 WHAT TO EXPECT

DIAGNOSTIC MEASURES
* Your own observation of symptoms. Be alert to hoarseness that persists beyond 2 weeks.
* Your health care provider will do a physical exam and ask questions about your symptoms.
* A variety of medical tests will be done to verify the exact type of cancer cells, the grade (fast or slow growing), and if the cancer has spread (called staging) to other places in the body.

APPROPRIATE HEALTH CARE
* Treatment will depend on the cancer type, grade and location, its stage, your health, age, and preferences. Preserving a good voice quality is a goal of treatment. Your health care provider will discuss your specific diagnosis and treatment recommendations with you.
* Surgery, radiation, and/or chemotherapy (anticancer drugs) are the usual treatment

steps. Other treatments being studied include photodynamic therapy (drugs plus light), biologic therapy (using the immune system to fight the cancer), or gene therapy.
* Advanced cancer often requires surgery. Part or all of the larynx may be removed (laryngectomy). A tracheostomy is performed. This is an opening (stoma) in the throat for breathing. It may be temporary or permanent. A "trach" tube or stoma button keeps it open.
* After larynx removal, therapy will help patients learn to breathe, swallow, eat, and talk. Talking will involve learning esophageal speech or use of a mechanical device.

POSSIBLE COMPLICATIONS
* Complications may arise from treatments (chemotherapy, radiation, and surgery) and affect voice, breathing, swallowing, and eating.
* Spread of cancer in the body; it can be fatal.
* Cancer may recur after treatment.

PROBABLE OUTCOME—Early diagnosis and treatment has the best outcome. Late diagnosis or spread of cancer has poorer outlook.

 HOW TO TREAT

GENERAL MEASURES
* Stop smoking. Find a way to quit that works.
* Use good mouth care on teeth and gums.
* Consider joining a cancer support group.
* To learn more: American Cancer Society, (800) ACS-2345; website: www.cancer.org or National Cancer Institute, (800) 4-CANCER; website: www.cancer.gov.

MEDICATION—Anticancer (chemotherapy) drugs may be prescribed.

ACTIVITY—Following larynx removal surgery, you should be able to do almost all the activities you did before. Straining and heavy lifting may be difficult since you cannot hold your breath. You can shower by using a shield over the stoma. Avoid swimming and water activities unless instructions and equipment are used.

DIET—Diet changes depend on the treatment. Surgery may require a liquid diet at first, then a soft diet. Learning to swallow again will take practice. Several small meals and snacks during the day may make eating easier.

 CALL YOUR DOCTOR IF

* You or a family member has symptoms of larynx (laryngeal) cancer.
* New symptoms occur during or after treatment.

LATEX ALLERGY

GENERAL INFORMATION

DEFINITION—Latex allergy involves reactions of the body to natural rubber latex. Latex is a milky fluid produced by rubber trees and is used in thousands of products. Rubber gloves are the main source of allergic reactions. There are three types of reactions: irritant dermatitis, allergic contact dermatitis, and immediate-type latex allergy.

BODY PARTS INVOLVED—Skin.

SEX OR AGE MOST AFFECTED—Both sexes; all ages.

SIGNS & SYMPTOMS
Irritant contact dermatitis:
* Dry, crusty, itchy, sore areas on the skin.
* Usually affects the hands.
Allergic contact dermatitis (chemical sensitive):
* Rash that starts 6 to 48 hours after exposure.
* Skin is dry and crusty. Blisters and sores occur.
* Usually affects the hands, but may spread.
Immediate type latex allergy:
* Normally occurs right away, but could take hours.
* Skin is red and itchy; may have hives.
* Eyes are red and watery.
* Runny nose, coughing, or sneezing.
* Chest feels tight; may be short of breath.
* Shock or a life-threatening reaction (rare).

CAUSES
* Irritant dermatitis is due to the skin being irritated.
* Allergic contact dermatitis is due to a chemical in the product, not latex. (This is like a poison ivy reaction.)
* In immediate-type latex allergy, the body's immune system reacts to repeated exposure to latex products.

RISK INCREASES WITH
* Health care workers or others who use latex gloves often, or are exposed to them.
* Having had many operations (where you were exposed to latex gloves).
* Other allergies, such as hay fever, asthma, and eczema.
* Food allergies.
* Rubber industry or latex manufacturing work.
* Certain disorders present at birth, such as spina bifida.

HOW TO PREVENT—For those diagnosed with the allergy, avoid latex.

WHAT TO EXPECT

DIAGNOSTIC MEASURES
* Your own observation of symptoms.
* Your health care provider will do a physical exam of the skin. A blood test may be done.
* Skin testing is rarely done, as it may result in a severe reaction.

APPROPRIATE HEALTH CARE—There is no treatment, except to avoid latex products.

POSSIBLE COMPLICATIONS
* Some people may need to change jobs due to latex exposure in their workplace.
* Rarely, anaphylaxis, a severe, life-threatening reaction occurs.

PROBABLE OUTCOME—There is no cure for latex allergy. Repeated exposure to latex can worsen the immune system response. Avoiding latex is the best action to take. Many products are made from latex, so this is not always an easy thing to do.

HOW TO TREAT

GENERAL MEASURES
* Find out which products in your home and work contain latex. Find substitutes you can use for those products. Read labels.
* Health care workers and others should wear powder-free latex gloves or non-latex gloves. Powder can get in the air, and if breathed in can cause a reaction.
* Most male condoms, as well as diaphragms and cervical caps, are latex. If you use them, ask your health care provider about options for birth control and safe sex.
* Wear a medical alert type tag or ID that lets others know you have this allergy.
* Advise any health care provider you consult that you have a latex allergy.
* Discuss your latex allergy with your employer to find ways to avoid latex exposure at work.
* If your allergy is severe, carry a kit with a self-injecting device that contains the drug epinephrine. Know how to use the device. Instruct your family or others as to how to give the injection if you are unable to.
* To learn more: Asthma and Allergy Foundation of America, 1125 15th Street, NW, Suite 502, Washington, DC 20005; (800) 7-ASTHMA; website: www.aafa.org or Latex Allergy Links website: www.latexallergylinks.org.

MEDICATION—Drugs may be prescribed for allergy symptoms.

ACTIVITY—No limits.

DIET—No special diet.

CALL YOUR DOCTOR IF

You or a family member has latex allergy symptoms.

LAXATIVE ABUSE

GENERAL INFORMATION

DEFINITION—Laxative abuse occurs when someone misuses or overuses laxatives. Laxative abuse is defined as (1) use of laxative for weight control, or (2) frequent use of laxatives over an extended period of time. It may result from a false belief that frequent bowel movements are necessary. Patients with eating disorders or binge eaters may abuse laxatives to get rid of large meals. Many individuals unintentionally develop the laxative habit.

BODY PARTS INVOLVED—Gastrointestinal system.

SEX OR AGE MOST AFFECTED—Both sexes; often occurs in adolescents or older adults.

SIGNS & SYMPTOMS
• Chronic constipation or chronic diarrhea.
• Gas and bloating.
• Laxative dependence (need laxatives to produce bowel movements).
• Dehydration due to excess loss of fluid.
• Electrolyte imbalance (minerals needed for body function), which causes tremors, muscle cramps, and spasms.
• Blood in the stools.
• Nausea or vomiting.
• Colon infection.

CAUSES—Short-term or long-term, laxatives create and perpetuate the very problem they were intended to correct. Laxatives induce constipation as the tissues become dried out, muscles become weak, and the delicate nerves lining the colon become damaged. Because of the damage that laxatives cause, ever-increasing dosages of laxatives may be required in order to achieve the desired effect. Where one laxative dose produced results, now two, then three doses a day are required. People who abuse laxatives for a long period of time may end up taking as many as 6 to 8 laxatives a day.

RISK INCREASES WITH
• Those with eating disorders or binge eaters. They believe they are losing weight and that they are thinner. What is lost is water weight. It comes back on within 48 hours.
• The false belief that frequent bowel movements are necessary.
• Preparation for competitions (sports, pageants, etc.).

HOW TO PREVENT
• Don't use laxatives regularly.
• Avoid constipation. Drink plenty of water with each meal and during the day. Eat more fresh fruits, vegetables, and whole grains to increase dietary fiber. Go to the bathroom when you feel the urge.
• Exercise regularly to stimulate bowel activity.
• Recognize and get treatment for eating disorders (anorexia or bulimia) or disordered eating (abnormal change in eating patterns).

WHAT TO EXPECT

DIAGNOSTIC MEASURES
• Your own observation of symptoms.
• Ask your health care provider about how to recover normal bowel function and what steps to use to begin to reverse the laxative habit.

APPROPRIATE HEALTH CARE
• Self-care is usually all that is needed.
• Counseling help may be useful for patients who are chronically abusing laxatives. This type of therapy is important for people with eating disorders.

POSSIBLE COMPLICATIONS—Depends on the type of laxatives abused, the amount abused, and how long they have been abused. Severe harm to the body, including death, could occur.

PROBABLE OUTCOME—Depend on the extent of the abuse and the motivation of the person. Withdrawal from laxatives can take days, weeks, or even months. Body functions should then return to normal.

HOW TO TREAT

GENERAL MEASURES
• Stopping laxatives may be done gradually or by going "cold turkey" (stopping in one day).
• Changing to products containing psyllium may help if you gradually withdraw from laxatives.
• Withdrawal symptoms may include nausea, constipation, bloating, and gas. They will stop as your body recovers and learns how to regulate itself again.

MEDICATION—No drugs are usually needed. If a drug you take causes constipation, a change in drug or dosage change may help.

ACTIVITY—Exercise daily. Being fit helps maintain bowel function.

DIET
• Be sure to eat enough food to promote regular bowel movements. Include high-fiber foods like fruits, vegetables, and whole grains.
• Drinking lots of water is important. Try to drink 8 to 10 glasses per day if possible. If you are constipated, warm/hot beverages can help.

CALL YOUR DOCTOR IF

You or a family member has a laxative abuse problem.

LEAD POISONING

GENERAL INFORMATION

DEFINITION—A high level of lead in the body. Lead is all around us. It is found in paint, batteries, drinking water, and pottery or other ceramic dishes. A little bit of lead finds its way into everyone and usually causes no problems. Too much lead in the body can cause serious problems, especially in infants and young children.

BODY PARTS INVOLVED—Gastrointestinal system; nervous system.

SEX OR AGE MOST AFFECTED—Both sexes; all ages, most common in young children.

SIGNS & SYMPTOMS
- Often no symptoms or they may be delayed.
- Pale skin, fatigue, feeling sluggish, sleeping problems.
- Behavior changes (such as being irritable).
- Child may be overly active.
- Stomach discomfort and poor appetite.
- Difficulty in concentrating.
- Headache; vomiting; weight loss.
- Constipation.
- Higher lead levels: severe stomach cramps; rigid abdomen, muscle weakness, seizures, or coma.

CAUSES—Breathing in of lead dust or fumes, or taking lead in by mouth (ingestion). Lead in the body interferes with normal body functions. It affects red blood cells and the nerve cells in the brain.

RISK INCREASES WITH
- Children under 3. Their brain and nervous systems are still developing and are more affected by lead.
- Childhood behaviors such as hand-to-mouth activity and pica (repeated eating of nonfood products) increase the risk of taking in lead.
- Homes with lead-based paint (its use stopped in the mid-1970s). Children eat, chew, or suck on the paint. During remodeling, lead paint dust can get into the air.
- Lead plumbing (its use stopped in 1986).
- Using lead-glazed ceramics for food or drink.
- Colored ink in newspapers, magazines, and plastic bags.
- Candy from Mexico with high lead levels.
- Hobbies such as glazed pottery making, lead soldering, painting, preparing lead shot, stained-glass making, car or boat repair, and others.
- Work or job exposure. Over 900 occupations have been connected with lead poisoning.
- Some cosmetics and folk remedies.
- Retained bullets or shrapnel.

HOW TO PREVENT
- Have children age 6 months to 6 years tested regularly for lead levels. Talk to your child's health care provider.
- Avoid risk factors where possible.
- Routine blood-lead tests for workers exposed to lead.
- Education about lead and ways to decrease lead exposure. Call (800) 424-LEAD; website: www.epa.gov/lead.

WHAT TO EXPECT

DIAGNOSTIC MEASURES
- Your health care provider may do a physical exam.
- Medical tests may include blood studies to measure lead levels, kidney and liver function testing, and x-rays of the abdomen.

APPROPRIATE HEALTH CARE
- Treatment involves avoiding any further exposure to the lead.
- For some patients, medical therapy will help the body excrete (get rid of) the lead. Hospital care may be needed for severe symptoms.

POSSIBLE COMPLICATIONS
- Damage to the nervous system, kidneys, liver, heart, and other body organ systems.
- Children may have mental retardation, behavior problems, learning disorders, aggressiveness, or delayed or slower growth. Seizures, coma, and death could occur.
- Adults may have loss of sex drive, impotence, or infertility. High lead levels in a pregnant woman can harm her unborn child.

PROBABLE OUTCOME—Lead poisoning without any apparent brain damage generally improves with treatment. Some problems may be long-lasting or permanent.

HOW TO TREAT

GENERAL MEASURES
- A report should be made to the local health department. An inspection of the home or workplace can be done to find the source of lead. Lead-level blood tests should be done for all family members.
- If the source is in the home, the patient needs to live elsewhere until lead source is removed.

MEDICATION—Chelating agents to excrete lead may be prescribed.

ACTIVITY—No limits.

DIET—To reduce lead levels, eat a diet that has plenty of iron, calcium, and zinc; avoid excess fat. Eat lean meat, eggs, raisins, greens, dairy, fruit, and potatoes.

CALL YOUR DOCTOR IF

You or a family member has symptoms of lead poisoning or you want lead levels tested.

LEGG-CALVÉ PERTHES DISEASE
(Slipped Femoral Epiphysis; Coxa Plana)

 GENERAL INFORMATION

DEFINITION—A hip disorder of childhood. It involves gradual weakening of the head of the thigh bone where it meets the pelvis.

BODY PARTS INVOLVED—Either leg at the hip joint (occasionally both).

SEX OR AGE MOST AFFECTED—It affects children ages 2 to 12 years (most often 4 to 8) of both sexes, but it is more common in boys (85% of the patients).

SIGNS & SYMPTOMS
• Pain and stiffness in the hip and thigh. Sometimes both sides are involved.
• Pain in the leg and often in the knee, even though the disorder is in the hip.
• Limping or other problems with walking.
• Symptoms usually begin slowly over time.

CAUSES—The bone becomes weak due to lack of a blood supply to the top of the bone. The weak bone is not able to handle weight. Why this occurs is unknown. It may involve growth hormones in the body or blood clotting problems. Injury is usually not a factor.

RISK INCREASES WITH
• Boys more than girls.
• Use of cortisone drugs for other disorders.
• Overweight persons.
• Periods of rapid growth.
• Children with low birth-weight and delayed development may be more at risk.

HOW TO PREVENT—No specific preventive measures.

 WHAT TO EXPECT

DIAGNOSTIC MEASURES
• Your own observation of symptoms, especially a limp or knee pain in your child.
• Your child's health care provider will do a physical exam and ask questions about the symptoms and activities.
• Medical tests usually include x-rays or other tests to determine how far the problem has progressed.

APPROPRIATE HEALTH CARE
• Treatment may not be needed for about half of the patients with the disorder. These children will be watched to see if any problems develop. This can include children younger than 6 with no hip motion problems, or older children who maintain good range of motion.

• Other treatment steps are aimed at maintaining the range of motion and keeping the hip-bone in the hip socket. They may include a cast, brace, physical therapy, or surgery.
• Surgery to reinforce the bone's attachment to the joint and prevent further problems (sometimes).
• A hospital stay may be needed for traction (a steady pull on the leg).

POSSIBLE COMPLICATIONS
• Delayed treatment may cause permanent bone injury.
• Osteoarthritis may develop later in life.

PROBABLE OUTCOME—Often curable in 2 to 3 years with early treatment. The blood supply to the bone becomes normal, and new bone cells start growing to replace the old bone.

 HOW TO TREAT

GENERAL MEASURES
• Youngsters often have difficulty accepting the need for rest, casts, braces, or other treatment. Help your child find activities and interests that don't involve a lot of movement or athletics.
• Use heat to relieve pain. Warm compresses, heating pads, or other methods are effective.

MEDICATION—For minor discomfort, you may use nonprescription drugs, such as acetaminophen or ibuprofen.

ACTIVITY—Bed rest may be necessary for 6 months to 1 year until the condition improves, or until after surgery. When the bones can bear weight, crutches, braces, or casts are usually necessary. After that, activities may be resumed gradually.

DIET—No special diet, unless the child is overweight.

 CALL YOUR DOCTOR IF

• Your child has hip or knee pain, stiffness, or a limp.
• The following occur during treatment:
  - Symptoms don't improve in 4 weeks, despite treatment.
  - Pain increases.

LEGIONNAIRE'S DISEASE
(Legionella Pneumophilia Bronchopneumonia)

 GENERAL INFORMATION

DEFINITION—A form of lung infection named after an epidemic that affected people attending an American Legion convention in 1976. The disease was probably around long before that, but was not recognized.

BODY PARTS INVOLVED—Bronchial tubes; lungs.

SEX OR AGE MOST AFFECTED—It can affect both sexes and all ages, but is more common in middle-aged persons.

SIGNS & SYMPTOMS
* General ill feeling.
* Headache and muscle aches.
* Chills and fever up to 105°F (40.6°C).
* Cough without sputum that progresses to one with gray or blood-streaked sputum.
* Nausea, vomiting, diarrhea, and tiredness.
* Mental changes such as disorientation or confusion.

CAUSES
* Infection from *Legionella* bacteria. The germs also cause a milder illness called Pontiac fever. The germs are breathed into the lungs. Symptoms begin 2 to 10 days after exposure. The germs are not known to spread from one person to another, or from drinking water. The risk of getting the infection is quite low, especially in healthy persons.
* The bacteria are found in wet or moist environments. They have been found in hot water tanks, in water from shower-heads or faucets, cooling towers, air conditioners, whirlpool spas, soil, potting soil, and other locations.

RISK INCREASES WITH
* Chronic illness, including diabetes, kidney failure, or emphysema.
* Weak immune system due to illness or drugs.
* Smoking increases the risk 3 to 4 times over.
* Drinking alcohol to excess.

HOW TO PREVENT
* No specific preventive measures. Take steps to reduce risk factors where possible.
* Though home cooling and heating systems don't usually carry the germs, it is important to keep them clean.
* Don't smoke.
* Avoid alcohol or limit it to 1 to 2 drinks a day.

 WHAT TO EXPECT

DIAGNOSTIC MEASURES
* Your health care provider will do a physical exam and ask about your symptoms and activities.

* Medical tests may include blood studies, sputum culture, and other testing to confirm the diagnosis.

APPROPRIATE HEALTH CARE
* Treatment is with antibiotics and supportive care.
* Hospital care may be needed for severe cases.

POSSIBLE COMPLICATIONS
* Shock or delirium.
* Congestive heart failure.
* Kidney failure.
* Heart-rhythm disturbances.
* If untreated, 15% of cases are fatal.

PROBABLE OUTCOME—Usually curable with prompt diagnosis and treatment.

 HOW TO TREAT

GENERAL MEASURES—The following apply to mild cases or to care after a hospital stay:
* Use a cool-mist humidifier to increase air moisture and thin lung secretions so that they can be coughed up more easily. Clean humidifier daily.
* Use warm compresses or a heating pad on the chest to relieve chest pain.
* Practice deep-breathing exercises as often as your strength allows.
* Avoid talking loudly, laughing, or singing. They may trigger excessive coughing.

MEDICATION
* Antibiotics. Be sure to finish all the dosage prescribed.
* If the cough is painful and doesn't produce sputum, you may use nonprescription drugs to suppress it. If the cough produces sputum, don't suppress it.
* You may take aspirin (not for children) or acetaminophen to reduce fever.

ACTIVITY—Rest in bed until symptoms improve. Allow 2 to 4 weeks for recovery.

DIET—No special diet. Drink plenty of fluids each day.

 CALL YOUR DOCTOR IF

* You or a family member has symptoms of Legionnaire's disease.
* The following occur during or after treatment:
  - Higher fever occurs.
  - Severe chest pain, despite treatment.
  - Increased shortness of breath.
  - Dark or bluish nails, lips, or skin.
  - Blood in the sputum.

ILLNESS & DISORDERS

LEUKEMIA, ACUTE

GENERAL INFORMATION

DEFINITION—Leukemia is cancer of blood cells. Three types of blood cells are formed in bone marrow. White blood cells fight infections, red blood cells carry oxygen, and platelets help control bleeding. Bone marrow is the soft material in the center of bones. With leukemia, the cancerous (abnormal) cells replace normal cells. The body then develops infections, anemia, or bleeds easily. Acute leukemia usually has a sudden onset and symptoms progress rapidly. Forms of acute leukemia are:
• Acute lymphocytic leukemia (ALL). It affects all ages, but is more common in children.
• Acute myeloid (myelogenous) leukemia (AML). It affects both children and adults (usually older adults).

BODY PARTS INVOLVED—Bone marrow and lymph tissue in early stages. The disease eventually affects all body tissues.

SEX OR AGE MOST AFFECTED—Both sexes and all ages depending on type of leukemia.

SIGNS & SYMPTOMS
• Low fever, chills, and sweating.
• Tiredness and weakness.
• Anemia (pale skin, fatigue).
• General ill feeling.
• Easy bruising or bleeding. Cuts heal slowly.
• Pin-head size spots on the skin.
• Repeated infections.
• Bone or joint pain.
• Loss of appetite and/or weight.
• Other symptoms if cancer cells collect in organs such as brain, lungs, genitals, digestive tract, or kidneys.

CAUSES—Exact cause unknown. It is believed to develop from a combination of genetic and environmental factors.

RISK INCREASES WITH
• Family history of leukemia.
• Men more than women; whites and Hispanics.
• Excess exposure to x-rays (radiation).
• Genetic disorder, such as Down syndrome.
• Exposure to benzenes or other toxic chemicals.
• Weak immune system due to illness or drugs.
• AML risks: smoking, history of blood disorder, or previous treatment for childhood ALL.

HOW TO PREVENT—Cannot be prevented. If you have a family history of leukemia, seek genetic counseling before starting a family.

WHAT TO EXPECT

DIAGNOSTIC MEASURES
• Your health care provider will do a physical exam and ask questions about your symptoms.

• Medical tests include blood studies. Samples of bone marrow (liquid and solid) will be taken for viewing with a microscope. Other tests are done to see if the cancer has spread.

APPROPRIATE HEALTH CARE
• Treatment depends on the leukemia type and other factors and involves 3 steps. Induction (remission), then consolidation (prevent relapse), and then maintenance. Treatment may include anticancer drugs (chemotherapy), radiation therapy, bone marrow transplant, stem cell transplant, surgery, and biologic therapy.
• Chemotherapy uses drugs, and radiation therapy uses radiation to attack the cancer cells. Biologic therapy uses the body's immune system to fight cancer.
• Bone marrow transplant involves replacing the leukemia-affected marrow with healthy bone marrow.
• Stem cell transplant replaces blood cells destroyed in treatment with stem cells (immature blood cells).
• Blood and platelet transfusions may be needed.
• Surgery may be done to remove the spleen.
• Counseling may help you cope with having cancer.

POSSIBLE COMPLICATIONS
• Hemorrhage or severe infection (can be fatal).
• Failure of leukemia to respond to treatment.
• Relapse (leukemia recurs after remission).

PROBABLE OUTCOME—Depends on the type of leukemia, the patient's health and response to treatment. Remission occurs when there is no evidence of leukemia in the blood or bone marrow. 5 years of remission can mean a cure.

HOW TO TREAT

GENERAL MEASURES
• Dental care (to avoid infections and bleeding).
• Avoid crowds and people with infections.
• To learn more: National Cancer Institute, 6116 Executive Blvd., MSC8322, Bethesda, MD 20892; (800) 422-6237; website: www.cancer.gov.

MEDICATION
• You will usually be prescribed anticancer drugs taken by mouth or by IV (through a vein).
• Antibiotics may be prescribed for infections.
• Biologic therapy drugs may be prescribed.

ACTIVITY—As tolerated.

DIET—A healthy diet helps you feel better.

CALL YOUR DOCTOR IF

• You or your child has symptoms of leukemia.
• During or after treatment, any symptoms cause you concern.

LEUKEMIA, CHRONIC

GENERAL INFORMATION

DEFINITION—Leukemia is cancer of blood cells in the bone marrow. Three types of blood cells are formed in bone marrow. White blood cells fight infections, red blood cells carry oxygen, and platelets help control bleeding. Bone marrow is the soft material in the center of bones. With chronic leukemia, the cancer (abnormal) cells do not fight infection as well as normal white blood cells do. Chronic leukemia develops over a long period of time. Forms of chronic leukemia include:
• Chronic lymphocytic leukemia (CLL). It affects adults only and is twice as common as CML.
• Chronic myeloid (myelogenous) leukemia (CML). It mostly affects adults (rare in children).

BODY PARTS INVOLVED—Blood-forming organs: bone marrow; lymph glands; liver; spleen.

SEX OR AGE MOST AFFECTED—Both sexes, usually adults.

SIGNS & SYMPTOMS
• Sometimes, no symptoms occur.
• Low fever, chills, and sweating.
• Tiredness and weakness.
• Anemia (pale skin, fatigue).
• General ill feeling.
• Easy bruising or bleeding or cuts that heal slowly.
• Pin-head size spots on the skin.
• Repeated infections.
• Bone or joint pain.
• Appetite and/or weight loss. Fullness in the stomach.
• Other symptoms if cancer cells collect in organs, such as brain, lungs, genitals, digestive tract, or kidneys.

CAUSES—Exact cause unknown. It is believed to develop from a combination of genetic and environmental factors.

RISK INCREASES WITH
• Family history of leukemia (such as brother or sister).
• Men more than women; whites and Hispanics.
• Excess exposure to radiation.
• Exposure to benzenes and other toxic chemicals.
• Weak immune system due to illness or drugs.
• Smoking.

HOW TO PREVENT—No specific preventive measures.

WHAT TO EXPECT

DIAGNOSTIC MEASURES
• Your health care provider will do a physical exam and ask questions about your symptoms.

• Medical tests include blood studies. Samples of bone marrow (liquid and solid) will be taken for viewing with a microscope. Other tests are done to see if the cancer has spread.

APPROPRIATE HEALTH CARE
• Treatment depends on the leukemia type and other factors. Treatment for CML may include anticancer drugs (chemotherapy), radiation therapy, bone marrow transplant, stem cell transplant, surgery, and biologic therapy. CLL patients may not need any immediate treatment. Follow-up exams are done. If disease progresses, then chemotherapy may be recommended.
• Chemotherapy uses drugs, and radiation therapy uses radiation to attack the cancer cells. Biologic therapy uses the body's immune system to fight cancer.
• A bone marrow transplant replaces leukemia-affected marrow with healthy bone marrow.
• Stem cell transplant replaces blood cells destroyed in treatment with stem cells (immature blood cells).
• Blood and platelet transfusions may be done.
• Surgery may be done to remove the spleen.
• Counseling may help you cope emotionally.

POSSIBLE COMPLICATIONS
• Hemorrhage or severe infection (can be fatal).
• Failure of leukemia to respond to treatment.
• Relapse (leukemia recurs after remission).

PROBABLE OUTCOME—Depends on the type of leukemia, the patient's health and response to treatment. Remission occurs when there is no evidence of leukemia in the blood or bone marrow. 5 years of remission can mean a cure.

HOW TO TREAT

GENERAL MEASURES
• Dental care (to avoid infections and bleeding).
• Avoid crowds and people with infections.
• To learn more: National Cancer Institute, 6116 Executive Blvd., MSC8322, Bethesda, MD 20892; (800) 422-6237; website: www.cancer.gov.

MEDICATION
• You will usually be prescribed anticancer drugs taken by mouth or by IV (through a vein).
• Antibiotics may be prescribed for infections.
• Biologic therapy drugs may be prescribed.

ACTIVITY—As tolerated.

DIET—A healthy diet helps you feel better.

CALL YOUR DOCTOR IF

• You or a family member has symptoms of leukemia.
• During or after treatment, any symptoms cause you concern.

LEUKOPLAKIA, ORAL

GENERAL INFORMATION

DEFINITION—Oral leukoplakia is a general term to describe a white patch on the mouth. Hairy leukoplakia is a different disorder, and it occurs in people who have a weak immune system due to drugs or illness. Another form of leukoplakia occurs in the genitals of women.

BODY PARTS INVOLVED—Inside of cheek; floor of mouth; tongue; palate; roof of mouth.

SEX OR AGE MOST AFFECTED— It affects all ages, but it is most common in adults over 60, and in men more than in women.

SIGNS & SYMPTOMS
• A white or off-white patch in the membranes of the mouth. The patch may be tiny or the size of a quarter. It can involve the lips, inside of the cheek, floor and roof of the mouth, tongue, or gums. It is not painful.
• The patch feels firm, rough and stiff. It can not be rubbed off.
• The area may be more sensitive when touched or when eating hot or spicy foods.
• It is sometimes first noticed by a dentist when doing a dental exam.

CAUSES—In some cases, the cause is unknown. Certain risk factors, such as smoking, may cause the disorder. It can not be spread from one person to another.

RISK INCREASES WITH
• Use of tobacco products, including cigarettes, chewing tobacco, snuff, pipes, or cigars.
• Repeated trauma to the mouth or tongue such as from a sharp or broken tooth or from dentures.
• Excess alcohol use.
• Infections such as candidiasis, syphilis, or Epstein-Barr virus.

HOW TO PREVENT
• No specific preventive measures.
• For many health reasons, don't smoke or use tobacco products, and avoid alcohol.

WHAT TO EXPECT

DIAGNOSTIC MEASURES
• Your own observation of symptoms.
• Your health care provider can diagnose the disorder with a physical exam of the mouth and tongue.
• A biopsy is usually done if a pre-cancerous risk is suspected. The biopsy involves the removal of a small amount of skin tissue to be viewed under a microscope.

APPROPRIATE HEALTH CARE
• Medical care may involve a wait-and-watch plan to see if any changes occur in the affected area.
• Drug therapy may be prescribed, or surgery may be recommended. Your health care provider will discuss the options with you.

POSSIBLE COMPLICATIONS
• Leukoplakia may recur if the problem causing it (such as tobacco use) is not stopped.
• In a small percent of cases, there is a cancer risk.

PROBABLE OUTCOME—Leukoplakia by itself does not cause any problems and does not require treatment. The concern is that it may be pre-cancerous, and that makes it important to have it diagnosed. In the majority of cases, cancer will not develop.

HOW TO TREAT

GENERAL MEASURES
• Stop any tobacco use and/or alcohol use (including alcoholic mouthwashes).
• Get treatment for any tooth problems or have any denture problems fixed.

MEDICATION
• Topical or oral forms of vitamin A may be prescribed.
• Other forms of treatment are currently undergoing study.

ACTIVITY—No limits.

DIET—No special diet.

CALL YOUR DOCTOR IF

You or a family member has symptoms of leukoplakia.

LICE
(Pediculosis; Head Lice; Body Lice; Crab Lice)

GENERAL INFORMATION

DEFINITION—Lice are tiny parasites that live on the body or in clothing. Pediculosis (lice infestation) is the medical term. Three types of lice affect humans: head lice, body lice, and crab (or pubic) lice. Head lice are common in school children.

BODY PARTS INVOLVED—Hairy areas anywhere, especially the scalp, eyebrows or genital area; skin, especially areas in which clothing is in close contact with skin, such as the shoulders, waist, genital area or buttocks.

SEX OR AGE MOST AFFECTED—Both sexes; all ages.

SIGNS & SYMPTOMS
- Itching and scratching of the head or other body parts. It may take 2 to 3 weeks or longer after being infected before itching symptoms start. The itching is more common at night.
- You may see eggs ("nits") on hair shafts.
- Scalp may be red and sore. The hair may be matted.

CAUSES—Tiny parasites that bite through skin to obtain nourishment (blood). The bites cause itching, redness, and soreness.

RISK INCREASES WITH
- Contact with an infected person.
- Contact with an infected object such as combs, hats, helmets, clothing, sheets, or pillowcases.
- Crowded living conditions.
- For crab lice, sexual intercourse with an infected person.
- Body lice are not common. They occur in the homeless, and those who can't bathe or change clothes often.

HOW TO PREVENT
- Bathe and shampoo hair often. However, good hygiene alone will not prevent head lice.
- Don't share combs, brushes, or hats with others. Wash combs and brushes carefully.
- Careful follow-up in schools and daycare centers where head lice have occurred.
- If head lice or nits are found on your child, notify the child's school or daycare.

WHAT TO EXPECT

DIAGNOSTIC MEASURES
- Self-diagnosis and self-treatment are sometimes all that is needed for head lice.
- When unsure if hair lice are the problem, or if body or crab lice are the cause, see your health care provider. Lice are diagnosed with a physical exam of the affected area.

- A sample of the lice or nit may be removed for viewing under a microscope.

APPROPRIATE HEALTH CARE
- Treatment may be done with a product to kill the lice and eggs.
- Manual removal may be the best option, even when an anti-lice product is used
- If the lice infect eyelashes, ask your health care provider about treatment.

POSSIBLE COMPLICATIONS—Infection at the site of scratching.

PROBABLE OUTCOME—Curable with treatment. Allow 5 days after treatment for symptoms to disappear. Lice often recur.

HOW TO TREAT

GENERAL MEASURES
- Uninfected family members do not need treatment.
- For manual removal, use a special nit comb. A magnifying glass may help you see the nits and lice. Live lice are hard to see as they move quickly. Part the hair in sections and examine each part carefully.
- Wash articles such as combs, curlers, hairbrushes, and barrettes in hot water.
- Vacuuming floors, furniture, car seats or other items may help remove any hairs with nits. Special lice sprays may be recommended.
- Machine-wash clothing and bedding in hot water. Dry in the dryer's hot-air cycle. Putting unwashable items in plastic bags for 2 weeks has been recommended in the past, but is probably not needed. Lice can't live longer than 24 hours unless they have blood for food.
- For more information, contact the National Pediculosis Association., 50 Kearney Rd., Needham, MA 02494; (781) 449-NITS; website: www.headlice.org.

MEDICATION
- Nonprescription anti-lice (pediculicide) products are available. One type is Nix which contains permethrin. Follow label instructions for use and follow-up care. Use a special nit comb to help rid the hair of nits. Repeat the treatment in 7 to 10 days (if advised).
- Your health care provider may prescribe, and give directions for using anti-lice products.

ACTIVITY—No limits.

DIET—No special diet.

CALL YOUR DOCTOR IF

- You or a family member has symptoms of lice that you are concerned about.
- Self-treatment for lice has not worked.

LICHEN PLANUS

GENERAL INFORMATION

DEFINITION—A chronic skin condition that is not cancerous or contagious.

BODY PARTS INVOLVED—It may involve the skin of the legs, trunk, arms, wrists, scalp or penis. The lining of the mouth or vagina, toenails, and fingernails (around or under the nailbed) may also be involved.

SEX OR AGE MOST AFFECTED—All ages, but most common in adults over 40.

SIGNS & SYMPTOMS
- Small, slightly raised bumps that itch. The bumps are purplish or reddish-purple with a whitish surface.
- An uneven, whitish line inside the mouth or vagina.
- Sudden hair loss in patches on the head.
- Bumps in the mouth may make it hard to eat.
- If the vagina is involved, it may cause a discharge, bleeding, or pain with intercourse.

CAUSES—Unknown. It may be a problem with the body's immune system.

RISK INCREASES WITH
- Stress (may make it worse).
- Adverse reaction to certain drugs.
- Hepatitis C.

HOW TO PREVENT—Cannot be prevented at present.

WHAT TO EXPECT

DIAGNOSTIC MEASURES
- Your own observation of symptoms.
- Your health care provider can usually diagnose the condition with an exam of the affected area.
- Medical skin tests or a biopsy may be done to confirm the diagnosis. A biopsy involves the removal of a small amount of skin tissue to be viewed under a microscope.

APPROPRIATE HEALTH CARE
- The goal of treatment is to relieve the symptoms; mainly the itching. This usually involves self-care and sometimes, drug therapy.
- A special treatment called PUVA using ultraviolet light combined with drugs may help some people.

POSSIBLE COMPLICATIONS
- Chronic condition where new bumps appear as old bumps clear up.
- Rarely, hair or nail problems, which can include permanent loss.
- Lichen planus in the mouth may slightly increase the risk of oral cancer. Your health care provider will follow-up on a regular basis to watch for any problems.

PROBABLE OUTCOME—There is no cure. Symptoms can be helped with treatment. Be patient and keep up with your treatment, even if results are slow. The bumps often go away on their own within a year. Once the bumps are gone, a brown area may remain on the skin. It will fade in time.

HOW TO TREAT

GENERAL MEASURES
- Use cool-water soaks to relieve itching.
- Reducing stress in your life may help with the symptoms as well as prevent a recurrence. Learn ways to help yourself relax.
- To learn more: American Academy of Dermatology, 930 E. Woodfield Rd., Schaumburg, IL, 60173-4927; website: www.aad.org.

MEDICATION
- You may use nonprescription antihistamines taken by mouth to help control itching.
- Nonprescription cortisone creams or ointments can help to reduce pain and itching. Follow directions on the label.
- Stronger drugs may be prescribed.

ACTIVITY—No limits.

DIET—No special diet.

CALL YOUR DOCTOR IF

- You or a family member has symptoms of lichen planus.
- New, unexplained symptoms develop. Drugs used in treatment may produce side effects.

LIPOMAS

GENERAL INFORMATION

DEFINITION—Benign (noncancerous), slow-growing tumors of fat cells. Lipomas grow under the skin (subcutaneous). In a few cases, lipomas may grow in deeper body tissues or in the body's organs.

BODY PARTS INVOLVED—Trunk; neck; back; upper thighs; arms.

SEX OR AGE MOST AFFECTED—They affect both sexes, and all ages, but are more common in adults.

SIGNS & SYMPTOMS
* Lumps are dome-shaped, and may be small or large.
* Lumps feel "doughy," smooth, and easily movable.
* One or many lipomas may occur on a person.
* Skin over the lump is normal in appearance.
* Most often, they cause no symptoms, such as itching or pain. However, a form of lipoma that contains blood vessels can cause pain.

CAUSES—Unknown, but the tendency is probably inherited. Minor injury may trigger their growth.

RISK INCREASES WITH—Family history of lipomas.

HOW TO PREVENT—Cannot be prevented at present.

WHAT TO EXPECT

DIAGNOSTIC MEASURES
* Your own observation of symptoms.
* Your health care provider can usually diagnose lipomas with an exam of the affected area.
* In a few cases, medical tests may be done to confirm the diagnosis or check for complications.

APPROPRIATE HEALTH CARE
* No treatment is needed for lumps that are stable in size.
* Surgical removal (if recommended) is usually done in a medical office. Lipomas can be removed with small incisions or removed by liposuction. Instructions for home care after surgery will be provided. (See Lipoma Removal in Surgery section.)

POSSIBLE COMPLICATIONS—For the majority of people, there are no complications. In rare cases, certain forms of lipomas may cause complications.

PROBABLE OUTCOME—These lumps are benign and require no treatment. They may be removed if they cause symptoms, are large and/or unattractive, or for medical testing.

HOW TO TREAT

GENERAL MEASURES—Follow medical advice about skin care after any surgical procedure.

MEDICATION—Drugs are not needed for this disorder.

ACTIVITY—No limits.

DIET—No special diet.

CALL YOUR DOCTOR IF

* You or a family member is concerned about skin growths.
* The following occur after lipoma surgery:
  - Fever.
  - Bleeding that does not respond to moderate pressure.
  - Signs of infection (warmth, swelling or redness), at the surgical site.

LIVER CANCER

GENERAL INFORMATION

DEFINITION—Growth of cancer cells in the liver. The liver is the largest internal organ in the body. It is located behind the ribs on the right side.

BODY PARTS INVOLVED—Liver; bile ducts.

SEX OR AGE MOST AFFECTED—Both sexes; all ages, but most common in men over 60.

SIGNS & SYMPTOMS
* The early stages may produce no symptoms.
* Loss of appetite and weight loss.
* Tender mass in the right upper abdomen.
* Pain in the upper abdomen.
* Low fever, usually less than 101°F (38.3°C).
* Yellow eyes and skin (from jaundice).
* Swollen abdomen from fluid retention.
* Nausea and vomiting.
* Feeling tired or weak.

CAUSES
* Unknown. People with certain risk factors are more likely to develop liver cancer than others.
* A primary cancer is when it begins in the liver.
* A secondary cancer is when it results from the spread (metastases) of cancer from another place in the body. The most common sources are cancers of the rectum, colon, lung, breast, pancreas, esophagus, or skin (malignant melanoma).

RISK INCREASES WITH
* Chronic viral hepatitis B or hepatitis C infection.
* Liver disease, such as cirrhosis of the liver.
* Long-term exposure to aflatoxin (a substance in fungus that grows on peanuts, corn, other nuts and grains).
* Age over 60; males more than females.
* Family history of liver cancer.
* Tobacco use.
* Certain inherited metabolic disorders.
* Anabolic steroid (male hormone) use.

HOW TO PREVENT
* No specific preventive measures. Get cancer screening and hepatitis B vaccine for high-risk persons.
* Avoid excess alcohol use (it can lead to cirrhosis).
* Avoid risk factors such as smoking and steroid use.

WHAT TO EXPECT

DIAGNOSTIC MEASURES
* Your own observation of symptoms.
* Your health care provider will do a physical exam and ask questions about your symptoms.

* Medical tests may include blood studies and liver function tests. Other tests are usually done in order to confirm the diagnosis and to determine if cancer has spread (called staging).

APPROPRIATE HEALTH CARE
* Treatment will depend on the stage of the cancer, your health and your preferences. The main treatments involve surgery, chemotherapy (anticancer drugs), and radiation (used less often). Since many liver tumors cannot be removed by surgery, other treatment forms are evolving. These include embolization, radiofrequency ablation, cryotherapy, and alcohol injections. Your health care provider will discuss the options with you.
* Surgery is done only for cancer found in an early stage. The cancer can still recur because cancer cells may have spread before surgery.
* Liver transplants have been done in a few select cases.
* Treatment may involve steps to relieve symptoms and make you comfortable, rather than treating the cancer.
* Counseling may help in coping with this disorder.

PROBABLE OUTCOME
* This condition can be cured only if it is caught early, has not spread, and surgery is successful. In other cases, it cannot be cured, but treatment can help relieve symptoms and help a person live longer.
* Scientific research into causes and treatment continues, so there is hope for effective treatment and cure.

HOW TO TREAT

GENERAL MEASURES—To learn more: American Cancer Society, (800) ACS-2345; website: www.cancer.org or National Cancer Institute, (800) 4-CANCER; website: www.nci.nih.gov.

MEDICATION
* For minor discomfort, you may use nonprescription drugs such as acetaminophen. Stronger pain relievers will be prescribed as needed.
* Anticancer drugs may be given.

ACTIVITY—Stay as active as your strength allows.

DIET—No special diet. Don't drink alcohol.

CALL YOUR DOCTOR IF

* You or a family member has symptoms of liver cancer, especially unexplained weight loss, low fever, or a mass is felt in the abdomen.
* New or unexpected symptoms develop during treatment.

LUNG ABSCESS

GENERAL INFORMATION

DEFINITION—An infected area of lung tissue, surrounded by lung inflammation. The infected lung tissue dies and is replaced with pus. The infection is not contagious from person to person.

BODY PARTS INVOLVED—Lung.

SEX OR AGE MOST AFFECTED—Both sexes; all ages.

SIGNS & SYMPTOMS
• Cough with sputum. The sputum is pus-like, often blood-streaked, and sometimes smells bad.
• Bad breath.
• Sweating.
• Fever up to 101°F (38.3°C) or higher.
• Chills.
• Weight loss.
• Chest pain (sometimes).

CAUSES—Lung abscesses are generally caused by a bacterial infection. They are usually a complication of pneumonia. A lung abscess may occur when an unconscious or sedated person inhales infected material from the upper-breathing passages. The patient may be unconscious from a head injury, or heavily sedated.

RISK INCREASES WITH
• Recent illness, especially pneumonia that has been slow to heal.
• Alcoholism.
• Periodontal disease.
• Recent general anesthesia or injury causing unconsciousness.

HOW TO PREVENT—No specific preventive measures. Be sure to seek prompt medical treatment for lung infections, especially pneumonia.

WHAT TO EXPECT

DIAGNOSTIC MEASURES
• Your own observation of symptoms.
• Your health care provider will do a physical exam.
• Medical tests may include blood tests, a culture of pus from the abscess, and x-rays of the lung. A bronchoscopy may be done if a foreign body is suspected. This test uses an optical instrument with a lighted tip that is passed into the windpipe, and then into the bronchi.

APPROPRIATE HEALTH CARE
• Hospital care is usually required.
• Treatment is with antibiotic drugs. Surgery may be needed if antibiotics are not helping the abscess heal.
• Other care in the hospital may involve breathing support with oxygen and procedures to help loosen secretions. Physical therapy can help strengthen the breathing muscles.
• Surgery (sometimes) to remove pus from the abscess or to remove the abscess and part of the lung, if the abscess does not heal.

POSSIBLE COMPLICATIONS
• Abscess may not respond well to antibiotic treatment.
• Rupture of the abscess, causing empyema or massive bleeding in the lung.
• Spread of infection to other body parts, especially the brain.

PROBABLE OUTCOME—Usually curable with antibiotic treatment (may last for 4 to 6 weeks or for several months).

HOW TO TREAT

GENERAL MEASURES
• Don't smoke. Find a way to quit that works.
• Practice deep-breathing exercises as often as possible.

MEDICATION—Antibiotics for prolonged periods of time to treat infection and prevent a recurrence. They are given through a vein (IV) at first, and then taken by mouth.

ACTIVITY—Reduced activity until tests show a healed abscess.

DIET—No special diet. Increase your fluid intake. By drinking extra liquids, the body is forced to eliminate part of the fluid through the lungs. This makes thick lung secretions thinner, so they can be coughed up more easily.

CALL YOUR DOCTOR IF

• You or a family member has symptoms of a lung abscess.
• Symptoms of a lung infection recur after treatment, especially a sputum-producing cough, fever, or general ill feeling.

ILLNESS & DISORDERS

LUNG CANCER
(Bronchogenic Carcinoma)

 GENERAL INFORMATION

DEFINITION—Malignant cell growth in the lungs. There are two major types, non-small cell (more common) and small cell. Lung cancer causes more deaths than any other form of cancer, and the number is increasing. It is related almost exclusively to smoking.

BODY PARTS INVOLVED—Bronchial tubes and lungs. Cancer spreads to the larynx, liver, brain, bones and kidneys.

SEX OR AGE MOST AFFECTED—Adults of both sexes between ages 40 and 70.

SIGNS & SYMPTOMS
- Usually there are no symptoms in the early stages.
- Persistent cough.
- Wheezing.
- Chest pain.
- Fatigue and weakness.
- Weight loss.
- Shoulder, arm, or bone pain.
- Coughing up blood.

CAUSES—Abnormal cells that grow and destroy healthy lung tissue. Primary lung cancer is one that begins in the lungs. It can spread (metastasize) to other places in the body. Secondary lung cancer is when cancer from another place in the body spreads to the lungs.

RISK INCREASES WITH
- Adults over 60.
- Smoking. Cigarettes (highest risk), pipes, and cigars.
- Secondhand smoke.
- Radon gas.
- Lung diseases.
- Environmental exposure to asbestos, uranium ore, nickel, chromates, bischloromethyl ether, or air pollution.

HOW TO PREVENT
- Don't smoke. Tumors don't develop for a long time, so smokers can quit at any time and greatly reduce the risk of developing lung cancer.
- Obtain regular health checkups if you are a smoker.
- Check your house for radon gas.

 WHAT TO EXPECT

DIAGNOSTIC MEASURES
- Your health care provider will do a physical exam and ask questions about your symptoms.
- A number of medical tests will be done. The tests first help diagnose the cancer and then determine if it has spread (staging).

APPROPRIATE HEALTH CARE
- Treatment varies and depends on location and size of tumor, any spread of the cancer, your health, age, and preferences. Treatment may include surgery, anticancer drugs (chemotherapy) and/or radiation therapy, and biologic therapy.
- Chemotherapy uses drugs and radiation therapy uses radiation to attack the cancer cells. Biologic therapy uses the body's immune system to fight cancer.
- Surgery to remove all of the lung (pneumonectomy) or part of the lung (lobectomy) may be recommended if cancer is at an early stage.
- Treatment may involve steps to relieve symptoms and make you comfortable, rather than treating the cancer.
- Counseling may help you cope with having cancer.

POSSIBLE COMPLICATIONS
- Complications from treatments.
- Lung collapse; fluid on the lung.
- Spread of cancer beyond the lung (which can be fatal).

PROBABLE OUTCOME—Outcome depends on the type of cancer, whether it has spread, patient's general health, and response to treatment. The outcome is more favorable with early diagnosis compared to diagnosis of advanced disease. Early diagnosis improves the success rate of treatment.

 HOW TO TREAT

GENERAL MEASURES— To learn more: American Cancer Society, (800) ACS-2345; website: www.cancer.org or National Cancer Institute, (800) 4-CANCER; website: www.nci.nih.gov.

MEDICATION
- For minor pain, use nonprescription drugs such as acetaminophen or ibuprofen.
- Stronger pain drugs and nausea or anti-anxiety drugs may be prescribed.
- Anticancer drugs or biologic therapy drugs may be prescribed.

ACTIVITY—Be as active as possible. Follow medical advice about resuming activities.

DIET—No special diet.

 CALL YOUR DOCTOR IF

- You or a family member has symptoms of lung cancer.
- Any symptoms occur that cause you concern.

LUPUS ERYTHEMATOSUS, DISCOID (DLE)

GENERAL INFORMATION

DEFINITION—Discoid lupus erythematosus (DLE) is a chronic skin disorder. Localized DLE (the more common form) involves the skin on the face, scalp, ears, and neck. Generalized DLE involves the skin on the arms and chest. DLE is different from systemic lupus erythematosus (SLE), which affects many different internal organs.

BODY PARTS INVOLVED—Skin.

SEX OR AGE MOST AFFECTED—Adults of both sexes. The peak incidence occurs in women in their 30s.

SIGNS & SYMPTOMS
• Coin-shaped (discoid), red, raised, scaly skin patches (they may be referred to as rashes, plaques or lesions). Erythematosus means reddening of the skin.
• The centers are lighter in color than the outside ring.
• Patches may appear anywhere on the face. The cheeks and jawline are the most common sites. Some people describe them as "butterfly" rash when they appear on both sides of the nose.
• The patches may sometimes appear on the scalp with patches of hair loss.
• Mucous membranes of the mouth may be affected.
• The affected skin is usually not itchy or painful.
• Scarring occurs as the rash heals.

CAUSES—Unknown. Both genetic (hereditary) and environmental factors may contribute. It is thought to be an autoimmune disorder. In these disorders, the immune system by mistake attacks the body itself. It cannot be spread from one person to another.

RISK INCREASES WITH—Family history of DLE.

HOW TO PREVENT—No specific preventive measures.

WHAT TO EXPECT

DIAGNOSTIC MEASURES
• Your own observation of symptoms.
• Your health care provider may do a physical exam and an exam of the affected skin.
• Medical tests may include blood studies and a skin biopsy. A biopsy involves removal of a sample of the affected skin for viewing under a microscope.

APPROPRIATE HEALTH CARE—Treatment involves drug therapy and sunscreens.

POSSIBLE COMPLICATIONS
• Scarring of the face.
• Systemic lupus erythematosus (about 10% of patients). If it does occur, it is usually not severe.

PROBABLE OUTCOME—Outcome is generally good. Symptoms of the disorder may come and go over years, but they are not life-threatening. Treatment can help improve the cosmetic appearance of the rash.

HOW TO TREAT

GENERAL MEASURES
• Sun exposure is a trigger for a flare-up. Don't go outdoors between 10 a.m. and 2 p.m., when the sun's ultraviolet light is strongest. If you can't avoid exposure to bright sunlight, wear protective clothing and maximum-protection sunscreen products.
• Regular checkups with your health care provider are important, even when in remission.
• To learn more: Lupus Foundation of America, 2000 L St., NW, Suite 710, Washington, DC 20036; (800) 558-0121; website: www.lupus.org.

MEDICATION
• Steroid skin creams or ointments are usually prescribed. Follow instructions carefully about their use.
• Plastic tape coated with steroid, injections of steroid into affected skin, or rarely, oral steroids may be prescribed (with more severe symptoms).
• Antimalaria drugs may be prescribed. They are taken by mouth and often help the symptoms of this disorder.
• Use sunscreens for sun protection.

ACTIVITY—No limit.

DIET—No special diet.

CALL YOUR DOCTOR IF

• You or a family member has symptoms of discoid lupus erythematosus.
• The following occur during treatment:
  - New skin symptoms.
  - Swelling, redness, or pain in joints.

ILLNESS & DISORDERS

LUPUS ERYTHEMATOSUS, SYSTEMIC (SLE)

GENERAL INFORMATION

DEFINITION—An inflammatory disease that affects various parts of the body. Lupus symptoms often flare up and then subside.

BODY PARTS INVOLVED—Connective tissue (collagen). Many body systems are affected, including joints, skin, kidneys, brain, heart and lungs.

SEX OR AGE MOST AFFECTED—All ages and both sexes, but 90% of cases occur in women between ages 30 and 50.

SIGNS & SYMPTOMS
- Joint aches or pain, with redness and swelling.
- Fever and fatigue.
- Skin rash. Butterfly-like rash on the cheeks.
- Anemia (pale skin and feeling weak).
- Chest pain (with deep breathing).
- Increased sensitivity to the sun.
- Hair loss.
- Ulcers (sores) in the mouth or the nose.
- Seizures.

CAUSES—Unknown. Both genetic (hereditary) and environmental factors may contribute. It is thought to be an autoimmune disorder. In these disorders, the immune system attacks the body itself by mistake. The disease cannot be spread from one person to another.

RISK INCREASES WITH
- Females.
- Family history of lupus.
- Having other autoimmune disorders.
- Smoking.
- Genetic factors. It occurs more often among African Americans, Hispanic Americans, Native Americans, and Asians.

HOW TO PREVENT—Cannot be prevented at present.

WHAT TO EXPECT

DIAGNOSTIC MEASURES
- Your health care provider will do a physical exam and ask questions about your symptoms and activities.
- Medical tests include samples of blood to measure specific antibodies. Patients with vague, recurrent symptoms may require long-term observation and repeated testing before a final diagnosis can be made.

APPROPRIATE HEALTH CARE
- Treatment steps depend on the extent and severity of the disorder.
- Drugs are usually prescribed to treat the condition, as well as the symptoms and complications.

POSSIBLE COMPLICATIONS
- Anemia (often due to iron deficiency).
- Blood disorders and blood vessel disorders.
- Complications may occur in the heart, lung, gastrointestinal system, kidneys, joint/muscle/bone, nervous system, and eyes.
- Unable to continue regular job; changes are needed in working conditions.
- Pregnancies in SLE patients are considered high-risk.

PROBABLE OUTCOME—SLE is currently considered incurable. 20% to 30% of the cases are mild and may have only a skin rash. The majority of cases have continued remissions, flares, and relapses. The flares or relapses may occur 2 to 3 times a year. Many patients lead a normal lifestyle while in remission. Symptoms can often be relieved or controlled with treatment.

HOW TO TREAT

GENERAL MEASURES
- Obtain prompt medical treatment for any infection.
- Avoid sun exposure or use protection of hats, sunglasses, sunscreens, and long-sleeved clothing.
- Apply heat or ice to relieve joint pain.
- Control the stress in your life. Learn relaxation techniques or obtain counseling if needed.
- Talk to your health care provider if you are thinking about becoming pregnant.
- Get regular medical and dental check-ups.
- To learn more: Lupus Foundation of America, 2000 L St., NW, Suite 710, Washington, DC 20036; (800) 558-0121; website: www.lupus.org.

MEDICATION—Drugs to suppress the immune system, steroid and nonsteroidal anti-inflammatory drugs, hormones, or antimalarial drugs may be prescribed. These relieve symptoms but don't cure the disease. Other drugs may be prescribed depending on specific complications.

ACTIVITY
- Remain as active as possible. Extra rest may be needed. Exercises can help to retain range-of-motion. Exercise does not improve joint aches or fatigue.
- Physical therapy may be recommended.

DIET—Eat a healthy diet. Reduce salt intake.

CALL YOUR DOCTOR IF

- You or a family member has symptoms of systemic lupus erythematosus.
- After diagnosis, any new symptoms occur, other symptoms get worse, or drugs cause side effects.

LYME DISEASE

GENERAL INFORMATION

DEFINITION—A disorder caused by a tick bite. Most people who get Lyme disease do not become seriously ill. It is named for Lyme, Connecticut, where it was first described. It has now occurred in 48 of the 50 states.

BODY PARTS INVOLVED—Skin of the thighs, buttocks or underarms; central nervous system; heart and blood vessels; large joints, especially in the knee.

SEX OR AGE MOST AFFECTED—Both sexes; all ages.

SIGNS & SYMPTOMS
Stage 1:
• A rash (called erythema migrans) that starts as a small red spot. The spot expands and becomes round or oval in shape with a clear center. It resembles a bulls-eye.
• Mild flu-like symptoms may occur (fever, headache, stiff neck, fatigue, muscle and joint pain).
Stage 2:
• Rash develops on other places of the body.
• Single-joint pain or body pain.
• Central nervous system symptoms that may range from headache to loss of consciousness.
Stage 3 (may occur months to years after first stage):
• The nerves, joints, heart, and brain may be seriously affected causing a number of new symptoms.

CAUSES—Infection with a spirochete (a specific type of germ), *Borrelia burgdorferi*, transmitted by an infected deer tick bite. The tick bite may occur 3 to 30 days prior to the rash. The infection cannot be spread from one person to another.

RISK INCREASES WITH—Work, play, or recreational activities in states and locations at high risk for ticks. States include those in the northeast, mid-Atlantic, upper north-central United States, and some California counties. Locations include grassy, brushy, or wooded areas.

HOW TO PREVENT
• Wear protective clothing with tight collars and cuffs.
• Use effective insect repellents, such as DEET, in areas with ticks.
• Have dogs and cats wear tick-repellent collars.
• Careful skin check and removal of any ticks. If the tick is removed from the skin within 36 hours, there is usually no infection.
• Vaccines are being studied.

WHAT TO EXPECT

DIAGNOSTIC MEASURES
• Your own observation of symptoms.
• Your health care provider will do a physical exam and ask questions about your symptoms and activities.
• Medical tests may include blood studies and others to help confirm the diagnosis.

APPROPRIATE HEALTH CARE—Early treatment with antibiotic drugs is important to prevent symptoms from getting worse.

POSSIBLE COMPLICATIONS
• Various degrees of persistent joint or nervous system pain, fatigue, memory problems, and other symptoms.
• Rarely, death may occur.

PROBABLE OUTCOME—The severity differs from one person to another. Mild cases clear up on their own, without treatment. Most other cases can be treated successfully with antibiotics. In a few cases, symptoms may not respond to antibiotics. Additional treatment may help or be ineffective.

HOW TO TREAT

GENERAL MEASURES
• Use crutches to keep weight off affected joints, if necessary.
• Heat relieves joint pain. Take warm baths or showers, or use heating pads.
• To learn more: Lyme Disease Association, PO Box 1438, Jackson, NJ 08527; (888) 366-6611; website: www.lymediseaseassociation.org or American Lyme Disease Foundation, 293 Route 100, Suite 204, Somers, NY 10589; (914) 277-6970 (not toll free); website: www.aldf.com.

MEDICATION—You may be prescribed:
• An oral antibiotic (usually for 14 to 21 days) for early stage of the disease.
• Antibiotics given through a vein (IV) for later stages.
• Nonsteroidal anti-inflammatory drugs.
• Steroid drugs to reduce the inflammatory response in the heart or central nervous system.

ACTIVITY—Get extra rest until symptoms improve. Then resume normal activities gradually.

DIET—No special diet.

CALL YOUR DOCTOR IF

• You or a family member has symptoms of Lyme disease.
• New, unexplained symptoms develop.

LYMPHOGRANULOMA VENEREUM
(LGV; Lymphogranuloma Inguinale)

GENERAL INFORMATION

DEFINITION—Lymphogranuloma venereum is a contagious venereal disease that involves the genitals and lymph glands. This disease is found mostly in tropical and subtropical areas. It is rare in the United States.

BODY PARTS INVOLVED—Genitals; lymph glands.

SEX OR AGE MOST AFFECTED—Both sexes of adults, often ages 20 to 40, and more common in men.

SIGNS & SYMPTOMS
* The following symptoms begin 1 to 4 weeks after exposure and progress in order.
* A painless blister on the genitals which ulcerates (becomes an open and runny sore) and then heals quickly.
* Enlarged lymph glands in the groin that form large, red, tender masses. These are called buboes.
* Multiple areas of deep infection that discharge thick pus and blood-stained material.
* Other symptoms include:
 - Fever.
 - Muscle aches and pain, including backache.
 - Headaches.
 - Joint pain.
 - Appetite loss.
 - Vomiting.

CAUSES—A bacteria, *Chlamydia*, which is transmitted by sexual activity. This includes direct sexual contact with the genitals, rectum, or mouth.

RISK INCREASES WITH
* Travel to and sexual activity in a country where the disorder occurs frequently.
* Anal intercourse.
* Unprotected sexual activity with new partners.

HOW TO PREVENT
* Use latex condoms during sexual intercourse with new partners.
* Don't engage in sexual activity with an infected person.

WHAT TO EXPECT

DIAGNOSTIC MEASURES
* Your own observation of symptoms.
* Your health care provider will do a physical exam including the genital and rectal areas.
* Medical tests may include blood studies, a culture of the discharge from the lesions and antibody tests for *Chlamydia*. Tests for other sexually transmitted diseases are often done.

APPROPRIATE HEALTH CARE
* Treatment may include drugs, surgery, and self-care.
* Surgery may be needed for some complications. Affected lymph glands (buboes) may be drained. An abscess (a pus-filled sore) may be drained. Fistulas (an abnormal passage between two organs or from an internal organ to the body surface) may be repaired.
* Your sexual contacts should be examined also.

POSSIBLE COMPLICATIONS
* Relapse or reinfection.
* Tissue damage, scarring, rectal or intestinal blockages, and extreme swelling of the genitals.
* In severe cases, it attacks the central nervous system.
* Newborns can contract the disease from infected mothers during birth.

PROBABLE OUTCOME—Usually curable with appropriate treatment.

HOW TO TREAT

GENERAL MEASURES
* Heat applied to affected area may help discomfort.
* To learn more: Centers for Disease Control & Prevention (CDC) National STD & AIDS Hotlines (800) 227-8922; website: www.cdc.gov/std.

MEDICATION
* Antibiotics for infection will be prescribed.
* For minor discomfort, you may use nonprescription drugs such as acetaminophen.
* Stronger pain relievers may be prescribed.

ACTIVITY—After treatment, resume normal activity as soon as symptoms improve. Don't resume sexual relations until completely healed.

DIET—No special diet.

CALL YOUR DOCTOR IF

* You or a family member has symptoms of lymphogranuloma venereum.
* The following occur during treatment:
 - Temperature rises to 101°F (38.3°C) or higher.
 - Pain cannot be relieved with simple pain drugs.
* New, unexplained symptoms develop. Drugs used in treatment may produce side effects.

LYMPHOMA, NON-HODGKIN'S
(Lymphosarcoma; Reticulum Cell Sarcoma)

 GENERAL INFORMATION

DEFINITION—Non-Hodgkin's lymphomas are a group of closely related cancers that affect the lymphatic system. Hodgkin's disease is another related, yet different type, of lymphoma. Lymphoma is a term that describes cancer of the body's lymphatic system. The lymphatic system is a part of the body's immune system that fights infections and diseases.

BODY PARTS INVOLVED
• Lymphocytes (white blood cells).
• Lymph glands (glands that fight infection and produce immune substances).
• Spleen (a large lymph gland).

SEX OR AGE MOST AFFECTED—Both sexes; all ages, but more common in older men.

SIGNS & SYMPTOMS
• Swollen, non-tender, rubbery, distinct lymph glands anywhere in the body, but most often in the armpit, neck, or groin.
• Weight loss.
• General ill feeling.
• Anemia.
• Bleeding from the gastrointestinal tract.
• Jaundice (yellow skin and eyes).

CAUSES—Generally unknown. There is an association with two types of viruses: Epstein-Barr virus (EBV), and human T-cell lymphoma/leukemia virus (HTLV-1). Genetics may be a factor. Other possible causes are being researched and studied.

RISK INCREASES WITH
• Adults over 40. Males more than females.
• Weak immune system due to illness or drugs.
• Previous treatment with radiation, chemotherapy, or immune suppressing, or antispasmodic drugs.
• Work that involves exposure to carcinogens (a substance known to cause cancer).

HOW TO PREVENT—No specific preventive measures.

 WHAT TO EXPECT

DIAGNOSTIC MEASURES
• Your own observation of symptoms.
• Your health care provider will do a physical exam and ask questions about your symptoms.
• A variety of medical tests will be done to verify the exact type of cancer cells, the grade (fast or slow growing), and if the cancer has spread (called staging) to other places in the body.

APPROPRIATE HEALTH CARE
• Treatment will depend on the cancer type, grade and location, its stage, your health, age and preferences. Your health care provider will discuss your specific diagnosis and treatment recommendations with you.
• Watchful waiting may be an option. This means monitoring the cancer cells for a period of time before deciding on treatment.
• Radiotherapy and/or chemotherapy (anticancer drugs) are often the first treatment steps.
• Bone marrow or stem cell transplantation may be considered if other methods fail.
• Other treatment options include phototherapy (using ultraviolet light), biologic therapy (using the immune system) to treat the cancer, and possibly new approaches now being studied.
• Surgery is less often used as a treatment.

POSSIBLE COMPLICATIONS
• Cancer spreads to other parts of the body.
• Cancer treatments can weaken the body's immune system, which increases the risk for infections.
• Anemia.
• Recurrence of tumors after treatment.
• Any of the complications could be fatal.

PROBABLE OUTCOME—The outcome varies according to the cancer cell type, if it is slow or fast growing, if it has spread, and the individual's age and response to treatment. If one treatment is not working, there may be other options that can be tried. Treatments are constantly improving, so there is hope for cure or remission.

 HOW TO TREAT

GENERAL MEASURES—To learn more: American Cancer Society, (800) ACS-2345; website: www.cancer.org or National Cancer Institute, (800) 4-CANCER; website: www.cancer.gov.

MEDICATION
• Chemotherapy (anticancer drugs) may be prescribed. Side effects from chemotherapy may improve once the body adjusts to the drug.
• Other drugs, such as steroids, may be prescribed.

ACTIVITY—Stay as active as possible.

DIET—No special diet.

 CALL YOUR DOCTOR IF

• You or a family member has symptoms of non-Hodgkin's lymphoma.
• Any new symptoms develop during treatment or other symptoms worsen.

MALABSORPTION
(Malabsorptive Syndrome)

GENERAL INFORMATION

DEFINITION—The body is not properly absorbing nutrients (vitamins, minerals, proteins, sugars, fats, etc.) from foods. Most nutrients are absorbed through the small intestine. Malabsorption is not a disease in itself. It is a result of some other condition.

BODY PARTS INVOLVED—Intestinal tract; liver; pancreas.

SEX OR AGE MOST AFFECTED—Both sexes; all ages.

SIGNS & SYMPTOMS
- Diarrhea.
- Weakness.
- Weight loss.
- Gas with stomach discomfort and swelling.
- Bad-smelling, bulky stools, often with mucus.
- Mild anemia (pale skin and feeling weak and tired).
- Bone pain.
- Swollen hands and feet.

CAUSES—A variety of health problems can cause malabsorption. The small intestine can be affected by infections, inflammation, irritation, structural defects, injury, surgery, faults in the digestive process, congenital defects, and others.

RISK INCREASES WITH
- Lactose intolerance.
- Celiac disease.
- Crohn's disease, ulcerative colitis, or chronic diarrhea.
- Chronic pancreatitis.
- Cystic fibrosis.
- Small intestine disorders such as diverticulosis, strictures, and partial obstruction.
- Bacteria or parasite infection.
- Short bowel syndrome (due to surgery that removed half or more of the small intestine).
- Stomach or bowel surgery or radiation.
- Liver disease.
- Excess use of laxatives or antacids.
- HIV infection.
- Imbalance of minerals in the body.

HOW TO PREVENT—No specific preventive measures. Avoid risk factors where possible.

WHAT TO EXPECT

DIAGNOSTIC MEASURES
- Your own observation of symptoms.
- Your health care provider will do a physical exam and ask questions about your symptoms and activities.

- Medical tests may include blood, stool, and urine studies and x-rays of the intestinal tract. Other tests may be done to help diagnose the cause.

APPROPRIATE HEALTH CARE
- Treatment depends on the underlying cause and the needs of each patient. Steps may include special feeding methods, diet changes, or drugs.
- Some patients may need feeding through a vein (IV). This is called total parenteral nutrition (TPN).
- Some patients may need tube feeding. A tube is inserted into the stomach or the bowel for feeding.

POSSIBLE COMPLICATIONS
- Prolonged illness.
- Failure to thrive in infants.
- Additional illness caused by nutritional, vitamin, or mineral deficiency.
- Anemia.

PROBABLE OUTCOME—The degree to which symptoms can be controlled depends on the cause, but many things are common to all malabsorptive disorders. The onset is usually slow and difficult to diagnose. Disorders may be present for months or years before being recognized. Treatment is long, complicated, and may need to be changed often.

HOW TO TREAT

GENERAL MEASURES—Patience and a positive attitude are important in cure.

MEDICATION—You may be prescribed enzymes to aid digestion, antidiarrheals, antibiotics, anti-inflammatory drugs, intestinal hormones, medium chain triglycerides, vitamins and other supplements, and antacids.

ACTIVITY—As tolerated by symptoms and physical condition.

DIET—Diet changes may be prescribed. They may include milk-free, gluten-free, low-fat, no-fat, or other restrictions. You will be advised about specific diet instructions.

CALL YOUR DOCTOR IF

- You or a family member has symptoms of malabsorption.
- Any of the following occur during treatment: black, tarry bowel movements, fever of 101°F (38.3°C) or higher, severe abdominal pain, or muscle cramps.

MALARIA

GENERAL INFORMATION

DEFINITION—A serious infection caused by malarial parasites. Malaria is transmitted by a mosquito bite. Most cases of malaria in the United States are in immigrants and travelers returning from malaria-risk areas. A few cases are transmitted by blood transfusion, from mother to fetus during pregnancy, or by mosquito bite that occurred in the United States.

BODY PARTS INVOLVED—Blood cells; blood vessels; liver; central nervous system.

SEX OR AGE MOST AFFECTED—Both sexes; all ages.

SIGNS & SYMPTOMS
* Symptoms usually occur about 10 to 28 days after infection (though it can be up to a year).
* Fatigue and general ill feeling.
* Muscle and joint pain.
* Symptoms may include headache, nausea, vomiting, and diarrhea.
* Shaking chills, with a fever. This is followed by heavy sweating, along with a drop in temperature.

CAUSES—The mosquito becomes infected with malaria after biting a person with the disease. The parasites multiply in the mosquito for a week, then enter the bloodstream of the next person the mosquito bites. Once in a person's bloodstream, the parasites travel to the liver, where they thrive and multiply rapidly. After several days, thousands re-enter the bloodstream and destroy red blood cells. Some parasites remain in the liver, continue to multiply, and are released again at intervals into the bloodstream.

RISK INCREASES WITH—Living in, or travel to, any country where malaria is a risk. It is most prevalent in rural tropical areas such as found in Latin America, Asia, and Africa.

HOW TO PREVENT
* Take antimalaria drugs before visiting an area where malaria is a risk. Continue to take the drugs after you return. A travel health clinic or your health care provider can give you instructions.
* In mosquito-infested areas, wear long-sleeved shirts and pants, especially from dusk to dawn. Use a DEET insect repellent on exposed skin. Sleep under a bednet that has been dipped in permethrin insecticide.
* Contact Centers for Disease Control (CDC) traveler information about malaria risks and prevention. Toll free voice (877) FYI-TRIP or toll free to get fax information (888) 232-3299, or website: www.cdc.gov/travel.

WHAT TO EXPECT

DIAGNOSTIC MEASURES
* Your own observation of symptoms.
* Your health care provider will do a physical exam and ask questions about your symptoms and recent travels.
* Medical tests will include blood studies. Other tests may be done if complications are a concern.

APPROPRIATE HEALTH CARE
* Treatment is with drugs.
* Hospital care may be needed with severe symptoms.

POSSIBLE COMPLICATIONS
* Anemia, jaundice, or brain or kidney damage.
* Bleeding, seizures, or coma.
* Severe hypoglycemia (low blood sugar).
* Pulmonary edema (fluid in the lungs).
* Hemoglobinuria (hemoglobin in the urine).

PROBABLE OUTCOME—Curable with treatment. Symptoms usually improve in about 48 hours and fever is gone in about 4 days. Children, persons with weak immune systems, and pregnant women are more at risk for complications.

HOW TO TREAT

GENERAL MEASURES
* Protect yourself from secondary bacterial infection while you are ill with malaria. Wash your hands often.
* All cases of malaria are reported to the local health department.

MEDICATION
* One or more antimalaria drugs to kill the parasite will be prescribed. It will depend on the type of malaria diagnosed.
* Take nonprescription acetaminophen for fever.

ACTIVITY—Rest in bed until fever and chills subside. Resume your normal activities gradually as symptoms improve.

DIET—No special diet.

CALL YOUR DOCTOR IF

* You or a family member has symptoms of malaria. Symptoms may begin up to one year after returning from travel in a malaria-risk area. During your travels, you should have the name of a medical person or center to contact if symptoms develop.
* After diagnosis, weakness lasts for a prolonged time. This may indicate anemia.
* Symptoms of malaria recur after treatment.

MARFAN SYNDROME

GENERAL INFORMATION

DEFINITION—A rare, inherited connective tissue disorder. Connective tissue supports and adds strength to other body tissue and body parts such as tendons and ligaments and heart valves. The severity of the symptoms varies greatly among patients.

BODY PARTS INVOLVED—Musculoskeletal; endocrine system and metabolic system.

SEX OR AGE MOST AFFECTED—Newborns of both sexes.

SIGNS & SYMPTOMS
- Tall and thin body shape.
- Long arms and legs.
- Long, thin fingers (arachnodactyly).
- Chest deformity (may be sunken in or protrude out).
- Curved spine (scoliosis).
- High palate in the mouth and crowded teeth.
- "Double jointed;" joint weakness or looseness.
- Dislocation of eye lens, usually upward.
- Myopia (nearsighted).
- Symptoms of heart problems (e.g., shortness of breath, tiredness, irregular or rapid heart beat).
- Stretch marks on the shoulders, hips and lower back.
- Easy bruising or bleeding (uncommon).

CAUSES—Inherited disorder in about 85% of cases. Other cases occur with no known cause. The disorder is present from birth and diagnosis can sometimes be made in newborns. However, signs or symptoms are often not seen until adolescence or young adulthood.

RISK INCREASES WITH
- Advanced paternal age may be a risk in those cases that are not clearly inherited.
- Family history of Marfan syndrome.

PREVENTIVE MEASURES
- No preventive measures. Prenatal diagnosis is possible in some cases.
- Each child has a 50% chance of inheriting the disorder from an affected parent. Children may be more or less severely affected.
- Get genetic counseling if you have Marfan syndrome or there is a family history of it.

WHAT TO EXPECT

DIAGNOSTIC MEASURES
- Your health care provider will do a physical exam and ask about family medical history.
- There is no one test to diagnose Marfan syndrome. Medical tests include echocardiogram (for diagnosing heart problems) and an eye exam. Genetic testing may be done.

APPROPRIATE HEALTH CARE
- Treatment will involve a team approach that involves eye, cardiac, orthopedic, and dental care. Drugs are used to prevent complications.
- Annual screening echocardiograms are recommended beginning in adolescence in order to detect the start of any complications. X-rays of spine are needed during growth years to detect scoliosis.
- Have annual eye exams. Special lenses and eye drops or surgery may be needed for lens dislocation.
- Surgery may be needed for cardiovascular problems.
- Scoliosis may require use of brace or surgery.
- Surgery may be needed for sunken chest.
- Pregnant women with Marfan syndrome are managed as high-risk patients. Outcome is usually excellent.

POSSIBLE COMPLICATIONS
- Cardiovascular problems can be life-threatening.
- Bacterial endocarditis (heart inflammation).
- Complications of the aorta (heart artery).
- Heart and lung problems.
- Depression and anxiety.
- Retinal detachment (rare).

PROBABLE OUTCOME—Early diagnosis and steps to prevent and treat complications have helped to improve the outlook for patients. Lifespan is about the same as an average person.

HOW TO TREAT

GENERAL MEASURES—To learn more: National Marfan Foundation, 22 Manhasset Ave., Port Washington, NY 11050; (800) 862-7326; website: www.marfan.org.

MEDICATION
- Beta-blockers may be prescribed for heart problems.
- Hormones may be given prior to puberty.
- Antibiotic therapy may be prescribed.

ACTIVITY
- Fully active unless limited by symptoms. Exercise helps physical and emotional well-being. Get medical advice before starting any exercise or sports activity.
- You may be advised to avoid contact sports, activities that risk head injury, rapid decompression (scuba diving), isometric exercises (weightlifting, pull-ups, etc.).

DIET—No special diet.

CALL YOUR DOCTOR IF

- You believe your child has signs or symptoms of Marfan syndrome.
- After diagnosis, symptoms change or worsen.

MASTITIS

GENERAL INFORMATION

DEFINITION—Mastitis is a breast disorder that usually occurs in a woman who has recently given birth. It develops in about 1 to 2% of new mothers and is more likely in women who are breast-feeding. However, it can occur even in women who are not breast-feeding or pregnant.

BODY PARTS INVOLVED—Breasts.

SEX OR AGE MOST AFFECTED—Females of childbearing age.

SIGNS & SYMPTOMS
• Symptoms may occur anytime while nursing, but usually begin 1 to 5 weeks after delivery.
• Tender or painful, swollen, hard, hot area of the breast(s).
• Redness of the breasts.
• General feeling of weakness, lack of well-being.
• Fever and chills.

CAUSES—Infection from bacteria germs that enter the mother's breast. Most mastitis occurs only on one side. It is unknown exactly why some women get mastitis and others do not. Germs may gain access to the breast through a crack in the nipple, but women without sore nipples also get mastitis.

RISK INCREASES WITH
• Major risks are breast-feeding and cracked nipples.
• Women with a very abundant milk supply may be more prone to getting mastitis.
• Women who are not breast-feeding but have diabetes, chronic illness, or weak immune system.

HOW TO PREVENT
• There are no specific preventive measures.
• Wash nipples before nursing. Wash hands before touching breasts.
• Regular emptying of the breasts. Breast-feed equally from both breasts.
• If a nipple becomes sore, apply lanolin cream or other skin care products as recommended.

WHAT TO EXPECT

DIAGNOSTIC MEASURES
• Your own observation of symptoms.
• Your health care provider will do a physical exam of the breasts.
• Medical tests may be done to be sure that there are no other problems that may be causing symptoms.

APPROPRIATE HEALTH CARE—Treatment includes adequate breast emptying, rest, drinking plenty of fluids, and drug therapy, if needed.

POSSIBLE COMPLICATIONS
• Without proper treatment, or with incomplete treatment, mastitis may lead to breast abscess. This is a pus-filled infection in the breast.
• Chronic mastitis may rarely occur in women who are breast-feeding.

PROBABLE OUTCOME—Usually curable in 10 days with treatment. Symptoms will start to get better in 1 to 2 days.

HOW TO TREAT

GENERAL MEASURES
• Apply a warm compress or an ice pack (whichever feels better) to the engorged breast after feeding. Don't use ice packs within 1 hour of nursing; instead use warm compresses.
• Wear a good support bra during treatment.
• Most often, you can continue to breast-feed, even though breasts are infected. Offer the affected breast first to promote complete emptying. If needed, use a breast pump to completely empty the breast.
• Take your temperature 1 to 3 times a day at first, to check for any fever.
• Massage nipples with cocoa butter or a cream, if recommended.

MEDICATION
• Pain relievers. For minor discomfort, you may use nonprescription drugs, such as acetaminophen or ibuprofen.
• Antibiotics for infection may be prescribed. Complete the entire dosage prescribed even if symptoms improve. Breast-feeding can usually be continued while taking the drug.

ACTIVITY—Get extra rest whenever you can.

DIET—No special diet. Eat regularly and drink extra fluids.

CALL YOUR DOCTOR IF

• You or a family member has symptoms of mastitis.
• During treatment, a fever occurs, you have nausea or vomiting, feel dizzy, or faint.
• You have signs of a breast abscess. An area with redness, pain, tenderness, and fluctuance (feels like pushing on an inflated inner tube).

ILLNESS & DISORDERS

MEASLES
(Red Measles; Rubeola)

GENERAL INFORMATION

DEFINITION—A viral illness that infects the respiratory tract (lungs, throat, and nasal passages) and skin. Measles is one of the most easily spread diseases. It can occur in all ages, but usually affects children. Measles was once very common, but it is now rare in the United States due to immunization. It is still common in certain other countries in the world. Cases that occur in the United States are often in people who have become infected in other countries.

BODY PARTS INVOLVED—Skin; eyes; upper-respiratory tract.

SEX OR AGE MOST AFFECTED—All ages, but most common in children.

SIGNS & SYMPTOMS—Measles symptoms usually occur in the following sequence:
• Fever, often high.
• Fatigue.
• Appetite loss.
• Sneezing and runny nose.
• Harsh, hacking cough.
• Red eyes and sensitivity to light.
• Tiny white spots in the mouth and throat.
• Rash on the forehead and around ears that spreads to the body.

CAUSES—Measles is caused by a virus. Germs are spread by contact with an infected person, breathing in germs in the air, or touching an object with germs on it. Symptoms first appear 7 to 14 days after exposure. An infected person can spread the germs to others 4 to 5 days prior to the start of the rash and 4 to 5 days after it starts.

RISK INCREASES WITH
• People who are not immunized.
• Areas of the world that don't offer immunizations.
• Reduced protective affect of the vaccine over time. A teenager or young adult could become infected with measles if exposed.

HOW TO PREVENT
• Immunize children against measles. Prevention is important because measles can have rare, but serious, complications.
• Careful hand washing helps prevent spread of any type of germs.

WHAT TO EXPECT

DIAGNOSTIC MEASURES
• Your health care provider will do a physical exam and ask questions about your symptoms and vaccine history. Measles is usually diagnosed by the symptoms.

• A blood test may be done to confirm the diagnosis.

APPROPRIATE HEALTH CARE—There is no specific treatment for measles. Home care involves rest, relief of symptoms, and keeping the patient away from other persons that are not immune to measles.

POSSIBLE COMPLICATIONS
• Ear and chest infections.
• Pneumonia.
• Encephalitis or meningitis.
• Complications can be life-threatening.

PROBABLE OUTCOME—Symptoms usually clear up after about 3 days.

HOW TO TREAT

GENERAL MEASURES
• The eyes are more sensitive to light. Avoid reading books or watching TV for a few days.
• Use a cool-mist humidifier (if advised) to ease the cough and thin lung secretions so they can be coughed up more easily. Clean the humidifier daily.
• Children who are old enough can suck on throat lozenges, cough drops, or hard candy to help ease throat discomfort.
• If fever is 101°F (38.3°C) or higher, take steps to lower it, if the child is uncomfortable, unable to sleep, or vomiting. Use drug therapy as advised by your child's health care provider. A lukewarm bath or sponge bath may help cool a febrile child.

MEDICATION
• Use acetaminophen or ibuprofen to relieve discomfort and reduce fever. Don't give aspirin if under age 18.
• An antihistamine or calamine lotion may help relieve the itchy rash. Follow instructions on label and be sure the product is approved for the age group.

ACTIVITY—Rest may help until the fever and rash get better. Children should not return to school or daycare until 4 to 5 days after the fever and rash disappear.

DIET—No special diet. Drink extra fluids, including water, tea, lemonade, and fruit juice.

CALL YOUR DOCTOR IF

• You or your child has symptoms of measles.
• Breathing difficulty, wheezing, chest or stomach pain, earache, or vision problems occur.

MELANOMA

GENERAL INFORMATION

DEFINITION—A skin cancer that can occur on any skin or mucosal surface of the body. Melanoma can spread to other areas of the body, such as the lymph nodes, liver, lungs, and central nervous system.

BODY PARTS INVOLVED—Usually in skin of the head, neck, legs or back. It appears rarely in the eye, mouth, vagina or anus.

SEX OR AGE MOST AFFECTED—It can affect any age, usually adults, and is rare in children. It is the most common cancer in women age 25 to 29, and second to breast cancer in women ages 30 to 34.

SIGNS & SYMPTOMS
• A changing mole is the most common symptom.
• Flat or slightly raised skin lesion. It can be black, brown, blue, red, white, or a mixture of colors. Borders are often irregular. Some may bleed, itch, or cause pain.

CAUSES—Cells (melanocytes) that give skin its brownish color change into melanoma cells. It is unclear why this occurs. Melanomas may appear on normal skin or arise from a mole (nevus) or other abnormal skin area that has changed in appearance. They tend to occur at sites of sun exposure. When the cells grow down into deep skin layers, they invade blood vessels and lymph vessels and are spread to other body areas.

RISK INCREASES WITH
• Moles (more so with large numbers of moles).
• Occupations or activities involving excessive sun exposure, such as farming, athletics, or sunbathing.
• Excess sun exposure and sunburns in childhood.
• Having atypical moles (dysplastic nevi).
• Increased age.
• Genetic factors. This is most common in fair-skin, blond people. It is rare in black people.
• Weak immune system due to illness or drugs.
• Personal or family history of melanoma.
• Sunny or high altitude climates.

HOW TO PREVENT
• Wear sunglasses, broad-rimmed hats, and protective clothing. Always use a sunscreen (15 SPF or higher).
• Examine your skin regularly for changes in pigmented areas (such as moles). Ask a family member to examine your back, scalp, and soles of the feet. Get medical advice about any skin lesion (especially brown or black) that becomes multicolored, develops irregular edges or surfaces, and bleeds or changes in any way.

WHAT TO EXPECT

DIAGNOSTIC MEASURES
• Your own observation of suspicious growths.
• Your health care provider will do an exam of the affected skin area.
• Biopsy (removal of a small amount of affected skin for viewing under a microscope) aids in diagnosis. Other tests may be done to see if the cancer has spread (staging).

APPROPRIATE HEALTH CARE
• Treatment varies and depends on location and size of affected area, stage of the cancer, your health, age, and preferences. Treatment may include surgery (most often), anticancer drugs (chemotherapy), and/or radiation therapy, and biologic therapy.
• Goal of surgery is to remove as much of the skin cancer as possible. Skin graft may be done if large areas of tissue are removed. Lymph nodes may also be removed.
• Chemotherapy uses drugs, and radiation therapy uses radiation to attack the cancer cells. Biologic therapy uses the body's immune system to fight cancer.

POSSIBLE COMPLICATIONS
• Cancer spreads (metastasis) to other places in the body, which can be fatal.
• Melanoma recurs (the same site or new site).

PROBABLE OUTCOME—Varies greatly. Early melanomas that have not spread are curable with surgical removal. Once the tumor has spread to distant organs, the prognosis is poor. Symptoms can be relieved or controlled.

HOW TO TREAT

GENERAL MEASURES
• Since there is a risk of melanoma recurring, be sure to have follow-up medical exams.
• To learn more: American Cancer Society, (800) ACS-2345; website: www.cancer.org or National Cancer Institute, (800) 4-CANCER; website: www.cancer.gov.

MEDICATION
• Anticancer (chemotherapy) drugs may be prescribed.
• Biologic therapy drugs may be prescribed.

ACTIVITY—No limits.

DIET—No special diet.

CALL YOUR DOCTOR IF

• You or a family member has symptoms of melanoma.
• During or after treatment, changes occur in the same or another skin area.

MÉNIÈRE'S DISEASE

GENERAL INFORMATION

DEFINITION—A disorder of the inner ear that causes a variety of symptoms. In most cases, only one ear is involved. Ménière's is named for the French doctor who described it in 1861.

BODY PARTS INVOLVED—Semicircular canals of the inner ear, usually on one side only (80-85%).

SEX OR AGE MOST AFFECTED—It usually affects adults between ages 30 and 60, and it is slightly more common in women than men.

SIGNS & SYMPTOMS
• Original symptoms often start suddenly, and recurrent attacks may come on with no warning. Attacks may occur daily, or in some persons, just once a year. Attacks may last 30 minutes to 2 hours, or longer. Symptoms may be mild to severe.
• Vertigo (feeling that you are spinning or everything around you is spinning).
• Noises in the affected ear (tinnitus), such as roaring, ringing, or buzzing.
• Hearing loss that comes and goes and often increases over time.
• Feeling pressure or pain in the affected ear.
• Nausea, vomiting, and sweating may occur with the vertigo. Stomach discomfort, headache, and diarrhea may occur also.

CAUSES—The exact cause is unknown. There is a variety of suggested causes, and research continues.

RISK INCREASES WITH—Unknown (mostly). Salty diets, exposure to excessive noise, stress, recent viral illness, allergies, immune disorders, ear infections, or genetic factors may play a role.

HOW TO PREVENT—No specific preventive measures.

WHAT TO EXPECT

DIAGNOSTIC MEASURES
• Your own observation of symptoms.
• Your health care provider will do a physical exam and and an exam of the ear.
• Medical tests may include blood studies, balance studies, various hearing tests, and other tests to rule out other disorders with similar symptoms.

APPROPRIATE HEALTH CARE
• Treatment usually consists of lifestyle changes (such as with your diet) and drugs, or sometimes surgery, to relieve the symptoms.
• Different types of surgery may be recommended for severe symptoms or to prevent further hearing loss.

POSSIBLE COMPLICATIONS
• Permanent hearing loss.
• Chronic tinnitus.
• The symptoms can affect all aspects of a person's life.

PROBABLE OUTCOME—There is no cure. Attacks of Ménière's disease recur and worsen over many years. Symptoms can often be relieved with one or more types of treatment. The disorder is frustrating, but not life-threatening.

HOW TO TREAT

GENERAL MEASURES
• During an attack, lie flat on a surface that does not move. Avoid bright lights. Focus eyes on an object that does not move. Don't eat or drink (to avoid nausea). Once the attack passes, get up slowly. You may feel sleepy and want to sleep for awhile.
• Learn techniques to control stress in your life. This helps some people with Ménière's.
• Avoid noisy places or situations.
• Quit smoking. Find a way to stop that works.
• To learn more: Ear Foundation/ Ménière's Network, 1817 Patterson St., Nashville. TN 37203; (800) 545-4327; website: www.earfoundation.com.

MEDICATION—You may be prescribed:
• Antinausea drugs, to reduce nausea and vomiting.
• Scopolamine patches, to treat nausea.
• Tranquilizers, to reduce dizziness.
• Antihistamines, to help lessen symptoms.
• Diuretics, to decrease fluid in the inner ear.
• Antibiotics placed in the middle ear.
• Drugs, to suppress the immune system.

ACTIVITY—Don't drive, climb ladders, or work around dangerous machinery.

DIET
• Salt causes the body to retain fluid. By decreasing salt in your diet, it will help to reduce the amount of fluid in the inner ear.
• Limit the use of caffeine and alcohol.

CALL YOUR DOCTOR IF

• You or a family member has symptoms of Ménière's disease.
• The following occur during treatment: decreased hearing in either ear, persistent vomiting, fever of 101°F (38.3°C) or higher.
• New, unexplained symptoms develop. Drugs used in treatment may produce side effects.

MENINGITIS, ASEPTIC
(Viral Meningitis)

 GENERAL INFORMATION

DEFINITION—An infection of the thin membranes that cover the brain and the spinal cord. Aseptic means it is nonbacterial. This infection can be spread from one person to another. It is more common in group settings such as young children in daycare, football team members, college students, and people who live in group care facilities.

BODY PARTS INVOLVED—Brain; spinal cord.

SEX OR AGE MOST AFFECTED—Both sexes; all ages.

SIGNS & SYMPTOMS
- Fever.
- Headache, sometimes severe.
- Irritability.
- Eyes become more sensitive to light.
- Stiff neck.
- Vomiting.
- Confusion, lethargy, and drowsiness.

CAUSES
- While this disorder is most often caused by a virus, other types of germs can be the cause. The most common cause is a group of viruses called enteroviruses. Less often, herpes virus, mumps virus, HIV, and other viruses may be the cause. Germs are spread by contact with an infected person, or touching an object with germs on it and then touching the mouth, nose, or eyes.
- Other causes include tuberculosis, various fungi, certain diseases, parasites, exposure to certain chemicals, and some drugs.

RISK INCREASES WITH
- Weak immune system due to illness or drugs.
- Group homes, daycare, or schools where outbreaks may occur.

HOW TO PREVENT
- Keep immunizations up-to-date against viruses such as mumps, measles, and chickenpox. Currently, there is no vaccine for the enteroviruses.
- Wash hands carefully to prevent the spread of any type of germs.

 WHAT TO EXPECT

DIAGNOSTIC MEASURES
- Your health care provider will do a physical exam and ask about your symptoms and activities.
- Medical tests may include blood studies, a stool culture, and others to confirm the diagnosis.

APPROPRIATE HEALTH CARE
- No specific drugs exist to treat aseptic meningitis caused by enteroviruses. The body defenses will normally cure the disorder. Treatment involves getting extra bed rest, drinking fluids, treating symptoms such as fever.
- If symptoms are severe, hospital care may be needed.

POSSIBLE COMPLICATIONS—Complications are rare. They may occur in those with weak immune systems or the very young.

PROBABLE OUTCOME—Most patients recover fully in 5 to 14 days. In some people, symptoms such as fatigue or lightheadedness may persist longer.

 HOW TO TREAT

GENERAL MEASURES—None specific.

MEDICATION
- Nonprescription drugs for fever, nausea, or minor pain may be used.
- Antibiotics may be given if there is a possibility the meningitis is caused by a bacterial infection.
- Drugs may be prescribed for other causes of the meningitis once they are identified.

ACTIVITY
- Get extra rest. Begin to resume your normal activities as soon as symptoms improve.
- Children should stay home from school or daycare until symptoms improve.

DIET—No special diet. Drink plenty of fluids daily, even if you don't feel like it.

 CALL YOUR DOCTOR IF

- You or a family member has symptoms of aseptic meningitis.
- Symptoms don't improve in a week.

MENINGITIS, BACTERIAL
(Spinal Meningitis)

 GENERAL INFORMATION

DEFINITION—Bacterial infection or inflammation of the thin membranes (meninges) and fluid surrounding the brain and spinal cord. It is a life-threatening disorder, and prompt treatment is vital.

BODY PARTS INVOLVED—Central nervous system.

SEX OR AGE MOST AFFECTED—Both sexes; all ages, but more severe in persons under age 2 or over age 60.

SIGNS & SYMPTOMS
* Fever, chills, and sweating.
* Headache.
* Irritability.
* Eyes sensitive to light; pupils may be of different sizes.
* Stiff neck.
* Vomiting.
* Red or purple skin rash (associated with one kind of bacteria).
* Confusion, lethargy, drowsiness, or unconsciousness.
* Sore throat or other signs of respiratory (nose, throat, and lungs) illness may occur before other symptoms.
* Poor feeding in infants.
* Seizures.

CAUSES—An infection usually caused by one of three types of bacteria. *Haemophilus influenzae type b* (Hib), *Neisseria meningitidis,* or *Streptococcus pneumoniae.* (Routine vaccines for children have lowered the risk of Hib infection.) Bacterial germs are spread by close contact with an infected person. The infection may start in another body part, such as the lung, ear, nose, throat, or sinus that spreads to the meninges.

RISK INCREASES WITH
* Newborns, infants, young people, and adults over 60.
* Ear, sinus, respiratory, or tooth infections.
* Weak immune system due to illness or drugs.
* Head injury.
* Close contact with a person with meningitis.
* People with cochlear implants (hearing devices).

HOW TO PREVENT
* Get medical care for treatment of any infection in your body to prevent its spread.
* Avoid contact with anyone who has meningitis (depending on bacterial type). Those who have had close contact with a person with meningitis may need preventive antibiotic treatment even if they have no symptoms.

 WHAT TO EXPECT

DIAGNOSTIC MEASURES
* Your health care provider will do a physical exam and ask questions about the symptoms.
* Medical tests may include blood studies, culture of cerebrospinal fluid, x-rays, CT, and others to confirm the diagnosis.

APPROPRIATE HEALTH CARE
* Hospital care is usually needed, sometimes in an intensive care unit.
* Treatment involves antibiotics, supportive care for symptoms, and steps to prevent complications.

POSSIBLE COMPLICATIONS—Permanent brain damage including paralysis, hearing loss, speech difficulty, seizures, and mental impairment. It could be fatal.

PROBABLE OUTCOME—Full recovery is likely in 2 to 3 weeks with prompt treatment and if no complications arise.

 HOW TO TREAT

GENERAL MEASURES—The family should stay in close contact with the patient's medical team and help by making their visits with the patient as supportive as possible.

MEDICATION
* Antibiotics will be give through a vein (IV).
* Steroids may be prescribed. They help prevent the risk of hearing loss.
* Anticonvulsants may be used to treat or prevent seizures.

ACTIVITY—After a 2 to 3-week period of recovery, you should be as active as your strength allows.

DIET—You may be given intravenous nutrients in the hospital. At home, eat a normal, well-balanced diet.

 CALL YOUR DOCTOR IF

* You or a family member has symptoms of bacterial meningitis. Get emergency help if needed.
* You have had contact with someone who has meningitis.

MENOPAUSE

GENERAL INFORMATION

DEFINITION—Menopause is the permanent cessation of menstruation. It can occur as early as age 40 or as late as early 60s. It usually spans 1 to 2 years. Menopause is only one event in the "climacteric." This is a biological change in all body tissue and body systems that occurs in both sexes between the mid-40s and mid-60s. Menopause that occurs before age 40 is termed premature. Menopause does not occur suddenly. Perimenopause usually begins a few years before the last menstrual cycle.

BODY PARTS INVOLVED—Female reproductive system, with secondary effects in other body parts.

SEX OR AGE MOST AFFECTED—Women, especially between ages 45 and 50.

SIGNS & SYMPTOMS
• Some women may go through menopause without having symptoms. In most women, both physical and emotional symptoms occur.
• Irregular menstrual periods.
• Hot flashes or flushes and night sweats. These are sensations of heat spreading from the waist or chest toward the neck, face, and upper arms. The medical term is vasomotor symptoms.
• Headaches.
• Dizziness.
• Rapid or irregular heartbeat.
• Vaginal itching, burning, or pain with intercourse.
• Bloating in the upper abdomen.
• Irritable bladder (urge to urinate).
• Tender breasts.
• Mood changes, including tension and anxiety.
• Sleeping difficulty.
• Changes in sex drive.
• Depression, feeling sad or down, and fatigue.

CAUSES
• A normal decline in ovary function. This results in decreased levels of the female hormones, estrogen and progesterone.
• Surgical removal of both ovaries.
• Medical treatment of endometriosis or cancer.

RISK INCREASES WITH—Menopause is a natural part of the aging process for women. Smoking and hysterectomy are risks for premature menopause.

HOW TO PREVENT—No prevention needed.

WHAT TO EXPECT

DIAGNOSTIC MEASURES—Your health care provider can determine if it is menopause by your age and symptoms. It is often diagnosed in females after 1 year of no menstrual periods.

APPROPRIATE HEALTH CARE
• No specific treatment is usually needed.
• Counseling may be helpful if emotional changes interfere with personal relationships or work.

POSSIBLE COMPLICATIONS
• Reduced skin elasticity and vaginal moisture.
• Higher risk of hardening of the arteries, heart disease, stroke, and osteoporosis after menopause.
• Changes in feelings of self-worth.

PROBABLE OUTCOME—Menopause is a normal process, not an illness. Most women adapt without major problems or concerns.

HOW TO TREAT

GENERAL MEASURES
• Continue to use birth-control measures until 12 months after your last menstrual period.
• Reduce stress in your life as much as possible. Acupuncture, meditation, and relaxation techniques are all helpful ways to reduce any stress of menopause.
• Women who smoke start menopause about two years earlier than nonsmokers do. If you smoke, talk to your health care provider about programs to help you quit.
• To learn more: The North American Menopause Society, P.O. Box 94527, Cleveland, OH 44101; (800) 774-5342; website: www.menopause.org.

MEDICATION
• Estrogen therapy alone or combination with progestogen are options for treating hot flashes. Hormone therapy has benefits as well as risks. The decision is made by a woman and her health care provider.
• Antidepressants may be prescribed for hot flashes.
• Herbal (or those termed natural remedies) help some women. Discuss these with your health care provider.
• Drugs to prevent and/or treat loss of bone density may be prescribed.
• Take calcium supplements and vitamin D if needed.
• For vaginal dryness, use nonprescription vaginal lubricants or vaginal moisturizers.

ACTIVITY—No limits. Exercise helps your well-being. Weight-bearing activities (such as walking) help bone strength.

DIET—Eat a well-balanced diet.

CALL YOUR DOCTOR IF

• You or a family member has menopause symptoms that cause concern.
• Bleeding 6 months or more after last period.

MENORRHAGIA

GENERAL INFORMATION

DEFINITION—Menorrhagia is a common disorder that involves heavy blood loss during menstruation. The average amount of blood loss during a normal menstrual period is about two ounces. With menorrhagia, a woman may lose three ounces or more. Menorrhagia is more a symptom of a disease or condition rather than a disorder in itself.

BODY PARTS INVOLVED—Female reproductive system.

SEX OR AGE MOST AFFECTED—Females from age 12 to 55.

SIGNS & SYMPTOMS
• Menstrual periods have been extra heavy for several months in a row.
• Menstrual periods last for more than 7 days.
• Passing of large clots of blood.
• Paleness and fatigue (anemia).

CAUSES—The menstrual cycle is a process (series of events) that occurs in a woman's body each month. Different factors can disrupt the process and lead to menorrhagia.

RISK INCREASES WITH
• Women near menopause or young women who do not have a regular menstrual cycle.
• Hormone imbalance (estrogen and progesterone).
• Infections of the genitals or urinary tract. This includes sexually transmitted diseases.
• Kidney, liver, or thyroid disease.
• Pituitary tumors, polycystic ovarian syndrome, or blood vessel problems.
• Ectopic pregnancy or a miscarriage.
• Ovarian dysfunction (ovaries do not produce eggs).
• Fibroids (benign uterine tumors).
• Endometriosis or endometrial hyperplasia.
• Cervical or uterine polyps.
• Intrauterine device (IUD).
• Bleeding disorders.
• Drugs (steroids, blood thinners or anticancer).
• Obesity or being overweight.
• Rarely, cancer of the uterus or cervix.

HOW TO PREVENT—No preventive measures.

WHAT TO EXPECT

DIAGNOSTIC MEASURES
• Your health care provider will do a physical exam and a pelvic exam and ask about your symptoms.
• Medical tests may include Pap smear, pregnancy test, blood test, ultrasound, and hysteroscopy (using an instrument to see inside the uterus). Liver, kidney, and thyroid function tests, and endometrial biopsy (removal of a small amount of tissue for microscope exam) may be done.

APPROPRIATE HEALTH CARE
• Treatment usually depends on the age of the woman, her desires for fertility, and any other medical disorder. Treatment steps may include drugs or surgery.
• Stop using an IUD. Use another birth control method.
• Surgery options may include endometrial ablation or endometrial resection, dilatation and curettage (D & C), uterine fibroid embolization, or hysterectomy. The options, risks, and benefits will be explained to you.

POSSIBLE COMPLICATIONS
• Anemia due to excess blood loss. Menorrhagia is a common cause of anemia in premenopausal women.
• Surgery may be required.
• Sometimes, bleeding is so severe that it interrupts normal daily routines like work, school, and social life.
• Other complications are related to the causes.

PROBABLE OUTCOME—Varies with cause of the bleeding. Treatment helps reduce the bleeding in most women.

HOW TO TREAT

GENERAL MEASURES—For self-care, wear extra sanitary pads during heavy flow. If a tampon is used, change tampon every 4 to 6 hours. Avoid scented pads and tampons. Don't douche.

MEDICATION
• Use nonsteroidal anti-inflammatory drugs, such as naproxen or ibuprofen, to relieve pain and possibly reduce bleeding. Avoid aspirin (may prolong bleeding).
• One or more types of hormones to control the bleeding may be prescribed.
• If hormones cannot be taken for some reason, other drugs to control the bleeding may be recommended.
• Iron replacement may be prescribed for anemia.
• If a drug you take is the cause, a change in drug or a change in dosage amounts may be recommended.

ACTIVITY—Resting with feet up may help during heavy periods.

DIET—No special diet.

CALL YOUR DOCTOR IF

• You or a family member has signs or symptoms of menorrhagia.
• Symptoms worsen or new symptoms develop after treatment begins.

MENTAL RETARDATION

GENERAL INFORMATION

DEFINITION—Below average, general intellectual functioning along with an inability to adapt to the normal aspects of daily life in a person under age 18. Intellectual functioning is typically measured by an intelligence quotient (IQ) test (if the person can take an IQ test). Those with mental retardation score 70 to 75 or below. The normal range is 80 to 130 (100 is average). Retardation is classified as mild (IQ 50 to 70), moderate (IQ 35 to 49), severe (20 to 34), or profound (IQ less than 20). Mild retardation is the most common form (over 80% of cases). Mildly retarded children may not be identified until they start school. Profoundly and severely retarded children are often diagnosed at birth. Males are affected more than females.

BODY PARTS INVOLVED—All.

SEX OR AGE MOST AFFECTED—Both sexes; all ages.

SIGNS & SYMPTOMS
- Failure to meet developmental milestones. These are physical and behavioral signs of development or maturation of infants and children.
- Persistence of infantile behavior.
- Lack of curiosity.
- Decreased learning ability.
- Inability to meet educational demands of school.
- Behaviors may include: being aggressive, dependent, passive, stubborn; having low self-esteem, injures self; frustrates easily; mood disorders; attention difficulties.
- Physical traits may include: shortness in size, malformed ears and eyes, seizures, and birthmarks.

CAUSES
- Genetic—Inborn errors of metabolism or chromosome disorders. Down syndrome is the most frequent genetic disorder causing mental retardation.
- Intrauterine—Congenital infections, placental-fetal malfunction, complications of pregnancy (infections, preeclampsia, eclampsia, maternal alcohol or drug abuse or poor diet).
- Perinatal (just before the birth)—Prematurity, postmaturity, birth injury, and metabolic disorders.
- Postnatal (after birth)—Endocrine or metabolic disorders, infection, trauma, toxic, and other causes of brain damage, or abuse.

RISK INCREASES WITH—Risk factors are related to the causes.

HOW TO PREVENT
- Genetic counseling and prenatal genetic testing for families with a history of mental retardation.
- During pregnancy, get good prenatal care; eat healthy; avoid smoking, alcohol, or other drugs of abuse.
- Screening of newborns for metabolic disorders.
- Protect children from injury, poisoning, or abuse.

WHAT TO EXPECT

DIAGNOSTIC MEASURES
- Your own observation of symptoms.
- Your child's health care provider will do a physical exam and certain mental tests (if the child is old enough) to help with the diagnosis. You will be asked about your own observation of signs in your child.

APPROPRIATE HEALTH CARE—Goals are to develop the child's potential to the fullest. Retardation cannot be reversed, but much can be done to help the child function as normally as possible. Beginning in infancy, special education with social and behavioral training can enhance the child's skills. Care of a retarded person is educational, not medical.

POSSIBLE COMPLICATIONS
- Child has emotional and behavioral problems.
- Stresses placed on the family.

PROBABLE OUTCOME
- Mildly retarded people can learn to lead independent, productive lives.
- Moderately retarded people are trainable, but often require protective care (e.g., group home).
- More severely and profoundly retarded people usually require continuous care.

HOW TO TREAT

GENERAL MEASURES
- The diagnosis has a profound effect on the family. It will affect every aspect of their lives. Counseling and/or spiritual support are both helpful for parents to learn to accept and cope. Joining a support group for families of children with mental retardation can help also.
- To learn more: The Arc of the United States, 1010 Wayne Ave., Suite 650, Silver Springs, MD 20910; (800) 433-5255; website: www.thearc.org.

MEDICATION—Drugs for medical problems, such as seizures may be prescribed.

ACTIVITY—As fully active as child's physical condition permits.

DIET—No special diet.

CALL YOUR DOCTOR IF

You are concerned about your child's development.

METABOLIC SYNDROME
(Insulin Resistance Syndrome; Syndrome X)

 GENERAL INFORMATION

DEFINITION—Metabolic syndrome is not just a specific disorder. Rather it is a group (or cluster) of five health risks. Having any three of these five health risks would mean that you have the syndrome. A person with metabolic syndrome is more likely to have heart disease, stroke, and diabetes in the future. The health risks include:
* Abdominal obesity.
* Elevated fasting blood triglycerides (a type of fat).
* Low levels of HDL, or "good" cholesterol.
* High fasting blood sugar (glucose) or high insulin.
* High blood pressure.

BODY PARTS INVOLVED—Heart and blood vessels (cardiovascular system) and others.

SEX OR AGE MOST AFFECTED—Both sexes, children, adolescents, and adults.

SIGNS & SYMPTOMS—Usually, there are no physical symptoms.

CAUSES—The exact cause of the syndrome is not known. It may be due to a combination of genetic makeup (that you inherit from your parents) and lifestyle choices of diet and physical activity.

RISK INCREASES WITH—Studies are ongoing to see who may be at risk for metabolic syndrome. It does occur more often in Hispanics than in whites or African Americans.

HOW TO PREVENT
* Eat a healthy diet.
* Exercise routinely.
* Don't use tobacco in any form.
* Maintain a healthy body weight.

 WHAT TO EXPECT

DIAGNOSTIC MEASURES—Your health care provider will order certain medical tests and go over the results with you. Metabolic syndrome is diagnosed if you have three or more of the following:
* Waistline of 40 inches or more for men and 35 inches or more for women (measured across the belly).
* Blood pressure of 130/85 mm Hg or higher.
* Triglyceride level above 150 mg/dL.
* Fasting blood glucose (sugar) level greater than 100 mg/dL.
* HDL, the "good" cholesterol, less than 40 mg/dL (men) or under 50 mg/dL (women).

APPROPRIATE HEALTH CARE—You and your health care provider can decide on an action plan to reduce your risks of heart disease and stroke. This may include changes in diet, getting more exercise, weight loss, stopping smoking, and perhaps drug therapy.

POSSIBLE COMPLICATIONS—If not treated, the syndrome often leads to early heart disease, stroke, and other vascular (blood vessel) problems, as well as diabetes. The more risk factors you have, the more likely you are to have complications.

PROBABLE OUTCOME—Lifestyle changes involving your diet, weight loss, exercise, and drugs (if needed) can usually reverse the risk factors.

 HOW TO TREAT

GENERAL MEASURES
* Diet and life-style changes do not mean you have to give up all the good things you enjoy. Even moderate changes can have a big impact on your risk factors.
* To learn more: American Heart Association, 7272 Greenville Ave., Dallas, TX 75231; (800) 242-8721; website: www.americanheart.org.

MEDICATION
* Drugs may be prescribed to lower cholesterol and lower high blood pressure.
* Weight loss drugs may be prescribed for a short time.

ACTIVITY—Increase physical activity. Try to get at least 30 minutes of aerobic exercise (such as walking) every day.

DIET
* Limit foods that contain saturated fats and high amounts of cholesterol. Read food labels carefully.
* Eat plenty of fruits and vegetables and high-fiber foods.
* Begin a weight-reduction diet if you are overweight.

 CALL YOUR DOCTOR IF

* You or a family member wants more information about the metabolic syndrome.
* You need help with diet and exercise planning.

METATARSALGIA

GENERAL INFORMATION

DEFINITION—Metatarsalgia is a general term for pain under the ball of the foot. The ball is the bottom, front part of the foot behind the toes. It is a common problem that can be very painful, but is usually not serious.

BODY PARTS INVOLVED—Muscles, ligaments, and bones of the foot.

SEX OR AGE MOST AFFECTED—Both sexes, usually adults ages 30-80.

SIGNS & SYMPTOMS
• Pain, dull ache, or burning feeling in the ball of one or both feet.
• It hurts when walking and feels better when you rest.
• It is described as feeling like "have a stone in your shoe" or "walking on pebbles."
• Toes may be painful, or feel numb and tingly.
• Foot may be swollen.

CAUSES—There are five metatarsal bones in the foot that run from the arch to the toe joint. These bones take a lot of pressure when you walk, jump, or run. Anything that puts extra pressure on the front of the foot can cause metatarsalgia.

RISK INCREASES WITH
• High-impact sports that involve running or jumping.
• Wearing shoes that do not fit correctly, are poorly made, or are worn-out.
• For women, wearing high heels, and shoes that are too tight across the ball of the foot.
• Certain foot shapes (such as high arches) or other foot problems.
• With aging, the fat pad in the foot tends to thin out.
• Certain medical problems, such as diabetes.
• Obesity.

HOW TO PREVENT
• Wear good shoes that fit well and are right for the activity.
• Start slowly with any new exercise or sports routines.
• Weight loss may help if overweight.

WHAT TO EXPECT

DIAGNOSTIC MEASURES
• Your own observation of symptoms.
• Consult your health care provider if self-treatment does not help to improve the symptoms. Your health care provider will examine the foot, and ask questions about symptoms, your activities, and the that shoes you wear.
• An x-ray may be taken to make sure there is no bone fracture.

APPROPRIATE HEALTH CARE
• Self care is often all that is needed.
• Special shoes, or special shoe inserts (called orthotics), may be prescribed.
• Surgery may help if there is a problem such as bunions, hammertoes, or a pinched nerve.

POSSIBLE COMPLICATIONS—Without treatment, the foot joint may be less flexible and grow stiff. Pain may increase.

PROBABLE OUTCOME—Lifestyle changes involving your diet, weight loss, exercise, and drugs (if needed) can usually reverse the risk factors.

HOW TO TREAT

GENERAL MEASURES
• Rest with your feet elevated (raised up) after periods of standing or walking.
• Rub an ice pack over the painful area for about 15 minutes at a time, several times a day.
• Switch to heat after a day or two if it feels better. Use a heating pad or soak your feet in warm water.
• Do simple stretches while seated:
  - Place heels on floor, swing toes in and then out.
  - Lift one leg straight and flex ankle by pointing toes up and then toward the floor; repeat with other leg.
• Wear adhesive felt, gel, or foam padding around toe area. Cushioned insoles, metatarsal pads, or arch supports may help. These can be found at most drug stores.
• Wear shoes that fit well and have plenty of toe room.

MEDICATION—For minor pain, you may use nonprescription pain drugs, such as ibuprofen.

ACTIVITY
• Limit activities until the symptoms improve.
• Try swimming or bicycling instead of running or walking while you have the symptoms.

DIET—No special diet.

CALL YOUR DOCTOR IF

• You or a family member has metatarsalgia symptoms that have lasted several days or are very painful.
• Pain or discomfort gets worse despite treatment.

ILLNESS & DISORDERS

MISCARRIAGE
(Spontaneous Abortion)

 GENERAL INFORMATION

DEFINITION—Loss of a pregnancy prior to the 20th week is generally considered a miscarriage. It happens in about 20% to 30% of first pregnancies. It may occur so early that the woman is unaware that she is pregnant. Many miscarriages are only "threatened." The pregnancy continues to term.

BODY PARTS INVOLVED—Reproductive system.

SEX OR AGE MOST AFFECTED—Women of childbearing age.

SIGNS & SYMPTOMS
- Uterine cramps.
- Vaginal bleeding (from slight to heavy).

CAUSES—There are many reasons pregnancy ends in miscarriage. Sometimes, no cause is found. Most miscarriages occur because a pregnancy is not developing normally.

RISK INCREASES WITH
The first trimester (first 12 weeks of pregnancy):
- Genetic defect (chromosomal disorder such as Down syndrome) or structural abnormalities of the fetus.
- Uterine abnormalities that prevent the fertilized egg from growing normally.
- Smoking.
The second trimester (13 to 28 weeks of pregnancy):
- Uterine abnormalities that cause detachment of the fetus and placenta.
- Severe stress (physical or emotional).
Anytime:
- Use of substance that harms fetus (cocaine, tobacco).
- Infections, such as viral infections.
- Trauma or severe medical conditions.
- Having certain chronic disorders.

HOW TO PREVENT—Cannot always be prevented. To reduce risk:
- Obtain regular medical checkups.
- Eat a normal, well-balanced diet.
- Avoid alcohol, smoking, or substances of abuse.
- Don't use nonprescription drugs or herbal products without medical advice.

 WHAT TO EXPECT

DIAGNOSTIC MEASURES—Ultrasound exam may be needed for diagnosis. If a fetal heartbeat can be seen, this means that there is a good chance that the pregnancy will proceed normally. When the ultrasound scan shows certain problems or abnormalities with the fetus, nothing can be done to save the pregnancy.

APPROPRIATE HEALTH CARE
- Surgery may be done to remove any remaining tissue or a dead fetus. D & C (dilatation and curettage), or D & E (dilatation and evacuation) may be needed.
- For a threatened miscarriage, follow your obstetric provider's orders. Bed rest at home may help stabilize the pregnancy. Bleeding may be severe, requiring hospital care and blood transfusion.
- Counseling for patient and partner may be helpful.

POSSIBLE COMPLICATIONS
- Uterine infection (fever, chills, and aching).
- Hemorrhaging (bleeding).
- "Incomplete" abortion, in which some placenta or fetal tissue remains in the uterus, or missed abortion, in which the fetus dies but remains in the uterus.

PROBABLE OUTCOME
- With treatment, a miscarriage is not life-threatening. It usually does not affect a woman's ability to carry a healthy baby to term in the future.
- Feelings of loss and grief are common. Feelings of guilt may also be present.

 HOW TO TREAT

GENERAL MEASURES—Following a miscarriage:
- Expect a small amount of vaginal bleeding or spotting for 8 to 10 days. Avoid tampons for 2 to 4 weeks.
- Wait through 2 or 3 normal menstrual cycles (or as advised) before attempting to become pregnant again.

MEDICATION
- A drug to control bleeding may be given.
- Pain relievers may be prescribed.
- Antibiotics may be prescribed for an infection.
- An Rh-negative female may be given RhoD (immune globulin).

ACTIVITY
- For a threatened miscarriage: Rest in bed until symptoms disappear. Avoid sexual intercourse.
- After a miscarriage: Reduce activity and rest often during the next 48 hours.

DIET—Usually no special diet. Follow any medical advice.

 CALL YOUR DOCTOR IF

- You or a family member has vaginal bleeding during pregnancy.
- Bleeding and cramps worsen, or you pass tissue, or fever and chills occur.

MITRAL VALVE PROLAPSE

 GENERAL INFORMATION

DEFINITION—A disorder in which a slight deformity of the mitral valve can produce a degree of leakage of blood. The mitral valve is located in the left side of the heart. Mitral valve prolapse (MVP) causes a heart "click" or murmur that may be heard through a stethoscope (an instrument used for listening to body sounds).

BODY PARTS INVOLVED—Heart.

SEX OR AGE MOST AFFECTED—Both sexes; all ages. In the past, more women than men were diagnosed. Recent studies show that it may affect men and women equally.

SIGNS & SYMPTOMS
• Often no symptoms are present (about 60% of cases) and the condition may be discovered on a routine physical exam. When symptoms do occur, they may vary from a few that are mild to having many symptoms. The symptoms are sometimes referred to as mitral valve prolapse syndrome (MVPS).
• Chest pain (sharp, dull, or pressing).
• Fatigue, shortness of breath.
• Dizziness.
• Lightheadedness when getting up from a chair or bed.
• Heart palpitations.
• Anxiety and panic attacks.
• Migraines.

CAUSES—The mitral valve is one of four heart valves that keep blood flowing in one direction. Prolapse means that openings (called leaflets) in the valve don't close as firmly as they should. This allows a small amount of blood to leak and cause the murmur. Why MVP occurs is unknown. The condition may be inherited or due to another disease.

RISK INCREASES WITH
• Family history of heart valve disorders.
• Connective tissue disorders (e.g., systemic lupus erythematosus, Marfan syndrome, and others).
• Other heart conditions and some muscle disorders.

HOW TO PREVENT—No preventive measures.

 WHAT TO EXPECT

DIAGNOSTIC MEASURES
• Your own observation of symptoms.
• Your health care provider may do a physical exam and listen to the sounds of the heart.
• Medical tests may include an echocardiogram (heart function test) to confirm the diagnosis.

APPROPRIATE HEALTH CARE
• Treatment is usually not needed. A medical follow-up may be done every few years to check for proper heart function.
• In some cases where there is more leakage, drugs and lifestyle changes may be recommended for treatment.
• Surgery for valve replacement may be recommended in a few cases.
• If other symptoms such as fatigue, anxiety, or panic attacks occur, your health care provider can discuss treatment options.

POSSIBLE COMPLICATIONS
• Excess blood may leak backward through the mitral valve (called mitral regurgitation).
• Endocarditis (inflammation of the heart valves and heart lining).
• Stroke.
• Sudden death.

PROBABLE OUTCOME—MVP is usually a benign disorder that needs no treatment and does not prevent a normal active life. Complications are rare.

 HOW TO TREAT

GENERAL MEASURES—Be reassured that for most people, the condition is benign and requires no treatment except follow-up evaluation.

MEDICATION
• Antibiotics may be recommended for some patients prior to any dental work or certain types of surgery.
• Other drugs may be prescribed depending on specific symptoms or to prevent complications.

ACTIVITY
• Daily aerobic exercise is helpful for most patients.
• Athletes with MVP who have many symptoms may be restricted from some types of sports.

DIET
• Weight-loss diet is suggested for overweight patients.
• Avoiding caffeine and alcohol may be recommended.

 CALL YOUR DOCTOR IF

• You or a family member has signs or symptoms of mitral valve prolapse.
• Symptoms worsen or new symptoms occur after diagnosis.

ILLNESS & DISORDERS

MOLLUSCUM CONTAGIOSUM

 GENERAL INFORMATION

DEFINITION—A contagious, viral infection of the skin.

BODY PARTS INVOLVED—Skin anywhere on the body. The virus usually occurs on the face in children. In adults, it usually occurs on the inner thighs, abdomen and genitals.

SEX OR AGE MOST AFFECTED—Both sexes; all ages.

SIGNS & SYMPTOMS
* Small, raised bumps (papules) on the skin.
* Bumps are firm, smooth, domed with a central pit, and skin-colored or white. The skin over the bumps is transparent and thin.
* Bumps cause eye irritation if they are on the eyelids.
* Affected area does not hurt or itch.

CAUSES—A virus of the pox group. The germs are spread by person-to-person contact. This virus may be spread sexually. The time period from being exposed to having symptoms is usually 2 to 7 weeks. It may also be spread by touching objects that have the germs on them, such as shared clothing, towels, wash cloths, and sports equipment.

RISK INCREASES WITH
* Other allergies or a family history of allergy.
* Use of drugs that cause a weak immune system.
* Outbreaks have been reported among children using swimming pools.

HOW TO PREVENT
* Practice good personal hygiene.
* Avoid sexual contact with infected people. It is unclear if condoms are effective in preventing spread.
* After diagnosis, to prevent spread to other parts of the body or to other people, don't scratch bumps.

 WHAT TO EXPECT

DIAGNOSTIC MEASURES
* Your own observation of symptoms.
* Your health care provider can diagnose the disorder by a skin exam of the affected area.
* If needed, the diagnosis can be confirmed with a skin scraping and microscopic study.

APPROPRIATE HEALTH CARE
* Treatment is not always needed. In some cases, drugs may be recommended for treatment.
* Bumps may be removed with surgery. Options include cutting, burning electrically or chemically, or by freezing.

POSSIBLE COMPLICATIONS—Usually none. Scarring or disfigurement are rare.

PROBABLE OUTCOME—Outcome is good. They heal on their own without treatment in otherwise healthy people. It will take about 10 to 24 months. Treatment helps to prevent their spread to other persons and to speed up the healing time.

 HOW TO TREAT

GENERAL MEASURES
* After treatment with liquid nitrogen, leave the blisters alone. The tops will come off spontaneously in 7 to 14 days.
* Keep blisters dry. Cover with small adhesive bandages any that may be irritated by clothing.

MEDICATION
* Painless, medicated drops may be applied by your health care provider.
* Other drugs may be prescribed that you can apply to the bumps yourself.

ACTIVITY—No limits, except to avoid sexual relations until the bumps disappear.

DIET—No special diet.

 CALL YOUR DOCTOR IF

* You or a family member has symptoms of molluscum contagiosum.
* A reinfection occurs after treatment.
* New unexplained symptoms develop. Drugs used in treatment may produce side effects.

MONONUCLEOSIS, INFECTIOUS

GENERAL INFORMATION

DEFINITION—An infectious viral disease that affects the lungs, liver and lymphatic system.

BODY PARTS INVOLVED—Lymph nodes; liver; spleen; throat; bronchial tubes.

SEX OR AGE MOST AFFECTED—It usually affects children and young adults (from 12 to 40 years of age) of both sexes.

SIGNS & SYMPTOMS
• Fever.
• Sore throat (sometimes severe).
• Appetite loss.
• Fatigue.
• Swollen lymph glands, usually in the neck, underarms, or groin.
• Enlarged spleen.
• Enlarged liver.
• Jaundice with yellow skin and eyes (sometimes).
• Headache.
• General aching.

CAUSES—A contagious virus (Epstein-Barr virus). It is passed from person to person by close contact, such as kissing, shared food or coughing.

RISK INCREASES WITH
• Fatigue or overwork. The high rate among college students and military recruits may result from too little rest and crowded living conditions.
• High school or college students.
• Weak immune system due to illness or drugs.

HOW TO PREVENT—Avoid close contact with persons having infectious mononucleosis.

WHAT TO EXPECT

DIAGNOSTIC MEASURES
• Your own observation of symptoms.
• Your health care provider will do a physical exam and ask questions about your symptoms.
• Medical tests may include blood studies.

APPROPRIATE HEALTH CARE—No specific cure or treatment is available. Extra rest and healthy diet are important. There is no need to keep away from other people. Do avoid close contact so the germs aren't spread.

POSSIBLE COMPLICATIONS
• Ruptured spleen, resulting in emergency surgery.
• Anemia.
• In rare cases, the heart, lungs, or central nervous system could become involved. The disease can prove serious, even fatal.

PROBABLE OUTCOME—It usually clears up on its own in 10 days to 6 months. Fatigue usually lasts for 3 to 6 weeks after other symptoms get better. A few patients have a chronic form in which symptoms last for months or years.

HOW TO TREAT

GENERAL MEASURES
• To relieve the sore throat, gargle frequently with warm or cold double-strength tea or warm salt water (mix one-half teaspoon of salt in one cup of water).
• Don't strain hard for bowel movements. This may injure an enlarged spleen.
• If you are a student, check on ways to continue school work while you are recovering.

MEDICATION
• For minor pain, you may use nonprescription drugs such as acetaminophen. Don't use aspirin in children under age 18.
• If symptoms are severe, you may be prescribed a short course of cortisone drugs.

ACTIVITY
• Rest in bed while you have fever. Resume activity gradually. Rest when you are tired.
• Don't join in contact sports until at least 1 month after complete recovery.

DIET—No special diet. You may not feel like eating while you are ill. Eat soft foods or drink milk shakes. Drink at least 8 glasses of fluids a day (or more) during periods of fever.

CALL YOUR DOCTOR IF

• You or a family member has symptoms of infectious mononucleosis.
• The following occur during treatment:
  - Fever over 102°F (38.9°C).
  - Constipation, which may cause straining.
  - Severe pain in the upper left abdomen (rupture of the spleen is a medical emergency!).
  - Yellowing of the skin.
  - Difficulty swallowing or breathing due to severe sore throat.

ILLNESS & DISORDERS

MOTION SICKNESS
(Car, Sea or Air Sickness)

 GENERAL INFORMATION

DEFINITION—An unpleasant, temporary disorder that often occurs while traveling.

BODY PARTS INVOLVED—The semicircular canals in the inner ear are affected. These fluid-filled canals normally maintain a person's sense of balance.

SEX OR AGE MOST AFFECTED—Both sexes; all ages.

SIGNS & SYMPTOMS
* Loss of appetite, nausea, and vomiting.
* Spinning sensation.
* Weakness and being unsteady.
* Confusion; anxiety; sweating.
* Paleness.
* Yawning.

CAUSES—Motion that may be from a plane, boat, car; amusement park ride, or swinging. The body, the inner ear, and the eyes send conflicting messages to the brain. The ears may sense motion that the eyes can not see, or the eyes may see movement that the body does not feel. People who suffer from motion sickness may have the symptoms just thinking about movement (such as when sitting on a plane waiting for take-off).

RISK INCREASES WITH
* Travel.
* Ear disorders such as allergies or infections.
* Smoky environment or poor ventilation.
* Drinking too much alcohol.
* Visual stimuli (moving horizon).

HOW TO PREVENT
* Avoid large meals and alcohol before and during trips.
* Sit in areas of the airplane (usually over the wings) or boat with the least motion.
* Recline in your seat, if possible.
* Breathe slowly and deeply. Don't read.
* Avoid areas where others are smoking, if possible.
* In a car, airplane, or bus, turn on the air vent to improve air movement.
* Take preventive drugs before a trip.
* There are behavior-modification techniques for those who are afraid to fly or have motion sickness. Contact the airline or your travel agent for information.
* Mental and emotional factors can add to motion sickness. Try to resolve concerns about travel before leaving home. Maintain a positive attitude.
* Consider preventive therapy. One technique involves special training for using your eyes that may help avoid the symptoms of motion sickness.

 WHAT TO EXPECT

DIAGNOSTIC MEASURES
* Your own observation of symptoms.
* If your symptoms persist or cause concern, see your health care provider. A physical exam may be done and medical tests may be recommended to rule out other disorders.

APPROPRIATE HEALTH CARE—Self-care is usually all that is needed.

POSSIBLE COMPLICATIONS—No serious complications are expected.

PROBABLE OUTCOME—Recovery once the trip is over or soon thereafter.

 HOW TO TREAT

GENERAL MEASURES
* If symptoms occur, try to rest in a dark room with a cool cloth over the eyes and forehead.
* Allowing yourself to vomit can help the nausea. However, don't make yourself vomit.
* Acupressure may help. This is done by placing pressure on a point three finger-widths above the wrist on the inner arm. Elastic wristband products can be purchased to put pressure on this area.
* A battery-operated wristband product is available that will apply a mild, electrical pulse to the area. It is used for prevention and treatment.

MEDICATION
* For minor discomfort, you may use nonprescription drugs, such as dimenhydrinate (Dramamine), or meclizine (Bonine) before and during travel. These can cause drowsiness.
* A scopolamine patch to control symptoms may be prescribed.
* Other drugs may be prescribed if simple treatment methods are not effective.

ACTIVITY—Limited only by the symptoms.

DIET
* Eat lightly or not at all before and during brief trips. For longer trips, sip frequently on beverages (tea and juices) to maintain your fluid intake. Avoid alcohol, carbonated drinks, and extra-cold beverages.
* Ginger helps some people. Take it on an empty stomach. It is available in a tea, capsules, or candied pieces.

 CALL YOUR DOCTOR IF

You or a family member plans to travel and has had disabling motion sickness in the past.

MOUTH OR TONGUE TUMOR, BENIGN

 GENERAL INFORMATION

DEFINITION—Abnormal new growth in the mouth or tongue that is unlikely to spread to other body parts. Benign mouth and tongue tumors usually occur alone and grow very slowly over a period of 2 to 6 years.

BODY PARTS INVOLVED—Lips; gums; palate; tongue; membrane covering the lips and cheeks; floor of the mouth.

SEX OR AGE MOST AFFECTED—Adults over 60.

SIGNS & SYMPTOMS
• A lump in any part of the mouth or tongue.
• It may become sore and bleed.
• It may interfere with the way dentures fit.
• It may interfere with speech or swallowing.

CAUSES—Unknown. It is most common in people who smoke cigarettes, cigars, or pipes, or use chewing tobacco or snuff. Benign tumors do not spread to other areas.

RISK INCREASES WITH
• Use of tobacco.
• Dentures that fit poorly.

HOW TO PREVENT
• Don't smoke or use tobacco products.
• See your dentist for annual dental exams and for problems with denture fit.

 WHAT TO EXPECT

DIAGNOSTIC MEASURES
• Your own observation of symptoms.
• Your health care provider will do a physical exam of the affected area.
• A biopsy may be done to confirm the diagnosis. A biopsy involves the removal of a small amount of skin tissue to be viewed under a microscope.

APPROPRIATE HEALTH CARE—Surgery to remove the tumor may be recommended.

POSSIBLE COMPLICATIONS
• Bleeding from the tumor.
• Infection in the tumor.

PROBABLE OUTCOME—Curable with surgical removal. They are not likely to recur.

 HOW TO TREAT

GENERAL MEASURES—After surgery, cleanse the mouth 3 to 4 times a day with a soothing salt water solution (mix one-half teaspoon of salt in one cup of warm water).

MEDICATION
• For minor discomfort, you may use nonprescription drugs such as acetaminophen or ibuprofen.
• Antibiotics will be prescribed if infection exists.

ACTIVITY—No limits.

DIET—A liquid diet may be necessary for a day or two after surgery. No special diet after recovery.

 CALL YOUR DOCTOR IF

• You or a family member has symptoms of a mouth or tongue tumor.
• The following occur after surgical treatment:
  - Fever.
  - Bleeding at the surgical site.
  - Pain.

MULTIPLE MYELOMA
(Plasma Cell Myeloma)

 GENERAL INFORMATION

DEFINITION—Cancer of the plasma cells of the bone marrow. Plasma cells normally help the body destroy germs and protect against infection. The cancer is called multiple because it usually occurs in many bones in the body.

BODY PARTS INVOLVED—Bone marrow of all bones, but most common in the thigh, back, pelvis or upper arms.

SEX OR AGE MOST AFFECTED—Both sexes, but most common in men between ages 50 and 70.

SIGNS & SYMPTOMS
* Pain in the affected bone. The pain is severe, boring, and deep. If the bone collapses, pain spreads to other parts of the body.
* Weight loss.
* Symptoms of anemia, such as weakness, paleness, tiredness, and breathlessness.

CAUSES—Unknown. The bone pain is caused by the cancerous plasma cells. The anemia is caused by damaged red blood cells and decreased platelets.

RISK INCREASES WITH
* Family history of myeloma.
* Older adults.
* Other plasma cell disease.
* Exposure to certain chemicals and high radiation doses may be risk factors.

HOW TO PREVENT—No specific preventive measures.

 WHAT TO EXPECT

DIAGNOSTIC MEASURES
* Your own observation of symptoms.
* Your health care provider will do a physical exam and ask questions about your symptoms and activities.
* Different medical tests are done to verify the diagnosis and to determine if the cancer has spread to other places in the body (called staging).

APPROPRIATE HEALTH CARE
* Treatment will depend on the stage of the disease, your health, age, and preferences. Your health care provider will discuss the options and their risks and benefits. All treatments have numerous side effects.
* Watchful waiting is usually recommended if there are no symptoms. This means monitoring the cancer cells for a period of time before deciding on treatment.

* Treatment may involve radiation, chemotherapy, surgery (for complications), biologic therapy (using body's immune system), stem cell transplantation, and plasmapheresis (using patient's blood for therapy).
* Treatment may involve steps to relieve symptoms and make you comfortable, rather than treating the cancer.

POSSIBLE COMPLICATIONS
* Recurrent infections.
* Kidney failure.
* Spontaneous bleeding.
* Bone fractures.
* Paralysis.

PROBABLE OUTCOME—Treatment can help with the symptoms and improve quality of life, but rarely produces a cure. Some patients live up to 5 years after symptoms appear. Temporary remissions may occur with treatment. Research into causes and treatment continues, so there is hope for more effective treatment and cure.

 HOW TO TREAT

GENERAL MEASURES
* The more you can learn and understand about this disorder, the more you will be able to make informed decisions about where to go for your care, the treatments available, the risks involved, side effects of therapy and expected outcome.
* To learn more: International Myeloma Foundation, 12650 Riverside Dr., Suite 206, North Hollywood, CA 91607; (800) 452-2873; website: www.myeloma.org or American Cancer Society, (800) ACS-2345; website: www.cancer.org.

MEDICATION—You may be prescribed:
* Anticancer and cortisone drugs (chemotherapy).
* Pain relievers.
* Antibiotics for infections.
* Blood transfusions, if anemia becomes severe.
* Drugs to treat hypercalcemia (too much calcium).

ACTIVITY—Stay as active as pain or bone complications allow.

DIET—No special diet.

 CALL YOUR DOCTOR IF

* You or a family member has symptoms of multiple myeloma.
* Fever, or any sign of infection, or unexplained bleeding occurs.
* Drugs used in treatment produce side effects.

MULTIPLE SCLEROSIS (MS)

GENERAL INFORMATION

DEFINITION—A chronic disorder that affects the central nervous system (brain, spinal cord, and optic nerve). Types include:
• Relapsing-remitting. Most common. Patients have flare ups followed by partial or complete recovery.
• Primary-progressive. Slow and continued worsening of symptoms. May be temporary minor improvements.
• Secondary-progressive. This type follows the relapsing-remitting type. Symptoms steadily worsen.
• Progressive-relapsing. Symptoms steadily worsen from the start. Has flare ups, with or without recovery.

BODY PARTS INVOLVED—Central nervous system.

SEX OR AGE MOST AFFECTED—It more often affects adults 20 to 50, and women twice as often as men.

SIGNS & SYMPTOMS
• Signs and symptoms may be mild, moderate, or severe. They vary from person to person and at times in the same person.
• Fatigue (called MS lassitude)
• Problems with walking. Lack of coordination.
• Bowel and bladder problems.
• Vision problems or hearing problems (less often).
• Vague loss of sensation or numbness and tingling.
• Mood swings and depression.
• Sexual problems.
• Difficulty with memory, concentration, attention, and problem solving.
• Speech or swallowing problems (sometimes).

CAUSES—Unknown. It is believed to be an autoimmune disorder. In these disorders, the immune system attacks the body itself by mistake and in different ways. Genetic and environmental (such as a virus) factors may contribute.

RISK INCREASES WITH
• Females more than males.
• People of Northern European descent.
• Family history of MS.
• Growing up in a cold climate (compared to tropical).

HOW TO PREVENT—No preventive measures.

WHAT TO EXPECT

DIAGNOSTIC MEASURES
• Your health care provider will do a physical exam and ask questions about your symptoms, activities, and medical history.

• No specific test is available to diagnose MS. Medical tests may include blood, urine, and spinal fluid studies. An MRI scan (see Glossary) of the brain and spinal cord will usually show typical changes that indicate multiple sclerosis. Often, a specialist called a neurologist is needed to make the diagnosis.

APPROPRIATE HEALTH CARE
• Treatment may include one or more drugs to treat symptoms, prevent complications, or slow progression of the disorder. Physical therapy may be recommended. Plasma exchange (a blood treatment) may be of help.
• Counseling may be helpful.

POSSIBLE COMPLICATIONS—Numerous complications can occur. They often result from problems such as immobility, chronic urinary-tract infections, difficulty with swallowing and breathing, and mental and emotional disorders.

PROBABLE OUTCOME—Multiple sclerosis is incurable. The course of the disorder will be different for each person. Some will be favorable and others unfavorable. Symptoms can often be relieved or controlled.

HOW TO TREAT

GENERAL MEASURES
• Multiple sclerosis will affect every aspect of your life. You will need to educate yourself about your specific symptoms and what to expect and how to adjust to the disease. The more you can learn, the better able you will be to cope with the changes in your life.
• Joining a support group is may help.
• To learn more: National Multiple Sclerosis Society, 733 Third Ave., New York, NY 10017, (800) 344-4867; website: www.nationalmssociety.org.

MEDICATION
• Drugs called disease-modifying agents are often prescribed.
• Cortisone drugs may be prescribed for inflammation.
• Drugs for specific symptoms will be prescribed as needed.

ACTIVITY—Get enough rest. Exercise to the extent possible. It helps physical and emotional well-being. It keeps muscles limber and strong, and helps balance and coordination.

DIET—Eat a healthy diet that is high in fiber to help prevent constipation.

CALL YOUR DOCTOR IF

• You or a family member has symptoms of multiple sclerosis.
• After diagnosis, any symptoms cause concern.

MUMPS

GENERAL INFORMATION

DEFINITION—A contagious viral disease that causes painful swelling of the glands located between the ear and jaw. Mumps infections are now rare because of the routine vaccines given to infants. About 10% of adults are susceptible to mumps.

BODY PARTS INVOLVED—Parotid glands (salivary glands that lie between the ear and jaw). Other organs, including the testicles, ovaries, pancreas, breasts, brain and meninges (membranes that cover the brain) sometimes become involved.

SEX OR AGE MOST AFFECTED—All ages, but most common in children (2 to 12 years). Approximately 10% of adults are susceptible to mumps.

SIGNS & SYMPTOMS
* Inflammation, swelling, tenderness, or pain of the glands. The glands feel firm, and discomfort increases with chewing or swallowing.
* Fever.
* Headache.
* Sore throat.
* Rarely, if complications develop, the following may occur:
  - Painful, swollen testicles.
  - Abdominal pain.
  - Severe headache, if the brain or meninges (lining of the brain) are involved.

CAUSES—Person-to-person transmission of the mumps virus (*paramyxovirus*). The virus can be passed anytime from 48 hours before symptoms begin to 6 days after symptoms appear. Virus incubation is 14 to 24 days after contact; the average is 18 days.

RISK INCREASES WITH
* Epidemics in unvaccinated countries or areas.
* Lack of immunization.

HOW TO PREVENT
* Obtain routine mumps vaccines for infants.
* If you have not had mumps or been vaccinated, and a close family member has mumps, seek advice from your health care provider.

WHAT TO EXPECT

DIAGNOSTIC MEASURES
* Your own observation of symptoms.
* Your health care provider can usually diagnose mumps by the signs and symptoms.
* Blood studies may be done to confirm the diagnosis.

APPROPRIATE HEALTH CARE
* Home care after diagnosis.
* Medical care for complications.

POSSIBLE COMPLICATIONS
* Complications are rare, and if they occur are usually in persons over age 19. Complications can involve the testicles, thyroid, brain, spinal cord, prostate, pancreas, and the breasts. Testicle involvement may rarely lead to infertility in males.
* Mumps in the first trimester of pregnancy may lead to miscarriage.
* Hearing loss in children.

PROBABLE OUTCOME—Recovery in about 10-12 days. After having it once, a person almost always has lifetime immunity to mumps.

HOW TO TREAT

GENERAL MEASURES
* You do not need to keep the infected person away from the family. By the time symptoms appear, the disease has usually already spread.
* Apply heat or ice, whichever feels better, to the swollen, painful glands. Use a hot-water bottle, hot towel, or ice-pack.
* Stay out of school, daycare, or work until no longer contagious (about 9 days after symptoms begin).

MEDICATION
* Once the infection begins, it must run its natural course. There is no safe or effective drug that can treat mumps.
* For minor pain, you may use nonprescription drugs such as acetaminophen or ibuprofen.
* If testicles are involved, stronger pain relievers and other drugs may be prescribed.

ACTIVITY—Allow as much activity as strength and feeling of well-being allow. Patients are no longer contagious when swelling disappears.

DIET—Soft food diet is helpful if chewing causes pain. Increase daily fluid intake to at least 6 to 8 glasses of liquid a day.

CALL YOUR DOCTOR IF

* You or a family member has symptoms of mumps.
* Fever rises above 101°F (38.3°C).
* The following occur during the illness:
  - Vomiting or abdominal pain.
  - Severe headache.
  - Drowsiness or inability to stay awake.
  - Swelling or pain in the testicles.
  - Twitching of the face muscles.
  - Convulsion.
  - Discomfort or redness in the eyes.

MUSCULAR DYSTROPHY

GENERAL INFORMATION

DEFINITION—A group of inherited disorders that cause muscle weakness and wasting (decrease in size). There are nine major types of muscular dystrophy (and some subtypes within those types). Duchenne is one of the most common types.

BODY PARTS INVOLVED—Different types affect different areas of the body, such as shoulders, hips or face.

SEX OR AGE MOST AFFECTED—The disorders are usually diagnosed in children (most often boys), and less often in teens or adults.

SIGNS & SYMPTOMS
Early symptoms:
• Weakness.
• Duck-like gait. Lack of coordination.
• Falling, with difficulty getting up.
• Muscles appear larger and stronger but are weaker than normal.
Later symptoms:
• Muscle loss severe enough to require use of a wheelchair by age 9 to 12.
• Severe distortion of the body.
• Recurrent respiratory infections.

CAUSES—Inherited. Muscular dystrophy is a genetic abnormality. It can be carried by a female who does not have symptoms, but passes it on to male children. In other cases, it may be passed on by one or both parents. In still other cases, there is no family history.

RISK INCREASES WITH—Family history of muscular dystrophy.

HOW TO PREVENT—If you have a family history of muscular dystrophy:
• Get genetic counseling before starting a family.
• If pregnant, consider testing to determine whether the fetus is male and the disorder is present.
• Carriers can be detected with medical tests because their blood contains high levels of a certain enzyme.

WHAT TO EXPECT

DIAGNOSTIC MEASURES
• Your child's health care provider will do a physical exam and ask questions about the symptoms.
• Medical tests may include blood studies and muscle biopsy. A biopsy involves removal of a small amount of tissue for viewing under a microscope. An electromyogram (measures electrical impulses in muscles) and nerve conduction study may be done.

APPROPRIATE HEALTH CARE
• There is no cure for muscular dystrophy. Treatment can help improve the symptoms and help prevent complications. A child will need to be assisted in many ways to make the most of his abilities and keep his independence to the extent possible.
• Your child will need a health care team. This may include physical, occupational, speech, and respiratory therapists as well as routine medical care. Illnesses are more common and need to be watched for and treated.
• Surgery may be needed to release tight, painful muscles. If heart problems develop, a pacemaker may be surgically implanted to help the heart beat normally.
• Counseling can help parents cope with the diagnosis. It can help children if emotional problems develop.

POSSIBLE COMPLICATIONS
• Muscle weakness (leads to wheelchair use).
• Fractures or injuries from falls.
• Spinal curvature due to weak spine muscles.
• Pneumonia.
• Heart problems.
• Muscle shortening and tightening (contractures).

PROBABLE OUTCOME—Outcome varies depending on the type of muscular dystrophy. Some types are more mild, progress slowly, and patients may have a normal lifespan. Other types progress more rapidly, lead to disability and a shortened lifespan. Research is ongoing.

HOW TO TREAT

GENERAL MEASURES
• Support groups may help you cope.
• To learn more: Muscular Dystrophy Association, 3300 E. Sunrise Drive, Tucson, AZ 85718; (800) 572-1717; website: www.mdausa.org.

MEDICATION—Drugs may be prescribed to slow muscle loss, improve lung function, treat heart problems, for constipation, to treat infections, or for other complications.

ACTIVITY—The patient should be as physically and mentally active as possible. Many devices can help overcome handicaps caused by weakness. Braces may help.

DIET—Eat a well-balanced diet. Being overweight should be avoided (it adds more burden to already weak muscles).

CALL YOUR DOCTOR IF

• Your child develops symptoms of muscular dystrophy.
• After diagnosis, symptoms develop that cause concern. Symptoms include fever, cough and chest pain.

ILLNESS & DISORDERS

MYASTHENIA GRAVIS

GENERAL INFORMATION

DEFINITION—A disorder of the muscles that causes muscle weakness of varying degrees.

BODY PARTS INVOLVED—It often involves the muscles around the eyes, mouth, and throat, and the arms and legs. It can affect the breathing muscles also.

SEX OR AGE MOST AFFECTED—Both sexes; all ages, but more common in adolescents and young adults and in females.

SIGNS & SYMPTOMS
* Drooping eyelids.
* Double vision.
* Loss of normal facial expression.
* Swallowing difficulty.
* Weakness of the arms and legs.
* Difficulty speaking clearly.
* Breathing difficulty.
* Most flare-ups appear after a brief period of normal muscle function and worsen as the muscle is used.

CAUSES
* One of a group of autoimmune disorders. In these disorders, the immune system attacks the body itself by mistake. With myasthenia gravis, there is a miscommunication between the nerves and the muscles.
* Tumor of the thymus (newborns only).

RISK INCREASES WITH
* Family history of myasthenia gravis.
* Newborns and infants of mothers with myasthenia gravis. They show symptoms in 2 to 3 weeks.

HOW TO PREVENT—Cannot be prevented at present.

WHAT TO EXPECT

DIAGNOSTIC MEASURES
* Your own observation of symptoms.
* Your health care provider will do a physical exam and ask questions about your symptoms and activities.
* Medical tests may include studies of blood antibodies, electrical tests on muscle, and x-rays of the chest.

APPROPRIATE HEALTH CARE
* Treatment will help control symptoms. It may involve extra rest, drug therapy, surgery, or plasmapheresis.
* Surgical removal (thymectomy) of the thymus gland may be recommended. It can improve symptoms in some patients, and even cure the disease in others.

* Plasmapheresis involves removal of blood from the patient, treating the blood, and reinjecting it.
* Acute flare-ups (myasthenia crises) may require emergency hospital care for breathing problems.

POSSIBLE COMPLICATIONS
* Choking from swallowing difficulty.
* Increased breathing difficulties.
* Pneumonia.

PROBABLE OUTCOME—Symptoms may get worse and then improve for a period of time. Symptoms can be helped with treatment. Patients usually live many years with the disease. Research into causes and treatment continues, so there is hope for effective treatment and cure.

HOW TO TREAT

GENERAL MEASURES
* Avoid exposure to infections and try to avoid stress.
* To learn more: Myasthenia Gravis Foundation, 1821 University Ave., W., Suite S256, St. Paul, MN 55104; (800) 541-5454; website: www.myasthenia.org.

MEDICATION
* Anticholinesterase drugs to help improve muscle function are usually prescribed.
* Immunosuppressive drugs may be prescribed at times when symptoms worsen.
* Intravenous immune globulin (IVIG) may be used for some patients to suppress the immune system.

ACTIVITY
* Plan activities to make the most of energy peaks. Frequent rest periods are important. Day-to-day changes in symptoms are common.
* Avoid strenuous activities and too much exposure to the sun or to cold weather.

DIET—Eat foods high in potassium (if advised). These include oranges, tomatoes, bananas, broccoli, and apricots. Soft diet may be helpful if chewing and swallowing are difficult.

CALL YOUR DOCTOR IF

* You or a family member has symptoms of myasthenia gravis.
* You develop swallowing or breathing difficulty.

MYOCARDITIS

GENERAL INFORMATION

DEFINITION—Inflammation of the heart muscle (myocardium). It can lead to poor heart function. Myocarditis usually occurs as a complication of another illness.

BODY PARTS INVOLVED—Heart muscle.

SEX OR AGE MOST AFFECTED—Both sexes; all ages; often affects middle-aged men.

SIGNS & SYMPTOMS
• No symptoms or symptoms may be mild and vague.
• Fatigue.
• Shortness of breath with physical activity.
• Irregular heartbeat.
• Fever.
• Chest pain or discomfort.
• Muscle aches.
• If myocarditis causes congestive heart failure, the following symptoms may also occur:
 - Swollen feet and ankles.
 - Distended (sticking out) neck veins.
 - Rapid heartbeat, even when at rest.
 - Breathing difficulty while resting or lying down.

CAUSES—The inflammation can result from numerous medical conditions. A viral infection is the most common cause.

RISK INCREASES WITH
• Viral infection, such as Coxsackie, adenovirus, measles, influenza, herpes simplex, hepatitis, varicella, HIV, or others.
• Bacterial infections, such as tetanus, gonorrhea, typhoid fever, tuberculosis, or diphtheria.
• Immune system disorders (lupus, arthritis, others).
• Parasitic infections.
• Radiation therapy.
• Certain drugs.
• Pregnancy.
• Rheumatic fever.
• Exposure to certain toxins or chemicals.

HOW TO PREVENT—No specific preventive measures. Avoid risk factors where possible.

WHAT TO EXPECT

DIAGNOSTIC MEASURES
• Your own observation of symptoms.
• Your health care provider will do a physical exam.
• Medical tests may include blood studies, chest x-ray, and heart function tests. A biopsy may be done. This involves removal of a small amount of tissue for viewing under a microscope.

APPROPRIATE HEALTH CARE
• There is no specific treatment for myocarditis. Treatment usually involves rest, treating symptoms, and drugs for a diagnosed infection.
• Hospital care may be needed for more severe symptoms.

POSSIBLE COMPLICATIONS
• Congestive heart failure.
• Pulmonary edema (fluid in the lungs).
• Heart rhythm problems.
• Inflammation of muscles (myositis).
• Sudden death due to abnormal heart rhythm.

PROBABLE OUTCOME—Mild cases caused by a virus usually clear up on their own in about 2 weeks. Mild cases from other causes are usually treated successfully. In more severe cases, the outcome will depend on the underlying cause, patient's health status, and treatment.

HOW TO TREAT

GENERAL MEASURES
• Compliance with your treatment plan is important for your recovery.
• To learn more: American Heart Association, 7272 Greenville Ave., Dallas, TX 75231; (800) 242-8721; website: www.americanheart.org.

MEDICATION—You may be prescribed:
• Antibiotics for a bacterial infection.
• Steroid drugs to reduce inflammation.
• Diuretics to reduce fluid build up.
• Digitalis to stimulate a stronger heartbeat.
• Anticoagulants to prevent clot formation.
• Pain remedies.
• Drugs to reduce the heart's workload.

ACTIVITY
• Rest in bed until symptoms improve. Recovery time varies, depending on the underlying cause.
• After recovery, resume normal activities gradually.

DIET—A low-salt diet may be recommended.

CALL YOUR DOCTOR IF

• You or a family member has symptoms of myocarditis.
• Symptoms get worse or don't improve with time or treatment.
• New, unexplained symptoms develop. Drugs used in treatment may produce side effects.

NARCOLEPSY

GENERAL INFORMATION

DEFINITION—A disorder of sleep that affects the control of sleep and wakefulness. Types of symptoms and their severity vary among different people who have the disorder. Often, it goes undiagnosed for years.

BODY PARTS INVOLVED—Central nervous system.

SEX OR AGE MOST AFFECTED—Both sexes. May begin in adolescence or young adulthood and continue throughout life.

SIGNS & SYMPTOMS
• Excessive daytime sleepiness (hypersomnia).
• Uncontrollable sleep attacks that may occur up to 10 times a day. They may last from 30 seconds up to 30 minutes or more. An attack leaves the person feeling refreshed, but another may occur again quickly. Attacks occur while driving, talking, working, or at social events.
• Hallucinations (seeing things that aren't there) when first going to sleep or waking up. This is called hypnagogic or hypnopompic.
• A short period of paralysis (sudden loss of muscle strength) when falling asleep or just before awakening.
• A few seconds of paralysis not related to sleep when feeling sudden emotion, such as anger, fear, or joy. This is called cataplexy.
• Nighttime sleep is disturbed by leg jerks, tossing and turning, nightmares, and frequent awakenings.

CAUSES—It is a neurologic (nervous system) disorder. The exact cause is being researched. A problem with certain brain chemicals that tell the body when to sleep and wake up appears to be a cause. There is also a genetic link.

RISK INCREASES WITH
• A family history of narcolepsy.
• Genetic factors.

HOW TO PREVENT—No known preventive measures.

WHAT TO EXPECT

DIAGNOSTIC MEASURES
• Your own observation of symptoms.
• Your health care provider will do a physical exam and ask about your symptoms and activities.
• You may be asked to keep a 2-week diary about your sleep patterns.
• An overnight study in a sleep clinic may be done.

APPROPRIATE HEALTH CARE—Treatment usually involves lifestyle changes along with drugs to help control the drowsiness. It may take several weeks or months to achieve the best results.

POSSIBLE COMPLICATIONS
• Accidental injury during a sudden sleep attack.
• The disorder may affect all aspects of one's life. This includes work, social life, personal relationships, and emotional health.

PROBABLE OUTCOME—The disorder appears to be life-long. There is no cure. Drugs and lifestyle changes can help improve the symptoms. Most people with the disorder can lead a near-normal lifestyle.

HOW TO TREAT

GENERAL MEASURES
• Schedule a regular time for going to bed and getting up. Stick to the schedule. Get at least 8 hours of sleep.
• Take regular naps 2 to 3 times during the day. One 15-minute nap after lunch and another at around 5:30 PM may help symptoms.
• Don't do shift work.
• Avoid over-stimulating activities, if possible.
• Wear a medical alert type bracelet or pendant to indicate you suffer from this disorder.
• To learn more: Narcolepsy Network, 10921 Reed Hartman Hwy., Ste. 119, Cincinnati, OH 45242; (513) 891-3522 not toll-free; website: www.narcolepsynetwork.org.

MEDICATION
• Stimulants that increase levels of daytime alertness may be prescribed.
• Modafinil (Provigil) for narcolepsy symptoms may be prescribed.
• Antidepressants or sodium oxybate (Xyrem) for cataplexy or other symptoms may be prescribed.
• New drugs for this disorder are being studied.

ACTIVITY
• Don't engage in any activity that carries the risk of injury from a sudden sleep attack. These include activities such as driving long distances, climbing ladders, or working around dangerous machinery.
• Exercise regularly, but not within 3 hours of bedtime.

DIET—No special diet.

CALL YOUR DOCTOR IF

• You or a family member has symptoms of narcolepsy.
• New, unexplained symptoms develop. Drugs used in treatment may produce side effects.

NASAL POLYPS

GENERAL INFORMATION

DEFINITION—A nasal polyp is a benign (noncancerous), soft tissue growth that develops inside the nose. Polyps look like small grapes and can grow alone, but usually occur in clusters. They often affect both sides of the nose.

BODY PARTS INVOLVED—Nasal mucous membranes.

SEX OR AGE MOST AFFECTED—Both sexes; all ages, but more common in adults.

SIGNS & SYMPTOMS
* Obstruction of air through the nose (chronic "stuffy-nose" feeling).
* Sense of smell is reduced.
* Nasal discharge.
* Sneezing.
* Facial pain or headaches.
* Feeling of fullness in the face.
* Itchy eyes.
* Large polyps may cause the nose to be deformed.

CAUSES—Chronic inflammation of the lining of the nose and sinuses. Inflammation is normally a reaction to injury, infection, or irritation. Why it occurs in the nose and sinuses and causes polyps is not clearly understood.

RISK INCREASES WITH
* Chronic sinus, nasal, or lung disorders. This can include asthma, allergic rhinitis, cystic fibrosis, sinusitis, fungal infections, and others.
* Aspirin sensitivity. This is not a true allergy, but it may cause allergy-like reactions (such as hives, swelling, and asthma). People with this sensitivity need to avoid aspirin and other nonsteroidal anti-inflammatory drugs.

HOW TO PREVENT—No specific preventive measures. Getting treatment for allergies, infections, or other nose and sinus problems may help reduce the risk factors.

WHAT TO EXPECT

DIAGNOSTIC MEASURES
* Your own observation of symptoms.
* Your health care provider will do an exam of the nasal passages.
* Medical tests may include a CT or endoscopy (small, lighted telescopic instrument) to see inside the nose. Allergy testing may be done in some cases.

APPROPRIATE HEALTH CARE
* Treatment may involve drugs to temporarily shrink the polyps and help relieve the symptoms.
* Surgery is often done to remove polyps. The type of surgery will depend on the location, size, and the number of polyps involved. Your health care provider will discuss the options, the risks, and benefits with you. See Nasal Polyps removal in Surgery Section.

POSSIBLE COMPLICATIONS
* Polyps may recur after surgery.
* Recurrent or chronic sinusitis.

PROBABLE OUTCOME—Treatment with drugs or surgery can help improve the symptoms.

HOW TO TREAT

GENERAL MEASURES
* Try to avoid any substances that you know you are allergic to, such as dust mites, pollen, mold, etc.
* For information about surgery and postoperative care, see Nasal Polyp Removal in surgery section.

MEDICATION
* For minor pain, you may use acetaminophen.
* Nonprescription antihistamines may help relieve symptoms, but they do not treat the polyps.
* Corticosteroid drugs in oral form may be prescribed for a short period to attempt to shrink the polyps.
* Corticosteroid drugs in nasal spray may be prescribed for treatment of smaller polyps. They are also prescribed following surgery to help prevent recurrence of polyps.
* Antibiotics or antifungal drugs may be prescribed for treatment of infection.

ACTIVITY—No limits.

DIET—No special diet. If you have food allergies, be sure to avoid those foods.

CALL YOUR DOCTOR IF

* You or a family member has symptoms of nasal polyps.
* Any new symptoms develop or other symptoms get worse after treatment is started.

NASAL SEPTUM, DEVIATED

GENERAL INFORMATION

DEFINITION—The septum is the structure that divides the nose into two parts. In some people it is significantly off-center, or deviated. This can result in the obstruction of normal airflow through the nasal passages. The septum is made up of cartilage (toward the tip) and bone (closer to the forehead). Ideally, the septum should divide the right and left side of the nose into two equal parts. It is estimated that 80% of all nasal septa are slightly off-center. These are usually not noticed and do not normally cause any problems.

BODY PARTS INVOLVED—Septum.

SEX OR AGE MOST AFFECTED—Both sexes; all ages.

SIGNS & SYMPTOMS
- An apparently crooked nose.
- Obstruction of air through one or both nostrils.
- Nasal congestion or discharge.
- Nosebleeds, headaches, or facial pain may occur.
- Sinus infections.
- Often, there are no symptoms.

CAUSES—Trauma to the nose, or it may be congenital (being born with a deviated septum).

RISK INCREASES WITH—None known.

HOW TO PREVENT—Protect yourself from nose injury. Wear protective headgear for contact sports or cycling. Buckle your auto seat belt.

WHAT TO EXPECT

DIAGNOSTIC MEASURES
- Your own observation of symptoms.
- Your health care provider can usually diagnose the problem by an exam of the nose. The exam involves the use of a bright light and nasal speculum (an instrument that spreads the nostril open).
- Medical tests may be done to confirm the diagnosis.

APPROPRIATE HEALTH CARE
- No treatment may be needed if there are no symptoms or if symptoms are mild.
- Surgery to correct the deviation may be recommended if the deviated septum is causing symptoms such as sinus infections or nosebleeds. Your health care provider will discuss the options with you. Surgery may involve:
  - Submucosal removal, which relieves obstruction.
  - Rhinoplasty, which corrects anatomical deformity.
  - Septoplasty, which relieves nasal obstruction and improves appearance.

POSSIBLE COMPLICATIONS
- Recurrent nosebleeds.
- Recurrent nasal or sinus infections.

PROBABLE OUTCOME—Usually treatable with surgery. If symptoms are not troublesome, surgery is usually not needed.

HOW TO TREAT

GENERAL MEASURES—For an explanation of one type of corrective surgery and postoperative care, see Rhinoplasty in Surgery Section.

MEDICATION
- For minor discomfort, you may use nonprescription drugs, such as decongestants, to decrease nasal secretions.
- Antibiotics to treat infection may be prescribed.
- Caution: Avoid over-the-counter nasal sprays.

ACTIVITY—No limits, unless surgery is needed. If so, resume your normal activities gradually.

DIET—No special diet.

CALL YOUR DOCTOR IF

- You or a family member has symptoms of a deviated nasal septum, especially recurrent nosebleeds, or nasal and sinus infections.
- New symptoms develop after surgery.

NAUSEA & VOMITING IN PREGNANCY
(Morning Sickness During Pregnancy)

 GENERAL INFORMATION

DEFINITION—50% to 80% of pregnant women suffer from nausea and vomiting in pregnancy. The symptoms often occur in the morning (from 6 to 9 a.m.), but they may occur at any time during the day.

BODY PARTS INVOLVED—Gastrointestinal system.

SEX OR AGE MOST AFFECTED—Females of childbearing age.

SIGNS & SYMPTOMS
* Mild, moderate, or somewhat severe nausea with or without vomiting.
* It usually occurs during the first 12 to 14 weeks of pregnancy.
* It may continue longer, and for some women, last throughout pregnancy.
* By the end of the third month, most women stop having most of the symptoms.

CAUSES—Exact causes of nausea and vomiting during pregnancy are unknown. Nausea may result from changes in the body or hormonal changes that take place for normal growth of the baby.

RISK INCREASES WITH—Being pregnant with more than one baby.

HOW TO PREVENT—It may help to not let your stomach get empty; eat something every 2 hours if needed.

 WHAT TO EXPECT

DIAGNOSTIC MEASURES
* Usually self diagnosis and self-care are all that are needed.
* Talk to your obstetric provider if the symptoms are a concern.

APPROPRIATE HEALTH CARE
* Self-care.
* Medical treatment is usually not needed.
* Acupuncture may be a helpful option for some women.

POSSIBLE COMPLICATIONS—Hyperemesis gravidarum. This is a rare condition of pregnancy that involves severe nausea, vomiting, and weight loss.

PROBABLE OUTCOME—The symptoms usually stop after the first 3 to 4 months of pregnancy. Your baby's well-being is not affected as long as you're able to keep food down, eat a well-balanced diet, and drink plenty of fluids.

 HOW TO TREAT

GENERAL MEASURES
* Try to identify odors or foods that are most upsetting, and avoid them. Many pregnant women discover what they can and cannot eat.
* Keep rooms well aired out to rid your home of cooking smells or other odors.
* Don't smoke. Avoid secondhand smoke.
* Try to keep a positive attitude. If you have problems that you cannot resolve, ask for help from family, friends, or counselors.
* Keep a daily record of your weight.
* Try acupressure bands. You can find these soft cotton wristbands at drugstores.
* Consider getting a device that regularly stimulates the underside of your wrist with a mild electric current. The devices are safe and they seem to work well for some women. One or more of these devices allow you to adjust the amount of stimulation (e.g., ReliefBand Device).

MEDICATION
* Drugs are not usually prescribed for this disorder. If the symptoms are severe, you may be prescribed certain drugs for the nausea.
* Nonprescription remedies (oral drugs or rectal suppositories) may ease the problem. Don't take or use any of these products without medical advice.
* A trial of vitamin B6 may be recommended, which appears safe at the present.
* If taking your pregnancy vitamin pill causes nausea, ask your obstetric provider about stopping it for a period of time.

ACTIVITY—No limits. Resting in a dark and quiet room often provides some relief.

DIET—The following may help lessen the nausea:
* At night, place a small, quick-energy snack, such as soda crackers, at your bedside. Eat it before getting up.
* Eat a small snack at bedtime and when you get up to go to the bathroom during the night.
* Eat a snack every hour or two during the day. Avoid large meals.
* Drink ginger ale or ginger tea.

 CALL YOUR DOCTOR IF

* You have morning sickness that does not improve, despite the self-help measures.
* You vomit blood or material that resembles coffee grounds.
* Abdominal pain, cramping, or fever occurs.
* You lose more than 1 or 2 pounds.

NEPHROTIC SYNDROME
(Nephrosis)

GENERAL INFORMATION

DEFINITION—A condition that results from damage to tiny blood vessels in the kidneys called glomeruli. Normally, the glomeruli filter the waste and excess water from blood and into urine. When they are damaged, they do not filter properly. This causes substances (proteins) in the blood and urine to become imbalanced. Fluid then builds up in the body, instead of being passed into the urine and out of the body.

BODY PARTS INVOLVED—Kidneys. Late or complicated stages involve all body cells.

SEX OR AGE MOST AFFECTED—It affects all age groups, and males more than females. In children, it is more common from ages 2 to 6.

SIGNS & SYMPTOMS
* Fluid retention (edema). At first, it causes puffy eyes and ankles, which is followed by general puffiness of the skin, and then, a swollen abdomen.
* Weight gain due to fluid retention.
* Less urination (as low as 20% of normal).
* Appetite loss, weakness, and general ill feeling.
* Frothy (foamy) urine.

CAUSES—The cause of the kidney damage is often unknown. It may be due to numerous underlying disorders. In children, it is usually due to minimal change disease.

RISK INCREASES WITH
* Disorders that affect kidney function. These include diabetes, lupus erythematosus, cancers, glomerulonephritis, autoimmune disorders, serum sickness and other severe allergic disorders, blood clot in the kidney, numerous types of infections, sickle cell anemia, congenital heart disease, severe high blood pressure, other disorders, and drugs that are toxic to the kidneys.
* Weak immune system due to illness or drugs.
* Family history of renal failure.
* Exposure to some chemical toxins.

HOW TO PREVENT
* Obtain medical treatment for any risk factors listed.
* Drugs may be prescribed to help prevent nephrotic disorder in persons at risk.

WHAT TO EXPECT

DIAGNOSTIC MEASURES
* Your health care provider will do a physical exam and ask about your symptoms and activities.

* Medical tests may include urine and blood studies. A kidney biopsy may be done to diagnose any kidney disorder. A biopsy involves removal of a small amount of kidney tissue or fluid for viewing under a microscope.

APPROPRIATE HEALTH CARE
* Treatment will be prescribed for any underlying disorder diagnosed. This may improve the symptoms of nephrotic syndrome.
* Treatment is usually with drugs and sometimes diet changes (if needed).

POSSIBLE COMPLICATIONS
* Infections, kidney failure, heart or lung disorders.
* Nutrients the body needs may be lost in urine and cause bone problems, brittle hair and nails, hair loss, and stunted growth in children.

PROBABLE OUTCOME—The outcome will depend on the underlying cause diagnosed. If it is treatable, such as an infection, the outcome is often good. In children with minimal disease, almost all respond to treatment. In other cases, the outcome may be less favorable and kidney failure and other complications may occur.

HOW TO TREAT

GENERAL MEASURES—To learn more: National Kidney Foundation, 30 E. 33rd St., Suite 1100, New York, NY 10016; (800) 622-9010; website: www.kidney.org.

MEDICATION—You may be prescribed:
* Cortisone or immunosuppressive drugs.
* Diuretics to reduce fluid retention.
* Drugs to treat infections.
* Angiotensin-converting enzyme (ACE) inhibitors to reduce protein loss.
* Drugs for high blood pressure or high cholesterol.
* Anticoagulants for blood clots.
* Stopping any drug that is the cause.

ACTIVITY—After the swelling decreases, be as active as your strength and condition allows.

DIET—You will be advised about any limits on fat, salt, protein, and fluid intake.

CALL YOUR DOCTOR IF

* You or a family member has symptoms of nephrotic syndrome.
* After diagnosis, any of the following occur:
  - Infection (fever, headache, sores on the skin, cough, or burning during urination).
  - Amount of urine decreases, or fluid retention, vomiting, diarrhea, or nausea occurs.

NOSE FRACTURE

 GENERAL INFORMATION

DEFINITION—Fracture or damage to the bones and cartilage of the nose. This often happens when other facial bones are also fractured. The injury may be to the front or the side of the nose.

BODY PARTS INVOLVED—Nose.

SEX OR AGE MOST AFFECTED—Older children (over age 8) and adults. Young children's noses have only cartilage. Males are more often affected than females.

SIGNS & SYMPTOMS
• Pain in the nose.
• Nosebleed.
• Swollen, discolored nose.
• Bruising around the eyes.
• Difficulty in breathing through the nose.
• Crooked or misshapen nose (sometimes).

CAUSES—Injury (trauma) to the nose. This is often from a motor vehicle accident, being hit on the nose, running into a hard object, or due to a fall.

RISK INCREASES WITH—Previous nose injury.

HOW TO PREVENT
• Wear protective headgear for contact sports or when riding motorcycles or bicycles.
• Use seat belts in motor vehicles.

 WHAT TO EXPECT

DIAGNOSTIC MEASURES
• Your own observation of symptoms.
• Your health care provider will do a physical exam of the face and nose.
• X-rays may or may not be needed depending on the type of injury.

APPROPRIATE HEALTH CARE
• A minor nose fracture with no displacement may not require further medical treatment. It will heal on its own. Rest at home. Apply ice several times a day until the swelling is gone. Use two pillows when lying down to keep the head above the heart. This helps with pain.
• Treatment may involve reduction (correction) of the fracture. This can be done right after the injury, before any swelling occurs. It can also be done days later, when the swelling is gone. A local or general anesthetic is used.
• The reduction may be done by manipulating the nose into place with finger pressure. It may require the use of two probes inserted into the nose to move the bones back into place. More severe fractures may require surgery. An incision (cut) is made on the front of the nose.

The bones are put back together with special tools. Wires, plates, or screws may be used to hold the bones in place. A splint may be needed.
• Plastic surgery can be done at a later date if there is a problem with the cosmetic appearance of the nose.

POSSIBLE COMPLICATIONS
• Infection of the nose and sinuses.
• Persistent breathing difficulty.
• Permanent change in appearance.
• Deviated nasal septum. This occurs when the structure that divides the nose in half is off-center.
• Septal hematoma. Blood becomes trapped in the septum. This can lead to complications if it is not drained.

PROBABLE OUTCOME—Minor fractures with no deformity usually heal on their own. Major fractures can be repaired with treatment. Most of the swelling will be gone in 10 to 20 days, but some swelling may last for months. The nose may feel tender for about a month.

 HOW TO TREAT

GENERAL MEASURES—First aid steps: Have the person sit down and lean forward to keep blood from going down the back of the throat. Have them breathe through the mouth. Apply cold compresses or an ice pack to the nose to reduce swelling. Do not try to move displaced bones in an attempt to straighten the nose. If a nosebleed is heavy or cannot be stopped, seek emergency medical care to get it under control.

MEDICATION
• For minor discomfort, you may use nonprescription drugs such as acetaminophen.
• Stronger pain relievers may be prescribed.
• Antibiotics may be prescribed to prevent or treat an infection.
• Decongestants may be prescribed, to reduce swelling.

ACTIVITY
• Rest until any bleeding stops.
• Most activities can be resumed right away.
• You can usually return to non-contact sports in two weeks, and contact sports in three weeks. Protective gear may need to be worn. Follow any medical advice.

DIET—No special diet.

 CALL YOUR DOCTOR IF

• You or a family member has symptoms of a fractured nose.
• New symptoms develop after treatment.

NOSEBLEED
(Epistaxis)

GENERAL INFORMATION

DEFINITION—Sudden bleeding from one or both nostrils. The bleeding involves blood vessels (arteries and veins) in the nose. Nosebleeds may occur close to the nose opening or deeper in the nose.

BODY PARTS INVOLVED—Nose.

SEX OR AGE MOST AFFECTED—All ages, but twice as common in children as adults.

SIGNS & SYMPTOMS
- Blood oozing from the nostril. If the broken vessel is close to the nostril, the blood is bright red. If the broken vessel is deeper in the nose, the blood may be bright or dark red.
- Lightheadedness from a large amount of blood loss (rare).
- Rapid heartbeat, shortness of breath, and pallor (with significant blood loss only).
- Black stool from swallowed blood.

CAUSES—Injury to the nose, breathing dry air, allergies, illnesses, or for no apparent reason.

RISK INCREASES WITH
- Injury to the nose.
- Nasal or sinus infection.
- A foreign body in the nose.
- Dry mucous membranes in the nose from any cause, such as low humidity.
- Bleeding tendencies associated with some illnesses.
- Allergic rhinitis (hay fever) or nonallergic rhinitis.
- Use of certain drugs, such as anticoagulants, aspirin, or prolonged use of nose drops.
- Exposure to irritating chemicals.
- Excess alcohol use.
- High altitude or dry climate.

HOW TO PREVENT
- Avoid injury if possible.
- Get medical treatment for sinus or allergy problems.
- Humidify the air if you live in a dry climate or at high altitude.
- Avoid picking at nose or vigorous nose blowing.
- Avoid aspirin if you have frequent nosebleeds.

WHAT TO EXPECT

DIAGNOSTIC MEASURES
- Your own observation of symptoms.
- Exam by a health care provider (sometimes).

APPROPRIATE HEALTH CARE
- Seek emergency treatment if self-care is not successful. Gauze packing may be inserted to absorb blood, stop the dripping, and exert pressure on the ruptured blood vessels.
- Continued or recurrent bleeding may require cauterization (use of heat to seal off blood vessels).
- Surgery (for severe bleeding only) to tie off the artery feeding the bleeding area.

POSSIBLE COMPLICATIONS—Bleeding may rarely be severe and require medical care.

PROBABLE OUTCOME—Most nosebleeds are harmless, even though it seems like a lot of blood is lost. They are usually controlled with self-care by applying pressure to the nose.

HOW TO TREAT

GENERAL MEASURES
Self-care:
- Sit up with your head bent forward.
- Clamp your nose closed with your fingers for 5 uninterrupted minutes. During this time, breathe through your mouth.
- If bleeding stops and recurs, repeat, but pinch your nose firmly on both sides for 8 to 10 minutes. Holding your nose tightly closed allows the blood to clot and seal the damaged blood vessels.
- You may apply cold compresses or an ice pack at the same time you are applying pressure.
- Don't blow your nose for 12 hours after bleeding stops to avoid dislodging the blood clot.
- Don't swallow blood. It may upset your stomach or make you "gag," causing you to inhale blood.
- Don't talk (also to avoid gagging).

MEDICATION—Drugs are not needed for a nosebleed. They may be prescribed to treat an underlying disorder.

ACTIVITY—Resume your normal activities as soon as symptoms improve.

DIET—No special diet.

CALL YOUR DOCTOR IF

- You or a family member has a nosebleed that won't stop with self-care steps.
- After the nosebleed, you become nauseous or vomit, or your temperature rises to 101°F (38.3°C) or higher.

OBESITY & OVERWEIGHT

 GENERAL INFORMATION

DEFINITION—*Obesity* is defined as having an unhealthy amount of body fat. *Overweight* is defined as an excess amount of body weight as compared to an acceptable weight. The common tool to measure obesity and overweight is the body mass index (BMI). It measures body weight in relation to height. Note: A BMI may indicate a person is overweight, but it could be due to lean muscle and not excess body fat (such as with an athlete).

BODY PARTS INVOLVED—Total body.

SEX OR AGE MOST AFFECTED—Both sexes; all ages.

SIGNS & SYMPTOMS
- Low energy levels.
- Breathing/snoring problems; sleep apnea.
- Appearance of large body size.
- Fatigue and joint pain from supporting excess weight.

CAUSES—Obesity and overweight occur when a person consumes more calories then he or she burns. Other risk factors can affect this imbalance in different people.

RISK INCREASES WITH
- Genetic factors. Obesity runs in families.
- Emotional feelings. People eat when they are depressed, upset, angry, sad, or bored.
- Eating disorder, such as binge eating.
- Metabolic and endocrine disorders.
- Steroids, some antidepressants, and other drugs.
- Rarely, neurologic disorders.

HOW TO PREVENT
- Proper diet and nutrition. Regular exercise.
- Behavior and lifestyle changes, as needed.

 WHAT TO EXPECT

DIAGNOSTIC MEASURES
- The body mass index (BMI) formula uses height and weight to measure weight status.
  - Adult BMI of 25 to 29.9 = overweight.
  - Adult BMI of 30 or more = obese.
  - BMI formula: *(weight, in pounds, times 703) divided by (height in inches squared).* Website to calculate BMI: www.cdc.gov/nccdphp/dnpa/bmi/bmi-adult.htm.
- Waist size (circumference) measures abdominal fat. Over 40 inches (102 cm) in men and over 35 inches (88 cm) in women indicates health and obesity risk factors.

APPROPRIATE HEALTH CARE
- Treatment steps depend on health status, age, degree of obesity or overweight, and motivation. Steps can include a combination of diet, exercise, behavior modification, and drugs. Gastrointestinal surgery may be recommended with severe obesity if other methods fail.
- You and your health care provider can develop a weight-loss plan based on your individual needs. Keep a food and activity diary to keep track of your progress.

POSSIBLE COMPLICATIONS
- High risk for many major physical health problems that can lead to disability and death.
- Emotional problems (depression, and feeling unattractive, rejected, and shameful).
- Prejudice or discrimination at work, school, social occasions, and travel.

PROBABLE OUTCOME—Obesity and overweight can be controlled if motivation is maintained for life.

 HOW TO TREAT

GENERAL MEASURES
- Books, websites, and weight-loss programs are available to help with weight-loss. Diet plans should provide proper nutrition, information on exercise and behavior changes, and maintaining the weight-loss long-term.
- Behavior changes start with identifying the behaviors that lead to overeating and being inactive. Then learn how to change and maintain the new behaviors. Support groups or a weight-loss counselor can help.
- To learn more: Weight Control Information Network, 1 Win Way, Bethesda, MD 20892-3665; (877) 946-4627; website: www.niddk.nih.gov/health/nutrit/nutrit.htm.

MEDICATION—Drugs for obesity may be prescribed on a trial basis to see if they help.

ACTIVITY—Increase physical activity. Start with a daily 10 minute walk. Aim for 20 to 30 minutes of activity 3 to 5 times a week, plus muscle strengthening 2 times a week.

DIET
- Choose an eating plan that will work for you. Diets need to be healthy, help you lose weight, and maintain the new weight. A dietitian can help you choose a plan.
- A realistic weight-loss rate is 1 pound per week. It is normal to have periods when no weight is lost on your plan. Don't stop; weight loss will begin again.

 CALL YOUR DOCTOR IF

You or a family member wants to lose weight.

OBSESSIVE COMPULSIVE DISORDER

 GENERAL INFORMATION

DEFINITION—A disorder that involves recurrent, intrusive, and unwanted thoughts (obsessions), and repetitive, ritualistic behaviors (compulsions). People with obsessive-compulsive disorder (OCD) realize that their behavior is excessive, disruptive, and unreasonable, but are unable to change it or explain it. It causes significant distress or impairment and can consume most of a person's time.

BODY PARTS INVOLVED—Nervous system.

SEX OR AGE MOST AFFECTED—Both sexes; It may begin gradually in childhood or early adult life; rarely starts after age 50.

SIGNS & SYMPTOMS
* Obsessions that recur. Trying to ignore or resist them is unsuccessful. Obsessions can include:
  - Fears of infection (from germs, dirt, etc.) and fear of serious illness.
  - Doubts (Is the door shut/locked? Is the iron on?).
  - Excessive orderliness or symmetry.
  - Fear that one's actions hurt other people or cause bad thing to happen.
  - Inappropriate sexual and aggressive thoughts.
* Compulsions are repetitive, purposeful behaviors to try to suppress the anxiety caused by obsessions. Compulsions include:
  - Asking for assurances.
  - Avoiding places or actions.
  - Doubts and checking (ovens, locks, doors, lights).
  - Excessive washing (hands or bathing).
  - Hoarding possessions.
  - Repeating behaviors such as dressing rituals.
  - Counting/cleaning/ordering/arranging.

CAUSES—The cause is unknown. It may be due to a low level of serotonin (a brain chemical). Serotonin is involved in sending impulses from one nerve cell to the next, and in regulating repetitive behavior.

RISK INCREASES WITH
* Problems with work, school, relationships, living situation, abuse, or illness.
* Family history of the disorder.

HOW TO PREVENT—No specific prevention methods known.

 WHAT TO EXPECT

DIAGNOSTIC MEASURES
* Your health care provider may do a physical exam and ask questions about the symptoms.

* No medical tests can diagnose the disorder. A patient's description of the behavior offers the best clues to diagnosis.

APPROPRIATE HEALTH CARE
* Treatment is aimed at reducing anxiety, resolving inner conflicts, relieving depression, learning ways of dealing with stress, building self-esteem, and gaining an understanding of the compulsive behavior.
* Behavioral therapy (usually a process known as "exposure and response prevention") is used in treatment. It is often combined with drugs to achieve satisfactory results.
* Family education about the disorder is important.
* Group therapy may be helpful for some patients.
* A patient who is severely affected (and who does not respond to drug therapy) may benefit from precise, localized brain surgery (rare).

POSSIBLE COMPLICATIONS
* Unable to develop and maintain normal work and personal relationships.
* Depression, anxiety, and panic episodes.
* Housebound and limited lifestyle due to symptoms.

PROBABLE OUTCOME—OCD continues for life. Symptoms may ease up for a while, or become more severe. Effective and specific therapy is now available. It may not lead to a cure, but can reduce symptoms.

 HOW TO TREAT

GENERAL MEASURES—To learn more: Obsessive-Compulsive Foundation, 676 State St., New Haven, CT 06511; (203) 401-2070 (not toll free); website: www.ocfoundation.org.

MEDICATION
* Antidepressants are often effective and may be prescribed. Complete benefits may not be seen for 3 weeks. About 10% of patients are unable to tolerate the side effects of the drugs, but an adverse response to one does not mean there will be problems with another.
* Antianxiety or tranquilizer drugs may also be prescribed.

ACTIVITY—No limits.

DIET—No special diet.

 CALL YOUR DOCTOR IF

* You or a family member has symptoms of obsessive-compulsive disorder.
* Symptoms continue or worsen after during treatment.
* Drugs used in treatment produce side effects.

ORAL CANCER

GENERAL INFORMATION

DEFINITION—Growth of malignant cells in the mouth or tongue. These are rare, but dangerous.

BODY PARTS INVOLVED—Lips; gums; palate; tongue; membranes inside the lip or cheek; floor of the mouth; tonsillar area.

SEX OR AGE MOST AFFECTED—Both sexes and adults over 40. It is increasing in young people who chew smokeless tobacco.

SIGNS & SYMPTOMS
• A pale lump, usually painless, with a hard rim that appears in any part of the mouth or tongue.
• Lump grows larger, becomes an open sore, and bleeds easily.
• Dentures may not fit properly.
• Lump may make the tongue stiff and difficult to control, causing speaking and swallowing difficulty.

CAUSES—Unknown.

RISK INCREASES WITH
• Use of tobacco in any form (including smokeless).
• Family history of oral cancer.
• Past history of oral cancer.
• Excess alcohol use.
• Sun exposure (cancer on the lower lip).
• Serious periodontal (gum) disease.

HOW TO PREVENT
• Don't use tobacco in any form; and drink alcohol in moderate amounts, if at all.
• To help diagnosis a cancer at an early stage, see your dental care provider or health care provider if you have any sore patches or lumps on the lips or in the mouth that do not heal in two weeks.
• Practice good oral hygiene and get regular dental checkups.

WHAT TO EXPECT

DIAGNOSTIC MEASURES
• Your own observation of symptoms.
• Your health care provider will do an exam of the mouth and neck area.
• Medical tests may include blood studies, x-rays of the head, a biopsy, and other tests. Biopsy involves removal of a small amount of tissue for viewing under a microscope. The larger the lump at the time of diagnosis, the greater the chance that it has metastasized (spread) to other places in the body.

APPROPRIATE HEALTH CARE
• Treatment will vary depending on location of the cancer (lips, tongue, palate, etc.), if the cancer has spread, and the patient's age and health.

• Surgery is a common treatment for oral cancer. If needed, a person's normal facial appearance can often be restored by plastic surgery.
• Radiation therapy and/or anticancer drugs may be recommended.
• Newer treatments such as hyperthermia (using heat on cancer cells) and gene therapy are being studied.
• Follow-up therapy may be needed to help adjust to new ways of eating and talking.

POSSIBLE COMPLICATIONS
• Slow healing after surgery.
• Spread to lymph nodes in the neck, requiring head and neck surgery.
• Speech and swallowing problems.
• Cancer may recur.
• The five-year survival rate is about 50% for those diagnosed with oral cancer.

PROBABLE OUTCOME—Recovery depends on where the cancer is located, if it has spread, and patient's general health. The outcome is more favorable with early diagnosis, as compared to diagnosis of advanced disease. Early diagnosis improves the success rate of treatment.

HOW TO TREAT

GENERAL MEASURES
• Discontinue use of tobacco in any form.
• To learn more: American Cancer Society, (800) ACS-2345; website: www.cancer.org or National Cancer Institute, (800) 4-CANCER; website: www.nci.nih.gov.

MEDICATION—You may be prescribed:
• Anticancer drugs (chemotherapy).
• Pain relievers after surgery.
• Antibiotics, if infection occurs.

ACTIVITY—Resume your normal activities gradually after surgery.

DIET
• Depends on the extent of the disease and your ability to chew or swallow. A soft diet may be required.
• A liquid diet may be needed for a few days after surgery.

CALL YOUR DOCTOR IF

• You or a family member has any signs of oral cancer.
• The following occur after treatment: increasing pain, fever, new lumps or sores, or excessive bleeding.

ILLNESS & DISORDERS

OSGOOD-SCHLATTER DISEASE
(Osteochondrosis)

 GENERAL INFORMATION

DEFINITION—A common, temporary condition involving the knee and tibia (shin bone). It occurs often in young athletes (boys more than girls). Osgood-Schlatter disease (OSD) is named for the two doctors who first described it.

BODY PARTS INVOLVED—Tibial tubercle, a prominence just below the knee cap attached to a large thigh muscle connecting the bone of the upper leg (femur) to the large bone in the lower leg (tibia). Usually, only one knee is affected.

SEX OR AGE MOST AFFECTED—It usually occurs during the pre-teen or teenage growing years. It is uncommon after age 16.

SIGNS & SYMPTOMS
• Swelling, pain, and tenderness below the knee joint and over the shin bone. The symptoms may be mild to severe.
• Pain worsens with activity and gets better with rest. Pain may occur with jumping, kneeling, running, climbing stairs, or anytime the knee is bent and extended.
• Bony bump may be felt just below the kneecap. It may feel tender, warm, and hurt when pressed.

CAUSES—A combination of rapid growth and stress on the knee joint due to overuse. The tendon in the kneecap that connects it to the tibia becomes inflamed due to constant pulling by the quadriceps muscles. The tendon may stretch and tear away (called avulsion) from the tibia and take a piece of bone with it.

RISK INCREASES WITH
• Sports and activities that involve running, jumping, cutting, or jogging.
• Boys between 11 and 18. As more girls participate in sports, their risk of OSD increases.
• Rapid skeletal growth.

HOW TO PREVENT—No specific preventive measures. Encourage a child to exercise moderately, avoiding extremes.

 WHAT TO EXPECT

DIAGNOSTIC MEASURES
• Your own observation of symptoms.
• Your health care provider will do a physical exam of the leg and ask questions about your symptoms and activities.
• Medical tests may include an x-ray or bone scan of the knee to confirm the diagnosis.

APPROPRIATE HEALTH CARE
• Treatment may involve using ice or heat, drugs (if needed for pain), rest, and limits on sports activities.
• Stretching exercises may be prescribed.
• Occasionally, other treatments may be recommended depending on symptoms. These may include using crutches, having a leg cast or splint, or wearing an elastic knee brace.
• Surgery (rarely) if other treatment fails.

POSSIBLE COMPLICATIONS
• In a few cases, chronic pain may occur.
• About 60% of adults who have had OSD have some pain when kneeling.

PROBABLE OUTCOME—Usually resolves on its own within 1 to 2 years. Some discomfort may persist for 2 to 3 years or until growth is completed. A permanent, painless bump may remain below the knee.

 HOW TO TREAT

GENERAL MEASURES
• Apply ice to the affected area several times a day for the first 2 to 3 days to reduce swelling and pain.
• After a few days, heat may help discomfort. Use warm compresses, a heating pad, or take warm baths.

MEDICATION—For minor discomfort, you may use nonprescription drugs such as ibuprofen.

ACTIVITY
• Your health care provider will advise you of the limits on sports and activities. Each individual case is different. The usual recommendation is to stop any sports or activities that cause pain. Participation may be permitted when it does not cause pain. Resuming some activities too quickly could make the symptoms worse.
• When you return to normal sports activities, recommendations may include wearing a knee brace, special insoles in your shoes, using heat before and ice on your knee after your activity, and stretching and strengthening exercises.

DIET—No special diet.

 CALL YOUR DOCTOR IF

• Your child has symptoms of Osgood-Schlatter disease.
• The following occur during treatment:
  - Pain increases.
  - Fever.
  - Other unexpected symptoms.

OSTEOARTHRITIS
(Degenerative Joint Disease)

 GENERAL INFORMATION

DEFINITION—Gradual deterioration (degeneration) of cartilage in a joint.

BODY PARTS INVOLVED—Osteoarthritis is most common in weight-bearing joints (feet, ankles, knees, hips). It also affects fingers, wrists, shoulders, and spine.

SEX OR AGE MOST AFFECTED—It can occur at any age in both sexes, but is more likely in adults over age 45.

SIGNS & SYMPTOMS
• Joint stiffness and pain, including backache. Weather changes, such as cold and damp, may increase aching.
• Limited movement and less flexibility in joints.
• No redness, heat, or fever in affected joints (usually).
• Swelling of affected joints, such as fingers.
• May have cracking or grating sounds in joints.

CAUSES—The cartilage normally forms a soft protective layer between the bones of a joint. When the cartilage deteriorates, it allows the bones to rub together. This causes the pain and limited movement.

RISK INCREASES WITH
• Age. 50% of people over age 60 have some signs of osteoarthritis.
• Obesity.
• Activities that stress joints (e.g., dancers, football players, instrumental musicians, carpet layers, and others).
• Injury to the joint.
• Family history of osteoarthritis.

HOW TO PREVENT
• Avoid obesity or being overweight.
• Be physically active, but avoid activities that lead to joint injury, especially after age 40. Try regular stretching or yoga exercises.

 WHAT TO EXPECT

DIAGNOSTIC MEASURES
• Your health care provider will do a physical exam and ask questions about your symptoms and activities.
• Medical tests may include studies of joint fluid (to rule out inflammatory forms of arthritis) and x-rays of joints.

APPROPRIATE HEALTH CARE
• Treatment goals are to control pain, slow progression of the disorder, and improve mobility and function. This may include lifestyle changes, drugs, self-care steps, and surgery.
• Lifestyle changes may involve diet (to maintain healthy weight), exercises, and using mechanical aids.

• Mechanical aids can include: shock-absorbing or orthopedic shoes, canes, crutches, or walkers. They may include splints, braces, or elastic supports to help joints; neck brace, collar, or corset to help back pain.
• Acupuncture may help some people.
• Surgery for osteoarthritis may be recommended for some patients. There are different options.

POSSIBLE COMPLICATIONS
• Crippling (sometimes).
• Symptoms can lead to limits in daily activities, affect the ability to work, may bring on stress and depression, and restrict social and recreational activities.

PROBABLE OUTCOME—Symptoms can usually be relieved, but joint changes are permanent. Pain may begin as a minor irritant, but it can become severe enough to interfere with daily activities and sleep. The disorder worsens over time.

 HOW TO TREAT

GENERAL MEASURES
• Heat can ease discomfort or pain. Use heating pads or warm soaks several times a day for 10 minutes at a time.
• Cold can help reduce swelling and inflammation. Use an ice pack several times a day for 20 to 30 minutes.
• Sleep on a firm mattress or place plywood (3/4-inch thick) between springs and mattress.
• Try to avoid outdoor activity in cold weather.
• To learn more: Arthritis Foundation, local chapter, or contact them at P.O. Box 7669, Atlanta, GA 30357-0669; (800) 283-7800; website: www.arthritis.org.

MEDICATION
• Nonsteroidal anti-inflammatory drugs. These drugs may be nonprescription or prescribed. All have some side effects. You may need to try more than one to see what works best for you.
• Glucosamine and chondroitin supplements may help. Take for at least 6 weeks as a trial.
• Cortisone joint injections may be prescribed.
• Other drugs may be prescribed as needed.

ACTIVITY—Exercise is beneficial. Your health care provider can advise you about an exercise program. Swimming or water aerobics are good. They don't stress the joints.

DIET—If overweight, weight loss will help joints.

 CALL YOUR DOCTOR IF

• You or a family member has joint problems.
• Symptoms worsen after treatment starts.

OSTEOMYELITIS

GENERAL INFORMATION

DEFINITION—Infection of the bone and bone marrow.

BODY PARTS INVOLVED—It can involve any bone in the body. In a child, it usually affects the femur (upper leg bone), tibia (lower leg bone), the humerus or radius (bones in the arm). In an adult, it usually affects the pelvis or spine.

SEX OR AGE MOST AFFECTED—It occurs in both sexes and all ages (often children and the elderly).

SIGNS & SYMPTOMS
• High fever.
• Pain, swelling, redness, warmth, and tenderness in the area over the infected bone, especially when moving a nearby joint. Nearby joints, such as the knee, may also be red, warm, and swollen.
• May have limited use or not be able to use an infected extremity (arm or leg).
• Child may guard or protect area from being touched.
• General ill feeling.
• Excessive sweating, chills, back pain (sometimes).

CAUSES—Bacterial infection is the most common cause. Fungal or other infections are more rare. Bones can be infected by: bacteria in the bloodstream from infection in another body part; bacteria in soft body tissue located next to the bone; and bacteria that directly infects the bone.

RISK INCREASES WITH
• Recent injury or surgery.
• Diabetes or sickle cell anemia.
• Infection that occurs in another part of the body.
• People on dialysis (hemodialysis).
• Weak immune system due to illness or drugs.
• Intravenous (IV) drug abuse.

HOW TO PREVENT—Obtain prompt medical treatment of any bacterial infection to prevent its spread to bone or other body parts.

WHAT TO EXPECT

DIAGNOSTIC MEASURES
• Your own observation of symptoms.
• Your health care provider will do a physical exam of the affected area.
• Medical tests include blood studies and cultures to identify the bacteria. Samples of pus, joint fluid, and infected bone may be removed and used for tests to confirm the diagnosis. Imaging studies such as bone scans or x-rays may be done.

APPROPRIATE HEALTH CARE
• Treatment usually involves hospital care, drug therapy, rest, and other supportive measures.
• The affected bone and joint may be immobilized (not allowed to move). Bracing may be used for the spine.
• Surgery may be done to drain an abscess, remove dead bone tissue or infected bone, and to stabilize the spine. Bone or skin grafts may be required.
• An artificial joint that is infected may need to be removed and replaced.
• A patient may be placed in a sealed chamber where high-pressure oxygen is used for treatment.

POSSIBLE COMPLICATIONS
• Chronic osteomyelitis. It may last for months or years and be difficult to treat. It can cause periodic bone pain, tenderness, and abscess (area of pus) that may drain through the skin. Treatment may require more surgery and drugs for an extended period of time.
• Reduced function in affected limb and joint.
• Recurrence of the infection.
• Rarely, treatment is unsuccessful and infection continues. Surgery may be done to fuse the joint or amputate the limb.

PROBABLE OUTCOME—Outcome will depend on severity of infection, effectiveness of drug treatment, results of surgical procedures, and general health of patient. Treatment success rates have increased and new therapies are being studied.

HOW TO TREAT

GENERAL MEASURES—Follow medical advice about home care after treatment.

MEDICATION
• Antibiotics will be prescribed to treat the infection. They are sometimes given through a vein (IV) while in the hospital. The drugs usually need to be continued at home after the hospital stay. This may be done by continuing the IV drugs or with drugs that are taken by mouth.
• Pain relievers may be prescribed.

ACTIVITY
• Rest in bed until symptoms get better. Resume your normal activities gradually.
• Physical therapy (sometimes) to help affected limbs and joints regain function and flexibility.

DIET—No special diet.

CALL YOUR DOCTOR IF

• You or a family member has symptoms of osteomyelitis.
• Symptoms persist or recur despite treatment.

OSTEOPOROSIS

GENERAL INFORMATION

DEFINITION—Loss of normal bone density, bone mass, and bone strength. Osteoporosis (it means porous bones) is a progressive disease that leads to increased thinning of bones and risk of fractures (broken bones).

BODY PARTS INVOLVED—Bones.

SEX OR AGE MOST AFFECTED—It occurs in both sexes, but is most common in women after menopause due to a decrease in the hormone estrogen. Estrogen protects against bone loss.

SIGNS & SYMPTOMS
- Osteoporosis does not cause pain, and there are usually no obvious symptoms. It is called a "silent" disease.
- People don't realize they have osteoporosis until they fall and suffer a fracture, or a spontaneous fracture occurs in a back-bone. Pain from fractures may be mild to severe. The pain may stop when the fracture heals or it may be chronic due to permanent bone damage.

CAUSES—Loss of bone mass and density occurs due to a decrease of calcium (a mineral) and other substances that are needed for maintaining bone strength. A number of risk factors can contribute to the decrease.

RISK INCREASES WITH
- Females; advanced age; Asian or white persons.
- Early menopause (either naturally or due to surgery).
- Lack of exercise (sedentary lifestyle).
- A broad range of diseases and drugs.
- Poor nutrition. Lack of calcium, protein, and vitamins.
- Women with a small body frame or quite thin.
- Eating disorders (bulimia or anorexia).
- Family history of osteoporosis.
- Smoking.
- Excess alcohol use.
- Men with low testosterone levels.

HOW TO PREVENT
- Prevention needs to start at a young age.
- Adequate calcium intake (1200 to 1500 mg a day) with milk and dairy products or calcium supplements.
- Regular exercise, such as walking (which is weight-bearing, and is better for bone strength).
- Avoid risk factors such as alcohol or smoking.
- Drugs may be prescribed in high-risk cases.

WHAT TO EXPECT

DIAGNOSTIC MEASURES—Medical tests may include bone x-rays, ultrasound, and bone density studies. The diagnosis may be that bone density is normal, or there is mild bone loss (osteopenia), or osteoporosis.

APPROPRIATE HEALTH CARE
- Treatment is aimed at stopping further bone loss, preventing fractures, relieving pain (if needed), and bone rebuilding. Treatment steps include drugs, lifestyle changes, and medical care for any underlying disorder. A treatment plan will be based on your individual case.
- Lifestyle changes may include diet changes, exercise, modifying behaviors, and home safety to prevent falls.
- If a drug you take is a risk factor for osteoporosis, the medical advice may be to stop the drug, reduce the dosage, or use an alternative drug.

POSSIBLE COMPLICATIONS
- Falls and bone fractures, such as hip, spine and wrist.
- Severe, disabling pain.
- Deformed spinal column and bent back (sometimes called Dowager hump). Loss of height.

PROBABLE OUTCOME—Treatment (no matter what age) can help halt and may reverse some bone loss. Pain symptoms can usually be helped with drugs.

HOW TO TREAT

GENERAL MEASURES
- Stop smoking. Find a way to quit that works.
- Stop excess alcohol use.
- To learn more: National Osteoporosis Foundation, 1150 17th St., Suite 500 NW, Washington, DC 20036, (800) 223-9994; website: www.nof.org.

MEDICATION
- Different prescription drugs are used to prevent and treat bone loss. If one drug causes problems or is not effective, another drug can be prescribed.
- For minor pain, use nonprescription drugs such as acetaminophen or ibuprofen. Stronger pain drugs may be prescribed.
- Calcium and vitamin D supplements may be needed.

ACTIVITY—Exercise strengthens muscles and bones and improves balance. Aerobic and weight-bearing exercises should be part of a daily 30-minute program.

DIET—Eat a healthy, well-balanced diet.

CALL YOUR DOCTOR IF

- You or a family member has symptoms of osteoporosis.
- Pain develops, especially after an injury.

OTOSCLEROSIS

GENERAL INFORMATION

DEFINITION—Slow formation of abnormal, spongy bone growth in the middle ear. The growth prevents one of the small bones in the middle ear from transmitting sound waves. This can lead to hearing loss. Otosclerosis usually affects both ears.

BODY PARTS INVOLVED—Middle-ear bones and nerves in the ear that allow us to hear. Otosclerosis usually affects both ears.

SEX OR AGE MOST AFFECTED—It occurs in all ages and both sexes, but is more common in females from ages 15 to 30.

SIGNS & SYMPTOMS
• Slow, continuing hearing loss. Early on, the disease is called otospongiosis.
• Ringing or other types of noises in the ears (tinnitus).
• Dizziness or imbalance if the vestibular portion of the ear is affected.

CAUSES—Appears to be an inherited disease. Sixty percent of those affected have a positive family history of the disorder. In other cases, the cause is unknown. A viral infection may be a factor.

RISK INCREASES WITH
• Family history of hearing loss.
• Genetics. Otosclerosis affects to some degree about 10% of all white persons.
• Pregnancy, which may trigger the onset.
• Osteogenesis imperfecta (a bone disease of the ear).

HOW TO PREVENT—Cannot be prevented at present. Obtain genetic counseling before starting a family if you or your spouse has otosclerosis.

WHAT TO EXPECT

DIAGNOSTIC MEASURES
• Your own observation of symptoms.
• Your health care provider will do a physical exam of the ears and ask questions about your symptoms and family history of hearing problems.
• Diagnosis is based on hearing tests such as an audiogram and Rinne test (study of bone conduction). A CT (an imaging study) of the head may be done to rule out other disorders.

APPROPRIATE HEALTH CARE
• Treatment will depend on the degree of hearing loss. It may involve surgery and/or hearing aids, and sometimes fluoride supplements.
• If the hearing loss is minor, no treatment is usually needed. Hearing tests will be given periodically to see if hearing loss is progressing.
• Treatment usually involves surgery (stapedectomy) to remove a part or all of the stapes (a bone in the middle ear) and replace it with a prosthesis (artificial substitute). The hearing is improved in almost all cases.
• Hearing aids will benefit many patients. Different types are available. A hearing specialist can help you choose what will work best for your individual needs.
• A bone anchored hearing aid (BAHA) may be recommended. It is an implantable hearing aid that takes minor surgery to put in place.

POSSIBLE COMPLICATIONS
• Without surgery, some degree of hearing loss may continue for years. Total deafness is a rare complication.
• Hearing loss can cause problems with work, social events, and family relationships. Emotional distress may occur.

PROBABLE OUTCOME—Surgical treatment can help restore or improve hearing in most patients. In patients not needing or unable to have surgery, hearing aids can be of benefit.

HOW TO TREAT

GENERAL MEASURES—To learn more: American Speech-Language-Hearing Association, 10801 Rockville Pike Rd., Rockville, MD 20852; (800) 638-8255; website: www.asha.org.

MEDICATION
• Antibiotics may be prescribed after surgery.
• Sodium fluoride may be prescribed to prevent further hearing loss by hardening the spongy bone. It won't, however, improve hearing.

ACTIVITY—After surgery, resume your normal activities gradually.

DIET—No special diet.

CALL YOUR DOCTOR IF

• You or a family member has symptoms of otosclerosis.
• Sudden hearing loss or dizziness occurs.
• New symptoms occur after surgery.

OVARIAN CANCER

 GENERAL INFORMATION

DEFINITION—A malignant growth in the ovary that is likely to spread to other body parts and threaten life. There are many different types of ovarian cancer. Epithelial tumors account for the majority, and they grow more rapidly. Other ovarian cancers are slow growing, or they have spread from other cancer in the body.

BODY PARTS INVOLVED—One or both ovaries. It may spread to the lungs and bone.

SEX OR AGE MOST AFFECTED—It affects females of all ages, but is most common after age 50.

SIGNS & SYMPTOMS
- Often no symptoms occur until late in the disease.
- Discomfort in the lower abdomen, gas, and indigestion.
- Pelvic pain, or swelling in the abdomen with no pain.
- Feeling of being constipated or unable to have a bowel movement.
- Irregular menstrual periods; bleeding from the vagina.
- Pain with intercourse.
- A need to urinate often.
- Excess hair growth.
- Nausea, loss of appetite, not being able to eat, and weight loss. Sometimes a weight gain occurs.

CAUSES—The exact cause is unknown.

RISK INCREASES WITH
- Personal history of breast cancer. A family history of breast and/or ovarian cancer, colon, lung, prostate, and uterine cancers.
- Women who carry mutated genes such as BRCA1 and BRCA2.
- Advancing age.
- Women who began to menstruate before age 12 and/or start menopause after age 50.
- Women who have used ovulation-stimulating fertility drugs have a slightly increased risk of ovarian cancer.
- Late pregnancies (over age 30).
- Never having had children.

HOW TO PREVENT
- No specific preventive measures. Having yearly pelvic exams may aid in earlier diagnosis and treatment.
- For women with a family history of ovarian cancer, screening tests and genetic counseling may be recommended. In some cases, ovary removal may be discussed if a woman has a strong family history of breast or ovarian cancer and pregnancy is not desired.
- Birth control pills may help with prevention.

 WHAT TO EXPECT

DIAGNOSTIC MEASURES
- Your health care provider will do a physical exam and ask questions about your symptoms.
- A number of medical tests will be done. The tests help diagnose the cancer and also determine if it has spread (staging).

APPROPRIATE HEALTH CARE
- Treatment varies and depends on the location and size of a tumor, any spread of the cancer, health, age and preferences of the patient. Treatment may include chemotherapy (anticancer drugs) and/or radiation therapy, surgery, and biologic therapy.
- Chemotherapy uses drugs and radiation therapy uses radiation to attack the cancer cells. Biologic therapy uses the body's immune system to fight cancer.
- The goal of surgery is to remove as many of the cancer cells as possible so that chemotherapy will be more effective. In patients who desire pregnancy, surgery may remove only the ovary and the fallopian tube.
- Treatment may involve steps to relieve symptoms and make you comfortable, rather than treating the cancer.
- Counseling may help you cope.

POSSIBLE COMPLICATIONS
- Pleural effusion (excess fluid in the lining of the lungs) or ascites (excess fluid in the peritoneal cavity).
- Spread of cancer to other places in the body (can cause pain, other complications, or death).
- Infertility if both ovaries are removed.
- Recurrence of cancer.

PROBABLE OUTCOME—Depends on the stage of the disease when it is first diagnosed. Other factors that affect outcome are a woman's age and her general health.

 HOW TO TREAT

GENERAL MEASURES—To learn more: American Cancer Society, (800) ACS-2345; website: www.cancer.org or National Cancer Institute, (800) 4-CANCER; website: www.nci.nih.gov.

MEDICATION—Anticancer drugs (chemotherapy) and pain relievers, as needed, may be prescribed.

ACTIVITY—Be as active as health permits.

DIET—Eat a normal, well-balanced diet.

 CALL YOUR DOCTOR IF

You or a family member has symptoms of ovarian cancer.

OVARIAN TUMOR, BENIGN

GENERAL INFORMATION

DEFINITION
• The ovaries are the female reproductive organs that hold and release eggs and produce female hormones. An abnormal growth in the ovary that is solid is called a tumor. It is different from a cyst. An ovarian cyst contains fluid. However, in the ovary, some tumors may have fluid areas within them and are called cystic tumors. Ovarian tumors are usually small, but in some cases, may grow large enough to make a woman appear pregnant.
• In some cases, the tumor may have features that suggest it will behave as a cancer, but over a long period of time (10 to 20 years). These are called low malignant-potential (LMP) ovarian tumors or borderline ovarian tumors.

BODY PARTS INVOLVED—One or both ovaries.

SEX OR AGE MOST AFFECTED—Females between puberty and menopause.

SIGNS & SYMPTOMS—May not cause symptoms. If symptoms occur, they may include:
• Mild pelvic pain.
• Pain in the lower back.
• Discomfort with sexual intercourse.
• Changes in menstrual flow, the length of periods, and time between periods.
• Excess hair growth, deep voice, and weight gain (sometimes).
• If a large ovarian tumor twists or ruptures, it can cause severe pain, rigid muscles, and swelling.

CAUSES
• Usually, unknown. It is likely to be related to problems of female hormone production and secretion.
• Endometriosis.

RISK INCREASES WITH—Unknown.

HOW TO PREVENT—No specific preventive measures. Use of oral contraceptives may decrease risk.

WHAT TO EXPECT

DIAGNOSTIC MEASURES
• Your own observation of symptoms.
• Your health care provider will do a physical and pelvic exam.
• Medical tests can include blood studies, ultrasound, and laparoscopy (a telescope-like tool is used to look inside the abdomen).

APPROPRIATE HEALTH CARE
• Treatment may not be needed, except to have regular pelvic exams. The tumor's growth can be monitored.
• Some tumors require surgery to diagnose accurately, rule out cancer, or for treatment purposes. If one ovary must be removed, normal conception and childbirth is possible as long as a normal ovary remains on the other side.

POSSIBLE COMPLICATIONS
• Complications from surgery may occur.
• Tumor may recur after treatment.

PROBABLE OUTCOME—Most ovarian tumors require no treatment and disappear on their own within a few months. In other cases, treatment usually provides a complete cure. Benign or noncancerous tumors do not invade nearby tissue the way cancerous tumors do.

HOW TO TREAT

GENERAL MEASURES
• If surgery is required, see Laparotomy (in Surgery section) for an explanation of surgery and postoperative care.
• To learn more: try the library or perform a web search. A good site to start with is www.4women.gov.

MEDICATION—Female hormones may be prescribed. These help shrink or destroy some tumors. Oral contraceptives are often used as the first step in treatment.

ACTIVITY—No limits unless surgery is necessary.

DIET—No special diet.

CALL YOUR DOCTOR IF

• You or a family member has symptoms of an ovarian tumor.
• Severe pain and abdominal distention occurs.
• New, unexplained symptoms develop. Drugs used in treatment may produce side effects.

PAGET'S DISEASE OF BONE
(Osteitis Deformans)

 GENERAL INFORMATION

DEFINITION—A gradual, progressive bone disease. It is named for an English doctor who first described the disease. Paget's disease of the breast is a different disorder.

BODY PARTS INVOLVED—It usually involves the bones of the skull, spine, legs, collar bone, and pelvis.

SEX OR AGE MOST AFFECTED—It can affect both sexes and is most common in middle-aged people.

SIGNS & SYMPTOMS
* Most often, there are no early symptoms.
* Bone pain (especially at night).
* Skin over the bones is warm.
* Joint pain or stiffness.
* Headaches.
* Hearing loss and tinnitus (noises in the ear).
* Fractures (may occur from minor trauma).
* Bowing (deformity) of extremities, such as of the legs.
* Nerve problems, from pressure on the nerves.

CAUSES—Unknown. It may involve genetics and/or a virus. The affected bone breaks down and then abnormal bone growth occurs. The new bone is weak, fragile, enlarged, and deformed.

RISK INCREASES WITH—Family history of Paget's disease.

HOW TO PREVENT
* No specific preventive measures.
* Those with family history should have a blood-screening test periodically to help with early diagnosis.

 WHAT TO EXPECT

DIAGNOSTIC MEASURES
* Your own observation of symptoms.
* Your health care provider will do a physical exam.
* Medical tests may include blood and urine studies, x-rays of affected bones, and a bone scan. Hearing and vision testing may be done if the skull is involved.

APPROPRIATE HEALTH CARE
* Treatment may include physical therapy, use of assistive devices, drugs, exercise, home care, and surgery.
* If there are no symptoms, treatment may not be needed. Follow-up exams will monitor the disease status.
* Physical therapy helps maintain and improve muscle strength, range of motion, flexibility, and endurance.

* Walkers, canes, crutches, special shoes, or shoe inserts may help if walking is a problem.
* Transcutaneous electrical nerve stimulation (TENS) or massage may help muscle pain and tightness.
* Rarely, splinting may be needed for severely affected areas to prevent fractures.
* Bone surgery may be needed to treat fractures, correct deformities, or treat arthritis.
* Hearing aid may be useful if hearing loss occurs.

POSSIBLE COMPLICATIONS—Many complications can occur that affect different organs and body parts. Complications include arthritis, heart disease, hearing loss, kidney stones, bone cancer, vision changes, spinal disease, enlarged head, loose teeth, and others.

PROBABLE OUTCOME
* There is no cure, but treatment can control or reduce symptoms. With early treatment (before major bone changes occur), the outlook is generally good.
* Research into cause and treatment continues.

 HOW TO TREAT

GENERAL MEASURES
* Use heat to relieve pain (warm compresses, or soaks).
* Accident-proof your home. Avoid throw rugs and slippery floors. Install hand rails next to the tub. Other changes may be needed depending on patient's needs.
* To learn more: Paget Foundation, 120 Wall St., Suite 1602, New York, NY 10005-4001; (800) 237-2438; website: www.paget.org.

MEDICATION
* Drugs will usually be prescribed that help slow the rate of bone turnover. Several options are available and their risks and benefits will be discussed with you.
* Nonprescription drugs for pain can be used. Stronger ones may be prescribed (if needed).
* Calcium and vitamin D are often recommended.

ACTIVITY—Home exercises will help maintain mobility. Avoid stress on affected bones. Follow instructions provided by your physical therapist or health care provider.

DIET—Eat a healthy diet. Avoid weight gain.

 CALL YOUR DOCTOR IF

* You or family member has symptoms of Paget's disease of bone.
* New or worsening symptoms occur during treatment.

PANCREAS CANCER

GENERAL INFORMATION

DEFINITION—Growth of cancer cells in the pancreas. The pancreas produces intestinal enzymes (juices) to help digest food, and insulin to control blood sugar.

BODY PARTS INVOLVED—Pancreas, an organ in the back of the upper abdomen.

SEX OR AGE MOST AFFECTED—It usually affects adults ages 35 to 70, and men more than women.

SIGNS & SYMPTOMS
• Usually no symptoms occur in early stages of cancer.
• Weight loss. Loss of appetite.
• Pain in the back or upper abdomen.
• Fatigue.
• Jaundice (yellow skin and eyes). Intense itching may occur with jaundice.
• Nausea, vomiting, and problems with digestion.
• Depression, though not caused by cancer, may occur.

CAUSES—Unknown. It may be to be a combination of hereditary factors and environmental factors.

RISK INCREASES WITH
• Chronic pancreatitis (inflammation of the pancreas).
• Diabetes.
• Genetic factors. It is more common in African-Americans than in whites, Asians, or American Hispanics.
• Smoking.
• Excess alcohol use.
• Diet high in fat and low in fruits and vegetables.
• Obesity and lack of physical activity.
• Exposure to industrial chemicals, such as urea, naphthalene, or benzidine.
• Certain hereditary disorders.

HOW TO PREVENT—No specific preventive measures. To reduce cancer risks: get recommended screening tests, maintain healthy weight, eat a healthy diet, exercise regularly, and don't smoke.

WHAT TO EXPECT

DIAGNOSTIC MEASURES
• Your own observation of symptoms.
• Your health care provider will do a physical exam and ask questions about any symptoms.
• A number of medical tests will be done. The tests help to diagnose the cancer, and then determine if it has spread (staging).

APPROPRIATE HEALTH CARE
• Treatment varies and depends on location and size of tumor, any spread of the cancer, your health, age, and preferences. Treatment may include chemotherapy (anticancer drugs) and/or radiation therapy, surgery, and biologic therapy.
• Chemotherapy uses drugs and radiation therapy uses radiation to attack the cancer cells. Biologic therapy uses the body's immune system to fight cancer.
• Surgery may be performed to remove the tumor if the cancer has not spread to other places in the body.
• Treatment may involve steps to relieve symptoms and make you comfortable, rather than treating the cancer.
• Counseling may help you cope.

POSSIBLE COMPLICATIONS
• Spread (metastasis) of cancer to other places in the body. This has often already occurred by the time of diagnosis.
• Surgical complications.
• Malnutrition (lack of nutrients the body needs).
• Increased pain.

PROBABLE OUTCOME
• The diagnosis often comes too late for effective treatment. Survival for more than 1 or 2 years is unlikely. However, symptoms can be relieved or controlled.
• Research into cause and treatment continues.

HOW TO TREAT

GENERAL MEASURES—To learn more: American Cancer Society, (800) ACS-2345; website: www.cancer.org, or National Cancer Institute, (800) 4-CANCER; website: www.nci.nih.gov.

MEDICATION—You may be prescribed:
• Pain relievers.
• Chemotherapy (anticancer drugs).
• Pancreatic enzymes to replace those that the pancreas cannot manufacture.
• Sedatives for sleep if needed.
• Vitamin supplements.

ACTIVITY—Remain as active as you can. It helps your quality of life.

DIET
• Low-fat diet may be recommended.
• Loss of appetite may make eating difficult. Try eating several small meals each day. Choose foods easy to digest and eat healthy snacks.

CALL YOUR DOCTOR IF

• You have symptoms of pancreatic cancer.
• New changed symptoms occur.

PANCREATITIS

GENERAL INFORMATION

DEFINITION—Inflammation of the pancreas. The pancreas supplies digestive juices and hormones for the body. Acute pancreatitis occurs suddenly and lasts for a short period. If injury to the pancreas occurs, chronic pancreatitis can develop.

BODY PARTS INVOLVED—Pancreas.

SEX OR AGE MOST AFFECTED—Adults of both sexes.

SIGNS & SYMPTOMS
Acute pancreatitis:
- Extreme abdominal pain.
- Vomiting.
- Abdominal swelling and gas.
- Fever.
- Muscle aches.
- Drop in blood pressure.

Chronic pancreatitis:
- Persistent mild or severe pain, often after meals, in the upper abdomen. Pain sometimes spreads to the back or over the entire body. Pain is aching, burning, gnawing, or stabbing. Pain episodes may last days or weeks, but rarely less than 1 day.
- Mild jaundice (yellow skin and eyes) in some.
- Rapid weight loss.

CAUSES—The inflammation is a reaction to injury, infection, or irritation of the pancreas. It can be brought on by a number of different factors. Sometimes the cause is unknown.

RISK INCREASES WITH
- Alcoholism.
- Disease of the gallbladder or bile ducts.
- Obstruction of the pancreatic duct by stones, scarring, or slow-growing cancer (rare).
- Abdominal injury.
- Viral, bacterial, or parasitic infection.
- Hyperlipidemia (high fat levels in the blood).
- Tumor.
- Trauma, surgery or some medical procedures.
- Peptic ulcer disease.
- Use of drugs, such as sulfa drugs, azathioprine, chlorothiazide, or cortisone drugs.

HOW TO PREVENT—Avoid risk factors where possible.

WHAT TO EXPECT

DIAGNOSTIC MEASURES
- Your own observation of symptoms.
- Your health care provider will do a physical exam and ask questions about your symptoms and activities.
- Medical tests may include blood, stool, and urine studies; x-rays of the abdomen; CT scan or ultrasound of the pancreas; and others.

APPROPRIATE HEALTH CARE
- Acute pancreatitis normally requires hospital care for intravenous (IV) fluids and control of pain and vomiting. Oxygen or breathing support with a machine may be needed for breathing problems. Surgery may be required for gallstones, perforated peptic ulcer, or to drain a source of infection.
- Chronic pancreatitis may be treated as an outpatient with drugs, diet controls, and avoidance of alcohol. In some cases, surgery may be needed to control pain.

POSSIBLE COMPLICATIONS—Complications may occur from acute and chronic pancreatitis. They can affect the heart, lungs, kidneys, and other body organs, and could be fatal in a few cases.

PROBABLE OUTCOME—Acute pancreatitis is often curable with treatment. Chronic pancreatitis may have recurrent attacks for years. Drugs and diet changes can help symptoms.

HOW TO TREAT

GENERAL MEASURES
- Follow medical instructions. Compliance with the treatment plan helps the outcome.
- To learn more: National Digestive Diseases Information Clearinghouse, 2 Information Way, Bethesda, MD 20892, (800) 891-5389; website: www.digestive.niddk.nih.gov.

MEDICATION—You may be prescribed:
- Pain relievers.
- Digestive enzymes that the damaged pancreas cannot manufacture.
- Antibiotics, if bacterial infection develops.
- Drugs to reduce stomach acid.
- Insulin, if diabetes is present.

ACTIVITY—For acute pancreatitis, bed rest or rest sitting in a chair, if that is more comfortable. Increase activities gradually as symptoms resolve. No limits for chronic pancreatitis.

DIET—Small, frequent, and low-fat meals. Abstain completely from drinking alcohol.

CALL YOUR DOCTOR IF

- You or a family member has symptoms of acute pancreatitis.
- Jaundice (yellow skin and eyes), fever of 101°F (38.3°C) or higher, continued weight loss, muscle cramps, or seizures occur.

PANIC DISORDER

GENERAL INFORMATION

DEFINITION—Repeated and unexpected episodes of irrational fear and panic. Panic disorder is a type of anxiety. It occurs with attack-like symptoms (often during sleep). Most attacks last 2 to 10 minutes, but some may extend as long as an hour or two. Many people may have one panic attack and never have another.

BODY PARTS INVOLVED—Central nervous system; heart; lungs; skin; hands; feet.

SEX OR AGE MOST AFFECTED—Twice as many females as males; young adults, ages 25-44.

SIGNS & SYMPTOMS
Physical symptoms:
• Pounding, racing or skipping heartbeat, chest pains, and shortness of breath.
• Choking feeling, lump in the throat feeling, weakness, faintness, dizziness, lightheaded, and sweating.
• Trembling, numbness, tingling, flushes, or chills.
• Muscle spasms or contractions in the hands and feet.
• Feeling of "butterflies" in the stomach. Nausea.
Emotional symptoms:
• Intense fear of losing one's mind (fear of going crazy), an urge to flee, fear of dying.
• Sense of terror, doom, or dread.
• Sense of unreality, loss of contact with people and objects, and fear of losing control.
• Fear of having another panic attack.

CAUSES—The brain's "alarm system" appears to be affected by a combination of biologic/genetic factors, illnesses, drugs, and one's personal history of traumatic events.

RISK INCREASES WITH
• Stress (emotional or physical); feelings of guilt, fatigue, or overwork; illness; alcohol or drug abuse.
• Personal history of other emotional problems and family history of panic disorder.

HOW TO PREVENT—No specific measures to prevent a first panic attack. Treatment helps prevent repeated attacks.

WHAT TO EXPECT

DIAGNOSTIC MEASURES
• Your health care provider will do a physical exam and ask questions about your symptoms and activities.
• Medical tests may be done to rule out other disorders. A variety of physical disorders can mimic panic attacks.

APPROPRIATE HEALTH CARE
• Treatment may involve psychotherapy (treatment of emotional and mental problems), self-care, and drugs.
• Cognitive-behavioral therapy may help. Cognitive therapy teaches how to change thoughts, behaviors or attitudes. Behavioral therapy teaches ways to reduce anxiety with deep breathing and muscle relaxation.

POSSIBLE COMPLICATIONS
• Without treatment, it can negatively affect all aspects of life (work, family, friends, social, and recreational).
• Chronic anxiety or depression; phobias, including agoraphobia (fear of being alone or in public places).
• People with this disorder often feel that there is a physical problem causing their symptoms. They will go from doctor to doctor to get a diagnosis. Despite assurances that they are in good health, they continue to believe otherwise.

PROBABLE OUTCOME—For many, this disorder gets better at times and worse at other times. Treatment can help reduce or prevent the attacks. Sometimes it recurs after treatment, but repeated treatment can be successful.

HOW TO TREAT

GENERAL MEASURES
• Talk to a friend or family member about your feelings. It may help lessen your anxiety.
• Keep a journal about anxious thoughts or emotions. Think about causes and solutions.
• Join a self-help group.
• Learn relaxation techniques.
• Reduce stress in your life, where possible.
• To learn more: National Institute of Mental Health; 6001 Executive Blvd, Bethesda, MD 20892-9663; (800) 647-2642; website: www.nimh.nih.gov.

MEDICATION—You may be prescribed an antidepressant, benzodiazepine, or beta-blocking agent. The drug may be slowly reduced or stopped, after 6 months to a year, to determine if the panic attacks will return. If they do not return, the drug can be discontinued.

ACTIVITY—Exercise daily; get enough sleep.

DIET
• Consider giving up caffeine (coffee, tea, soft drinks). You may have withdrawal symptoms but they will stop in a few days.
• Don't use alcohol to numb your feelings.

CALL YOUR DOCTOR IF

• You or a family member has panic attacks.
• Symptoms return after treatment.

PARALYSIS

GENERAL INFORMATION

DEFINITION—The loss of ability to move a part of the body caused by the inability to contract one or more muscles. The condition varies in degree and severity from paralysis of one small muscle to paralysis of almost the total body. The paralysis may be temporary or permanent. Types include: paraplegia (partial or complete paralysis of both legs), quadriplegia (partial or complete paralysis of both arms and legs), and hemiplegia (partial or complete paralysis of one side of the body).

BODY PARTS INVOLVED—Brain; spinal cord; nervous system; muscles.

SEX OR AGE MOST AFFECTED—Both sexes; all ages.

SIGNS & SYMPTOMS—The following vary, depending on the site and extent of damage:
- Loss of movement and sensation in affected arms or legs.
- Loss of urinary and bowel control; impaired sexual function; loss of normal blood pressure; loss of body-temperature control; constipation.
- Difficulty speaking, understanding or recognizing words.
- Blurred, double or decreased vision.

CAUSES—Normally, the brain originates the impulses for muscle movement. These impulses travel via the spinal cord and peripheral nerves to the muscles. Paralysis occurs when there is an injury or disruption in this nerve pathway. Causes include:
- Stroke (most common). Stroke may be caused by bleeding in brain, or blood clot or obstruction of blood vessel to brain.
- Brain: tumor, abscess, hemorrhage, infection (encephalitis).
- Spinal cord: injury (from an accident); pressure on the spinal cord (disk prolapse, cervical osteoarthritis), decompression sickness.
- Disease: multiple sclerosis, poliomyelitis, myelitis, Friedreich's ataxia, meningitis, motor neuron disease.
- Nerve disorders (neuropathies): secondary to disorders such as diabetes mellitus, vitamin deficiency, liver disease, alcoholism, cancer and toxic effects of drugs or metals.
- Muscle disorders such as muscular dystrophy and sometimes, myasthenia gravis.

RISK INCREASES WITH
- Any activity with a high risk of injury.
- Excess alcohol consumption or drug use.

HOW TO PREVENT
- Observe safety precautions; don't take risks.
- Don't dive into shallow water.
- Wear protective headgear during contact sports and while riding a bicycle or motorcycle.
- Obtain medical treatment to control any chronic medical condition.

WHAT TO EXPECT

DIAGNOSTIC MEASURES—Diagnosis with emergency care may be needed. Medical tests will be determined by the cause of the paralysis.

APPROPRIATE HEALTH CARE
- Treatment of any underlying cause.
- Hospital care in intensive unit if paralysis affects the breathing muscles.
- Surgery to limit further spinal-cord damage or to remove bones or a tumor.
- Time in an extended-care facility or special rehabilitation facility (sometimes).
- Physical and occupational rehabilitation.
- Psychotherapy or counseling for depression or for sexual problems.

POSSIBLE COMPLICATIONS—Kidney infections, especially if a urinary catheter is needed; lung infections; constipation; fecal impaction; pressure sores; deep-vein blood clot; depression; limb deformities.

PROBABLE OUTCOME—Depends on the extent of injury. Damaged spinal cord and nerves are limited in their ability to recover.

HOW TO TREAT

GENERAL MEASURES—The more you can learn and understand about your disorder, the more you will be able to make informed decisions about where to go for your care, the treatments available, the risks involved, side effects of therapy and expected outcome.

MEDICATION—You may be prescribed:
- Antibiotics to treat infection.
- Drugs to control hypertension, diabetes, or other underlying disorders.
- Anticoagulants to prevent blood clot.
- Stool softeners and laxatives.

ACTIVITY—Resume activities gradually to the extent possible. With rehabilitation, many lost functions can be compensated for or restored. Use passive exercise for paralyzed or partially paralyzed muscles to prevent contractures.

DIET
- Eat a high-fiber diet to prevent constipation.
- If you have a urinary catheter, drink plenty of fluids a day to prevent bladder stones and urinary-tract infections.

CALL YOUR DOCTOR IF

After diagnosis, any symptoms cause concern.

PARKINSON'S DISEASE

 ## GENERAL INFORMATION

DEFINITION—A chronic disease of the central nervous system that affects the movements of the body. It is named for the doctor who first described it.

BODY PARTS INVOLVED—Area of the brain that regulates movement; muscles.

SEX OR AGE MOST AFFECTED—Parkinson's usually starts after age 50, but can occur in younger adults.

SIGNS & SYMPTOMS
* Tremors (worse with rest; better with moving).
* General muscle stiffness and slowness.
* Shuffling, wide-based walk, and balance problems.
* Stooped posture.
* Loss of facial expression.
* Voice changes (weak and high pitched).
* Swallowing difficulty, drooling.
* Mental functioning can slowly decrease.
* Depression and nervousness.

CAUSES
* Dopamine is a brain chemical that helps control normal muscle movement. With primary (or idiopathic) Parkinson's disease, less dopamine is produced due to a loss of nerve cell function. It is unknown why this loss of nerve cell function occurs.
* Secondary Parkinson's disease can be due to drugs, brain injury, tumors, encephalitis, slow-virus infection, some toxins, and carbon-monoxide poisoning.

RISK INCREASES WITH
* Unknown for the primary type.
* For secondary type, risk factors are listed in Causes.

HOW TO PREVENT—No preventive measures for primary type. For secondary type, avoid risk factors, where possible.

 ## WHAT TO EXPECT

DIAGNOSTIC MEASURES
* Your health care provider will do a physical exam and ask questions about your symptoms and activities.
* There is not a special test to diagnose the disorder. Medical tests may be done to rule out other disorders. If symptoms get better with the drug levodopa, it usually means a person has Parkinson's disease.

APPROPRIATE HEALTH CARE
* Treatment options may involve various types of therapy, exercise, self-care, drug therapy, and surgery. Individual treatment will vary depending on a person's age, stage of the disease, and symptoms.

* Counseling can help treat emotional symptoms such as depression, anxiety, stress, anger, and frustration.
* Physical therapy, occupational therapy (help with daily activities), and speech therapy may be helpful.
* Surgery may be an option for severe symptoms or when drugs are not helping. It is not a cure, but it may relieve symptoms.

POSSIBLE COMPLICATIONS
* Dementia.
* "Freezing" (sudden, but temporary inability to move).
* Falls and fractures.
* Debilitation (weakness and loss of strength).

PROBABLE OUTCOME
* There is no cure for primary type. It is progressive, but unpredictable. There may be good days and bad days. It is not a fatal disease in itself. Symptoms can generally be relieved or controlled with treatment.
* Secondary type outcome depends on cause.

 ## HOW TO TREAT

GENERAL MEASURES
* Accident-proof your home to help prevent falls and injuries. Install handrails, remove area rugs, keep cords out of the way, and carry a cordless phone with you.
* Getting dressed can be a problem. Choose clothes that are easy to slip on. Wear clothes and shoes that have Velcro fasteners. Allow plenty of time to dress.
* To learn more: American Parkinson Disease Association, 1250 Hylan Blvd., Suite 4B, Staten Island, NY 10305; (800) 223-2732; website: www.apdaparkinson.org or National Parkinson Foundation, 1501 NW 9th Ave., Miami, FL 33136; (800) 327-4545; website: www.parkinson.org.

MEDICATION
* One or more drugs can be prescribed to treat the symptoms. If one does not help or stops being effective, others can be tried.
* Vitamins or other supplements may be prescribed.

ACTIVITY—Exercises will help maintain mobility, balance, range of motion, and well-being. Follow instructions provided by your physical therapist or health care provider.

DIET—Eat a healthy diet. Add fiber to the diet and increase fluid intake to prevent constipation. If chewing is a problem, take small bites, eat slowly, and chop up food.

 ## CALL YOUR DOCTOR IF

You or a family member has symptoms of Parkinson's disease or symptoms worsen.

PARONYCHIA

GENERAL INFORMATION

DEFINITION—Inflammation of tissue folds that surround a nail. The inflammation can be from bacterial or fungal infection, and is not contagious.

BODY PARTS INVOLVED—It usually occurs on the hands and less often on the feet.

SEX OR AGE MOST AFFECTED—Both sexes; all ages.

SIGNS & SYMPTOMS
Bacterial paronychia:
* Pain or tenderness, redness, warmth, and swelling of tissue adjacent to the fingernail.
* Central whitish area produced by pus.
Fungal paronychia:
* Redness and swelling around the fingernail.
* No pain, warmth, itching, or pus.

CAUSES
* Bacterial paronychia is preceded by injury, such as a torn hangnail. The infecting bacteria are usually *Staphylococcus*.
* Fungal paronychia is caused by a fungus or yeast infection.

RISK INCREASES WITH
* Injury around the nail.
* Work exposure to constant wetness (dishwashers, bartenders, housewives).
* Diabetes.
* Nail biting or finger sucking.
* Artificial nails.
* Shoes that bind or pinch the toes.

HOW TO PREVENT
* Protect hands from wetness.
* Leave hangnails alone.
* Avoid fingertip injury.
* Avoid tight shoes.

WHAT TO EXPECT

DIAGNOSTIC MEASURES
* Your own observation of symptoms.
* Your health care provider will do an exam of the affected nail.
* Medical studies, such as a culture of the discharge, may be done to identify the germ.

APPROPRIATE HEALTH CARE
* Treatment involves avoiding factors that may be the cause, self-care, and drug therapy.
* Sometimes part, or all, of a toenail may need to be removed.

POSSIBLE COMPLICATIONS—If untreated, may permanently damage the fingernail and nail bed. Rarely, the infection may enter bone or bloodstream.

PROBABLE OUTCOME
* Bacterial paronychia is curable with treatment in 2 weeks.
* Fungal paronychia is chronic and may require 6 months to heal.
* Recurrence is common with both forms.

HOW TO TREAT

GENERAL MEASURES
* Use warm-water soaks several times a day.
* If an abscess (pus-filled area) occurs, it may require incision (cutting) and drainage.
* Wear heavy-duty vinyl gloves to prevent contact with irritating substances, such as water, soap, detergent, metal scrubbing pads, scouring pads, scouring powder, and other chemicals.
* Dry the insides of gloves after use. Discard gloves if they develop a hole. A glove with a hole harms the hand more than not wearing a glove.
* Wear vinyl gloves when you peel or squeeze lemons, oranges, grapefruit, tomatoes, or potatoes.
* Wear leather or heavy-duty fabric gloves for housework or gardening.
* Avoid contact with irritating chemicals, such as paint, paint thinner, turpentine, and polish for cars, floors, shoes, furniture, or metal.
* Use lukewarm water and very little mild soap to shower or bathe. All soaps are irritating. Expensive soaps offer no more protection against irritation than less-expensive ones.

MEDICATION
* For minor pain, you may use nonprescription drugs, such as ibuprofen or acetaminophen.
* Antibiotics may be prescribed for bacterial infection.
* Topical antifungals and topical steroids may be prescribed for fungal infection.

ACTIVITY—No limits.

DIET—No special diet.

CALL YOUR DOCTOR IF

* You or a family member has symptoms of paronychia.
* Pain is not helped by treatment.

PELVIC INFLAMMATORY DISEASE (PID)

 ## GENERAL INFORMATION

DEFINITION—Pelvic inflammatory disease (PID) is an infection of the upper genital area. Any sexually active female may be affected. PID is one of the most common and serious complications of sexually transmitted diseases (STDs) in women. Up to 40% of untreated genital infections progress to PID. Salpingitis (fallopian tube inflammation) is another term.

BODY PARTS INVOLVED—Fallopian tubes; cervix; uterus; ovaries; urinary bladder.

SEX OR AGE MOST AFFECTED—Sexually active females after puberty. The peak incidence occurs in late teens and early 20s.

SIGNS & SYMPTOMS
- Some women have no symptoms.
- Pain or cramps in the lower abdomen.
- Vaginal discharge (may have a foul odor).
- Painful intercourse or pain when urinating.
- Irregular menstrual bleeding.
- Fever, nausea, and vomiting.

CAUSES—Bacterial infection (usually chlamydial or gonorrheal). The bacteria infection starts in the vagina and cervix and then spreads to the upper genital area. PID usually develops from 2 days to 3 weeks after exposure to the bacteria, but can take months to develop. The infection may be transmitted by an infected sexual partner.

RISK INCREASES WITH
- Women who have a sexually transmitted disease.
- Teenagers (more at risk than older women).
- Multiple sexual partners, or exposure to a single partner who is infected.
- Use of an intrauterine contraceptive device (IUD).
- Prior episode of PID.
- Abortion.
- Pelvic surgery.
- Women who douche once or twice a month. This may push bacteria into the upper genital area.

HOW TO PREVENT
- Use latex (rubber) condoms to help prevent sexually transmitted infections.
- Oral contraceptives may help to decrease the risk.
- Get routine medical check-ups for sexually transmitted diseases if you have multiple sexual partners.
- Get medical care for abnormal vaginal discharge, unusual odor, fever, and bleeding between periods.
- Have your sexual partner tested and treated if needed. Don't resume sexual activity with your partner until tests show no infection, or it has been treated.

 ## WHAT TO EXPECT

DIAGNOSTIC MEASURES
- Your health care provider will do a physical and a pelvic exam.
- Medical tests may include blood studies, culture of the vaginal discharge, and pregnancy test. Other tests may be done to confirm the diagnosis, and rule out other disorders.

APPROPRIATE HEALTH CARE
- Treatment is with drugs and hospital care (if needed).
- Treatment may be done on an outpatient basis if infection is mild. It is important to follow your treatment schedule. Close medical follow-up care is needed.
- Hospital care may be needed for severe illness, more diagnostic tests, an abscess, pregnancy, HIV infection, or if drugs are to be given in a vein (IV).
- Surgery to drain an abscess may be needed.
- Surgery may help chronic PID or pelvic pain.
- Counseling can be helpful if infertility occurs.

POSSIBLE COMPLICATIONS
- Chronic pelvic pain.
- Infertility or ectopic pregnancy.
- Recurrent PID.
- Abscess (pus-filled area). It can be life threatening.

PROBABLE OUTCOME—With early diagnosis and treatment, most women recover with no complications. Late treatment or incomplete treatment can lead to serious complications.

 ## HOW TO TREAT

GENERAL MEASURES
- If you have a sexually transmitted disease (STD), your partner needs treatment (even if he has no symptoms).
- Use sanitary pads to absorb the discharge or menstrual flow. Don't douche during treatment.
- To learn more: National STD Hotline (800) 227-8922; website: www.ashastd.org/NSTD/index.html.

MEDICATION—Antibiotics (by injection or taken by mouth) for bacterial infection will be prescribed. Finish taking all the drug prescribed for a complete cure.

ACTIVITY—You will be advised when it is safe to resume sexual intercourse.

DIET—No special diet.

CALL YOUR DOCTOR IF

You or a family member has symptoms of pelvic inflammatory disease or symptoms recur after treatment.

PENIS CANCER

GENERAL INFORMATION

DEFINITION—Malignant tumor of the penis. Penis cancer is uncommon.

BODY PARTS INVOLVED—Penis, including the glans (tip), corona (rounded border of the glans) or prepuce (foreskin covering the glans).

SEX OR AGE MOST AFFECTED—Men over age 50.

SIGNS & SYMPTOMS
• A small, circular lesion (resembles a pimple) or persistent, painless sore on the penis. The lesion is easily visible in a circumcised male, but it may go unnoticed in an uncircumcised male.
• Pain, bleeding, or discharge.
• Discomfort with urination.
• Enlarged lymph nodes in the groin.

CAUSES—Unknown. A human papillomavirus (HPV) may play a role in the cause. The virus can be sexually transmitted.

RISK INCREASES WITH
• Cigarette smoking.
• Having unprotected sexual relations with multiple partners. This increases the risk of HPV infection.
• AIDS (acquired immunodeficiency syndrome).
• Psoriasis (skin disorder) treatment that uses drugs along with ultraviolet light.

HOW TO PREVENT
• No specific preventive measures. Avoid risk factors where possible. Practice good genital hygiene to reduce risks of infection or irritation. If uncircumcised, retract the foreskin and clean the entire penis when bathing.
• Do a self-exam of the penis and testicles monthly. This can help detect cancers early, when treatment is most successful. See your health care provider for any sign of infection or sores on the penis.

WHAT TO EXPECT

DIAGNOSTIC MEASURES
• Your own observation of symptoms.
• Your health care provider will do a physical exam of the penis and ask questions about any symptoms.
• A number of medical tests will be done. The tests help to diagnose the cancer and then determine if it has spread (staging).

APPROPRIATE HEALTH CARE
• Treatment varies and depends on the location and size of tumor, any spread of the cancer, health, age, and preferences. Treatment may include chemotherapy (anticancer drugs) and/or radiation therapy, surgery, and biologic therapy.

• Chemotherapy uses drugs and radiotherapy uses radiation to attack the cancer cells. Biologic therapy uses the body's immune system to treat cancer.
• Surgery to remove the tumor. Local tumors of the foreskin may require circumcision only. Invasive tumors require part or total removal of the penis and some lymph nodes. Urine will still be able to exit the body.
• Treatment may involve steps to relieve symptoms and make you comfortable, rather than treating the cancer.
• Counseling may help you cope with having cancer.

POSSIBLE COMPLICATIONS—Men may delay treatment due to denial, fear of surgery, and loss of sexual function. Treatment delay increases the risk of the cancer spreading.

PROBABLE OUTCOME—Will depend on the extent of the cancer at diagnosis. Early diagnosis and treatment has a more favorable outcome. Recurrence is possible after treatment.

HOW TO TREAT

GENERAL MEASURES
• The more you can learn and understand about this disorder, the more you will be able to make informed decisions about where to go for your care, the treatments available, the risks involved, side effects of therapy and expected outcome.
• To learn more: American Cancer Society, (800) ACS-2345; website: www.cancer.org or National Cancer Institute, (800) 4-CANCER; website: www.nci.nih.gov.

MEDICATION—Anticancer drugs may be prescribed. They may be used on the skin, taken by mouth, or given by injection.

ACTIVITY—Resume normal activities as soon as possible after treatment. Sexual relations are possible if enough penile tissue remains after surgery. If the total penis is removed, sexual pleasure is still possible using special techniques.

DIET—No special diet.

CALL YOUR DOCTOR IF

• You or a family member has any lump or sore on the penis.
• Excessive bleeding occurs at the surgical site.
• New, unexplained symptoms develop. Drugs used in treatment may produce side effects.

PERICARDITIS

GENERAL INFORMATION

DEFINITION—Inflammation of the pericardium. The pericardium is a sac (thin membrane) around the heart. It has two layers, with a small amount of "lubricating" fluid between them. The fluid lets the heart move around within the sac. With inflammation, the heart can become squeezed inside the sac.

BODY PARTS INVOLVED—Pericardium.

SEX OR AGE MOST AFFECTED—Both sexes; all ages (more often in men ages 20 to 50).

SIGNS & SYMPTOMS
* Dull or sharp pain in the front of the chest. The pain moves to the neck, arm, and shoulder. The pain worsens with movement and eases when sitting up or leaning forward.
* Rapid breathing.
* Cough.
* Fever, sweating, and chills.
* Weakness.
* Anxiety.

CAUSES—The inflammation is a reaction to injury, infection, or irritation of the heart lining. It can be caused by a number of different factors. In many cases, the cause is unknown.

RISK INCREASES WITH
* Rheumatic fever and other diseases of connective tissue, such as lupus erythematosus.
* Complication of a heart attack.
* Complication following heart surgery.
* Complication of a chest injury.
* Viral, bacterial, tuberculous, amebic, toxoplasmotic, or fungal infection.
* Chronic kidney failure.
* Spread of cancer to the pericardium.
* Radiation therapy.

HOW TO PREVENT—No specific preventive measures. To avoid risk factors, get treatment for disorders that may lead to pericarditis.

WHAT TO EXPECT

DIAGNOSTIC MEASURES
* Your own observation of symptoms.
* Your health care provider will do a physical exam and ask questions about your symptoms and activities.
* Medical tests may include blood studies, chest x-ray, heart tests (electrocardiogram and echocardiogram), and others.

APPROPRIATE HEALTH CARE
* Treatment is aimed at relieving symptoms and treating the underlying disorder. Treatment may include drugs and, sometimes, hospital care.
* Home care is usually sufficient.
* Hospital care may be needed if there are complications. A needle may be used to draw off excess fluid if it is causing problems for heart function. Rarely, surgery may be needed on the pericardium.

POSSIBLE COMPLICATIONS
* Pericarditis becomes chronic if it lasts for 6 to 12 months following the initial (acute) episode.
* Excess fluid in the pericardial sac impairs heart function.
* Pericardium becomes thick and scarred.
* Blood circulation problems.

PROBABLE OUTCOME—Usually curable with treatment. Allow 2 to 3 weeks for healing. It may recur one or more times in the next 6 to 12 months.

HOW TO TREAT

GENERAL MEASURES
* Apply a heating pad or warm compresses to the chest to relieve pain.
* To learn more: American Heart Association, 7272 Greenville Ave., Dallas, TX 75231; (800) 242-8721; website: www.americanheart.org.

MEDICATION
* Nonsteroidal anti-inflammatory drugs to reduce pain and inflammation are usually prescribed.
* Steroid drugs for severe forms of pericarditis may be prescribed.
* Stronger pain drugs may be prescribed.
* Drugs to treat any infection (bacterial, fungal, etc.) will be prescribed.

ACTIVITY
* Rest in bed until fever and pain subside.
* Resume your normal activities gradually.
* Resume sexual relations once fever and pain are gone (or when medically advised).

DIET—No special diet.

CALL YOUR DOCTOR IF

* You or a family member has symptoms of pericarditis.
* The following occur during treatment: Fever, shortness of breath and rapid heartbeat, cough (with blood), unexplained weight loss, or increased pain.

PERIODONTITIS
(Gum Inflammation)

 GENERAL INFORMATION

DEFINITION—Inflammation and infection of the gums, causing loss of bone around the teeth. Periodontitis is responsible for more tooth loss than tooth decay.

BODY PARTS INVOLVED—Gums; jaw bones.

SEX OR AGE MOST AFFECTED—Both sexes; usually adults over age 20.

SIGNS & SYMPTOMS
* There may be no symptoms.
* Unpleasant taste in the mouth and bad breath.
* Bleeding of the gums.
* Loosening of teeth in the sockets.
* Aching teeth and gums when eating hot, cold, or sweet food.

CAUSES—Plaque (a sticky deposit of food, bacteria, and mucus) builds up on the teeth. It turns hard and becomes tartar (calculus). Bacteria in the plaque and tartar can cause a gum infection called gingivitis. If untreated, gingivitis infection spreads to the bones that support the teeth causing periodontitis. Pockets of infection occur around the roots of the teeth.

RISK INCREASES WITH
* Poor dental hygiene.
* Clenching or grinding teeth.
* Weak immune system due to illness or drugs.
* Smoking.
* Certain drugs.
* Pregnancy.
* Diabetes.
* Poor nutrition (not eating a healthy diet).
* Family history of gum disease.
* Tongue or lip piercing.

HOW TO PREVENT
* Practice good oral hygiene daily. Visit your dental care provider on a regular basis for dental exams and cleaning of teeth to remove plaque and tartar.
* To brush teeth: Scrub the clear, sticky plaque off teeth daily with a soft toothbrush. A soft brush is less likely to damage teeth and gums than a hard brush. Place the brush at the gum line and gently rotate it, pointing the bristles toward the gum. Brush one section of teeth at a time.
* To floss teeth: Wind waxed or unwaxed dental floss around one finger on each hand. Force the dental floss between teeth. Gently clean the tooth surfaces with a back-and-forth, sawing motion at the gum line. Floss between all lower teeth, using your fingers as guides. Next, loosen the floss and place it on the tops of your thumbs. Floss between all upper teeth, using your thumbs as guides.

 WHAT TO EXPECT

DIAGNOSTIC MEASURES
* Your own observation of symptoms.
* Your dental care provider will do an exam of the teeth, gums, and supporting bones.
* X-rays may be done to check for bone loss.

APPROPRIATE HEALTH CARE
* Treatment may involve correcting dental problems, scaling, planing, and surgery. Your dental care provider will discuss a treatment plan with you.
* Dental work may be done for rough or jagged teeth.
* Dental appliances may need to be repaired.
* Scaling and root planing involves cleaning of deep pockets and smoothing the roots of the teeth.
* Gum surgery may be needed. Pockets of infection may need to be cut open and cleaned. Loose teeth may need to be removed. Bone and tissue grafts may be needed to help support the teeth.
* Dental implants may be recommended for lost teeth.

POSSIBLE COMPLICATIONS
* Without treatment, teeth loosen so much that they may fall out or need to be removed.
* Recurrence of periodontitis.
* Tooth abscess (pus-filled area).
* Mouth infections.

PROBABLE OUTCOME—Usually curable with a combination of dental treatment and maintaining a good oral hygiene program.

 HOW TO TREAT

GENERAL MEASURES—To learn more: American Dental Association, 211 E. Chicago Ave., Chicago, IL 60611-2678; (800) 947-4746; website: www.ada.org.

MEDICATION
* For minor pain, you may use nonprescription drugs such as acetaminophen.
* Antibiotics may be prescribed for infection.

ACTIVITY—No limits.

DIET—No special diet.

 CALL YOUR DENTIST IF

You or a family member has symptoms of periodontitis.

ILLNESS & DISORDERS

PERIPHERAL NEUROPATHY
(Peripheral Neuritis)

GENERAL INFORMATION

DEFINITION—A group of symptoms caused by damage to sensory nerves or motor nerves in the peripheral nervous system.
• Sensory nerve damage affects sensations (such as heat, cold, and pain). The sensations may be abnormal, decreased, or lacking.
• Motor nerve damage affects muscle movement or function. It results in muscle weakness, decreased movement, or loss of control of movement.

BODY PARTS INVOLVED—The peripheral nervous system is made up of nerves that branch out of the spinal cord and go to all parts of the body. Peripheral neuropathy usually affects the fingers, toes, hands, feet, lower arms, and legs. It may affect bladder or bowel control.

SEX OR AGE MOST AFFECTED—Adults of both sexes.

SIGNS & SYMPTOMS
• Burning, tingling, and numbness in a localized area, frequently in the hands and feet.
• Shooting pain that is often worse at night. Pain is made worse by touch or temperature changes.
• Muscle weakness throughout the body on one or both sides. It is often in the same place on both sides.
• Painless ulcers on the toes or fingers.
• Pale, dry skin that becomes sensitive to touch.
• Severe back pain or loss of bladder or bowel control, if caused by back disk disease.

CAUSES—Damage may be from nerve destruction, pressure, or degeneration. The damage may be to one nerve or nerve group. Nerves become damaged due to a number of causes. Sometimes, no cause is found.

RISK INCREASES WITH
• Adults over 60.
• Exposure to certain chemicals or toxic substances.
• Certain drugs.
• Poor nutrition (not eating a healthy diet).
• Poor control of diabetes.
• Alcoholism.
• Family history of neuropathies.
• Nerve disorders, nerve injury, or pressure on nerves.
• Autoimmune disorder or connective tissue disease.
• Infections, kidney or liver failure, and some cancers.
• Bone fractures or ruptured disk.
• Some hereditary disorders.

HOW TO PREVENT—No specific preventive measures.

WHAT TO EXPECT

DIAGNOSTIC MEASURES
• Your health care provider will do a physical exam and ask questions about your symptoms and activities.
• Medical tests may be done to discover any underlying medical disorder.

APPROPRIATE HEALTH CARE
• The most important part of treatment is to identify any underlying cause and treat it.
• Other treatments may include drugs, physical and occupational therapy, diet and exercise, assistive devices, relaxation techniques (such as biofeedback training), surgery to relieve pressure, and others.
• Your health care provider will discuss your diagnosis and a specific treatment plan with you. No one plan works for everyone.

POSSIBLE COMPLICATIONS—Complications can cause chronic pain, disability, and may sometimes be life-threatening.

PROBABLE OUTCOME—Mild cases may be cured if nerve damage is limited and the underlying cause is diagnosed and treated. More severe cases may be incurable, but treatment can often help symptoms improve.

HOW TO TREAT

GENERAL MEASURES—For self-care: Inspect hands and feet daily for unnoticed wounds. Keep feet clean and toenails trimmed properly. Wear shoes that fit well. Take measures to make your home a safe place for you.

MEDICATION
• For minor pain, use nonprescription ibuprofen or acetaminophen. Other pain drugs may be prescribed.
• A variety of drugs can be used to treat the symptoms or underlying disorder. Your health care provider will discuss the options and the risks and benefits.

ACTIVITY—Physical therapy and exercises to do at home may be recommended. If you have difficulty maintaining balance, walk with a cane or other support.

DIET—If poor nutrition is a cause, eat a healthy diet.

CALL YOUR DOCTOR IF

• You or a family member has symptoms of peripheral neuropathy.
• Symptoms persist or worsen despite treatment.

PERITONITIS

GENERAL INFORMATION

DEFINITION—A serious inflammation of part or all of the lining of the abdominal cavity (peritoneum).

BODY PARTS INVOLVED—The abdominal cavity contains such organs as the stomach, intestines, spleen, gallbladder, liver, appendix, kidneys, and pancreas.

SEX OR AGE MOST AFFECTED—Both sexes; all ages.

SIGNS & SYMPTOMS
* Pain in one area of, or all through, the abdomen. Pain usually starts suddenly and becomes more severe with time. Pain may be cramp-like at first and then steady. The patient often prefers to lie quietly on the back because movement or pressure on the abdomen increases pain.
* Shoulder pain (sometimes).
* Chills and fever (often high).
* Dizziness and weakness.
* Rapid heartbeat and rapid breathing.
* Low blood pressure.
* Nausea and vomiting.

CAUSES—The inflammation is a reaction to infection (most often), injury, or irritation of the abdominal lining. It can be caused by a number of different factors involving any of the organs in the abdomen.

RISK INCREASES WITH
* Infection inside the abdomen (e.g., appendicitis or bowel infection).
* Inflammation of the stomach, gallbladder, or pancreas.
* Penetrating injury to the abdominal wall, such as from a knife or bullet wound.
* Peptic ulcer.
* Pelvic inflammatory disease.
* Rupture of an ectopic pregnancy.
* Recent abdominal surgery.
* Bowel obstruction.
* Advanced liver disease.
* Hernia.
* Tuberculosis.
* Ovarian cyst or abscess.

HOW TO PREVENT—No specific preventive measures. Get medical treatment for any disorder that could lead to peritonitis.

WHAT TO EXPECT

DIAGNOSTIC MEASURES
* Your health care provider will do a physical exam and ask questions about your symptoms.
* Blood tests, x-rays, and other medical tests are usually done to help diagnose the underlying disorder.

APPROPRIATE H
* Hospital care is n
and any underlying
treatment for dehydra
drugs injected into a v
transfusions, and surge
* Surgery may be neede
cause of the inflammatio
damage or injury.

POSSIBLE COMPLICATI
* Shock.
* Blood poisoning (septicem
* Intestinal obstruction cause
(bands of scar tissue).
* Kidney or liver failure.

PROBABLE OUTCOME—Usu
early diagnosis and treatment. T
and complications can be fatal. C
depends on age, length of illness,
any pre-existing condition(s).

HOW TO TREAT

GENERAL MEASURES—Early diagn
treatment of the underlying disorder, su
appendicitis, ulcer or ectopic pregnancy
essential. If abdominal pain develops, do
waste valuable time with home treatment
especially laxative use. Laxatives may cau
inflamed abdominal organs to rupture.

MEDICATION
* Antibiotics to treat infection are usually prescribed.
* Pain relievers (sometimes) after diagnosis or surgery.

ACTIVITY—Rest in bed, after treatment, until symptoms disappear. If surgery is needed, resume your activities gradually after surgery.

DIET—While in the hospital, fluids and nutrients may be given through a vein. Oral feedings will resume when your gastrointestinal system can tolerate them.

CALL YOUR DOCTOR IF

* You or a family member has symptoms of peritonitis. This is an emergency! Early diagnosis and treatment of the underlying disorder are essential.
* Any new symptoms occur after treatment.

PERS

DEFINIT
not illnes
conditio
Persons
abnorm
These
person
functio
patter
may l

SEX
all ag

SIG
* Pa
sus
def
* S
(er
re
or

i

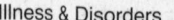

...SONALITY DISORDERS

GENERAL INFORMATION

...ION—A group of conditions that are ...ses, but ways of behaving. Each ... is defined by its main symptoms. ... with these conditions have patterns of ...al behavior, thought, and emotion. ...patterns interfere with daily activity, ...al relationships, and social and work ...ning. The person feels their behavior ...s are "normal" and "right." The behaviors ...ad to trouble with the law.

...OR AGE MOST AFFECTED—Both sexes; ...es.

...S & SYMPTOMS
...ranoid—Shows unwarranted ...piciousness and distrust of others; is ...ensive, oversensitive.
...chizoid and schizotypal—Cold ...notionally); has difficulty forming ...ationships; is withdrawn, shy, superstitious, ...socially isolated.
...Compulsive—Perfectionist, rigid in habits, ...decisive; needs control.
• Histrionic—Dependent, immature, excitable, ...ain; constantly craves stimulation and ...attention; communicates by appearances or ...ehavior (not verbally).
• Narcissistic—Has an exaggerated sense of one's own importance; is preoccupied with power; lacks interest in others; demands attention; feels entitled to special consideration.
• Avoidant—Fears and overreacts to rejection; has low self-esteem; is socially withdrawn; dependent.
• Dependent—Passive, overaccepting, unable to make decisions; lacks confidence.
• Passive-aggressive—Stubborn, sulking; fears authority; procrastinates; is chronically late, argumentative, helpless, clinging.
• Antisocial—Selfish, callous, promiscuous, impulsive, reckless; unable to learn from experience; fails at school and work.
• Borderline—Impulsive; has unstable and intense interpersonal relationships; displays inappropriate anger, fear, and guilt; lacks self-control; has identity problems; may self-mutilate (cut or burn oneself to relieve tension); is suicidal (sometimes).

CAUSES—Unknown. May be multiple factors, including genetics, type of parenting in childhood, one's own personality traits, and early social experiences (such as abuse).

RISK INCREASES WITH
• History of abuse as a child.
• Family history of mood disorders.

HOW TO PREVENT—No specific preventive measures.

WHAT TO EXPECT

DIAGNOSTIC MEASURES
• Diagnostic measures may include observation of symptoms by other people.
• Diagnosis may include medical history, behavioral history, physical exam, and psychological evaluation by a health care provider.

APPROPRIATE HEALTH CARE
• Treatment requires a trusting relationship between the therapist and patient. This can be difficult, as motivation for treatment often comes from someone other than the person with the disorder.
• Psychotherapy provides help with thoughts, feelings, and behavior. It may include:
  - Family and group therapy, group living situations, and self-help groups.
  - Behavior-changing techniques involve the learning of social skills, reinforcement of appropriate behavior, setting limits on inappropriate behavior, learning to express feelings, self-analysis of behavior, and accepting accountability for actions.

POSSIBLE COMPLICATIONS
• Difficulty maintaining personal relationships and jobs; anxiety and depression.
• Drug and alcohol abuse.
• Noncompliance with treatment.
• Suicide.

PROBABLE OUTCOME—Treatment can be effective for some patients, bringing about a gradual change in behavior. For others, prognosis is guarded; and for some, the outcome is poor.

HOW TO TREAT

GENERAL MEASURES—None specific.

MEDICATION—No drugs will cure a personality disorder. Drugs may be prescribed for treatment of specific symptoms such as:
• Antidepressants or antianxiety drugs.
• Antipsychotic drugs for psychoses.

ACTIVITY—No limits.

DIET—No special diet.

CALL YOUR DOCTOR IF

• A family member has symptoms of a personality disorder.
• Symptoms continue or worsen during treatment.

PHARYNGITIS

GENERAL INFORMATION

DEFINITION—Inflammation or infection of the pharynx. The pharynx is the hollow passage at the back of the throat. It is made up of the nasopharynx, which leads to the nose and oropharynx which leads to the mouth. The larynx (voice box) is located below the pharynx.

BODY PARTS INVOLVED—Throat area.

SEX OR AGE MOST AFFECTED—It occurs in all age groups, but most often affects children.

SIGNS & SYMPTOMS
• Sore throat.
• Swallowing difficulty.
• Tickle or "lump" in the throat.
• Fever.
• Swollen glands in the neck (sometimes).
• Throat may be red or covered with a white or grayish membrane (sometimes).
• Body aches (sometimes).

CAUSES—Viral infection (most common cause) or bacterial infection (such as streptococcus). The germs are spread by person-to-person contact. Rarely, there may be other causes, such as irritation.

RISK INCREASES WITH
• Common cold, flu, or seasonal allergies.
• Weak immune system due to illness or drugs.
• Smoking or second-hand smoke.
• Chronic illness, such as diabetes.
• Close quarters, such as with military recruits, in schools, and daycare centers.

HOW TO PREVENT
• Avoid close contact with anyone with a sore throat.
• Avoid germs. Wash hands often, especially children.

WHAT TO EXPECT

DIAGNOSTIC MEASURES
• Your own observation of symptoms.
• Your health care provider will do an exam of the throat, ears, nose, neck, and lungs.
• Medical tests may include blood study and throat culture (from a swab of the throat), or rapid strep test find the type of infection.

APPROPRIATE HEALTH CARE—Treatment will include self-care measures and antibiotic drugs for bacterial infections. Antibiotics will not help viral infections.

POSSIBLE COMPLICATIONS
• Airways may become blocked.
• Abscess (pus-filled area of infection).
• Rheumatic fever, scarlet fever, or glomerulonephritis, if pharyngitis is caused by streptococcal bacteria and does not receive adequate antibiotic treatment.

PROBABLE OUTCOME—Most cases of viral infection clear up on their own in a week. Antibiotic drugs can successfully treat bacterial infections. Complications are rare.

HOW TO TREAT

GENERAL MEASURES
• To relieve the sore throat, gargle frequently with warm or cold double-strength tea or warm salt water (mix one-half teaspoon of salt in one cup of water).
• Wash hands often to help prevent the spread of germs to other family members. Avoid kissing or sharing cups or other utensils.

MEDICATION
• For minor discomfort, you may use nonprescription drugs such as ibuprofen. Don't give aspirin to a child under age 18.
• Nonprescription throat lozenges (for patients over age 3) may help ease discomfort.
• Antibiotic drugs are usually prescribed for bacterial infection. Finish entire course of drugs even if symptoms improve.

ACTIVITY—Return to normal activities as symptoms improve. A person can no longer spread the germs if they have taken the antibiotic drug for at least 24 hours.

DIET—Drink plenty of fluids. If swallowing solid food is painful, try a liquid or soft diet for a few days.

CALL YOUR DOCTOR IF

• You or a family member has symptoms of pharyngitis.
• The following occur during treatment:
  - Breathing/swallowing difficulty or chest pain.
  - Fever worsens or severe headache develops.
  - Thick mucus drainage from the nose.
  - Cough that produces colored or bloody sputum.
  - Skin rash.
  - Dark urine.

PHEOCHROMOCYTOMA

 ## GENERAL INFORMATION

DEFINITION—A rare type of tumor of the adrenal glands. There are two adrenal glands, each located above a kidney. They produce hormones for important body functions. The tumor usually affects one adrenal gland. In some cases, it may develop outside the glands. This type of tumor is most often benign (90%), but can be cancerous.

BODY PARTS INVOLVED—Adrenal glands.

SEX OR AGE MOST AFFECTED—Adults of both sexes between ages 30 and 50.

SIGNS & SYMPTOMS
* Episodes of at least some of these symptoms may occur several times a day or may occur less often (up to 2 months apart). Symptoms increase as tumor grows.
* High blood pressure episodes.
* Severe headaches.
* Rapid heartbeat following exercise, emotional upset, or exposure to cold.
* Tremors and nervousness.
* Feelings of doom.
* Feelings of hunger.
* Episodes of flushing.
* Sweating, paleness.
* Weakness and fatigue.
* Unexplained weight loss.
* Nausea and vomiting.

CAUSES—Hormones produced by adrenal glands work with the central nervous system to control heart rate, blood pressure, and other vital body functions. When a tumor (the pheochromocytoma) exists, even though it is benign, excess hormones are produced. The excess hormones cause symptoms. Cause of the tumor is unknown.

RISK INCREASES WITH
* Unknown for most cases.
* A disorder called multiple endocrine neoplasia (MEN) syndrome.

HOW TO PREVENT—No specific preventive measures.

 ## WHAT TO EXPECT

DIAGNOSTIC MEASURES
* Your own observation of symptoms.
* Your health care provider will do a physical exam.
* Medical tests may include studies of urine and blood to measure hormone production, x-ray, CT, MRI, (see Glossary for all) and other studies. These help diagnose the tumor and also determine if it is benign or cancer, and any spread of the cancer.

APPROPRIATE HEALTH CARE
* Treatment will depend on the diagnosis. It may include surgery, chemotherapy (anticancer drugs), and radiation.
* Surgery is usually done to remove the tumor.

POSSIBLE COMPLICATIONS
* Tumor may recur.
* Stroke, caused by very high blood pressure.
* High blood pressure may continue after surgery. It can be treated with drugs.
* Kidney, brain, heart damage, and death caused by unrecognized and untreated pheochromocytoma.

PROBABLE OUTCOME—The outlook is generally good for those with benign tumors removed by surgery. For those tumors that are cancerous, the outlook is more guarded.

 ## HOW TO TREAT

GENERAL MEASURES—For a description of abdominal surgery and postoperative care, see Laparotomy in Surgery section.

MEDICATION
* Drugs are sometimes prescribed before surgery to suppress the effect of hormones.
* Drugs to treat high blood pressure may be needed.
* Anticancer (chemotherapy) drugs may be prescribed.

ACTIVITY—Usually, no limits after recovery from surgery.

DIET—Prior to surgery, a high-salt diet may be recommended to increase blood volume.

 ## CALL YOUR DOCTOR IF

* You or a family member has symptoms of pheochromocytoma.
* Symptoms recur after treatment.

PHOBIAS

GENERAL INFORMATION

DEFINITION—A type of anxiety disorder involving intense and/or unrealistic fears. The fears may involve an object, situation, activity, event, or even a bodily function. When fears are real (due to danger or a threat to life), the body's alarm system switches on and is ready to help protect us. With phobias, this alarm system switches on when there is no real threat or danger. Phobias can cause minor or major problems in a person's life. Most people with phobias recognize that the fear is not appropriate to the situation. Phobias are classified as:
• Social—fear of embarrassment in social situations, such as public speaking or using a public bathroom.
• Agoraphobia—fear of being in crowds or fear of public places.
• Specific (simple)—fear of a specific object or situation, such as animals, insects, heights, flying, or closed places.

BODY PARTS INVOLVED—Nervous system.

SEX OR AGE MOST AFFECTED—Females more than males; usually late adolescent or young adulthood.

SIGNS & SYMPTOMS—The following anxiety symptoms occur when exposed to, or thinking of the phobic stimulus:
• Palpitations (irregular and rapid heartbeat).
• Desire to flee.
• Sweating, tremors.
• Flushing.
• Nausea.
• Negative thoughts and scary images.

CAUSES—Exact cause is unknown. It may involve genetics, family influence, traumatic events, medical conditions, or imbalance of certain brain chemicals.

RISK INCREASES WITH
• Family history of anxiety.
• Persons with other anxiety disorders.
• Women more than men.

HOW TO PREVENT—No specific preventive measures to prevent the phobia. After diagnosis, treatment can help prevent or control the reaction.

WHAT TO EXPECT

DIAGNOSTIC MEASURES
• Your own observation of symptoms.
• Your health care provider will usually do a physical exam and ask about your symptoms and activities.
• Medical tests may be done to rule out other disorders.

APPROPRIATE HEALTH CARE
• Treatment may involve psychotherapy, drug therapy, and self-help methods. No treatment may be needed if the phobia is not interfering with daily life.
• Cognitive-behavioral therapy may help. Cognitive therapy teaches how to change thoughts, behaviors or attitudes. Behavioral therapy teaches ways to reduce anxiety with deep breathing and muscle relaxation.

POSSIBLE COMPLICATIONS
• Limits in lifestyle due to avoiding the phobic stimulus. Agoraphobia, especially, restricts a person's activities and is severely disabling.
• Overuse of drugs or alcohol to relieve anxiety.

PROBABLE OUTCOME
• Specific phobias—some stop on their own as the person ages. Others do not cause any problems if the object can be avoided (such as snakes). Some get better as people go through their fearful situations (such as flying). Others can be cured or helped with treatment.
• Social phobias—usually can be resolved with treatment. Drugs are often helpful.
• Agoraphobia—it is more difficult to treat because the person has so many fears, but treatment can help.

HOW TO TREAT

GENERAL MEASURES
• Self-help suggestions if you feel your fear taking hold:
  - Shift your thought from the negative ("The dog will bite") to one that is real and positive ("The dog is on a leash").
  - Do something you can control—count backward from 1000, read a book, talk aloud, or take deep, measured breaths.
  - Shift your thoughts to pleasant ones.
  - Practice relaxation techniques.
• Joining a support group is helpful for some patients.
• To learn more: Anxiety Disorders Association of America, 8730 Georgia Ave., Suite 600, Silver Spring, MD 20910; (240) 485-1001 (not toll free); website: www.adaa.org.

MEDICATION—Drugs are sometimes helpful. Your health care provider will discuss the options, the risks, and benefits.

ACTIVITY—No limits.

DIET—No special diet. Avoid caffeine and alcohol.

CALL YOUR DOCTOR IF

• You or a family member has symptoms of a phobia.
• Symptoms of the phobia return after treatment.

PHOTOSENSITIVITY

 GENERAL INFORMATION

DEFINITION—Skin that reacts abnormally to light. A reaction may occur after only a few minutes of exposure. This is likely to be a problem for those taking part in hot-season sports such as swimming, surfing, sailing, tennis, or water skiing. The most common form is called polymorphous light eruption (PMLE), or sun poisoning.

BODY PARTS INVOLVED—Skin in areas most exposed to sunlight.

SEX OR AGE MOST AFFECTED—Both sexes; all ages.

SIGNS & SYMPTOMS
• Red or pink skin rash, sometimes with small blisters, in areas exposed to sunlight.
• Rash may itch or burn.

CAUSES—Symptoms are triggered by exposure to sun (ultraviolet light). It is not known why the body develops this reaction. The sunlight exposure may come through glass (such as in an automobile) or thin clothing. Some people react to winter daylight as well as summer sun. Tanning booths are a source of ultraviolet light.

RISK INCREASES WITH
• Use of drugs, herbs, or products that cause increased sensitivity to ultraviolet light. The most common drugs include tetracycline antibiotics, thiazide diuretics, antihistamines, sulfa drugs, nonsteroidal anti-inflammatory drugs, and birth control pills. The herb St. John's Wort can also cause the problem.
• Some sunscreens and some cosmetics, including lipstick, perfume, and soaps.
• Skin disorders such as porphyria.
• Previous episodes of photosensitivity.
• Systemic lupus erythematosus (an immune disorder).
• Weak immune system due to drugs or illness.

HOW TO PREVENT
• Stay out of the sun when possible if you have a history of photosensitivity. Avoid tanning booths.
• Wear dark colored clothing that is tightly woven when in sunlight. Wear a hat with a wide brim.
• Sunscreen may help. Use with care. Some sunscreens cause a reaction in photosensitive persons.
• Avoid the drugs or products known to cause photosensitivity. Not all individuals who use these drugs will have a photosensitive reaction. Also, a reaction will be different in different people. A person may have a one time reaction and not experience it again.

 WHAT TO EXPECT

DIAGNOSTIC MEASURES
• Your own observation of symptoms.
• See your health care provider if you have concerns about the symptoms or they are severe. A physical exam of the affected skin area will be done. Questions will be asked about your sun exposure, products you use, and drugs that you take.
• A medical test may be done to check your skin's reaction to ultraviolet light.

APPROPRIATE HEALTH CARE
• Switching temporarily to different drugs or skin care products may be recommended. This will help determine a cause for the reaction.
• In some cases, phototherapy may be prescribed. This treatment (done in a medical office) gradually exposes your skin to ultraviolet light. This is done over several weeks and helps to lessen the skin's sensitivity.
• PUVA therapy may be recommended. This treatment involves use of a drug, along with ultraviolet light.

POSSIBLE COMPLICATIONS—Chronic rash or other symptoms when exposed to the sun (even short periods) especially in spring and summer.

PROBABLE OUTCOME—In most cases, it takes up to 1 week for recovery if further sun exposure is avoided. If a drug or other product is the problem, symptoms usually stop after it is discontinued. In other photosensitivity cases, symptoms may come and go depending on sun exposure.

 HOW TO TREAT

GENERAL MEASURES
• Apply cool, moist compresses to affected skin.
• Stay out of the sun during the hours of strongest ultraviolet light (10 a.m. to 2 p.m.).

MEDICATION
• Use aspirin (if over age 18), acetaminophen, or an antihistamine to relieve mild pain or itching.
• Beta-carotene taken orally may help some.
• You may be prescribed steroid drugs for severe cases, or other drugs which can reduce the photosensitivity.

ACTIVITY—Avoid prolonged sun exposure.

DIET—No special diet.

 CALL YOUR DOCTOR IF

You or a family member has symptoms of photosensitivity and self-care does not help.

PICA

GENERAL INFORMATION

DEFINITION—Craving, eating, or mouthing items that are not food. Pica does occur in adults, but usually affects children between ages 2 and 6, and persons with developmental disorders.

BODY PARTS INVOLVED—Brain; gastrointestinal tract.

SEX OR AGE MOST AFFECTED—Both sexes; adults and children.

SIGNS & SYMPTOMS
• Eating non-food substances, such as starch, clay, ice, plaster, paint, cigarette ashes, hair, gravel, chalk, needles, string, pencil erasers, and others.
• Stomach pain (sometimes).

CAUSES—The exact cause is unknown. Factors that may contribute to the cause include physical, emotional, nutritional, family, social, economic, and cultural factors.

RISK INCREASES WITH
• Family history of pica.
• Poor nutrition or a vitamin deficiency.
• Poverty.
• Developmental disorders.
• Anemia.
• Pregnancy.
• Cultures where clay eating is a common practice.
• People on diets who try to ease hunger with nonfood items.

HOW TO PREVENT—There are no specific preventive measures. To reduce risks, provide a well-balanced diet for yourself and your children.

WHAT TO EXPECT

DIAGNOSTIC MEASURES
• Your own observation of symptoms.
• Your health care provider will usually do a physical exam.
• Medical tests may include blood studies, x-rays, and other tests to rule out medical disorders. There is no diagnostic test for pica.

APPROPRIATE HEALTH CARE
• Treatment usually includes behavior and diet changes, if needed.
• Several different types of behavioral training are used to treat pica. Your health care provider will discuss the options with you depending on your individual situation.

POSSIBLE COMPLICATIONS
• Lead poisoning from paint or plaster.
• Intestinal infections from parasites in soil.
• Anemia.
• Malnutrition (not getting enough nutrients).
• Intestinal obstruction.

PROBABLE OUTCOME
• It may go on for years with no harmful effects.
• It may stop on its own in a few months.
• In some cases, it can be helped with treatment.
• For others, it may continue (even with treatment) into the teenage years. This occurs more often with developmental disorders.
• Pica during pregnancy usually ends with childbirth.

HOW TO TREAT

GENERAL MEASURES—Childproof your home by removing nonfood substances the child is eating. Repaint homes in which lead-base paints have been used. Don't use older baby cribs painted with lead-base paint.

MEDICATION—Drugs are usually not needed for this disorder.

ACTIVITY—No limits.

DIET—A well-balanced diet will be prescribed. A dietitian may help plan meals if any nutritional deficiency is diagnosed.

CALL YOUR DOCTOR IF

• You or a family member has symptoms of pica.
• You are pregnant and have symptoms of pica.
• Pica does not improve in 2 weeks, despite treatment.

PILONIDAL DISEASE

 GENERAL INFORMATION

DEFINITION—An infection in the skin, just above the crease of the buttocks. It starts with a pilonidal cyst (a sac) under the skin. The cyst can become infected and form an abscess (pus-filled area). An opening (sinus) may also develop that goes from the abscess to the outside skin.

BODY PARTS INVOLVED—Skin.

SEX OR AGE MOST AFFECTED—The disease affects both sexes, but is more common in males, from teenagers to age 40.

SIGNS & SYMPTOMS
* Symptoms may go unnoticed in mild cases.
* Pain, redness, tenderness, and swelling in the area.
* Fever and chills.
* Discharge of pus.
* Sitting or walking may be difficult.

CAUSES—It was thought for many years that people were born with the cysts. Now the theory is that they are acquired. There is still much unknown about them. In some cases, hairs growing inside the cyst may lead to infection. In other cases, no hair is found in the cyst and the cause is unknown.

RISK INCREASES WITH
* Obesity.
* Men more than women.
* Family history of pilonidal disease.
* Sedentary lifestyle (lack of exercise).
* Repeated trauma (injury) to the tailbone area.
* Work that requires a lot of sitting.
* Activities such as biking or motorcycle riding that can cause sweating and friction to the tailbone area.
* Heavy growth of body hair.

HOW TO PREVENT
* Bathe or shower daily to keep the area clean. Warm tub baths seem more effective in preventing infection of the cyst than showers.
* Avoid risk factors where possible.

 WHAT TO EXPECT

DIAGNOSTIC MEASURES
* Your own observation of symptoms.
* Your health care provider will do a physical exam of the cyst.
* Medical tests may include blood studies and a culture of the discharge from the cyst.

APPROPRIATE HEALTH CARE
* Treatment may involve self-care, incision and drainage of the cyst, drugs, and surgery. Your health care provider will discuss the options with you.
* Treatment may not be needed for mild disease. Use extra care in keeping that area of the body clean. You may be advised to shave or use a hair remover product to keep the area free of hair.
* Incision and drainage may be recommended. This involves opening the cyst so that any hair or pus can be removed. The opening is then packed with gauze. Healing may take several weeks.
* Surgical removal (excision) of the cyst or sinus may be recommended. Several different surgical methods can be used. Healing time will depend on the procedure. You will be advised about follow-up home care. See Pilonidal Cyst Removal in Surgery Section.

POSSIBLE COMPLICATIONS—The disease recurs in about 40% of the patients after the initial treatment. It may clear up on its own after age 40.

PROBABLE OUTCOME—Mild cases may need no treatment. In cases of abscess or recurrence of the disease, treatment can help. Healing time may take weeks to months, depending on treatment procedure.

 HOW TO TREAT

GENERAL MEASURES
* If the cyst is infected, take warm baths to relieve pain. Sit in a tub of warm water for 10 to 15 minutes as often as it feels good.
* If surgery is necessary, see Pilonidal Cyst Removal (in Surgery section) for an explanation of the surgery and postoperative care.

MEDICATION—Antibiotics may be prescribed for infection.

ACTIVITY—No limits, unless the cyst becomes infected. Then, limit activities until the infection is cured. Use a special doughnut cushion if sitting is uncomfortable.

DIET—No special diet.

 CALL YOUR DOCTOR IF

* You or a family member has symptoms of a pilonidal disease.
* Symptoms recur after treatment.

PINWORMS (Enterobiasis; Seatworm; Threadworm; Oxyuriasis)

GENERAL INFORMATION

DEFINITION—Infestation with intestinal parasites, a common occurrence in children. Pinworms are more a nuisance than a major health problem.

BODY PARTS INVOLVED—Cecum (pouchlike beginning of the large intestine on the right side to which the appendix is attached); large intestine; anus; skin around the anus.

SEX OR AGE MOST AFFECTED—Both sexes; all ages, but most common in children.

SIGNS & SYMPTOMS
* Some people may be infected and have no symptoms.
* Skin irritation and painful itching around the anus, especially during sleep.
* Restless sleep.
* Vaginal discharge, itching and discomfort if pinworms migrate into the vaginal opening.

CAUSES
* Infestation of the intestine by a very small worm about 1/4 to 1/2 inch long. Pinworms travel from the intestine to the rectum to lay eggs around the anus and buttocks. If a person scratches the area, the eggs can get under the fingernails and be passed to anything or anyone that person touches.
* Pinworms are easy to catch from someone who is infected. Eggs are passed to others on toilet seats or by hand-to-hand or hand-to-mouth contact. They may drift in the air, where they are inhaled or swallowed. Eggs hatch and the larvae travel to the large intestine, where they mature, mate, and repeat the cycle.

RISK INCREASES WITH—Groups of children, as in daycare, school, or at camps.

HOW TO PREVENT
* Wash hands carefully before meals and after using the toilet.
* Keep the nails short and clean.
* Bathe daily, right after waking up. This helps rid the body of any eggs before they can be spread.
* Have children wear clean underwear and pajamas daily.
* Don't scratch the anus or put fingers near the nose or mouth.
* Vacuum children's play area frequently.
* Wash bedding and pajamas on a regular basis.

WHAT TO EXPECT

DIAGNOSTIC MEASURES
* You may help diagnose the pinworms yourself.

* They look like small pieces of white or yellow thread.
* They may sometimes be seen on a child's stool.
* Since they are active at night, check your child a few hours after bedtime. Shine a flashlight on the rectal area and you may see the worms in action.
* Perform a tape test for the eggs:
  - Your health care provider may give you a tongue depressor with clear tape on it and a glass slide. If you do not have this, use your own clear (scotch) tape.
  - Place tape against your child's anal skin first thing in the morning (before washing or activity) to collect eggs.
  - Then place the sticky side of the tongue depressor tape on the glass slide. If your own tape is used, place it in a plastic bag and seal it.
  - Take slide or bag to the medical office for viewing under a microscope to check for pinworm eggs.

APPROPRIATE HEALTH CARE—Once the pinworm diagnosis is confirmed, the infection is usually treated with a drug to kill the worms. All family members should be treated even if they have no symptoms.

POSSIBLE COMPLICATIONS—No serious complications expected.

PROBABLE OUTCOME—The infection is curable in two weeks with treatment. If worms reappear soon after treatment, it usually means a new infection, not treatment failure. A second treatment can be effective.

HOW TO TREAT

GENERAL MEASURES—On the day of treatment, wash sheets, towels, and clothing, especially bedclothes, in hot water. Cut and clean fingernails.

MEDICATION
* A two-dose course of an antiworm drug is usually prescribed. The second dose is taken 2 weeks after the first dose.
* Nonprescription creams or lotions to relieve itching may be helpful.

ACTIVITY—No limits.

DIET—No special diet.

CALL YOUR DOCTOR IF

* Anyone in your family has symptoms of pinworms.
* Pinworms reappear after treatment.

PITUITARY GLAND, UNDERACTIVE
(Hypopituitarism)

 GENERAL INFORMATION

DEFINITION—The pituitary is a small, dime-sized gland located just below the brain. It works with the hypothalamus in the brain to regulate body functions. Hormones released by the pituitary are used in many of these functions. An underactive pituitary fails to release enough of one or more of these hormones. If all hormones are absent, it is called panhypopituitarism. Hormones include:
• Growth hormone—for growth of tissue and bones.
• Prolactin hormone—for female breast development and milk production.
• Thyroid-stimulating hormone—used by the thyroid gland for metabolism functions.
• Adrenocorticotropic hormone—used by the adrenal gland to control blood pressure.
• Luteinizing hormone and follicle-stimulating hormones—control sexual function in males and females.
• Antidiuretic hormone—affects the kidneys in the production of urine.
• Oxytocin—for contractions of the uterus during childbirth and the release of milk during breast-feeding.

BODY PARTS INVOLVED—Pituitary gland and body parts mentioned above.

SEX OR AGE MOST AFFECTED—Both sexes; all ages.

SIGNS & SYMPTOMS
• Decrease in appetite and weight loss.
• Abdominal pain; nausea.
• More sensitive to cold or heat.
• Persistent headaches.
• Mental changes.
• Changes in vision.
• Women may have menstrual period changes, failure to produce milk, hot flashes, and infertility.
• Men may have decreased sexual interest.
• Severe thirst and lack of urination.
• Failure of growth (seen after age 6 months).
• Lack of secondary sexual features that develop in puberty. These include voice changes, breast development, and growth of pubic hair.

CAUSES—Usually caused by disorders that affect the pituitary, the hypothalamus, or surrounding structures. Sometimes the cause is unknown.

RISK INCREASES WITH
• Tumors.
• Head injury.
• Infection (tuberculosis, syphilis, or meningitis).
• Blocked blood supply to the pituitary.
• Immune system problem.

• Pregnancy and delivery.
• Radiation or surgery.
• Congenital defect (a problem present at birth).

HOW TO PREVENT—None specific. Obtain medical care for any risk factors.

 WHAT TO EXPECT

DIAGNOSTIC MEASURES
• Your own observation of symptoms.
• Your health care provider will do a physical exam and ask about your symptoms and activities.
• Medical tests may include blood studies of hormone levels and hormone function. CT or MRI scans (see Glossary for all) may be done.

APPROPRIATE HEALTH CARE
• Treatment is aimed at treating the cause of the pituitary failure (which may include drugs or surgery) and hormone replacement as needed.
• Surgery to remove underlying tumors or blood clots, if needed.

POSSIBLE COMPLICATIONS—Hormonal failure and possible death without treatment. Other complications depend on the underlying cause.

PROBABLE OUTCOME—It is usually a lifelong disorder. Outcome is generally favorable if an underlying disorder is successfully treated and hormone-replacement therapy is continued.

 HOW TO TREAT

GENERAL MEASURES
• This disorder requires close medical supervision and continuing treatment.
• Wear a medical alert-type bracelet or neck pendant indicating your hormone deficiencies and their proper treatment.

MEDICATION
• Hormones are usually prescribed to replace those the pituitary is not producing.
• Drugs may be prescribed for treatment of an underlying disorder.

ACTIVITY—Stay as active as your condition allows.

DIET—No special diet.

 CALL YOUR DOCTOR IF

• You or a family member has symptoms of an underactive pituitary gland.
• After surgery, signs of infection develop, such as fever, lethargy, and muscle aches.
• New, unexplained symptoms develop.

PITUITARY TUMOR

GENERAL INFORMATION

DEFINITION—Pituitary tumors are usually benign (noncancerous) tumors called adenomas. Other, less-common types may be cancerous. Tumors are also classed as functioning (producing hormones) or nonfunctioning (not producing hormones). Hormones released by the pituitary include:
• Growth hormone—for growth of tissue and bones.
• Prolactin hormone—for female breast development and milk production.
• Thyroid-stimulating hormone—used by the thyroid gland for metabolism functions.
• Adrenocorticotropic hormone—used by the adrenal gland to control blood pressure.
• Luteinizing hormone and follicle stimulating hormones—control sexual function in males and females.
• Antidiuretic hormone—affects the kidneys in the production of urine.
• Oxytocin—for contractions of the uterus during childbirth and the release of milk during breast-feeding.

BODY PARTS INVOLVED—The pituitary is a small, dime-sized gland located just below the brain. It works with the hypothalamus to regulate body functions from within the brain. Hormones released by the pituitary are used in many of these functions.

SEX OR AGE MOST AFFECTED—Both sexes and all ages, but most common between ages 30 and 50.

SIGNS & SYMPTOMS
• Symptoms may occur due to tumor growth. It can put pressure on eye nerves causing vision problems, headaches, and other symptoms.
• Numerous symptoms may occur due to an over-production or under-production of any of the hormones listed above. No symptoms are specific for diagnosing a tumor. Often, symptoms may go unnoticed, fail to cause alarm, or be attributed to another illness.

CAUSES—Unknown. Some types are part of a hereditary disorder.

RISK INCREASES WITH—Unknown.

HOW TO PREVENT—No preventive measures.

WHAT TO EXPECT

DIAGNOSTIC MEASURES
• Your own observation of symptoms.
• Your health care provider will do a physical exam and ask about your symptoms.
• Medical tests may include cerebrospinal fluid and blood studies, x-rays of the skull, CT scan or MRI of the brain, and vision tests.

APPROPRIATE HEALTH CARE
• Treatment may involve a combination of surgery to remove the tumor, radiation treatment, hormone therapy, or other drugs.
• Different types of surgery are used to treat the tumors. The procedure depends on the type of tumor, its location and its size. Your health care provider will explain the options with you.
• Radiation therapy may be used in combination with surgery. It may also be used for people who, for medical or other reasons, are not able to have surgery.

POSSIBLE COMPLICATIONS
• Spread of the tumor to other parts of the brain.
• Blindness due to pressure from tumor.
• Recurrence of tumor after treatment.

PROBABLE OUTCOME—Outcome will depend on the type of tumor, and the patient's age and general health status. Early diagnosis and treatment offer the most favorable outcome.

HOW TO TREAT

GENERAL MEASURES
• If surgery is required, the family should maintain an optimistic outlook, stay in close contact with the patient's doctor and help by making their visits with the patient as supportive as possible.
• Wear a medical alert-type bracelet or neck pendant indicating your hormone deficiencies and their proper treatment.

MEDICATION
• Pain relievers may be prescribed.
• Hormone-replacement drugs may be prescribed. They may require frequent dosage adjustments.
• Drugs may be prescribed that reduce hormone production.
• Anticancer drugs may be prescribed.

ACTIVITY—Resume your normal activities gradually after surgery.

DIET—Restricted while you are in the hospital; after surgery, you may return to a regular diet.

CALL YOUR DOCTOR IF

• You or a family member has symptoms of a pituitary tumor.
• The following occur after surgery:
  - Bleeding at the surgical site.
  - Signs of general infection, such as fever, chills, headache, and muscle aches.
  - Clear discharge from the nose.
  - There is a recurrence of any symptoms.

PITYRIASIS ALBA

 GENERAL INFORMATION

DEFINITION—A common disorder of the skin. It causes a temporary loss of pigmentation (coloring) in patches found usually on the cheeks and sometimes, the neck and shoulders. *Pityriasis* means "scaly" and *alba* means "white" in Latin.

BODY PARTS INVOLVED—Skin.

SEX OR AGE MOST AFFECTED—It occurs mostly in children of both sexes, but may appear in adults up to ages 20 to 30.

SIGNS & SYMPTOMS
• Small white or light-pink patches with vague borders. They sometimes have pinpoint-sized white papules (small, raised bumps). Patches feel smooth.
• Patches are most apparent in summer because the areas do not tan. Tanning increases the contrast between the areas.
• There may be 1 to 20 patches at a time.
• Patches may itch occasionally, but they are not painful.

CAUSES—Unknown. The tendency may be inherited.

RISK INCREASES WITH
• Family history of allergies of any kind.
• Skin that is extra dry and/or sun exposure may be risk factors.

HOW TO PREVENT—No specific preventive measures.

 WHAT TO EXPECT

DIAGNOSTIC MEASURES
• Your own observation of symptoms.
• Your health care provider can usually diagnose the disorder by an exam of the affected skin.
• Medical tests are generally not needed.

APPROPRIATE HEALTH CARE—No truly effective therapy is available. Some skin-care products may help the dry skin.

POSSIBLE COMPLICATIONS—None expected.

PROBABLE OUTCOME—Patches may come and go for years. Between ages 20 and 30, they disappear completely.

 HOW TO TREAT

GENERAL MEASURES—Use sunscreen or protective clothing to prevent sunburn in affected areas.

MEDICATION
• Moisturizers may improve roughness or dryness, but do not improve the color.
• Prescription or nonprescription topical steroid drug(s) to control itching may be recommended.

ACTIVITY—No limits.

DIET—No special diet.

 CALL YOUR DOCTOR IF

You or a family member has symptoms of pityriasis alba.

PITYRIASIS ROSEA

GENERAL INFORMATION

DEFINITION—A common skin disorder with a faint rash that lasts weeks to months. *Pityriasis* means "scaly" and *rosea* means "pink" in Latin.

BODY PARTS INVOLVED—Skin, especially of the chest and abdomen.

SEX OR AGE MOST AFFECTED—It affects all ages, but is most common in adolescents and young adults. Women are affected more often than men are.

SIGNS & SYMPTOMS
* A faint rash (often found in skin creases) of oval or round, pale-pink or light-brown areas. One larger patch (the "herald patch") may appear first. They may evolve into a "Christmas tree" pattern on the chest or back.
* Mild fatigue.
* Itching, usually mild.
* Occasional slight fever and headache.

CAUSES—Unknown, but may be caused by a virus or autoimmune disorder. It does not appear to be highly contagious (easily spread from one person to another).

RISK INCREASES WITH
* Fall and spring seasons.
* Weak immune system due to illness or drugs.

HOW TO PREVENT—Cannot be prevented at present.

WHAT TO EXPECT

DIAGNOSTIC MEASURES
* Your own observation of symptoms.
* Your health care provider can usually diagnose the disorder by an exam of the affected skin.
* Medical tests may include blood studies. A scraping of the skin or a sample of the skin may be removed for viewing under a microscope.

APPROPRIATE HEALTH CARE
* No specific treatment will cure the disorder.
* Treatment can help relieve the itching. In more severe cases, treatment with ultraviolet light or moderate exposure to sunlight may be recommended.

POSSIBLE COMPLICATIONS
* Affected skin areas may have color changes in darker-skinned persons.
* Rarely, bacterial infection may occur in affected skin.

PROBABLE OUTCOME—Pityriasis rosea usually runs its natural course in 5 weeks to 4 months. No drug or treatment is available to shorten its course, but itching and discomfort can be relieved. New rash areas continue to break out for several weeks. Once over, it is unlikely to recur.

HOW TO TREAT

GENERAL MEASURES—Bathe as usual with a mild soap. Use warm water, as hot water may increase the itching. Oatmeal baths may help.

MEDICATION
* For minor discomfort, you may use nonprescription drugs, such as:
  - Calamine lotion, to decrease itching.
  - Steroid cream, to control more severe itching.
  - Acetaminophen, to reduce fever.
* Other topical or oral steroids and antihistamines may be prescribed.

ACTIVITY—Avoid activities that cause excess sweating. This can make the rash worse.

DIET—No special diet.

CALL YOUR DOCTOR IF

You or a family member has symptoms of pityriasis rosea.

PLACENTA PREVIA

GENERAL INFORMATION

DEFINITION—The placenta normally attaches high on the uterus wall, away from the cervix. In placenta previa, the placenta is covering or near the cervical opening (os). It can block the cervical opening to the vagina (birth canal). Placenta previa carries a risk of excessive bleeding, which can threaten the well-being of the mother and the baby. A low-lying placenta diagnosed in early pregnancy usually self-corrects as the uterus enlarges. Types of placenta previa include:
• Total placenta previa: The placenta completely covers the opening of the cervix. This type presents the most serious risk to the mother.
• Partial placenta previa: The placenta partially covers the opening of the cervix.
• Marginal placenta previa: The placenta just reaches the cervix.

BODY PARTS INVOLVED—Uterus; placenta (the organ that transfers nourishment and oxygen from mother to fetus); cervix (opening to the uterus).

SEX OR AGE MOST AFFECTED—Pregnant women.

SIGNS & SYMPTOMS
• Sudden, painless bleeding during the second or third trimester of pregnancy. Bleeding may be mild at the start and become severe. Bleeding may not occur until labor begins in some cases.
• Cramping may occur in some patients.

CAUSES—Exact cause of placenta previa is unknown. A number of factors may be involved.

RISK INCREASES WITH
• Previous uterine surgery involving the lining of the uterus. This includes dilation and curettage (D & C) and cesarean section.
• Smoking.
• Prior induced abortion.
• Multiple previous pregnancies and births.
• Pregnancy with twins or other multiples.
• Pregnant women over age 35.
• Previous placenta previa.

HOW TO PREVENT—Placenta previa cannot be prevented. Good prenatal care during pregnancy can help identify it early.

WHAT TO EXPECT

DIAGNOSTIC MEASURES
• Your own observation of symptoms, especially of vaginal bleeding during pregnancy.
• If bleeding occurs, medical tests may include blood studies and ultrasound to determine the exact location of the placenta. Rarely, a vaginal exam may be done.

APPROPRIATE HEALTH CARE
• Treatment will depend on the type of previa, amount of bleeding, fetal age, condition and presentation, and the presence or absence of labor.
• Hospital care that includes blood transfusions, intravenous (IV) fluids, and oxygen may be needed with severe bleeding.
• If the bleeding is heavy or the pregnancy is at term, delivery is usually done. There may be a trial of labor for vaginal delivery or a cesarean delivery.
• If the pregnancy is between 34 and 37 weeks and the mother and fetus are stable, amniocentesis may be done to check fetal lung maturity. With mature lungs, the newborn will not need breathing support.
• If the baby's lungs are immature or the pregnancy is less than 34 weeks, the treatment may involve medical observation for a period. You may be placed on bed rest at home. Follow your obstetric provider's instructions carefully.

POSSIBLE COMPLICATIONS
• Poor fetal growth, due to an abnormal placenta providing a decrease in blood flow and oxygen delivery.
• Premature delivery, or (possibly) fetal death.
• Rarely, blood loss could lead to maternal shock and death.

PROBABLE OUTCOME—With prompt care, the outcome for mothers and term infants is good. Outcome for premature baby will depend on number of weeks of gestation and the baby's condition at birth.

HOW TO TREAT

GENERAL MEASURES—Follow all medical instructions.

MEDICATION
• Steroids may be prescribed to help fetal lungs mature.
• Drugs to delay labor may be used in some cases.

ACTIVITY—Rest in bed until bleeding stops or you deliver your child. Avoid sexual intercourse or douching.

DIET—No special diet.

CALL YOUR DOCTOR IF

You or a family member has symptoms of placenta previa. Report any bleeding immediately. This is an emergency!

PLANTAR FASCIITIS

GENERAL INFORMATION

DEFINITION—Plantar fasciitis is an inflammation (red, sore, swollen) of the plantar fascia. The plantar fascia is a thick band of tissue on the bottom of the foot. It extends from the heel bone to the base of the toes. Plantar refers to the sole of the foot. Fascia describes thin, fibrous, supportive tissue. It is a common foot problem, and is different from heel spurs. But, a person may have both of these foot problems at the same time.

BODY PARTS INVOLVED—Foot.

SEX OR AGE MOST AFFECTED—It can affect anyone, of any age, no matter their fitness level.

SIGNS & SYMPTOMS
* Pain and tenderness in the heel and sole of the foot under the heel bone.
* Pain often occurs after resting or after rising in the morning. There may be no pain when sitting.
* One or both feet can be affected.
* It hurts worse when running faster or when weight is on the ball of the foot.

CAUSES—Overuse or stress to the foot causes the plantar fascia to become stretched, irritated, and inflamed.

RISK INCREASES WITH
* People over age 40. Women more often than men.
* Athletes who overtrain, wear improper shoes, or fail to warm up.
* Running, jumping, or walking on hard surfaces.
* Having flat feet or high arches.
* Previous foot or ankle injury.
* Wearing high heeled, poorly fitting, or worn-out shoes.
* Being on the feet for many hours a day.
* Overweight.

HOW TO PREVENT
* Wear proper footwear for sports, exercise, and work.
* Do stretching exercises for the Achilles tendon (tendon from the heel to the calf).
* With any new exercise or sport, build up your pace gradually. Warm up before exercise.
* Maintain a healthy weight for your height.

WHAT TO EXPECT

DIAGNOSTIC MEASURES
* Your own observation of symptoms.
* Your health care provider will examine your foot and ankle and ask about your symptoms. The bottom of your foot will be touched and pressed to identify the cause of the pain.
* X-rays and other tests may be done to check for other disorders.

APPROPRIATE HEALTH CARE
* There are a variety of treatment options that involve self-care.
* If other treatments fail after 6 months, shock wave therapy (nonsurgical) or surgery may be options.

POSSIBLE COMPLICATIONS
* Affected skin areas may have color changes in darker-skinned persons.
* Rarely, bacterial infection may occur in affected skin.

PROBABLE OUTCOME—Usually curable for most people. Different types of treatment work for different people. Complete healing may take from weeks to months. Other methods of treatment are being studied and may be available in the future.

HOW TO TREAT

GENERAL MEASURES—Follow your health care provider's advice. Basic ideas are listed here.
* Massage an ice pack over the painful area. Do this for 15 minutes, 3 or 4 times a day, and after activities.
* Before getting out of bed, use a towel to pull toes back toward the ankle. Count to 10, and do it 10 times.
* While sitting, grab a towel with your toes or roll your foot back and forth over a can of frozen juice. Stand on the ball of your foot on the edge of a step and raise and lower leg.
* Try heel cushions or arch supports. Use them in both shoes so other problems don't develop. Custom orthotics (special shoe inserts) may be prescribed.
* Taping helps some people. Apply athletic tape as directed on the product's instructions.
* Night splints are products that keep the muscles stretched while sleeping. They may help.
* Buy shoes that fit well. Sandals help some people.

MEDICATION
* For minor pain and inflammation, use nonprescription drugs, such as ibuprofen.
* Steroids may be injected into the foot.

ACTIVITY—Stay off your feet as much as possible until symptoms are better. Try swimming or cycling for exercising.

DIET—If your weight is a problem, begin a weight-loss diet.

CALL YOUR DOCTOR IF

* You or a family member has symptoms of plantar fasciitis.
* Symptoms don't improve despite treatment.

PLEURAL EFFUSION
(Hemothorax)

 GENERAL INFORMATION

DEFINITION—An abnormal accumulation of fluid in the pleural space. It is not a disease in itself, but a complication of some disorder or injury. Pleura are the thin membranes that line the lungs and chest cavity. Normally the fluid in this area provides lubrication and allows smooth, uniform contractions of the lungs during breathing. The fluid may be termed exudate (often cloudy) or transudate (watery). Special types of pleural effusion include: empyema, (pus is present), hemothorax (blood is present), pneumothorax (air is present), and chylothorax (milky fluid made up of lymph and fat is present).

BODY PARTS INVOLVED—Lung; pleura.

SEX OR AGE MOST AFFECTED—Both sexes; all ages.

SIGNS & SYMPTOMS
• No symptoms sometimes (with small effusion). It may be discovered on a routine health exam.
• Chest pain. Pain varies from vague discomfort to stabbing pain. It is often worse with coughing or breathing. Pain may extend to the lower chest wall or abdomen.
• Shortness of breath.
• Dry cough.
• Other symptoms may be associated with an underlying disease. Symptoms can include edema (e.g., swollen feet and ankles), night sweats, fever, weight loss, bloody sputum.

CAUSES—Many conditions can cause pleural effusion, and sometimes, no cause is found. The effusion results from too much fluid being produced, too little fluid draining out, or an excess accumulation of fluid.

RISK INCREASES WITH
• Congestive heart failure.
• Lung or chest infections, such as pneumonia, tuberculosis or lung abscess.
• Cancer.
• Collapsed lung or chest injury (trauma).
• Pulmonary embolism (blood clot in the lung).
• Viral or fungal infection.
• Pleurisy (lung inflammation).
• Benign (noncancerous) tumor.
• Kidney or liver disorders.
• Adverse drug reaction.
• Vascular disease (e.g., rheumatoid arthritis).
• Surgery complication.

HOW TO PREVENT—Not usually preventable. To reduce risk, get medical care for any problem that may lead to pleural effusion.

 WHAT TO EXPECT

DIAGNOSTIC MEASURES
• Your own observation of symptoms.
• Your health care provider will do a physical exam.
• Medical tests may include culture of pleural fluid obtained by thoracentesis (needle inserted into the chest to withdraw fluid), x-ray, MRI, CT, ultrasound (see Glossary for all), or biopsy (removal of tissue sample for viewing under a microscope).

APPROPRIATE HEALTH CARE
• Small effusions may need treatment only for the cause.
• With larger effusions, the fluid may be removed via a needle or a tube placed in the chest. A fibrinolytic drug may be added to the space to help prevent fluid accumulation.
• Surgery may be needed to remove fibrous material from the lung.
• Treatment will be provided for any disorder that caused pleural effusion.

POSSIBLE COMPLICATIONS—Will depend on the underlying cause.

PROBABLE OUTCOME—A pleural effusion can be treated successfully, but the outcome of the underlying disorder depends on diagnosis and treatment. If a drug is the cause, stopping the drug usually resolves the problem.

 HOW TO TREAT

GENERAL MEASURES—Follow medical instructions for any home care.

MEDICATION
• You may be prescribed antibiotic or antifungal drugs.
• Different drugs including anticancer drugs (chemotherapy) may be prescribed once an underlying disorder is diagnosed.

ACTIVITY—Reduce activity until treatment is complete. Gradually return to normal activity.

DIET—No special diet.

 CALL YOUR DOCTOR IF

• You or a family member has symptoms of pleural effusion.
• Symptoms recur after treatment.
• New symptoms develop. They may be due to the underlying disorder.

PLEURISY

GENERAL INFORMATION

DEFINITION—Inflammation and irritation of the pleura. The pleura is a thin, two-layered membrane that lines the lung and chest cavity. Pleurisy is not a disease, but may be a symptom of many different disorders. Fluid (pleural effusion) may develop at the site of inflammation, between the two membrane layers. This is called wet pleurisy. If there is no fluid build up, it is dry pleurisy.

BODY PARTS INVOLVED—Pleura.

SEX OR AGE MOST AFFECTED—Both sexes; all ages.

SIGNS & SYMPTOMS
* Sudden chest pain that worsens with breathing and coughing. The pain varies from vague discomfort that occurs only with deep breathing or coughing to intense, stabbing pain. Pain is usually over the area of pleural inflammation, but it may also occur in the lower chest or abdomen.
* Fever (sometimes).
* Discomfort on moving the affected side.
* Rapid, shallow breathing.
* Breathing difficulty if pleural effusion develops.

CAUSES—Pleurisy can be caused by infection (e.g., bacterial, fungal, or viral), injury, irritation, blood clot, or disease. Sometimes, no cause is found.

RISK INCREASES WITH
* Lung or chest infection (e.g., pneumonia, bronchitis, tuberculosis).
* Blood clot in the lung.
* Injury to the chest or rib fracture.
* Cancer in other parts of the body.
* Collagen vascular disease, such as systemic lupus erythematosus or rheumatoid arthritis.
* Collapse of a part of the lung.
* Kidney, liver, or pancreas disorders.
* Weak immune system due to illness or drugs.
* Smoking.

HOW TO PREVENT—No specific preventive measures. Obtain medical treatment for any causes listed above to reduce the risk of pleurisy.

WHAT TO EXPECT

DIAGNOSTIC MEASURES
* Your own observation of symptoms.
* Your health care provider will do a physical exam and ask about your symptoms and activities.
* Medical tests may include blood and pleural fluid studies, x-rays of the chest, and others to diagnose the cause.

APPROPRIATE HEALTH CARE
* The main treatment is aimed at the underlying cause. Other treatment may help the symptoms of pleurisy.
* Excess fluid in the pleura may need to be removed. This is done with a needle inserted into the pleura to draw out the fluid.

POSSIBLE COMPLICATIONS
* Fluid build up (pleural effusion).
* Pneumonia.
* Scar tissue (adhesions) may form that cause pain and shortness of breath.

PROBABLE OUTCOME—Outcome depends on successful treatment of the disorder causing it. Sometimes, pleurisy symptoms clear completely on their own in 1 to 2 weeks.

HOW TO TREAT

GENERAL MEASURES
* Lie with the sore side down, on a firm surface. This will help ease the pain.
* Holding a pillow firmly against the chest wall helps ease the pain when coughing.
* For chest pain, you may try loosely wrapping the entire chest with two or three nonadhesive, 6-inch-wide elastic bandages. Unwrap it several times a day.
* Quit smoking. Find a way to stop that works.

MEDICATION
* Take nonsteroidal anti-inflammatory drugs, such as aspirin (adults) or ibuprofen, to relieve pain and inflammation.
* Antibiotics, bronchodilators, or stronger pain relievers may be prescribed.
* Other drugs may be prescribed depending on the cause of the pleurisy.

ACTIVITY—Reduce activity until pain and cough get better. Then resume normal activities gradually.

DIET—No special diet.

CALL YOUR DOCTOR IF

* You or a family member has symptoms of pleurisy.
* The following occur during treatment:
  - Fever.
  - Increased pain.
  - Increased breathlessness.
  - Cough that is dry and non-productive.
  - Blue or dark fingernails, toenails, or lips.
  - Blood in the sputum.

PNEUMOCONIOSIS

GENERAL INFORMATION

DEFINITION—Lung inflammation caused by breathing industrial dusts. Inhaling such particles for many years may cause little patches of irritation to form in one or both lungs. The scar tissue formed by the irritation may make the lungs less flexible and porous. Pneumoconiosis is not contagious. It usually takes at least 10 years of exposure and sometimes up to 25 years for it to develop. Only a few persons exposed to the dusts actually become ill.

BODY PARTS INVOLVED—Lungs.

SEX OR AGE MOST AFFECTED—Men over age 40.

SIGNS & SYMPTOMS
Early symptoms:
• Shortness of breath.
• Cough that produces little or no sputum.
• General ill feeling.
Late symptoms:
• Restless sleep.
• Appetite and weight loss.
• Chest pain.
• Hoarseness; coughing up blood.
• Bluish nails.

CAUSES—Exposure to small particles of industrial dusts cause the following forms of pneumoconiosis:
• Coal dust causes black-lung disease (coal miner's pneumoconiosis, anthracosis).
• Beryllium and its compounds (once used in manufacturing fluorescent lamp bulbs, ceramics, and chemicals) cause berylliosis.
• Talc, iron, cotton, synthetic fiber, and aluminum dusts cause a rare form of pneumoconiosis.
• Asbestos and silica cause asbestosis and silicosis.

RISK INCREASES WITH
• Smoking.
• Greater amounts of dust inhaled over the years.

HOW TO PREVENT
• Practice safety during exposure to industrial dusts. Wear a protective mask or external-air-supplied hood. Get an x-ray once a year.
• Don't smoke. Avoid second hand smoke.

WHAT TO EXPECT

DIAGNOSTIC MEASURES
• Your health care provider will do a physical exam and ask questions about your symptoms and activities. Be sure to tell your provider about your work history and any exposure to industrial dusts.

• Medical tests may include a chest x-ray, pulmonary function tests, and others to confirm diagnosis and check for complications.

APPROPRIATE HEALTH CARE
• Drugs and lung therapy may help the symptoms and treat complications.
• Chest physical therapy (such as controlled coughing) and bronchial drainage help clear secretions. You will be given special training about doing these procedures.

POSSIBLE COMPLICATIONS
• Congestive heart failure.
• Lung collapse, pleurisy, or other lung disease.
• Tuberculosis (in the late stages).
• Lung cancer.

PROBABLE OUTCOME—This condition is currently considered incurable. Symptoms can be relieved or controlled. It reduces life span, but many patients live into their 60s and 70s.

HOW TO TREAT

GENERAL MEASURES
• Avoid any further exposure to industrial dusts.
• Quit smoking. Find a way to stop that works for you.
• Get medical care for any respiratory infection (such as a cold). Get influenza and pneumococcal vaccines.
• To learn more: American Lung Association, 61 Broadway, 6th Floor, New York, NY 10006, (800) 586-4872; website: www.lungusa.org.

MEDICATION
• Antibiotics may be prescribed for infections.
• Bronchodilators (inhaled or oral) with inhalation therapy may be prescribed. This is supervised at first by an inhalation therapist.
• For minor discomfort, you may use nonprescription drugs, such as acetaminophen or aspirin.

ACTIVITY—No limits, except those caused by symptoms.

DIET—No special diet.

CALL YOUR DOCTOR IF

• You or a family member has symptoms of pneumoconiosis.
• The following occur during treatment:
  - Temperature of 101°F (38.3°C) or more.
  - Increased chest pain or shortness of breath.
  - Blood in sputum.
  - Continuing weight loss.
  - Unexplained symptoms develop.

PNEUMOCYSTIS JIROVECI PNEUMONIA
(Pneumonia Pneumocystis Carinii)

GENERAL INFORMATION

DEFINITION—Inflammation of the lungs caused by infection. (It was previously called pneumonia *pneumocystis carinii*.) It occurs in children (including infants) and adults with a weakened immune system. They are usually AIDS patients. Most people have been exposed to these germs by age four, but their immune systems are able to fight off any infection.

BODY PARTS INVOLVED—Lower-respiratory system (bronchial tubes and lungs).

SEX OR AGE MOST AFFECTED—All ages, both sexes, but most common in adult men.

SIGNS & SYMPTOMS
• There may be no symptoms in the early stage.
• Dry, nonproductive cough. Smokers may have a productive cough.
• Shortness of breath and wheezing.
• Fever.
• Fatigue.
• Weight loss.
• Night sweats.
• Tightness in the chest.

CAUSES—*Pneumocystis jiroveci* believed to be a fungus. It is most likely transmitted through the air. It is unknown if it lives in soil or other places. It is also unknown how long it takes symptoms to start after exposure. Person to person spread is a possibility, but is not proven.

RISK INCREASES WITH
• HIV (human immunodeficiency virus) and AIDS (acquired immunodeficiency syndrome).
• People with weak immune systems due to illness or drugs.
• Current fungal infection, such as thrush.
• Cancer chemotherapy (anticancer drugs).
• Long-term steroid drug use.
• Severe malnutrition (any disorder of nutrition).
• Previous infection with this disorder.

HOW TO PREVENT—It is almost entirely preventable with drugs. Preventive drugs can be prescribed for those at risk.

WHAT TO EXPECT

DIAGNOSTIC MEASURES
• Your own observation of symptoms.
• Your health care provider will do a physical exam and ask questions about the symptoms.
• Medical tests may include x-rays, a study of a specimen of sputum, and high resolution CT scan. A bronchoscopy may be done. This involves inserting a tube down the throat to view the lungs and to get a sample of tissue for diagnosis.

APPROPRIATE HEALTH CARE
• Treatment is with drugs given by mouth or given through a vein (IV).
• Treatment may be done at home for mild cases. For more severe infection, hospital care may be needed.

POSSIBLE COMPLICATIONS
• Prolonged illness, sometimes fatal.
• Side effects of drugs, especially skin rash and low white blood cell count.

PROBABLE OUTCOME—With prompt diagnosis and treatment, the outlook is generally good for mild cases. With more severe cases, the risk of complications is higher.

HOW TO TREAT

GENERAL MEASURES—To learn more: American Lung Association, 61 Broadway, 6th Floor, New York, NY 10006, (800) 586-4872; website: www.lungusa.org.

MEDICATION
• Antibiotics, such as trimethoprim-sulfamethoxazole, pentamidine (oral or aerosol), or others will be prescribed.
• Corticosteroids may be prescribed.
• Cough medicine may be recommended.

ACTIVITY—Bed rest is recommended until fever subsides. Normal activities should be resumed gradually.

DIET—No special diet.

CALL YOUR DOCTOR IF

• You or a family member has symptoms of *Pneumocystis jaroveci*.
• The following occur during treatment:
  - Higher fever.
  - Pain becomes worse.
  - Increased shortness of breath.
  - Dark or bluish fingernails, toenails, or skin.
  - Blood in the sputum.
  - Nausea, vomiting, or diarrhea.
• New, unexplained symptoms develop. Drugs used in treatment may produce side effects.

PNEUMONIA, BACTERIAL

GENERAL INFORMATION

DEFINITION—Infection and inflammation of the lungs with bacterial germs. It causes fluid to collect in the air sacs (alveoli), making it difficult to breathe. Bacterial pneumonia is not usually contagious.

BODY PARTS INVOLVED—Lungs; bronchial tubes.

SEX OR AGE MOST AFFECTED—Both sexes; all ages, but most severe in young children and adults over age 60.

SIGNS & SYMPTOMS
* High fever (over 102°F or 38.9°C) and chills.
* Shortness of breath.
* Cough with sputum that may contain blood or blood streaks.
* Rapid breathing.
* Chest pain that worsens with inhalations.
* Abdominal pain.
* Fatigue.
* Bluish lips and nails (rare).
* Loss of appetite and weight loss.

CAUSES—Infection with bacteria, such as *Pneumococci, Haemophilus, Streptococci* or *Staphylococci.* The germs are usually breathed in, but may be spread in other ways.

RISK INCREASES WITH
* Age (newborns, infants, and adults over 60).
* Use of anticancer drugs.
* Smoking.
* Chronic diseases.
* Recent surgery.
* Poor general health from any cause.
* Weak immune system due to illness or drugs.
* Hospital care, for any reason.

HOW TO PREVENT
* Obtain prompt medical care for respiratory infections.
* Arrange for pneumococcal and influenza vaccines.
* Avoid risk factors where possible.

WHAT TO EXPECT

DIAGNOSTIC MEASURES
* Your own observation of symptoms.
* Your health care provider will do a physical exam and ask questions about your symptoms.
* Medical tests may include sputum culture, a blood study, x-rays of lungs, and lung scan.

APPROPRIATE HEALTH CARE
* Hospital care is often needed for more severe cases. Treatment may include breathing support, fluids and/or drugs injected into a vein (IV), and removing excess fluids from the lung.
* Some cases may be treated at home.

POSSIBLE COMPLICATIONS
* Pleurisy and pleural effusion (problems of the membrane layers that cover the lung).
* Bronchiectasis (damaged airways in the lungs).
* Spread of infection.
* Pulmonary abscess (pus-filled area).
* Complications, including death, are more likely in older persons who have other respiratory disorders or serious diseases.

PROBABLE OUTCOME—Usually curable, in otherwise healthy persons, in 1 to 2 weeks with treatment. It may take longer for the very young, elderly, or those with other disorders.

HOW TO TREAT

GENERAL MEASURES
* Don't suppress the cough with a drug if the cough produces sputum or mucus. It is useful in ridding the body of lung secretions.
* Use a heating pad on low heat or warm compresses to relieve chest pain.
* Quit smoking. Find a way to stop that works.
* To learn more: American Lung Association, 61 Broadway, 6th Floor, New York, NY 10006, (800) 586-4872; website: www.lungusa.org.

MEDICATION
* Antibiotics for infection will be prescribed.
* You may use nonprescription drugs, such as acetaminophen, to relieve minor discomfort.

ACTIVITY—Rest in bed, until fever is gone and pain and shortness of breath disappear. Then resume normal activities gradually.

DIET—No special diet. Increase fluid intake. Extra fluid may help thin the lung secretions so they are easier to cough up.

CALL YOUR DOCTOR IF

* You or a family member has symptoms of pneumonia.
* The following occur during treatment:
  - Fever, pain or shortness of breath increases.
  - Dark or bluish fingernails, toenails, or skin.
  - Blood in the sputum.
  - Nausea, vomiting, or diarrhea.

PNEUMONIA, MYCOPLASMA
(Atypical Pneumonia; Walking Pneumonia)

 GENERAL INFORMATION

DEFINITION—A lung inflammation caused by infection with *Mycoplasma pneumoniae*, an organism (germ) that is similar to bacteria. The disorder is also called walking pneumonia, because a patient is usually not confined to bed or in need of hospital care. Some people may not even realize they have pneumonia, as the symptoms are often mild.

BODY PARTS INVOLVED—Upper-respiratory system.

SEX OR AGE MOST AFFECTED—Can affect all ages, but is more common in ages 5 to 20 and males more than females.

SIGNS & SYMPTOMS
* Cough that is dry at first and then produces sputum.
* Fever.
* Sore throat.
* Stuffy nose.
* Chest or ear pain may occur.
* Headache.
* Wheezing.
* Muscle aches and fatigue.

CAUSES—Mycoplasma pneumonia is infectious and is spread through close contact with an infected person. Germs are spread into the air when the infected person coughs or sneezes. Symptoms may begin 15 to 25 days after being exposed to the germs.

RISK INCREASES WITH
* Close living conditions (military barracks, college dorms, and families).
* Weak immune system due to illness or drugs.

HOW TO PREVENT—No specific preventive measures. Avoid exposure to persons who are ill with respiratory infections. Wash hands often to prevent spread of any type of germs.

 WHAT TO EXPECT

DIAGNOSTIC MEASURES
* Your own observation of symptoms.
* Your health care provider will do a physical exam and ask questions about your symptoms.
* Medical tests may include blood studies, sputum culture, and chest x-rays.

APPROPRIATE HEALTH CARE
* Treatment may include extra rest, treatment of symptoms, and antibiotics. For most patients, treatment can be done at home.
* Hospital care may be needed for someone with severe symptoms or complications.

POSSIBLE COMPLICATIONS
* Skin rash.
* Ear infection or sinus inflammation.
* Asthma.
* Hemolytic anemia (lack of red blood cells).
* Severe pneumonia.
* Other, less common complications may occur.

PROBABLE OUTCOME—Symptoms usually clear up in about two weeks. Some symptoms, such as cough or fatigue, may persist for 4 to 6 weeks. The disorder will heal on its own, but treatment with antibiotics can help speed recovery. Once a person has had the infection, there is some immunity, but it is not life-long.

 HOW TO TREAT

GENERAL MEASURES
* Use a heating pad on low heat or warm compresses to relieve chest pain.
* To learn more: American Lung Association, 61 Broadway, 6th Floor, New York, NY 10006, (800) 586-4872; website: www.lungusa.org.

MEDICATION
* Antibiotics, such as erythromycin, clarithromycin, azithromycin, or tetracycline (for ages over 8), may be prescribed. They will shorten the duration of fever and other symptoms, but you can carry the germs for weeks in spite of treatment.
* Cough medicine, nose drops, sprays or oral decongestants may be recommended.
* You may use acetaminophen or ibuprofen for fever or minor pain.

ACTIVITY—Get extra rest until symptoms improve. Normal activities should be resumed gradually. Children may return to school once symptoms improve.

DIET—No special diet. Extra fluid may help thin lung secretions so they can be coughed up more easily.

 CALL YOUR DOCTOR IF

* You or a family member has symptoms of mycoplasma pneumonia.
* The following occur during treatment:
  - High fever, increased pain, or shortness of breath.
  - Dark or bluish fingernails, toenails, or skin.
  - Blood in the sputum, nausea, vomiting or diarrhea.
  - Rash or earache.
  - Severe headache.

PNEUMONIA, VIRAL

GENERAL INFORMATION

DEFINITION—Lung inflammation caused by a virus infection. It causes fluid to collect in the air sacs (alveoli) making it difficult to breathe.

BODY PARTS INVOLVED
• Lower respiratory tract (bronchial tubes, bronchioles and lungs).
• Upper respiratory tract (nose, throat, tonsils, sinuses, trachea and larynx).

SEX OR AGE MOST AFFECTED—Both sexes; all ages, but can be more severe in young children and adults over age 60.

SIGNS & SYMPTOMS
• Fever, chills, and sweating.
• Muscle aches and fatigue.
• Cough, with or without sputum, or "croup."
• Rapid, difficult (sometimes) breathing.
• Sore throat.
• Loss of appetite.
• Enlarged lymph glands in the neck.

CAUSES—Viral infection. These include influenza, chickenpox, and respiratory syncytial virus (especially in adults); respiratory viruses, measles, and cytomegalovirus (especially in infants).

RISK INCREASES WITH
• Newborns and infants.
• Adults over 60.
• Weak immune system due to illness or drugs.
• Persons with chronic diseases.
• Smoking.
• Crowded living conditions.
• Recent upper respiratory infection.

HOW TO PREVENT
• No specific preventive measures.
• Measles vaccines for children, chickenpox vaccine, and annual flu vaccines can help prevent infections that can lead to pneumonia.
• Wash hands often to prevent spread of any germs.

WHAT TO EXPECT

DIAGNOSTIC MEASURES
• Your own observation of symptoms.
• Your health care provider will do a physical exam and ask questions about your symptoms.
• Medical tests may include a sputum culture, blood studies, and x-rays.

APPROPRIATE HEALTH CARE
• Treatment may involve drug therapy and providing relief for the symptoms.
• Most patients can be treated at home.
• Hospital care may be needed for more severe cases.

POSSIBLE COMPLICATIONS
• Bacterial infection of the lungs.
• Other lung disorders such as bronchitis.

PROBABLE OUTCOME—Usually clears up on its own in 1 to 3 weeks. In more severe cases, recovery may take longer. Some people are fatigued and weak for up to 6 weeks after recovery.

HOW TO TREAT

GENERAL MEASURES
• Coughing and deep breathing is recommended to help clear secretions. Dispose of tissues carefully.
• Use a heating pad on low heat or warm compresses to relieve chest pain.
• Use a cool-mist ultrasonic humidifier (if advised) to increase air moisture and loosen lung secretions. Use pure water; don't put drugs in the humidifier. Clean the humidifier daily.
• Quit smoking. Find a way to stop that works.
• To learn more: American Lung Association, 61 Broadway, 6th Floor, New York, NY 10006, (800) 586-4872; website: www.lungusa.org.

MEDICATION
• Antiviral drugs may be prescribed depending on the virus and how long it's been since symptoms started.
• For minor pain, fever, and congestion, you may use nonprescription drugs, such as acetaminophen or decongestant nose drops, nasal sprays, or tablets.
• Antibiotics do not cure viral infections. They may be prescribed to prevent or treat a complicating bacterial infection.

ACTIVITY—Bed rest is helpful until fever, pain, and shortness of breath have been gone at least 48 hours. Then normal activity may be resumed slowly.

DIET—No special diet. Drink plenty of fluids. This helps to thin lung secretions so they are easier to cough up.

CALL YOUR DOCTOR IF

• You or a family member has symptoms of viral pneumonia.
• The following occur during treatment:
  - Temperature rises over 102°F (38.9°C).
  - Pain gets worse.
  - Nausea, vomiting, or diarrhea.
  - Increasing shortness of breath.
  - Blood in the sputum.
  - Increasingly bluish nails and skin.

PNEUMOTHORAX

GENERAL INFORMATION

DEFINITION—Air in the chest between the two layers of the pleura (thin membranes that cover the lung). When air gets into the pleural space, the pressure becomes greater than the pressure in the lung. This causes a partial or a complete collapse of the lung. Types of pneumothorax include:
- Spontaneous—it occurs without a cause. It is common in young men age 20 to 40.
- Secondary spontaneous—complication of lung disease.
- Traumatic—caused by an injury to the chest.
- Tension—excessive pressure builds up around lung. Air gets in, but cannot get out. It can be life-threatening.

BODY PARTS INVOLVED—Lung; pleura.

SEX OR AGE MOST AFFECTED—All ages, but most common in active young men (ages 20 to 40).

SIGNS & SYMPTOMS
- The symptoms vary according to the degree of lung collapse and extent of other lung disease. Symptoms may be less acute if the pneumothorax develops slowly.
- Sharp chest pain. Pain may extend to a shoulder or across the chest or abdomen.
- Shortness of breath and rapid breathing.
- Anxiety.
- Dry, hacking cough (sometimes).
- Bluish nails.
- Coughing bloody sputum (sometimes).
- Rapid pulse.
- Fainting and shock (tension pneumothorax).

CAUSES—Air may get into the pleural space due to a rupture of the small air or fluid sacs in the lungs. Air may also enter the chest from the outside, such as with a chest wound. The air may result from medical procedures performed on the chest cavity. The air may result from damaged lungs due to chronic lung disease, other diseases, or injury.

RISK INCREASES WITH
- Physical exertion in a healthy person, with no obvious injury, infection, or disease. Activities most likely to produce pneumothorax include:
  - Ascent while scuba diving.
  - Diving or high-altitude flying.
  - Activities that require stretching the chest and rib cage, such as track and field events, throwing sports, and bowling.
- Asthma, emphysema, chronic bronchitis, lung abscess, empyema or other lung disease.
- A wound to the chest area, which permits outside air to rush into the pleural space.
- Removing fluid from the lung (thoracentesis).
- Smoking.
- Family history of pneumothorax.
- Use of ventilator for breathing support.

HOW TO PREVENT—No specific preventive measures. Get medical care for chronic lung disorders. Don't smoke.

WHAT TO EXPECT

DIAGNOSTIC MEASURES
- Your own observation of symptoms.
- Your health care provider will do a physical exam and ask about your symptoms and activities.
- X-rays of the chest help to confirm the diagnosis and determine the size of the pneumothorax.

APPROPRIATE HEALTH CARE
- Treatment depends on the size of the pneumothorax and the condition of the lungs.
- No treatment may be needed in some cases. Small amounts of air are reabsorbed naturally and the lung will re-expand on its own.
- Hospital care may be needed for treatment.
  - A small needle may be inserted into the chest cavity to relieve excess pressure.
  - A tube may be placed in the chest and attached to a special vacuum bottle. This allows the air to be slowly removed and the lung to re-expand.
  - Surgery may be needed if the pneumothorax has recurred or if the lung does not re-expand after 5 days.

POSSIBLE COMPLICATIONS
- Repeated pneumothorax.
- Critical illness and death with tension pneumothorax.

PROBABLE OUTCOME—Most patients recover fully in 2 to 4 weeks.

HOW TO TREAT

GENERAL MEASURES
- Don't smoke; try not to cough; avoid loud talking, laughing, or singing.
- Rest in a sitting position. It may be more comfortable.

MEDICATION—You may use nonprescription drugs, such as acetaminophen, for minor pain. Stronger pain relievers may be prescribed if needed.

ACTIVITY—Rest often. Allow two or more weeks for recovery.

DIET—No special diet.

CALL YOUR DOCTOR IF

You or a family member has symptoms of pneumothorax.

POISON IVY, OAK, SUMAC

 GENERAL INFORMATION

DEFINITION—Poison ivy, oak, and sumac are three types of plants that cause a skin reaction (contact dermatitis). The reaction results from contact with an oily substance (resin) produced by these plants. This particular allergic reaction is the most common in the United States. About 50% of the total population has developed an allergy to these plants.

BODY PARTS INVOLVED—Skin.

SEX OR AGE MOST AFFECTED—Both sexes; all ages.

SIGNS & SYMPTOMS
Skin rash with the following signs:
- Bright red spots that develop 24 to 48 hours (sometimes may take several days) after contact.
- Weeping, crusting, and swelling.
- Intense itching and burning.
- Blisters (the fluid in blisters is not contagious).
- Enough of the oily resin remains on hands or clothing so that the rash is carried to other body parts, such as the face or genitals.

CAUSES—Contact with any part of the poison ivy, poison oak, or poison sumac plants. They grow as vines or bushes and have three leaves (poison ivy and poison oak), or a row of paired leaves (poison sumac). They produce a potent resin (urushiol) that is the cause of the problem. A reaction may also occur from touching the poison substance when it is on clothing, equipment (hunting, golfing, or athletic), or animals, such as pets. It can also come from any smoke these plants give off if they are burned. This may affect the face, eyelids, throat, and lungs.

RISK INCREASES WITH
- Spring and summer (though plants are dangerous year round).
- Not wearing protective clothing.

HOW TO PREVENT
- Learn to identify and avoid contact with these plants.
- When walking in areas where these plants grow, wear shoes, socks, long pants, long-sleeved shirts, and, sometimes, gloves. Wash this clothing right after you return if possible. Use a product that prevents the poison from getting on your skin.
- If you are exposed, washing the skin immediately with soap and water and sponging with rubbing alcohol may prevent the rash.

 WHAT TO EXPECT

DIAGNOSTIC MEASURES
- Your own observation of symptoms.
- Consult your health care provider if rash is severe or does not improve. The diagnosis can be confirmed

APPROPRIATE HEALTH CARE
- Self-care at home.
- If needed, drugs may be prescribed.

POSSIBLE COMPLICATIONS—A skin infection may develop.

PROBABLE OUTCOME—Itching, redness, and swelling are often improved by the second day, and complete healing occurs within 7 to 14 days.

 HOW TO TREAT

GENERAL MEASURES
- Sweating and heat make the itching worse, so try to stay cool.
- Apply cool compresses to the affected area.
- A soothing bath helps. Use Aveeno (a product made of oatmeal) or baking soda (about a half cup) per bath.
- Wash all clothing and shoes, and any equipment that came in contact with the plant oils, with soap and water.
- Give pets a warm, soapy bath to remove any oil from the fur.

MEDICATION
- You may use calamine lotion to relieve the itching.
- Oral antihistamines may be helpful also.
- Your health care provider may prescribe topical or oral steroid drugs for severe symptoms.

ACTIVITY—No limits. Avoid activities that can cause sweating. This can worsen itching.

DIET—No special diet.

 CALL YOUR DOCTOR IF

- You or a family member has a severe rash.
- If swelling or pain develops around the eyes, nose, or genitals.
- Rash gets worse or doesn't improve with self-care methods.

POLYARTERITIS NODOSA
(Polyarteritis; Necrotizing Angiitis)

GENERAL INFORMATION

DEFINITION—Inflammation of small and medium size arteries in the body. This decreases the blood supply to the body organs supplied by the affected arteries.

BODY PARTS INVOLVED—Can affect the muscles, joints, skin, heart, brain, intestinal tract, nerves, liver, kidneys, and genitals

SEX OR AGE MOST AFFECTED
* Both sexes, but more common in men.
* All ages, but most common in adults under age 50.

SIGNS & SYMPTOMS
* General symptoms include weight loss, fever, fatigue, general ill feeling, muscle and joint aches, weakness, high blood pressure, and headache.
* Other symptoms may be due to the affected organ:
  - Blood in the urine (kidney involved).
  - Chest pain (heart involved).
  - Abdominal pain (intestinal tract and liver involved).
  - Numbness and tingling of the hands and feet (nerves involved).
  - Purplish rash and other skin disorders (skin involved).
  - Testicle pain (testicles involved).

CAUSES—It is considered an autoimmune disease, although the cause is unknown. Hepatitis B appears to be a factor.

RISK INCREASES WITH
* Having hepatitis B and sometimes hepatitis C.
* Other autoimmune diseases.
* Methamphetamine abuse.
* Smoking.
* Use of certain drugs, including penicillin, antithyroid drugs, thiazide diuretics, and some vaccines.

HOW TO PREVENT—No specific preventive measures.

WHAT TO EXPECT

DIAGNOSTIC MEASURES
* Your own observation of symptoms.
* Your health care provider will do a physical exam and ask questions about your symptoms.
* Medical tests may include blood and urine studies, x-ray, biopsy, and MRI (see Glossary for all). Angiography may be done—a dye is injected into the arteries to highlight the affected areas and x-rays taken.

APPROPRIATE HEALTH CARE
* Treatment is with drugs to reduce the inflammation.
* Hospital care may be needed for severe cases and complications.
* Surgery may be needed if there are complications involving the intestinal tract.

POSSIBLE COMPLICATIONS
* Kidney failure.
* Heart attack or heart failure.
* Stroke.
* Nervous system disorders.
* Intestinal perforation.
* Aneurysm rupture.
* Side effects of drugs used in treatment.

PROBABLE OUTCOME
* The disorder is chronic and progressive. Symptoms may be relieved or controlled. With treatment, about 80% of patients survive 5 years or more. Without treatment, few patients live beyond 5 years.
* Research into causes and treatment continues, so there is hope for more effective treatment and cure.

HOW TO TREAT

GENERAL MEASURES—To learn more: National Institute of Arthritis & Musculoskeletal & Skin Disorders, 1 AMS Circle, Bethesda, MD, 20892-3675, (877) 226-4267; website: www.nih.gov/niams or Polyarteritis Nodosa Research & Support Network, website: www.pansupport.org.

MEDICATION
* Cortisone drugs and immunosuppressive drugs are usually prescribed. They need to be continued even after symptoms improve. The dosage may be reduced once the symptoms are controlled. Some patients want to stop the drugs because of side effects. Without drugs, however, the disorder will progress and cause complications.
* Drugs to treat other disorders such as hepatitis B, heart drugs, or drugs for high blood pressure may be prescribed.

ACTIVITY—Resume your normal activities gradually as symptoms improve.

DIET—No special diet unless advised by your health care provider.

CALL YOUR DOCTOR IF

* You or a family member has symptoms of polyarteritis nodosa.
* New, unexplained symptoms develop. Drugs used in treatment may produce side effects.

POLYCYSTIC OVARIAN SYNDROME
(Stein-Leventhal Syndrome)

GENERAL INFORMATION

DEFINITION—Polycystic ovarian syndrome (PCOS) is an endocrine (hormone) condition. It is not a disease itself. It is a set of signs and symptoms, that when combined, make up the condition.

BODY PARTS INVOLVED—Ovaries, but can affect the entire body.

SEX OR AGE MOST AFFECTED—PCOS affects 5% to 10% of all women of childbearing age. It may begin during puberty and become more severe with time.

SIGNS & SYMPTOMS
* Irregular menstrual bleeding. This results in periods of light flow along with heavy flow. There is increased time between periods, often up to several months.
* Hirsutism—increased hair growth on the face, arms, legs, and from pubic area to navel.
* Thinning of the scalp hair (alopecia).
* Overweight or obesity.
* Trouble getting pregnant; miscarriages.
* Acne.
* Dark patches of skin or skin tags (small skin growths).
* Polycystic ovaries. These are fairly common and involve enlarged ovaries from many small cysts.
* Anovulation (absence of ovulation). The monthly release of the egg from the ovary fails to take place.

CAUSES—The cause of PCOS is unclear. Hormone imbalances, insulin production, and hereditary factors all seem to play a role.

RISK INCREASES WITH
* Lifestyle factor such as obesity, poor diet, and physical inactivity.
* Family history of PCOS or diabetes.

HOW TO PREVENT—Cannot be prevented at present.

WHAT TO EXPECT

DIAGNOSTIC MEASURES
* Your own observation of symptoms.
* Your health care provider will usually do a physical exam and a pelvic exam. Questions will be asked about your symptoms, menstrual cycle, and pregnancies.
* Medical tests may include studies of blood for levels of hormones, glucose, insulin, and fats (cholesterol and triglyceride). Other tests such as an ultrasound may be done to rule out other disorders. There is no specific test to diagnose PCOS.

APPROPRIATE HEALTH CARE
* Treatment goals: regulate menstrual cycle, reduce hair growth and acne problems, help with fertility (if pregnancy desired), and prevent long-term problems.
* A diet and exercise program for overweight or obese women will help improve physical and mental health.
* Infertility is usually treated successfully through diet and exercise, weight loss, and drug therapy. If these steps are not successful, other options are available.
* Counseling may help you cope with emotional stress.

POSSIBLE COMPLICATIONS
* Infertility (unable to get pregnant) or miscarriages.
* Depression and anxiety.
* High cholesterol and triglyceride levels.
* Heart and blood vessel disease; high blood pressure.
* Diabetes.
* Cancer of the breast or uterus.

PROBABLE OUTCOME—Treatment, along with weight control and exercise, can relieve or eliminate symptoms. Pregnancy (if desired) can be achieved in many patients.

HOW TO TREAT

GENERAL MEASURES
* Options for removing excess hair from your face, arms, and legs include drugs, bleaching, electrolysis, laser therapy, plucking, waxing, and depilation.
* Quit smoking. Find a way to stop that works.
* More information is available from a variety sites on the Internet dedicated to PCOS.

MEDICATION
* Diabetic drugs (such as metformin), birth-control pills, or other drugs may be prescribed.
* Drugs to help with fertility may be prescribed.
* Vaniqa (eflornithine cream) for excess facial hair) or spironolactone for excess body hair may be prescribed.

ACTIVITY—No limits on activity, including sexual intercourse. Physical activity is important. Exercise daily.

DIET—Low-carbohydrate diet may be recommended. Begin a weight-loss diet if you are overweight.

CALL YOUR DOCTOR IF

* You or a family member has symptoms of polycystic ovarian syndrome.
* New symptoms occur with treatment.

POLYCYTHEMIA

GENERAL INFORMATION

DEFINITION—An increase of red blood cells in the body. The disease has 3 forms:
• Polycythemia vera, which involves overproduction of red blood cells, white blood cells, and platelets.
• Secondary polycythemia (reactive polycythemia), which is a complication of diseases or factors other than blood-cell disorders.
• Stress polycythemia (pseudopolycythemia), which involves decreased blood plasma.

BODY PARTS INVOLVED—Blood-forming organs: bone marrow; spleen; lymph glands; lymph channels.

SEX OR AGE MOST AFFECTED—It more often affects adults over age 50 (but has a range of ages from 15 to 90), and it is more common in men.

SIGNS & SYMPTOMS—Some patients have no symptoms. Others may have any of the following:
• Fatigue, headache, drowsiness, or dizziness.
• Itching or flushed skin.
• Enlarged spleen.
• Unexplained bleeding.

CAUSES
• Polycythemia vera: unknown.
• Secondary polycythemia: congenital heart disease, chronic lung disease, cigarette or cigar smoking, living at high altitude.
• Stress polycythemia: use of diuretic drugs, smoking, or dehydration.

RISK INCREASES WITH
• Some anticancer drugs used to treat cancer.
• Jewish ancestry.
• Exposure to radiation.
• Family history of polycythemia.

HOW TO PREVENT—Polycythemia cannot be prevented at present.

WHAT TO EXPECT

DIAGNOSTIC MEASURES
• Your own observation of symptoms.
• Your health care provider will do a physical exam and ask questions about your symptoms.
• Medical tests may include studies of bone marrow and blood (red-blood cell count, hematocrit), x-ray of the kidneys, and others to confirm the diagnosis.

APPROPRIATE HEALTH CARE
• Treatment steps will depend on the age of patient, disease duration, type of polycythemia, complications, disease activity, and response to treatment.
• Treatment steps to keep the red blood cell range near normal and prevent clotting or hemorrhage include phlebotomy (withdrawal of excess blood) and drug therapy.
• For secondary or stress polycythemia, proper treatment of the underlying cause is important. Drug therapy or surgery may be recommended.

POSSIBLE COMPLICATIONS
• Blood clots in veins or arteries.
• Gout.
• Stroke.
• Heart attack.
• Peptic ulcer.
• Kidney stones.
• Leukemia.

PROBABLE OUTCOME
• Polycythemia vera is incurable, but symptoms can be controlled. With treatment, average survival ranges from 7 to 15 years, with some patients living 20 or more years.
• Other forms of polycythemia can usually be cured if the causes can be eliminated.

HOW TO TREAT

GENERAL MEASURES
• Stop smoking. Consult your doctor about recommendations for a cessation program.
• Adherence to your treatment plan brings about improved survival and well-being.

MEDICATION—You may be prescribed:
• Drugs to suppress production of red blood cells and platelets.
• Allopurinol if uric acid levels are high.
• Low-dose aspirin for ages over 18 (sometimes).
• Anti-itching drugs, such as antihistamines.
• Drugs for stomach acidity.

ACTIVITY—Resume normal activity when symptoms improve.

DIET—No special diet. Drink enough fluids to help maintain adequate body fluid.

CALL YOUR DOCTOR IF

• You or a family member has symptoms of polycythemia.
• Symptoms recur after treatment.
• New, unexplained symptoms develop. Drugs used in treatment may produce side effects.

POLYMYALGIA RHEUMATICA & GIANT CELL ARTERITIS

GENERAL INFORMATION

DEFINITION—Polymyalgia rheumatica (PMR) and giant cell arteritis (GCA) seem to be related inflammatory disorders. They often occur together. In PMR, inflammation affects the whole body. In GCA, certain arteries, such as those in the head and neck, are inflamed.

BODY PARTS INVOLVED—Muscles; temporal arteries; eyes; connective tissue.

SEX OR AGE MOST AFFECTED—Adults over 50. The disease occurs more often in women than men.

SIGNS & SYMPTOMS
- The symptoms may resemble those of an infection such as influenza. Symptoms can come on suddenly.
- Low fever and weakness.
- Muscle stiffness or aches and pains, especially in the morning. The muscles involved are usually those of the trunk, upper arms, and legs.
- Headache (usually in one temple).
- Pain in the temples or scalp, and sometimes, the jaw and tongue.
- Blurred or double vision; loss of vision in one eye.
- Appetite loss and weight loss.

CAUSES—Exact cause of the inflammation is unknown. It may involve the immune system, or be due to viral, genetic, or environmental factors.

RISK INCREASES WITH—White adults over age 50, especially women.

HOW TO PREVENT—No specific preventive measures.

WHAT TO EXPECT

DIAGNOSTIC MEASURES
- Your own observation of symptoms.
- Your health care provider will do a physical exam and ask questions about your symptoms.
- There is no specific diagnostic test for either disorder. Medical tests may include blood studies, tests for anemia, CT or MRI (see Glossary for both), and a biopsy. Biopsy involves the removal of a small amount of tissue or fluid for viewing under a microscope.

APPROPRIATE HEALTH CARE—Treatment involves drug therapy and exercise.

POSSIBLE COMPLICATIONS
- PMR may recur. It can be successfully treated again with drugs. GCA rarely recurs after treatment.

- Without treatment for GCA, there is a risk for loss of vision, stroke, heart failure, chest pain, and aneurysm.
- Adverse effects of steroid treatment (osteoporosis, high blood pressure, cataracts, and others).

PROBABLE OUTCOME—With treatment, the symptoms can clear up quickly and complications are unlikely. Treatment with drugs needs to continue for months to years depending on each individual patient. An active lifestyle is expected.

HOW TO TREAT

GENERAL MEASURES
- For headache relief, apply heat to the painful side of the head. For muscle stiffness, apply heat directly to the affected area or take warm baths.
- To learn more: Arthritis Foundation, P.O. Box 7669, Atlanta, GA 30357-0669, (800) 283-7800; website: www.arthritis.org.

MEDICATION
- Cortisone drugs in high doses until the acute phase ends. These relieve symptoms by reducing inflammation. Adverse effects may occur. For ongoing treatment with cortisone, the dosage will be reduced as low as possible to keep symptoms under control.
- Methotrexate may be prescribed.
- Nonsteroidal anti-inflammatory drugs may be prescribed for polymyalgia rheumatica. They may not completely control symptoms.

ACTIVITY—Exercise regularly. Swimming, walking, biking, and stretching exercises will help keep muscles strong, flexible, and functional. Avoid straining the muscles (such as doing heavy lifting). Adequate rest is also important. Don't overdo physical activities.

DIET—No special diet.

CALL YOUR DOCTOR IF

- You or a family member has symptoms of polymyalgia rheumatica or giant cell arteritis.
- The following occur during or after treatment:
  - Any changes in vision. Call immediately!
  - Temperature of 101°F (38.3°C).
  - Blood in the urine.
  - Shortness of breath.
  - Chest pain.
  - Bloody bowel movements.
  - Severe abdominal pain.
  - Any illness with fever.
- New, unexplained symptoms develop. Drugs used in treatment may produce side effects.

POLYMYOSITIS & DERMATOMYOSITIS

 GENERAL INFORMATION

DEFINITION—Polymyositis is muscle inflammation that leads to a gradual weakening of the muscles. When the disorder involves the skin, it is called dermatomyositis.

BODY PARTS INVOLVED—Muscles, including large muscles of the skeleton and tiny muscles that control small arteries; skin; connective tissue.

SEX OR AGE MOST AFFECTED—Women are affected more often than men. It usually begins between ages 30 and 60. It may also occur in children.

SIGNS & SYMPTOMS
• Symptoms vary from person to person and may be mild to severe. Their onset may be sudden or slow.
• Muscle weakness that often begins in the hip, thighs, and shoulder muscles. Other muscles may be affected.
• Frequent falls and difficulty in getting up.
• Muscle pain.
• Skin rash that may itch on the face, shoulders, arms, and over joints. The rash may be red or violet.
• Cold hands and feet.
• Speaking or swallowing difficulty.

CAUSES—Exact cause is unknown. They may be autoimmune disorders. In these disorders, the immune system by mistake attacks the body. Other factors may be involved such as viral, genetic, or environmental causes.

RISK INCREASES WITH
• Females over age 30.
• Family history of autoimmune disorders.

HOW TO PREVENT—No known preventive measures.

 WHAT TO EXPECT

DIAGNOSTIC MEASURES
• Your health care provider will do a physical exam and an exam of any affected skin.
• Medical tests may include blood studies, heart tests, x-ray, and MRI (see Glossary for both). A biopsy may be done, which involves removal of a small amount of muscle tissue for viewing under a microscope. An electromyogram may be done. This test studies the electrical activity of muscles.

APPROPRIATE HEALTH CARE—Treatment usually involves drugs, physical therapy, and other therapy to help with activities of daily living.

POSSIBLE COMPLICATIONS
• Progressive muscle weakness.
• Heart, gastrointestinal, and lung problems.
• Adverse effects of drugs.
• Skin ulcers (open sores), infections, and scarring.
• Cancer.

PROBABLE OUTCOME—The outcome varies. Symptoms can improve at times and get worse at other times. Earlier diagnosis and treatment improves the outcome. Some patients recover completely. Others have persistent symptoms, such as weakness. Others may have complications that can lead to disability and be life threatening.

 HOW TO TREAT

GENERAL MEASURES
• Cool-water compresses may relieve itching.
• To learn more: Myositis Society of America. 1233 20th St. NW, Suite 402, Washington, DC 20036; (202) 887-0088 (not toll free); website: www.myositis.org.

MEDICATION—You may be prescribed:
• Cortisone drugs, in high doses until acute symptoms diminish, then in lower doses.
• Drugs to suppress the immune system.
• Drugs to help control itching.
• Drugs for pain.
• Drugs for bone building.

ACTIVITY
• Physical therapy may be prescribed. It helps keep muscles flexible, strong, and functional. Follow instructions for exercises to do at home.
• Swimming is a good exercise.
• Don't overdo any activity. Rest as needed.

DIET—No special diet. Avoid weight gain.

 CALL YOUR DOCTOR IF

• You or a family member has symptoms of polymyositis or dermatomyositis.
• Symptoms don't improve or recur despite treatment.
• New, unexplained symptoms develop. Drugs used in treatment may produce side effects.

PORPHYRIA

GENERAL INFORMATION

DEFINITION—Any of a group of disorders in which the body has too much porphyrin. Porphyrin is a chemical that works with enzymes in the body to make heme. Heme is the part of blood that makes it red and carries the oxygen. Types include:
* Acute intermittent porphyria (AIP).
* Variegate porphyria (VP).
* Hereditary coproporphyria (HCP).
* ALAD dehydratase porphyria (ADP).
* Porphyria cutanea tarda (PCT).
* Erythropoietic porphyria (EPP).
* Congenital erythropoietic porphyria (CEP).
* Hepatoerythropoietic porphyria (HEP).

BODY PARTS INVOLVED—Central nervous system; skin; liver; digestive system.

SEX OR AGE MOST AFFECTED—Both sexes; all ages.

SIGNS & SYMPTOMS
* Symptoms vary and can appear over hours or days. A variety of factors can trigger an attack. Symptoms usually affect the nervous system or the skin.
* Chest, abdominal, or leg pain.
* Muscle cramps and weakness.
* Numbness and tingling in the feet and hands.
* Emotional and mental changes including depression, mania, anxiety, agitation, confusion, and others.
* Skin changes, including itching, blistering, and sensitivity to the sun.
* Excessive hair growth.
* Urine turns color (dark-red, purplish, or brown).

CAUSES—Porphyrin builds up in the body due to enzyme deficiencies. Enzymes are required to complete the porphyrin-heme process. There are several different types of enzyme deficiencies. Most types are inherited. Others develop during a person's life.

RISK INCREASES WITH—Family history of porphyria.

HOW TO PREVENT
* Cannot be prevented at present.
* Porphyria attacks may result from drugs, alcohol, smoking, infection, reduced calorie intake, stress (physical and emotional), excess iron, hepatitis C, pregnancy, and before a menstrual period. Talk to your health care provider about avoiding these factors where possible.

WHAT TO EXPECT

DIAGNOSTIC MEASURES
* Your own observation of symptoms.

* Your health care provider will do a physical exam and ask questions about your symptoms and activities.
* Medical tests are done to measure porphyrins in the urine, blood, and stool.

APPROPRIATE HEALTH CARE
* Treatment involves medical care during attacks, preventing attacks, and counseling if needed. Specific treatment will depend on the type of porphyria.
* Phlebotomy may be done. A unit of blood is removed on a regular basis to get rid of excess iron in the body.
* Hospital care may be required for severe symptoms.
* Genetic counseling before starting a family is advised.

POSSIBLE COMPLICATIONS—A variety of complications may occur that cause physical problems as well as psychological problems.

PROBABLE OUTCOME—There is no cure. Some people with porphyria never have symptoms. In others, the symptoms may be mild to severe. Symptoms can usually be relieved with treatment. A few patients may have complications.

HOW TO TREAT

GENERAL MEASURES
* Don't take any drugs, herbs, or supplements without medical advice.
* Avoid bright sunlight. If you must be in bright sun, use a hat and protective clothing.
* To learn more: American Porphyria Foundation, P.O. Box 22712, Houston, TX 77227, (713) 266-9617 (not toll free); website: www.porphyriafoundation.com.

MEDICATION—You may be prescribed:
* Intravenous (IV) glucose or heme to help prevent or treat acute attacks.
* Drugs for depression or anxiety.
* Drugs to reduce nausea and vomiting.
* Drugs to reduce the porphyrin in the body.
* Drugs to help reduce premenstrual attacks.
* Drugs for anemia (if needed).
* Beta carotene for skin symptoms.

ACTIVITY—No limits except for the sunlight restrictions.

DIET—Eat a normal diet or as advised.

CALL YOUR DOCTOR IF

* You or a family member has symptoms of porphyria.
* Any symptoms of an attack occur.
* New, unexplained symptoms develop.

POSTMENOPAUSAL BLEEDING

GENERAL INFORMATION

DEFINITION—Unexpected bleeding from the vagina that begins 6 to 12 or more months after menopause. This is not a normal condition and can be a symptom of a serious medical problem.

BODY PARTS INVOLVED—Reproductive system.

SEX OR AGE MOST AFFECTED—Females after menopause.

SIGNS & SYMPTOMS
• Vaginal bleeding. It may be a light-brown discharge or heavy, red bleeding (with or without clots).
• Mucus may be a part of the bleeding.
• Bleeding episodes vary in length.
• Pelvic pain (sometimes).

CAUSES
• Atrophy of the lining of the uterus (endometrium) or the vagina. Atrophy means shrinking or wasting away of tissue.
• Hormone therapy. Using estrogens (female hormones).
• Cancer.
• Endometrial hyperplasia (the uterine lining becomes overgrown).
• Endometrial or cervical polyps (benign growths).
• Myoma (benign fibroid tumor in the uterus).
• Trauma (injury) to the vagina.

RISK INCREASES WITH
• Women over 60, due to fragile blood vessels and thin vaginal or uterine lining.
• Obesity.
• Hormone therapy. Women are likely to have some bleeding the first year.

HOW TO PREVENT—No specific preventive measures.

WHAT TO EXPECT

DIAGNOSTIC MEASURES
• Your own observation of symptoms.
• Your health care provider will usually do a physical exam, including a pelvic exam. (Be sure to tell your health care provider about nonprescribed substances that you take, such as soy protein.) Unexplained postmenopausal bleeding requires further medical testing. Tests start with blood studies and a Pap smear.

Additional tests may include:
- Biopsy of a small amount of tissue removed from the uterine lining. This is done with a thin suction device.
- Ultrasound of the pelvic area.
- Sonohystogram, an ultrasound with a saline (salt-water solution) injected into the uterus.
- A hysteroscopy. A telescopic instrument with a special light is used to look inside the uterus.
- A dilatation and curettage, referred to as D & C (dilatation of the cervix and a scraping out of the uterus with a curette). It may be both diagnostic and a treatment to relieve the bleeding.

APPROPRIATE HEALTH CARE
• Specific therapy, usually drugs or surgery, is dependent on the cause. Sometimes, even after testing, no clear-cut reason for the bleeding is found.
• Surgery (hysterectomy) to remove the uterus may be needed.

POSSIBLE COMPLICATIONS—Depends on the cause. If cancer is the cause, the outcome will depend on the type of cancer and the stage at which it is diagnosed. Many of these cancers are caught early, when treatment is more effective.

PROBABLE OUTCOME—The outcome will depend on the cause of the bleeding. In the majority of cases, the cause is not cancer. Benign conditions can usually be treated and bleeding symptoms should clear up.

HOW TO TREAT

GENERAL MEASURES—Follow medical advice about home care after any treatment.

MEDICATION
• If hormone drugs are currently being taken, the dose may need to be adjusted. In other cases, hormones may be prescribed.
• Drugs may be prescribed to treat any underlying disorder diagnosed.

ACTIVITY
• No limits unless advised by your health care provider.
• Sexual relations may be resumed as soon as desired after diagnosis and treatment.

DIET—No special diet.

CALL YOUR DOCTOR IF

You or a family member has unexplained bleeding after menopause or bleeding persists, despite treatment.

ILLNESS & DISORDERS

POSTPARTUM MOOD DISTURBANCES
(Postpartum Blues, Depression, & Psychosis)

 GENERAL INFORMATION

DEFINITION—Mood disturbances following the birth of a baby affect nearly half of all new mothers. The symptoms are most common 3 to 10 days following delivery, but can occur anytime in the first 6 months. Types include:
* Postpartum blues (baby blues), which involves mild symptoms that last a short time.
* Postpartum depression symptoms are sometimes described as baby blues that deepen and last longer.
* Postpartum psychosis is a rare and severe depression.

BODY PARTS INVOLVED—Brain.

SEX OR AGE MOST AFFECTED—Females of childbearing age.

SIGNS & SYMPTOMS
The symptoms vary, but can include:
* Mild sadness, crying spells, and mood swings.
* Appetite loss and weight loss, or weight gain.
* Sleep problems; unable to sleep when baby is sleeping, or waking up and having trouble returning to sleep.
* Loss of energy; fatigue.
* Irritability; anxiety, or feelings of tension or anger.
* Slow speech and thought, unable to make decisions.
* Headaches and other physical discomfort.
* Confusion about one's ability to improve life.
* Feelings of hopelessness, worthlessness, or gloom.
* Fears about your health and infant's health.
* Poor personal hygiene.

CAUSES—Exact cause is unknown. It may involve physical, emotional, social, genetic, and hormone factors.

RISK INCREASES WITH
* Personal or family history of depression.
* Postpartum depression after prior pregnancy.
* Physical and emotional stress, lack of sleep; poor nutrition, or problems with baby's health.
* Pregnancy problems (e.g., preterm birth).
* Lack of support from partner, family, or friends.

HOW TO PREVENT
* There is no sure way to prevent depression. Screening test may help identify women at risk.
* Get medical advice on ways to guard against a recurrence if you had depression before.

 WHAT TO EXPECT

DIAGNOSTIC MEASURES
* Your own or other's observation of symptoms.
* Your health care provider will ask questions about your symptoms and history to help with diagnosis.
* A depression screening test may be given. Blood tests may be done to check for any physical problems.

APPROPRIATE HEALTH CARE—Treatment may involve counseling (psychotherapy) and/or group therapy, drugs, self-help, and education. Individual treatment depends on the type and degree of the symptoms. Rarely, hospital care is needed.

POSSIBLE COMPLICATIONS
* Lack of bonding between mother and baby.
* Children of depressed mothers are more at risk for developmental problems.
* Relationship problems with partner.
* Depression may become chronic or recurrent.
* Postpartum psychosis. A mother may harm herself or her baby.

PROBABLE OUTCOME
* It's common for mothers to have some degree of baby blues. It normally resolves on its own within about 10 days.
* For most women, postpartum depression is temporary and treatable. It may last a few weeks to months.

 HOW TO TREAT

GENERAL MEASURES
* Don't feel guilty if you have mixed feelings about motherhood. Adjustment and bonding take time. Find time for you and your partner to be alone. Go on outings, such as walks or short visits with friends or family so you don't feel alone. Get help from family or friends who will shop for you or care for the baby while you rest.
* Share your feelings with your partner, friends, other mothers, or a support group.
* To learn more: Depression After Delivery; (800) 944-4773; website: www.depressionafterdelivery.com.

MEDICATION—Antidepressant drugs may be prescribed. These are effective when used for 3 to 4 weeks. Breast-feeding mothers should get medical advice before using drugs.

ACTIVITY—Try to get some exercise each day.

DIET—Eat a well-balanced diet. Avoid alcohol.

 CALL YOUR DOCTOR IF

* You or a family member has symptoms of a postpartum mood disturbance.
* You have thoughts of hurting yourself or the baby, hear voices, see things, or feel unable to cope, or if a new mother talks of these feelings. Seek help promptly!

POST-TRAUMATIC STRESS DISORDER (PTSD)

GENERAL INFORMATION

DEFINITION—A type of anxiety sometimes seen in people who have experienced an event that is extremely distressing. Such events (e.g., natural disasters, murder, rape, war, torture, imprisonment, accidents) produce psychological (emotional) stress in everyone. PTSD involves a persistent re-experiencing of the trauma and other symptoms. The symptoms may begin right after the event or develop months or years later.

BODY PARTS INVOLVED—Nervous.

SEX OR AGE MOST AFFECTED—Both sexes; all ages (more common in women than men).

SIGNS & SYMPTOMS
- Recurrent, intrusive, and distressing memories of the event. A sense of reliving the event (flashbacks).
- Recurrent dreams or nightmares relating to the event.
- Chronic anxiety.
- Insomnia.
- Inability to concentrate; memory problems.
- A sense of personal isolation (feeling alone).
- Lack of interest in activities once enjoyed.
- Phobic (fearful) reactions to situations or avoiding activities that recall memory of event.
- Emotional effects (irritability, restlessness, tearfulness, explosive outbursts of behavior including violence, a numbness of feelings, or painful guilt feelings).

CAUSES—Exact cause is unknown. Exposure to an overwhelming, distressing event is a main factor. Other factors may involve a person's personality type, chemical imbalance in the brain, environmental stresses, and genetics.

RISK INCREASES WITH
Event:
- The type, severity, and duration of the event.
- Proximity of event (direct involvement or witness).
Personal:
- Emotional problems (e.g., low self-esteem).
- Lack of support from family, friends, or community.
- Childhood history of alcoholic parents, abuse, neglect, parents divorce, poverty, or violence.
- Previous experience with trauma.
- Personal or family history of mental disorders.
- Alcohol or drug abuse.

HOW TO PREVENT
- Counseling and crisis intervention right after a traumatic event may prevent the development of PTSD.
- Debriefing soon after an event. Persons involved discuss the event, their emotions and their reactions.

WHAT TO EXPECT

DIAGNOSTIC MEASURES
- Your own or other's observation of symptoms.
- Your health care provider will do a physical exam and ask questions about your symptoms and exposure to a traumatic event.
- Medical tests may be done to rule out physical disorders. Mental health tests may be done.

APPROPRIATE HEALTH CARE
- Treatment may include medical care (for injuries or substance abuse), counseling (psychotherapy), drugs, education, self-help, and support groups. Individual treatment depends on your situation (safety from harm), your symptoms, and your health status.
- Cognitive-behavioral therapy is often recommended. Cognitive therapy teaches how to change thoughts, behaviors or attitudes. Behavioral therapy teaches ways to reduce anxiety with deep breathing and muscle relaxation. Other therapies can be effective.

POSSIBLE COMPLICATIONS
- Marriage and family conflicts, difficulty in parenting children effectively, loss of friends, and unemployment.
- Depression, anxiety, phobias, drug or alcohol abuse, self-inflicted violence, and suicide.

PROBABLE OUTCOME—For some, the symptoms go away on their own after 6 months. Most patients can be helped with treatment. In others, the disorder may become chronic.

HOW TO TREAT

GENERAL MEASURES
- Learn relaxation techniques.
- Talking about the event may help. Talk to family, friends, clergy, or join a support group.
- To learn more: National Institute of Mental Health; 6001 Executive Blvd, Bethesda, MD 20892-9663; (800) 647-2642; website: www.nimh.nih.gov.

MEDICATION—Antidepressant, antianxiety drugs, or drugs to treat insomnia may be prescribed (for a short time).

ACTIVITY—Exercise is helpful for physical and mental well-being. 30 minutes each day is a good goal. Try to get enough sleep at night.

DIET—No special diet.

CALL YOUR DOCTOR IF

- You or a family member has symptoms of post-traumatic stress disorder.
- Symptoms don't improve or become worse.

ILLNESS & DISORDERS

POTASSIUM IMBALANCE

GENERAL INFORMATION

DEFINITION—Higher or lower than normal levels of potassium in the blood, body fluids, and body cells. Important electrolytes, including potassium, sodium, and calcium, maintain normal heart rhythm and regulate the body's water balance. They also help control muscle contractions and nerve impulses.

BODY PARTS INVOLVED—Blood, which affects all body cells and body fluids.

SEX OR AGE MOST AFFECTED—Both sexes; all ages.

SIGNS & SYMPTOMS
For above-normal levels (hyperkalemia):
• Tingling in hands and feet. Weakness and numbness.
• Extreme weakness and paralysis.
• Dangerously rapid, irregular heartbeat or heart attack.
For below-normal levels (hypokalemia):
• Mild weakness and muscle cramps, often following or during exercise.
• Discomfort in the legs while sitting.
• Confusion and disorientation.
• Extreme weakness and paralysis.
• Life-threatening rapid, irregular heartbeat.

CAUSES—Electrolytes need to be in a certain balance to maintain the health and proper functioning of the body. A high or low potassium level results in an electrolyte imbalance and can cause the heart and muscle symptoms.

RISK INCREASES WITH
Hyperkalemia:
• Kidney or renal disease.
• Severe burns, infections, or crushing muscle injuries.
• Acidosis (high acid concentration in the blood).
• Rhabdomyolysis (involves muscle and kidney injury).
• Chemotherapy (anticancer drugs).
• Adrenal gland disorders.
• Certain drugs that decrease potassium excretion.
• Rarely, strenuous exercise.
Hypokalemia:
• Use of diuretic drugs for medical or other purposes. Athletes may use diuretics to meet certain weight limits before competing (e.g., jockeys, boxers, wrestlers).
• Excessive, sweating vomiting, or diarrhea.
• Eating disorders; laxative abuse.
• Prolonged fasting or starvation.
• Alcoholism (poor diet may cause low potassium).
• Hyperaldosteronism, Cushing's syndrome, inherited kidney defects, and eating too much black licorice.

HOW TO PREVENT—If you take diuretics or have renal or kidney disease, have frequent blood studies to check potassium levels.

WHAT TO EXPECT

DIAGNOSTIC MEASURES
• Your own observation of symptoms, especially muscle weakness and heart-rhythm changes.
• Your health care provider may do a physical exam.
• Medical tests may include blood and urine studies of potassium and other electrolytes. An ECG (electrocardiogram) may be done. It measures the electrical activity of the heart.

APPROPRIATE HEALTH CARE
• Treatment usually involves drugs to correct the potassium imbalance.
• Most cases are treatable at home. Hospital care and intravenous (IV) therapy may be needed for severe cases of hypokalemia or hyperkalemia. Dialysis (a way to clean the blood) may be required if kidneys fail.

POSSIBLE COMPLICATIONS
• Treatment of hypokalemia may result in hyperkalemia and vice versa.
• Cardiac arrest and death.

PROBABLE OUTCOME—Some potassium imbalances are temporary and correct themselves. Treatment can help other imbalances.

HOW TO TREAT

GENERAL MEASURES—If you take diuretics and digitalis, your family members should learn cardiopulmonary resuscitation (CPR). Learn to count your own pulse at the wrist or neck.

MEDICATION—You may be prescribed:
• Oral or intravenous (IV) potassium supplements to raise low levels.
• Diuretics to increase urination and decrease high potassium levels.
• Intravenous (IV) fluids (electrolytes) to correct a serious imbalance.
• Drugs to treat an underlying disorder.
• Changes in your current drugs if they are causing the potassium imbalance.

ACTIVITY—Resume normal activities once symptoms improve.

DIET—You may be advised to eat more or less high-potassium foods.

CALL YOUR DOCTOR IF

You or a family member has symptoms of a potassium imbalance.

PREECLAMPSIA & ECLAMPSIA
(Pregnancy-Induced Hypertension; Toxemia)

GENERAL INFORMATION

DEFINITION—A serious problem of pregnancy. Preeclampsia (also called pregnancy-induced hypertension) typically occurs from the 20th week of pregnancy until 7 days after delivery. If seizures occur, it is considered eclampsia.

BODY PARTS INVOLVED—It involves blood pressure, kidney function, and the central nervous system.

SEX OR AGE MOST AFFECTED—Pregnant females.

SIGNS & SYMPTOMS
Mild preeclampsia:
• Significant blood pressure rise, even if still in the normal range.
• Puffiness in the face, hands, and feet that is worse in the morning.
• Excessive weight gain (more than a pound a week during the last trimester).
Preeclampsia that is more severe:
• Continued blood pressure rise.
• Continued swelling and puffiness.
• Blurred vision.
• Headache.
• Irritability.
• Abdominal pain.
Eclampsia:
• Seizures; worsening of above symptoms.
• Coma.

CAUSES—Unknown. A dysfunction of the placenta may start the process that leads to other problems.

RISK INCREASES WITH
• Diabetes before pregnancy or gestational diabetes.
• High blood pressure before pregnancy.
• Kidney, renal, or blood vessel disease.
• First pregnancy or first pregnancy with a new partner.
• Preeclampsia in a previous pregnancy.
• Family history of preeclampsia or eclampsia, heart disease, or high blood pressure.
• Obesity.
• Multiple gestation (twins, triplets, etc.).
• Mother's age over 40 or less than 20.
• African American women.

HOW TO PREVENT—None specific. A urine test may help detect women at risk. Research is ongoing. Regular prenatal care will help find abnormal blood pressure early.

WHAT TO EXPECT

DIAGNOSTIC MEASURES—Diagnostic tests may include blood pressure tests, blood studies, 24-hour urine study (to check the protein levels), and ultrasound (to assess fetal development).

APPROPRIATE HEALTH CARE
• Treatment will depend on the severity of the symptoms and the maturity of the fetus.
• Mild symptoms may be treated at home.
• Hospital care is needed if the condition worsens or for early delivery.
• Eclampsia, because of seizure activity, usually requires hospital care and rapid delivery. A cesarean section may be required.

POSSIBLE COMPLICATIONS
• Mother: Stroke, kidney failure, seizures, high blood pressure, hemorrhage, pulmonary edema, heart failure, and death.
• Baby: Premature birth, low birth weight, intrauterine growth restriction, and stillbirth.

PROBABLE OUTCOME—The cure is to deliver the baby. Complications for mother and baby can often be prevented with prompt diagnosis and treatment. The symptoms usually resolve days to weeks after delivery. If premature labor occurs, the newborn's survival chances depend on its maturity.

HOW TO TREAT

GENERAL MEASURES
• If you are at home, weigh daily and keep a record. Use a home test to check for protein in the urine (instructions will be provided).
• To learn more: Preeclampsia Foundation, 12727 NE 20th St., Suite 16, Bellevue, WA 98005; (800) 665-9341; website: www.preeclampsia.org.

MEDICATION
• Antihypertensive (blood pressure) drugs may be prescribed.
• Anticonvulsants to prevent seizures. Magnesium sulfate may be prescribed or given by vein (IV) if labor has started.

ACTIVITY—Rest often. This is important to control preeclampsia. Rest on your left side to help blood circulation.

DIET—No special diet (unless advised).

CALL YOUR DOCTOR IF

• You or a family member has symptoms of preeclampsia at any stage of pregnancy.
• The following occur during treatment: Severe headache or vision changes, weight gain of 3 or more pounds in 24 hours, nausea, vomiting, diarrhea, cramping abdominal pains, excessive irritability, or other symptoms cause concern.

PREMATURE EJACULATION

GENERAL INFORMATION

DEFINITION—Male orgasm and ejaculation prior to the wishes of both sexual partners. There is no precise duration (or time) for sexual relations and reaching a climax. There are many variables that affect individual couples. Premature ejaculation (PE) is a common problem. It is called primary if a male has always had the problem. It is called secondary if a male was previously able to have ejaculatory control and is now not able.

BODY PARTS INVOLVED—Brain and central nervous system; reproductive system.

SEX OR AGE MOST AFFECTED—Male adolescents and adults.

SIGNS & SYMPTOMS
• Repeated episodes of premature ejaculation.
• Feelings of self-doubt, inadequacy, and guilt.

CAUSES—The exact cause is unknown. It may involve psychological (mental or emotional) factors (most likely) or physical factors (less likely).

RISK INCREASES WITH
• Poor relationship with sexual partner or poor communication (not able to talk things over).
• Fear of pregnancy of sexual partner.
• Fear of contracting a sexually transmitted disease.
• Anxiety about sexual performance.
• Cultural or religious conflicts.
• Belief that sex is sinful or dirty.
• May be due to underlying physical disorder (such as prostatitis).

HOW TO PREVENT—No specific preventive measures.

WHAT TO EXPECT

DIAGNOSTIC MEASURES
• Your own observation of signs.
• Your health care provider may do a physical exam and ask questions about your symptoms and sexual history.
• Medical test results are usually normal, as most males with this problem are healthy individuals.

APPROPRIATE HEALTH CARE
• Treatment may involve counseling for the patient and his partner, and drug therapy.
• Your health care provider may have you try the following methods. They are recommended by sex researchers and therapists Masters and Johnson. These measures often lead to ejaculatory control for 5 to 10 minutes or longer.
  - Sensate-focus exercises, in which each partner caresses the other's body without intercourse to learn relaxed, pleasurable aspects of touching.
  - Mutual physical exam of each other's bodies to acquaint both partners thoroughly with anatomy. This helps reduce shameful feelings about sex.
  - Stop-and-start technique, in which the man is stimulated through controlled intercourse or masturbation until he feels an impending ejaculation. Stimulation is stopped and then resumed in 20 to 30 seconds.
  - Squeeze technique, in which the woman squeezes her partner's penis with her thumb and forefinger when he feels an impending ejaculation. When ejaculatory feelings pass, intercourse is resumed. This is repeated as often as needed until the man can control ejaculation to the satisfaction of both partners.
• Counseling from a qualified sex therapist may be recommended if other methods are not successful.

POSSIBLE COMPLICATIONS
• Low self-esteem.
• The problem can recur after successful treatment.
• Stress with the marriage or other personal relationship.

PROBABLE OUTCOME— The couple, and not just the man, needs to work on the problem together. It is usually curable in most people within 6 months with treatment.

HOW TO TREAT

GENERAL MEASURES—Work on ways to improve communication with your partner and try to reduce your performance anxiety.

MEDICATION
• There is no specific drug to treat the problem. A class of antidepressants called selective serotonin reuptake inhibitors (SSRIs) helps some men delay sexual climax. Your health care provider may prescribe one of these drugs for you. It may be used as a single dose prior to sexual intercourse or taken on a daily basis.
• A topical anesthetic agent may be recommended. It may help to reduce penile sensitivity and delay ejaculation. An example is lidocaine. It can be applied to the penis under a condom about 30 minutes before intercourse. Follow instructions provided with the product.

ACTIVITY—No limits.

DIET—No special diet.

CALL YOUR DOCTOR IF

• You or a family member has repeated episodes of premature ejaculation.
• Problem continues despite treatment.

PREMATURE LABOR & PREMATURE BIRTH

 ## GENERAL INFORMATION

DEFINITION—Premature labor is labor that begins before the 37th week of pregnancy. Premature birth may follow premature labor.

BODY PARTS INVOLVED—Female reproductive system.

SEX OR AGE MOST AFFECTED—Pregnant females.

SIGNS & SYMPTOMS
• Uterine contractions at regular intervals that begin before the 37th week of gestation (3 weeks prior to due date) and premature opening (dilation) of the cervix.
• Passage of mucus (may be bloody).
• Feeling of pelvic pressure; low back pain; cramping.
• Flow of fluid (amniotic fluid) from the uterus (sometimes). This may occur with a gush or may be only a steady watery discharge.
• Some degree of vaginal bleeding or spotting.

CAUSES—In most cases, the exact problems that cause premature labor are not well-known. Many obstetric, medical, and anatomic disorders are factors for premature labor.

RISK INCREASES WITH
• Premature rupture of the membranes ("water breaks").
• Small fetus relative to gestational age.
• Large fetus or more than one fetus.
• Illness of the mother, including preeclampsia, high blood pressure or diabetes.
• Abnormal shape or size of the uterus; weak cervix.
• Hormone imbalance.
• Vaginal infection that spreads to the uterus.
• Placenta problems, such as placenta previa.
• Excessive amniotic fluid (polyhydramnios).
• Poor nutrition (more so if weight loss occurs).
• Previous premature labor.
• Smoking, excess alcohol use, or drug abuse.
• Injury to the uterus.
• Urinary-tract infection, such as kidney infection (pyelonephritis).
• Mother-to-be is under age 18, older than 40, or seriously underweight before pregnancy.

HOW TO PREVENT
• Obtain good prenatal care during pregnancy.
• Don't smoke, abuse drugs, or drink alcohol.
• Eat a normal, well-balanced diet during pregnancy. Take prescribed prenatal vitamins.
• Don't use drugs of any kind, including nonprescription drugs, without medical advice.
• If you have a weak cervix (sometimes evident before pregnancy), get medical advice about a minor operation to strengthen the cervix.
• Rest more and decrease activity in the 3rd trimester, especially if you have bloody spotting or irregular contractions.

 ## WHAT TO EXPECT

DIAGNOSTIC MEASURES
• Your own observation of watery vaginal drainage or regular uterine contractions.
• Diagnostic tests may include amniocentesis to determine fetal maturity and to check for infection inside the uterus that could be causing the symptoms. Ultrasound is used to determine fetal weight, age, growth, and position. Blood and urine studies will check for infection.

APPROPRIATE HEALTH CARE
• Hospital care may be necessary for any underlying risk factors (such as infections or dehydration).
• Immediate cesarean delivery may be needed.
• Treatment may continue until the 36th or 37th week of pregnancy when there is less risk for the baby.

POSSIBLE COMPLICATIONS
• Premature infant.
• Uterine infection after delivery.
• Fetal death.

PROBABLE OUTCOME
• In about 50% of cases, the premature labor ceases, either on its own or with treatment.
• Labor can often be stopped with treatment to allow more time for the fetus to mature.
• In some cases delivery must proceed; sometimes by cesarean section. Outcome depends on fetal maturity.

 ## HOW TO TREAT

GENERAL MEASURES—Follow medical advice.

MEDICATION
• Drugs to stop labor may be prescribed.
• Antibiotics if an infection develops. Antibiotics may also be used to help protect the fetus from infection.
• Corticosteroid therapy may be considered to help fetal lung maturity.

ACTIVITY—Complete bed rest is needed once signs of premature labor begin. Discontinue work or other physical activities. Avoid any sexual activity.

DIET—If labor starts, drink only clear liquids until you deliver.

 ## CALL YOUR DOCTOR IF

• You or a family member has symptoms of premature labor. Call immediately. This is an emergency!
• Any symptoms develop that cause concern.

PREMENSTRUAL DYSPHORIC DISORDER (PMDD)

GENERAL INFORMATION

DEFINITION—Premenstrual dysphoric disorder (PMDD) is a severe form of premenstrual syndrome (PMS). Symptoms of PMDD interfere with daily activities, and can cause problems with personal relationships. PMDD is also called late-luteal dysphoric disorder.

BODY PARTS INVOLVED—Gastrointestinal system; central nervous system; skin; reproductive system; breasts.

SEX OR AGE MOST AFFECTED—Females who have menstrual periods.

SIGNS & SYMPTOMS
• The symptoms occur 5 to 14 days before, and go away a few days after, the start of menstruation.
• Symptoms vary for every woman, and vary at times in the same woman. Most of the symptoms involve emotional or behavioral factors. Symptoms may include:
 - Being irritable or angry.
 - Feeling depressed, sad, and hopeless.
 - Feelings of tension or anxiety.
 - Mood swings marked by periods of crying.
 - Lack of interest in daily activities and relationships.
 - Trouble paying attention and unable to concentrate.
 - Fatigue or lack of energy.
 - Food cravings or overeating.
 - Trouble sleeping.
 - Feeling out of control.
 - Physical symptoms,e.g., bloating, breast tenderness, headache, and joint or muscle pain.

CAUSES—No single cause has been found. It may be a response to hormone changes related to the menstrual cycle or low levels of serotonin, a chemical in the brain. Research into the cause is ongoing.

RISK INCREASES WITH
• Women with a personal or family history of mood disorders, such as depression or postpartum depression.
• Stressful life events.

HOW TO PREVENT—No preventive measures for the first episode.

WHAT TO EXPECT

DIAGNOSTIC MEASURES
• Your own observation of the symptoms.
• Your health care provider will do a physical exam (including a pelvic exam). Questions will be asked about your symptoms and lifestyle.

• To aid in the diagnosis, you may be asked to keep a symptom diary for two or more months. List the dates of your period and which symptoms you have (and their severity) on the days before and after your period.

APPROPRIATE HEALTH CARE
• Treatment options for PMDD include lifestyle changes, counseling, drug therapy, and use of alternative therapies. No single treatment works for every woman.
• Lifestyle changes include diet changes, stopping smoking, aerobic exercise, and steps to reduce stress.
• Counseling may help a woman find ways to cope with the PMDD symptoms.
• Biofeedback, acupuncture, and massage may help some women. Relaxation techniques may be used as treatment for stress. Phototherapy (treatment with light) may help in some cases.

POSSIBLE COMPLICATIONS—The symptoms may get worse over time and last until menopause (when menses ceases).

PROBABLE OUTCOME—Treatment can help reduce some PMDD symptoms. Treatment may be needed for at least a year. There are a variety of treatment options. It may take time to find what works best for you.

HOW TO TREAT

GENERAL MEASURES
• Join a support group. Talking about your PMDD symptoms with others can help.
• To learn more, do an Internet search or visit a library.

MEDICATION
• Antidepressant drugs may be prescribed. These help the symptoms of PMDD.
• Other drugs may be prescribed for specific symptoms such as headaches, anxiety, pain, and bloating.
• Vitamins and supplements may be recommended.

ACTIVITY—Do aerobic exercise (20 to 30 minutes) daily, or at least three times per week.

DIET
• Eat a healthy diet. Try eating frequent, small meals.
• Reduce or eliminate salt, caffeine, sugar, and alcohol.

CALL YOUR DOCTOR IF

• You or a family member has symptoms of PMDD.
• Symptoms get worse or new ones develop despite treatment.

PREMENSTRUAL SYNDROME (PMS)

 GENERAL INFORMATION

DEFINITION—Premenstrual syndrome (PMS) involves symptoms that begin 7 to 14 days prior to a menstrual period and usually stop when menstruation begins. About half of all women experience PMS at some time, some very frequently.

BODY PARTS INVOLVED—Gastrointestinal system; central nervous system; skin; reproductive system; breasts.

SEX OR AGE MOST AFFECTED—It most often affects women ages 25 to 40.

SIGNS & SYMPTOMS
- Depressed mood.
- Nervousness and irritability.
- Dizziness or fainting.
- Fatigue.
- Emotional instability; mood swings.
- Increased or decreased sex drive.
- Headaches.
- Tender, swollen breasts.
- Bloating, constipation, or diarrhea.
- Other digestive disturbances.
- Fluid retention (edema) in ankles, hands, and face.
- Increase of minor infections, such as colds.
- Acne outbreaks.
- Decreased urination.
- Many other symptoms (over 150) have been attributed to PMS.

CAUSES—Unknown, but may be due to changes in the level of hormones (especially estrogen and progesterone). These changes cause retention of sodium in the bloodstream, resulting in edema in body tissues including the brain. Increased levels of prostaglandin (a chemical) in the bloodstream may be a factor. More theories about the basis of PMS include emotional, diet, changes in brain chemicals, and other factors.

RISK INCREASES WITH
- Increased levels of emotional stress.
- Caffeine and high fluid intake may worsen symptoms.
- Smoking may also intensify or increase symptoms.
- PMS risk increases with age.
- Other disorders such as depression.

HOW TO PREVENT—No specific preventive measures. Try to avoid stressful situations at the expected time of PMS. Share your feelings and needs with a close friend or spouse.

 WHAT TO EXPECT

DIAGNOSTIC MEASURES
- Your own observation of symptoms.

- Your health care provider may do a physical exam to rule out other disorders. Diagnosis usually depends on a history of symptoms. Keep a menstrual diary. Write down your symptoms and when they occur, your physical and emotional changes, and the pain involved.

APPROPRIATE HEALTH CARE
- Treatment steps involve education about PMS, diet, exercise, lifestyle changes, and drug therapy (if needed).
- Individual or couple counseling helps some patients.

POSSIBLE COMPLICATIONS
- Severe emotional stress that disrupts a woman's life.
- Premenstrual dysphoric disorder (symptoms are more severe than with PMS).

PROBABLE OUTCOME—Treatment may be effective. Drugs can sometimes help control some symptoms. PMS stops with menopause.

 HOW TO TREAT

GENERAL MEASURES
- Reduce stress where possible. Learn relaxation techniques. Reduce activities on days you have symptoms.
- Quit smoking. Find a way to stop that works.
- Join a support group. Talking about your PMS symptoms with others can help.
- To learn more, do an Internet search or visit a library.

MEDICATION—These are used with varying success:
- Nonsteroidal anti-inflammatory drugs (NSAIDs) to decrease prostaglandin levels.
- Antidepressants or antianxiety drugs.
- Diuretics to reduce fluid retention.
- Pain drugs (acetaminophen or ibuprofen).
- Vitamin B6, vitamin E, magnesium, or calcium.
- Hormones to suppress ovarian function.
- Herbal products, e.g., evening primrose oil.
- Oral contraceptives.

ACTIVITY
- Begin a regular exercise program. It can help relieve or reduce PMS symptoms.
- Try to get enough sleep at night.

DIET—Eat a low-fat, low-salt, high complex carbohydrate diet with frequent small meals. Limit use of caffeine.

 CALL YOUR DOCTOR IF

- You or a family member has symptoms of PMS that interfere with normal activities or relationships.
- Symptoms don't improve, despite treatment.

PRIAPISM

GENERAL INFORMATION

DEFINITION—A persistent erection of the penis without sexual arousal or desire. It is a serious condition that requires medical care to prevent complications.

BODY PARTS INVOLVED—Penis.

SEX OR AGE MOST AFFECTED—Males; all ages, it can affect children.

SIGNS & SYMPTOMS—A prolonged, usually painful erection. The erection may last hours to days.

CAUSES—It may be associated with certain diseases or use of drugs. Sometimes, no cause is found. Two types occur:
* Low-flow: blood becomes trapped in the penis causing its engorgement.
* High-flow (rarer): occurs when the blood in the penis does not circulate properly. It is usually due to an injury.

RISK INCREASES WITH
* Drugs that are used to treat impotence.
* Blood disease (sickle-cell disease or thalassemia).
* Cancer (leukemia or multiple myeloma).
* Certain drugs used to treat other disorders (such as chlorpromazine, prazosin, trazodone, some corticosteroids, anticoagulants, and antihypertensives).
* Spinal tumor, injury, or anesthesia.
* Carbon monoxide poisoning,
* Black widow spider bite.
* Malaria.
* Cocaine, marijuana, ecstasy, and alcohol abuse.
* Use of anabolic steroids.
* Prolonged sexual activity.

HOW TO PREVENT—No specific preventive measures. Avoid risk factors where possible.

WHAT TO EXPECT

DIAGNOSTIC MEASURES
* Your own observation of symptoms.
* Emergency treatment is necessary because of the risk of permanent damage to the penis. Your health care provider will do a physical exam and an exam of the penis. Questions will be asked about your symptoms, activities, and drug use.
* Medical tests may include a small amount of blood taken from the penis for study. Ultrasound or angiogram (special type of x-ray) tests may be done.

APPROPRIATE HEALTH CARE
* Treatment may include drug therapy, aspiration of the blood, or surgery. Any underlying cause will also need treatment. Patients with sickle-cell disease may need a blood transfusion. Spinal anesthesia is sometimes helpful.
* As a temporary measure, ice packs may be applied to the penis and perineum to help reduce swelling. Walking up a flight of stairs may help divert blood flow.
* Aspiration involves using a needle to remove blood from the penis. This will reduce pressure and swelling.
* Surgery may be needed if other treatment measures are not effective. A shunt (passageway) may be inserted to divert the blood flow. In high-flow priapism, surgery may be done to tie off an injured artery to restore normal blood flow.

POSSIBLE COMPLICATIONS
* Impotence.
* Recurrence of priapism.
* Infection.
* Complications from surgical procedures may occur.

PROBABLE OUTCOME—With prompt, effective medical care, the outcome is generally good. Delayed treatment can lead to increased risk of erectile dysfunction.

HOW TO TREAT

GENERAL MEASURES—No measures other than medical care.

MEDICATION
* Decongestant drugs may be prescribed. They are injected into the penis or taken by mouth. They narrow the veins in the penis and cause the swelling to subside.
* If a drug you take is the cause of priapism, it may be discontinued. An alternative drug may be prescribed.

ACTIVITY—Rest until erection is relieved.

DIET—No special diet.

CALL YOUR DOCTOR IF

You or a family member has an erection that persists for no apparent reason. Do not waste time trying to get it down with cold compresses. Go immediately to an emergency room.

PRICKLY HEAT
(Miliaria Rubra)

 GENERAL INFORMATION

DEFINITION—A skin disorder caused by obstructed sweat-gland ducts.

BODY PARTS INVOLVED—Skin.

SEX OR AGE MOST AFFECTED—All ages, but most common in infants.

SIGNS & SYMPTOMS—Clusters of vesicles (small, fluid-filled skin blisters that may come and go within a matter of hours) or red rash without vesicles in areas of heavy sweating.

CAUSES—Obstruction of sweat-gland ducts for unknown reasons.

RISK INCREASES WITH
- Obesity.
- Hot, humid weather.
- Genetic factors, such as fair, sensitive skin.
- Plastic bedsheets.
- High fever.

HOW TO PREVENT—Avoid risk factors.

 WHAT TO EXPECT

DIAGNOSTIC MEASURES
- Your own observation of symptoms.
- See your health care provider if skin symptoms cause concern.

APPROPRIATE HEALTH CARE—Self-care is usually all that is needed.

POSSIBLE COMPLICATIONS—A bacterial skin infection may develop.

PROBABLE OUTCOME—Usually curable with treatment. Recurrence is common.

 HOW TO TREAT

GENERAL MEASURES
- Take frequent cool showers or tub baths.
- Apply lubricating ointment or cream to skin 6 or 7 times a day.
- Use cool-water soaks to relieve itching and hasten healing. Pat skin dry, and dust with cornstarch after and between soaks.
- Wear cotton socks and leather-soled footwear rather than shoes made of synthetic materials.
- Expose the affected skin to air as much as possible.
- Don't use binding materials, such as adhesive tape, or wear tight clothing.
- Change diapers on infants as soon as they are wet.
- Avoid sunburn once you have had prickly heat. The body's inflammatory reaction to sunburn may trigger a new outbreak of prickly heat.
- Provide a cool, dry environment.

MEDICATION
- Nonprescription steroid cream applied 2 or 3 times a day (use only upon recommendation of your health care provider).
- Oral antibiotics may be prescribed if there is a secondary bacterial infection.

ACTIVITY—Decrease activity during hot, humid weather or until skin heals.

DIET—No special diet.

 CALL YOUR DOCTOR IF

Prickly heat doesn't improve in 10 days, despite home care.

ILLNESS & DISORDERS

PROCTITIS

GENERAL INFORMATION

DEFINITION—Inflammation of the rectum and tissues around the anus. It may be acute (short term) or chronic (long term).

BODY PARTS INVOLVED—Anus; rectum.

SEX OR AGE MOST AFFECTED—Adults and adolescents and of both sexes, but more common in males around age 30.

SIGNS & SYMPTOMS
* Rectal pain.
* Constant urge to have a bowel movement, often when little or no stool is present.
* Blood or mucus discharge from the rectum.
* Cramping pain in the left lower abdomen.
* Fever.

CAUSES—The inflammation may be due to diseases, side effects of medical treatments, rectal injury, infections, allergies, and problems of the nerves in the rectum. In some cases, the cause is unknown.

RISK INCREASES WITH
* Gonorrhea.
* Syphilis (usually secondary).
* Herpes simplex virus.
* Candidiasis.
* Chlamydia.
* Papilloma virus.
* Amebiasis.
* Nonspecific sexually transmitted infection.
* Radiation therapy.
* Male-to-male sexual activity.
* Use of laxatives.
* Rectal injury, rectal medications.
* Radiation therapy.
* Endocrine disorders.
* Ulcerative colitis (early stages).
* Crohn's disease.
* Chronic constipation.
* Cancer of the rectum.
* Food allergy.
* Vascular disease.

HOW TO PREVENT
* Practice safe sex methods. Unsafe sexual activity may increase the risk of an HIV infection. Avoid anal intercourse.
* To prevent constipation, establish a regular pattern for bowel movements. Eat a high-fiber diet and drink plenty of fluids each day.
* Don't use laxatives regularly.
* Don't eat foods to which you are allergic.
* Sexually transmitted diseases, such as gonorrhea and syphilis, must be reported to the local health department to prevent their spread. Information is kept confidential.

WHAT TO EXPECT

DIAGNOSTIC MEASURES
* Your own observation of symptoms.
* Your health care provider will do a physical exam.
* Medical tests may include blood studies, stool cultures, tests for gonorrhea, syphilis, and other sexually transmitted diseases and stool cultures. Diagnostic tests such as proctoscopy or sigmoidoscopy may be done to rule out other disorders. These procedures use a telescope-like instrument to look inside the rectum, colon, and bowels.

APPROPRIATE HEALTH CARE
* Treatment will usually be with drug therapy for the underlying cause.
* Rarely, surgery may be needed.

POSSIBLE COMPLICATIONS
* Anal scarring and stricture (permanent narrowing of the anus).
* Abscess, perforation, or fistula.
* Chronic ulcerative colitis.

PROBABLE OUTCOME—The outcome of proctitis depends on successful treatment of the underlying cause. Infections can usually be cured with antibiotics. Other disorders can be relieved or controlled with treatment.

HOW TO TREAT

GENERAL MEASURES
* Keep the anal area clean with frequent bathing.
* Take sitz baths often to relieve pain. Sit in a tub of warm water for 10 to 15 minutes as often as necessary.

MEDICATION
* You may be prescribed:
  - Antibiotics for sexually transmitted infections. If the cause is a gonorrheal infection, drugs may need to be injected into a muscle.
  - Acyclovir for herpes simplex infection.
  - Steroid suppositories or rectal foam to reduce inflammation from other causes.
* You may use nonprescription topical anesthetics to relieve discomfort.

ACTIVITY—No limits.

DIET
* You may be advised to eat a high-fiber diet.
* Drink plenty of fluids each day.

CALL YOUR DOCTOR IF

* You or a family member has symptoms of proctitis, or symptoms recur after treatment.
* New, unexplained symptoms develop.

PROSTATE CANCER

GENERAL INFORMATION

DEFINITION—Growth of malignant (cancerous) cells in the prostate gland. The prostate is about the size of a walnut and is located just below the urinary bladder in men. It helps form semen. This cancer often grows very slowly and may never cause symptoms. In some cases, it grows more rapidly, such as in younger men.

BODY PARTS INVOLVED—Prostate.

SEX OR AGE MOST AFFECTED—Men over age 50.

SIGNS & SYMPTOMS
• No symptoms (usually). Most prostate cancers are discovered during a routine rectal exam.
• Difficult, frequent, weak, or painful urination.
• Pain in the low back or pelvis from spread of cancer.
• Painful ejaculation.

CAUSES—Unknown.

RISK INCREASES WITH
• Males over age 50.
• Family history of prostate cancer.
• High-fat diet.
• African American more than whites or others.

HOW TO PREVENT—No specific preventive measures. A yearly rectal exam and other testing may help detect early prostate cancer. A healthy diet may have some preventive benefit, but it has not yet been proven.

WHAT TO EXPECT

DIAGNOSTIC MEASURES
• Your own observation of symptoms, especially urinary obstruction.
• Your health care provider will do a digital rectal exam (DRE). During a DRE, a gloved, lubricated finger is inserted into the rectum to check the prostate gland for lumps.
• Blood levels of prostate-specific antigen (PSA) will be checked. PSA, a protein produced by the prostate, is higher than normal in prostate diseases.
• Ultrasound, biopsy, CT, and other tests may be done to confirm the cancer diagnosis and to see if it has spread to other places in the body (staging).

APPROPRIATE HEALTH CARE
• Treatment depends on the cancer stage, age, the health status and personal preferences of the patient.
• Treatment may include surgery, radiation, hormone therapy, chemotherapy (sometimes), and watchful waiting. It helps to discuss your options with family and friends and/or support groups. Other treatments are being studied.

• Watchful waiting. This means monitoring the disorder for a time before deciding on treatment. Some prostate cancers grow quite slowly.
• Surgery to remove the prostate gland and surrounding tissues, if the cancer has not spread. Other surgery may just remove the cancerous area and not the entire prostate. Your health care provider will explain the options, the risks and benefits.
• Cryosurgery may be recommended. It treats cancer that has not spread by freezing the cancer cells.
• Radiation or hormone treatment if the cancer has spread or for patients unable to undergo surgery.
• Tiny "seeds" may be inserted in the prostate. They deliver a dose of radiation over 3 to 6 months.
• Counseling, if sexual difficulties occur after treatment.

POSSIBLE COMPLICATIONS
• Cancer may recur after treatment.
• Urinary incontinence.
• Sexual impotence after surgery (sometimes).
• Spread to bone, bladder, and other organs (which can be fatal).

PROBABLE OUTCOME—Often curable with if treated before cancer spreads. If the cancer has spread, treatment can relieve symptoms and prolong life.

HOW TO TREAT

GENERAL MEASURES—To learn more: American Cancer Society, (800) ACS-2345; website: www.cancer.org or National Cancer Institute, (800) 4-CANCER; website: www.nci.nih.gov.

MEDICATION
• One or more types of hormones may be prescribed to slow cancer growth.
• Chemotherapy (anticancer drugs) may be prescribed if the cancer has spread.
• Drugs for pain may be prescribed.

ACTIVITY—Resume your normal activities gradually after any treatment. Follow medical advice about resuming sexual relations.

DIET—A low-fat diet may be recommended.

CALL YOUR DOCTOR IF

• You or a family member has symptoms of prostate cancer.
• During treatment, any sign of urinary-tract infection occurs, such as frequent, difficult, or painful urination, fever and chills, aching around the genitals or rectum, or backache.
• Drugs used in treatment cause side effects.

ILLNESS & DISORDERS

PROSTATIC HYPERPLASIA, BENIGN (BPH; Prostate Hypertrophy)

GENERAL INFORMATION

DEFINITION—Enlargement of the prostate gland. The prostate is about the size of a walnut and is located just below the urinary bladder in men. An enlarged prostate presses against the urethra (tube that carries urine outside) making it narrower. The bladder muscle becomes thicker and more sensitive, causing a need to urinate more often.

BODY PARTS INVOLVED—Prostate gland; bladder; urethra.

SEX OR AGE MOST AFFECTED—Men over age 50.

SIGNS & SYMPTOMS
* Increased urinary urgency and frequency, especially at night.
* Weak urinary stream.
* Stopping and starting again while urinating.
* Straining and dribbling during urination.
* Feeling that the bladder cannot be emptied completely.
* Leaking of urine and sometimes blood in the urine.

CAUSES—Exact cause unknown. It is common for the prostate to enlarge as a man ages.

RISK INCREASES WITH—Aging.

HOW TO PREVENT—No specific prevention measures are known.

WHAT TO EXPECT

DIAGNOSTIC MEASURES
* Your own observation of symptoms.
* Your health care provider will do a digital rectal exam (DRE). During a DRE, a gloved, lubricated finger is inserted into the rectum to feel the prostate gland's size and check for lumps.
* Blood levels of prostate-specific antigen (PSA) will be checked. Other medical tests may include urine flow rate study, urinalysis, urine culture, x-ray of the urinary tract, and ultrasound.
* A question and answer interview is done about your symptoms. This can help in making treatment decisions. After treatment, it provides a good idea of how much the symptoms have improved.

APPROPRIATE HEALTH CARE
* Treatment may include watchful waiting, nonsurgical treatment, surgery, or drug therapy. Emergency treatment may be needed if all urine output is blocked.
* Watchful waiting is an option. This means monitoring the symptoms for a time before deciding on treatment.

* Several types of nonsurgical procedures are available. They include balloon dilation, prostatic stents, microwave therapy, needle ablation using radiofrequency, electrovaporization, and laser therapy. Your health care provider will explain and discuss these options.
* Surgery may be recommended if there are more severe symptoms, complications occur, or there is a health risk. Several surgical options are available. The choice usually depends upon the size of the enlarged prostate. Surgery removes the enlarged part of the prostate. The rest is left intact.

POSSIBLE COMPLICATIONS
* Urinary retention.
* Urinary stones.
* Urinary-tract infections.
* Reduced kidney function.

PROBABLE OUTCOME—Symptoms may improve, worsen, or stay the same. A variety of treatments are available that can help to relieve the symptoms.

HOW TO TREAT

GENERAL MEASURES
* Urinate as soon as you feel the urge. Don't let the bladder become too full before emptying it.
* For an explanation of surgery and postoperative care, see Prostate Gland Removal in Surgery section.

MEDICATION
* Drugs called 5-alpha reductase inhibitors may be prescribed to shrink the prostate.
* Alpha-adrenergic blockers may be prescribed. They help relax the muscles in the prostate.
* Antibiotics will be prescribed if you develop a urinary-tract infection.
* Read labels on all nonprescription drugs. Avoid those that state "not recommended if you have prostatic hypertrophy." Examples are antidiarrheals and antihistamines.

ACTIVITY—No limits on activities.

DIET—No special diet. Avoid spicy foods and pepper, which irritate the urethra.

CALL YOUR DOCTOR IF

* You or a family member has symptoms of BPH.
* During treatment, any sign of urinary-tract infection occurs. This includes frequent, difficult, or painful urination, fever and chills, aching around the genitals or rectum, or backache.
* New, unexplained symptoms develop after treatment.

PROSTATITIS

GENERAL INFORMATION

DEFINITION—Inflammation of the prostate. The prostate is about the size of a walnut and is located just below the urinary bladder in men. Inflammation causes swelling of the prostate. The swelling can occur gradually or come on suddenly. Symptoms occur when the swollen prostate presses against the urethra. This is the tube that carries urine from the bladder outside. Prostatitis is a common disorder in adult males. Types include:
- Acute bacterial prostatitis.
- Chronic bacterial prostatitis.
- Chronic nonbacterial prostatitis/chronic pelvic pain syndrome.
- Asymptomatic prostatitis.

BODY PARTS INVOLVED—Prostate gland.

SEX OR AGE MOST AFFECTED—Male adolescents and adults.

SIGNS & SYMPTOMS
- Urgency to urinate. Burning or pain with urination.
- Frequent urination. Waking at night to urinate.
- Difficulty starting urination and emptying the bladder completely.
- Fever, chills, tiredness, and muscle and joint aches.
- Pain between the scrotum and anus.
- Blood in the urine (sometimes) or in the semen.
- Low back pain.
- Not enjoying sex; unable to get and keep an erection.

CAUSES
- Acute and chronic bacterial types are caused by bacteria infection. In some cases, it is sexually transmitted.
- In nonbacterial types, the causes are unclear. It is not contagious, nor infectious, and does not cause cancer.

RISK INCREASES WITH
- Urinary-tract infection or sexually transmitted disease.
- Diabetes.
- Weak immune system due to illness or drugs.
- A catheter used to remove urine after surgery.

HOW TO PREVENT—None specific. Avoid infections and sexually transmitted diseases.

WHAT TO EXPECT

DIAGNOSTIC MEASURES
- Your own observation of symptoms.
- Your health care provider will do a digital rectal exam (DRE). With DRE, a lubricated, gloved finger is inserted into the rectum to feel the prostate gland's size and check for lumps.
- Medical tests may include urinalysis and culture of secretions obtained during the DRE.

APPROPRIATE HEALTH CARE
- Treatment may include drug therapy, lifestyle changes, hospital care, counseling, and rarely, surgery.
- Counseling may help with stress or sexual dysfunction problems. Support groups may help some patients.
- Hospital care for severe symptoms.
- Rarely, surgery to drain an abscess of the prostate or to remove the prostate if other treatment fails.

POSSIBLE COMPLICATIONS
- Prostatitis recurs or may become chronic.
- Abscess (pus-filled infection).
- Bladder obstruction and urinary retention.
- Urinary-tract infection.
- Infertility.
- Blood poisoning.

PROBABLE OUTCOME—Outcome is generally good for bacterial prostatitis. Treatment may take weeks or longer and different drugs may be tried. Other types can be more difficult to treat, and the outcomes vary.

HOW TO TREAT

GENERAL MEASURES
- To relieve discomfort, sit in a tub with 6 to 8 inches of warm water for 15 minutes at least 3 times a day.
- Use an inflatable donut cushion for sitting.
- Ejaculating every 3 days or prostatic massage may help drain excess prostate fluid. Ask your health care provider about these options.

MEDICATION—You may be prescribed:
- Antibiotics for bacterial infection. In severe cases, they may be given through a vein (IV). Take the full course of antibiotics to help prevent recurrence.
- Nonsteroidal anti-inflammatory drug for pain.
- Steroids for inflammation.
- Drugs to help improve bladder or prostate function.
- Tranquilizer, if stress is a concern.
- Stool softener to avoid constipation.

ACTIVITY—Stay active. Walking is a good exercise if it doesn't cause pain. You will be advised about sexual activity limits.

DIET—Avoid alcohol, coffee, and spicy foods. These irritate the urethra. Drink plenty of fluids.

CALL YOUR DOCTOR IF

- You or a family member has symptoms of prostatitis.
- Symptoms don't improve after treatment.

PRURITUS ANI
(Anal Itching)

GENERAL INFORMATION

DEFINITION—Itching or burning around the anus and, sometimes, the genitals.

BODY PARTS INVOLVED—Anus.

SEX OR AGE MOST AFFECTED—Both sexes; all ages. It is much more common in men than in women.

SIGNS & SYMPTOMS
* Itching, often intense and worse at night.
* There may be some seepage from the anus.

CAUSES
* Unknown (often).
* Yeast infection.
* Pinworms, scabies, or lice.
* Contact dermatitis caused by soaps, contraceptive foam or jelly, perfumed toilet paper, deodorant sprays, douches, or underwear made of synthetic fabric.
* Various skin disorders, including psoriasis or seborrheic dermatitis.
* Fissures, fistulas, proctitis, prolapsing hemorrhoids, skin tags, and dysfunction of the sphincter muscle.
* Vaginal discharge or skin atrophy in women caused by low estrogen levels.
* Chronic diarrhea.
* Excessive coffee intake.

RISK INCREASES WITH
* Diabetes.
* Excessive sweating.
* Antibiotic drug use.
* Food allergy.
* Overweight.

HOW TO PREVENT—None specific. Avoid causes and risk factors where possible.

WHAT TO EXPECT

DIAGNOSTIC MEASURES
* Your own observation of symptoms.
* Your health care provider will do an exam of the affected area.
* Medical tests may include studies, such as cultures for fungi, or a microscopic exam for pinworm eggs, or scabies in skin burrows.

APPROPRIATE HEALTH CARE—Treatment will be provided for any specific infection or problem that is diagnosed and for the itching.

POSSIBLE COMPLICATIONS
* Skin damage, allowing a bacterial infection to develop.
* Skin-thickening and chronic inflammation.
* Recurrence is common.

PROBABLE OUTCOME—Symptoms can be controlled with treatment, even if the cause cannot be found. It may take weeks to months for the itching to stop.

HOW TO TREAT

GENERAL MEASURES
* Keep showers or baths brief to reduce dryness and soap irritation. Don't overclean the anal area by rubbing or using too much soap. Use plain, unscented soap, or avoid soap entirely.
* Keep the rectal area clean, dry, and cool. Clean carefully after bowel movements. Use moist wipes or moistened toilet paper. Dry toilet paper can be irritating.
* Avoid contact with substances to which you are sensitive.
* Wear loose clothing and underclothing. Wear underwear with a cotton crotch or underwear made of cotton, rather than nylon or other synthetics.
* Women may be more comfortable using tampons for menstrual periods rather than sanitary napkins.
* Wear soft mittens on your hands at night, if you are scratching while asleep.

MEDICATION
* You may try nonprescription cortisone ointment or cream. Apply 3 times a day, and rub in gently until it disappears. Discontinue use once itching stops.
* Stronger topical cortisone drugs may be prescribed.
* Drugs to treat an infection or other medical problem may be prescribed.

ACTIVITY—Avoid activities that cause excess sweating.

DIET—Avoid spicy or highly-seasoned foods and coffee. These irritate mucous membranes of the anus. Eat plenty of high-fiber foods to help avoid constipation.

CALL YOUR DOCTOR IF

* You or a family member has symptoms of pruritus ani that persist, despite self-care.
* The skin area seems infected.

PRURITUS VULVAE

GENERAL INFORMATION

DEFINITION—Pruritus vulvae is an acute or chronic itching of the skin around the vulva (the vaginal lips) and anus. It is not contagious.

BODY PARTS INVOLVED—Vulva and skin surrounding the vulva and anus.

SEX OR AGE MOST AFFECTED—Female adolescents and adults, especially after menopause.

SIGNS & SYMPTOMS
* Itching that may be severe and burning. The itching may be continuous or come and go.
* Sensitivity and irritation in the genital area.
* The skin may be dry.
* Thin, white vaginal discharge (sometimes).
* Discomfort during sexual intercourse.

CAUSES—It may be a symptom of an infection or other health problem. It may develop without any known cause.

RISK INCREASES WITH
* Skin disease, such as psoriasis or lichen planus.
* Systemic disease, such as diabetes.
* Atrophy and dryness caused by lack of estrogen.
* Skin reaction to irritants such as toilet tissue, sanitary pads, soap, douches, deodorants, powders, perfume, and fabric.
* Systemic allergies, including food allergies.
* Disorder of the vagina or rectum, such as vaginitis or hemorrhoids.
* Genital warts.
* Vulvar cancer (rare).
* Days prior to menstruation.
* Hot, humid weather.
* Obesity.
* Lack of urinary control (incontinence).

HOW TO PREVENT—No specific preventive measures. Obtain medical care for any underlying disorders to reduce risk factors.

WHAT TO EXPECT

DIAGNOSTIC MEASURES
* Your own observation of symptoms.
* Your health care provider will do an exam of the affected area and ask questions about your symptoms and activities.
* Medical tests may include study of vaginal discharge and, if needed, a biopsy of the vulva (removal of a small amount of tissue for viewing under a microscope. In some cases, the exact cause is not found.

APPROPRIATE HEALTH CARE—Treatment for the underlying cause and topical skin-care products are usually recommended.

POSSIBLE COMPLICATIONS
* Bacterial infection of the inflamed skin.
* Pruritus may be chronic (persists for long time).

PROBABLE OUTCOME—Treatment can help symptoms, but it may be long term.

HOW TO TREAT

GENERAL MEASURES
* Avoid the irritants listed among the risk factors.
* Wear cotton underpants rather than nylon or other synthetic material.
* Keep the area as dry and cool as possible. Wear loose clothing. Don't douche.
* Don't scratch the itchy area. Scratching will aggravate soreness and cause more irritation.
* Wash the genital area with water and unscented soap only once a day.
* Use a lubricant, such as K-Y Lubricating Jelly or petroleum jelly, during intercourse. Avoid intercourse if it is painful.
* After urinating or having a bowel movement, clean the genital area gently with moist cotton or antiseptic wipes. Wipe from front to back (vagina to anus).
* During menstruation, insert tampons carefully. Change sanitary napkins frequently.
* Sit in bathtub of warm (tepid, not hot) water several times a day to help relieve itching.

MEDICATION
* Drugs may be prescribed for any infection.
* Use nonprescription steroid creams or ointments. Follow instructions on the label.
* Stronger steroid creams or lotions, or hormone ointment may be prescribed.
* Hormone therapy or topical application of estrogen is sometimes recommended for postmenopausal women.
* Sedating antihistamines may be recommended to help in sleeping at night.

ACTIVITY—Avoid excess sweating.

DIET—Avoid foods that produce allergic reactions. Avoid or limit caffeine beverages. Also avoid tomatoes and peanuts.

CALL YOUR DOCTOR IF

* You or a family member has symptoms of pruritus vulvae.
* Symptoms don't improve in 2 weeks, despite treatment or if scratching leads to skin infection.

PSEUDOGOUT

GENERAL INFORMATION

DEFINITION—An inflammatory form of arthritis that usually involves the large joints of the body. It usually occurs in acute (rapid onset) attacks, but often the disease may progress without the attacks.

BODY PARTS INVOLVED—Large joints (most often, the knee, wrist, ankle).

SEX OR AGE MOST AFFECTED—Elderly; more common in men than women.

SIGNS & SYMPTOMS
* Attacks of swelling, pain, and warmth in one or more of the joints.
* Joints involved most often are the knee (50% of the time), ankle, wrist, and shoulder.
* Attacks may last for 2 or more days.
* Freedom from pain or less severe pain between attacks.
* Limited range of motion of the joints.
* Fever.

CAUSES—Pseudogout, like gout, involves deposits of calcium crystals in and around the joints. The medical term is calcium pyrophosphate dihydrate (CPPD). Why the crystals form is unknown. The joint becomes inflamed leading to problems with cartilage, tendons, ligaments, and muscles that all connect to the joint.

RISK INCREASES WITH
* Stroke, heart attack, or surgery.
* Aging.
* Metabolic diseases (e.g., hypothyroidism, hyperthyroidism, gout, and amyloidosis).
* Family history of pseudogout.
* Eating too much calcium is not a risk factor.

HOW TO PREVENT—None known.

WHAT TO EXPECT

DIAGNOSTIC MEASURES
* Your own observation of symptoms.
* Your health care provider will do a physical exam of the affected area and ask questions about your symptoms and activities.
* Medical tests may include blood studies, a microscopic exam of a sample of joint fluid, and x-rays.

APPROPRIATE HEALTH CARE
* Treatment may include drugs, physical therapy, exercise, and self-care.
* Drainage of fluid from the inflamed joint if needed.
* Rarely, joint surgery may be recommended.

POSSIBLE COMPLICATIONS
* Recurrences of the attacks.
* Permanent joint damage.
* Depression or other emotional problems may occur.

PROBABLE OUTCOME—There is no cure. Treatment can usually help relieve the symptoms.

HOW TO TREAT

GENERAL MEASURES
* Apply ice to the affected area several times a day for the first 2 to 3 days to reduce swelling and pain.
* After a few days, heat may help discomfort. Use warm, moist compresses, heating pad, or take warm baths.

MEDICATION
* Nonsteroidal anti-inflammatory drugs (NSAIDs) may be prescribed for pain and inflammation.
* Stronger pain medicine may be prescribed.
* A corticosteroid injection into the joint may help relieve symptoms.
* A colchicine injection may be prescribed to reduce inflammation.

ACTIVITY
* Rest as needed during an acute attack.
* If an affected joint cause pain when walking, use a cane, crutches, or a walker temporarily.
* Physical therapy may be prescribed to help maintain range of motion. You may be taught exercises to do at home. These will help keep joints and muscles flexible, strong, and functioning as well as possible.
* Swimming, water aerobics, or riding an exercise bike are good forms of exercise.
* Avoid heavy lifting or other tasks that put too much stress on your joints.

DIET—Avoid gaining weight. If your weight is a problem, a weight-loss diet may be recommended.

CALL YOUR DOCTOR IF

* If you or a family member has symptoms of pseudogout.
* Symptoms worsen after treatment begins.
* New or unexplained symptoms develop. Drugs used in treatment may cause side effects.

PSEUDOMEMBRANOUS ENTEROCOLITIS

GENERAL INFORMATION

DEFINITION—A rare, severe illness that involves the bowels. It affects the lining and deeper layers of the intestines. It is normally caused by an overuse of antibiotics.

BODY PARTS INVOLVED—Large and small intestines.

SEX OR AGE MOST AFFECTED—Adults, especially those over age 60.

SIGNS & SYMPTOMS
- Symptoms may be mild to severe.
- Watery diarrhea (sometimes bloody) with stomach cramps.
- Fever.
- Drop in blood pressure, sometimes to shock levels, with weak pulse and rapid heartbeat.
- Nausea and vomiting.
- Disorientation.
- Symptoms usually begin 3 to 9 days after starting antibiotic treatment. In some cases, they may appear days to weeks after treatment has stopped.

CAUSES—Most often the bacterial germ, *Clostridium difficile*. This germ is found in about 5% of healthy persons and normally causes no problems. It lives in a delicate balance in the bowels with other bacteria. When antibiotics are used for treating bacterial infections, they can upset this bacterial balance of the intestinal tract. This allows *Clostridium difficile* to grow rapidly and produce a toxin that damages the intestinal wall.

RISK INCREASES WITH
- Adults over age 60.
- Recent surgery.
- A stay in a hospital.
- Cancer treatment.
- Poor general health.
- Use of antibiotics, especially lincomycin, clindamycin, ampicillin, chloramphenicol, cephalosporins, penicillin, or sulfa drugs.

HOW TO PREVENT—No specific preventive measures. Maintaining good health can help prevent the need for treatment with antibiotics.

WHAT TO EXPECT

DIAGNOSTIC MEASURES
- Your own observation of symptoms.
- Your health care provider will do a physical exam.
- Medical tests may include blood studies, stool cultures, and x-rays. An endoscopy with biopsy may be done. This involves using a lighted, tube-like instrument to see inside the intestines. It is also used to remove a small bit of tissue for viewing under a microscope.

APPROPRIATE HEALTH CARE
- Treatment usually involves drug therapy, supportive care, hospital care if needed, and discontinuing or changing the antibiotic causing the problem.
- Mild cases can be treated at home.
- Hospital care for moderate to severe cases. Fluids given through a vein (IV) may be required to prevent dehydration.
- In rare cases, surgery may be needed due to complications of the bowels and to prevent or treat a perforation (a tear in the wall of the intestine).

POSSIBLE COMPLICATIONS
- Shock and severe dehydration.
- Peritonitis caused by perforation of the intestine.
- In people who are elderly and have a serious illness, it can sometimes be fatal.

PROBABLE OUTCOME—Symptoms will usually disappear in 1 to 2 weeks with treatment. Some may have a relapse, which can be treated successfully.

HOW TO TREAT

GENERAL MEASURES—Follow medical advice for any home care.

MEDICATION
- Vancomycin, metronidazole, or other drugs may be prescribed to treat the *Clostridium difficile* infection. They may be taken by mouth or given by injection. Sometimes, repeat treatments may be needed.
- Don't take drugs for the diarrhea unless prescribed. They can prolong the infection.
- Supplements (such as lactobacilli capsules) that help healthy bacteria grow in the intestines may be recommended.

ACTIVITY—Rest in bed until symptoms of the illness get better. Move legs often while in bed to reduce the risk of deep-vein blood clots. Resume normal activities gradually.

DIET
- Patients in the hospital may need nutrition given through a vein (IV) for a few days. Then a soft diet may be prescribed until intestinal tract is back to normal.
- Patients at home need to drink plenty of fluids.

CALL YOUR DOCTOR IF

- You or a family member has symptoms of pseudomembranous enterocolitis.
- Symptoms return after treatment.

PSITTACOSIS
(Parrot Fever; Ornithosis)

 GENERAL INFORMATION

DEFINITION—An infection transmitted by birds. The infection may be mild to severe. It is primarily a lung disease, but it may affect other organs.

BODY PARTS INVOLVED—Lungs.

SEX OR AGE MOST AFFECTED—Both sexes; all ages.

SIGNS & SYMPTOMS
- Fever and chills.
- General ill feeling.
- Appetite loss.
- Cough without sputum that progresses to a cough with occasional discolored sputum.
- Shortness of breath.

CAUSES—Infection by the germ, *Chlamydia psittaci*, a special type of bacteria. Psittacosis is found in psittacine birds (parrots, parakeets, and lovebirds), poultry, pigeons, canaries, and some sea birds. Birds may not appear to be sick. Germs enter the human body by breathing in air that contains the germ or by a bite from an infected bird. Symptoms start 5 to 14 days after exposure. Human to human transmission is rare but possible.

RISK INCREASES WITH
- Bird owners.
- Pet shop employees.
- Veterinary clinic employees.
- Poultry farmers or ranchers.
- Zoo workers.
- Working in poultry processing plants.

HOW TO PREVENT
- Avoid dust from bird feathers and cage contents.
- Don't handle any sick bird. Imported psittacine birds must be treated for 45 days with feed that contains chlortetracycline. This eliminates the germs from the birds' blood and feces.

 WHAT TO EXPECT

DIAGNOSTIC MEASURES
- Your own observation of symptoms.
- Your health care provider will usually do a physical exam and ask questions about your exposure to birds.
- Medical tests may include blood studies or a sputum culture, and x-rays of the lungs.

APPROPRIATE HEALTH CARE
- Treatment usually involves drugs and supportive care for symptoms.
- Hospital care may be needed in severe cases. Breathing support may be required and fluids may be given through a vein (IV).
- Public health agencies will be notified about cases of psittacosis.

POSSIBLE COMPLICATIONS
- Hepatitis.
- Heart inflammation.
- Nervous system complications.
- Infection may recur.
- Kidney failure.
- Severe or fatal pneumonia (rare).

PROBABLE OUTCOME—Usually curable in 7 to 14 days with treatment.

 HOW TO TREAT

GENERAL MEASURES
- Use a heating pad or warm, moist compresses on the chest to relieve pain.
- Don't smoke.

MEDICATION
- Doxycycline, tetracycline, or other antibiotic drug will be prescribed. They may be taken by mouth or given through a vein (IV). Take the full course of drugs prescribed, even if symptoms improve in a day or two.
- For minor pain, take nonprescription drugs such as acetaminophen or ibuprofen.

ACTIVITY—Usually no limits unless hospital care is needed. Fatigue and weakness may persist for several weeks for some patients.

DIET—No special diet. Increase fluid intake to help thin lung secretions so they can be coughed up more easily.

 CALL YOUR DOCTOR IF

- You or a family member has symptoms of psittacosis.
- Symptoms get worse or do not improve despite treatment.

PSORIASIS

GENERAL INFORMATION

DEFINITION—A chronic, scaly skin disorder. There are several types. The most common is plaque (discoid) psoriasis.

BODY PARTS INVOLVED—It affects the skin of the scalp, elbows, knees, chest, back, arms, legs, toenails, fingernails, and the fold between the buttocks.

SEX OR AGE MOST AFFECTED—Begins in late childhood or young adulthood and continues throughout life.

SIGNS & SYMPTOMS
- Skin areas that are slightly raised, have red borders, and are covered with large white or silver-white scales. The areas crack and become painful.
- Itching (sometimes).
- Joint pain.

CAUSES—Unknown. It is thought to be one of a group of autoimmune disorders. In these disorders, the immune system by mistake attacks the body itself.

RISK INCREASES WITH
- Family history of psoriasis.
- Rheumatoid arthritis.
- Injury to the skin.
- Infections (viral and bacterial) elsewhere in the body.
- Smoking or alcohol use.
- Genetic factors. People with psoriasis have HLA antigens, and the incidence is highest among white people.

HOW TO PREVENT
- Cannot be prevented at present.
- After diagnosis, avoid trigger factors (such as smoking, stress, or too much sun) to help prevent a flare-up.

WHAT TO EXPECT

DIAGNOSTIC MEASURES
- Your own observation of symptoms.
- Your health care provider can diagnose the disorder with an exam of the affected skin.
- A biopsy may sometimes be done. It involves removing a small amount of skin tissue for viewing under a microscope.

APPROPRIATE HEALTH CARE
- No permanent cure exists. Steps in treatment depend on the type of psoriasis, extent of the disease, your response to it, and the effect on your lifestyle.
- Treatment steps include drugs to be used on the skin or taken by mouth, phototherapy, and self-care.

- Phototherapy may be prescribed. It involves use of sunlight or artificial light. Expose skin to moderate amounts of sunlight as often as possible. Artificial light may be used. This can be done at a medical office, or, in some cases, patients may have a unit they use at home.
- Counseling if needed for emotional problems.

POSSIBLE COMPLICATIONS
- It can cause embarrassment and self-consciousness about one's appearance.
- Drugs used cause adverse effects.
- Pustular psoriasis (skin has pus-filled blisters).
- Psoriatic arthritis (inflammation in the joints).

PROBABLE OUTCOME—Symptoms can be controlled, but not cured. There may be long periods of inactivity.

HOW TO TREAT

GENERAL MEASURES
- Maintain good skin hygiene with daily baths or showers. Avoid skin injury, including harsh scrubbing, which can trigger new outbreaks.
- Avoid skin dryness to decrease the risk of recurrences. To reduce scaling, use nonprescription, waterless cleansers and hair products that contain coal tar or cortisone. Use a moisturizer after bathing.
- Oatmeal baths may loosen scales. Use one cup of oatmeal to a tub of warm water.
- To learn more: National Psoriasis Foundation, 6600 SW 92nd Ave., Suite 300, Portland, OR 97223, (800) 723-9166; website: www.psoriasis.org.

MEDICATION—No one drug therapy works for everyone. You may be prescribed one or more of the following:
- Topical drugs including corticosteroids, forms of vitamin D-3, coal tar, anthralin, retinoids, or salicylic acid. Some of these may be combined into one product.
- Drugs to suppress the immune system (more severe cases). They may be taken by mouth or by injection.
- PUVA (combines use of a psoralen drug and exposure to ultraviolet light–wavelength A).
- Combination of tar baths with UVB (ultraviolet therapy wavelength B).
- Antihistamines to relieve itching.

ACTIVITY—No limits.

DIET—No special diet.

CALL YOUR DOCTOR IF

- You or a family member has symptoms of psoriasis.
- Symptoms do not improve with treatment.
- New, unexplained symptoms develop. Drugs used in treatment may produce side effects.

PSORIATIC ARTHRITIS

 GENERAL INFORMATION

DEFINITION—Joint inflammation that occurs along with psoriasis (a skin disorder). Psoriatic arthritis can affect joints in any part of the body. The disorder is usually mild.

BODY PARTS INVOLVED
• Joints in any part of the body, but most likely in finger joints and low-back and neck joints in the spine.
• Skin or nails that have psoriasis lesions and are close to the affected joint. Sometimes additional skin sites include the scalp, navel, underarm and groin.

SEX OR AGE MOST AFFECTED—Both sexes; usually begins between ages 30 and 35 and continues intermittently throughout life.

SIGNS & SYMPTOMS
• Pain, swelling, limited movement, tenderness, and warmth in the affected joints.
• Psoriasis. Skin areas that are slightly raised, have red borders, and are covered with large white or silver-white scales. The areas crack and become painful. (Rarely, a person may have psoriatic arthritis without obvious signs of psoriasis.)
• Tiredness and fever (sometimes).

CAUSES—Unknown. It is thought to be one of a group of autoimmune disorders. In these disorders, the immune system by mistake attacks the body itself. Genetic (family) factors may be involved. In some cases, it may be linked to an infection.

RISK INCREASES WITH
• Psoriasis.
• Family history of psoriasis.

HOW TO PREVENT—No specific preventive measures.

 WHAT TO EXPECT

DIAGNOSTIC MEASURES
• Your own observation of symptoms.
• Your health care provider will do a physical exam and ask about your symptoms.
• There is no one test that will diagnose the disorder. Medical tests may include blood studies, joint fluid studies, x-rays, CT, or MRI (see Glossary for these three tests).

APPROPRIATE HEALTH CARE
• Treatment may include drug therapy, physical therapy, exercise, and self-care. Psoriasis therapy will continue also.
• Ultrasound or diathermy (heat therapy) may be prescribed.
• Splints for the affected joints may be recommended.
• Physical therapy can help with joint range of motion, flexibility, stretching, and muscle strength.
• In some cases, surgery may be recommended for severe joint problems or for joint replacement.

POSSIBLE COMPLICATIONS
• May progress to chronic arthritis and severe crippling may occur (rare).
• Drugs used in treatment may have adverse effects.

PROBABLE OUTCOME—There is no cure for this disorder. The symptoms often go away and then return. Symptoms can be relieved or controlled with treatment.

 HOW TO TREAT

GENERAL MEASURES
• Use heat to relieve joint pain. Warm soaks, heating pads, or warm compresses may help. If heat does not help, try cold compresses.
• To learn more: National Psoriasis Foundation, 6600 SW 92nd Ave., Suite 300, Portland, OR 97223, (800) 723-9166; website: www.psoriasis.org.

MEDICATION
• For minor discomfort, you may use nonprescription drugs such as nonsteroidal anti-inflammatories (aspirin or ibuprofen).
• Prescription strength nonsteroidal anti-inflammatory drugs, cortisone injections into inflamed joints, and drugs to suppress the immune system may be prescribed to reduce joint inflammation.
• Drugs will be prescribed for psoriasis at the same time as treatment for the arthritis symptoms.

ACTIVITY—Rest during flare-ups, then resume your normal activities gradually. Exercise regularly to help maintain your strength and flexibility. Swimming is a good exercise.

DIET—No special diet.

 CALL YOUR DOCTOR IF

• You or a family member has symptoms of psoriatic arthritis.
• Symptoms do not improve with treatment.
• Drugs used in treatment produce side effects.

PTOSIS
(Blepharoptosis)

GENERAL INFORMATION

DEFINITION—Drooping of the upper eyelid, partially or completely covering the eye. It is pronounced as TOE-sis. The disorder may be acquired (most common type) or present at birth (congenital).

BODY PARTS INVOLVED—Upper eyelid; eye.

SEX OR AGE MOST AFFECTED—Both sexes; all ages (usually occurs in adults over age 30).

SIGNS & SYMPTOMS—Drooping of one or both eyelids, accompanied by poor blinking reflexes. The extent of droop may vary at different times of the day.

CAUSES
- The acquired type is usually due to the muscles that elevate the eyelid becoming weak, thin, or stretched. This is often due to aging, but may be caused by disease, injury, or other medical problem.
- The congenital type is usually due to lack of development in the eyelid muscles (levators).

RISK INCREASES WITH
- Aging.
- Family history of ptosis.
- Paralysis of nerve fibers to the eyelids.
- Myasthenia gravis.
- Muscular dystrophy.
- Diabetes.
- Stroke.
- Brain tumor.
- Horner's syndrome.
- Birth injury.
- Head or eyelid injury.
- Tumor in the upper lobe of a lung.
- Eye surgery (such as cataract).

HOW TO PREVENT—No specific preventive measures.

WHAT TO EXPECT

DIAGNOSTIC MEASURES
- Your own observation of symptoms.
- Your health care provider can diagnose the disorder by an exam of the affected eyelid.
- Medical tests may be done to determine the cause of acquired ptosis.

APPROPRIATE HEALTH CARE
- No treatment may be needed if the symptoms are mild and no cause is found.
- Specific treatment will be directed toward any underlying disease that is diagnosed.
- Surgery to tighten the muscles of the eyelid may be done to prevent interference with vision or to improve appearance.
- Special glasses with a crutch attachment to hold up the eyelid may be an option.

POSSIBLE COMPLICATIONS
- If uncorrected in a child, it can lead to amblyopia (lazy eye).
- In some uncorrected cases, there may be decreased field of vision and headaches.
- Complications may occur from surgery. Ptosis may recur after surgery or the muscle can be overtightened.

PROBABLE OUTCOME—If surgery is performed, it is usually successful in improving appearance and eyelid function. The outcome may depend on treatment of the cause.

HOW TO TREAT

GENERAL MEASURES—Follow medical advice about home care after surgery or other treatments.

MEDICATION—Drugs are usually not needed for ptosis, but it may be prescribed for the underlying disorder.

ACTIVITY—No limits (unless advised).

DIET—No special diet.

CALL YOUR DOCTOR IF

- You or a family member has symptoms of ptosis.
- Ptosis worsens or vision is affected.

PUERPERAL INFECTION
(Puerperal Fever; Postpartum Infection)

 GENERAL INFORMATION

DEFINITION—Bacterial infection following delivery of a baby. Infection most often occurs in the uterus and causes inflammation (endometritis).

BODY PARTS INVOLVED—Any or all: vagina; vulva; perineum (area between the vagina and rectum); cervix, uterus; peritoneum (membrane that covers abdominal organs).

SEX OR AGE MOST AFFECTED—Females of childbearing age.

SIGNS & SYMPTOMS
• Fever and chills for two or more days after the first postpartum day (first day after delivery).
• Headache and muscle aches.
• Appetite loss.
• Vaginal discharge with a foul odor.
• Stomach (abdominal) pain.
• General ill feeling.

CAUSES—Infection by bacteria normally found in a healthy vagina.

RISK INCREASES WITH
• Cesarean delivery.
• Genital or urinary tract infection before delivery.
• Use of a fetal scalp electrode during labor.
• Anemia, either before pregnancy, or from loss of blood during delivery.
• Poor nutrition during pregnancy.
• Long delay between water break (rupture of the placental membranes) and delivery (more than 24 hours).
• A small part of the placenta left in the uterus.
• Extra-long labor.
• Multiple vaginal exams.
• Obesity.
• Diabetes.

HOW TO PREVENT—No specific preventive steps. To reduce risk:
• Avoid anyone with an active infection for the last 2 weeks of pregnancy.
• Notify your obstetric provider as soon your water breaks. Don't have sexual intercourse after this occurs.
• Wash the genital area often during the first week after delivery.

 WHAT TO EXPECT

DIAGNOSTIC MEASURES
• Your health care provider will do a physical exam including a pelvic exam.
• Medical tests may include blood and urine studies and studies of the vaginal discharge. Other tests may be done if drug treatment fails.

APPROPRIATE HEALTH CARE
• Treatment usually involves antibiotics for the infection. Hospital care may be needed for severe infection.
• Surgery may be done to remove fragments of placenta or to treat an abscess or blood clot. An infected episiotomy (incision made during delivery) may need to be opened and drained.

POSSIBLE COMPLICATIONS
• Deep-vein blood clot in the pelvis.
• Pelvic abscess.
• Shock.
• Scarring
• Infertility.
• Blood poisoning (although rare, could be fatal).

PROBABLE OUTCOME—Usually curable in 7 to 10 days with treatment.

 HOW TO TREAT

GENERAL MEASURES
• To relieve pain, place a heating pad or hot-water bottle on the abdomen or back. Take frequent, warm baths to relax muscles and help relieve pain.
• Use sanitary pads, rather than tampons, for the vaginal discharge.
• If you breast-feed, ask your health care provider about continuing to do so during treatment.

MEDICATION
• One or more antibiotics for infection will be prescribed. They may be taken by mouth or given through a vein (IV).
• Drugs to reduce fever and relieve pain may be prescribed.
• Anticoagulants may be prescribed to prevent blood-clots from forming.

ACTIVITY
• Rest in bed, except to use the bathroom, until fever and other signs of infection clear up. You will probably be more comfortable if you lie on your left side.
• Abstain from sexual relations until signs of infection have been gone for 7 days.

DIET—Drink lots of fluids to prevent dehydration.

 CALL YOUR DOCTOR IF

• You or a family member has symptoms of a puerperal infection, even several hours after delivery.
• Symptoms of infection recur after treatment.

PULMONARY EDEMA

GENERAL INFORMATION

DEFINITION—A condition of excess fluid (edema) in the lungs.

BODY PARTS INVOLVED—Lungs and heart.

SEX OR AGE MOST AFFECTED—Both sexes; it more often affects middle-aged and elderly adults.

SIGNS & SYMPTOMS
• Sometimes, the symptoms begin suddenly in the middle of the night and worsen rapidly.
• Extreme shortness of breath, sometimes with wheezing.
• Rapid breathing.
• Restlessness and anxiety.
• Paleness and sweating.
• Bluish nails and lips.
• Weakness and fatigue.
• Swollen feet and ankles.
• Cough. This may be unproductive at first, but later it can produce frothy, blood-stained sputum.
• Fever (sometimes).

CAUSES—Lungs are normally air-filled. They take in oxygen and pass it on to the blood for transport to all cells in the body. When fluid builds up in the lungs, it interferes with oxygen intake. This can affect all body functions. Pulmonary edema can be caused by a number of different disorders, but heart disorders are the most likely.

RISK INCREASES WITH
• Heart disorders (such as heart failure or heart attack) can cause fluid to build up in veins in the lungs. Pressure causes the veins to leak excess fluid into the lungs.
• Pneumonia (lung infection).
• Pulmonary embolism (blood clot).
• Drug overdose (such as from heroin or narcotics).
• Shock.
• High altitude illness.
• Drowning.
• Pancreatitis (inflammation of the pancreas).
• Kidney problems, liver problems, or thyroid disease.
• Inhaled toxins.

HOW TO PREVENT—Get treatment for any illness or disease that could be a risk factor for pulmonary edema.

WHAT TO EXPECT

DIAGNOSTIC MEASURES
• Your own observation of symptoms.
• Your health care provider will do a physical exam and ask questions about your symptoms.

• Medical tests may include blood studies, blood-oxygen levels, chest x-ray, pulmonary function studies, and heart function studies.

APPROPRIATE HEALTH CARE
• Treatment is designed to reduce the excess fluid, improve lung and heart function, and treat any underlying disorder.
• Hospital care is almost always needed. Emergency treatment is often required.
• Hospital treatment may include supplemental oxygen, breathing support with a ventilator (breathing machine), fluids given through a vein (IV), drugs, and special diet. Patients are sometimes more comfortable sitting with legs dangling over the side of the bed.

POSSIBLE COMPLICATIONS—Heart attack, heart rhythm problems, shock, adverse effect of drugs, or death (if treatment is delayed or unsuccessful).

PROBABLE OUTCOME—In most cases, symptoms can be controlled with treatment. The underlying disease causing pulmonary edema may require lifelong treatment.

HOW TO TREAT

GENERAL MEASURES—Self-care is not appropriate for pulmonary edema.

MEDICATION—You may be prescribed:
• Narcotics to relieve anxiety, decrease blood flow to the lung, and reduce oxygen demand of the body.
• Diuretics to help remove excess fluid from the bloodstream and the lungs.
• Drugs such as beta-blockers, ACE inhibitors, nitrates, calcium-channel blockers, digoxin, and others to reduce workload on the heart.
• Drugs to treat any underlying disorder.

ACTIVITY—Rest in bed until your symptoms get better. After treatment, resume your normal activities gradually. Walking is a good activity to help increase strength. Resume sexual relations when you have medical approval.

DIET—In the hospital, sodium and fluids are usually restricted. After recovery, a low-salt, low-fat diet and reduced fluid intake may be recommended.

CALL YOUR DOCTOR IF

You or a family member has symptoms of pulmonary edema that appear suddenly. This is an emergency! Call 911 first.

PULMONARY EMBOLISM

 GENERAL INFORMATION

DEFINITION—A blood clot in one of the arteries carrying blood to the lungs. The blood clot usually begins in a deep vein of the leg, or less often, another place in the body. The clot moves through the bloodstream, passing through the heart and into an artery in the lungs. The blockage reduces breathing ability and can destroy lung tissue. Rarely, other types of clots form that are made up of fat, air bubbles, tissue from a tumor, or bacteria.

BODY PARTS INVOLVED—Veins, especially veins in the legs; pulmonary artery and smaller artery branches that nourish the lungs; broken bone.

SEX OR AGE MOST AFFECTED—Both sexes; all ages, but most common in adults.

SIGNS & SYMPTOMS
• Sudden shortness of breath.
• Faintness or fainting.
• Pain in the chest.
• Cough (sometimes with bloody sputum).
• Rapid heartbeat.
• Low fever.
• These symptoms are often preceded by swelling and pain in the leg.

CAUSES—Deep-vein thrombosis, which can occur anytime blood pools in a vein.

RISK INCREASES WITH
• Previous embolism or deep-vein thrombosis.
• Any injury or illness that requires prolonged bed rest.
• Sitting for long periods, as on car or plane trips.
• Recent surgery.
• Heart disease, high blood pressure, or lung disorders.
• Bone fractures, such as hip fracture.
• Overweight.
• Pregnancy.
• Use of birth-control pills; risk increases with smokers.
• Cancer.
• Smoking.
• Family history of tendency to form blood clots.

HOW TO PREVENT
• Avoid prolonged bed rest during illnesses. Wear compressive stockings during recovery (in or out of bed).
• Start moving legs and walking as soon as possible after surgery.
• Don't smoke, especially if you are a woman age 35 or older who takes birth-control pills.
• When traveling, be sure to take breaks and stand and walk every 1 to 2 hours.

 WHAT TO EXPECT

DIAGNOSTIC MEASURES
• Your own observation of symptoms.
• Your health care provider will do a physical exam and ask questions about your symptoms and activities.
• Medical tests may include chest x-ray, lung scan, pulmonary angiogram (a special x-ray study of blood flow), CT, blood studies, and other tests as needed.

APPROPRIATE HEALTH CARE
• Treatment is aimed at maintaining heart, blood vessel, and lung functions as well as preventing clot recurrence.
• Hospital care is necessary. Supplemental oxygen will be provided, and drugs will be given through a vein (IV).
• Surgery may be necessary to tie off the big vein leading to the heart and lungs (vena cava) or to insert a filter to trap recurrent clots.

POSSIBLE COMPLICATIONS
• High blood pressure in the lungs (pulmonary hypertension).
• Heart damage (condition called cor pulmonale).
• Death (from a large clot blocking the artery).

PROBABLE OUTCOME—Usually curable with treatment. Embolism may recur.

 HOW TO TREAT

GENERAL MEASURES—Self-care steps (or follow any medical advice): Wear elastic or compressive stockings or leg wraps with elastic bandages. Don't sit with your legs or ankles crossed. Keep your feet higher than your hips if sitting for long time. Raise the foot of your bed.

MEDICATION
• Anticoagulant drugs will be prescribed. You may need indefinite treatment with these drugs to prevent a recurrence.
• Clot-dissolving (clot buster) drugs may be prescribed. They break down the blood clots.
• Drugs for other disorders may be prescribed.

ACTIVITY—Rest in bed until all symptoms of the clot improve. While in bed, move legs often.

DIET—No special diet.

 CALL YOUR DOCTOR IF

• You or a family member has symptoms of pulmonary embolism. This is an emergency! Call 911.
• Chest pain, coughing up blood, shortness of breath, or increased swelling and pain in the leg develops.

PURPURA, ALLERGIC
(Anaphylactoid purpura;
Henoch-Schönlein purpura)

 ## GENERAL INFORMATION

DEFINITION—An allergic disorder involving sudden bleeding into the skin or intestines.

BODY PARTS INVOLVED—It can involve the joints (usually knees, ankles, hips, wrists, and elbows); the gastrointestinal tract; kidneys; and the skin of the legs, thighs, and abdomen.

SEX OR AGE MOST AFFECTED—It usually affects children ages 2 to 11, most often boys. Adults are rarely affected.

SIGNS & SYMPTOMS
- Headache, fever, and loss of appetite may occur first.
- Itching, red skin rash that seems to be just beneath the skin surface. The rash usually consists of large hives with small bruises or blood spots in the centers. The rash is most often on the legs, thighs, and lower abdomen, but it may be scattered over the body. The rash turns a bruised, purple color. (That is why the name purpura is given to the disorder.)
- Joint pain and swelling at the knees, ankles, hips, wrists, or elbows.
- Cramping stomach (abdominal) pain and vomiting.
- Blood in urine or stools.

CAUSES—Purpura is probably an autoimmune reaction in the inflamed small blood vessels in the body. The allergic trigger is not known. Attacks often follow an upper respiratory infection or the use of some drugs.

RISK INCREASES WITH
- Recent illness such as cold or flu. Both viral and bacterial infections have preceded allergic purpura.
- Use of certain drugs. These include antibiotics such as penicillin and ampicillin, and some vaccines, such as typhoid, measles, yellow fever, and cholera.
- Bee stings, some chemical toxins, cold exposure, and food allergies have also preceded allergic purpura.

HOW TO PREVENT—No specific preventive measures. Avoid any of the risk factors where possible.

 ## WHAT TO EXPECT

DIAGNOSTIC MEASURES
- Your own observation of symptoms.
- Your health care provider will do a physical exam and ask questions about the symptoms.
- Medical tests may include blood and urine studies. X-rays or CT testing may be done to assess complications.

APPROPRIATE HEALTH CARE
- Most patients require hospital care. This is important to help watch for, and prevent, complications.
- Treatment involves discontinuing any drugs or trigger factors that could be the cause, along with supportive therapy to relieve symptoms.

POSSIBLE COMPLICATIONS
- Kidney damage. It may occur years later.
- The disorder can cause complications in almost every organ system. These include gastrointestinal, cardiovascular (heart and blood vessels), and the lungs.

PROBABLE OUTCOME—Most children recover completely. Mild cases may last a few days. Usually, recovery takes 1 to 4 weeks. In about 50% of cases, the disorder will recur.

 ## HOW TO TREAT

GENERAL MEASURES—At home, use warm soaks to relieve joint pain.

MEDICATION
- There is no specific drug to treat the disorder. Drugs to reduce inflammation (such as ibuprofen or naproxen), or to treat an infection may be prescribed.
- In some cases, corticosteroids may be prescribed.

ACTIVITY—When fever and pain are gone, the child may gradually resume normal activities as strength and well-being will allow.

DIET—Eat a normal, healthy diet.

 ## CALL YOUR DOCTOR IF

- Your child has symptoms of allergic purpura.
- The following symptoms occur after treatment:
  - Increased abdominal pain.
  - Blood in the stool or black, tarry stools.
  - New bleeding under the skin.
  - Blood in the urine.

ILLNESS & DISORDERS

PYLORIC STENOSIS, CONGENITAL
(Hypertrophic Pyloric Stenosis)

 GENERAL INFORMATION

DEFINITION—A condition of infancy in which encircling muscles at the end of the stomach enlarge and cause obstruction.

BODY PARTS INVOLVED—It affects the pylorus (a muscular tube that carries food from the stomach to the small intestine).

SEX OR AGE MOST AFFECTED—It is more common in firstborn males and usually begins between 2 and 5 weeks of age, but can occur as late as 4 months.

SIGNS & SYMPTOMS
• Recurrent vomiting after feedings that becomes increasingly forceful.
• Muscular, olive-sized mass in the upper abdomen (sometimes).
• No pain or fever. Infant seems happy, but hungry, after vomiting.
• Constipation.
• Gradual weight loss and dehydration.

CAUSES—The muscular band that encircles the pylorus thickens and eventually closes off the outlet from the stomach.

RISK INCREASES WITH—Family history of pyloric stenosis.

HOW TO PREVENT—Cannot be prevented at present.

 WHAT TO EXPECT

DIAGNOSTIC MEASURES
• Your child's health care provider will do a physical exam.
• A barium-swallow x-ray or ultrasound may be done to confirm the diagnosis.

APPROPRIATE HEALTH CARE—Treatment is with surgery to cut the thickened muscle (pyloromyotomy).

POSSIBLE COMPLICATIONS—Without treatment, weight loss, dehydration, shock, and/or death.

POSSIBLE OUTCOME—Curable with surgery. The child usually recovers quickly.

 HOW TO TREAT

GENERAL MEASURES—After surgery:
• A firm ridge will appear at the incision site. This is a healthy sign and requires no treatment.
• Wash the incision site gently several times a day.
• If the baby seems uncomfortable, apply warm compresses to the incision site.

MEDICATION—Fluids and electrolytes will be given through a vein (IV) until the baby is ready for surgery. Drugs are usually not needed after surgery.

ACTIVITY—You will be advised of any limits.

DIET—The baby may tolerate small feedings of half-strength formula while awaiting surgery. If not, formula will be given by stomach tube.

 CALL YOUR DOCTOR IF

• Your baby vomits repeatedly.
• The following occur after surgery:
- Pain, swelling, redness, bleeding, or drainage at the surgical site.
- Temperature rises to 101°F (38.3°C).

RABIES
(Hydrophobia)

 GENERAL INFORMATION

DEFINITION—A serious viral infection of the central nervous system, transmitted by the bite of infected animals. In two-thirds of patients, symptoms may appear 1 to 3 months after the bite. Sometimes they may appear in as short as 5 days or as long as 5 years.

BODY PARTS INVOLVED—Brain and central nervous system; body parts bitten by the rabid animal.

SEX OR AGE MOST AFFECTED—Both sexes; all ages.

SIGNS & SYMPTOMS
Early symptoms are:
• Restlessness and irritability.
• Fatigue.
• Slight fever.
• Cough.
• Sore throat.
• Increased saliva and tears.
2 to 10 days later:
• Violent spasms of throat muscles that make swallowing impossible.
• Hyperactivity and violent behavior.
• Confusion.
• High fever.
• Irregular heartbeat.
• Irregular breathing.

CAUSES
• A virus in the saliva of infected animals passes to humans through broken skin or a mucous membrane. The virus travels slowly from the bite area to the brain.
• Animals that are commonly infected include dogs (especially wild dogs), bats, skunks, foxes, coyotes, and raccoons. Other animals can also be infected, so consult your local health department after any animal bite.

RISK INCREASES WITH—Professions or activities that may involve exposure to wild animals (cave exploration, hunting, farm or ranch workers, forest rangers, some laboratory workers, and veterinarians).

HOW TO PREVENT
• Vaccinate your dog or cat against rabies.
• Report stray animals in the neighborhood, and teach children to avoid them.
• Have a rabies immunization if your work involves animals.
• Keep tetanus immunizations current.
• Avoid wild animals. In the United States, bats, skunks, and raccoons are the most likely to be infected, but any carnivore can carry the disease.

 WHAT TO EXPECT

DIAGNOSTIC MEASURES
• Your health care provider will examine the wound.
• Medical tests may include blood tests and fluid and electrolyte studies.
• An exam of the animal's tissue (if available) will be done. Your own observation of the animal's behavior is important. Determine if the animal was provoked. Animals that attack without reason are more likely to be infected.

APPROPRIATE HEALTH CARE
• Treatment will be determined by type of exposure (bite or nonbite), the risk of rabies in the type of animal, circumstances of the biting incident, and vaccination status of animal.
• Hospital care is needed for serious wounds. Surgery may be done to clean and repair the bite wound.

POSSIBLE COMPLICATIONS—Once symptoms begin, survival is rare.

PROBABLE OUTCOME—Rabies can be prevented with early treatment following exposure to animal bites.

 HOW TO TREAT

GENERAL MEASURES—For animal bites or scratches:
• Wash the bite area for 10 minutes with soap and water to remove all saliva.
• Cover the wound with a clean bandage.
• Immediately call your health care provider's office or emergency room for advice.
• Call your local animal-control center to catch the animal, if possible.
• Get medical care if you have been exposed to a bat (such as waking up and finding one in the room) even if you have no bite or scratch marks.
• Don't panic. The incubation period allows time for diagnosis and treatment.

MEDICATION—You may be prescribed:
• Injections of rabies-immune globulin. (Painful injections in the abdomen are no longer used.)
• Injections of human-diploid-cell-strain vaccine, if the animal is proven rabid.
• Tetanus booster if needed.

ACTIVITY—No limits.

DIET—No special diet.

 CALL YOUR DOCTOR IF

Anyone is bitten by an animal or has other exposure to an animal that may have rabies.

RADIATION SICKNESS

GENERAL INFORMATION

DEFINITION—Side effects that develop from radiation treatment for cancer or after accidental exposure to radiation. Symptoms vary widely and are often temporary, depending on the radiation dosage and area radiated.

BODY PARTS INVOLVED—Depends on the location of treatment or exposure. See Signs & Symptoms below.

SEX OR AGE MOST AFFECTED—Both sexes; all ages.

SIGNS & SYMPTOMS
Symptoms may include:
* Nausea, vomiting and diarrhea.
* Headache.
* Fatigue and shortness of breath.
* Rapid heartbeat.
* Yeast infection in the mouth.
* Dry mouth and loss of taste.
* Swallowing difficulty.
* Worsening of tooth or gum disease.
* Hair loss; dry cough.
* Heart inflammation with chest pain.
* Burning, inflammation, or scarring of the skin.
* Permanent skin darkening.
* Bleeding spots anywhere under the skin.
* Anemia; sexual impotence.

CAUSES—Radiation damage to the immune system and to healthy tissues.

RISK INCREASES WITH
* Dose and rate of radiation treatment exposure.
* Amount of body area exposed to radiation treatment.

HOW TO PREVENT
* If you work around radiation, learn and follow all safety regulations for yourself and patients.
* Avoid unnecessary radiation exposure.

WHAT TO EXPECT

DIAGNOSTIC MEASURES
* Your health care provider may do a physical exam.
* Medical tests may include blood studies of hemoglobin, platelet counts and white-blood-cell counts, x-rays of treated areas, and dosimetry (a test to detect and measure exposure to radiation).

APPROPRIATE HEALTH CARE
* Hospital care is usually needed. Treatment is aimed at controlling symptoms and preventing infections. Treatment may include drugs, fluids given through a vein (IV), blood transfusions, and surgery.
* Surgery to treat wounds or bone-marrow transplant may be needed for severe exposure.

POSSIBLE COMPLICATIONS
* Increased risk of infections due to poor immune system function.
* Sterility or birth defects may occur.
* Increased risk of cancer especially bone-marrow cancer or leukemia.
* With radiation treatment, other complications depend upon the area involved. Modern radiation equipment makes serious complications unlikely.

PROBABLE OUTCOME
* With radiation treatment, most side effects or complications disappear gradually afterward.
* With radiation accidents not severe enough to cause immediate death, side effects may not appear for years.

HOW TO TREAT

GENERAL MEASURES
* During radiation treatment, keep medical personnel informed of how you are feeling. Treatments can sometimes be adjusted or interrupted until you feel better.
* If you lose your hair, consider wearing a wig until hair growth resumes.
* Use effective birth-control measures to prevent pregnancy until it is determined that it is safe to have children.

MEDICATION—You may be prescribed:
* Antinausea drugs.
* Pain relievers.
* Blood transfusions for anemia.
* Antibiotics to treat infections.
* Antidiarrheal drugs.
* Sedatives if sleeping is a problem.

ACTIVITY—Be as active as your strength allows. Rest often.

DIET—Eat a healthy diet. You may need a liquid diet for a short time or you may want to prepare food in a blender if you have trouble swallowing. Intravenous (IV) feeding or use of a small stomach tube is also possible until you can resume normal eating.

CALL YOUR DOCTOR IF

* You or a family member is accidentally exposed to radiation.
* Feelings of illness occur during radiation treatment, especially if there are unexpected symptoms.
* Signs of infection develop, such as fever and chills, muscle aches, headache, and dizziness, during or after exposure or treatment.

RAPE TRAUMA SYNDROME

GENERAL INFORMATION

DEFINITION—The physical and emotional effects of rape. The term rape refers to forcible sexual intercourse with an unwilling partner. Rape involves varying degrees of physical and emotional trauma. In most cases, the rapist is a man and the victim is a woman.

BODY PARTS INVOLVED—Genitals; rectum; mouth; brain.

SEX OR AGE MOST AFFECTED—All ages and both sexes, but more common in females.

SIGNS & SYMPTOMS
Right after the rape:
• Physical injuries such as cuts, bruises, or other injuries, including vaginal and rectal tears.
• Fear, anger, crying, or unusual behavior such as laughter.
• No outward emotional signs (sometimes).
Later effects (may be weeks to months):
• Feelings of self-blame and guilt.
• Depression and withdrawal, even from family and friends.
• Mood swings; feelings of grief, shame, and revenge.
• Loss of appetite.
• Fear of intercourse; fear of men.
• Nightmares and sleep disorders.
• Fear of being alone.
• Anxiety.

CAUSES—Rape is extremely traumatizing. All rape victims will suffer physical and emotional effects.

RISK INCREASES WITH—Any victim of rape or attempted rape.

HOW TO PREVENT
• There is no specific prevention for rape trauma syndrome.
• The scope of rape prevention is complex. It involves individuals, society, and the government.

WHAT TO EXPECT

DIAGNOSTIC MEASURES—See Appropriate Health Care below.

APPROPRIATE HEALTH CARE
• Emergency medical care will be provided for your physical injuries. A general physical exam and pelvic exam will be done according to specific medical guidelines. A report is normally made to local law agencies.
• Ask for help from a rape crisis center (or similar agency). They provide support and help you through the medical, emotional, and legal necessities.

• Medical personnel will usually discuss:
- Risks of pregnancy, sexually transmitted diseases, HIV/AIDS, hepatitis B, and other infections.
- The measures available to prevent such risks and what follow-up tests may be required.

POSSIBLE COMPLICATIONS
• Sexually transmitted diseases.
• Emotional trauma that may last years.
• Pelvic injury.
• Pregnancy.

PROBABLE OUTCOME
• It takes most rape victims a long time to feel like they've returned to a normal existence. Some never do, and some say that they are completely changed people.
• Length of recovery time varies depending on the individual and previous life experiences. Recovery may involve two stages:
- *Acute.* This involves dealing with the immediate physical and emotional effects.
- *Reorganization.* This involves reorganizing life after the rape and learning to cope again. The personality of the individual, support system, existing life-problems, and prior sexual assaults, are all factors in recovering.

HOW TO TREAT

GENERAL MEASURES
• Get counseling help. It is important for your emotional recovery. Don't just try to put the matter out of your mind or try to "go it alone." Suppressing feelings can increase distress.
• Keeping a journal or diary about your feelings, thoughts, and reactions may be helpful. Talk over your feelings with family or a good friend.
• Prepare yourself as much as possible for legal proceedings that force you to relive the trauma.
• To learn more: National Sexual Assault Hotline (800) 656-HOPE (4673) which connects callers to a nearby rape crisis center; website: www.rainn.org.

MEDICATION—You may be prescribed:
• Antibiotic, if infection is suspected or diagnosed.
• Emergency contraception.
• Sedatives or tranquilizers to reduce anxiety.
• Drug therapy to prevent other diseases.
• Tetanus prevention.

ACTIVITY—No limits.

DIET—No special diet.

CALL YOUR DOCTOR IF

• You or someone you know has been raped.
• Emotional and/or physical problems become worse.

RAYNAUD DISEASE & PHENOMENON

GENERAL INFORMATION

DEFINITION
• Primary Raynaud (or Raynaud disease) is a disorder of the circulatory system. It is more common in females ages 20 to 40.
• Secondary Raynaud (or Raynaud phenomenon) is a circulatory system disorder. It occurs as a complication of other disease. It can affect anyone who has the underlying disease.

BODY PARTS INVOLVED—Both types involve small blood vessels in the body. They usually affect blood circulation to the fingers, but they may affect the toes, and rarely, nose, lips, nipples, knees, and ears.

SEX OR AGE MOST AFFECTED—Primary Raynaud is more common in females under 40; secondary is more common in adults over 40.

SIGNS & SYMPTOMS
• Symptoms may develop over a period of years. In secondary Raynaud, symptoms may begin suddenly.
• When exposed to cold or after emotional stress, fingers turn pale followed by a bluish tinge, then redness.
• Numbness and tingling occur along with the color changes. Pain is not common, but can occur.
• Warmth helps relieves these symptoms. Hands may become swollen and painful when warmed.

CAUSES—The exact cause is unknown. The blood vessels may constrict (narrow) due to cold or emotional stress, or there may be increased thickness to the blood.

RISK INCREASES WITH
• Smoking; it hurts circulation to hands and feet.
• Autoimmune disorder (scleroderma, lupus erythematosus, rheumatoid arthritis, or others).
• Environmental factors (use of vibrating tools or exposure to certain chemicals or toxins).
• Infections, such as hepatitis B and C.
• Cancers, such as leukemia and lymphoma.
• Metabolic disorders, such as diabetes.
• Heart, blood vessel, or nerve disorders.
• Certain drugs.

HOW TO PREVENT
• Don't smoke. Raynaud is rare among nonsmokers. Avoid secondhand smoke.
• Get medical care for disorders listed as risks.

WHAT TO EXPECT

DIAGNOSTIC MEASURES
• Your own observation of symptoms.
• Your health care provider will do a physical exam of the affected areas and ask questions about your symptoms and activities.

• Medical tests may include blood studies and a cold challenge test (putting hands in cold water). A nailfold capillary test may be done to check tiny blood vessels in the skin at the base of a fingernail.

APPROPRIATE HEALTH CARE
• Treatment involves treating any underlying cause, lifestyle changes, and drug therapy.
• Biofeedback training to teach you how to raise skin temperature may be helpful.
• Surgery to sever (cut) sympathetic nerves to the involved hands or feet (rare).

POSSIBLE COMPLICATIONS
• Fingertip or toe ulcers (open sores).
• Smooth skin on fingertips or toes.
• Gangrene and amputation (rare).

PROBABLE OUTCOME
• Most persons cope well with Raynaud disorder and live a normal life span. In about half of the patients, the disease may improve or disappear after several years.
• Secondary Raynaud may be curable if the underlying cause can be cured.

HOW TO TREAT

GENERAL MEASURES
• Stop smoking. Symptoms will improve.
• Avoid trigger factors, such as vibrating tools.
• Avoid exposure to cold if possible. Wear mittens or gloves outdoors and when handling ice or frozen foods. Wear comfortable, roomy shoes and wool socks.
• Avoid drugs which can worsen symptoms (beta-blockers, ergot drugs, and clonidine)
• Use caution in handling iced drinks or being in air-conditioned rooms.
• Avoid stressful situations. Learn relaxation techniques.
• To learn more: Raynaud's Association, 94 Mercier Ave., Hartsdale, NY 10530; (800) 280-8055; website: www.raynauds.org.

MEDICATION
• Vasodilator drugs may be prescribed. They help dilate (widen) blood vessels to improve blood circulation.
• Topical drugs to be applied to the fingertips may be prescribed (protect against skin ulcers).

ACTIVITY—Keep warm. Regular exercise is recommended. Exercise improves circulation.

DIET—No special diet.

CALL YOUR DOCTOR IF

• You or a family member has symptoms of Raynaud.
• Discomfort worsens or ulcers appear on skin.

RECTAL PROLAPSE
(Procidentia)

GENERAL INFORMATION

DEFINITION—Protrusion (bulging) of rectal tissues outside the anus. Partial prolapse is protrusion of the mucosa alone. Complete prolapse (procidentia) is protrusion of the entire thickness of the rectum.

BODY PARTS INVOLVED—Anus and rectum.

SEX OR AGE MOST AFFECTED—It can affect adults of both sexes, usually over age 60, and children ages 1 to 3. Rectal prolapse in infants can be a sign of cystic fibrosis.

SIGNS & SYMPTOMS
- A vague sense of fullness in the lower abdomen or rectal area.
- A mucus discharge sometimes tinged with blood from the rectum.
- A firm mass of tissue that can be felt at the anus after a bowel movement.
- Pain when having bowel movements.

CAUSES—Exact cause is unknown. There are certain known risk factors.

RISK INCREASES WITH
- Cystic fibrosis (children).
- Aging.
- Weak pelvic or rectal muscles.
- Weak anal sphincter.
- Previous surgery on the rectum or vagina.
- Constipation and straining to have bowel movements.
- Multiple sclerosis.
- Stroke, paralysis, or spinal tumor.
- Lower back or pelvic injury; lumbar disc disease.
- Chronic obstructive pulmonary disease.
- Pelvic floor dysfunction.
- Multiple pregnancies.
- Benign prostatic hypertrophy.
- Parasitic infections.
- Congenital (born with) rectal structure problems.

HOW TO PREVENT
- Women can practice pelvic-strengthening exercises (Kegel exercises) to prevent recurrences.
- Do not strain when having bowel movements. Avoid constipation and diarrhea.

WHAT TO EXPECT

DIAGNOSTIC MEASURES
- Your own observation of symptoms.
- Your health care provider will do an exam of the rectal area.

- Medical tests may include barium enema (special x-ray) and exam of the rectal area by colonoscopy or proctosigmoidoscopy. These two are visual exams of the anus and colon with the lighted tip of an optical instrument. Cystic fibrosis testing may be done in children.

APPROPRIATE HEALTH CARE
- Treatment varies according to underlying cause. Causes of straining need to be corrected.
- In children, prolapse is usually temporary.
- Occasionally, minor prolapse can be reversed by gently pushing the protruding tissue back into the rectum.
- For most patients, surgery is usually needed to repair the prolapse. There are several different options available. Your health care provider will explain them to you and discuss the risks and benefits. Surgery is usually done under a general anesthetic.

POSSIBLE COMPLICATIONS
- Ulceration (sores) and bleeding in tissue that protrudes.
- Bowel incontinence.
- Rectal prolapse may occur with another prolapse, such as the uterus or the bladder.
- Rectal prolapse may recur.

PROBABLE OUTCOME—Good prognosis with treatment. In children, there is usually complete recovery.

HOW TO TREAT

GENERAL MEASURES—Use sanitary napkins or absorbent pads to absorb the mucus discharge.

MEDICATION—To prevent constipation, bulk-formers or stool softeners may be prescribed.

ACTIVITY
- Recovery from surgery may take 4 to 6 weeks. Then resume normal activities gradually.
- Practice pelvic-strengthening exercises to prevent a recurrence.

DIET—Drink plenty of fluids each day and eat a diet high in fiber to help prevent constipation.

CALL YOUR DOCTOR IF

- You or a family member has symptoms of rectal prolapse.
- Rectal pain or bleeding occur.
- Fever or chills develop, indicating infection.
- Symptoms return after treatment.

REFLEX SYMPATHETIC DYSTROPHY SYNDROME

 GENERAL INFORMATION

DEFINITION—A chronic disorder that often affects the arms or legs, and rarely, other parts of the body. Symptoms vary in severity and how long they last.

BODY PARTS INVOLVED—It involves the nerves, skin, muscles, blood vessels, and bones.

SEX OR AGE MOST AFFECTED—It occurs in both sexes at any age, but is more common in ages 40 to 60. The number of cases among teens and young adults is increasing.

SIGNS & SYMPTOMS
• Pain (may be burning or aching) and swelling. These symptoms may increase over time.
• Changes in skin. It may be sweaty or cold. Color may change from pale to purple/blue or gray. Affected area may be tender, thin, and shiny.
• Hair and nail growth is increased. These symptoms may decrease with time.
• Stiff joints and muscle spasms.

CAUSES—The exact cause is unknown. It usually occurs after major or minor injuries to an arm or leg. It can occur following an illness, such as a heart attack. The pain that occurs is more severe than would be expected from the injury. The sympathetic nervous system that controls blood flow and sweat glands appears to play a role in the cause.

RISK INCREASES WITH
• Genetic factors may increase the risk.
• A tendency towards increased sympathetic activity. This includes cold hands, excessive sweating, or a history of fainting.
• Major or minor injury to an arm or leg.
• Heart attack, stroke, pancreatic cancer, herpes zoster, arthritis, or nerve compression disorder.
• Chest, neck, or shoulder injury.
• The period following surgery.
• Prolonged time in a cast or splint.

HOW TO PREVENT—No specific preventive measures.

 WHAT TO EXPECT

DIAGNOSTIC MEASURES
• Your own observation of symptoms.
• Your health care provider will do a physical exam and ask questions about your symptoms and activities. This is often enough for diagnosis.
• An anesthetic injection may be given and if relief of symptoms occurs within 30 minutes, it helps to confirm the diagnosis. Other tests may be done to check for complications.

APPROPRIATE HEALTH CARE
• There is no cure, but there is a variety of treatment options. These include drugs, counseling, physical therapy, splinting, surgery, spinal cord stimulation, implanted drug pumps, and others. Your health care provider will devise a treatment plan based on your symptoms.
• TENS (transcutaneous electrical stimulation) may be recommended. It uses brief pulses of electricity applied to nerve endings under the skin to relieve pain.
• Massage therapy often helps with symptoms.
• Biofeedback may help. It is a technique that involves learning to become more aware of your body to help you relax and to relieve painful symptoms.
• Counseling may help you learn ways to cope with the chronic pain.

POSSIBLE COMPLICATIONS
• Disabling pain. It may affect entire arm or leg.
• Muscle wasting (atrophy) and severe joint damage.
• Skin damage that cannot be reversed.
• Tightening of the muscles as they lose their tone. Hand and fingers or foot and toes may contract into a fixed position.
• Depression and anxiety due to chronic pain.

PROBABLE OUTCOME—Outcome will vary in different people. Some are helped with treatment, some cases clear up on their own, and others have ongoing pain despite treatment.

 HOW TO TREAT

GENERAL MEASURES
• Applying cold may relieve swelling and sweating. If the affected area is cool, applying heat may offer relief.
• Joining a support group may help.
• To learn more: Reflex Sympathetic Dystrophy Syndrome Association, P.O. Box 502, Milford, CT 06460; (877) 662-7737; website: www.rsds.org.

MEDICATION
• You may take nonprescription drugs for pain and inflammation such as ibuprofen.
• Steroids to reduce swelling and inflammation, drugs to widen blood vessels, injections of local anesthetic, or pain drugs may be prescribed.

ACTIVITY
• Keep up usual daily activities as best you can.
• Physical therapy may be prescribed to help keep muscles flexible, strong, and mobile.

DIET—Eat a healthy diet.

 CALL YOUR DOCTOR IF

You or a family member has symptoms of reflex sympathetic dystrophy or pain continues despite treatment.

REITER'S SYNDROME

GENERAL INFORMATION

DEFINITION—A disorder that can include inflammation of the joints (arthritis), the urinary tract (urethritis), the eye (conjunctivitis), and may also involve the skin. Two forms are:
• A sexually transmitted form (most often *Chlamydia* infection). It usually affects male adolescents and young adults (12 to 40 years).
• A form that follows a gastrointestinal bacterial infection (such as *Salmonella*, *Shigella*, *Yersinia* and *Campylobacter*). It affects men and women equally and can occur in children.

BODY PARTS INVOLVED—Joints; eyes, including white eye covering; urethra and head of the penis; skin.

SEX OR AGE MOST AFFECTED—Male adolescents and young adults (12 to 40 years).

SIGNS & SYMPTOMS
• Symptoms may or may not appear at the same time.
• Inflammation of the urethra (tube that takes urine from the bladder to the outside).
• Discharge from the penis or vagina. It often occurs 1 to 2 weeks after sexual contact.
• Pain or discomfort when urinating.
• Painful, swollen joints, especially in the knees, ankles, feet, and wrists.
• Stiffness and pain in the back and neck due to inflammation of the spine.
• Small ulcers (sores) inside the mouth, tongue, and on the penis tip.
• Red, itchy, burning and tearing of the eyes.
• Skin rash similar to psoriasis on the soles, palms, and around fingernails and toenails.
• Diarrhea may occur before other symptoms.
• General ill feeling.

CAUSES—Unknown. It appears to be a combination of genetic factors and various disease agents. A genetic marker (the HLA-B27 gene) is found in numerous patients.

RISK INCREASES WITH
• Recent gastrointestinal illness with diarrhea.
• Previous sexually transmitted infections.
• Family history of Reiter's syndrome.
• Weak immune system due to illness or drugs.
• Genetic factors.

HOW TO PREVENT—Men can use rubber (latex) condoms during sexual intercourse or abstain from sex.

WHAT TO EXPECT

DIAGNOSTIC MEASURES
• Your own observation of symptoms.
• Your health care provider will do a physical exam and ask questions about your symptoms and activities.

• Medical tests may include blood studies (to look for the genetic marker) and a culture of the urethral discharge. X-rays may be done.

APPROPRIATE HEALTH CARE
• There is no treatment to cure Reiter's. Symptoms are managed with drug therapy and physical therapy.
• Physical therapy is often recommended to help maintain range of motion of the joints.
• Usually, no treatment is needed for eye symptoms, unless they are severe or chronic.

POSSIBLE COMPLICATIONS
• Chronic or recurrent symptoms that lead to disability.
• Heart, lung, or nervous system problems (rare).
• Severe eye disease that could lead to blindness.
• Ankylosing spondylitis (arthritis of the spine).
• Deformities of the feet.

PROBABLE OUTCOME—Symptoms may range from mild to severe. Arthritis symptoms may continue up to 4 months, others may clear up sooner. Most patients recover in 2 to 16 weeks. Many patients have recurrences over the years.

HOW TO TREAT

GENERAL MEASURES
• Use a firm mattress on your bed.
• If joint impairment is chronic, get medical advice about occupational therapy.

MEDICATION
You may be prescribed:
• Nonsteroidal anti-inflammatory drugs for arthritis symptoms.
• Antibiotics, such as tetracyclines, for urethritis.
• Corticosteroid injections for painful joints.
• Corticosteroid eye drops if eye symptoms are severe.
• Topical corticosteroid drugs for skin problems.
• Drugs that suppress the immune system.
• Drugs called tumor-necrosis factor inhibitors that are used for other forms of arthritis.

ACTIVITY
• After inflammation improves, exercise the affected joints daily with stretching and strengthening routines. Follow medical instructions. Maintain good posture.
• To relieve foot pain, wear cushion pads and arch supports in your shoes.

DIET—No special diet.

CALL YOUR DOCTOR IF

• You or a family member has symptoms of Reiter's syndrome.
• Symptoms recur or new symptoms develop.

RENAL FAILURE, ACUTE
(Kidney Failure, Acute)

 GENERAL INFORMATION

DEFINITION—Sudden failure of the kidneys to function. Kidneys have several important roles. They produce certain hormones and help rid the body of waste products. When kidneys fail, the waste products build up and cause symptoms that vary in severity. This disorder usually has a short, sometimes severe course.

BODY PARTS INVOLVED—Kidneys.

SEX OR AGE MOST AFFECTED—Both sexes; all ages.

SIGNS & SYMPTOMS
Early stages:
- Reduced urine output and increased thirst.
- Fatigue and listlessness.

Later stages:
- Little or no urine output.
- Nausea, vomiting, diarrhea, and appetite loss.
- Mental changes, including irritability, stupor, or coma.
- Convulsions.
- Severe itching.
- High or low blood pressure.
- Unexplained bruising, bleeding spots under the skin or unexpected bleeding.
- The symptoms of the underlying cause (see below) will also be present.

CAUSES—Conditions in the kidney, or in other areas of the body, that cause the kidneys to stop functioning. This leads to a buildup of waste products in the blood and tissues. Underlying conditions include:
- Shock with very low blood pressure.
- Blood poisoning (septicemia).
- Congestive heart failure.
- Fluid and electrolyte imbalance.
- Blood-transfusion reaction.
- Severe accident with severe muscle injury.
- Glomerulonephritis (kidney inflammation).
- Multiple myeloma (bone cancer).
- Obstruction of the blood vessels to the kidney.
- Kidney stones (obstruct the ureters or the urethra).
- Prostate enlargement.
- Use of certain medications.
- Overdose of poisons or drugs, such as drugs of abuse.

RISK INCREASES WITH
- People with one kidney.
- Recent surgery.
- Accidents with severe injuries.
- Medical history of conditions that affect the kidney, such as diabetes or gout.

HOW TO PREVENT—No specific preventive measures. Seek medical care for causes and risk factors when possible.

 WHAT TO EXPECT

DIAGNOSTIC MEASURES
- Your health care provider will do a physical exam and ask questions about your symptoms and activities.
- Medical tests may include blood and urine studies that measure kidney function, and fluid and electrolyte balance. Ultrasound, x-ray, heart studies, and other tests may be done to diagnose any complications.

APPROPRIATE HEALTH CARE
- Emergency hospital care may be needed to provide fluid and electrolyte therapy and dialysis.
- Treatment is directed at the failure's cause.
- Surgery, if the cause can be corrected by surgery.
- Dialysis (artificial method of removing waste products from the blood) may be required until the kidneys recover their function.

POSSIBLE COMPLICATIONS—Shock, infections, uremia, seizures, coma, heart or lung problems, chronic kidney failure, or death.

PROBABLE OUTCOME—If the underlying condition can be controlled and the kidney failure can be treated promptly, complete recovery is likely. Recovery time may take days to weeks.

 HOW TO TREAT

GENERAL MEASURES
- Follow medical instructions. Compliance with your medical treatment plan is essential.
- To learn more: National Kidney Foundation, 30 E. 33rd St., New York, NY 10016; (800) 622-9010; website: www.kidney.org.

MEDICATION—Diuretics (to remove excess fluid) and drugs to treat the underlying condition may be prescribed.

ACTIVITY—Rest in bed until the condition is cured. Then resume your normal activities as soon as symptoms improve.

DIET—Food and water intake is controlled to stop fluid and electrolyte imbalance and to reduce buildup of body wastes. A diet high in carbohydrates and low in protein (main source of waste products), to reduce kidneys' work load, may be a part of the treatment.

 CALL YOUR DOCTOR IF

- You or a family member has renal failure symptoms.
- Symptoms recur after treatment.

RENAL FAILURE, CHRONIC
(Kidney Failure, Chronic)

 GENERAL INFORMATION

DEFINITION—Gradual failure (over months to years) of the kidneys to function. Kidneys have several important roles. They produce certain hormones and help rid the body of waste products. When kidneys fail, the waste products build up and cause symptoms that vary in severity.

BODY PARTS INVOLVED—Kidneys, which eventually affect all body systems.

SEX OR AGE MOST AFFECTED—Both sexes; all ages (often the elderly).

SIGNS & SYMPTOMS
• None or few symptoms until 60% to 75% of the kidney function fails. The symptoms listed may then occur.
• Listlessness, mental confusion, and drowsiness.
• Mild shortness of breath.
• Sudden weight loss
• Nausea and vomiting.
• Itching, dry skin, and easy bruising.
• Headaches.
• Frequent hiccups.
• Changes in urine flow.
• Muscle cramps, twitches, or pain. Bone or joint pain.
• Numbness or tingling in hands or feet.
• Anemia with paleness and fatigue.
• Unusual bleeding.
• High blood pressure.

CAUSES—Many conditions (in the kidney, or in other areas of the body) can cause the kidneys to slowly lose their ability to function normally.

RISK INCREASES WITH
• High blood pressure.
• Diabetes or gout.
• Disorders that cause kidney inflammation such as systemic lupus erythematosus.
• Glomerulonephritis (kidney inflammation).
• Polycystic kidneys; other hereditary disorders.
• Chronic kidney stones and infections.
• Certain drugs that are toxic to the kidneys.
• Blood-vessel diseases and various cancers.
• Previous kidney surgery.
• HIV, sickle-cell disease, and amyloidosis.
• Heroin abuse.

HOW TO PREVENT—None specific. Avoid risks where possible.

 WHAT TO EXPECT

DIAGNOSTIC MEASURES
• Your health care provider will do a physical exam and ask questions about your symptoms and activities.

• Medical tests may include blood and urine tests that measure kidney function and fluid and electrolytes. Ultrasound, x-ray, heart studies, and other tests may be done to diagnose underlying disorder or complications.

APPROPRIATE HEALTH CARE
• Treatment is aimed at slowing the progress of the disease, treating the underlying disorder, treating complications, and replacing kidney function.
• Treatment steps may include hospital care, drugs, diet changes, dialysis, and kidney transplant.
• Hospital care may be needed for severe symptoms.
• Dialysis to filter and remove waste products from the blood may be needed for advanced kidney failure. Hemodialysis uses a machine. Peritoneal dialysis uses the body's abdominal lining as a filter.
• A kidney transplant may be recommended.

POSSIBLE COMPLICATIONS
• Kidney failure can affect almost any body function.
• End stage renal disease (ESRD).

PROBABLE OUTCOME—Kidney failure is a condition that worsens gradually. Treatment can help slow the progress. Kidney dialysis or kidney transplant will eventually be needed.

 HOW TO TREAT

GENERAL MEASURES—To learn more: National Kidney & Urologic Diseases Information Clearinghouse, 3 Information Way, Bethesda, MD 20892, (800) 891-5290; website: www.kidney.niddk.nih.gov.

MEDICATION—You may be prescribed:
• Diuretics to reduce fluid build up in the body.
• Drugs to lower high blood pressure, treat anemia, treat an underlying disorder, prevent bone loss, treat symptoms (such as itchy skin), or treat complications.
• Changes in drugs you now take that may be toxic to the kidneys.

ACTIVITY—Reduce activity as needed. Get adequate sleep.

DIET—Limits on protein, salt, and fluids are usually needed. A dietitian can be helpful in providing instructions.

 CALL YOUR DOCTOR IF

• You or a family member has symptoms of chronic renal failure.
• Symptoms develop that cause you concern.

RESPIRATORY SYNCYTIAL VIRUS (RSV)

 GENERAL INFORMATION

DEFINITION—A common, viral infection of the nose, throat, and lungs that is easily spread from one person to another. It occurs mainly in the winter and spring months. Most children have had an infection by age three. Symptoms are usually mild, but can be quite serious, especially in infants. A person can get it more than once, but symptoms tend to be milder.

BODY PARTS INVOLVED—Upper and lower respiratory tracts.

SEX OR AGE MOST AFFECTED—Both sexes; all ages; most common in infants and children (it is the major cause of respiratory tract infections in this age group).

SIGNS & SYMPTOMS
Early symptoms (are like a common cold):
* Runny nose and low-grade fever.
* Feeling tired and loss of appetite.
* Cough, sometimes with wheezing.
Later symptoms:
* Infant or child refuses to eat.
* There is an increase in coughing and wheezing.
* Ear-ache.
* Much less active and sleeping more than usual.
* Serious breathing problems. Skin color may be bluish.
* Spells of apnea (breathing stops for 10 to 15 seconds).

CAUSES—The virus is spread by close contact with an infected person, such as holding hands. It is also spread by touching a surface or object, such as a toy, that an infected person has handled. The germs can live on an object, a hard surface, or on used facial tissues for several hours and on hands for 30 minutes or longer.

RISK INCREASES WITH
* Infants and young children.
* Daycare centers. Both children and teachers.
* Living, working, or being in crowded places.

HOW TO PREVENT
* Fight germs by washing your hands often.
* Take care to throw away used facial tissues.
* Cover your mouth with your elbow when coughing or sneezing.
* Avoid crowds and tobacco smokers during seasonal outbreaks.
* Avoid close contact with people with cold symptoms.
* Preventive injections may be prescribed for young children at risk of a severe RSV illness.

 WHAT TO EXPECT

DIAGNOSTIC MEASURES
* If you have concerns about the symptoms, see your health care provider. They may confirm an RSV diagnosis with a physical exam. Generally they know when there is an outbreak of RSV in the community.
* Medical tests are normally not required for healthy patients. They may be done for people who have a risk of complications.

APPROPRIATE HEALTH CARE
* Most people with mild symptoms, or have a child with the symptoms, treat it as a cold.
* Hospital care may rarely be needed for those with more severe symptoms. Oxygen, special drugs, and fluids to prevent dehydration may be required.

POSSIBLE COMPLICATIONS
* Ear infection.
* Pneumonia or bronchiolitis, which are serious lung disorders. They are more likely to occur in premature infants, or children and adults who have heart or lung problems. Most everyone recovers, but they can be life threatening.

PROBABLE OUTCOME—Most cases are mild, require no specific treatment, and last about 7 to 10 days.

 HOW TO TREAT

GENERAL MEASURES
* Treatment of mild symptoms in otherwise healthy people is the same as for a cold. Get extra rest and drink plenty of fluids until the symptoms are better. Watch for complications.
* Avoid being around cigarette smoke.

MEDICATION
* Children may be given acetaminophen. Get medical advice before using other drugs.
* Use salt (saline) nose drops for a stuffy nose.
* A child in a hospital may be given drugs for severe symptoms of the virus.
* Adults may take nonprescription drugs for pain or cold remedies.
* Antibiotics don't help a virus infection. They may be given if a bacterial infection occurs.

ACTIVITY—Reduce daily activity while ill.

DIET—No special diet. Drink plenty of fluids.

☎ **CALL YOUR DOCTOR IF**

You or your child has symptoms of respiratory syncytial virus that cause you concern.

RESTLESS LEGS SYNDROME

 GENERAL INFORMATION

DEFINITION
• Restless legs syndrome (RLS) is a disorder that causes unpleasant sensations in the legs.
• More than 80% of people with RLS also have a more common condition known as periodic limb movement disorder (PLMD). PLMD involves involuntary leg twitching or jerking movements during sleep. They typically occur every 10 to 60 seconds, sometimes throughout the night. People have no control over them.

BODY PARTS INVOLVED—Legs.

SEX OR AGE MOST AFFECTED—RLS occurs more often in women than in men. It may begin at any age, even infancy. Patients with severe symptoms are usually middle-aged or older.

SIGNS & SYMPTOMS
• The main symptom of RLS involves sensations in the legs. They are often described as burning, creeping, tugging, or like insects crawling inside the legs.
• They usually occur deep inside the leg, between the knee and ankle. More rarely, they occur in the feet, thighs, arms, and hands. The sensations usually affect both sides of the body.
• The sensations range in severity from uncomfortable, to irritating, to painful. They may come and go.
• Lying down and trying to relax causes the symptoms.
• Symptoms may be less during the day and more severe in the evening or at night. They cause difficulty in falling, and staying, asleep.
• Long car trips, sitting in a movie theater, long airplane trips, or relaxation exercises can trigger the symptoms.

CAUSES—In most cases, the cause of RLS is unknown. In others, there are certain factors or conditions that may be related to RLS, but it is unknown if they actually cause it.

RISK INCREASES WITH
• Family history of RLS.
• Low iron levels or anemia.
• Chronic diseases such as kidney failure, diabetes, Parkinson's disease, and peripheral neuropathy.
• Pregnancy.
• Certain drugs.

HOW TO PREVENT—No preventive measures.

 WHAT TO EXPECT

DIAGNOSTIC MEASURES
• Your own observation of symptoms.
• Your health care provider will do a physical exam and ask questions about your symptoms and activities.

• Medical tests may be done to identify any medical disorder that may be a factor in the symptoms.

APPROPRIATE HEALTH CARE
• Treatment will be provided for any disorder diagnosed.
• Treatment options for RLS may include lifestyle changes and drugs or supplements.

POSSIBLE COMPLICATIONS
• Left untreated, the condition can lead to exhaustion and daytime fatigue.
• Symptoms may gradually worsen with age.

PROBABLE OUTCOME
• There is no cure. Symptoms may disappear for weeks or months, but usually return. Treatment can reduce the symptoms and increase periods of restful sleep.
• With pregnancy, RLS usually stops by 4 weeks after delivery.

 HOW TO TREAT

GENERAL MEASURES
• Don't smoke. Tobacco may aggravate or trigger symptoms in some patients. Find a way to quit that works.
• A regular sleep pattern can help reduce symptoms. Try to go to bed and get up at the same times each day.
• Taking a hot bath, massaging the legs, or using a heating pad or ice pack may help relieve symptoms.
• To learn more: Restless Legs Syndrome Foundation, 819 Second Street, SW, Rochester, MN 55902-2985; (507) 287-6465 (not toll free); website: www.rls.org.

MEDICATION
• No one drug works for everyone with RLS. There are several options and your health care provider will discuss their benefits and side effects with you. If one type doesn't help, another can be tried.
• Diet supplements may be recommended.
• If a drug you take could be a cause of RLS, you may be advised to change the dose or take a different drug.

ACTIVITY—A program of regular, moderate exercise may help you sleep better. Excessive exercise may worsen symptoms.

DIET—Avoid caffeine and alcohol. They may trigger symptoms.

 CALL YOUR DOCTOR IF

• You or a family member has symptoms of restless legs syndrome.
• Symptoms continue despite treatment.

ILLNESS & DISORDERS

RETINAL DETACHMENT

GENERAL INFORMATION

DEFINITION—A separation or tear of the retina (the light-receptive tissue at the back of the eye) from the remainder of the eye. Retinal detachment is a medical emergency.

BODY PARTS INVOLVED—Eye.

SEX OR AGE MOST AFFECTED—All ages (most often ages 40 to 70) and both sexes.

SIGNS & SYMPTOMS—The following symptoms usually affect one eye, but sometimes both are affected:
* Light flashes in the field of vision.
* Floating spots in the field of vision.
* Blurred vision.
* Wavy visual images (sometimes).
* Gradual loss of vision. This may not be noticed because it is so gradual.
* No pain.

CAUSES—Retinal detachments may develop in eyes with retinas weakened by a hole or a tear. This allows fluid to seep underneath and weaken the attachment, so that the retina then becomes detached.

RISK INCREASES WITH
* Aging.
* Eye injury.
* Diabetes (can lead to diabetic retinopathy).
* Vascular disease.
* Previous retinal detachment.
* Family history of retinal detachment.
* Extreme nearsightedness (myopia).
* Complications of eye surgery.
* Tumors or inflammation.
* Glaucoma.

HOW TO PREVENT
* No specific preventive measures.
* Patients at risk need regular eye exams.
* If you have diabetes or vascular disease, obtain medical care to control the disorder.

WHAT TO EXPECT

DIAGNOSTIC MEASURES
* Your own observation of symptoms.
* Your eye doctor (ophthalmologist) diagnoses the detachment by an exam of the eye.
* An ultrasound may be done in some cases.

APPROPRIATE HEALTH CARE
* Treatment will depend on location and severity of the detachment. There are several procedures available. Sometimes, a combination of one or more procedures is used. The procedures are most often done as an outpatient, but hospital care may be needed for surgery. A local or general anesthetic may be used. Your eye doctor will explain the procedures to you.

* The retina may be reattached using special lasers or cryotherapy (using below-freezing temperatures).
* A gas bubble may be injected into the eye. It holds the retina in place while, over a period of days, the fluid that seeped in is resolved. The gas bubble is eventually absorbed by the body. This procedure may require the head to remain in a certain position for days to weeks.
* More advanced detachments may require surgery. Scleral buckle or vitrectomy are two types of surgery that may be recommended.

POSSIBLE COMPLICATIONS
* Without treatment, partial or complete blindness in the affected eye may occur.
* With delayed treatment, detachment may extend to the macula (the area of most detailed vision). This can cause permanent loss of detailed (central) vision.
* Detachment may recur. This can occur within a few months of surgery. Treatment will need to be repeated.

PROBABLE OUTCOME—Usually curable with prompt treatment. Recovery of vision may take weeks to months. If vision was good before the detachment, good vision should return. If vision was poor prior to the detachment, the return may be slow and remain poor.

HOW TO TREAT

GENERAL MEASURES—Follow medical advice about home care after any eye surgery.

MEDICATION—Drugs are usually not needed for this disorder.

ACTIVITY—You will be advised about limits on activity depending on the type of procedure used. Follow all instructions carefully.

DIET—No special diet.

CALL YOUR DOCTOR IF

* You or a family member has flashes or floating spots in your field of vision. Do not delay in getting medical help. This can be an emergency.
* Any sign of infection occurs (bleeding, redness, pain, swelling, or fever) or vision worsens after surgery.

REYE'S SYNDROME

GENERAL INFORMATION

DEFINITION—A rare disease that involves the brain, liver, and other major organs.

BODY PARTS INVOLVED—Brain; liver; kidneys; heart.

SEX OR AGE MOST AFFECTED—It can occur at any age, but most often affects children and young teenagers.

SIGNS & SYMPTOMS
- Vomiting.
- Lethargy.
- Drowsiness.
- Confusion.
- Delirium.
- Personality changes (such as irritability).
- Seizures.
- Arm or leg weakness, or unable to move them.
- Double vision.
- Speech problems.
- Coma.

CAUSES—Unknown. Reye's syndrome usually occurs following a virus infection. Studies link most cases to the use of salicylate drugs, such as aspirin, during a viral illness, especially chickenpox and influenza.

RISK INCREASES WITH
- Recent illness, such as chickenpox, influenza, or other respiratory illness.
- Use of aspirin with the viral illness.

HOW TO PREVENT—Don't give a child under the age of 18 aspirin for fever until it has been diagnosed. If the illness is diagnosed as viral, never use aspirin.

WHAT TO EXPECT

DIAGNOSTIC MEASURES
- Your own observation of symptoms.
- Your health care provider will do a physical exam.
- Medical tests may include blood studies of liver function and a study of cerebrospinal fluid (CSF). An EEG (electroencephalogram, which measures electrical activity of the brain) may be done.

APPROPRIATE HEALTH CARE
- There is no specific treatment that will cure the disorder. Hospital intensive care is needed.
- Treatment steps are aimed at preventing complications such as swelling of the brain. This may involve inserting a feeding tube, intravenous (IV) fluids, urinary catheter, mechanical breathing support, kidney dialysis, blood transfusion, cardiovascular (heart and blood vessel) monitoring, and therapies to reduce pressure on the brain.

POSSIBLE COMPLICATIONS
- Pneumonia.
- Respiratory failure.
- Heart rhythm problems or heart attack.
- Seizures.
- Permanent brain damage, coma, or death caused by pressure on the brain.

PROBABLE OUTCOME—Some patients will have a mild illness with complete recovery. Others may have more severe symptoms and develop varying degrees of brain damage. Early diagnosis is important to help prevent complications.

HOW TO TREAT

GENERAL MEASURES—To learn more: National Reye's Syndrome Foundation, 426 N. Lewis, P.O. Box 829, Bryan, OH 43506, (800) 233-7393; website: www.reyessyndrome.org.

MEDICATION—You may be prescribed:
- Steroids or other drugs to reduce pressure and swelling of the brain.
- Diuretics to help remove excess fluid from the body.
- Glucose solutions to maintain normal levels of glucose.

ACTIVITY—Bed rest is needed until the symptoms improve. Normal activities may then be resumed gradually.

DIET—Nothing by mouth initially. After recovery, no special diet required.

CALL YOUR DOCTOR IF

- Your child has symptoms of Reye's syndrome. Call at the first sign of confusion, lethargy, or other mental changes!
- After hospital care, any symptoms of Reye's syndrome recur or the child develops a fever.
- New, unexplained symptoms develop. Drugs used in treatment may produce side effects.

RH ISOIMMUNIZATION
(Erythroblastosis Fetalis)

GENERAL INFORMATION

DEFINITION—Incompatibility between an infant's blood type and that of its mother. This results in the destruction of the infant's red blood cells during pregnancy and after birth by antibodies from its mother's blood.

BODY PARTS INVOLVED—Blood of pregnant mother and fetus.

SEX OR AGE MOST AFFECTED—Newborn infants only.

SIGNS & SYMPTOMS
Signs during pregnancy:
* Decreased fetal growth.
* Decreased fetal movement.
Signs in a newborn:
* Paleness.
* Jaundice (yellow skin and eyes) that begins within 24 hours after delivery.
* Unexplained bruising or blood spots under the skin.
* Tissue swelling (edema).
* Breathing difficulty.
* Seizures.
* Lack of normal movement.
* Poor reflex response.

CAUSES—The baby of an Rh-negative (blood type) mother and an Rh-positive father may be Rh-positive. If the father is known to be Rh negative, there is no concern. During pregnancy, but more commonly during delivery, a small amount of the infant's blood is absorbed by the mother through the placenta, stimulating her body to produce antibodies against Rh-positive blood. The antibodies are produced after delivery, so the first infant is not affected. With each subsequent pregnancy, anti-Rh antibodies cross the placenta and may destroy fetal blood cells. The resulting anemia can be severe enough to cause fetal death. If the fetus survives, antibodies can cross to the baby during birth, causing jaundice and other symptoms shortly after birth.

RISK INCREASES WITH—Each pregnancy after the first one that involved different blood types.

HOW TO PREVENT—Medical care early in pregnancy is important to determine the risk of Rh incompatibility and provide treatment if needed.

WHAT TO EXPECT

DIAGNOSTIC MEASURES
* Blood tests are done to type the mother's, father's, and infant's blood, measure the mother's Rh-positive antibodies, and to detect anemia in the infant's blood.
* Amniocentesis may be done. A small amount of amniotic fluid is withdrawn from the amniotic sac surrounding the unborn child in the uterus for a diagnostic procedure. It can be used sometimes to determine the fetal blood type.
* Cordocentesis (percutaneous umbilical blood sampling [PUBS]) may be recommended. It is done to determine fetal blood type and the degree of anemia.

APPROPRIATE HEALTH CARE
* Intrauterine blood transfusions (sometimes).
* Transfusion to completely exchange the infant's blood after birth.
* Hospital care. The newborn child will remain in the hospital up to 2 weeks after an exchange transfusion.

POSSIBLE COMPLICATIONS
* Complications may develop from procedures such as amniocentesis or cordocentesis.
* Emergency delivery of the baby may be required.
* Hydrops fetalis in the newborn. This involves severe edema (swelling), heart, lung, and liver problems.

PROBABLE OUTCOME—With prompt diagnosis, monitoring, and treatment, the outcome is generally good.

HOW TO TREAT

GENERAL MEASURES—If you have an Rh-negative blood type:
* Tell any doctor or medical professional who treats you. Make sure this information is in your medical records.
* Wear a medical alert type bracelet or pendant to identify your medical problem.

MEDICATION—If you are pregnant and have Rh-negative blood type, you will be prescribed an anti-Rh gamma globulin injection (RhoGAM) at 28 weeks and again within 72 hours after delivery or at the end of a pregnancy for any reason. You may have an antibody titer drawn during pregnancy to see if you are producing anti-Rh antibodies. You do not need RhoGAM if your fetus is Rh-negative.

ACTIVITY—No limits after treatment.

DIET—No special diet.

CALL YOUR DOCTOR IF

You have further questions about RH isoimmunization.

RHEUMATIC FEVER

GENERAL INFORMATION

DEFINITION—An inflammatory disorder that affects many parts of the body, especially the joints and heart. It occurs following group A streptococcal pharyngitis (strep throat). Strep infections are contagious, but rheumatic fever is not.

BODY PARTS INVOLVED—Joints; heart and heart valves; skin and brain (sometimes).

SEX OR AGE MOST AFFECTED—Children and adults of both sexes.

SIGNS & SYMPTOMS
* Joint inflammation that causes pain, redness, swelling, and warmth. Wrists, elbows, knees, or ankles are most often affected. The symptoms may move from one joint to another.
* Fever; fatigue; paleness.
* Appetite loss; general ill feeling.
* Stomach (abdominal) pain; chest pain.
* Mild skin rash on the chest, back, and abdomen.
* Small, painless bumps just under the skin in bony areas such as the elbows or knees.
* Uncontrolled arm and leg movement (chorea).
* If the heart is involved:
  - Shortness of breath.
  - Fluid build up that causes swelling of legs and back.
  - Rapid heartbeat, especially when lying down.

CAUSES—Rheumatic fever is caused by a preceding strep infection in the throat that occurs 1 to 6 weeks prior to the start of symptoms. It is probably an autoimmune disorder in which antibodies produced by the body to attack the strep bacteria also attack tissues of the joints or heart.

RISK INCREASES WITH
* Family history of rheumatic fever.
* Children ages 5 to 15, especially those that have frequent strep throat infections.
* Crowded or unclean living conditions.
* Poor nutrition.
* Surgery, including dental surgery.

HOW TO PREVENT—Obtain prompt antibiotic treatment of any strep infection, including those of the skin. Strep infections must be treated with antibiotics.

WHAT TO EXPECT

DIAGNOSTIC MEASURES
* Your own observation of symptoms.
* Your health care provider will do a physical exam and ask questions about your symptoms and previous illnesses.

* Medical tests may include blood studies, a throat culture, and x-rays of the chest and heart. An ECG (electrocardiogram) may be done. This test measures electrical activity of the heart. No test is specific to diagnose rheumatic fever.

APPROPRIATE HEALTH CARE
* Treatment includes rest and drugs to treat the symptoms and to prevent rheumatic fever from recurring.
* Home care is recommended for many cases. Hospital care may be required for more severe cases.

POSSIBLE COMPLICATIONS
* Rheumatic heart disease. In some cases, rheumatic fever may damage the heart valves. It may take 10 to 30 years for symptoms of valve damage to appear. A damaged valve can usually be replaced with surgery.
* Chronic heart disease (may lead to disability).
* Rheumatic fever may recur following reinfection with strep.

PROBABLE OUTCOME—Rheumatic fever is treatable, but not curable. It usually resolves in 2 to 12 weeks. Some cases may take 15 weeks.

HOW TO TREAT

GENERAL MEASURES—To learn more: American Heart Association, 7272 Greenville Ave., Dallas, TX 75231; (800) 242-8721 website: www.americanheart.org.

MEDICATION—You may be prescribed:
* Antibiotics for strep bacteria. Once rheumatic fever reaches the inactive stage, low-dose antibiotics may be continued indefinitely to prevent recurrence. They may be taken by mouth or given as an injection.
* Drugs to reduce inflammation.
* Diuretics to reduce fluid build-up in the body.
* Drugs to control leg or arm movements.
* Drugs for congestive heart failure if it occurs.

ACTIVITY—Bed rest normally (or very limited activity) until studies show the disease has subsided. Then return to normal activities gradually. Your health care provider will advise when to return to school.

DIET
* A liquid or soft diet in the early stages. Then provide a normal diet.
* A low-salt diet may be recommended if patient has carditis (inflammation of the heart).

CALL YOUR DOCTOR IF

* You or a family member has symptoms of rheumatic fever.
* Symptoms occur with treatment that cause concern.

RINGWORM
(Tinea)

GENERAL INFORMATION

DEFINITION—Fungal (tinea) infection of the skin.

BODY PARTS INVOLVED—Ringworm can involve the scalp (tinea capitis), skin (tinea corporis), groin skin (tinea cruris), nails (tinea unguium), feet (tinea pedis), and skin with beard (tinea barbae).

SEX OR AGE MOST AFFECTED—It affects children and adults and is more common in males than females.

SIGNS & SYMPTOMS
* Lesions (sores) that itch (sometimes).
* On the scalp—lesions cause patchy hair loss and scaling scalp.
* On body skin—lesions are red, circular, flat, scaling, and have well-defined borders.
* On the bearded area of the face—lesions cause an itchy, scaling rash under the beard.
* On the feet—in the skin between the toes, a soft scaling (may be blistered), itchy rash.
* Of the nails—thickened, yellow, dull nails with crusting at the free edge.

CAUSES—Fungal infection with one or more of 5 different fungi. They are found almost everywhere. Transmission is by person-to-person contact or by contact with infected surfaces, such as towels, shoes, or shower stalls. Worms have nothing to do with the infection.

RISK INCREASES WITH
* Crowded living conditions.
* Contact with infected persons or animals.
* Daycare centers or schools.
* Weak immune system due to illness or drugs.
* Chronic moisture and irritation of the skin.
* Warm, humid climates.

HOW TO PREVENT—The fungi are so prevalent that total prevention is impossible. To reduce risk:
* Get treatment for pets with skin problems.
* Carefully dry feet after bathing in a tub or shower or after swimming. Apply antiperspirant to your feet if they perspire excessively.
* Good personal hygiene.
* Don't share headgear (hat, comb, brush).
* Avoid tight shoes or underwear that may rub or irritate the skin.

WHAT TO EXPECT

DIAGNOSTIC MEASURES
* Your own observation of symptoms.
* See your health care provider if self-care does not help. An exam of the affected skin usually confirms the diagnosis.

* Medical tests may include microscopic exam of skin scrapings and exam with ultraviolet light (Wood's lamp) for ringworm on the scalp.

APPROPRIATE HEALTH CARE—Treatment is usually with topical drugs. Other specific care depends on location of infection.

POSSIBLE COMPLICATIONS
* Bacterial infection of ringworm lesions.
* Recurrence is common and ringworm becomes chronic in 20% of cases.

PROBABLE OUTCOME—Usually curable with treatment. It may take weeks to months depending on the location.

HOW TO TREAT

GENERAL MEASURES
* For infection on the body: Carefully launder all clothing, towels, or bed linens that have touched the lesions.
* Keep the skin dry. If the area is red, swollen, and weeping, use compresses made of 1 teaspoon salt to 1 pint water. Apply 4 times a day for 2 to 3 days before starting the local antifungal medication.
* For infection of the scalp, shampoo the hair daily.
* For infected feet, expose feet to air whenever possible. Wear sandals or leather shoes, wear cotton socks. Wash and dry your feet at least twice a day.
* For an infected beard, let the beard grow. If necessary to shave, use an electric shaver and not a blade.
* For nail infection, keep nails short.

MEDICATION
* Use topical antifungal drugs in the form of creams, lotions, or ointments. Treatment may continue after symptoms clear up to help prevent a recurrence.
* In widespread infections or nail infections, an oral antifungal may be prescribed.
* Topical steroids may be prescribed for itching or inflammation.
* Antibiotics may be prescribed for a bacteria infection.

ACTIVITY—No limits.

DIET—No special diet.

CALL YOUR DOCTOR IF

* You or a family member has symptoms of ringworm.
* Symptoms don't improve in 3-4 weeks or lesions become redder, painful, and ooze pus.

ROCKY MOUNTAIN SPOTTED FEVER
(Tick Typhus)

 GENERAL INFORMATION

DEFINITION—An acute illness with fever caused by a germ transmitted by infected ticks. This is not contagious from person to person. The disease gets its name from the area where it was first identified.

BODY PARTS INVOLVED—Skin; central nervous system; gastrointestinal tract; muscles.

SEX OR AGE MOST AFFECTED—Both sexes; all ages, more likely to occur in children and young adults.

SIGNS & SYMPTOMS—The following occur 3 to 12 days after a tick bite:
- Fever, often high, with chills.
- Red skin rash that begins on hands and feet and spreads to ankles, wrists, legs, trunk, and abdomen.
- Headache that may be severe.
- Muscle aches and weakness; stiff back.
- Nausea and vomiting.
- Mental confusion; coma.

CAUSES—*Rickettsia* germs that live inside ticks. People are infected through tick bites, usually in the spring or summer. *Rickettsia* also infect rodents, squirrels, and chipmunks. The disease occurs in all states of the United States, especially on the East coast from Georgia to Maryland, and in heavy brush areas, such as Long Island.

RISK INCREASES WITH
- Outdoor activities in tick-infested areas.
- Contact with dogs.

HOW TO PREVENT
- Wear protective clothing in tick-infested areas, and use insect repellent.
- During outdoor activity, carefully inspect the body frequently to remove ticks. If ticks are removed within 4 hours, it will reduce the risk of infection. Remove the tick with tweezers by grabbing as close to the skin as possible. Disinfect the bite site and wash hands with soap and water. Do not remove ticks by squeezing, using petroleum jelly (Vaseline), or burning them with a match. Save the tick in a plastic bag in a freezer. If illness occurs, it may be used to help with diagnosis.

 WHAT TO EXPECT

DIAGNOSTIC MEASURES
- Your own observation of symptoms.
- Your health care provider will do a physical exam and ask questions about your symptoms and activities.
- Medical tests may include blood studies and skin biopsy (small piece of skin is removed to view under a microscope). The history of a tick bite or travel to a tick-infested area helps confirm diagnosis.

APPROPRIATE HEALTH CARE
- Treatment is with drugs and supportive care.
- Patients with mild disease may be treated at home.
- Moderate to severe infections require hospital care. Treatment may include mechanical breathing support, blood transfusions, and close watch for complications such as kidney failure.

POSSIBLE COMPLICATIONS
- Brain infection.
- Seizures.
- Kidney failure.
- Hepatitis.
- Rocky Mountain spotted fever can be fatal if untreated (due to pneumonia or heart failure).

PROBABLE OUTCOME—Curable, if treatment is begun in the early stages. Those with severe illness are more likely to develop complications.

 HOW TO TREAT

GENERAL MEASURES
- Good mouth care is important.
- To learn more: Centers for Disease Control & Prevention, 1600 Clifton Rd, Atlanta, GA 30333; (800) 311-3435; website: www.cdc.gov/ncidod/dvrd/rmsf/.

MEDICATION—Antibiotics, such as doxycycline, tetracycline, or chloramphenicol will be prescribed.

ACTIVITY—Rest in bed until fever and other symptoms improve.

DIET—No special diet. Very ill patients may require intravenous (IV) feedings. For others, small frequent meals may be needed.

 CALL YOUR DOCTOR IF

- You or a family member has symptoms of Rocky Mountain spotted fever.
- New, unexplained symptoms develop. Drugs used in treatment may produce side effects.

ILLNESS & DISORDERS

ROSEOLA INFANTUM
(Exanthem Subitum)

 GENERAL INFORMATION

DEFINITION—A common, contagious childhood disease.

BODY PARTS INVOLVED—Skin; central nervous system.

SEX OR AGE MOST AFFECTED—It usually affects infants and young children (ages 1 to 3 years). 90% of cases occur before age two.

SIGNS & SYMPTOMS
* Fever, often high, for several days. It may be the only symptoms until the rash appears.
* Flat, reddish skin rash after 3 to 5 days of high fever. When the rash appears, fever disappears. Some children may never develop the rash.
* Irritability.
* Drowsiness.
* Loss of appetite.
* Diarrhea.

CAUSES—It is caused by a type of herpes virus. It is related to, but not the same herpes virus that causes cold sores. The fever begins 5 to 15 days (usually 9 days) after exposure. A child is infectious during the fever phase of the illness. It is not known exactly how the infection is spread from one person to another.

RISK INCREASES WITH
* Day care centers.
* Exposure to others in public places.

HOW TO PREVENT—There is no specific way to prevent the infection. Take general precautions such as frequent hand washing and not exposing your child to someone who is sick.

 WHAT TO EXPECT

DIAGNOSTIC MEASURES
* Your own observation of symptoms.
* Call your child's health care provider if you have any concern about the symptoms. The disorder can usually be diagnosed without any medical tests, but a blood or urine study may be done.

APPROPRIATE HEALTH CARE
* There is no specific treatment for roseola.
* Rest at home, drink extra fluids, and drug therapy to reduce the fever if needed.

POSSIBLE COMPLICATIONS
* Rarely, convulsions caused by high fever. They will not cause brain damage and will stop after the fever subsides.
* Infection of the brain or hepatitis (both very rare).

PROBABLE OUTCOME—The illness heals on its own in about 1 week. The rash will fade and clear up without leaving scars.

 HOW TO TREAT

GENERAL MEASURES
* it is usually unnecessary to keep the patient away from other people in the family. Everyone should wash their hands often to help prevent spreading germs.
* Lukewarm water bath or a warm sponge bath may be used to help reduce fever. Don't use ice or cold water or a fan (they can cause chills).

MEDICATION
* For relief from minor discomfort and to reduce fever, you may use nonprescription drugs such as acetaminophen or ibuprofen. Don't give aspirin to children under age 18.
* Antibiotics will not help a virus infection.
* Anticonvulsant drugs (if child has seizure) may be prescribed.
* Antiviral drugs may be prescribed for persons with weak immune systems.

ACTIVITY—The child should rest in bed until the fever disappears. Return to day care or school once temperature is normal.

DIET—The child should eat a normal, well-balanced diet. Encourage extra fluid intake. Continue baby-vitamin supplements if the child is accustomed to taking them.

 CALL YOUR DOCTOR IF

* Your child has symptoms of roseola.
* High fever occurs.
* Twitching or other signs of a convulsion begin.
* The child refuses liquids.
* The child cries loudly and persistently, and does not stop when picked up.
* The child is listless and has a stiff neck.

ROUNDWORMS
(Ascariasis)

 GENERAL INFORMATION

DEFINITION—Roundworms thrive in the gastrointestinal tract (and sometimes in the lungs). They are contagious.

BODY PARTS INVOLVED—Gastrointestinal tract; lungs (sometimes).

SEX OR AGE MOST AFFECTED—Both sexes; all ages, but most common in children.

SIGNS & SYMPTOMS
* Often, there may be no symptoms.
* Irritability.
* Restlessness at night.
* Erratic or poor appetite.
* Frequent fatigue.
* Weight loss or lack of weight gain.
* Stomach (abdominal) discomfort.
* Diarrhea (sometimes).
* Cough and wheezing (rare).
* Worms may sometimes be seen in bowel movements or in the child's bed. Rarely, one may be vomited.
* Fever.

CAUSES—There are several types of roundworms (or nematodes). Some can be seen by the human eye, and others can only be seen with a microscope. Their eggs can enter the human body through contaminated water, food, or soil-contaminated hands. In some types, the larvae (young worms) enter through the skin.

RISK INCREASES WITH
* Crowded or unclean living conditions.
* Using human feces as a fertilizer.

HOW TO PREVENT
* Wash hands often, and always before eating and after using the bathroom.
* Keep fingers away from the mouth.
* Have pets treated for worms. Avoid strange animals.

 WHAT TO EXPECT

DIAGNOSTIC MEASURES
* Your own observation of symptoms.
* Your health care provider may do a physical exam.
* Medical tests may include studies of the stool or a study of an adult worm, if passed, to identify the worm. X-ray of the lungs or an ultrasound may be done in some cases.

APPROPRIATE HEALTH CARE
* Treatment can be given at home and involves anti-worm drug therapy.
* In rare cases, surgery may be needed for complications, such as a bowel perforation (tear).

POSSIBLE COMPLICATIONS—If untreated:
* Worms migrate to other body parts.
* Intestinal obstruction (rare).

PROBABLE OUTCOME—Usually curable in one week with treatment.

 HOW TO TREAT

GENERAL MEASURES—Wash hands carefully after using the toilet or before meals. Keep fingers away from the mouth. Keep nails short and clean.

MEDICATION—Drugs called anthelmintics that kill roundworms will be prescribed. Follow the instructions provided for taking the drug.

ACTIVITY—No limits.

DIET—No special diet.

 CALL YOUR DOCTOR IF

* You or a family member has symptoms of roundworms.
* Roundworms reappear after treatment.
* Drugs used for treatment cause side effects.

ILLNESS & DISORDERS

RUBELLA
(German Measles)

 GENERAL INFORMATION

DEFINITION—A mild, contagious, viral illness. Use of the rubella vaccine has reduced the number of cases in the United States by 99%. Rubella is likely to cause serious birth defects in the unborn baby of a pregnant woman who develops the disease in the first 3 or 4 months of pregnancy.

BODY PARTS INVOLVED—Skin; lymph glands behind the ears and in the neck.

SEX OR AGE MOST AFFECTED—Both sexes; all ages, but most common in children.

SIGNS & SYMPTOMS
* Fever.
* Muscle aches and stiffness, especially in the neck.
* Fatigue and headache.
* Reddish rash on the head and body after the 2nd or 3rd day. The rash lasts 1 or 2 days.
* Swollen lymph glands, especially behind the ears and at the back and sides of the neck.
* Joint pain (adults).

CAUSES—The rubella virus is spread by person-to-person contact. It takes 14 to 23 days after exposure before symptoms appear. Patients are contagious from one week before the rash appears until one week after it started.

RISK INCREASES WITH
* Young, unimmunized adults.
* Crowded living conditions.
* School or daycare.
* Weak immune system due to illness or drugs.

HOW TO PREVENT
* Vaccination:
  - For children, rubella vaccine is usually given with the measles and mumps vaccine (MMR).
  - Nonpregnant women of childbearing age should be vaccinated if they have not had rubella or have not been vaccinated before. Pregnancy should be prevented for one month after vaccination. A blood test can be done if a woman is unsure about her rubella immunity.
  - Health care workers and daycare workers should get vaccinated if they have not been, or if their vaccination history is unknown. Young adults, such as college students should get two doses of MMR if not previously vaccinated.
* A person should not be vaccinated if he or she has a weak immune system, as occurs with cancer patients, currently takes cortisone or anticancer drugs, is receiving radiation therapy, or has a serious illness.
* A person, especially a pregnant woman, who is exposed to rubella and has not had it, or been vaccinated against it, should consult their health care provider right away.

 WHAT TO EXPECT

DIAGNOSTIC MEASURES
* Your own observation of symptoms.
* Your health care provider can usually diagnose the disorder with a physical exam.
* Medical tests are normally not done for rubella. If needed, cultures of the throat, blood, urine, or cerebrospinal fluid can confirm the presence of the virus.

APPROPRIATE HEALTH CARE—Home care is usually all that is needed.

POSSIBLE COMPLICATIONS
* Encephalitis (brain inflammation).
* Thrombocytopenia (a blood disorder).
* Agranulocytosis (reduction in white blood cells).
* Rubella infection in a pregnant woman may cause miscarriage or birth defects. The baby may have growth restriction; mental retardation; deafness; or liver, spleen, and bone marrow problems.

PROBABLE OUTCOME—No specific treatment is needed. The illness will heal on its own in one week in children, sometimes longer in adults. Complications are rare.

 HOW TO TREAT

GENERAL MEASURES—Be sure to contact any pregnant woman who has been exposed to the patient. Exposure includes contact with the infected person 1 week prior to, during or 1 week after the infection. This woman should consult her obstetric provider immediately.

MEDICATION—For minor discomfort, you may use nonprescription drugs such as acetaminophen or ibuprofen. Don't give aspirin to children under age 18.

ACTIVITY—Get extra rest until the symptoms get better.

DIET—No special diet.

 CALL YOUR DOCTOR IF

* You or a family member has symptoms of rubella.
* The following occur during treatment: high fever, red eyes, cough, shortness of breath, severe headache, drowsiness, lethargy, or convulsion.
* Unusual bleeding occurs 1 to 4 weeks after the illness (from gums, nose, uterus, or blood specks on the skin).

SALIVARY GLAND INFECTION

GENERAL INFORMATION

DEFINITION—An infection of a salivary gland. The salivary glands are located around the mouth and they produce saliva. Saliva is the moisture in the mouth that helps with chewing and swallowing. There are three pairs of salivary glands and the largest is called the parotids.

BODY PARTS INVOLVED—Salivary glands and ducts.

SEX OR AGE MOST AFFECTED—Adults of both sexes.

SIGNS & SYMPTOMS
• Pain and swelling of parotid gland (behind ear) or sublingual (under tongue) salivary gland.
• Dry mouth.
• May be hard to open mouth wide.
• Food may taste strange.
• There may be a bitter tasting pus, which is a creamy fluid, in the mouth caused by the infection.
• Fever.

CAUSES
• Bacterial infection, which may result from poor mouth care.
• The gland (or duct) could become blocked by tiny, stone-like substances.
• Mumps or other virus can infect the glands. Mumps is much less common now because of the childhood vaccine against it.

RISK INCREASES WITH
• Poor oral hygiene.
• Adults over age 60.
• Smoking.
• Dehydration.
• Poor eating habits, especially a lack of vitamins.
• Recent or chronic illness, such as a mouth infection, that lowers the body's germ-fighting ability.
• Diabetes.
• Use of certain drugs that cause a dry mouth.

HOW TO PREVENT—In many cases, the infection cannot be prevented. Good oral hygiene will help reduce the risk.

WHAT TO EXPECT

DIAGNOSTIC MEASURES
• Your own observation of symptoms.
• Your health care provider will do a physical exam of the head, neck, mouth, and throat.
• Tests may be done on a sample of the fluid from the infected gland.

APPROPRIATE HEALTH CARE
• Infections are usually treated with antibiotics.
• Medical care may involve opening a blocked duct with a special instrument.
• Home care may be all that is needed.

POSSIBLE COMPLICATIONS
• Abscess (pus-filled sore).
• Spread of infection to other parts of the body.
• Infection may recur.

PROBABLE OUTCOME—Usually can be cured in two weeks with treatment. Symptoms should improve within a few days of starting treatment. Complications are rare.

HOW TO TREAT

GENERAL MEASURES
• For pain control, apply warm soaks or use a heating pad on low setting. Massaging the area may help.
• Rinse mouth with warm salt water a few times a day. Use one-half teaspoon of salt in one cup of warm water. This may help ease the pain.
• Suck on hard candy, such as lemon drops to increase moisture in the mouth.
• Brush teeth and floss twice daily. This may help with healing and prevent spread of the infection.
• Avoid smoking. This will help in recovery.

MEDICATION
• Antibiotics will be prescribed for any bacterial infection.
• For minor pain, you may use nonprescription drugs such as acetaminophen.

ACTIVITY—No limits.

DIET—No special diet. Drink plenty of fluids each day.

CALL YOUR DOCTOR IF

• You or a family member has symptoms of a salivary gland infection.
• The infection does not improve in four days or symptoms get worse despite treatment.
• Fever persists or recurs after treatment.
• There is pain or swelling in the mouth.

ILLNESS & DISORDERS

SALIVARY GLAND TUMOR

GENERAL INFORMATION

DEFINITION—A type of growth in the salivary glands. The salivary glands are located around the mouth and they make saliva, the moisture in the mouth that helps you chew and swallow. Most salivary-gland tumors are benign (do not have cancer cells) and take several years to grow. Even cancer cell tumors rarely spread to other places in the body. The tumors can involve the parotid glands, which are the salivary glands in the jaw or other salivary glands in the floor of the mouth.

BODY PARTS INVOLVED—Salivary glands and ducts.

SEX OR AGE MOST AFFECTED—Adults of both sexes.

SIGNS & SYMPTOMS
• A soft or firm mass in the jaw or in the floor of the mouth.
• There may be pain or swelling.
• There may be general symptoms, such as weight loss, fever, or cough.

CAUSES—Unknown.

RISK INCREASES WITH
• Dehydration.
• Poor oral hygiene.
• Smoking.
• Salivary duct stone.
• False teeth.

HOW TO PREVENT—Most can't be prevented, but the risk may be reduced by:
• Not smoking.
• Keeping the mouth healthy with careful brushing and flossing of the teeth. Drink plenty of fluids each day and suck on hard candy to stop dry mouth.

WHAT TO EXPECT

DIAGNOSTIC MEASURES
• Your own observation of symptoms.
• Your health care provider will do a physical exam of the head, neck, mouth, and throat.
• Medical tests may include x-ray, MRI, CT, fine-needle aspiration (see Glossary for all), and/or biopsy (tissue or tumor is removed and examined under a microscope). These help to determine if the tumor is cancerous or benign.

APPROPRIATE HEALTH CARE
• For benign tumors, no treatment may be needed. Repeat medical exams will be done to monitor for any changes.
• In some cases, benign tumors may be surgically removed.
• If the tumor is cancerous, the treatment will depend on the type of cancer and if it has spread. A portion of the gland or the entire gland may be removed. Nearby lymph nodes and other tissue in the neck may also be removed. Radiation treatment and/or anticancer drugs (chemotherapy) may be recommended.

POSSIBLE COMPLICATIONS
• Infection at the surgical site.
• Facial nerve may be damaged during surgery.
• Cancer cells spread to other places in the body.
• Tumor may recur.

PROBABLE OUTCOME—Tumors that are benign (not cancerous) are usually cured with surgery. For cancerous tumors, the outcome depends on successful treatment and whether the cancer has spread or not.

HOW TO TREAT

GENERAL MEASURES
• After surgery, keep the mouth clean with salt water mouthwashes. At least three or four times a day, rinse the mouth with a solution of one-half teaspoon salt in one cup of warm water.
• Suck on hard candy, such as lemon drops to increase moisture in the mouth.
• Avoid smoking. This will help in recovery.

MEDICATION
• Drugs for pain or infection may be prescribed.
• Anticancer drugs to help destroy cancer cells may be prescribed.

ACTIVITY—Resume your normal activities as soon as possible after surgery.

DIET—No special diet. Drink plenty of fluids each day. After surgery, a liquid diet may be needed for a short time until your mouth heals.

CALL YOUR DOCTOR IF

• You or a family member has symptoms of a salivary gland tumor.
• After surgery, signs of infection occur in your mouth, such as feeling warmer or tender, redness, pain, and swelling.

SALMONELLA INFECTIONS

GENERAL INFORMATION

DEFINITION—An illness caused by a bacteria named *Salmonella*. This is a type of germ sometimes found in food or drinks. The illness can cause symptoms that affect the stomach and the intestines (digestive tract). A group of people may get sick at the same time if they all eat the same infected food at a picnic, a party, or at a restaurant. A mild *Salmonella* illness may feel like a simple upset stomach for some people.

BODY PARTS INVOLVED—Gastrointestinal tract; lymphatic system.

SEX OR AGE MOST AFFECTED—Both sexes; all ages.

SIGNS & SYMPTOMS
• Diarrhea, often with stomach cramps. Diarrhea is an abnormal increase in the number and looseness of stools or bowel movements a day.
• Nausea, vomiting, and fever.
• Blood in the stool (sometimes).
• Headache.
• Some people may have a rash.

CAUSES
• Symptoms start 6 to 72 hours after eating food such as meat, chicken, eggs, or drinking raw (unpasteurized) milk, or water that contains the *Salmonella* germs. Germs can stay alive even in frozen foods, but careful cooking will kill them.
• Illness can also be passed from person to person.
• Pet turtles, lizards, and other pets or animals can carry the germ and cause illness in humans.

RISK INCREASES WITH
• Living in a place with many other people such as a school dorm, or living in a place that is not kept very clean.
• People older than age 60, young children, and infants.
• Weak immune system due to illness or drugs.

HOW TO PREVENT
• Keep the kitchen area where you prepare meals very clean. Kill germs on knives and other items you use for cooking by washing them with hot water and soap.
• Stay away from sick pets or animals.
• Drink only milk that is pasteurized.
• Always wash your hands after you go to the bathroom, before you handle any food, and if you have touched an animal or pet.
• Avoid being around someone who has this illness.

WHAT TO EXPECT

DIAGNOSTIC MEASURES
• Your own observation of symptoms.
• Your health care provider may do a physical exam and may want to have a medical test done on a sample of the stool (bowel movement).

APPROPRIATE HEALTH CARE
• Most patients recover by just getting extra rest and replacing the fluids lost from the body due to the diarrhea.
• Hospital care if symptoms are severe (rare).

POSSIBLE COMPLICATIONS
• Dehydration from diarrhea and vomiting. This can be serious for infants and older persons.
• People who have a severe case of this illness or have complications may need treatment in a hospital.

PROBABLE OUTCOME—In most cases, the illness is mild and over in 2 to 7 days.

HOW TO TREAT

GENERAL MEASURES
• Keep the ill person away from other people in the house, if possible.
• Use a heating pad or hot-water bottle to relieve abdominal cramps.
• If diarrhea is severe, use a bedside commode.

MEDICATION
• Drugs are not needed for mild cases, but may be prescribed for severe cases and for patients who have other health problems.
• Do not use any drugs for the diarrhea unless your health care provider tells you to do so. The diarrhea is the way your body gets rid of the germs.

ACTIVITY—Get extra rest in bed until the symptoms get better. Then begin your normal routine slowly, day by day.

DIET—Replace the fluids lost from the body due to diarrhea with sports drinks such as Gatorade or a special children's product such as Pedialyte. Begin to eat regular food within 12 to 24 hours or when you feel better.

CALL YOUR DOCTOR IF

• You or a family member has symptoms of a *Salmonella illness*.
• An infant has signs of dehydration (dry, wrinkled skin, less urine output, or dark urine).
• A patient has a fever 102°F (38.9°C) or higher, yellow skin or eyes, cough with blood, or diarrhea gets worse.

SCABIES

GENERAL INFORMATION

DEFINITION—A skin disorder caused by little bugs called mites (the "itch" mite). Scabies is very contagious and can be spread from person-to-person or by sharing clothing, towels, or bedding. It may take as long as four to six weeks after you have been exposed for the rash to first appear.

BODY PARTS INVOLVED—Skin of the finger webs and folds under the arms, breasts, elbows, genitals and buttocks.

SEX OR AGE MOST AFFECTED—Both sexes; all ages.

SIGNS & SYMPTOMS
• A rash with small, very itchy, red bumps or blisters. They may look like pimples. Scabies usually infects the skin of the finger webs, and folds under the arms, breasts, elbows, genitals, and buttocks.
• Sores can form on the skin where it has been scratched.

CAUSES—A mite that burrows into deep skin layers, where the female mite lays her eggs. Eggs grow into adult mites in three weeks. Mites are so tiny that they can only be seen under a microscope. If you scratch the skin area, the mites and eggs get under the fingernails and then get spread to other places in the body.

RISK INCREASES WITH
• Living in a place with many other people such as a school dorm, or living in a place that is not kept very clean.
• Children in child care centers.
• Standing close to or touching the skin of a person who has scabies. It can also be spread by sexual contact.

HOW TO PREVENT
• Avoid being close to persons or linen and clothing that you suspect may be infected with scabies.
• Keep yourself as clean as possible:
  - Bathe daily, or at least two to three times a week.
  - Wash hands before eating.
  - Wash clothes often.

WHAT TO EXPECT

DIAGNOSTIC MEASURES
• Your own observation of symptoms.
• Your health care provider can diagnose scabies by looking at the affected skin area.
• Sometimes the skin may be scraped to gather the mites so they can be viewed under a microscope.

APPROPRIATE HEALTH CARE—Treatment is with a drug to be used on the skin.

POSSIBLE COMPLICATIONS
• Sores from scratching the itchy skin may become infected with bacteria.
• You can be reinfected with scabies.

PROBABLE OUTCOME—The skin will usually heal in about two weeks with treatment. The itching can last for up to four weeks even after treatment.

HOW TO TREAT

GENERAL MEASURES—Use hot water to wash all clothes, towels, bedding and washable toys used two days before and during treatment. Put items you can't wash in plastic bags for two weeks to kill the mites. You don't need to clean furniture or floors with special care.

MEDICATION
• Several different lotions or creams can be used for treatment. Infants and pregnant women may need a milder lotion than that used for other family members. These are general directions (follow your health care provider's instructions or read the directions that come with the product):
  - Take a bath or shower before applying the lotion.
  - Apply from the neck down, and cover the entire body. Wait 15 minutes before dressing.
  - Leave lotion on the skin for 8 to 12 hours, then take a bath or shower to remove it.
  - Your family or other close contacts should be treated at the same time.
  - You may need to repeat the lotion treatment if the rash does not go away in a few weeks or if it gets worse after being treated.
• In some cases, an anti-itching drug may be prescribed.

ACTIVITY—No limits.

DIET—No special diet.

CALL YOUR DOCTOR IF

• You or a family member has symptoms of scabies.
• After treatment, the skin shows signs of infection (redness, pus, swelling, or pain).

SCARLET FEVER

GENERAL INFORMATION

DEFINITION—Scarlet fever is a childhood skin rash disorder caused by a streptococcal (strep) bacteria infection. It is very contagious.

BODY PARTS INVOLVED—Throat; tonsils; skin.

SEX OR AGE MOST AFFECTED—Children and adolescents, especially between ages 2 and 10.

SIGNS & SYMPTOMS—Symptoms may vary in different children. The following is the usual course of the disease:
- Day 1—Fever as high as 104°F (40°C); a red sore throat, swollen tonsils (tonsils may have a whitish coating), enlarged lymph glands in the neck, cough, vomiting.
- Day 2—Bright red rash on the face, except around the mouth.
- Day 3—Reddened tongue ("strawberry tongue") and rash in body creases, which spreads to the neck, chest, back, and then the entire body. The rash looks like a sunburn with bumps.
- Day 6—The rash fades and skin may begin peeling, which can go on for 10 to 14 days.

CAUSES
- Streptococcal or strep infection caused by a type of germ that produces a scarlet fever toxin (poison). Germs are spread by contact with an infected person, breathing in germs in the air, or touching an object with germs on it.
- Very few strep infections lead to scarlet fever. Not everyone is susceptible to the toxin that produces the rash. In a family, one child may get scarlet fever, a second may have only a strep throat, and a third may carry the germ and spread it to others, but not be sick.

RISK INCREASES WITH
- Strep infections that recur often.
- Living in a place with many other people such as a school dorm.
- Exposure to others in public places.
- Children ages 2 to 10.

HOW TO PREVENT—Cannot be prevented completely, because some healthy persons will carry the strep germ without being ill. However, some ways to help prevent it include:
- Antibiotic drug for 10 days for strep infection.
- Avoid persons with sore throats.

WHAT TO EXPECT

DIAGNOSTIC MEASURES
- Your own observation of symptoms.
- Your health care provider will do a physical exam.
- Medical tests may include throat culture or blood test for strep bacteria. Testing may be done on other family members if they have symptoms.

APPROPRIATE HEALTH CARE—Treatment is with drug therapy. Care may be given at home.

POSSIBLE COMPLICATIONS—Without treatment, infections that are more serious can occur.

PROBABLE OUTCOME—With treatment, it is usually cured in about 10 days.

HOW TO TREAT

GENERAL MEASURES
- Keep the ill person away from other people, including family members. After the patient has taken the antibiotic drug for 24 hours, they are no longer contagious and can return to school or child-care. The rash is not contagious.
- Rinse mouth and gargle with warm salt water a few times a day. Use one-half teaspoon of salt in one cup of warm water. This may help ease the pain.
- Use a cool-mist, ultrasonic humidifier (if advised) to relieve the sore throat. Clean the humidifier daily.

MEDICATION
- Antibiotics will be prescribed. Be sure to take all the doses even if the symptoms improve.
- Use acetaminophen for pain relief and fever. Do not give aspirin to children under age 18.

ACTIVITY—Extra rest is a good idea until symptoms improve.

DIET—No special diet. Drink plenty of fluids.

CALL YOUR DOCTOR IF

- You or your child has symptoms of strep throat or scarlet fever.
- The following occur during treatment:
  - Fever goes away and then returns.
  - New symptoms begin, such as nausea; vomiting; earache; cough; headache; thick, colored, nasal drainage; chest pain; or difficulty breathing.

ILLNESS & DISORDERS

SCHIZOPHRENIC DISORDERS

GENERAL INFORMATION

DEFINITION—A group of disabling mental disorders. Schizo means "split" and phrenia refers to the mind. The person can't tell fact from fantasy, and therefore does not behave rationally. Symptoms may begin in the early teen years or early adulthood. Symptoms may take months or years to become apparent.

BODY PARTS INVOLVED—Brain.

SEX OR AGE MOST AFFECTED—Both sexes; all ages.

SIGNS & SYMPTOMS
- Delusions (fixed false, unreal beliefs).
- Hallucinations (hearing voices or seeing things that are not there).
- Becomes more withdrawn and wants to be alone.
- Lack of energy and desire to do things.
- Showing few emotions, or showing emotions that are not appropriate.
- Disordered thoughts that are shown in disorganized or disjointed speech.
- A belief that other people hear and "steal" one's thoughts or that one is being controlled by others.
- Suspicious and paranoid behavior (in paranoid schizophrenia).

CAUSES—Exact cause is unknown. It may involve abnormal amounts of some chemicals in the brain. Research is ongoing to find the cause and a possible cure.

RISK INCREASES WITH—Family history of schizophrenia.

HOW TO PREVENT—No specific preventive measures are known.

WHAT TO EXPECT

DIAGNOSTIC MEASURES
- Other's observation of symptoms.
- Your health care provider will do a physical exam and ask questions about the symptoms and activities. Some information about behavior may be supplied by family members.
- There is no specific test to diagnose schizophrenia. At times, it is difficult to tell one mental disorder from another. Medical tests will be done to rule out other medical problems.

APPROPRIATE HEALTH CARE
- The goal of therapy is to help the person get back in touch with reality. Treatment often begins with drugs to reduce the symptoms.

- Once symptoms are improved, treatment continues to help the person learn to cope with daily aspects of life. Treatment depends on the patient's needs and the severity of their symptoms. It may include social and work skills training, self-help groups, and counseling.

POSSIBLE COMPLICATIONS
- Life-long disability.
- Drugs may not be effective in treatment.
- Patients stop taking the drugs because of side effects, impaired thinking, or they because they feel they don't need them.
- Self-inflicted injuries; suicide.
- Hostile behavior toward others.
- Relapse, neglect, homeless, or ending up in prison.

PROBABLE OUTCOME—Treatment is effective for many patients and helps them to return to varying degrees of independence. About 30% return to normal lives and work. Sometimes the condition completely disappears. The majority of people with the disorder are not prone to violence.

HOW TO TREAT

GENERAL MEASURES
- The family or other important persons in the patient's life should also be involved in the therapy. This will help them understand the problem and what they can do to help the patient. Schizophrenia patients are sometimes difficult to live with.
- To learn more: National Alliance for the Mentally Ill, (800) 950-6264; website: www.nami.org or National Institute of Mental Health, (301) 443-4513 (not toll free); website: www.nimh.nih.gov.

MEDICATION—Antipsychotic drugs are usually prescribed. Some are taken by mouth. Others may be injected. If side effects are too severe with one drug or the symptoms are not controlled, a different drug is prescribed. The dose is reduced as symptoms improve. For most patients, the drugs may need to be taken for life.

ACTIVITY—Normally no limits. unless directed by your health care provider.

DIET—Eat a regular healthy diet.

CALL YOUR DOCTOR IF

- You or a family member has symptoms of schizophrenia.
- Symptoms continue or worsen after treatment is started.
- New, unexplained symptoms develop. Drugs used in treatment may produce side effects.

SCLERITIS

GENERAL INFORMATION

DEFINITION—Deep, localized inflammation of the sclera, the outermost white layer of tissue covering the eyeball. Scleritis is not contagious.

BODY PARTS INVOLVED—Sclera, which includes the conjunctiva and cornea. Scleritis may affect one or both eyes.

SEX OR AGE MOST AFFECTED—Adults ages 40 to 60 and women more than men.

SIGNS & SYMPTOMS
* Eye pain (may be severe and wake a person at night). The pain may radiate (spread) to the forehead, cheek, or behind the eye.
* Tearing.
* Photophobia (extra sensitivity to light).
* Purple-red, inflamed areas in one or more areas of the white of the eye.
* Partial vision loss (rare).

CAUSES—It is often associated with an autoimmune disorder (such as rheumatoid arthritis). It is believed that certain persons with autoimmune disorders are more susceptible to scleritis. Infection, foreign object in the eye, chemicals, or trauma may be factors also.

RISK INCREASES WITH
* Connective tissue disease (rheumatoid arthritis, ankylosing spondylitis, systemic lupus erythematosus, Reiter's syndrome, and others).
* Vascular disease (polyarteritis nodosa, Wegener's granulomatosis, giant cell arteritis, and others).
* Herpes zoster (shingles).
* Gout.
* Tuberculosis.
* Syphilis.
* Infections (bacterial, fungal, or viral).
* Prior eye surgery.
* Eye trauma (injury).

HOW TO PREVENT—No specific preventive measures.

WHAT TO EXPECT

DIAGNOSTIC MEASURES
* Your own observation of symptoms.
* Your health care provider may do a physical exam and an eye exam and ask about other symptoms.
* Medical tests will include a visual exam, eye pressure, slit lamp evaluation (this uses a microscope with a strong light to examine the eye). Other medical tests may be done depending on what underlying disorder may be suspected or involved.

APPROPRIATE HEALTH CARE
* Treatment usually involves drug therapy to treat the inflammation and underlying cause.
* Rarely, surgery may be needed.

POSSIBLE COMPLICATIONS—Eye problems including keratopathy, uveitis, cataracts, glaucoma, or perforation of the eyeball.

PROBABLE OUTCOME—It usually responds to treatment, but it may recur. In some cases, the outcome depends on treating the underlying cause.

HOW TO TREAT

GENERAL MEASURES—Follow medical advice.

MEDICATION—You may be prescribed nonsteroidal anti-inflammatories, oral cortisone drugs, cortisone eye drops, or immuno-suppressive drugs to reduce inflammation.

ACTIVITY—Reduce normal activity until inflammation subsides.

DIET—No special diet.

CALL YOUR DOCTOR IF

* You or a family member has symptoms of scleritis.
* Symptoms don't improve in 48 hours with treatment.
* Temperature rises to 100°F (37.8°C) or higher.
* Pain becomes worse.
* Vision is affected.

SCLERODERMA
(Progressive System Sclerosis)

GENERAL INFORMATION

DEFINITION—A disease in which the skin and other body parts change gradually, becoming thick, stiff, and hard. Scleroderma has two main classes, localized and systemic. Localized affects only certain parts of the body such as the skin and its tissues. Systemic affects the whole body, including blood vessels and major organs. There are subgroups defined within these two classes.

BODY PARTS INVOLVED—Skin; joints; digestive system, especially the esophagus; intestinal tract; heart; kidneys; lungs; blood vessels; fingers; toes.

SEX OR AGE MOST AFFECTED—Adults of both sexes, but more common in women between ages 30 and 50.

SIGNS & SYMPTOMS
* Patches on the skin that start in one place and spread.
* Fingers, toes, cheeks, nose, and ears may have numbness, pain, and color changes. Symptoms may be brought on by cold weather or emotional upset. This is called Raynaud's phenomenon.
* Skin—hardening and thickening, especially in the face, which becomes tight, losing elasticity.
* Digestive system problems—swallowing difficulty, poor food absorption, bloating after eating, weight loss, heartburn, and a feeling that food sticks in the chest.
* Feet and hands may be swollen.
* Feeling weak and tired.
* Joint pain, stiffness, and swelling.

CAUSES—The exact cause is unknown. It appears that the body's immune system, which normally protects the body against germs, becomes faulty. With scleroderma, it produces too much collagen, a fibrous type of protein found in connective tissues.

RISK INCREASES WITH—Unknown.

HOW TO PREVENT—Cannot be prevented.

WHAT TO EXPECT

DIAGNOSTIC MEASURES
* Your own observation of symptoms.
* Your health care provider will do a physical exam and check the affected skin. Questions will be asked about your symptoms.
* Medical tests may include blood studies and a biopsy. With a biopsy, a small amount of tissue is removed and viewed under a microscope. Other tests may be done to confirm the diagnosis or to check for any complications.

APPROPRIATE HEALTH CARE
* There is no cure for the disorder. The goals of treatment are to help with the symptoms and stop the progression of the disease. Follow the prescribed treatment plan (this list is general).
* Physical therapy and occupational therapy (to help with day-to-day living activities) may be prescribed.

POSSIBLE COMPLICATIONS—It is often slowly progressive and affects the gastrointestinal system, heart, lungs, and kidneys.

PROBABLE OUTCOME—The course of the disorder is variable and unpredictable.

HOW TO TREAT

GENERAL MEASURES
* Wear warm clothing, such as heavy socks, and gloves if going out in the cold. Cover your head and face.
* Sleep on 2 or 3 pillows, or raise the head of your bed 5 to 8 inches to prevent digestion problems.
* Stop smoking. Find a way to quit that works.
* Use heat to relieve joint stiffness.
* Seek counseling to help adjust to living with the disease. Joining a support group may help.
* To learn more: Scleroderma Foundation, 12 Kent Way, Suite 101, Byfield, MA 01922; (800) 722-4673; website: www.scleroderma.org.

MEDICATION
* Different drugs may be prescribed, depending on your symptoms. Drugs can improve circulation, help with joint stiffness and pain, improve the immune system, aid digestive problems, and lower high blood pressure.
* Use skin lotions, lubricants, and bath oils to soften skin.

ACTIVITY
* Be as active as your strength permits; avoid fatigue.
* Regular exercise (or movement) helps keep skin flexible, helps blood circulation, and prevents fixed joints.

DIET—Eat frequent, small meals to minimize bloating, heartburn, and stomach discomfort. A soft diet is sometimes helpful. Drink extra fluids to help with swallowing. A dietitian can help plan a nutritious diet.

CALL YOUR DOCTOR IF

* You or a family member has symptoms of scleroderma.
* Any sign of infection occurs.
* Symptoms get worse or new ones develop.

SCOLIOSIS
(Curvature of the Spine)

GENERAL INFORMATION

DEFINITION—A sideways curve (or twisting) of the spinal column.

BODY PARTS INVOLVED—It can involve the thoracic (middle) spine, the lumbar (lower) spine, or the thoracolumbar (between the two areas).

SEX OR AGE MOST AFFECTED—It most often affects children after age 10, and is more common in girls than in boys.

SIGNS & SYMPTOMS
Early stages:
* No obvious symptoms or signs. It comes on gradually. Scoliosis can be detected by a health care provider with a simple screening test. Schools sometimes have scoliosis screening programs.
Later stages:
* Visible curving of the upper body. The spine becomes S-shaped or C-shaped.
* Shoulders become uneven and rounded.
* Sunken chest.
* Swayback.
* One side of the pelvis thrusts forward.
* Back pain.

CAUSES—Most often the cause is unknown. Scoliosis is sometimes a result of:
* A disease of the central nervous system, such as cerebral palsy or muscular dystrophy.
* Congenital (being born with) defects of the spine.
* Uneven leg length.

RISK INCREASES WITH—Family history of scoliosis.

HOW TO PREVENT—Cannot be prevented at present.

WHAT TO EXPECT

DIAGNOSTIC MEASURES
* Your own observation of symptoms.
* Your child's health care provider can diagnose scoliosis with a physical exam.
* An x-ray may be done to confirm the diagnosis. The amount of curve in the spine is measured by degrees.

APPROPRIATE HEALTH CARE
* Treatment will depend on the age of the child, how severe the curve is, and how much it is progressing.
* Many cases of scoliosis are minor (less than 20 degrees) and require no treatment. Follow up medical exams will be done to see if the problem is progressing.
* For children with more of a curve (usually 25 to 40 degrees), treatment often involves wearing an orthopedic back brace. Sometimes this is needed for several years. Some braces are less visible and permit the person to wear regular clothes.
* Surgery to correct scoliosis is usually advised if the curve is more than 40 to 50 degrees or bracing is not helping. Surgery helps improve posture and back function.
* For adults with scoliosis, physical therapy or exercises to strengthen back muscles are sometimes helpful. Talk to your health care provider.

POSSIBLE COMPLICATIONS
* Severe curving of the spine and ribs.
* Social embarrassment, due to wearing a brace.
* Complications such as lung and heart damage, loss of bone strength, and back pain may occur. These are more likely when scoliosis is more severe and goes untreated.

PROBABLE OUTCOME—Mild curves may not require treatment. If treatment is done, the outcome is usually successful.

HOW TO TREAT

GENERAL MEASURES—To learn more: National Scoliosis Foundation, 5 Cabot Place, Stoughton, MA 02072; (800) 673-6922; website: www.scoliosis.org.

MEDICATION—Drugs will not correct this disorder.

ACTIVITY—Special exercises may be part of therapy. If a brace is necessary, sports participation will be restricted. Some activities, such as swimming, may help since they tone and strengthen the back.

DIET—No special diet.

CALL YOUR DOCTOR IF

You suspect your child is developing scoliosis.

SEASONAL AFFECTIVE DISORDER (SAD)

 GENERAL INFORMATION

DEFINITION—A mood disorder that occurs during the winter months and stops when spring begins. Light plays a major part in its origin and in its treatment. In rarer instances, the seasonal disorder symptoms occur in the summer months and may be caused by intolerance to heat.

BODY PARTS INVOLVED—Nervous system.

SEX OR AGE MOST AFFECTED—Adults and children and is more common in women.

SIGNS & SYMPTOMS
• Symptoms usually begin in September when days begin to shorten, and last through the winter into March when the days begin to get longer again.
• Depression.
• Feeling tired, sluggish, and needing more sleep.
• Increased appetite (especially for carbohydrates).
• Weight gain.
• Irritability and feeling less cheerful.
• Being less social.
• Decreased interest in sex and physical contact.
• Joint aches, stomach problems, and more infections.

CAUSES—It is thought that the lack of bright light in winter months causes changes in the brain chemistry. Melatonin, a substance produced at night by the pineal gland, normally helps with sleep. When too much melatonin is produced due to longer nights, it can cause symptoms of depression.

RISK INCREASES WITH
• The area of the country where a person lives. People in northern latitudes are more susceptible to SAD.
• Persons with other depressive illnesses.

HOW TO PREVENT—No measures are known to prevent the disorder.

 WHAT TO EXPECT

DIAGNOSTIC MEASURES
• Your own observation of symptoms.
• Your health care provider will do a physical exam and ask questions about your symptoms and activities. Diagnosing SAD can be difficult. The same symptoms can arise from other types of depression.
• Blood tests may be done to rule out other medical disorders. Diagnosis usually requires a three-year pattern of mood changes that begin in the autumn and stop in the spring.

APPROPRIATE HEALTH CARE
• Treatment may involve light therapy (phototherapy). Duration and intensities of this therapy will vary for each person. It is recommended that light therapy not be used without medical advice. Examples include:
- Sitting in a very bright light (equal to 10 or more 100-watt bulbs) for a period in the morning and, sometimes, in the evening. The term lux (Latin for light) is the unit of measure for the light therapy.
- Installing a computerized system of lighting in a patient's bedroom that creates an artificial dawn. The light goes from very dim to bright like a sunrise.
• Other forms of treatment include drug therapy or counseling to help cope with the symptoms.

POSSIBLE COMPLICATIONS—Problems in coping with life as a result of the symptoms.

PROBABLE OUTCOME—With correct diagnosis and treatment, symptoms can be helped.

 HOW TO TREAT

GENERAL MEASURES
• Mild symptoms may be helped with simple measures. Keep drapes and blinds open in your house and sit near windows and gaze outside often. Turn on bright lights on cloudy days. Keep a diary or journal of your mood changes so that any changes or patterns can be tracked.
• Stay social, visit friends, and stay busy with activities.
• To learn more: National Organization for Seasonal Affective Disorder, P.O. Box 40133, Washington, DC 20016; website: www.nosad.org.

MEDICATION—Antidepressants may be prescribed.

ACTIVITY
• Stay as active as your energy permits. Physical activity is almost always good for mood disorders.
• Get outside as much as possible, especially in the early morning light.
• Take vacations in the winter months to places that are warm and sunny.

DIET—Eat a normal well-balanced diet to maintain good health.

 CALL YOUR DOCTOR IF

• You or a family member has symptoms of seasonal affective disorder.
• Symptoms continue or worsen, despite treatment.

SEBACEOUS CYST
(Epidermoid Cyst; Wens)

 GENERAL INFORMATION

DEFINITION—A cyst is a closed sac beneath the skin. A sebaceous cyst is filled with a soft substance made up of oil and dead cells. It may occur with acne.

BODY PARTS INVOLVED—Skin of the trunk, face, neck and scalp.

SEX OR AGE MOST AFFECTED—Both sexes; all ages, but most common in adolescents and adults.

SIGNS & SYMPTOMS—A cyst with the following features:
• The cyst has sloped sides or is dome-shaped, is firm, and has a smooth surface. It normally does not hurt.
• The cyst is whitish or skin-colored.
• If the cyst becomes injured or infected, it may become bright red and painful.

CAUSES—Sebaceous cysts are caused by clogged hair follicles. They may enlarge from hormone changes or injury.

RISK INCREASES WITH—No specific risk factors.

HOW TO PREVENT—Cannot be prevented at present.

 WHAT TO EXPECT

DIAGNOSTIC MEASURES
• Your own observation of symptoms.
• Your health care provider will diagnose the cyst based on its appearance.

APPROPRIATE HEALTH CARE
• If needed, cysts can be removed through a simple incision in the skin lying over the cyst. The sac is removed and the incision closed with stitches. If the entire cyst wall is removed, it should not recur.
• For infected cysts, an incision may be needed to drain the pus.

POSSIBLE COMPLICATIONS
• Infection of a cyst can turn into an abscess (be filled with pus).
• Cysts can recur after treatment.

PROBABLE OUTCOME
• Most cysts do not cause symptoms and do not require any medical treatment. Some may disappear on their own.
• Sometimes cysts can be irritated by clothes rubbing against them or by shaving. Cysts that are causing problems, are infected, or are injured can be treated.

 HOW TO TREAT

GENERAL MEASURES—Before surgery, apply warm compresses to the cyst to reduce inflammation and size.

MEDICATION
• Drugs are usually not necessary for this disorder.
• If a cyst becomes infected, antibiotics may be prescribed.
• For some small, infected cysts, treatment may include an injection of a steroid drug.

ACTIVITY—No limits.

DIET—No special diet.

 CALL YOUR DOCTOR IF

• You or a family member has new skin growths or there is a change in any existing skin growth.
• After treatment, the treated skin becomes hot, red, and painful.
• The treated area does not appear to be healing well within one week.

SEVERE ACUTE RESPIRATORY SYNDROME (SARS)

 ## GENERAL INFORMATION

DEFINITION—Severe acute respiratory syndrome (SARS) is a type of respiratory illness. Respiratory refers to the lungs and breathing. In 2003, SARS was first diagnosed in Asia and then spread to other countries, including the United States.

BODY PARTS INVOLVED—Respiratory system.

SEX OR AGE MOST AFFECTED—Adults and children of both sexes.

SIGNS & SYMPTOMS
• Fever higher than 100.4°F (38.0°C). The fever starts 2 to 7 days after being infected.
• May include headache, an overall feeling of discomfort, and body aches.
• Some people also have mild breathing problems.
• After 2 to 7 days, patients may develop a dry cough and have more trouble breathing.

CAUSES
• The cause is a new form of the coronavirus. It is one of a family of viruses that in humans usually cause mild infections like common colds. How the new type came into being is unknown.
• SARS germs spread by close, person-to-person contact. A cough or sneeze can spread the germs into the nearby air and be breathed in by someone. They are also spread if you touch the skin of an infected person or objects that have the germs on them, and then touch your eyes, nose, or mouth. SARS may spread more broadly in the air or by other ways that are not now known. Also unknown is the time period that an infected person can spread the germs to others.

RISK INCREASES WITH
• Travel to an area where the infection is present.
• Close contact with an infected person.

HOW TO PREVENT
• Check for any travel precautions for the area you plan to visit. The Centers for Disease Control & Prevention has updated information about travelers health; website: www.cdc.gov or toll free hotline (877) 394-8747.
• If you are in an area where this infection is present, wash your hands often or use alcohol-based hand wipes. Avoid crowds if possible.
• Wearing a facemask or other protective device may be helpful.

 ## WHAT TO EXPECT

DIAGNOSTIC MEASURES
• The symptoms for SARS are like those for other viral illnesses, such as cold and flu. If you have been exposed to SARS or have recently been traveling, and symptoms occur, seek medical help right away. Advise any health care provider in advance of your visit about the SARS exposure. Arrangements can be made, as needed, to prevent the spread of germs to others.
• Your health care provider will do a physical exam and have blood and urine studies done.
• An x-ray and other medical tests may be needed. Specific tests to diagnose SARS are still being developed.

APPROPRIATE HEALTH CARE
• Once a SARS infection is diagnosed, hospital treatment is needed. This may be in an intensive care unit.
• Treatment is aimed at assistance with the breathing problems. Oxygen is provided through a facemask. Some patients require breathing support with a ventilator (a device to help the lungs).
• Research is ongoing to develop a rapid diagnostic test, effective drug therapies, and a vaccine for the disease.

POSSIBLE COMPLICATIONS
• Severe breathing problems (may lead to death).
• It is unknown if people who recover from SARS suffer permanent lung damage.

PROBABLE OUTCOME—Outcome varies depending on the severity of the symptoms. Most people will recover from the infection.

 ## HOW TO TREAT

GENERAL MEASURES—None specific.

MEDICATION—Drugs are not available to cure the infection. Drugs to treat the symptoms will be given while in the hospital.

ACTIVITY—Resume normal activities slowly once symptoms improve.

DIET—May require feeding through a vein (IV) while in the hospital. Then return to a regular diet with recovery.

 ## CALL YOUR DOCTOR IF

You or a family member has symptoms of SARS. You should seek emergency care. Be sure to advise any health care providers in advance of your visit about the SARS exposure.

SEXUAL DYSFUNCTION, FEMALE

 GENERAL INFORMATION

DEFINITION—Female sexual dysfunction is not a disease. It is a term used to describe problems with sexual desire, arousal, orgasm, and sexual pain in women. It can affect women of any age. Over 40% of women have sexual problems at some time in their lives.

BODY PARTS INVOLVED—Brain and central nervous system; autonomic nervous system.

SEX OR AGE MOST AFFECTED—Sexually active women.

SIGNS & SYMPTOMS
- Lack of sexual desire or no interest in sex.
- Not able to feel aroused. There may be no sexual response in the body, or response may start, and then stop.
- Failure to achieve orgasm (climax), even when sexually aroused.
- Pain with sexual intercourse.

CAUSES—Sexual dysfunction is usually due to a variety of factors involving a woman's mind, body, and sexual partner.

RISK INCREASES WITH
- Depression, stress, or anxiety. Worries about family problems, finances, career, childcare, marital problems.
- Previous sexual abuse or trauma.
- Feelings of shame or guilt about sex.
- Pregnancy (during and after); fear of pregnancy.
- Lack of experience or knowledge about sex on the part of either partner.
- Male partner is having sexual problems.
- Not enough or ineffective foreplay. Feeling boredom with the same sexual routine.
- Couples differ in what they expect from sex, and their attitude toward sex.
- Other people close by in the home (children, mother-in-law).
- Fatigue (e.g., working or caring for children).
- Medical conditions such as cancer, diabetes, heart or thyroid disease, arthritis, and others.
- Drug abuse, including alcohol.
- Heavy smoking.
- Gynecology factors (infection or other disorders).
- Side effects of some drugs.
- Intercourse causes pain.
- Hysterectomy with removal of ovaries.
- Menopause (reduced estrogen levels affect sexual function).

HOW TO PREVENT
- Avoid the risk factors where possible.
- Get counseling for any anxieties or fears about sex.
- Maintain good communication with sexual partner.

 WHAT TO EXPECT

DIAGNOSTIC MEASURES
- Your health care provider will do a physical exam and ask questions about your symptoms and sexual history. It may be difficult to discuss your sexual concerns, but it is important to be open and honest.
- One or more medical tests may be done to check for any health problems.

APPROPRIATE HEALTH CARE
- Treatment will depend on the type(s) of dysfunction and the causes. The options for treatment steps will be discussed with you.
- Treatment will be provided for any medical disorder. This includes vaginal dryness or other problems that may cause painful intercourse.
- Counseling may be suggested for emotional problems such as stress, anxiety, depression, or sexual fears.
- Sex education may be needed for the woman and her partner. Learning about the female anatomy, sexual response, and arousal can help both partners.
- Treatment with a sex therapist may be helpful. Partners can learn techniques to help stimulate each other, perform self-stimulation, use sexual aids, new sexual routines, and communicate about sexual desires.
- A small vacuum device to improve blood flow to the clitoris may be prescribed. It may help sexual arousal.

POSSIBLE COMPLICATIONS
- Ongoing inability to enjoy sex.
- Relationship problems with partner.

PROBABLE OUTCOME—Some sexual problems go away on their own. Others are helped with treatment and the support of a caring partner. Some problems are more difficult to resolve.

 HOW TO TREAT

GENERAL MEASURES—None specific.

MEDICATION—Nonprescription vaginal lubricants may help. Hormone therapy may be prescribed. Other drugs are currently being tested for female sexual problems.

ACTIVITY—Exercise daily. It can reduce stress, improve your physical well-being, and may lead to better sexual health.

DIET—Eat a well-balanced diet.

 CALL YOUR DOCTOR IF

You or a family member has sexual dysfunction problems and wants help in resolving them.

SHIN SPLINTS
(Medial Tibia Stress Syndrome)

GENERAL INFORMATION

DEFINITION—Pain in the lower leg brought on by exercise or athletic activity. *Shin splints* is a common term that has been used to describe a variety of different leg injuries and it is generally being replaced by more specific diagnostic terms. The most common shin pain is caused by medial tibia stress syndrome (MTSS). The tibia (shin bone) is the larger of the two bones between the knee and the ankle. Medial refers to the inside part of the tibia (the most common injury site).

BODY PARTS INVOLVED—Legs.

SEX OR AGE MOST AFFECTED—Both sexes and almost all ages, from young children to older adults.

SIGNS & SYMPTOMS
• Pain, dull ache, or tenderness, and sometimes swelling, redness, and warmth, in the inner side (medial), back side (posterior), or outer side (anterior) of the lower leg.
• Pain may come and go as activity continues.

CAUSES—It is an overuse condition that can be caused by several factors. This shin problem usually develops gradually over weeks to months or could occur after a single excessive or intense training session. The problem is exercise-induced, but the specific cause of the pain is difficult to pinpoint. It may be periostitis (inflammation of the outer layer of the bone), myositis (muscle inflammation), tendinitis (inflammation of the muscle-tendon complex) or a combination of two of these. Faulty foot mechanics contribute to the injury.

RISK INCREASES WITH
• Sports involving running (e.g., runners and sprinters, football, basketball, soccer, and rugby players); jumping activities such as gymnastics or figure skating.
• Training too quickly, too hard, and too long.
• Training that involves switching from one type of sport to another (e.g., a triathlon).
• High impact aerobics or aerobic dancing.
• Poorly fitting or worn-out running shoes.
• Foot arches that are flat (pronated) or high (supinated), or imbalance in leg muscles.

HOW TO PREVENT
• Stretch and strengthen the leg muscles.
• Stretch before and after running.
• Avoid hard and uneven surfaces. Use soft surfaces such as dirt or grass for jogging, running, and walking.
• Warmup before an activity; avoid overtraining.
• Well-fitting shoes with good arch support.
• Try sports activities, such as swimming or biking that have less impact on the shins.

WHAT TO EXPECT

DIAGNOSTIC MEASURES
• Your own observation of symptoms.
• See your health care provider if self-care does not help. A physical exam and x-ray or bone scan may be done to rule out a stress fracture.

APPROPRIATE HEALTH CARE
• Self-care is all that is usually needed.
• Medical care (if needed) may involve drug therapy, physical therapy, and other treatments.

POSSIBLE COMPLICATIONS
• May progress to stress fracture.
• Shin splints may recur.

PROBABLE OUTCOME—Healing time may range from a few days to two weeks to two months.

HOW TO TREAT

GENERAL MEASURES
• Use ice massage over the painful area (in a circle about the size of a softball). Do this for 15 minutes at a time three or four times a day.
• After a few days, apply heat if you want. Use hot soaks, hot showers, or heating pads.
• Massage area gently and often to provide comfort and decrease swelling.

MEDICATION
• For minor discomfort, use nonprescription anti-inflammatory drugs such as aspirin (not for children) or ibuprofen.
• Other nonsteroidal anti-inflammatory drugs may be prescribed.

ACTIVITY
• Discontinue sports or exercise until the pain is gone. Return to pre-injury activity level slowly.
• In some cases, severe pain may require the use of crutches for a short period of time.
• If foot mechanics are a problem, such as excessive pronation, special shoes, heel lifts, or orthotics (inserts for the shoes) may be prescribed. Orthotics can be nonprescription products. In some cases, custom-made orthotics are recommended.
• Try different exercises (cross-training) such as swimming or walking in water, bicycle riding, or regular walking.

DIET—No special diet.

CALL YOUR DOCTOR IF

• You or a family member has painful shin splints.
• Mild symptoms don't improve in 2 to 3 weeks.

SHOCK

GENERAL INFORMATION

DEFINITION—The heart and blood vessels are unable to supply enough blood and oxygen to meet the demands of the body. Shock can be caused by several different conditions and is a medical emergency.

BODY PARTS INVOLVED—Whole body.

SEX OR AGE MOST AFFECTED—Both sexes; all ages.

SIGNS & SYMPTOMS
• Cold hands and feet.
• Fast, weak pulse.
• Not knowing where you are or confusion.
• Anxiety with feelings of impending doom.
• Skin that is pale, moist and sweaty.
• Shortness of breath and rapid breathing.
• Lack of urination.
• Low blood pressure.

CAUSES
• Hypovolemic shock is a sudden loss of blood or body fluids. The bleeding may be visible, or bleeding that occurs inside the body. Sudden fluid loss occurs with severe burns, severe vomiting, and/or diarrhea.
• Cardiogenic shock is due to damaged heart function.(includes heart attack or heart failure).
• Anaphylactic shock is an adverse reaction to a substance to which the body is sensitive. These can include drugs such as penicillin, insect bites, or food allergies.
• Septic shock is caused by blood poisoning or major infections in the body.
• Neurogenic shock is caused by damage to the nervous system, such as a spinal cord injury.
• Shock can be caused by exposure to extreme heat or cold for too long.

RISK INCREASES WITH
• Serious injury, illness, or surgery.
• Heart disorders.
• Contact with a substance you are allergic to.
• Overdose of mind-altering drugs.
• Excess alcohol consumption.

HOW TO PREVENT
• You can't prevent shock. You can avoid the risk factors where possible.
• You may be able to help someone in shock, or prevent shock, until emergency medical help is available if you are prepared. To prepare yourself:
  - Take a first-aid course.
  - If you or a family member has a severe allergy, be sure there is an emergency kit available and that you know how to give the injection.
  - Carry emergency supplies, such as a first-aid kit, in your car or truck.
• Wear a medical alert tag if you have a serious medical or allergy problem.

WHAT TO EXPECT

DIAGNOSTIC MEASURES—A careful physical exam will be done.

APPROPRIATE HEALTH CARE
• Emergency care in the hospital will include fluids given through a vein, oxygen for breathing support, and drug therapy.
• Treatment will be provided for the injuries or other causes of the shock. The patient will be watched closely for any complications until the risk is over.

POSSIBLE COMPLICATIONS
• Heart or lungs are unable to function.
• Permanent brain damage.
• Death.

PROBABLE OUTCOME—The outcome will depend on how severe the symptoms are and receiving prompt treatment.

HOW TO TREAT

GENERAL MEASURES—Get emergency help right away. Shock requires immediate medical care.

MEDICATION
• If shock is from blood or fluid loss, treatment includes blood transfusion or fluids given through a vein.
• If blood pressure is at a dangerous low level, drugs to raise blood pressure may be given.
• If infection is present, antibiotics will be used.

ACTIVITY—Rest in bed until completely recovered. Move legs actively while in bed to decrease the likelihood of blood clots.

DIET—Diet will depend on your medical condition.

CALL YOUR DOCTOR IF

You or a family member has symptoms of shock or observe them in someone else. Call 911 immediately. This is a life-threatening emergency!

ILLNESS & DISORDERS

SHOULDER, FROZEN
(Adhesive Capsulitis)

GENERAL INFORMATION

DEFINITION—A general term used to describe pain and stiffness in the shoulder joint that leads to loss of shoulder movement. Adhesive capsulitis is the medical term. It can last a few months to a year or longer.

BODY PARTS INVOLVED—It affects the shoulder capsule (tissues surrounding the ball and socket joint) and the ligaments that attach the shoulder bones to each other. Sometimes both shoulders are affected.

SEX OR AGE MOST AFFECTED—It occurs more often in people over age 40, and in women more than men.

SIGNS & SYMPTOMS
• Stage 1 (painful)—Ache or pain in the shoulder, often mild. It progresses to severe pain that interferes with sleep and normal activities. Pain gets worse with shoulder movement. This stage may last for 2 to 9 months.
• Stage 2 (adhesive)—Less pain occurs, but stiffness increases in the shoulder. This prevents normal range of motion movement. Reduced movement increases stiffness. This stage may last 4 to 12 months.
• Stage 3 (recovery)—Healing starts. For most patients, the range of motion begins to increase. This stage may last for 12 months or up to several years.

CAUSES—The cause is unknown. It may be due to an inflammatory process. Some cases may result from an injury that leads to lack of use due to pain. Adhesions (type of scar tissue) grow between the joint surfaces, causing limited motion. There is less synovial fluid (normally it lubricates the shoulder joint to help it move).

RISK INCREASES WITH
• Shoulder injury, fracture, or trauma (could be very minor).
• Diabetes.
• Heart disease, stroke or lung conditions, thyroid problems, Parkinson's disease, and depression.
• Being immobile (prolonged inactivity) due to trauma, overuse injuries, or surgery.

HOW TO PREVENT
• Obtain early medical treatment for any shoulder injury, pain, or stiffness.
• Do regular stretching exercises.

WHAT TO EXPECT

DIAGNOSTIC MEASURES
• Your own observation of symptoms.

• Your health care provider will do an exam of the affected shoulder and ask questions about your symptoms and activities.
• X-rays or other tests may be done to confirm the diagnosis.

APPROPRIATE HEALTH CARE
• Exercises and drugs (sometimes) are used to help restore joint movement and reduce pain.
• Physical therapy and stretching exercises will help improve joint movement. They may be uncomfortable to do, but should not cause excess pain. You will be instructed about exercises to do at home.
• Other treatments may include acupuncture, ultrasound therapy, and electrical stimulation.
• Manipulation may help some patients. This procedure can be done under a local or general anesthesia. The shoulder joint capsule is stretched to break up scar tissue. It helps right away, but exercise is still needed.
• If other treatment does not help the symptoms after several months, shoulder surgery may be an option. It is usually done with an arthroscope (small instrument) through tiny incisions.

POSSIBLE COMPLICATIONS—Some permanent shoulder disability and pain may occur despite treatment.

PROBABLE OUTCOME—Most patients can expect increased shoulder mobility and function with time and treatment. It may take many months to see the improvement. You may need help in performing daily activities that require lifting your arms.

HOW TO TREAT

GENERAL MEASURES—Apply heat (warm compresses or heating pad) to the affected area or apply ice packs if it feels better.

MEDICATION
• Nonsteroidal anti-inflammatory drugs or muscle relaxers may be prescribed. Injections of cortisone or local anesthesia into joints may help to reduce severe pain.
• For minor pain, you may use nonprescription drugs such as ibuprofen.

ACTIVITY
• Follow instructions for home exercises.
• Start to resume athletic or fitness activities as symptoms ease.

DIET—No special diet.

CALL YOUR DOCTOR IF

• You or a family member has symptoms of a frozen shoulder.
• Symptoms get worse after treatment starts.

SICKLE CELL ANEMIA & SICKLE CELL TRAIT

 GENERAL INFORMATION

DEFINITION—Sickle cell anemia is an inherited blood disorder. It causes chronic anemia, periods of severe pain, high risk of infections, and general poor health. People with the sickle cell trait usually have no symptoms of the disorder, but may pass it onto their children.

BODY PARTS INVOLVED—Bone marrow; lymph glands; spleen; liver; thymus.

SEX OR AGE MOST AFFECTED—Usually begins around 6 months of age and lasts a lifetime.

SIGNS & SYMPTOMS
- Swollen hands or feet, fever, and paleness.
- Shortness of breath; rapid heartbeat; fatigue.
- Episodes of pain in any organ or joint.
- Frequent infections, especially pneumonia.
- Eye problems.
- Delayed growth and development in children.
- Jaundice (yellow skin and/or eyes).

CAUSES—A gene that causes defective hemoglobin (blood cells). The gene occurs mostly in African Americans (about 8% are carriers) and some Hispanics. Defective hemoglobin changes blood cells from smooth and round to a stiff, sickle shape. These abnormal cells cause blood flow in blood vessels to become blocked. This leads to the symptoms and sickle crisis (severe pain episode). A chronic short supply of red blood cells causes anemia.

RISK INCREASES WITH—Family history of sickle cell anemia. If both parents have the gene, their child may have sickle cell anemia. If one parent has the gene, the child will not get the disorder, but may carry the sickle cell trait.

HOW TO PREVENT
- If you have a family history of sickle cell anemia, ask for testing. If the condition is present, obtain genetic counseling before starting a family.
- Early pregnancy test to see if the baby has inherited the double-dose gene (both parents are carriers).

 WHAT TO EXPECT

DIAGNOSTIC MEASURES
- Blood tests can diagnose sickle cell anemia.
- Screening tests are done on newborns in most states. If the screening test shows sickle hemoglobin, a second test is done to confirm diagnosis.

APPROPRIATE HEALTH CARE
- A health care provider with special knowledge of this disorder may be recommended for ongoing health care.

- Counseling may be helpful in adapting to this condition, especially for children. Support groups may help.
- Hospital care may be required at times of severe attacks for intravenous (IV) therapy and oxygen therapy and, sometimes, blood transfusions.
- Bone marrow transplants may be an option.

POSSIBLE COMPLICATIONS—Infections, other medical problems, stroke, and death.

PROBABLE OUTCOME—There is no cure for sickle cell anemia. Life span is reduced, but has gradually increased to over 40 years. More effective treatments are helping.

 HOW TO TREAT

GENERAL MEASURES
- Home treatment involves good nutrition and hygiene, rest as needed, and steps to avoid infection and stress. Encourage a child to lead as normal a life as possible.
- Some things may worsen symptoms. These include an injury or infection, pregnancy, surgery, traveling to high altitudes (as in driving up a mountain, or an airplane trip).
- See your health care and dental care providers on a regular basis. Keep all vaccines and flu shots up to date.
- Wear a medical alert type bracelet or pendant to identify the medical disorder.

MEDICATION
- No drugs are effective for the disease. Drugs are prescribed to treat symptoms and prevent complications. Adults should get prompt treatment for infections.
- Use nonsteroidal anti-inflammatory drugs or acetaminophen for pain.
- Penicillin started in infancy helps prevent infection.
- Hydroxyurea helps reduce frequency of painful crisis. It may be prescribed for certain patients.
- Daily vitamin supplements are often needed.

ACTIVITY
- Avoid strenuous exercise. Avoid being out in very hot or cold temperatures. Rest in bed during acute attacks.
- Activity may be somewhat limited due to chronic anemia and poor muscular development.

DIET—Eat a healthy diet. Drink plenty of fluids.

 CALL YOUR DOCTOR IF

- After diagnosis, any signs of infection occur, pain increases, or symptoms develop that cause concern.
- You want to know if you have sickle cell gene.

SILICOSIS

GENERAL INFORMATION

DEFINITION—A chronic lung condition due to breathing silica (quartz) dust. Silicosis is the most common form of pneumoconiosis. This is a group of lung diseases caused by inhaling certain mineral dusts.

BODY PARTS INVOLVED—Lungs.

SEX OR AGE MOST AFFECTED—It usually affects men (due to occupational exposure).

SIGNS & SYMPTOMS
Early symptoms:
- Shortness of breath.
- Cough that produces little or no sputum.
- General ill feeling.

Later symptoms:
- Fitful sleep.
- Appetite loss.
- Chest pain.
- Hoarseness.
- Coughing blood.
- Symptoms of heart failure.
- Bluish nails.

CAUSES—Chronic breathing in of small particles of free crystalline silica dust. The dust may be invisible to the naked eye. It is so light that it can remain in the air for a long time. The disorder causes lung inflammation and then scarring of lung tissues. It usually takes 20 to 30 years of exposure to develop silicosis. If exposure is extremely high, it may take less than 10 years.

RISK INCREASES WITH
- Work such as mining, granite-cutting, concrete mixing and drilling, manufacturing pottery, metal-grinding, tunneling, sand-blasting, and others.
- Smoking adds to possible lung damage.

HOW TO PREVENT
- Be aware of the risks and follow all training and preventive instructions provided for your work. Get health screenings on a regular basis.
- Employers are required to take certain preventive measures to reduce exposure for workers.
- Don't smoke.

WHAT TO EXPECT

DIAGNOSTIC MEASURES
- Your health care provider will do a physical exam and ask questions about your symptoms and activities. Be sure to tell your provider about your work history and any exposure to silica.
- Medical tests may include x-ray of the chest, pulmonary function tests, and others to confirm the diagnosis and check for complications.

APPROPRIATE HEALTH CARE
- No specific treatment is known for silicosis. Drugs and lung therapy may help the symptoms and treat complications.
- Chest physical therapy (such as controlled coughing) and bronchial drainage help clear secretions. Get medical training about these procedures.

POSSIBLE COMPLICATIONS
- Pulmonary tuberculosis (late stages of silicosis).
- Chronic obstructive pulmonary disease (COPD).
- Lung fibrosis (scar tissue).
- Cor pulmonale.

PROBABLE OUTCOME—There is no cure and silicosis causes increasing lung problems. Outcome will vary for each individual depending on amount of lung damage. Symptoms can sometimes be relieved or controlled.

HOW TO TREAT

GENERAL MEASURES
- Avoid any further exposure to silica dust.
- Quit smoking. Find a way to stop that works.
- Obtain medical treatment for any respiratory infection, including the common cold.
- Get influenza and pneumococcal vaccines.
- Consider moving to a warm, dry climate if you have advanced disease.
- To learn more: American Lung Association, 61 Broadway, 6th Floor, New York, NY 10006, (800) 586-4872; website: www.lungusa.org.

MEDICATION
- Antibiotics may be prescribed for infections.
- Bronchodilators (inhaled or oral) with inhalation therapy may be prescribed. This is supervised at first by an inhalation therapist.
- For minor discomfort, you may use nonprescription drugs, such as acetaminophen or aspirin.

ACTIVITY—No limits, except those caused by symptoms.

DIET—No special diet. Maintain high fluid intake.

CALL YOUR DOCTOR IF

- You or a family member has symptoms of silicosis.
- Fever, increased chest pain or breathing problems, blood in the sputum, or other new symptoms develop.

SINUSITIS

GENERAL INFORMATION

DEFINITION—Infection or inflammation (redness and soreness) of the sinuses. Sinuses are air-filled spaces that make mucus to help clean the air we breathe. They are located behind the eyebrows, inside each cheekbone, and between the eyes. Sinuses open into the nose for mucus and air exchange. Sinusitis can be acute (short illness), or chronic if it continues for several weeks or recurs often.

BODY PARTS INVOLVED—The 8 sinuses (mucosa-lined air pockets) located within the facial bone structure and connected to the nose. Usually involved are the ethmoidal sinuses, located between the eyes; and the maxillary sinuses, located in the cheekbone.

SEX OR AGE MOST AFFECTED—Both sexes; all ages.

SIGNS & SYMPTOMS
• Nasal congestion with white or greenish-yellow (sometimes blood-tinged) discharge.
• Feeling of pressure inside the head.
• Eye pain.
• Headache that is worse in the morning or when bending forward.
• Cheek pain that may resemble a toothache.
• Post-nasal drip.
• Cough (sometimes) that is usually non-productive.
• Disturbed sleep (sometimes).
• Fever (sometimes).
• Swelling of the sinus openings, blocking the discharge, and increasing pain.

CAUSES
• Bacterial infection. A common cold or allergic reaction can cause the sinuses to swell and increase the amount of mucus they produce. Bacteria begin to grow in the excess mucus in the swollen sinuses and causes the symptoms.
• Fungal infection, such as aspergillosis, may occur in people who have a weakened immune system.
• Allergies that cause swelling of sinuses.

RISK INCREASES WITH
• Common cold or other viral illness.
• Weak immune system due to illness or drugs.
• Swimming or diving.
• Using nasal decongestant sprays too often.
• Growths (polyps) in the nose or a deviated septum.
• People with asthma or an allergic disease.
• Smoking.
• People with cystic fibrosis.
• Dental problems.

HOW TO PREVENT—Prompt treatment of any cold or other viral infection may reduce the risk.

WHAT TO EXPECT

DIAGNOSTIC MEASURES
• Your own observation of symptoms.
• Your health care provider will do a physical exam and ask questions about your symptoms and recent illnesses, such as a cold. Diagnosis can usually be made based on this information.
• Medical tests may be done in certain cases, such as repeated infections.

APPROPRIATE HEALTH CARE
• Drug treatment is aimed at improving symptoms and curing the infection.
• Sinusitis not responding to drug treatment may require surgery to drain blocked sinuses.
• Surgery may be done for polyps or a deviated septum.
• Sinusitis due to a fungus may require surgery.

POSSIBLE COMPLICATIONS
• Sinusitis may become chronic.
• Rarely, infection may spread into bones, eyes, or brain.

PROBABLE OUTCOME—Will often clear up on its own, but may be treated with drugs, or surgery if needed.

HOW TO TREAT

GENERAL MEASURES—Apply moist heat to relieve pain in the sinuses and nose. Take a warm shower once or twice a day.

MEDICATION
• For stuffy nose, use nonprescription nasal decongestants. Limit use to 3 days in a row. Saline nasal sprays may be used several times a day. Nonprescription antihistamines are sometimes helpful.
• For minor pain, you may use drugs such as acetaminophen.
• Drugs to reduce congestion may be prescribed.
• Antibiotics for a bacterial infection may be prescribed.

ACTIVITY—Resume your normal activities gradually. Exercise can help to clear your head.

DIET—No special diet, but drink extra fluids to help thin secretions.

CALL YOUR DOCTOR IF

• You or a family member has symptoms of sinusitis.
• The following occur during treatment:
  - Fever; bleeding from the nose; severe headache.
  - Swelling of the face (forehead, eyes, side of the nose, or cheek).

SJÖGREN'S SYNDROME

GENERAL INFORMATION

DEFINITION—One of a group of autoimmune disorders. In these disorders, the immune system by mistake attacks the body itself. Sjögren's syndrome mainly affects the glands that produce moisture, but it can affect the body as a whole. Symptoms may be mild or severe.

BODY PARTS INVOLVED—May involve only the exocrine (mucus secreting) glands or involve other organs, such as the lung or kidneys.

SEX OR AGE MOST AFFECTED—It occurs mostly in women (about 90% of cases) with an average age of 50.

SIGNS & SYMPTOMS
* Dry eyes. It may cause foreign body sensation, gritty feeling, redness, burning, sensitivity to light, itching, feeling that there is a "film" across the field of vision, and eye discharge.
* Dry mouth, nose, and throat. This can cause problems in swallowing and talking, changes in taste, thirst, ulcers (sores), or dental cavities. Nosebleeds, hoarseness, chronic nonproductive cough, ear infection, other infections may occur.
* Vaginal dryness can cause painful intercourse.
* Dry skin.
* Severe fatigue.
* Parotid glands become enlarged (sometimes referred to as "chipmunk face" or "chipmunk cheeks").
* Joint pain and stiffness.
* Other symptoms include hair loss, low-grade fever, itching skin, and muscle aches or pain.

CAUSES—Unknown. Genetic, immunologic, hormonal and environmental factors may contribute to its cause. Viral infection may trigger the disorder in some people. It may occur alone or along with other autoimmune disorders such as rheumatoid arthritis, scleroderma, systemic lupus erythematosus, or polymyositis.

RISK INCREASES WITH
* Family history of autoimmune disorders.
* Having other autoimmune disorders.

HOW TO PREVENT—No specific measures.

WHAT TO EXPECT

DIAGNOSTIC MEASURES
* Your health care provider will do a physical exam and ask questions about your symptoms.
* Medical tests of blood, tear production, saliva production, an eye exam, and others may be done to confirm the diagnosis.

APPROPRIATE HEALTH CARE
* Treatment is directed to relieving the dryness symptoms and preventing complications.
* Home care is usually all that is needed.

POSSIBLE COMPLICATIONS
* Damage to the kidneys, blood vessels, lungs, liver, eyes, pancreas, and brain may occur.
* Children born to some younger women with the disorder may be at risk for heart defects.

PROBABLE OUTCOME—Sjögren's syndrome is a chronic disorder. Symptoms sometimes stay the same, worsen, or sometimes disappear for a period. Treatment can relieve symptoms and help prevent complications.

HOW TO TREAT

GENERAL MEASURES
* Brush and floss teeth daily. Use a fluoride mouthwash. See the dentist for frequent checkups.
* Wear sunglasses when outside to help protect eyes from dust, wind, and strong light. See your eye care provider for regular exams.
* Warm compresses or heating pad may help ease joint pain or swollen gland discomfort.
* To learn more: Sjögren's Syndrome Foundation, 8120 Woodmont Ave., Suite 530, Bethesda, MD 20814; (800) 475-6473 (voice mail); website: www.sjogrens.org.

MEDICATION
* Use artificial tears for dry eyes. Use an eye ointment at night. Other drugs for dry eyes may be prescribed.
* Use nonprescription saliva substitutes and mouth-coating products for dry mouth.
* Vaginal lubricant (not petroleum jelly) will help vaginal dryness.
* Use aspirin or other nonsteroidal anti-inflammatory drugs for joint pain and muscle aches.
* Avoid decongestants and antihistamines. They can cause dry mouth or eyes.
* Steroids and other drugs may be prescribed.

ACTIVITY—Mild exercise daily helps keep joints flexible.

DIET
* Chew sugarless gum or suck on sugarless candies.
* Drink or sip fluids all during the day.
* If mouth soreness prevents eating regular foods, drink high-calorie, high-protein liquid supplements.

CALL YOUR DOCTOR IF

* You or a family member has symptoms of Sjögren's syndrome.
* Symptoms don't improve with treatment.

SKIN CANCER, BASAL-CELL

GENERAL INFORMATION

DEFINITION—Skin cancer in the skin's basal layer. The basal layer is at the bottom of the skin's outer layer (epidermis). It is the most common type of skin cancer.

BODY PARTS INVOLVED—Usually the skin of face, ears, backs of hands, shoulders and arms.

SEX OR AGE MOST AFFECTED—Adults over age 40, and men more often than women.

SIGNS & SYMPTOMS
• A sore that does not heal within 3 weeks. It may bleed, ooze, or have a crust.
• An area or patch of skin that is reddish or irritated. It might have a crust.
• A shiny, pearly looking bump on the skin. The color is usually pink, red, or white. On some people, the color may be tan, black or brown, and look like a mole.
• A skin growth that is pink with a slightly raised, rolled border. The center is crusted and is lower than the border. Tiny blood vessels may be seen, as it grows larger.
• An area that looks like a white or yellow scar. The skin is shiny and looks tight. This type is more rare.

CAUSES—Chronic sun exposure. The ultraviolet light in sunlight damages the skin, and causes the cells to change and grow into skin cancers.

RISK INCREASES WITH
• Excess sunlight exposure from work or play.
• People with fair skin and blue eyes.
• Living in an area where there is lots of sunlight.

HOW TO PREVENT
• Limit exposure to sunlight. Protect skin with a hat, clothing, and sunscreen with SPF of 15 or more. Reapply sunscreen every 2 hours during sun exposure.
• Perform a skin self-exam once a month. Check for new growths or changes in growths already present.

WHAT TO EXPECT

DIAGNOSTIC MEASURES
• Your own observation of symptoms.
• Your health care provider will examine the affected skin area.
• All or part of the affected skin tissue may be removed for biopsy. The tissue is viewed under a microscope to see if it is cancerous.

APPROPRIATE HEALTH CARE
• Treatment varies with appearance, extent, and location of the skin cancer. The treatment method chosen will often be decided by you and your health care provider together. Some

options that may be discussed are:
- Curettage and electrodesiccation—local anesthetic applied, then cutting out or shaving of the cancer, followed by high-frequency electrical current to destroy tissue with heat.
- Surgical excision—local anesthetic is applied, then skin is marked for surgery, and a scalpel is used for the excision.
- Moh's surgery—a special type of surgery is used to treat high-risk cancers, especially on the head and face.
- Cryosurgery—use of liquid nitrogen to freeze and kill the cells. A local anesthetic is sometimes used.
- Laser treatment—is sometimes used.
- Radiation treatment—used if cancer location requires it, such as locations near lips and eyelids.
- Photodynamic therapy uses drugs and special light.
• Healthy skin from elsewhere on the body may be used to replace skin removed in surgery (skin graft).

POSSIBLE COMPLICATIONS
• Skin cancer may recur in the same place after surgery.
• Scarring from the surgery.

PROBABLE OUTCOME—The cancer seldom spreads beyond the skin and is almost always harmless. It is curable in just about all cases. People who have had skin cancer are at higher risk for new skin cancers elsewhere on the skin.

HOW TO TREAT

GENERAL MEASURES
• Your health care provider will advise you of any follow-up care needed after the procedure.
• To learn more: American Cancer Society, (800) ACS-2345; website: www.cancer.org or National Cancer Institute, (800) 4-CANCER; website: www.nci.nih.gov.

MEDICATION
• Use nonprescription pain-relief drugs for minor pain.
• Skin cancer drugs (chemotherapy) applied to the skin may be prescribed.
• Antibiotic for the skin to prevent infection may be prescribed.

ACTIVITY—No limits.

DIET—No special diet.

CALL YOUR DOCTOR IF

• You or a family member has signs of skin cancer.
• After treatment, the treated skin becomes hot, red, and painful, or previous symptoms recur.

SKIN CANCER, SQUAMOUS-CELL

GENERAL INFORMATION

DEFINITION—A skin cancer in the squamous cells that make up the skin's outer layer (epithelium). It is the second most common type of skin cancer.

BODY PARTS INVOLVED—The cancer usually involves the skin of the face, ears, backs of hands, shoulders, and arms.

SEX OR AGE MOST AFFECTED—Adults over age 40 and men more than women.

SIGNS & SYMPTOMS
• A sore that does not heal within 3 weeks. It may bleed or ooze or have a crust.
• An area or patch of skin that is reddish or irritated. It might have a crust.
• A shiny, pearly looking skin bump. The color is usually pink, red, or white. On some people, the color may be tan, black, or brown and look like a mole.
• A skin growth that is pink with a slightly raised, rolled border. The center is crusted and is lower than the border. Tiny blood vessels may be seen as it grows larger.
• An area that looks like a white or yellow scar. The skin is shiny and looks tight. This type is more rare.

CAUSES—Chronic sun exposure. The ultraviolet light in sunlight damages the skin and causes the cells to change and grow into skin cancers.

RISK INCREASES WITH
• Excess sunlight exposure from work or play.
• People with fair skin and blue eyes.
• Living in an area where there is lots of sunlight.

HOW TO PREVENT
• Limit exposure to sunlight. Protect skin with a hat, clothing and sunscreen with SPF of 15 or more. Reapply sunscreen every 2 hours during sun exposure.
• Perform a skin self-exam once a month. Check for new growths or changes in growths already present.

WHAT TO EXPECT

DIAGNOSTIC MEASURES
• Your own observation of symptoms.
• Your health care provider will examine the skin growth for any abnormal appearance.
• All, or part, of the skin tissue may be removed for biopsy. The tissue is viewed under a microscope to see if it is cancerous.

APPROPRIATE HEALTH CARE
• Treatment varies with appearance, extent, and location of the skin cancer. The treatment method chosen will often be decided by you and your health care provider together. Some options that may be discussed are:
  - Curettage and electrodesiccation—local anesthetic applied, then cutting out, or shaving, of the cancer, followed by high-frequency electrical current to destroy tissue with heat.
  - Surgical excision—local anesthetic is applied, then skin is marked for surgery, and a scalpel is used for the excision.
  - Moh's surgery—a special type of surgery is used to treat high-risk cancers, especially on the head and face.
  - Cryosurgery—use of liquid nitrogen to freeze and kill the cells. A local anesthetic is sometimes used.
  - Laser treatment—is sometimes used.
  - Radiation treatment—used if cancer location requires it, such as locations near the lips and eyelids.
  - Photodynamic therapy uses drugs and special light.
• Healthy skin from elsewhere on the body may be used to replace skin removed in surgery (skin graft).

POSSIBLE COMPLICATIONS
• Skin cancer may recur in the same place after surgery.
• Scarring from the surgery.
• Cancer may spread to nearby lymph nodes.

PROBABLE OUTCOME—It is curable in just about all cases. People who have had skin cancer are at higher risk for new skin cancers elsewhere on the skin.

HOW TO TREAT

GENERAL MEASURES
• Your health care provider will advice you of any follow up care needed after the procedure.
• To learn more: American Cancer Society, (800) ACS-2345; website: www.cancer.org or National Cancer Institute, (800) 4-CANCER; website: www.nci.nih.gov.

MEDICATION
• Use nonprescription pain-relief drugs for minor pain.
• Skin cancer drugs (chemotherapy) applied to the skin may be prescribed.
• Antibiotic for the skin to prevent infection may be prescribed.

ACTIVITY—No limits.

DIET—No special diet.

CALL YOUR DOCTOR IF

• You or a family member has signs of skin cancer.
• After treatment, the treated skin becomes hot, red, and painful or previous symptoms recur.

SKIN LESIONS, BENIGN

GENERAL INFORMATION

DEFINITION—Noncancerous growths or areas of pigment or color change on the skin.

BODY PARTS INVOLVED—Skin.

SEX OR AGE MOST AFFECTED—Both sexes; all ages.

SIGNS & SYMPTOMS—Benign skin lesions fall into the following categories:
• Tags—Soft, flesh-colored buds, often on stalks, found on the neck, armpits or groin.
• Moles—Flat or raised lesions with clearly defined borders. Moles may be black, blue, red, yellow or brown.
• Cherry spots—Pinhead-sized, bright-red lesions on the chest or back.
• Strawberry marks—Bright-red raised areas in infants that grow until they are removed.
• Keloids—Thick, pale, irregular growths that begin at the site of a scar and gradually increase in size.
• Dermatofibromas—Rounded nodules, usually brownish and usually on the legs.
• Freckles—Flat, brownish spots of pinhead-size or larger.

CAUSES—Unknown, but most people have a few benign skin lesions.

RISK INCREASES WITH
• Family history of benign skin lesions.
• Pregnancy or use of oral contraceptives (brownish, freckle-like patches only).

HOW TO PREVENT—To decrease freckles, avoid excessive sun exposure. Other forms cannot be prevented.

WHAT TO EXPECT

DIAGNOSTIC MEASURES
• Your own observation of symptoms.
• Your health care provider will examine the skin growth for any abnormal appearance.
• Rarely, all, or part, of the skin tissue may be removed for biopsy. The tissue is viewed under a microscope to see if it is cancerous.

APPROPRIATE HEALTH CARE
• Usually, no treatment is needed.
• Surgery to remove lesions that enlarge, bleed, change color, are slow to heal or are unsightly. (See Skin Lesion Removal in Surgery section.)

POSSIBLE COMPLICATIONS—None expected for benign lesions.

PROBABLE OUTCOME—Treatment is usually unnecessary because most skin lesions are harmless. Suspicious or unsightly lesions can be removed surgically. If the affected area is large or in a prominent place, plastic surgery may be necessary after removal.

HOW TO TREAT

GENERAL MEASURES
• Examine skin lesions—especially those that are constantly rubbed or irritated by clothing—regularly for signs of growth, color change, pain, infection or bleeding.
• Makeup may be helpful in covering unsightly blemishes.
• If a lesion is removed, cover the area with a clean dressing and protect against injury. Ointments are rarely needed.

MEDICATION—Drugs are usually not needed.

ACTIVITY—No limits.

DIET—No special diet.

CALL YOUR DOCTOR IF

You or a family member has a skin lesion that enlarges, bleeds, changes color, is painful or doesn't heal.

ILLNESS & DISORDERS

SLEEP APNEA

GENERAL INFORMATION

DEFINITION—Episodes during sleep in which breathing stops for 10 seconds, or longer. In most cases, the person is unaware of the condition.

BODY PARTS INVOLVED—Central nervous system, upper airways (soft palate and tongue).

SEX OR AGE MOST AFFECTED—Both sexes; all ages. It is more common in men.

SIGNS & SYMPTOMS
* Periods of not breathing while asleep. This can happen hundreds of time each night. This causes less oxygen to get to the lungs and eventually triggers the lungs to suck in air. The person may make a gasping or snorting sound, but is usually not fully awake.
* Snoring and restless sleep.
* Daytime sleepiness and fatigue.
* Sexual dysfunction.
* Morning headaches.
* Mental or emotional problems such as memory loss, feeling irritable, poor judgment, or depression.

CAUSES
* Obstructive apnea. Breathing stops because the airway collapses and prevents air from getting into the lungs. Airway collapse may be due to several factors. There may be excess tissue at the back of the throat (large tonsils). The tongue may fall back and close off the airway. The muscles controlling the airway have become weakened.
* Central sleep apnea. Less common; caused by a problem in the central nervous system.
* Mixed apnea. The two types occur together.

RISK INCREASES WITH
* Overweight.
* Family history of sleep apnea.
* Persons having a large neck, recessed chin, or abnormal structure of the upper airway.
* Smoking.
* Use of alcohol or sedative drugs.
* African Americans, Pacific Islanders, and Mexicans.
* Acid reflux may contribute to sleep apnea.

HOW TO PREVENT—No specific preventive measures. Avoid risk factors such as smoking and alcohol.

WHAT TO EXPECT

DIAGNOSTIC MEASURES
* A bed partner may be the first to notice the symptoms.
* Your health care provider may do a physical exam and ask questions about your symptoms and lifestyle.

* Tests to check your airways may be done. An overnight study at a sleep center may be prescribed. Diagnostic devices that can be used at home may be recommended.

APPROPRIATE HEALTH CARE
* Treatment will depend on severity of apnea, other health problems, and daytime sleepiness.
* Steps should be taken to treat any underlying medical problems, such as heart or lung disorders. Lifestyle changes (such as weight loss) may be recommended.
* A special dental device may be prescribed.
* Devices to keep the airway open may help. Continuous positive airway pressure (CPAP) is often prescribed. A mask is worn over the nose and mouth during sleep. A small air-compressor forces air into the nasal passages to keep airway open.
* For severe apnea, surgery may be an option. Your health care provider will discuss options and the risks and benefits.

POSSIBLE COMPLICATIONS
* Heart failure, high blood pressure, and stroke. Other health effects may occur. It is unclear if apnea is the cause.
* Emotional problems; reduced quality of life.
* May affect bed partner's sleep quality, which leads to sleepiness and fatigue for that person.

PROBABLE OUTCOME—Outcome depends on the individual and how severe the symptoms are. Treatment can help improve apnea.

HOW TO TREAT

GENERAL MEASURES
* Sleep on your side, not your back. Pillows may help. Or sew a pocket on the back of your pajama top. Place a tennis ball in it.
* Quit smoking. Find a way to stop that works.
* To learn more: American Sleep Apnea Association, 1424 K St. NW. Ste. 302, Washington, DC 20005; (202) 293-3650 (not toll free); website: www.sleepapnea.org.

MEDICATION
* Specific drugs are not available for apnea. Drugs may be prescribed for depression, acid reflux, or other medical problems.
* Avoid drugs like sedatives, hypnotics, barbiturates, narcotics, and alcohol. Nasal strips do not treat apnea.

ACTIVITY—Exercise daily, but not right before bedtime.

DIET—Lose weight, if you are overweight.

CALL YOUR DOCTOR IF

You suspect you have sleep apnea or observe signs of sleep apnea in another family member.

SLEEP DISORDERS

 GENERAL INFORMATION

DEFINITION—Difficulty falling asleep or remaining asleep, being awake off and on, early-morning awakening, or a combination of these. Over 70 sleep disorders have been identified. The main one is insomnia.

BODY PARTS INVOLVED—Brain; may affect whole body.

SEX OR AGE MOST AFFECTED—Both sexes; all ages; more common in the elderly.

SIGNS & SYMPTOMS
* Feeling restless when trying to fall asleep.
* Brief sleep followed by wakefulness.
* Normal sleep until very early in the morning (such as 3AM to 4AM), then being wide awake (often with frightening thoughts).
* Periods of no sleep that alternate with periods of excess sleep.
* Feeling sleepy and tired during the day.

CAUSES—Sleep is a normal and natural function of the human body. Nerve cells in the brain control whether you are asleep or awake. When something affects the balance or normal rhythm of these nerve cells, changes in sleep patterns can occur.

RISK INCREASES WITH
Emotional problems:
* Depression.
* Anxiety.
* Stress.
Physical problems:
* Sleep apnea (a breathing problem), restless leg syndrome, or narcolepsy (daytime sleepiness).
* Allergies and early-morning wheezing. Other health problems that cause shortness of breath.
* Heartburn or gastroesophageal reflux disease (GERD).
* Painful disorders, such as fibromyalgia or arthritis.
* Medical problems that require urination or bowel movements during the night.
* Alcoholism.
* Use of certain drugs, such as decongestants.
* Drug abuse; includes overuse of sleep-inducers.
* Stimulants, such as coffee, tea, or cola drinks.
* Withdrawal from addictive substances.
* Obesity.
Lifestyle problems:
* Erratic work hours.
* New environment or location.
* Jet lag after travel.
* Noisy environment (includes a snoring partner).
* Lack of physical exercise.

HOW TO PREVENT—Maintain a healthy lifestyle that includes good sleep habits. Avoid risk factors of sleep disorders.

 WHAT TO EXPECT

DIAGNOSTIC MEASURES
* Your own observation of symptoms.
* If self-help fails, see your health care provider. A physical exam and medical tests may be done to help find the cause. An overnight sleep study may be prescribed.

APPROPRIATE HEALTH CARE—Your treatment plan will depend on the cause. It may include lifestyle changes, drugs, medical devices, or counseling.

POSSIBLE COMPLICATIONS
* Short-term sleep disorders may become chronic.
* Excess daytime sleepiness can affect all aspects of life.

PROBABLE OUTCOME—Most persons can establish good sleep patterns if the underlying cause of the problem is treated or stopped.

 HOW TO TREAT

GENERAL MEASURES
* Sometimes, self-care steps are all that is needed.
* Set a routine schedule of going to bed and waking up.
* Try to find ways to reduce stress in your life.
* Relax in a warm bath before bedtime.
* Create a comfortable sleep setting. It should be dark, cool, and quiet. Don't turn your bedroom into an office.
* Turn off your mind. Focus on peaceful and relaxing thoughts. Play soft music or relaxation tapes.
* Use ear plugs, eye shades, or an electric blanket.

MEDICATION
* You may be prescribed sleep-inducing drugs for a short period of time.
* Melatonin, a nonprescription product, may help some people. Ask your health care provider.
* Drugs may be prescribed if a specific disorder is diagnosed.

ACTIVITY—Exercise regularly, but not within 2 hours of bedtime.

DIET—Don't eat within 3 hours of bedtime if indigestion is a problem. A glass of warm milk before bedtime may help. Avoid caffeine.

 CALL YOUR DOCTOR IF

* You or a family member has symptoms of sleep a disorder and self-care does not help.
* Sleep problems don't improve, despite treatment.

ILLNESS & DISORDERS

SMALL-INTESTINE TUMOR
(Small-Bowel Neoplasms)

GENERAL INFORMATION

DEFINITION—Abnormal new growth in the small intestine or spread of abnormal cell growth from surrounding body structure. Most are benign; only 10% of small-intestine tumors are cancerous. Small-intestine tumors are uncommon compared to large intestine tumors.

BODY PARTS INVOLVED—Small intestine.

SEX OR AGE MOST AFFECTED—All ages, but most likely in adults.

SIGNS & SYMPTOMS
• No symptoms in many cases.
• Constipation.
• Tiredness and/or paleness.
• Blood in stools or black, tarry stools.
• Unexplained weight loss.
• nausea and vomiting.
• Jaundice (yellow skin and eyes).

CAUSES—Unknown.

RISK INCREASES WITH
• Celiac disease.
• Regional enteritis.
• Gardner syndrome.
• Peutz-Jeghers syndrome.
• Immunosuppression due to illness or drugs.

HOW TO PREVENT—No specific preventive measures.

WHAT TO EXPECT

DIAGNOSTIC MEASURES
• Your own observation of symptoms.
• Your health care provider will do a physical exam and ask about your symptoms.
• Medical tests may include blood studies for anemia, x-rays of the intestinal tract (upper and lower GI series), ultrasound and CT scan; endoscopy and enteroscopy. Tests are done to determine any cancerous growth and spread.

APPROPRIATE HEALTH CARE
• Surgery to remove the tumor if it is benign and causing symptoms and for malignant tumors.
• If the tumor is cancerous, radiation treatment. anticancer drugs (chemotherapy), or biologic therapy may be recommended.
• Chemotherapy uses drugs and radiation therapy uses radiation to attack the cancer cells. Biologic therapy uses the body's immune system to fight cancer.

POSSIBLE COMPLICATIONS
• Intestinal obstruction. Symptoms are: distended abdomen; severe colicky pain; nausea, vomiting; fever.
• Surgery complications may occur.
• Cancer may recur or spread to other parts of the body.

PROBABLE OUTCOME—With surgery the prognosis for benign tumors is good; with cancer, the prognosis depends on the type of cancer found and the success of treatment.

HOW TO TREAT

GENERAL MEASURES
• You will be advised of the follow-up care needed after surgery or other treatment.
• To learn more: American Cancer Society, (800) ACS-2345; website: www.cancer.org or National Cancer Institute, (800) 4-CANCER; website: www.nci.nih.gov.

MEDICATION
• Anticancer drugs may be prescribed.
• Cortisone drugs to reduce bowel inflammation that may cause obstruction.

ACTIVITY—No limits. Resume normal activities as soon as possible after surgery.

DIET—You may be prescribed a special diet following surgery or during treatment with radiation or anticancer drugs.

CALL YOUR DOCTOR IF

• You or a family member has symptoms of a tumor of the small intestine.
• After diagnosis, you have symptoms of intestinal obstruction.
• New, unexplained symptoms develop during treatment.

SNAKEBITE

GENERAL INFORMATION

DEFINITION—Bite from a venomous snake, such as a rattlesnake, copperhead, water moccasin, or coral snake. Bites on the legs and feet are more common. Bites on the head and trunk are more dangerous. Snakes are more likely to bite runners, joggers, walkers, hikers, backpackers, fishers, boaters, and campers or anyone playing or working where snakes live.

BODY PARTS INVOLVED—Exposed skin; blood; lymphatic system.

SEX OR AGE MOST AFFECTED—Both sexes; all ages.

SIGNS & SYMPTOMS
• If the bite is from a coral snake, it will have multiple fang marks and small cuts; symptoms may not appear for 3 to 4 hours. If the bite is from another snake, it will have deep single or double fang marks. Symptoms begin quickly.
• Severe pain and swelling around the bite.
• Skin color around the bite looks bruised.
• Bleeding spots under the skin, all over the body.
• Numbness and tingling around the mouth and in the hands and feet.
• Excessive sweating; fever.
• Low blood pressure and life-threatening shock.
• Breathing difficulty.
• Blurred vision; headache.
• Seizures; coma.

CAUSES—Snakes use their fangs to bite a person. Venomous snakes inject a venom through the fangs.

RISK INCREASES WITH—Bites from venomous snakes occur during outdoor activities in warm months in areas where snakes are known to live. People handling snakes or trying to capture snakes put themselves at risk.

HOW TO PREVENT
• Wear protective shoes, boots and clothing for hiking, camping, fishing, and hunting. Consider taking a snakebite kit with instructions with you.
• Don't try to pick up or handle snakes.

WHAT TO EXPECT

DIAGNOSTIC MEASURES—Emergency care will include a physical exam, blood studies, urinalysis and other tests as needed to monitor vital signs.

APPROPRIATE HEALTH CARE—In the hospital, the treatment may include:
• Breathing support with a machine if needed.
• Treatment to prevent any complications.
• Surgical debridement (removal of dead or infected tissue) after 3 or 4 days. Skin grafts may be needed.

POSSIBLE COMPLICATIONS
• Wound infection and skin loss.
• Heart, lung, blood, or kidney complications.
• Compartment syndrome (loss of blood circulation to muscles in a closed body space).
• Reaction to the antivenin includes anaphylaxis (severe allergic) and delayed serum sickness.
• Death from snakebite is rare.

PROBABLE OUTCOME—Usually curable with rapid medical care. Skin tissue affected by the bite may take weeks to months to heal.

HOW TO TREAT

GENERAL MEASURES—After a snakebite:
• If possible, identify the snake, but don't waste time looking for it.
• Don't panic! Venom spreads more quickly in the body if the victim runs or gets excited.
• Call 911 for emergency help. If help cannot get there right away, go to the nearest emergency center.
• Follow snakebite kit instructions if one is handy.
• Some basic first aid steps include: Remain calm. Keep bitten area below or at heart level, if possible. Remove jewelry and tight clothing. Do not cut or suction the bite. Cover area with a clean, dry pad. Do not use a tourniquet. If elastic bandage is available, wrap firmly around the area. Don't use ice on the area (cool compresses may be used). Cover victim with a blanket. Don't give victim food or drink, especially alcohol.

MEDICATION—You may be prescribed:
• Antivenin to counter the snake poison.
• Tetanus booster injection.
• Antibiotics to prevent infection.
• Pain relievers. Narcotics cannot be used for coral snake bites. They may cause shock.

ACTIVITY—Resume normal activities as soon as symptoms improve.

DIET—No special diet.

CALL YOUR DOCTOR IF

• You or someone you are with receives a snakebite.
• New, unexplained symptoms develop after snakebite treatment.

SODIUM IMBALANCE

GENERAL INFORMATION

DEFINITION—Above-normal sodium level (hypernatremia) or below-normal sodium level (hyponatremia) in the blood. Sodium helps regulate the body's water balance and maintains normal heart rhythm. It is responsible for the conduction of nerve impulses, and the contraction of muscles.

BODY PARTS INVOLVED—All body cells.

SEX OR AGE MOST AFFECTED—Both sexes; all ages.

SIGNS & SYMPTOMS
- Confusion.
- Restlessness and anxiety.
- Weakness.
- Muscle cramps (usually in the legs).
- Changes in pulse rate and blood pressure.
- Tissue swelling (edema).
- Stupor or coma (if severe imbalance).
- Sodium imbalance may be part of a disease with other symptoms, such as fever, vomiting, diarrhea, or excessive sweating.

CAUSES
Hyponatremia (below-normal sodium):
- Prolonged loss of body fluids from vomiting or diarrhea.
- Addison's disease.
- Congestive heart failure.
- Prolonged, excessive drinking of water. This is usually a psychiatric condition.
- Some cancers of the adrenal glands.
- Infections with high fever.
Hypernatremia (above-normal sodium):
- Inability to drink water, as with stroke or gastrointestinal diseases.
- Use of cortisone drugs.
- Excess intake of salty food or liquid, as in near drowning in salt water.
- Inappropriate secretion of antidiuretic hormone.

RISK INCREASES WITH
- Diabetes.
- Congestive heart failure.
- Use of diuretics (drugs to remove excess fluid).
- Kidney diseases. Healthy kidneys can usually control sodium levels.

HOW TO PREVENT
- Sodium imbalance is the result of an underlying disease. Medical treatment for that disorder will help prevent sodium imbalance.
- If you have a disorder or take drugs that affect sodium balance, learn as much as possible about your drugs and your condition. Learn how to prevent a sodium imbalance.

WHAT TO EXPECT

DIAGNOSTIC MEASURES
- Your own observation of symptoms.
- Your health care provider may do a physical exam.
- Medical tests may include blood and urine studies of sodium and other electrolytes.

APPROPRIATE HEALTH CARE
- Treatment will depend on the underlying cause.
- If a drug is the cause for sodium imbalance (above or below normal), it may be stopped or the dose lowered.
- For below-normal sodium levels, water restriction is usually the therapy. This will increase the sodium levels in the body. It is important that the treatment not overcorrect the sodium levels, as that can be dangerous.
- For above-normal levels of sodium, providing fluids (such as dextrose in water) to return sodium levels to normal is the usual therapy.

POSSIBLE COMPLICATIONS—Shock, which can be life threatening.

PROBABLE OUTCOME—Usually, the imbalance can be corrected and the underlying disorder treated to prevent a recurrence.

HOW TO TREAT

GENERAL MEASURES—If you have a disorder or take drugs that affect sodium balance, learn as much as possible about your drugs, your condition and how to prevent a sodium imbalance.

MEDICATION—You may be prescribed:
- Intravenous (IV) sodium, if sodium levels are low.
- Diuretics to decrease high sodium levels.
- Drugs to correct underlying disorders.

ACTIVITY—Bed rest until stable, or underlying condition resolved or controlled. Resume normal activities after recovery.

DIET—No special diet for low sodium levels. Most persons with high sodium levels benefit from a low-salt diet. Low-salt diets contain enough sodium to prevent hyponatremia. However, sodium levels are not influenced by diet alone.

CALL YOUR DOCTOR IF

- You or a family member has symptoms of a sodium imbalance.
- You are having problems with a disorder that affects sodium levels.

SORES, PRESSURE
(Bed Sores; Decubitus Ulcers)

 GENERAL INFORMATION

DEFINITION—Sores that affect the skin over pressure points in the lower back, buttocks, elbows, knees, shoulders, heels, ankles and other areas with bony prominences.

BODY PARTS INVOLVED—Skin; body tissue.

SEX OR AGE MOST AFFECTED—Both sexes; all ages, but most likely in the elderly.

SIGNS & SYMPTOMS—Spots of the skin that are red and shiny. Spots progress to blisters, then ulcers (deep sores), leading to a breakdown of tissue under the ulcer.

CAUSES—Constant pressure on the skin, especially over bony areas. Pressure reduces the blood supply, causing death in the tissue layers. Pressure sores usually develop in persons who cannot move because of chronic illness or disability that confines them to bed.

RISK INCREASES WITH
• Elderly people who are frail, disabled, ill, or immobile.
• Being confined to bed or a chair for long, or even short periods of time. Sores can start within 24 hours.
• Poor nutrition and low body weight.
• Impaired mental status.
• Skin that is too dry or too moist.
• Illness that reduces blood flow in the body.

HOW TO PREVENT
• Provide good nursing care for the disabled.
• Daily skin inspection in good light.
• Frequent changes of position in bed or wheelchair (hourly may be needed).
• Keep skin clean. Clean the skin of any urine or fecal matter as soon as possible. Apply moisturizers.

 WHAT TO EXPECT

DIAGNOSTIC MEASURES
• Your own observation of symptoms.
• Your health care provider can diagnose pressure sores by an exam of the affected area.

APPROPRIATE HEALTH CARE
• Treatment involves relieving the pressure, treating the sores, and improving nutrition, or other conditions.
• A water mattress, egg-crate rubber mattress, alternating-pressure mattress, or special airbed may be recommended.
• Special dressings for pressure sores, such as Gelfoam or Duoderm, may be prescribed.
• Dead skin and tissue may need to be removed. This can be done in different ways and can be painful to the patient.

POSSIBLE COMPLICATIONS—Infection develops in the pressure sores. Infection of bone (osteomyelitis) next to the ulcer. Complications can be life-threatening.

PROBABLE OUTCOME—Curable with treatment. Sores heal in 2 to 4 weeks, or sometimes longer. Healing time varies with the site and size of the ulcer and the patient's general health.

 HOW TO TREAT

GENERAL MEASURES
• Relieve pressure by not lying on the sores. Other options include protective, soft padding, such as gel flotation pads or sheepskin, over the affected area.
• Clean the area with mild soap and warm water and pat dry. Avoid harsh soaps, tincture of benzoin, or hexachlorophene. Cover the sore with bandage or dressing.
• Apply a skin product if prescribed. Apply a thin layer of the cream, ointment, or lotion 3 or 4 times daily. Rub in gently for several minutes, until it disappears.

MEDICATION
• Antibiotics will be prescribed if infection develops.
• Ointments, dressings, and drying agents may be prescribed.
• Drugs for pain may be needed when dead skin tissue is removed.
• Vitamin and mineral supplements may be needed.

ACTIVITY
• Change the position of an immobilized patient every 1 to 2 hours. A wheelchair patient should change position every hour.
• Passive or active exercises (if the patient is able). Instructions will be provided by your health care provider or physical therapist.

DIET—Normal, well-balanced diet that includes extra protein. Good nutrition is important in prevention and healing.

 CALL YOUR DOCTOR IF

• You or a family member has symptoms of pressure sores or you observe them in someone else.
• The following occur during treatment:
  - Skin sores become worse or don't improve.
  - Signs of infection, such as pain, redness, tenderness, swelling, or increased warmth of the affected area.
  - Fever.

SPINAL-CORD TUMOR

GENERAL INFORMATION

DEFINITION—An abnormal growth that presses on the spinal cord or its nerve roots. The growth may be benign (noncancerous) or malignant (cancerous). A benign tumor may be as damaging as a malignant tumor if it is not treated.

BODY PARTS INVOLVED—Spinal cord; nerves below the level of the spinal-cord tumor.

SEX OR AGE MOST AFFECTED—Both sexes; all ages, but most common in adults.

SIGNS & SYMPTOMS
- Symptoms may come on gradually and then suddenly be more severe.
- Dull, burning, or aching pain due to tumor putting pressure on the spinal cord. Pain may be constant and, sometimes, severe. It may feel like it's coming from various parts of the body.
- Pain may be located near the level of the tumor on the spinal cord. Midway affects the chest, higher affects arms and neck, and lower affects the back and legs.
- A loss of sensation that may include a feeling of numbness and skin being less sensitive to heat and cold.
- Muscle weakness or stiffness.
- Urination problems or incontinence (unable to control urination or bowel movements).
- If not treated, muscle wasting (loss of tissue) and paralysis may occur.

CAUSES
- A spinal cord tumor usually comes from cancer that has spread from another part of the body. The cancer may have started in the lung, breast, intestinal tract, prostate, kidney, thyroid, or lymphatic system.
- Tumors that start first (primary tumors) in the spinal cord are more rare, especially in childhood or old age. Their cause is often unknown. A few may result from a genetic disease or radiation exposure.

RISK INCREASES WITH—Cancer in any of the body parts listed above.

HOW TO PREVENT—No specific preventive measures. Steps to help reduce your cancer risk or diagnose the cancer early include:
- Not smoking.
- Eating healthy diet. Maintain healthy weight.
- Get recommended cancer screening exams.
- Learn cancer warning signs and symptoms.

WHAT TO EXPECT

DIAGNOSTIC MEASURES
- Your own observation of symptoms.
- Your health care provider will do a physical exam and ask questions about your symptoms.

This exam may include checking: your eye movement, reflexes, hearing, sense of touch and balance.
- Medical tests may include x-ray, CT, MRI, and others to help confirm the diagnosis.

APPROPRIATE HEALTH CARE
- Treatments include monitoring (no treatment right away), surgery, radiation and/or chemotherapy (anticancer drugs). It depends on the tumor type, your health, other cancer treatment, and your preferences.
- A slow-growing, benign tumor may be monitored for a period of time. It may have been found on a routine exam and not be causing symptoms, or the symptoms are mild.
- Surgery is often the first option if the tumor can be removed without damage to the spinal cord or nerves. Several different types of surgery are available. If the tumor is benign, surgery can provide a cure.
- Radiation therapy is usually done after surgery for a cancerous tumor. Radiation may also be done if the tumor cannot be removed with surgery.
- Research is ongoing for improved treatment options.

POSSIBLE COMPLICATIONS—Paralysis, spread of cancer to other body organs, surgery complications, infections, and other medical problems.

PROBABLE OUTCOME—Early diagnosis and early treatment offer the most favorable outcome for cancerous tumors. Many benign tumors are cured with surgery.

HOW TO TREAT

GENERAL MEASURES—To learn more: American Cancer Society, (800) ACS-2345; website: www.cancer.org or National Cancer Institute, (800) 4-CANCER; website: www.nci.nih.gov.

MEDICATION
- Pain relievers may be prescribed.
- Cortisone drugs to decrease swelling around the tumor and reduce pressure on spinal cord.
- Anticancer drugs, if the tumor is malignant.

ACTIVITY—Activity levels will depend on your condition. Be as active as your energy permits.

DIET—Eat a normal, well-balanced diet.

CALL YOUR DOCTOR IF

- You or a family member has any symptoms of a spinal cord tumor.
- new or unexpected symptoms occur during or after treatment.

SPONDYLITIS, ANKYLOSING
(Marie-Strümpell Disease)

GENERAL INFORMATION

DEFINITION—A chronic, progressive, rheumatic disease of the joints. Ankylosing means "fusing together." Spondylitis means "inflammation of the vertebrae" (bones in the spine).

BODY PARTS INVOLVED—Joints.

SEX OR AGE MOST AFFECTED—Males are affected more often than females. The onset is usually in the late teens or early twenties.

SIGNS & SYMPTOMS
Early stages:
• Recurrent episodes of low backache. Pain can also occur along the sciatic nerve (along the leg).
• Stiffness in the spine. It may be worse in the morning.
• The symptoms can be mild and a person may think it is just a common backache.
Later stages:
• Symptoms gradually become worse. Pain often spreads from the lower back to the middle back, or higher in the neck. Joints in the arms, legs, feet, and hands may be affected.
• It can bring about a "bent forward" posture caused by stiffening of the spine and support structures.
• Muscle stiffness.
• Fatigue; weight loss.
• Iritis (eye redness and soreness).

CAUSES—Unknown. It may be genetic or an autoimmune disorder (immune system goes wrong). The disorder causes some or all the bones of the spine to fuse together.

RISK INCREASES WITH
• Family history of ankylosing spondylitis.
• Having a certain gene called HLA-B27.

HOW TO PREVENT—No specific preventive measures. Consult your health care provider if you have a family history of the disorder and have ongoing back or joint pain.

WHAT TO EXPECT

DIAGNOSTIC MEASURES
• Your own observation of symptoms.
• Your health care provider will do a physical exam and ask questions about your symptoms.
• Medical tests may include blood studies and x-rays of the spine.

APPROPRIATE HEALTH CARE
• Treatments includes physical therapy, exercise, and drugs can help delay or prevent deformity, ease pain, and maintain function.

• Physical therapy includes exercises for breathing techniques, to maintain proper posture, and to build up muscle groups (to oppose the direction of possible deformities)
• Surgery to replace a damaged hip or to insert bone grafts in the spine (advanced stages only).

POSSIBLE COMPLICATIONS
• Heart and lung problems.
• Eye inflammation.
• Difficulty walking and standing.
• Osteoporosis and fractures of the spine.
• Anemia.
• Permanent disability.

PROBABLE OUTCOME—There is no cure for this disorder. Symptoms change with mild or moderate flare-ups and they may stop for periods of time. With treatment, symptoms can be relieved or controlled. Most patients can lead normal, productive lives. For some, the disease is severe and incapacitating due to deformities.

HOW TO TREAT

GENERAL MEASURES
• Sleep on your back on a firm mattress. Use a small pillow or none at all.
• Take hot baths or use heat compresses before exercising or to relieve pain. Get regular massages, if possible.
• Quit smoking. Find a way to stop that works.
• See your eye care provider for regular exams.
• To learn more: Spondylitis Association of America, PO Box 5872, Sherman Oaks, CA 91413; (800) 777-8189; website: www.spondylitis.org.

MEDICATION
• Use nonprescription, nonsteroidal anti-inflammatory drugs to help ease discomfort.
• Drugs to treat arthritis symptoms, stronger pain drugs, and muscle relaxants may be prescribed.

ACTIVITY
• Exercise to maintain good posture and retain as much upright carriage as possible.
• Swim regularly, if possible. Being in water lets you move stiff, painful areas more easily.
• Avoid activity that puts stress on the back. Avoid contact sports (risk of spinal injury).

DIET—No special diet.

CALL YOUR DOCTOR IF

• You or a family member has symptoms of ankylosing spondylitis.
• Increasing back pain or stiffness, or eye pain occur.

SPOROTRICHOSIS

 GENERAL INFORMATION

DEFINITION—A fungal infection that affects the skin. Sporotrichosis is not contagious from person to person.

BODY PARTS INVOLVED—Skin; lymph system; lungs; joints; bones (rare).

SEX OR AGE MOST AFFECTED—Adults of both sexes.

SIGNS & SYMPTOMS
• A small, movable, non-tender bump (nodule) usually on the fingers, hands, or arms. It starts at the place where the fungus entered the skin. The color may be pink, red, or purple.
• More bumps occur around the same area.
• The bumps may ulcerate (become open sores).
• The skin infection can spread in a line-like formation up the fingers, hands or arms. They spread along what is called lymphatic channels.

CAUSES
• Infection by a fungus, *Sporotrichum schenckii*, that lives in soil, sphagnum moss, weeds, baled hay, and decaying organic vegetation. It enters the skin through small cuts or punctures, such as from thorns. The infection may appear on the skin 1 to 12 weeks after exposure.
• Research has shown that a pet cat may have the infection and pass it to a human through a bite or scratch.

RISK INCREASES WITH
• Farm laborers, plant nursery workers, gardeners, and others who handle rosebushes, sphagnum moss, hay bales, or barberry bushes.
• Kids playing among hay bales.
• Those with weak immune system due to illness or drugs are more at risk for complications.

HOW TO PREVENT
• Wear gloves and long sleeves when working with plants with thorns, hay bales, pine seedlings, or other materials that could cause minor skin breaks.
• Avoid skin contact with sphagnum moss. It has been the cause of some outbreaks.

 WHAT TO EXPECT

DIAGNOSTIC MEASURES
• Your own observation of symptoms.
• Your health care provider will do a physical exam of the affected skin.
• Medical tests may include a culture of fluid from the sores or a small bit of tissue is removed for viewing under a microscope.

APPROPRIATE HEALTH CARE
• The disorder is treated with antifungal drugs.
• Rarely, hospital care may be needed if complications occur.

POSSIBLE COMPLICATIONS—Spread of the fungal infection to joints, lungs, and central nervous system. This is rare, but may occur in those who have diabetes or weak immune systems.

PROBABLE OUTCOME—Curable with treatment, but it can take several months to heal completely.

 HOW TO TREAT

GENERAL MEASURES
• You may be advised to apply warm compresses or a heating pad to the affected skin for 40 to 60 minutes a day. This can help control the skin symptoms.
• Cover lesions with loose-fitting bandages to prevent secondary infection with bacteria.

MEDICATION—Oral (taken by mouth) antifungal drugs are usually prescribed. Drugs may be continued for 1 to 2 months or more after the skin symptoms have cleared up.

ACTIVITY—No limits.

DIET—No special diet.

 CALL YOUR DOCTOR IF

• You or a family member has symptoms of sporotrichosis.
• Any new sores occur after treatment starts.
• New, unexplained symptoms develop.
Antifungal drugs used in treatment may produce side effects.

SPRAINS & STRAINS

GENERAL INFORMATION

DEFINITION—A sprain is a stretched or torn ligament. A strain is a stretched or torn muscle or tendon. Sprains occur most often in ankles, knees, or fingers, although any joint can be sprained. Strains often occur in the back or hamstring muscles (at the back of the thigh). It is sometimes difficult to know if the injury is a sprain and strain.

BODY PARTS INVOLVED—Muscles, tendons and any ligament attached to any joint. Ligaments are the fibrous, elastic connective bands that attach bone to bone (tendons connect muscle to bone).

SEX OR AGE MOST AFFECTED—Both sexes; all ages.

SIGNS & SYMPTOMS
• Pain or tenderness in the area of injury; severity varies with the extent of injury.
• Swelling of the affected joint.
• Redness or bruising in the area of injury, either right away, or several hours after injury.
• Loss of normal mobility in the injured joint.

CAUSES
• Sprains usually occur as a result of trauma (fall, twisting injury, or automobile accident). The ankle is injured most often because of its normal weakness, its exposed position and the stress it sustains in sports and other activities.
• Strains are often caused by twisting, pulling, or overuse injuries. Pulled muscle is another term used.

RISK INCREASES WITH
• Sports requiring running, jumping, and change of direction.
• High-risk activities such as skateboarding, contact sports, ice and roller skating, mountain biking, skiing and, rock climbing.
• Overweight.
• Trauma.
• Excessive exercise.
• Poor conditioning.
• Poor fitting shoes and high-heeled shoes.

HOW TO PREVENT
• Maintain good level of physical fitness.
• Maintain a healthy weight.
• To avoid injury:
  - Wear proper shoes and other protective gear for the sport or activity.
  - Stretch muscles before and after exercise.
  - Strengthen weak muscles with exercises.
  - Accident-proof your home.

WHAT TO EXPECT

DIAGNOSTIC MEASURES
• Your health care provider will do an exam of the injured area. Questions will be asked about your symptoms and activities that lead to the injury.
• Tests may include x-rays or other special scans of the injured area.

APPROPRIATE HEALTH CARE
• Treatment for a sprain or strain will depend on how mild or severe the injury is. It may range from simple self-care, to wearing a cast or brace, to having surgery.
• Rehabilitation for a sprain or strain starts after the pain and swelling improve. The goals are to restore complete joint function and a return to full activity levels. You and your health care provider will work out a recovery and exercise plan for your individual needs.

POSSIBLE COMPLICATIONS
• Joint may remain unstable.
• Arthritis may develop later on in the joint.

PROBABLE OUTCOME—With treatment and rest, it takes 6 to 8 weeks for recovery. It may take longer if the injury is severe.

HOW TO TREAT

GENERAL MEASURES—Use RICE therapy— Rest, Ice, Compression, Elevation.
• Rest and reduce activities as needed. Crutches or a cane may be required to get around.
• Apply ice. Place ice in a plastic bag and separate it from the skin with a thin towel. Continue the ice treatment for 20 minutes at a time at 2-hour intervals. After 24 hours, continue ice treatment or switch to heat.
• Compression may be done with elastic wrap. Also, special boots, casts, or splints may be prescribed.
• Elevate the injured area on a pillow, above the heart level if possible, to help reduce swelling.

MEDICATION—You may take pain relievers such as acetaminophen. If the sprain is severe, a stronger pain reliever may be prescribed. Avoid aspirin, as it may increase the tendency to bleed.

ACTIVITY—You may be taught exercises to do several times a day at home. Physical therapy may be needed. Don't return to previous activity level until advised to do so. You risk a re-injury and chronic joint problems.

DIET—No special diet.

CALL YOUR DOCTOR IF

• You or a family member has a joint injury.
• Pain, swelling or bruising, increases.

STOMACH CANCER
(Gastric Carcinoma)

 GENERAL INFORMATION

DEFINITION—Growth of cancer cells in the stomach. Most people do not have symptoms until the disease is advanced.

BODY PARTS INVOLVED—Stomach.

SEX OR AGE MOST AFFECTED—Adults over age 40 and is twice as common in men as women.

SIGNS & SYMPTOMS
Early stages:
• Vague symptoms of indigestion, such as fullness, burping, nausea, and poor appetite.
Later stages:
• Unexplained weight loss.
• Loss of appetite.
• Vomiting blood.
• Black stools.
• Fullness after eating small amounts.
• Pain in the stomach.
• Mass in the stomach that can be felt (sometimes).

CAUSES—Exact cause is unknown. *Helicobacter pylori* infection, a bacteria infection of the stomach, appears to be a factor. Dietary factors are believed to play a role.

RISK INCREASES WITH
• Age over 50. Men are more at risk than women.
• Excess alcohol or tobacco use.
• Previous stomach surgery.
• Diet that includes high amounts of smoked, pickled, and salted foods; and low amounts of protein, fresh fruits, and green, leafy vegetables.
• Pernicious anemia (unable to absorb vitamin B12).
• Family history of stomach cancer.
• Being overweight.
• People with type A blood.

HOW TO PREVENT
• There are no specific preventive measures. Changing some lifestyle behaviors can help lower the risks.
• Eat a nutritious, well-balanced diet with plenty of fresh fruits and vegetables. Lose weight if overweight.
• Decrease alcohol use if you drink more than 1 or 2 drinks a day. Don't smoke. If you do smoke, try to quit.
• To help find stomach cancer early, don't ignore symptoms of indigestion that last more than a few days. Do a yearly home test for blood in the stool.
• Treatment for ongoing *Helicobacter pylori* infection as a cancer-preventive step is being researched.

 WHAT TO EXPECT

DIAGNOSTIC MEASURES
• Your health care provider will do a physical exam and ask questions about your symptoms.
• Medical tests may include blood studies, CT, and x-rays of the stomach, esophagus, and small intestine. The stomach may be examined with a endoscope (a viewing tube passed down the esophagus to the stomach). A small amount of tissue may be removed for a biopsy.

APPROPRIATE HEALTH CARE
• Treatment options depend on the location of the cancer, how advanced it is, your overall health, and your own preferences.
• Surgery to remove part or all of the stomach may be an option, if the cancer has not spread.
• Drugs to treat the cancer or radiation therapy may achieve a temporary response.
• Treatment may involve steps to relieve symptoms and make you comfortable, rather than treating the cancer.

POSSIBLE COMPLICATIONS
• Excess fluid in the abdomen (ascites).
• Spread of cancer to lymph nodes, liver, pancreas, and colon.
• The 5-year survival rate is poor, even with treatment.

PROBABLE OUTCOME—Often, the cancer is diagnosed too late for effective treatment. New developments in treatment may offer hope in some cases. If the cancer is found early, and surgery removes the entire tumor, recovery may be complete.

 HOW TO TREAT

GENERAL MEASURES—To learn more: American Cancer Society, (800) ACS-2345; website: www.cancer.org or National Cancer Institute, (800) 4-CANCER; website: www.nci.nih.gov.

MEDICATION
• Anticancer (chemotherapy) drugs may be prescribed.
• Pain relievers may be prescribed.

ACTIVITY—As tolerated by your energy level.

DIET—Eat frequent small meals of soft foods. Try to maintain high calorie intake.

☎ **CALL YOUR DOCTOR IF**

• You or a family member has symptoms of stomach cancer.
• New symptoms occur during treatment.

STOMATITIS

GENERAL INFORMATION

DEFINITION—A common, and painful condition that affects the lining of the mouth. The two main types are acute herpetic stomatitis and aphthous stomatitis (canker sore), which is the most common. Stomatitis may be a sign of a more serious, underlying disorder.

BODY PARTS INVOLVED—It may involve the cheeks, gums, lips, tongue, roof, and floor of the mouth.

SEX OR AGE MOST AFFECTED—Both sexes; all ages.

SIGNS & SYMPTOMS
- Inflammation (redness, swelling, and soreness) of the mouth.
- Mouth sores that are shallow, usually red, and may have a white coating over them.
- Mild to severe pain.
- Bleeding (sometimes).
- Bad breath.

CAUSES—The condition can be caused by a variety of factors. For canker sores, the exact cause is unknown.

RISK INCREASES WITH
- Infection.
- Trauma (injury) and burns, such as from hot food or drink.
- Dryness of the mouth and nasal passages.
- Irritants.
- Toxic agents.
- Autoimmune conditions.
- Vitamin deficiency.
- Anemia.
- Allergies to food or drugs.
- Smoking.
- Dentures, jagged or sharp teeth.
- Emotional stress, anxiety.
- Poor nutrition.
- Radiation or chemotherapy (anticancer drugs).
- Excess alcohol.
- Excess eating of hot foods or spices.
- Sensitivity to mouthwashes, candy dyes, or lipstick.
- Side effect of certain drugs.
- Diseases such as HIV, Behçet's, Crohn's, and others.
- Family history of canker sores.

HOW TO PREVENT—No specific preventive measures. Avoid risk factors where possible.

WHAT TO EXPECT

DIAGNOSTIC MEASURES
- Your own observation of symptoms.
- See your health care provider if sores persist or cause pain so that you can't eat. An exam of the mouth will be done.
- Medical tests such as smears or cultures of the sores may be done to check for infection or other cause.

APPROPRIATE HEALTH CARE
- Most people will let the sores heal on their own or use self-treatment methods.
- Medical care will depend on the cause.
- Infections may be treated with drugs.

POSSIBLE COMPLICATIONS
- May recur after treatment.
- Underlying disorder may have complications.

PROBABLE OUTCOME
- Usually heals in 1 or 2 weeks, or longer. Some may require treatment, and others heal on their own.
- Some outcomes will depend on underlying disorders.

HOW TO TREAT

GENERAL MEASURES
- Careful oral hygiene is important. Use a soft-bristled toothbrush. Brush teeth and gums gently.
- Avoid mouthwash or toothpaste that may be a cause.
- Quit smoking. Find a way to stop that works.
- Have your dental care provider correct problems with jagged or sharp teeth, or ill-fitting dentures.

MEDICATION
- Drugs may be prescribed for the underlying cause, where it can be determined.
- Mouth rinses or oral lozenges may be prescribed.
- Nonprescription drugs for canker sores that are applied to the sores may help some people.
- Vitamins, iron, or folate will be prescribed if needed.
- Use ibuprofen or acetaminophen for minor pain.

ACTIVITY—No limits.

DIET
- Avoid spicy foods or foods that are hard, sharp, or dry (such as potato chips, tacos, or peanuts).
- Avoid any foods that cause an allergic reaction.
- Drink plenty of fluids.

CALL YOUR DOCTOR IF

- You or a family member has signs or symptoms of stomatitis.
- Symptoms don't improve with treatment.

STRABISMUS

GENERAL INFORMATION

DEFINITION—The eyes are not aligned together, and eyes point in different directions. One or both eyes may turn inward (crossed eyes), outward ("walleye"), upward, or downward. The ability of the eyes to focus is not fully mature at birth. Strabismus may be constant (occurs all the time) or intermittent (occurs some of the time).

BODY PARTS INVOLVED—Eyes; brain area that controls vision.

SEX OR AGE MOST AFFECTED—A true eye problem shows up from 3 or 4 months of age. It also may occur in childhood or later.

SIGNS & SYMPTOMS
* Eye movement that is not coordinated.
* Child may look at you with one eye closed, squint, or with the head turned to one side.
* Adults may have double vision, eyestrain, headaches, and/or an abnormal head position (from trying to see properly).

CAUSES—Eye movement is controlled by brain signals to six muscles around each eye. Loss of coordinated movement may result from:
* Muscle imbalance between the eyes.
* Lack of equal focusing ability in the eyes. The brain gets a different picture from each eye, so it blocks the one from the weaker eye. The weaker eye becomes more useless from disuse, and a "lazy," or wandering eye results.
* Brain damage or head injury (rare).

RISK INCREASES WITH
* Family history of strabismus.
* Down syndrome.
* Cerebral palsy.
* Eye tumor.
* Damage to fetal central nervous system.
* Birth trauma (injury).
* In adults, thyroid disease, stroke, myasthenia gravis, diabetes, brain tumor, other neurological disease.

HOW TO PREVENT—No specific preventive measures.

WHAT TO EXPECT

DIAGNOSTIC MEASURES
* Your own observation of symptoms. Note particularly if a young child covers one eye— this may indicate the eyes are not focusing together.
* Your health care provider will do an exam of the eyes.
* Medical tests may include a visual acuity test, a retina exam, and others.

APPROPRIATE HEALTH CARE
* Treatment has three goals: to obtain the best possible vision, gain the best eye alignment, and provide the best chance for binocular (both eyes) vision.
* Glasses or an eye patch may be used over the stronger eye to correct focusing imbalance. These force the weak eye to work. This treatment may be done for only a few hours a day or all waking hours (full-time).
* Eye-muscle exercises (called orthoptics) will improve the eye muscles to help straighten the eyes.
* Vision therapy involves exercises that help the eye and brain learn to work together better.
* Surgery to correct the condition of the eye muscles may be recommended. Sometimes a second operation is required. Your eye care provider will explain the risks and benefits of the surgery.
* A therapy for adults involves the use of eyeglasses overlaid with thin plastic prisms. These are used by a patient prior to surgery. They help determine the amount of adjustment needed on the eye muscles.

POSSIBLE COMPLICATIONS—Loss of normal vision in one eye.

PROBABLE OUTCOME
* With early diagnosis and treatment, strabismus can be corrected. It can take many months or even years. Without prompt care, vision loss in one eye may become permanent.
* Many persons adapt well to single-eye vision and learn to drive a car as well as other activities. If vision is lost in one eye, take extra care against injury in the other eye. Wear goggles for sports and other activities, such as carpentry, or welding, that have risk of injury.

HOW TO TREAT

GENERAL MEASURES —To learn more: American Academy of Ophthalmology, PO Box 7424, San Francisco, CA 94120; website: www.aao.org/aao/public.

MEDICATION—Botulinum toxin injections may sometimes be recommended for adults. They are injected into an eye-turning muscle, outside the eye, by using a special needle.

ACTIVITY—Protect your child against falls or injury while he or she adjusts to an eye patch.

DIET—No special diet.

CALL YOUR DOCTOR IF

* You or a family member has symptoms of strabismus.
* Any new symptoms develop during or after treatment.

STREP THROAT
(Streptococcal Sore Throat)

GENERAL INFORMATION

DEFINITION—Infection of the throat (the pharynx) by group A streptococcus (GAS) bacteria. Strep throat can spread from person to person. Infection can be present in someone with no symptoms, but who can still spread the germs (carrier state).

BODY PARTS INVOLVED—Throat; tonsils.

SEX OR AGE MOST AFFECTED—Both sexes; all ages, but most common in children.

SIGNS & SYMPTOMS
* Rapid onset of throat pain.
* Throat pain that is worse when you swallow.
* Headache, fever, general ill feeling.
* Children may have nausea and vomiting.
* Tender, swollen glands in the neck.
* Bright-red tonsils that may have specks of pus.

CAUSES—Streptococcal bacteria. Germs are spread by contact with an infected person, breathing in germs in the air, or touching an object with germs on it. A person usually has symptoms in 2 to 5 days of exposure. Strep throat is one of the most common types of infection caused by group A streptococcus. It can also cause skin infections and other health problems.

RISK INCREASES WITH
* Recent strep infection in a family member.
* Crowded living conditions such as a dorm.
* Being in daycare center or attending school.

HOW TO PREVENT
* Not always preventable. Avoid close contact with anyone with strep throat.
* Avoid germs. Wash hands often, especially children.

WHAT TO EXPECT

DIAGNOSTIC MEASURES
* Your own observation of symptoms.
* Your health care provider will examine the throat. A sore throat (pharyngitis) can also be caused by virus infection, allergies, or other problems. Further tests are usually needed.
* A throat culture or rapid strep test can confirm a strep infection.

APPROPRIATE HEALTH CARE—Treatment for strep infection is with antibiotic drugs and self-care.

POSSIBLE COMPLICATIONS
* Ear infection.
* Sinusitis.
* Rheumatic fever or scarlet fever.
* Glomerulonephritis (a kidney disorder).

PROBABLE OUTCOME—Curable with treatment. Symptoms are usually better within the first few days of treatment. Any complications are rare.

HOW TO TREAT

GENERAL MEASURES—To relieve the sore throat, gargle frequently with warm or cold double-strength tea or warm salt water (mix one-half teaspoon of salt in one cup of water).

MEDICATION
* Penicillin or another antibiotic will be prescribed. Complete the course prescribed, even if symptoms get better. This helps prevent any complications or having the infection recur.
* Use nonprescription pain medicine, such as ibuprofen if needed. Don't give aspirin to children under age 18.
* Throat lozenges for sore throats are available from drugstores and may help with pain relief.

ACTIVITY—Return to normal activities as symptoms improve. A person can no longer spread the germs if they have taken the antibiotic drug for at least 24 hours.

DIET—A liquid diet may be helpful while the throat is sore. Drink plenty of fluids, including milk shakes, soups, tea, carbonated drinks, or iced coffee. Any type and amount of solid food is fine as long as you can swallow it without too much pain.

CALL YOUR DOCTOR IF

* You or a family member has symptoms of strep throat.
* The following occur during treatment:
  - Fever recurs after being normal for a few days.
  - New symptoms appear, such as nausea, vomiting, earache, cough, swollen glands, skin rash, severe headache, nasal drainage, or shortness of breath.
  - Joints become red or painful.

ILLNESS & DISORDERS

STRESS

GENERAL INFORMATION

DEFINITION—Stress is the physical, mental, and emotional reactions you experience due to changes and demands in your life. The changes and demands can be large or small and each person will respond to them differently. Some people are more prone than others to stressful situations. Positive stress can be a motivator. Negative stress occurs when these changes and demands are overwhelming to you.

BODY PARTS INVOLVED—Almost all.

SEX OR AGE MOST AFFECTED—Both sexes; all ages.

SIGNS & SYMPTOMS
* Physical symptoms include muscle tension, headache, chest pain, upset stomach, diarrhea or constipation, racing heartbeat, cold clammy hands, fatigue, profuse sweating, rashes, rapid breathing, shaking, tics, jumpiness, changes in appetite, weakness, tiredness, and dizziness.
* Emotional reactions include anger, low self-esteem, depression, lack of interest, irritability, fear and phobic responses, difficulty concentrating, guilt, worry, agitation, anxiety, and panic.
* Behavioral reactions may lead to alcohol or drug abuse, an increase in smoking, sleep disorders, overeating, memory loss, or confusion.

CAUSES—During stressful times, the body increases the production of certain hormones. These cause changes in the heart rate, blood pressure, metabolism, and physical activity.

RISK INCREASES WITH—Some risk factors for stress include:
* Loss of a loved one (spouse, child, or friend).
* Holidays, such as Christmas.
* Injuries or severe illnesses.
* Problems with work or school.
* Recent move to a new city or state.
* Sexual difficulties between you and partner.
* Business or financial problems; buying a new home.
* Regular conflict between you and a spouse or family member, close friend, or business associate.
* Constant fatigue.
* Demands on your time and energy levels by other family members.
* World or national events such as war or disasters.

HOW TO PREVENT
* Try to take charge of those aspects of your life that you can control. Ask for help if needed.
* Since stress cannot always be prevented, learn coping techniques to protect your mental and physical health.

WHAT TO EXPECT

DIAGNOSTIC MEASURES
* Diagnosis is often by your own or other's observation of symptoms.
* Medical tests may be done to rule out medical problems that could cause the symptoms. A person may not realize they are stressed.

APPROPRIATE HEALTH CARE
* Counseling may be helpful. Talking about your problems is one way of relieving stress.
* Drug therapy may be recommended.

POSSIBLE COMPLICATIONS—Chronic stress can cause problems with your work and family relationships. Stress can also lead to high blood pressure, and risk of stroke and heart attack.

PROBABLE OUTCOME—Usually resolved with time, self-treatment, or medical care.

HOW TO TREAT

GENERAL MEASURES
* Here are some tips to help reduce stress:
  - Learn a meditation or relaxation technique and practice it regularly, daily if possible.
  - Share your feelings with a close friend.
  - Arrange daily schedules to make them less stressful.
  - Decide what is important and has to get done and what can be put off, left undone or passed on to others.
  - Take a short time away from any stressful situation you encounter during a day. A short walk can help.
  - Learn and practice a muscle-tensing and muscle-relaxing technique. Take warm baths.
  - Make lists of what needs to be done each day. Cross the items off as they are completed.
  - Take time for enjoyable recreation.
  - Avoid taking problems home or to bed with you. At the end of the day, take a few minutes and review the day. Let go of negative emotions. Decide about undone activities. Release mental or muscular tension.
* To learn more: National Mental Health Association, (800) 969-6642; website: www.nmha.org.

MEDICATION—If symptoms are severe, drug therapy may be recommended.

ACTIVITY—Exercise 20 to 30 minutes daily. It helps relieve stress.

DIET—No special diet. Don't skip meals.

CALL YOUR DOCTOR IF

You or a family member has symptoms of stress.

STROKE
(Brain Attack)

GENERAL INFORMATION

DEFINITION—A sudden decrease in the blood supply to part of the brain. This causes damage to the brain so it cannot function normally.

BODY PARTS INVOLVED—Central nervous system; musculoskeletal system.

SEX OR AGE MOST AFFECTED—Both sexes (men more than women); adults over 60 are most often affected.

SIGNS & SYMPTOMS—The symptoms may vary in different people:
* Inability to speak.
* Inability to move part of the body.
* Loss of consciousness.
* Sudden heavy feeling in an arm or leg, or feeling numb and unable to control muscles.
* Headache.
* Vision changes.
* Confusion.
* Dizziness.
* Loss of bowel and bladder control.

CAUSES
* Blood flow to the brain is blocked. It may be from a blood clot that forms in the brain itself due to narrowed arteries. It may be from a blood clot that forms elsewhere in the bloodstream and travels to the brain.
* Hemorrhage (bleeding) due to ruptured blood vessel. The bleeding may occur in the brain or in the space between the brain and the skull.

RISK INCREASES WITH
* Age over 55. Males.
* Diabetes.
* Prior stroke.
* Family history of stroke.
* Cigarette smoking.
* High blood pressure.
* Heart disease.
* Prior transient ischemic attacks (mini strokes).
* Alcohol abuse and some types of drug abuse.

HOW TO PREVENT
* Not always preventable.
* Exercise regularly, eat a healthy diet, and don't smoke.
* Get treatment for diabetes, heart disease, or other chronic disorders.
* Have your blood pressure checked regularly. If it is high, see your health care provider.
* Get medical advice about taking aspirin daily.

WHAT TO EXPECT

DIAGNOSTIC MEASURES
* Call 911 if you think you might be having a stroke or have someone take you to an emergency center. The first few hours are critical for effective treatment.

* Emergency care will include a physical exam and medical tests to check heart, brain, and other body functions.

APPROPRIATE HEALTH CARE
* Treatment may include drugs, oxygen to help with breathing, techniques to remove or breakup blood clots, and sometimes, surgery. Hospital care is needed until symptoms improve. Long-term care may be needed for some patients.
* Early rehabilitation after a stroke will help improve physical abilities. Outcome will depend on the extent of the brain injury. Physical therapy, occupational therapy, and speech therapy may be needed. Patient attitude and family support are important in the success.

POSSIBLE COMPLICATIONS
* Serious physical and mental health problems.
* Major lifestyle changes that affect work, family, and social life.

PROBABLE OUTCOME—Stroke causes death, permanent damage, or disability in two-thirds of all cases. The long-term outlook depends on the extent of brain damage. In some cases, complete recovery without long-term disability is possible.

HOW TO TREAT

GENERAL MEASURES—To learn more: American Stroke Association, 7272 Greenville Ave., Dallas, TX 75231; (888) 478-7653; website: www.strokeassociation.org.

MEDICATION
* Drugs to break up clots, control brain swelling, and prevent complications may be given in the hospital.
* Drugs for high blood pressure, clot prevention, and other preventive drugs may be prescribed.

ACTIVITY—If you have lost muscle control, physical therapy will help you learn to use affected limbs. You can often regain basic skills, such as eating, dressing, and toilet functions.

DIET—At first, you may require feeding tube, then progress to a pureed, soft, and then to a regular diet.

CALL YOUR DOCTOR IF

* You or a family member has symptoms of a stroke or observe them in someone else. This is an emergency!
* New, unexpected symptoms develop during or after treatment.

STYE
(Hordeolum)

 GENERAL INFORMATION

DEFINITION—A stye is an infection or inflammation (red, sore, swollen) of the upper or lower eyelid. It is typically harmless. The medical term for stye is hordeolum.

BODY PARTS INVOLVED—Eyelid; eyelashes; conjunctiva (white of the eye).

SEX OR AGE MOST AFFECTED—Both sexes; all ages.

SIGNS & SYMPTOMS
• A bump on the edge of the eyelid.
• The eyelid area is red, swollen, painful, or tender. The head of the stye is usually on the outside, but it may be on the underside of the lid.
• Eye may be sensitive to bright light.
• A gritty feeling in the eye.
• Eye may water.

CAUSES—Bacterial infection (most often, staphylococcal) in a hair follicle or a gland in the corner of the eye. The infection may be limited to the eyelid or may have spread from somewhere else in the body.

RISK INCREASES WITH
• Having diabetes or other health problem.
• Blepharitis (infection of eyelid margin).
• High cholesterol.
• History of styes.
• Certain chronic skin problems.

HOW TO PREVENT—There are no specific preventive measures. Use a mild shampoo on eyelashes when bathing or washing face. Don't share eye makeup with anyone.

 WHAT TO EXPECT

DIAGNOSTIC MEASURES
• Your own observation of symptoms.
• Consult your health care provider if the stye does not drain or is spreading. Your eye will be examined to make sure there is not another eye problem.

APPROPRIATE HEALTH CARE
• Self-care and time is usually all that is needed.
• Drug therapy may be prescribed.
• Sometimes minor surgery to drain the stye or drugs may be needed to help heal the infection.

POSSIBLE COMPLICATIONS
• Spread of infection to other glands in the eyelid.
• Ongoing infection that may not respond to treatment.

PROBABLE OUTCOME—The infection usually heals on its own. It will drain in about two days. Styes often recur, even with treatment.

 HOW TO TREAT

GENERAL MEASURES
• Use warm-water soaks to relieve pain and inflammation and hasten healing. Apply soaks for 10 minutes. Repeat as often as needed.
• Don't squeeze the stye. It will soon open and release the pus, bringing relief from the pain.
• Do not wear contact lenses until the infection is resolved.

MEDICATION—Antibiotic ointments or creams may be prescribed. Apply according to package instructions.

ACTIVITY—No limits.

DIET—No special diet.

 CALL YOUR DOCTOR IF

• You or a family member has a stye that does not drain on its own.
• Pain occurs in the eye.
• Vision changes.

SUBARACHNOID HEMORRHAGE

 GENERAL INFORMATION

DEFINITION—Sudden bleeding into the subarachnoid space (the area between 2 of the membranes that cover the brain). The space is normally filled with cerebrospinal fluid.

BODY PARTS INVOLVED—Brain; meninges (membranes that cover the brain); blood vessels to the brain.

SEX OR AGE MOST AFFECTED—Both sexes; all ages; most common in adults aged 25 to 50.

SIGNS & SYMPTOMS
* Acute, severe headache, often followed by unconsciousness.
* Stiff neck with pain on movement.
* Eye pain with extreme sensitivity to light.
* Drowsiness, dizziness, convulsions, or coma.
* Vomiting.
* Rapid heartbeat and breathing.
* Fever.
* Numbness, weakness or inability to move an arm or leg.

CAUSES
* Rupture of an aneurysm (weakened part of a blood vessel that causes a bulge or sac-like projection).
* Arteriovenous malformations (abnormalities in arteries or veins) may rupture.
* Head injury (such as from accident or fall).

RISK INCREASES WITH
* Atherosclerosis (hardening of the arteries) or high blood pressure.
* Family history of bleeding disorders.
* Cerebral aneurysms (run in families).
* Polycystic disease of the kidneys.
* Infection in any part of the central nervous system.
* Bleeding disorder, such as sickle-cell anemia, leukemia or any bleeding that is a side effect of prescription drugs.

HOW TO PREVENT
* No specific preventive measures.
* Avoid head injury. Use seat belts in cars, protective head gear in contact sports and helmets while biking.
* Obtain medical treatment for an existing aneurysm or arteriovenous malformation.

 WHAT TO EXPECT

DIAGNOSTIC MEASURES
* Your own observation of symptoms.
* Your health care provider will do a physical exam and ask about symptoms and activities.
* Medical tests may include studies of blood and cerebrospinal fluid, x-rays of the skull, CT, MRI, myelography (special x-ray), heart studies, and lumbar puncture (see Glossary for all tests).

APPROPRIATE HEALTH CARE
* Intensive care is required with treatment directed toward preventing complications.
* Surgery may be done to stop bleeding and remove collected blood.
* Drug therapy for treatment and preventing complications will be prescribed.

POSSIBLE COMPLICATIONS—Permanent disability or death due to complications or delay in diagnosis.

PROBABLE OUTCOME—With prompt medical treatment, recovery chances are increased. Outcome also depends on the patient's age, smoking history, location of an aneurysm, and severity of symptoms.

 HOW TO TREAT

GENERAL MEASURES
* Partial paralysis, weakness or numbness, and speech and visual difficulties may remain in some cases. The damaged area of the brain cannot be restored. However, undamaged areas of the brain often can be taught the lost functions. This usually requires rehabilitation, including physical therapy, occupational therapy or speech therapy. Determination and a positive attitude greatly affect the success of the rehabilitation process.
* Ongoing care may be provided at home or the patient may need to be cared for in an extended care facility.

MEDICATION—You may be prescribed:
* Drugs to control vasospasms (blood vessel spasms).
* Antiseizure drugs.
* Stool softeners to prevent constipation.
* Drugs for high blood pressure.
* Sedatives, antinausea drugs, drugs for pain, and others as needed.

ACTIVITY
* Strict bed rest until source of hemorrhage is eliminated.
* If you have lost some motor functions, occupational and physical therapists will help you use the affected limbs to regain basic skills, such as eating, dressing, and toilet functions.
* After recovery, resume the former activities that your strength and sense of well-being allow. Allow 6 to 12 months for recovery.

DIET—As tolerated at first. May require feeding tube or intravenous feedings.

 CALL YOUR DOCTOR IF

You or a family member has symptoms of a subarachnoid hemorrhage. Get emergency help!

SUBCONJUNCTIVAL HEMORRHAGE

 GENERAL INFORMATION

DEFINITION—Sudden appearance of blood in the white area of the eye. Although the bleeding may seem alarming, it is not serious. The bleeding is from the thin, clear membrane (conjunctiva) that covers the white of the eye (the sclera). Often, a person discovers the problem after waking up in the morning.

BODY PARTS INVOLVED—Eye.

SEX OR AGE MOST AFFECTED—Both sexes; all ages, including newborns.

SIGNS & SYMPTOMS
• A small, usually painless spot of bright red blood in the white of the eye. It may first appear as a patch, but may spread to cover the entire white area of the eye.
• Swelling may occur in that part of the eye.
• There are no vision problems.

CAUSES—When one of the tiny, unseen blood vessels in the conjunctiva breaks, it can bleed and cause the problem. There is often no obvious reason why the vessel breaks. It may follow coughing, sneezing, vomiting, heavy lifting, diving under water, or rubbing of the eyes.

RISK INCREASES WITH—Certain disorders such as high blood pressure, diabetes, or use of blood thinner drugs can be risk factors.

HOW TO PREVENT—No specific preventive measures.

 WHAT TO EXPECT

DIAGNOSTIC MEASURES—Your own observation of symptoms.

APPROPRIATE HEALTH CARE—No treatment is necessary, except time.

POSSIBLE COMPLICATIONS—None expected.

PROBABLE OUTCOME—The blood will go away by itself. It should be absorbed in 1 to 3 weeks. The blood may change color from red to yellow before disappearing.

 HOW TO TREAT

GENERAL MEASURES—Cool compresses may be applied at first. After 24 hours, you may use warm compresses applied to the eye to help hasten the removal of the blood.

MEDICATION
• Drugs are usually not needed for this disorder.
• Nonprescription artificial tears may help if there is any irritation.

ACTIVITY—No rest is needed and you may continue with your regular activities.

DIET—No special diet.

 CALL YOUR DOCTOR IF

• You or a family member has symptoms of subconjunctival hemorrhage with eye pain, your vision changes, or both eyes are affected.
• Your subconjunctival hemorrhage does not get better within 3 weeks, or it recurs often.

SUBDURAL HEMORRHAGE & HEMATOMA

 GENERAL INFORMATION

DEFINITION—Bleeding (hemorrhage) that causes blood to collect and clot (hematoma) beneath the outermost of 3 membranes that cover the brain (meninges). There are 2 types of subdural hematomas. An acute subdural hematoma occurs soon after a severe head injury. A chronic subdural hematoma is a complication that may develop days or weeks after a head injury. The injury may have been so minor that the patient does not remember it.

BODY PARTS INVOLVED—Brain; meninges; blood vessels to the brain.

SEX OR AGE MOST AFFECTED—Both sexes; all ages.

SIGNS & SYMPTOMS
* Recurrent headaches that worsen each day.
* Drowsiness or tiredness, dizziness, mental changes, or confusion.
* Weakness or numbness on one side.
* Slurred speech.
* Vision disturbances.
* Nausea and vomiting.
* Pupils of different size.
* Loss of consciousness after original injury.
* Seizures (convulsions).
* An infant may have increased head size, bulging fontanelles (soft spots in the skull), irritability, high-pitched cry, or seizures. Skull fracture can occur with child abuse.

CAUSES—Injury causes the blood vessels (located between the surface of the brain and its outer covering) to tear and spill blood into the subdural space.

RISK INCREASES WITH
* Head injury.
* Excess alcohol use.
* Drugs that thin the blood (anticoagulants).
* Very young or the elderly.
* Child abuse, such as shaken baby syndrome.

HOW TO PREVENT
* Use seat belts in motor vehicles. Don't drink alcohol or use mind-altering drugs and drive.
* Wear protective head gear during contact sports, or while riding a bicycle or motorcycle.
* Use of safety gear at work, such as hard hats.
* Safety measures at home to prevent falls.
* Report any suspected child abuse.
* Get medical care for illnesses that affect consciousness or balance.

 WHAT TO EXPECT

DIAGNOSTIC MEASURES
* Your own or other's observation of symptoms.
* Your health care provider will do a physical exam and ask questions about the symptoms and any recent head injury.

* Medical tests may include studies of blood and cerebrospinal fluid. X-ray, arteriography, MRI, and/or CT scan are different tests that may help determine the extent of injury.

APPROPRIATE HEALTH CARE
* Hospital care for emergency treatment.
* Treatment steps include lifesaving therapy, controlling symptoms, and preventing permanent brain damage.
* Emergency surgery may be needed to reduce pressure within the brain. This can involve drilling a hole in the skull to let the hematoma drain. Solid clots may be removed through a larger hole (craniotomy).
* Drug therapy may be required.
* In some cases, the hematoma may be small and not as serious. Blood will be absorbed in a few weeks.

POSSIBLE COMPLICATIONS—Death or permanent brain damage, including partial or complete paralysis, behavioral and personality changes, and speech problems.

PROBABLE OUTCOME—The degree of recovery depends upon general health, age, severity of the injury, rapidity of the treatment, and extensiveness of the bleeding or clot. After the clot is removed, brain tissue that has been compressed usually expands slowly to fill its original space. The outlook is good under the best circumstances.

 HOW TO TREAT

GENERAL MEASURES—There is no self-treatment. Follow medical advice about home care after treatment.

MEDICATION—You may be prescribed:
* Drugs to reduce swelling inside the skull.
* Anticonvulsant drugs for seizures.
* Other drugs for specific symptoms.

ACTIVITY—During recovery stay as active as your strength allows. Work and exercise moderately. Rest when you tire. If your speech or muscle control has been damaged, you may need physical therapy or speech therapy.

DIET—Most likely will require intravenous or tube feeding during acute phase and then shift to regular food as tolerated.

 CALL YOUR DOCTOR IF

* You or someone else has a head injury (even if it seems minor) and develops any symptoms of subdural hemorrhage. This is an emergency!
* Fever, surgical wound becomes infected (red, swollen, or tender), headache recurs, or other symptoms occur during or after treatment.

SUBSTANCE ABUSE

 GENERAL INFORMATION

DEFINITION—The continuing misuse of any mind altering substances or chemicals. There is a loss of self-control and a compulsion to continue despite adverse personal, physical, mental, and social outcomes that may result.

BODY PARTS INVOLVED—Whole body.

SEX OR AGE MOST AFFECTED—Males more than females; adolescents and young adults.

SIGNS & SYMPTOMS
Depends on the substance of abuse. Most produce:
* A temporary pleasant mood.
* Relief from anxiety.
* False feelings of self-confidence and being in control.
* Increased sensitivity to sights and sounds (including hallucinations).
* Altered activity levels—either lethargy and sleeplike states, or frenzied states (very active).
* Unpleasant or painful symptoms when abused substance is no longer used (withdrawal).
* Tolerance (need more of substance for high).
* People may observe new and odd behaviors.

CAUSES—Substances of abuse may produce addiction or dependence. Substances of abuse include:
* Nicotine and alcohol.
* Marijuana.
* Amphetamines; barbiturates; cocaine.
* Opiates. These include codeine, heroin, opium, morphine, methadone, hydrocodone, and oxycodone.
* Psychedelic or hallucinogenic drugs (club drugs), including PCP ("angel dust"), mescaline, GHB, and LSD.
* Volatile substances, such as glue, solvents, and paints that are inhaled.
* Abuse of cough remedy dextromethorphan.

RISK INCREASES WITH
* Family history of drug or alcohol abuse.
* Family problems (conflict, stress, lack of closeness, poor parenting, loss of job, physical or sexual abuse).
* Genetic factors (more prone to addiction).
* Peer pressure, especially in teenagers.
* Fatigue or overwork; work or school problems.
* Ease of obtaining the substances of abuse.
* Emotional problems, including depression, dependency, poor self-esteem, anxiety, and stress.

HOW TO PREVENT
* Don't socialize with persons who abuse drugs.
* Get medical help for emotional or mental problems. Don't turn to drugs or alcohol.
* Caring parents can help kids stay drug free.
* Drug education and prevention programs.

 WHAT TO EXPECT

DIAGNOSTIC MEASURES
* Your own or other's observation of symptoms.
* Your health care provider may do a physical exam.
* Medical tests may include blood studies and substance abuse screening studies.

APPROPRIATE HEALTH CARE
* Treatment can be voluntary or involuntary. Family, legal, or job factors may lead a person into treatment.
* No single treatment works for everyone. A plan needs to address the person's type of abuse, their physical and emotional health, and job, social, and legal aspects. A person is rarely able to quit without some help.
* The plan may require a combination of counseling, drug therapy, other medical services, family therapy, parenting instruction, job training, social and legal services. Treatment may take 3 months, or up to a year.
* Counseling (group or alone) is important in recovery.
* Physical symptoms of withdrawal will be treated.
* You may be monitored for use of the substance of abuse during treatment.

POSSIBLE COMPLICATIONS
* Accidents, infections and other health problems.
* Loss of job or family. Legal problems.
* Relapse to using substance of abuse.
* Death caused by overdose.

PROBABLE OUTCOME—Successful recovery from substance abuse can improve all aspects of one's life. It is not easy, but it can be done.

 HOW TO TREAT

GENERAL MEASURES
* Join a a local support group.
* Learn more: National Clearinghouse for Alcohol & Drug Information, (800) 729-6686; website: www.health.org.

MEDICATION—You may be prescribed drugs to help you through withdrawal symptoms. Other drugs may be prescribed to treat emotional or mental problems.

ACTIVITY—Exercise on a regular basis.

DIET—No special diet.

☎ CALL YOUR DOCTOR IF

* You or a family member has a problem with, or has symptoms of, substance abuse.
* Substance abuse continues despite treatment.

SUNBURN

GENERAL INFORMATION

DEFINITION—Redness and soreness of the skin that follows excess exposure to the sun or tanning devices.

BODY PARTS INVOLVED—Exposed skin.

SEX OR AGE MOST AFFECTED—Both sexes; all ages.

SIGNS & SYMPTOMS
• Sunburn symptoms develop 2 to 4 hours after exposure.
• Red, swollen, and (sometimes) blistered skin. Pain occurs and is worse in the first 6 to 48 hours.
• Fever, nausea, and feeling faint (sometimes).

CAUSES—Melanin, a pigment, in the skin helps to protect the skin from exposure to the ultraviolet light from the sun. When there is overexposure, the melanin is unable to keep up the protection, and sunburn occurs.

RISK INCREASES WITH
• Being of fair skin, blue eyes, and red or blonde hair.
• Exposure to the sun from 10:00 a.m. to 3:00 p.m.
• Certain drugs, soaps, or cosmetics may cause a photosensitive reaction. This causes the skin to be even more sensitive to the sun.

HOW TO PREVENT
• Avoid the sun from noon to 3 p.m. Sunburn can occur even on cloudy days. Ultraviolet light is not blocked by thin clouds on overcast days. It is partially screened by smoke and smog. A great deal of ultraviolet light can reflect from snow, water, sand, and sidewalks.
• Use sunscreen daily. Use products with a sun-protective factor (SPF) of 15 or more. Some of these resist water and perspiration. Reapply them every 2 hours or after swimming. Baby oil, mineral oil, or cocoa butter offer no protection from the sun.
• For the best protection, use a physical barrier agent such as zinc-oxide ointment. Reapply after swimming and at frequent intervals during exposure. Barrier agents are helpful on skin areas that are more likely to burn. These include the nose, ears, backs of the legs, and back of the neck.
• Wear clothing that covers your whole body. Protect your face with a wide-brimmed hat. Wear sunglasses.
• If you feel you must get a tan, do it very gradually.

WHAT TO EXPECT

DIAGNOSTIC MEASURES—See your health care provider for severe sunburn or if you have other symptoms such as nausea, vomiting, or swelling. An exam of the affected area will be done and treatment prescribed for any complications.

APPROPRIATE HEALTH CARE—Self-care is usually all that is needed. Medical care may rarely be required for severe symptom.

POSSIBLE COMPLICATIONS
• Blisters may become infected.
• Years of over-exposure to the sun can lead to wrinkled, saggy and leathery skin. The risk of skin cancer is greatly increased.

PROBABLE OUTCOME—Recovery in 3 days to 3 weeks. Tanning or peeling of the skin usually occurs, depending on how severe the burn was.

HOW TO TREAT

GENERAL MEASURES
• To reduce heat and pain, dip gauze or towels in cool water and lay these on the burned areas. Take cool showers.
• Soak in a tub of cool water to which an oatmeal product (Aveeno) or baking soda has been added. Pat skin dry, do not rub. Use a moisturizer to keep the skin from feeling dry.

MEDICATION
• Use nonprescription drugs, such as antihistamines, aspirin (not for children), or acetaminophen to help relieve discomfort.
• Ask your health care provider about using nonprescription burn remedies that contain local anesthetics such as benzocaine or lidocaine. They can produce allergic reactions in some persons.
• Drugs for pain or cortisone drugs to use briefly may be prescribed.

ACTIVITY—Rest in any comfortable position until symptoms get better. Cover yourself with an upside-down "cradle" or tent of cardboard or other material. This will keep bed linens off the burned skin.

DIET—No special diet. Increase fluid intake.

CALL YOUR DOCTOR IF

You or a family member has sunburn that seems severe or there are other symptoms from sun exposure.

SURGICAL WOUND INFECTION

GENERAL INFORMATION

DEFINITION—Infection that develops after a surgical procedure. Infections after surgery occur in 1.5% to 30% of cases, depending on the type of procedure. The medical term is surgical site infections (SSIs).

BODY PARTS INVOLVED—Surgery site.

SEX OR AGE MOST AFFECTED—Both sexes; all ages.

SIGNS & SYMPTOMS
• Symptoms usually begin within 5 to 10 days after surgery, but in some cases, they begin weeks later.
• Pain, redness, and heat around the surgical wound.
• Pus and other collections of fluid around the incision.
• Red streaks in the skin around the wound.
• Fever, chills (sometimes).

CAUSES—Infection with bacteria, including *streptococci*, *staphylococci*, or other germs. These sometimes cause infection, in spite of careful preventive measures.

RISK INCREASES WITH
• Very young and very old persons.
• Poor nutrition (weakness from not being able to eat).
• A pre-existing illness, such as diabetes.
• Weak immune system due to illness or drugs.
• Obese patients.
• Smoking.
• Other infection at the time of surgery.
• Type of surgery being performed.
• Type of surgery wound. It may range from clean to contaminated, depending on several medical factors.
• Increased length of time for the surgery.
• Emergency surgery.

HOW TO PREVENT
• Surgery team members need to follow all medical guidelines for preventing wound infections.
• In some cases, antibiotic drugs may be given prior to surgery to help prevent infections.

WHAT TO EXPECT

DIAGNOSTIC MEASURES
• Your own or other's observation of symptoms.
• Your health care provider will do a physical exam of the surgical wound area.
• Medical tests may include a culture of pus or blood from the infection site.

APPROPRIATE HEALTH CARE
• Treatment may include antibiotic drugs and wound-cleaning procedures.
• Surgery to open the wound and remove infected or damage tissue or treat an abscess may be required.

POSSIBLE COMPLICATIONS
• Delayed healing.
• Sepsis (also called blood poisoning) is a bloodstream infection.
• Chronic infection in some patients.

PROBABLE OUTCOME—In most patients, surgical wound infections heal in about 2 weeks.

HOW TO TREAT

GENERAL MEASURES
• After treatment, relieve pain with heat. Use a heating pad or warm compress 3 or 4 times a day for 30 to 40 minutes.
• Change wound dressings as directed.

MEDICATION
• Antibiotics may be prescribed for an infection. They may be taken by mouth or injected intravenously (into a vein).
• Vitamin and mineral supplements may be recommended.
• Pain relievers. You may use nonprescription drugs, such as acetaminophen, for minor pain.

ACTIVITY—Rest in bed until signs of infection disappear.

DIET—Usually, no special diet required.

CALL YOUR DOCTOR IF

• You or a family member has symptoms of a surgical-wound infection.
• High fever occurs and a general ill feeling, or infection seems to worsen after treatment.
• New, unexplained symptoms develop. Drugs used in treatment may produce side effects.

SYPHILIS

GENERAL INFORMATION

DEFINITION—A sexually transmitted disease. Syphilis is known as the "great mimic," because its symptoms are like those of many other diseases. There are two types. Congenital form occurs in babies (age 0 to 2 weeks) born to mothers with syphilis. Contagious form is the type that affects persons of all ages and both sexes who get it by sexual contact. There may be no symptoms or very mild ones. A person may not know they are infected.

BODY PARTS INVOLVED—Genitals; skin; central nervous system.

SEX OR AGE MOST AFFECTED
• Newborns (0 to 2 weeks) born to mothers with syphilis (congenital form).
• Persons of all ages and both sexes who have sexual contact (contagious form).

SIGNS & SYMPTOMS
• *Primary stage* (contagious; begins 9 to 90 days after exposure; usually at about 3 weeks):
 - A painless, red sore (chancre) on the genitals, mouth, or rectum. The sore usually affects the penis in males and vagina or cervix in females.
• *Secondary stage* (occurs if not treated; contagious; begins 2 to 8 weeks after the chancre appears):
 - Enlarged lymph glands in the neck, armpit, or groin.
 - Headache, sore throat, and feeling tired.
 - Rash on skin and mucous membranes of the penis, vagina, or mouth. The rash has small, red, scaly bumps.
 - Fever (sometimes).
• *Latent stage or hidden stage* (can be 2 to 30 years after second stage; may be contagious):
 - There are no signs or symptoms.
• *Tertiary stage* (rare; not contagious; may appear 2 to 30 years after other stages):
 - The infection can seriously damage the heart, brain, nervous system, eyes, skin, bones, and joints.

CAUSES—A germ (bacteria) called *Treponema pallidum*.
• Contagious form is spread by sexual contact (vaginal, anal, or oral sex) with someone who has the sores or rash. Germs cannot be spread from toilet seats, towels, or other objects.
• Congenital form passes to baby by infected mother.

RISK INCREASES WITH—Unsafe sex.

HOW TO PREVENT
• Latex male condoms used during sexual contact reduces risk, but not 100% protection.
• Avoid sexual contact with infected person or a person whose health history you don't know.
• Obtain blood test for syphilis early in pregnancy. If infected, get treated right away.

WHAT TO EXPECT

DIAGNOSTIC MEASURES
• Your own observation of symptoms.
• Your health care provider will do a physical exam.
• Blood tests and microscope studies of material from a sore are usually done to confirm the diagnosis. Tests for other sexually transmitted diseases are often performed.

APPROPRIATE HEALTH CARE
• Syphilis is treated with drugs.
• Be sure that all your sexual partners obtain treatment. The public health department will help you if needed.
• After drug treatment, blood tests will be done at regular intervals to verify that you are no longer infectious.
• The tertiary stage of syphilis generally requires treatment in a hospital.

POSSIBLE COMPLICATIONS
• After penicillin treatment, a Jarisch-Herxheimer reaction may occur. Previous symptoms get worse (for about 24 hours).
• Treatment in a few patients may need to be repeated.
• Syphilis sores makes it easier to get an HIV infection.
• Without treatment, the disease may progress to the next stage. A number of medical problems and death may occur with tertiary syphilis.

PROBABLE OUTCOME—Curable with antibiotic treatment.

HOW TO TREAT

GENERAL MEASURES—To learn more: Sexually Transmitted Diseases Hotline (800) 227-8922 or the Centers for Disease Control and Prevention (CDC) website: www.cdc.gov.

MEDICATION—Penicillin will be given by injection for all stages. If someone is allergic to penicillin, other antibiotics can be equally effective.

ACTIVITY—Avoid sexual activity until cured.

DIET—No special diet.

CALL YOUR DOCTOR IF

• You or a family member has symptoms of syphilis.
• The following occur during or after treatment: fever, skin rash, sore throat, or swelling in any joint, such as the ankle or knee.
• You have had sexual contact with someone who has syphilis.

TAPEWORM

GENERAL INFORMATION

DEFINITION—A parasitic infection of the digestive tract or other organs. Tapeworms are typically acquired from eating undercooked meat or fish.

BODY PARTS INVOLVED—Intestinal tract.

SEX OR AGE MOST AFFECTED—Both sexes; all ages.

SIGNS & SYMPTOMS
* Most people with this problem have no symptoms.
* Pain in the upper abdomen.
* Diarrhea.
* Unexplained weight loss.
* Symptoms of anemia (weakness, fatigue, and shortness of breath).
* Bowel movements containing worm eggs and worm body parts.

CAUSES
* Parasites: *Taenia saginata* from beef, *Taenia solium* from pork, and *Diphyllobothrium* from fish. People become infected by eating improperly cooked or raw food infected with the parasite.
* *Echinococcus* tapeworm is found in dogs and some livestock (often in sheep). Humans can get an infection (echinococcosis) from this tapeworm. Infected dogs leave feces in soil or water. Humans are infected by eating food grown in the soil or drinking the water. It can also be spread by handling an infected dog or livestock. The infection causes cysts (sores), usually in the liver. Symptoms may not develop for 10 to 20 years after exposure.

RISK INCREASES WITH—Travel to places such as Asia, Africa, or Latin America. This disorder is uncommon in the United States.

HOW TO PREVENT
* Cook beef, pork, and fish thoroughly. Additional information available from the National Center for Nutrition (800) 366-1655 or the Department of Agriculture Meat and Poultry Hotline (800) 535-4555.
* Buy only meat that has been inspected.
* Wash hands after handling raw meat or fish.
* Keep pet dogs clean and dewormed. Wash hands after handling pets or livestock.

WHAT TO EXPECT

DIAGNOSTIC MEASURES
* Your own observation of symptoms.
* Your health care provider may do a physical exam.
* Medical tests usually include a study of a stool sample to check for eggs or worms. If echinococcosis is suspected, an x-ray or blood study may be done.

APPROPRIATE HEALTH CARE
* The usual treatment is with drugs.
* Cysts from echinococcosis infection may need to be removed surgically.
* Have all family members examined for possible infection.

POSSIBLE COMPLICATIONS
* Cysticercosis, a more widespread infection from tapeworm larvae (rare).
* Obstruction of intestine (rare).
* Echinococcosis can cause severe health problems including death.

PROBABLE OUTCOME—Usually curable with appropriate treatment.

HOW TO TREAT

GENERAL MEASURES—Follow medical advice.

MEDICATION—Anthelmintic drug to kill the parasite will be prescribed. The drug can cure with a single dose. Medical tests should be repeated in 3 to 6 weeks to make sure the disorder is cured.

ACTIVITY—No limits.

DIET—No special diet.

CALL YOUR DOCTOR IF

* You or a family member has symptoms of a tapeworm.
* New, unexplained symptoms develop. Drugs used in treatment may produce side effects.

TAY-SACHS DISEASE

 GENERAL INFORMATION

DEFINITION—An inherited, rare disorder of the central nervous system in infants and young children. The classic form causes progressive impairment and early death. Less than 100 children are born with the disease each year in the United States.

BODY PARTS INVOLVED—Brain and central nervous system.

SEX OR AGE MOST AFFECTED—Infants and young children (up to age 5).

SIGNS & SYMPTOMS
• The child seems normal at birth. Symptoms begin to appear before 6 months.
• Loss of alertness and retarded mental development.
• Loss of muscle strength, such as difficulty sitting up or turning over.
• Deafness.
• Blindness.
• Severe constipation caused by an impaired nerve supply to the colon.
• Seizures.

CAUSES
• An inherited disease resulting from a recessive gene that causes enzyme deficiency. If both parents have the gene, they have a 25% chance of having a child with Tay-Sachs disease. If only one parent is a carrier, the children will not have the disease. The gene occurs in 1 out of 60 people of Ashkenazi Jewish or French Canadian ancestry.
• Other forms of Tay-Sachs include:
  - Juvenile form which appears about ages 2 to 5. Symptoms are like the classic form and death occurs by age 15.
  - Chronic form may appear at age 5. Symptoms are like the classic form but are milder.
  - Adult form, which appears between teens and 30s. Symptoms are like chronic the form.

RISK INCREASES WITH—Genetic factors. Many parents who carry the recessive gene are of Eastern European Jewish (Ashkenazi) or French Canadian origin.

HOW TO PREVENT
• A simple blood test can identify Tay-Sachs carriers. It can not be used in pregnant women. For pregnant women, an amniocentesis or chorionic villus testing can be done.
• Obtain genetic counseling if you or your spouse have a family history of Tay-Sachs or are of Ashkenazi or French Canadian background.
• Assisted reproductive technologies can be used to help at-risk couples have a non-affected baby.

 WHAT TO EXPECT

DIAGNOSTIC MEASURES
• Your own observation of symptoms.
• To make the diagnosis, your baby's health care provider will do a physical exam and an eye exam. A cherry-red spot at the back of the eye occurs in a baby with Tay-Sachs disease.
• A blood test will be done to confirm the diagnosis.

APPROPRIATE HEALTH CARE
• Treatment consists of providing comfort and support for the baby.
• Counseling may help parents and siblings to learn to cope with the distress produced by this condition.

POSSIBLE COMPLICATIONS—Symptoms progress to loss of all voluntary movement, which eventually causes death.

PROBABLE OUTCOME—There is no cure or treatment. Death usually occurs before age 5 with the classic form. Research is ongoing.

 HOW TO TREAT

GENERAL MEASURES
• Seek out support groups for families of Tay-Sachs victims.
• To learn more: National Tay-Sachs and Allied Disease Association, 2001 Beacon St., Suite 204, Brookline, MA 02146; (800) 906-8723; website: www.ntsad.org.

MEDICATION—Your health care provider may prescribe:
• Anticonvulsants to control seizures.
• Stool softeners and laxatives to relieve constipation.
• Other drugs to help with complications as they arise.

ACTIVITY—In the early stages, encourage the child to be as active as possible. Increasing loss of mental, nervous, and muscular functions will eventually confine the child to bed much of the time.

DIET—Provide plenty of fluids and a normal, high-fiber diet to reduce constipation. Feeding by tube usually becomes necessary as the disease progresses.

 CALL YOUR DOCTOR IF

• You are concerned about your infant's mental and physical development.
• You think you or any member of your family carries the abnormal gene. A genetic counselor can advise you on how to prevent having children with this disease.

ILLNESS & DISORDERS

TEAR DUCT INFECTION OR BLOCKAGE
(Dacryocystitis; Dacryostenosis)

 GENERAL INFORMATION

DEFINITION—An infected or blocked tear duct causes tears to gather or pool in the eyes and then run down the cheeks even though the person is not crying. Infection of the tear duct is called dacryocystitis. A blocked tear duct is called dacryostenosis.

BODY PARTS INVOLVED—Eye; tear (nasolacrimal) gland, sac or duct.

SEX OR AGE MOST AFFECTED
• Inherited blockage of the tear duct usually appears in infants at 3 to 12 weeks.
• Infection of the tear duct or sac occurs in all ages, but it is most common in children.
• Blockage caused by infection can occur at any age following an infection.

SIGNS & SYMPTOMS
• Increased tearing of one or both eyes.
• Mucus and pus drains out of the tear duct. It may drain on its own or come out when pressure is put on the area.
• Pain, redness, or swelling of the eye area.
• Fever (sometimes).

CAUSES—Tears are stored in a sac (lacrimal sac) and are released into the eyes to help keep them clean, for protection, and to provide lubrication. The tears drain out of the eyes through small pinpoint openings in the corner of the eyes. They then flow through a duct or tube into the nose. The duct is called the nasolacrimal duct. When infection or blockage occurs in the duct, the tears can not drain normally and they back up.

RISK INCREASES WITH
• Tear duct is not fully developed or formed properly in a newborn.
• Bacterial infection of the duct.
• Sinus or nasal infection, or abnormal growths or tumors.
• Surgery on the face, nose, or sinuses.
• Eye injury.
• Conjunctivitis (pink eye).
• Fracture of the nose or facial bones.
• Thickening of tear duct lining as person ages.

HOW TO PREVENT—No specific preventive measures. Get prompt medical care for eye, nose, or sinus infections. For contact sports, wear helmet and facemask to protect the face.

 WHAT TO EXPECT

DIAGNOSTIC MEASURES
• Your own observation of symptoms.
• Your health care provider will do a physical exam of the eye area.

• A sample of the discharge may be tested to check for the germs causing the infection. To confirm the diagnosis, a harmless dye may be placed in the eye. This helps determine if tears are flowing normally. Other tests may be needed in adults.

APPROPRIATE HEALTH CARE
• Treatment may involve drugs for infection, massaging the area, and, for some, surgery to open the duct. In some cases, no treatment is needed.
• If there is excessive tearing, surgery may be recommended to probe the tear duct. A thin wire is passed through the duct to open any obstruction.
• Other surgery options involve placing tubes in the tear duct that stay in for about 6 months or inserting a balloon to stretches the tear duct and then is removed.
• In adults, tear ducts damaged by chronic infection may need to be surgically replaced by creating a new passage or inserting an artificial duct. Tumors or nasal polyps may need to be treated.

POSSIBLE COMPLICATIONS—A blocked tear duct may cause chronic infection. Minor surgery is sometimes needed.

PROBABLE OUTCOME—Infected or blocked tear ducts are usually cured with treatment. Blocked tear ducts in an infant are usually outgrown when they are 9 to 12 months of age.

 HOW TO TREAT

GENERAL MEASURES
• Clean any drainage from the eye with a cotton ball or washcloth moistened with warm water. Gently wipe away any pus or crusted areas.
• For a child with a blocked duct, massage can help. Do it several times a day for 2 months, or as directed. Wash your hands carefully. Place your index finger along side the nose and firmly massage down toward the corner of the nose. Use a warm compress on the eye area to provide comfort and promote drainage.

MEDICATION—Antibiotics for infection may be prescribed. These may be eyedrops, eye ointment, or drugs taken by mouth.

ACTIVITY—No limits unless advised.

DIET—No special diet.

 CALL YOUR DOCTOR IF

• You or a family member has symptoms of a tear duct infection or blockage.
• Symptoms don't improve or vision changes.

TEETHING
(Cutting Teeth; Tooth Eruption)

GENERAL INFORMATION

DEFINITION—The process of the appearance of baby teeth and adult teeth. New teeth erupt continually from around age 6 months to 3 years. Between ages 6 and 12, children lose baby teeth, which are replaced with adult teeth. On average, the first set of teeth is complete soon after the second birthday.

BODY PARTS INVOLVED—Mouth; teeth.

SEX OR AGE MOST AFFECTED—Both sexes of children from ages 6 months to 3 years and 6 to 12 years.

SIGNS & SYMPTOMS
• Excess saliva production, drooling, and chewing on anything the baby can hold.
• Pain. (This symptom cannot be proven, but probably does occur.)
• Gums may become red or swollen.
• Irritability.
• Fretful and clinging.
• Difficulty in sleeping.
• Crying more than usual.
• Teething should never be considered the cause of fever, vomiting, diarrhea, prolonged loss of appetite, earache, convulsions, cough, or diaper rash. These are symptoms of an illness.

CAUSES—Teething is normal. There are 20 baby (or primary) teeth and 32 permanent teeth.

RISK INCREASES WITH—Teething problems are not related to any known risk factor.

HOW TO PREVENT
• Teething problems cannot be prevented, but the symptoms can be relieved.
• The timing of teeth eruption is highly variable. However, the sequence of normal tooth eruption in children is:
  - First teeth (lower front teeth) at about 6 months, sooner in girls than boys. Teething may start as early as one month or as late as one year. Rarely, a baby is born with one or more teeth.
  - Complete set of baby teeth by about age two and a half.
  - First adult teeth at about age 6.
  - Bicuspids (side teeth) ages 10 to 12.
  - Permanent molars at about age 12.

WHAT TO EXPECT

DIAGNOSTIC MEASURES
• Your own observation of teething symptoms.
• Your baby's health care provider will examine the baby's mouth and gums and any new teeth at well-baby check ups.

APPROPRIATE HEALTH CARE—Home care is all that is needed. Follow any special medical instructions if advised.

POSSIBLE COMPLICATIONS—None expected.

PROBABLE OUTCOME—Teething discomfort can be partially relieved.

HOW TO TREAT

GENERAL MEASURES
• Rub the child's gums with a clean finger; this is very comforting.
• Freeze a wet washcloth for the baby to chew on.
• Offer the child a safe, one-piece teething ring. It can be cooled in the refrigerator (don't freeze the ring).
• Don't put anything into the baby's mouth that might cause choking. Don't tie anything around the neck.
• Sucking a thumb, finger, or pacifier will not harm the baby's teeth. If sucking continues after age four, talk to your child's dentist to see if there are any concerns.
• Clean new teeth and gums with your finger using a soft washcloth. When the teeth are bigger, start brushing them with a baby's toothbrush.
• Begin regular dental visits at about age one.
• At age five, explain to the child that losing baby teeth is normal. This prevents the child from becoming concerned when tooth loss begins.

MEDICATION
• Drugs are not usually needed for teething.
• Your baby's health care provider may suggest:
  - Acetaminophen for the pain.
  - A cream or ointment rubbed on the gums to ease discomfort.

ACTIVITY—No limits.

DIET
• Don't let your baby go to bed or walk around with a bottle with milk in it. Milk that stays in contact with the teeth for a long time can cause decay.
• Start your baby or toddler off to a healthy diet that will promote healthy teeth. Avoid too many sweets, sticky foods, or constant snacks during the day.

CALL YOUR DOCTOR IF

You are unsure if teething is causing the symptoms.or signs of infection occur (such as pain, pus, a lot of swelling, or very red gums).

TELOGEN EFFLUVIUM

GENERAL INFORMATION

DEFINITION—A common hair loss disorder in which numerous, scattered hair follicles simultaneously change from the growth phase (called anagen) to the resting phase (called telogen) of the hair-growth cycle. The disorder can be acute (short term) or chronic (long term). Persons with telogen effluvium rarely progress to significant baldness and it is not contagious.

BODY PARTS INVOLVED—Scalp hair usually. It can cause hair loss on all parts of the body.

SEX OR AGE MOST AFFECTED—Both sexes (somewhat more common in females) and all ages; even infants can be affected.

SIGNS & SYMPTOMS
• Hair loss at much more than the normal rate. Normal hair loss is about 100 hairs a day (on a comb or brush, on a pillow, or in the sink).
• No itching or pain.

CAUSES—Psychological stress that can be due to a variety of factors (or events). The hair loss may begin several months after the event (such as childbirth) occurred.

RISK INCREASES WITH
• Illness (acute or chronic).
• Major surgery.
• Severe trauma.
• Severe emotional stress.
• High fever.
• Thyroid gland problems.
• Changes in diet (such as crash dieting, low protein intake, anorexia, and iron deficiency).
• Hormonal changes (such as those that occur during adolescence, following childbirth or starting or discontinuing use of oral contraceptives).
• Certain drugs (such as beta blockers, anticoagulants, and others, and immunizations).

HOW TO PREVENT—No specific preventive measures.

WHAT TO EXPECT

DIAGNOSTIC MEASURES
• Your own observation of symptoms.
• Your health care provider will do a physical exam of the scalp and ask questions about your symptoms and activities.
• Medical tests may be done to check for any underlying medical disorder.
• You may be asked to collect all hairs that are shed for a 24 hour period. This test may be repeated 3 to 4 times over several weeks. If the number shed decreases, then the disorder is resolving itself.

APPROPRIATE HEALTH CARE—No specific treatment is usually needed.

POSSIBLE COMPLICATIONS—None expected.

PROBABLE OUTCOME—Spontaneous recovery in 6 to 12 months.

HOW TO TREAT

GENERAL MEASURES—Continue to wash and brush your hair as usual. A change of hair style may disguise the hair loss and improve cosmetic appearance.

MEDICATION
• Drugs are usually not necessary for this disorder. They may be prescribed if an underlying disorder is diagnosed.
• Nonprescription hair growth products for the scalp may be tried if desired.
• If a drug you take is the cause, your health care provider will discuss other options.

ACTIVITY—No limits. Engage in a regular exercise program at 3 or more times a week to reduce stress and maintain good overall fitness.

DIET—If diet problems are involved, consult a dietician. Steps can be taken to to be sure a healthy diet is a part of your lifestyle.

CALL YOUR DOCTOR IF

• Hair loss doesn't improve in 4 months.
• Signs of infection (pain, redness, tenderness, swelling) begin at the site of hair loss.

TEMPOROMANDIBULAR JOINT (TMJ) DISORDER

GENERAL INFORMATION

DEFINITION—Pain in the temporomandibular joint. This is the joint on either side of the lower jaw that opens and closes the mouth.

BODY PARTS INVOLVED—Temporo-mandibular joint; facial muscles; sensory nerves.

SEX OR AGE MOST AFFECTED—Adults of both sexes, but more common in women.

SIGNS & SYMPTOMS
• Symptoms may come on slowly; they may begin suddenly if there is an injury to the area.
• Dull, aching pain on one side of the jaw. It occurs below or in front of the ear, in the temples, in back of the head, and along the jaw line.
• It may hurt to chew.
• "Clicking" or "popping" joint sounds.
• Unable to open the jaw all the way or rarely, jaw may "lock" in open position.
• Headache, dizziness, and toothache.
• Ears feel pressured, clogged, aching, or you may hear ringing.
• Tired facial muscles from yawning, speaking, or when waking up. Head, shoulder, and neck muscles may ache.

CAUSES—Normally the jaw, the skull, the muscles that attach to and move the jaw, and the involved nerves work together in a smooth relationship. For a variety of reasons, an imbalance occurs in the way one or more of these parts function. This brings about the symptoms.

RISK INCREASES WITH
• Physical and emotional stress.
• Joint is affected by jaw, head, or neck injuries.
• Grinding or clenching teeth (sometimes during sleep).
• Chewing gum or biting nails.
• Tension of the masticatory (chewing) muscles.
• Faulty alignment ("bite") between the upper and lower jaws (disk derangement).
• Osteoarthritis, rheumatoid arthritis, or gout.
• Work habits such as holding a phone between shoulder and ear.

HOW TO PREVENT—No specific preventive measures. Avoid risk factors where possible.

WHAT TO EXPECT

DIAGNOSTIC MEASURES
• Your own observation of symptoms.
• Your health care provider will do a physical exam of the jaw area and ask questions about your symptoms and habits.
• Medical tests may include jaw range-of-motion studies, x-rays, and others.

APPROPRIATE HEALTH CARE
• Treatment plans may include lifestyle changes, drug therapy for pain, diet changes, and simple jaw exercises. For tooth or denture problems, see a dental care provider.
• Counseling may be helpful for stress problems.
• Simple jaw exercises may help. You will be instructed on how to do stretching and relaxing exercises.
• You may be fitted with a special splint or biteplate that will help reduce clenching or teeth grinding.
• A procedure to wash out the joint or inject pain drugs may be done in a medical office with local anesthesia.
• Severe cases that do not respond to simpler measures may need surgery to reconstruct the joint (rare).

POSSIBLE COMPLICATIONS
• Arthritis of the joint.
• Chronic pain of the face.

PROBABLE OUTCOME—The symptoms often clear up on their own in about 2 weeks. In most other cases, simple treatment measures can relieve symptoms.

HOW TO TREAT

GENERAL MEASURES
• Try to limit jaw movements and learn to relax the jaw. Don't open it wide. Block a yawn by putting your fist under your chin. Don't chew gum.
• Ice and/or heat may be of benefit in relieving discomfort. Try one and then the other to see what works best for you. Massage the TMJ muscle area.
• To learn more: TMJ Association, PO Box 26770, Milwaukee, WI 53226; (414) 259-3223 (not toll free); website: www.tmj.org.

MEDICATION
• For pain and inflammation, use nonprescription drugs such as aspirin (not for children) or ibuprofen.
• Muscle relaxants, drugs for pain, or steroids may be prescribed for a short time.

ACTIVITY—No limits.

DIET—Eat a soft diet until symptoms subside. Avoid hard or chewy foods (such as bagels).

CALL YOUR DOCTOR IF

• You or a family member has symptoms of temporomandibular joint disorder.
• Symptoms do not improve with treatment.

TENDINITIS & TENOSYNOVITIS

GENERAL INFORMATION

DEFINITION—Inflammation of a tendon (tendinitis) and the lining of the tendon sheath (tenosynovitis). They often occur at the same time. Tendons are made up of tough, fibrous, cord-like tissue. A typical skeletal muscle has a tendon on each end that attaches to the bone.

BODY PARTS INVOLVED—Common sites are the shoulder (rotator cuff), elbow, heel (Achilles' tendon), knee or hamstring.

SEX OR AGE MOST AFFECTED—Both sexes; adolescents and adults.

SIGNS & SYMPTOMS
• Limited movement, tenderness, pain, and swelling around the inflamed tendon. Common sites are the shoulder, elbow, Achilles' tendon (heel), or hamstring.
• Weakness in the tendon caused by calcium deposits that often accompany tendinitis.

CAUSES—Inflammation or a small tear in a tendon. The tendons become inflamed for a variety of reasons. Inflammation is a reaction of the body's tissues to injury, infection, or irritation. The four signs of inflammation are redness, swelling, heat, and pain.

RISK INCREASES WITH
• Injury or overuse, usually from an athletic activity, exercising, or during work.
• Incorrect movement and strain during activity. For example, repeatedly holding and swinging a tennis racket incorrectly may cause tendinitis at the elbow (tennis elbow).
• Certain joint diseases (rheumatoid arthritis, scleroderma, gout, and Reiter's disease).
• Aging (tendons are more prone to injury).

HOW TO PREVENT
• Gradually build up the intensity and frequency of an activity.
• Avoid overuse of muscles and tendons. Maintain strength and flexibility. Warm up before each workout and stretch afterwards.
• Learn the proper techniques for any exercise or sport you intend to do regularly.
• Wear proper gear for any sport or exercise activity including well-fitting shoes.

WHAT TO EXPECT

DIAGNOSTIC MEASURES
• Your own observation of symptoms.
• See your health care provider if symptoms persist or are more severe. A physical exam of the affected area will be done and questions asked about your symptoms and activities.
• X-rays do not show tendon problems, but they may be done if an injury occurred.

APPROPRIATE HEALTH CARE
• Treatment usually involves self-care.
• Steps include rest, ice or heat, drug therapy, range-of-motion exercises, and plans to prevent recurrence.
• Surgery may be recommended in chronic tendinitis.
• Physical therapy may be needed to help regain strength and flexibility.

POSSIBLE COMPLICATIONS
• Chronic disability.
• Tendon rupture.
• Tendinitis may recur.

PROBABLE OUTCOME—Usually curable with self-care and rest of the affected tendon area. Pain and swelling usually decrease in a few days. Allow 6 weeks for complete healing.

HOW TO TREAT

GENERAL MEASURES
• When resting, sleeping, or sitting, place the injured area on a pillow (at or above heart level).
• Wrap the area in a compressive (Ace) elastic bandage to help reduce swelling.
• Apply ice packs to the affected area. Do this several times a day for the first 24 to 48 hours. Then, apply them twice a day until pain is gone. You can apply heat if it feels good. Take hot showers, soak in a warm bath, apply warm compresses, or use a heating pad.
• You may want to use a sling or splint for an arm or shoulder to limit movement. Use crutches, a cane or a brace, for affected leg, knee, or heel if needed.

MEDICATION
• Use nonprescription nonsteroidal anti-inflammatory drugs and pain relievers such as ibuprofen.
• Steroid injection for painful tendons may be prescribed. This reduces pain and inflammation and allows movement. Injections are done just a few times because steroids can weaken the tendon.

ACTIVITY
• After a few days, begin range-of-motion exercises to prevent stiffness in the area. Do them 3 to 4 times a day.
• Resume normal activities as symptoms improve.

DIET—No special diet.

CALL YOUR DOCTOR IF

• You or a family member has symptoms of tendinitis are more severe or symptoms don't improve with self-care.
• Pain and swelling increase despite treatment.

TENNIS ELBOW
(Epicondylitis, Lateral)

 GENERAL INFORMATION

DEFINITION—A disorder that involves the tendons on the outside of the elbow at the epicondyle. The epicondyle is the bony area on the outside of the elbow. This is where muscles of the forearm attach to the bone of the upper arm. When the muscles and bones of the elbow are involved as well as the tendons, it is called epicondylitis.

BODY PARTS INVOLVED—Elbow muscles, tendons, and epicondyle.

SEX OR AGE MOST AFFECTED—Both sexes; adults (20 to 40 years).

SIGNS & SYMPTOMS
• Pain and tenderness over the bony part of the elbow.
• Unable to straighten the arm completely.
• Stiffness in elbow in the morning.
• Pain when bending or twisting the hand and arm.
• Weak grip (even when grabbing a light object such as a coffee cup).

CAUSES—An overuse injury. Small tears occur in the tendon and inflammation develops. It is called tennis elbow, but can be due to numerous other activities.

RISK INCREASES WITH
• Work or an activity that requires repetitive forearm movement such as hedge clipping or tennis.
• Work or an activity that requires excessive, constant gripping or squeezing.
• Poor physical condition.
• Sudden strain on the forearm.

HOW TO PREVENT
• For work or sports activity requiring elbow movement, warm up the arm for 5 to 10 minutes. Take frequent breaks. Use ice pack on elbow if pain develops.
• Do flexibility and strength exercises for the arm and elbow.
• Don't play sports, such as tennis, for long periods until you are in good condition. Learn proper playing techniques. Tennis racquets can aggravate tennis elbow. Choosing a different size or type (larger, more flexible, larger grip) may help.

 WHAT TO EXPECT

DIAGNOSTIC MEASURES
• Your own observation of symptoms.
• See your health care provider if symptoms persist or are more severe. A physical exam of the affected area will be done and questions asked about your symptoms and activities.

• X-rays do not show tendon problems, but they may be done if an injury occurred.

APPROPRIATE HEALTH CARE
• Mild cases may be self-treated if desired.
• Treatment may involve rest, ice or heat, massage, drugs, exercises, and steps to prevent recurrence.
• Surgery possibly (if other methods of treatment fail).

POSSIBLE COMPLICATIONS
• Chronic disability.
• Tendon rupture.
• Tennis elbow may recur.

PROBABLE OUTCOME—Usually curable, but it takes time. Healing may require 3 to 6 months or longer.

 HOW TO TREAT

GENERAL MEASURES
• When resting, sleeping, or sitting, place the injured area on a pillow—at or above heart level.
• Wrap the thickest portion of the forearm in a compressive (Ace) bandage to reduce swelling. Massage the area several times a day.
• Apply ice packs to the affected area (several times a day) for the first 24 to 48 hours. Then, apply heat if it feels good. Take hot showers, soak in a bath, apply hot compresses, or a heating pad.
• You may need to wear a forearm splint to immobilize the elbow. Do the following exercise 3 or 4 times a day while wearing the splint. Stretch your arm, flex your wrist, and then press the back of your hand against a wall. Hold for 1 minute.

MEDICATION
• Use nonprescription nonsteroidal anti-inflammatory drugs and pain relievers such as ibuprofen or aspirin (not for children).
• Steroid injection for painful tendons may be prescribed. This reduces pain and inflammation and allows movement. Injections are done just a few times as steroids can weaken the tendon.

ACTIVITY—Don't repeat the activity that caused tennis elbow until symptoms clear up. Stretching and strength exercises are often prescribed to do at home.

DIET—No special diet.

 CALL YOUR DOCTOR IF

• You or a family member has symptoms of tennis elbow.
• Symptoms don't improve in 2 weeks with treatment.

TESTICLE, UNDESCENDED (Cryptorchidism)

 GENERAL INFORMATION

DEFINITION—While in the uterus, a baby boy's testicles grow in his abdomen and then move down (descend) into his scrotum. Sometimes at birth, one or both testicles have not descended into the scrotum. Over 3% of full-term newborn males, and 30% of premature newborn males have undescended testes. The medical term for the condition is cryptorchidism.

BODY PARTS INVOLVED—One or both testes (testicles); scrotum; spermatic cord.

SEX OR AGE MOST AFFECTED—Male infants and children.

SIGNS & SYMPTOMS—One or both testicles can't be felt in the normal position in the scrotum. "Testes" is another name for testicles.

CAUSES—Unknown. It may be related to a hormone deficiency in the mother or fetus.

RISK INCREASES WITH
• Family history of undescended testicle.
• Premature birth.
• Low birth weight.

HOW TO PREVENT—No specific preventive measures.

 WHAT TO EXPECT

DIAGNOSTIC MEASURES
• Your own observation of symptoms.
• Your child's health care provider will do a physical exam. One or both testicles will not be in the scrotum, but they can often be felt above it. If they cannot be located, medical testing may be needed. Follow-up exams are done to check if they have descended.

APPROPRIATE HEALTH CARE
• If the testicle lies in the scrotum at times and then occasionally retracts, the problem normally resolves itself by puberty. No treatment is needed.
• Surgery (called orchiopexy) to move the testicles into the scrotum is usually recommended. Surgery is normally performed between 6 and 24 months of age and is successful in most cases. Your child may have the surgery, which takes about one hour, and go home the same day. Follow-up care instructions will be provided.
• In cases where a testicle is missing or cannot be moved surgically, artificial ones (implants) are available.
• Adult men with undescended testicles may have them removed or left in place. Your health care provider will discuss options with you.

POSSIBLE COMPLICATIONS
• Inguinal hernia (weak area in wall of abdomen where intestines may protrude).
• Increased risk of testicular cancer as an adult.
• Sterility or reduced fertility rate.
• Emotional problems, about the physical appearance of an empty scrotum, may develop as a boy gets older.
• Testicular torsion (twisting).

PROBABLE OUTCOME—Most testicles will descend without treatment by 3 to 6 months of age. If they remain undescended, treatment can usually correct the problem.

 HOW TO TREAT

GENERAL MEASURES—None specific.

MEDICATION
• Hormone therapy may be prescribed in some cases. It helps increase male hormones, which may cause the testicles to descend.
• Pain relief drugs may be prescribed following surgery.

ACTIVITY—No limits, except those following surgery.

DIET—No special diet.

 CALL YOUR DOCTOR IF

Your child has undescended testicle. Call as soon as you find symptoms of this problem.

TESTICULAR CANCER

GENERAL INFORMATION

DEFINITION—Growth of malignant cells in the testicle. Testicles are the male sex glands and are located in the scrotum. It is the most common form of cancer in young men.

BODY PARTS INVOLVED—Testicles (usually one only).

SEX OR AGE MOST AFFECTED—It can affect all ages, but it is found more in ages 18 to 32.

SIGNS & SYMPTOMS
- A firm swelling in one testicle discovered by accident or by self-examination.
- No pain (90% of cases).
- Sense of fullness in the scrotum.
- A rarer type of the cancer may cause breast tenderness or swelling and loss of sexual desire.
- If cancer has spread, there may be back or chest pain, cough, and shortness of breath.

CAUSES—Unknown. There are several types of testicular cancer depending on the cells where it develops. The most common type is called germ cell. It develops in cells that produce sperm. Rarely are both testicles affected.

RISK INCREASES WITH
- Undescended testicles in infancy even if the testicle was surgically moved into the scrotum.
- Caucasian race.
- Being a younger male. Men over age 40 are less likely to get this form of cancer.
- Personal or family history of testicular cancer.
- Klinefelter's syndrome (a congenital disorder).
- Testicles that did not develop normally.

HOW TO PREVENT—Males should examine testicles routinely at least once a month. This will not prevent the cancer, but the self-exam may detect a tumor early enough for effective treatment. Your health care provider can give you instructions on how to do a self-exam.

WHAT TO EXPECT

DIAGNOSTIC MEASURES
- Your own observation of symptoms. Testicular self-examination is an important diagnostic measure.
- Your health care provider will do a physical exam of the genital area.
- Different medical tests are usually done to verify the diagnosis and to determine if cancer has spread (called staging).

APPROPRIATE HEALTH CARE
- Treatment often involves surgery (called orchidectomy) to remove the cancerous testicle. Radiation therapy and/or chemotherapy (anticancer drugs) may be prescribed depending on the type and stage of the cancer. Bone marrow transplantation is another form of treatment.
- Some patients may want to arrange to have their sperm frozen in a sperm bank before treatment. This will allow them to produce children (if fertility is lost).
- Testicular prosthesis (implants) may be a choice of some patients after surgery. They are made of saline and are implanted in the scrotum to look and feel natural.

POSSIBLE COMPLICATIONS
- Without treatment, cancer may spread to other places in the body.
- Cancer may recur or develop in the other testicle.
- Infertility.
- Impotence.

PROBABLE OUTCOME—Most types of testicular tumors are curable with early diagnosis and treatment. Removal of one testicle does not interfere with normal sexual function or the ability to have children.

HOW TO TREAT

GENERAL MEASURES—To learn more: American Cancer Society, (800) ACS-2345; website: www.cancer.org or National Cancer Institute, (800) 4-CANCER; website: www.nci.nih.gov.

MEDICATION
- Chemotherapy may be prescribed.
- Pain medicine if needed.

ACTIVITY
- Resume your normal activities as soon as possible. Radiation and chemotherapy may cause temporary fatigue requiring extra rest.
- Resume sexual relations when you are able.

DIET—No special diet.

CALL YOUR DOCTOR IF

- You or a family member has a firm swelling or mass in the scrotum.
- New, unexplained symptoms develop due to a treatment procedure.

ILLNESS & DISORDERS

TESTICULAR TORSION

GENERAL INFORMATION

DEFINITION—Twisting of the spermatic cord of the testicle. This may damage the testicle. Testicle torsion usually occurs on one side only. Prompt treatment is necessary to save the affected testicle.

BODY PARTS INVOLVED—Testicle; spermatic cord; blood supply to each.

SEX OR AGE MOST AFFECTED—Males of all ages, but most common in ages 12 to 20 years.

SIGNS & SYMPTOMS
* Sudden pain in one testicle. it often starts in the night. Some prior pain may have been felt off and on, but it went away on its own.
* Swelling, redness, and tenderness of the scrotum.
* Nausea and vomiting.
* Sweating.
* Fever (sometimes).
* More frequent urination.

CAUSES—Usually unknown. It may be a problem of weak connective tissue whereby the testicle is not attached firmly within the scrotum. The testicle is more movable and more likely to become twisted.

RISK INCREASES WITH
* Undescended testicles.
* Trauma to the scrotum.
* Strenuous exercise.

HOW TO PREVENT—No specific preventive measures. Wear an athletic supporter or cup when participating in contact sports to prevent genital injury.

WHAT TO EXPECT

DIAGNOSTIC MEASURES
* Your own observation of symptoms.
* Your health care provider will do a physical exam of the scrotum area and ask questions about your symptoms and activities. This is usually all that is needed for diagnosis.
* Medical tests are normally not needed, but may be done to confirm the diagnosis.

APPROPRIATE HEALTH CARE
* Immediate surgery is the usual treatment.
* In some cases, gentle manipulation by hand may undo the twisting. This is a temporary measure and is usually followed up with surgery to stop recurrence.
* Surgery is done to untangle the twisted spermatic cord. The affected testicle is attached to the inside scrotal wall, which prevents recurrence. The surgery will probably also include treatment on the unaffected testicle to prevent torsion.

POSSIBLE COMPLICATIONS
* Loss of testicle. The testicle may be injured beyond repair unless surgery is done within about 6 hours after symptoms begin. If one testicle must be removed, the remaining healthy testicle should provide enough hormones for normal male growth, sex life, and fertility.
* Cosmetic deformity.
* Infection in the scrotum and testicle.

PROBABLE OUTCOME—Curable with prompt diagnosis and treatment.

HOW TO TREAT

GENERAL MEASURES—After surgery, use ice packs to relieve pain and swelling. Wrap the ice in plastic. Apply it to the affected side, separating the ice from the skin with a cloth towel. Apply ice 5 to 10 minutes at a time. Repeat as often as necessary.

MEDICATION—After surgery, pain relievers may be prescribed.

ACTIVITY—Resume your normal activities gradually after surgery.

DIET—No special diet.

CALL YOUR DOCTOR IF

* You or a family member has symptoms of testicular torsion. This is an emergency!
* Signs of infection begin after surgery. These include fever, chills, muscle aches, headache, dizziness, and a general ill feeling.
* Excessive bleeding occurs at the surgical site.

TETANUS
(Lockjaw)

GENERAL INFORMATION

DEFINITION—An infection in a wound that causes severe muscle spasms and can lead to death. Tetanus cannot be spread from person to person. It is now rare, due to tetanus immunization.

BODY PARTS INVOLVED—Injured tissue; muscles throughout the body, especially the jaw, neck, back and abdomen.

SEX OR AGE MOST AFFECTED—Both sexes; all ages.

SIGNS & SYMPTOMS
* Stiffness of the jaw.
* Muscle pain and frequent, severe spasms.
* Headache.
* Sore throat and difficulty in swallowing.
* Difficulty using chest muscles to breathe.
* Fast pulse.
* Profuse sweating.
* Stiff neck, arms, and legs.

CAUSES—Bacteria (*Clostridium tetani*) that are present almost everywhere, especially in soil, manure, or dust. Bacteria may enter through any break in the skin, including burns or puncture wounds. The wound can be tiny such as with a splinter. Toxins produced by the bacteria travel to nerves that control muscle contraction, producing muscle spasms and seizures.

RISK INCREASES WITH
* Lack of up-to-date tetanus immunization.
* Newborn infants born to non-immunized mothers.
* Use of street drugs with unclean needles and syringes.
* Burns, surgical wounds, and skin ulcers.
* Outdoor work or outdoor sports activity.

HOW TO PREVENT
* Obtain tetanus vaccination. It is given in a series of shots in combination with a diphtheria and pertussis vaccine in children. Booster shots are recommended every 10 years thereafter.
* An additional booster shot may be needed at the time of an injury.

WHAT TO EXPECT

DIAGNOSTIC MEASURES
* Your own observation of symptoms.
* Your health care provider will do a physical exam and ask questions about your symptoms and activities.
* Medical tests may include blood studies and culture of the wound site.

APPROPRIATE HEALTH CARE
* Hospital care is required. A quiet, dark room may be recommended. Treatment may include the use of breathing support with a respirator (machine to help breathing), intravenous (IV) fluid support, and drug therapy.
* Surgery to remove infected tissue may be needed.

POSSIBLE COMPLICATIONS
* Pneumonia.
* High blood pressure.
* Severe pain with muscle spasms.
* Irregular heartbeat.
* Bone fractures.
* Coma.
* Infection.
* Brain damage.
* Respiratory paralysis and death.

PROBABLE OUTCOME—With early diagnosis and treatment, full recovery is likely in mild or moderate tetanus. Allow 4 weeks for recovery. The death rate from severe tetanus is about 50%.

HOW TO TREAT

GENERAL MEASURES—Provide the patient with reassurance and emotional support. Despite the seriousness of tetanus, patients are usually conscious.

MEDICATION—You may be given:
* Antitoxins to neutralize the nerve toxin.
* Muscle relaxants to control spasms.
* Sedatives to relieve anxiety.
* Anticonvulsants.
* Antibiotics.
* Tetanus combination vaccine.

ACTIVITY—During hospital time, bed rest is needed with as little disturbance as possible. During recovery, activities should be resumed gradually.

DIET—During treatment, intravenous (IV) fluids will be needed because of difficulty in swallowing.

CALL YOUR DOCTOR IF

* You or a family member has symptoms of tetanus or observes them in someone else. Call immediately. This is an emergency!
* You or someone in your family needs basic or booster tetanus immunizations.
* You have a puncture wound or injury that breaks the skin, and you have not had a tetanus immunization or booster in 5 years.

THALASSEMIA
(Mediterranean Anemia)

 GENERAL INFORMATION

DEFINITION—Inherited blood disorders in which red blood cells contain less hemoglobin than normal. Types are:
- Alpha-thalassemia—Found in populations from the Chinese subcontinent (Malaysia, Indochina, Africa). It is less common than the beta type.
- Beta-thalassemia—Found in Mediterranean area and Africa. If a person inherits one defective gene, it is called beta thalassemia minor (or trait); with two defective genes (one from each parent), it is called beta thalassemia major (or Cooley's anemia) and is a more serious disorder; a milder form also exists, betathalassemia intermedia.

BODY PARTS INVOLVED—Blood.

SEX OR AGE MOST AFFECTED—Both sexes; all ages.

SIGNS & SYMPTOMS—The minor form may produce no symptoms. When symptoms occur, they may include:
- Fatigue.
- Paleness.
- Breathlessness.
- Irregular heartbeat, especially with exertion.
- Bloody or dark urine.
- Jaundice (yellow skin and eyes).
- Deformed bones.
- Enlarged spleen.

CAUSES—Inherited cause by various gene mutations. The gene affects hemoglobin production. Hemoglobin in healthy people has two pairs of protein chains (alpha and beta); with thalassemia, one of the protein chains is reduced and causes an imbalance between the two chains in the hemoglobin produced.

RISK INCREASES WITH
- Family history of thalassemia.
- Genetic factors, including absence of the gene necessary to manufacture hemoglobin-A. The disorder first appeared in persons of Mediterranean heritage; it also affects people from the Middle East and Far East.

HOW TO PREVENT
- Cannot be prevented at present. If you have a family history of thalassemia, obtain genetic counseling before having children.
- Prenatal screening is available.

 WHAT TO EXPECT

DIAGNOSTIC MEASURES
- Your health care provider will do a physical exam and ask questions about your symptoms.
- Medical tests will include blood studies.

- A number of other medical tests may be done to verify the diagnosis or to determine if there are any complications.

APPROPRIATE HEALTH CARE
- Patients with thalassemia trait normally require no treatment. Genetic counseling is usually recommended.
- The main form of treatment for severe thalassemia is blood transfusions along with iron chelation (therapy to remove excess iron in the blood).
- Bone marrow transplantation or stem cell transplantation may be options for some.
- Research continues into finding new and effective treatments, such as gene therapy.
- Surgery to remove the spleen may be recommended.

POSSIBLE COMPLICATIONS
- Infections, worsening of anemia, jaundice, leg ulcers, cholelithiasis (gallstones), pathologic fractures, impaired growth rate, delayed or absent puberty, cardiac disease, and iron overload.
- Transfusion or chelation complications.
- It can cause death by early adulthood or middle age, depending on severity.

PROBABLE OUTCOME—Varies. This condition is currently considered incurable. However, symptoms can be relieved or controlled. Some forms are consistent with a normal or nearly normal lifespan.

 HOW TO TREAT

GENERAL MEASURES—To learn more: Cooley's Anemia Foundation, 129-09 26th Ave., Ste 203, Flushing, NY 11354; (800)522-7222; website www.thalassemia.org.

MEDICATION—You may be prescribed:
- Antibiotics for infections.
- Folic acid, vitamin C, and vitamin E.
- Deferoxamine by injection for iron chelation therapy.
- Drugs to prevent blood transfusion reactions.

ACTIVITY—Activity levels are usually not limited unless there are heart problems. You will be advised of any recommended limits.

DIET
- Try to avoid foods rich in iron.
- Drinking coffee or tea may help reduce the iron in the body.

 CALL YOUR DOCTOR IF

You or a family member has symptoms of anemia (fatigue, paleness, irregular heartbeat, breathlessness) or you want genetic counseling.

THORACIC-OUTLET SYNDROME
(Cervical-Rib Syndrome)

 GENERAL INFORMATION

DEFINITION—Thoracic outlet syndrome (TOS) is a general term used to describe symptoms that occur due to pressure on nerves and blood vessels in the neck area. The thoracic outlet is a space between the rib cage and the collar-bone.

BODY PARTS INVOLVED—Nerves and blood vessels that supply the neck, shoulders, arms and hands.

SEX OR AGE MOST AFFECTED—Adults between ages 35 and 55, usually women.

SIGNS & SYMPTOMS
• Numbness, tingling, or prickling feelings in the neck, shoulders, arms, and hands.
• There may be no pain or mild to more severe pain.
• Weakness and tiredness in the arms and hands.
• Poor blood flow that causes coldness, swelling, and blueness in the hands and fingers (rare).
• Sense of touch may be lost.

CAUSES—Nerves and blood vessels that supply the shoulder, arms, and hands begin in the neck. They then pass as a bundle near the cervical ribs and collarbone. Pressure on this nerve and blood vessel bundle creates symptoms. There are multiple problems that can lead to the pressure.

RISK INCREASES WITH
• An extra rib in the body. It may have fiber-like bands attached to it.
• Overextending arm or shoulder or repeated overhead arm movements. This may be due to work activities or exercise.
• Carrying heavy loads.
• Fracture of clavicle (collarbone) or first rib.
• Muscle weakness and drooping shoulders or head.
• Tumor or blood clots.
• Other health or emotional disorders may make a person more at risk for TOS.

HOW TO PREVENT—No specific preventive measures. Try to avoid repetitive arm and shoulder activities and overhead arm tasks. Exercise daily to maintain good physical fitness.

 WHAT TO EXPECT

DIAGNOSTIC MEASURES
• Your own observation of symptoms.
• Your health care provider will do a physical exam and ask questions about your symptoms and activities.

• You may be asked to make certain movements with the head, arm, and shoulders to help find the cause of the symptoms. Other medical tests may be done to rule out problems that could cause similar symptoms.

APPROPRIATE HEALTH CARE
• Treatment may involve physical therapy, stretching and strengthening exercises, drugs, ultrasound therapy, electrical stimulation, manipulation, or (rarely) surgery. Your health care provider will discuss an individual plan for you depending on your symptoms.
• Surgery may be a final option when other treatments are not helpful. It may relieve pressure on the nerves and blood vessels.

POSSIBLE COMPLICATIONS
• Problem can recur.
• If surgery is performed, it may have complications.
• Chronic pain syndrome, disability, and depression may occur in some patients.
• Some loss of function in arm and shoulders.

PROBABLE OUTCOME—Symptoms can be relieved in most patients with treatment.

 HOW TO TREAT

GENERAL MEASURES—Use heat to help relieve pain. Use a heating pad, warm showers, or warm, moist compresses.

MEDICATION
• You may use nonprescription drugs, such as acetaminophen or aspirin, to relieve pain. Drugs cannot correct the underlying condition.
• Other drugs or injections for specific symptoms may be prescribed.

ACTIVITY
• Physical therapy and exercise will be prescribed to promote shoulder muscle function and improve any posture faults. These are usually recommended for 2 to 3 months.
• Avoid straining or heavy activity for 3 months.

DIET—No special diet. If weight is a problem, a weight-loss diet is recommended.

 CALL YOUR DOCTOR IF

• You or a family member has symptoms of thoracic outlet syndrome.
• Symptoms don't improve in 2 weeks, despite treatment.

THROMBOCYTOPENIA

GENERAL INFORMATION

DEFINITION—A decrease in the number of platelet cells in the blood. Platelets (thrombocytes) play a vital role in the control of bleeding at the site of an injury. With thrombocytopenia, there is a tendency to bleed, mainly from the smaller blood vessels. This causes abnormal bleeding into the skin and other body places. There are several forms of the disorder, including idiopathic thrombocytopenic purpura (ITP) and thrombotic thrombocytopenic purpura (TTP).

BODY PARTS INVOLVED—Blood, which affects all body parts.

SEX OR AGE MOST AFFECTED—Both sexes; all ages.

SIGNS & SYMPTOMS
* Petechiae. These are small round, nonraised, purple-red spots on the skin.
* Bruising easily.
* Bleeding in the mouth and nosebleeds.
* Heavy or prolonged menstrual periods.
* Blood in the urine or stool.

CAUSES—Platelets are normally produced in the bone marrow and are removed or destroyed by the spleen when not needed. A number of underlying conditions may interfere with the production, function, and destruction of the platelets. If no underlying condition is found, it is called idiopathic.

RISK INCREASES WITH
* Infections, including HIV infection.
* Taking aspirin or other nonsteroidal anti-inflammatory drugs.
* Taking drugs such as quinidine, sulfa preparations, oral antidiabetic agents, gold salts, rifampin, etc.
* Hypersplenism (a disorder of the spleen).
* Hypothermia (exposure to cold temperatures).
* Blood transfusion or blood poisoning.
* Excess alcohol use.
* Preeclampsia (a disorder of pregnancy).
* Disorders such as systemic lupus erythematosus, anemia, leukemia, cirrhosis, certain cancers, and others.
* Exposure to x-ray or radiation.
* Children ages 2 to 4 (for idiopathic thrombocytopenic purpura).

HOW TO PREVENT
* Avoid drugs that are risk factors.
* For patients with thrombocytopenia, avoid trauma, and get medical care if trauma occurs.

WHAT TO EXPECT

DIAGNOSTIC MEASURES
* Your own observation of symptoms.

* Your health care provider will usually do a physical exam and ask questions about your symptoms and activities.
* Medical tests may include blood studies and other tests to check for an underlying disorder.

APPROPRIATE HEALTH CARE
* Treatment will be provided for any specific disorder that is diagnosed.
* Watchful waiting is an option. This means monitoring the symptoms for a time before deciding on treatment.
* Stop using any drug that could be the cause. An alternative drug may be prescribed. Avoid aspirin products.
* Surgery to remove the spleen (splenectomy) may be recommended for persistent cases.
* Pregnant women may require special treatment.
* Platelet transfusions may be prescribed. This may be for patients with serious bleeding, those planning major surgery, and those with chronic thrombocytopenia.

POSSIBLE COMPLICATIONS
* Severe blood loss.
* Anemia due to blood loss.
* Adverse effects of drug therapy.

PROBABLE OUTCOME
* Will depend on the underlying condition. Recovery occurs within two months for most cases of idiopathic thrombocytopenic purpura.
* Symptoms may come and go in chronic case.

HOW TO TREAT

GENERAL MEASURES
* Wear a medic alert type bracelet or neck tag that indicates your medical problem and any drugs you take.
* To learn more: Platelet Disorder Association, PO Box 61533, Potomac, MD; (877) 528-3538; website: www.itppeople.com.

MEDICATION—A number of drugs are used for treatment. Your health care provider will discuss the options, risks, and benefits before prescribing them.

ACTIVITY—If platelet counts are very low, bed rest and reduced activity to avoid injury may be recommended.

DIET—No special diet.

CALL YOUR DOCTOR IF

* You or a family member has symptoms of thrombocytopenia.
* Symptoms worsen during treatment. Severe blood loss is an emergency situation.
* New or unexplained symptoms develop.

THROMBOPHLEBITIS, SUPERFICIAL
(Phlebitis; Phlebothrombosis)

 GENERAL INFORMATION

DEFINITION—Inflammation (redness and swelling) and blood clots in a superficial vein. Superficial means the vein is near the surface of the skin.

BODY PARTS INVOLVED—Veins, usually in the legs. It sometimes occurs in the arms.

SEX OR AGE MOST AFFECTED
* Both sexes, but more common in females.
* All ages, but most common in adults.

SIGNS & SYMPTOMS
* Tenderness, redness, and pain in the affected area. The symptoms usually come on slowly.
* Vein may feel like a tender hard cord under the skin.
* Fever (sometimes).
* In some cases, there are no symptoms.

CAUSES—When a vein is damaged due to injury, surgery, or infection, the normal flow of blood is slowed down or blocked. Blood clots can then form.

RISK INCREASES WITH
* Illness or surgery with a lot of time spent in bed.
* Long car rides or airplane trips where you are sitting for long periods.
* Smoking.
* Elderly.
* Use of birth control pills.
* Overweight.
* Varicose veins.
* Injuries, burns, or infections.
* Pregnancy.
* Chronic illnesses, heart problems, and some cancers.
* Intravenous (IV) drug abusers.

HOW TO PREVENT
* Avoid risk factors where possible.
* On long trips, walk when you can, move legs often, and wear support stockings to prevent swollen legs. Ask your health care provider about taking aspirin before a long trip.

 WHAT TO EXPECT

DIAGNOSTIC MEASURES
* Your health care provider will examine the affected area of the leg and ask questions about your symptoms.
* Medical tests may be done to make sure there are no other medical problems. These include blood tests and ultrasound (using sound waves to check the blood flow).

APPROPRIATE HEALTH CARE
* Treatment usually involves rest and elevation of the affected leg (or arm) and, sometimes, drugs (depending on the cause).
* If varicose veins are a problem, they may need treatment.

POSSIBLE COMPLICATIONS—Serious complications are rare. The main concern is about blood clots forming in deep veins (deep venous thrombosis). They can have serious complications.

PROBABLE OUTCOME—Usually curable in several days to 3 weeks.

 HOW TO TREAT

GENERAL MEASURES
* Apply heat with warm compresses. Wet a towel in hot water, wring it out, and place it on the affected area.
* Wearing support stockings may help. Some types can be purchased at a drugstore. Your health care provider may prescribe prescription-type support stockings.
* If you smoke, this is a good time to stop. Talk to your health care provider about programs to help you quit.

MEDICATION
* Use nonsteroidal anti-inflammatory drugs, such as aspirin (adults) or ibuprofen, to decrease swelling, redness, and pain.
* Anticoagulants (drugs to prevent blood clots) may be prescribed.
* Antibiotics may be prescribed if there is an infection.

ACTIVITY—Rest with the affected leg or arm elevated as much as possible for 1 or 2 days. Move the feet, ankles, and legs often. When the symptoms begin to get better, resume normal activity slowly. Rest often. Don't sit or stand for prolonged periods, and don't cross your legs.

DIET—No special diet.

 CALL YOUR DOCTOR IF

* You or a family member has symptoms of superficial thrombophlebitis.
* The following occur during treatment: Fever of 102°F (38.9°C) or higher, pain gets worse, coughing blood, shortness of breath, chest pain, or swelling of leg or foot.
* New, unexplained symptoms develop. Drugs used in treatment may produce side effects.

ILLNESS & DISORDERS

THROMBOSIS, DEEP-VEIN

GENERAL INFORMATION

DEFINITION—A blood clot (thrombus) that forms inside a deep vein. It may partially or completely block blood flow, or it could break off and travel to the lung.

BODY PARTS INVOLVED—It often occurs in the lower legs (calves). Less often it occurs in the arm or pelvis.

SEX OR AGE MOST AFFECTED—Both sexes (slightly more common in men) and usually occurs in persons over age 40.

SIGNS & SYMPTOMS
• Sometimes no symptoms occur.
• Swelling, tenderness, or pain in the leg, especially the calf muscle.
• Warmth or redness of the leg.
• Soreness or pain when walking. The soreness does not disappear with rest.
• Pain when raising the leg and flexing the foot.
• Fever (sometimes).

CAUSES—Pooling of blood in the vein, which triggers blood-clotting mechanisms. The pooling may occur after prolonged bed rest, following surgery, or from long-lasting illness, such as heart attack, stroke, or bone fracture.

RISK INCREASES WITH
• Persons over 40.
• Obesity.
• Smoking.
• Estrogen use in birth control pills or for replacement after menopause. More of a risk with smokers.
• Surgery and surgery recovery.
• Long (e.g., over 4 hours) auto or plane trips.
• During pregnancy and right after childbirth.
• Cancer, heart failure, stroke, and polycythemia.
• Bed rest for an extended time, burns, or injuries.
• Intravenous (IV) drug abuse.
• Some blood disorders have risk of blood clots.

HOW TO PREVENT
• Avoid prolonged bed rest if possible. Move legs as often as possible after surgery or during a long illness.
• On long auto or airplane trips, move your legs at least once every hour. Elevate legs when possible. Drink plenty of fluids. Avoid alcohol.
• Stop smoking, especially if you take estrogen.
• Wear special compression stockings.

WHAT TO EXPECT

DIAGNOSTIC MEASURES
• Your health care provider will do a physical exam of the affected area. Questions will be asked about your symptoms and activities.

• Medical tests, such as ultrasound, may be done to confirm the diagnosis.

APPROPRIATE HEALTH CARE
• Small clots located in the calf may not need treatment right away. These clots often clear up on their own.
• In many cases, hospital care is required for drug injections and to watch for complications.
• A surgical procedure may be done to insert a filtering device ("umbrella") into the vena cava (main vein to the lungs). It will trap clots before they reach the lungs.
• Special compression stockings may be recommended. They help prevent pain, swelling, and complications.

POSSIBLE COMPLICATIONS
• Pulmonary embolism (blood clot travels to the lung) or embolism to another part of the body.
• Post-thrombotic syndrome due to vein damage. Blood pools in lower leg, causing swelling and pain in leg.
• Excessive bleeding from blood-thinner drugs.

PROBABLE OUTCOME—Usually curable with treatment.

HOW TO TREAT

GENERAL MEASURES—Follow medical advice.

MEDICATION
• Usually, an intravenous (IV) anticoagulant (blood thinner) drug is prescribed. This stops a clot from growing and prevents new clots. Blood tests will be ongoing to check the anticoagulant level. Oral anticoagulants may be prescribed for 6 months or longer.
• Thrombolytic drugs, which dissolve the clots, may be prescribed in more severe cases.

ACTIVITY
• Rest at home or as advised by your health care provider. While resting, make it a habit to move leg muscles, bend ankles, and wiggle toes.
• Elevate the feet higher than the hips when sitting or when in bed. Place a cushion under the feet or raise the foot of bed higher.

DIET—No special diet.

CALL YOUR DOCTOR IF

• You or a family member has symptoms of deep vein thrombosis.
• The following occur during treatment: Unexpected bleeding anywhere, chest pain, coughing up blood, shortness of breath, continued or increased swelling, and pain.

THROMBOSIS & EMBOLUS, ARTERIAL

 GENERAL INFORMATION

DEFINITION—Thrombosis is a blood clot that forms in an artery. If all or part of the clot breaks away and travels to another part of the artery, it is an embolus.

BODY PARTS INVOLVED—Clots may occur in the large or medium arteries anywhere in the body. The arteries in the neck or the arteries that go to the brain, intestine, legs, arms, or kidney are more often affected.

SEX OR AGE MOST AFFECTED—Adults of both sexes.

SIGNS & SYMPTOMS
Symptoms depend on where the embolus lodges:
• Brain: Temporary blindness, speaking difficulty, partial paralysis, hearing-loss, headache, and dizziness.
• Arms or legs: Pain in the arm or calf after exercise; weakness, numbness, burning and tingling sensations; or weak or absent pulse beyond the blocked blood flow. Symptoms ease up with rest.
• Intestine: Abdominal pain, nausea, vomiting, and shock.

CAUSES—Clots may form with any condition that damages the smooth lining of the heart or a blood vessel. As the clot grows—small or large portions break away and are carried by the bloodstream to the brain, abdomen, arms, legs, or other areas. Conditions that damage the blood-vessel lining include:
• Atherosclerosis (hardening of the arteries).
• Injury to a blood vessel from an accident or from surgery.
• Heart valve disease.
• Heart attack.
• Atrial fibrillation.

RISK INCREASES WITH
• Adults over 60.
• Smoking.
• High blood pressure.
• Diabetes.
• Previous transient ischemic attacks.

HOW TO PREVENT
• No specific preventive measures.
• If you have high blood pressure or diabetes, adhere to your treatment plan to control the disease.
• Anticoagulant (blood thinner) drugs may be prescribed for a short time after injury or surgery to prevent blood clots.
• Exercise regularly to help keep blood vessels healthy.

 WHAT TO EXPECT

DIAGNOSTIC MEASURES
• Your own observation of symptoms.
• Your health care provider will usually do a physical exam.
• Medical tests may include x-rays of the blood vessels after injection of a special substance.

APPROPRIATE HEALTH CARE
• Early treatment is needed and usually requires drugs or surgery (embolectomy).
• Surgery may be required to repair or replace damaged blood vessels or to remove an embolus by suction or bypass.

POSSIBLE COMPLICATIONS—When blood flow is blocked in an artery, it can cause damage and death to the body tissues involved.

PROBABLE OUTCOME—Depends on the organs affected, size of the affected blood vessel, and size of the clot. Clots in the arms or legs can be removed with surgery, to relieve symptoms. Clots to the brain, kidney, and intestines may cause death or permanent disability before they can be removed.

 HOW TO TREAT

GENERAL MEASURES—Follow medical advice.

MEDICATION
• Drugs to break up the clot may be given through a catheter (tube) directly into the artery involved.
• Anticoagulants to thin the blood and reduce the chance of clots forming may be prescribed.
• Vasodilators (drugs to widen blood vessels) may be prescribed.

ACTIVITY—Complete rest is necessary until blood flow is re-established by surgery or other treatment.

DIET—No special diet.

 CALL YOUR DOCTOR IF

• You or a family member has symptoms of arterial thrombosis or embolus. This is an emergency! Get medical help immediately.
• Symptoms return after surgery.
• New, unexplained symptoms develop. Drugs used in treatment may produce side effects.

ILLNESS & DISORDERS

THRUSH

GENERAL INFORMATION

DEFINITION—A fungal infection of the mouth. It is common in newborns and infants. In adults, it is usually a result of an underlying condition.

BODY PARTS INVOLVED—Mouth; gums; tongue; soft palate; cheeks; lips.

SEX OR AGE MOST AFFECTED—Newborns and infants, but may also affect older children and adults.

SIGNS & SYMPTOMS
• Patches (plaques) appear in the mouth.
• Patches are white to creamy-yellow, and slightly raised. They are similar to milk curds, but they don't wipe off.
• Usually no pain, but may have mild discomfort.
• If patches are rubbed off, they can leave small, painful ulcers (sores).
• The mouth is dry.
• Infant may have trouble feeding.

CAUSES
A fungus called *Candida albicans.* It is usually present in small numbers in the mouth. Certain factors may cause it to multiply out of control:
• Treatment with antibiotics. This may upset the natural balance of germs in the mouth and allow thrush to develop.
• Birth. Newborns may acquire the infection during passage through the birth canal, especially if the mother has a vaginal yeast infection. Thrush can appear within hours or up to 7 days after birth.
• Aging. Older persons develop thrush because of their lower natural resistance.

RISK INCREASES WITH
• Infants.
• People with poor nutrition.
• AIDS. Thrush in adults is part of the criteria used to diagnose AIDS.
• Diabetes.
• Dentures.
• Weak immune system due to illness or drugs.
• Chronic steroid drug use (oral or inhaled).

HOW TO PREVENT
• Good oral hygiene.
• Avoid antibiotics, unless prescribed for you.
• People at risk for thrush may be prescribed a preventive drug.

WHAT TO EXPECT

DIAGNOSTIC MEASURES
• Your own observation of symptoms.
• Your health care provider will do a physical exam of the mouth and ask questions about your symptoms and recent use of antibiotics or other drugs.
• Medical tests may include a scraping of the patch for viewing under a microscope.

APPROPRIATE HEALTH CARE
• Treatment is aimed at improving an underlying condition and relieving the symptoms of thrush.
• If an infant has the infection, sterilize any objects that may be placed in the baby's mouth.

POSSIBLE COMPLICATIONS—Complications are rare. They are more likely to occur in those with underlying conditions.

PROBABLE OUTCOME—Usually clears up in a few days, but it has a tendency to recur.

HOW TO TREAT

GENERAL MEASURES—Brush teeth with a soft toothbrush.

MEDICATION
• Nystatin oral suspension may be prescribed. Follow instructions that are provided with the product. Mothers who are nursing an infant with thrush should use the prescribed drug on her nipples. This prevents the infection from being spread back to the infant.
• Other antifungal drugs are effective and may be prescribed for adults.

ACTIVITY—No limits.

DIET—No changes in infants. Older children and adults should maintain a good fluid intake with milk, liquid gelatin, ice cream, custard, water, tea, or other beverages and foods that are easy to swallow. Use a straw for drinking if the patches are painful.

CALL YOUR DOCTOR IF

• You or a family member has symptoms of thrush.
• Signs of dehydration (sunken eyes, poor elasticity of the skin, and lethargy) appear in a child.
• Fever develops.

THUMB-SUCKING

GENERAL INFORMATION

DEFINITION—Placing the finger or thumb on the roof of the mouth behind the teeth and sucking with lips and teeth closed. Thumb sucking is common in infants and young children and is a behavior, not a disorder.

BODY PARTS INVOLVED—Mouth; teeth; tongue; pharynx; finger or thumb.

SEX OR AGE MOST AFFECTED—Children of both sexes up to age 12, but most common in young children.

SIGNS & SYMPTOMS—Sucking of the thumb. It is most likely to occur before going to sleep, watching TV, or when hungry, ill, or tired.

CAUSES—Thumb sucking is one of the first acts that an infant can do that brings pleasure. The need to suck is present in all babies. They will suck on almost anything that they can bring into contact with their mouths.

RISK INCREASES WITH—None known.

HOW TO PREVENT
• Thumb sucking is normal and does not need to be prevented. The behavior is calming and soothing to a baby.
• Provide pacifiers early in infancy if you desire. They cause no health problems. Once your child no longer needs a pacifier for their sucking need, you can start to wean them from pacifier use.

WHAT TO EXPECT

DIAGNOSTIC MEASURES—None needed.

APPROPRIATE HEALTH CARE—No treatment or action is usually necessary. Talk to your child's health care provider if you have any questions or concerns about thumb sucking.

POSSIBLE COMPLICATIONS—Thumb sucking that continues past age 6. It could cause problems with your child's mouth or teeth. Also, the child may get teased by others about the baby-like behavior. Parents should work with the child to change the habit for the sake of appearance and dental health.

PROBABLE OUTCOME—Some babies stop thumb sucking by age one. In most cases, the habit is given up by the time a child is 3 or 4 years old.

HOW TO TREAT

GENERAL MEASURES—For a child over age 6 or 7 who sucks the thumb or fingers, follow the advice of your child's health care provider, or try the suggestions listed here:
• Give the child extra attention.
• Watch the child's behavior to see if conflicts or anxiety seems to provoke sucking. Help the child explore other ways to cope with stress.
• If the child decides to try to stop sucking, help the child set goals. Give rewards for any progress toward the goal. Reward is not a bribe, but something earned through effort.
• Methods such as scolding, shaming, and nagging are usually of no avail. Other methods do not always work either. These include mittens, bad-tasting substances on the thumb, elbow splints, and others.
• Consult your child's dentist for help as well. The dentist may fit a training device in the child's mouth to prevent the thumb from touching the roof of the mouth.

MEDICATION—Drugs are not needed.

ACTIVITY—No limits.

DIET—No special diet.

CALL YOUR DOCTOR IF OR DENTIST IF

Your child wishes to stop thumb sucking and self-help methods are not working.

ILLNESS & DISORDERS

THYROID NODULE

GENERAL INFORMATION

DEFINITION—Nodules (lumps) involving the thyroid gland located in the front of the neck. Most often, the nodules are benign. Less than 10% are malignant (cancerous). Nodules are a common disorder.

BODY PARTS INVOLVED—Thyroid gland.

SEX OR AGE MOST AFFECTED—Both sexes (women more than men) and all age groups.

SIGNS & SYMPTOMS
• Most nodules have no symptoms. They are sometimes found during routine physical exams.
• Swelling or lump in the throat.
• Pain and tenderness in the thyroid gland.
• Difficulty swallowing if a large nodule is pressing on the windpipe or esophagus.
• Hyperthyroidism (overactive thyroid) symptoms if the nodule produces too much thyroid hormone. Symptoms can include weight loss, sleep problems, and being irritable.
• Hoarseness (rare).

CAUSES—The thyroid gland produces hormones that help regulate different body functions. For unknown reasons, the tissue in the thyroid develops into the nodules. There are several different types of nodules that develop. They may be cystic (fluid filled) or solid. There may be one nodule or many. Thyroid nodules can cause a goiter (an enlarged thyroid).

RISK INCREASES WITH
• Radiation treatment during childhood, even in small doses, to the head, neck, and upper chest.
• Exposure to nuclear radiation.
• Family history of thyroid tumors.

HOW TO PREVENT—No specific preventive measures.

WHAT TO EXPECT

DIAGNOSTIC MEASURES
• Your own observation of any symptoms.
• Your health care provider will do a physical exam and ask about your symptoms and history of radiation exposure.
• Medical tests are usually done to rule out cancer.

APPROPRIATE HEALTH CARE
• Treatment will depend on the type of nodules.
• Watchful waiting is an option if the nodule is benign. This means monitoring the thyroid with testing for a time before deciding if treatment is needed.
• Drug treatment may be prescribed to help shrink benign nodules.
• Surgery (thyroidectomy) is usually performed for malignant nodules. It is usually done also for larger benign nodules or nodules where the diagnosis is unclear if they are or are not cancerous. Thyroid hormone replacement therapy will be required for life after the thyroid is removed.

POSSIBLE COMPLICATIONS
• Side effects of treatment can lead to hypothyroidism or hyperthyroidism.
• Rarely, spread of a malignant tumor to other places in the body.
• Injury to the vocal cords during surgery.
• Permanent hoarseness or loss of voice following surgery.

PROBABLE OUTCOME
• Benign nodules can be treated successfully.
• Most thyroid cancers are curable.

HOW TO TREAT

GENERAL MEASURES—To learn more: American Thyroid Association, 6066 Leesburg Pike, Suite 650, Falls Church, VA 22041; (800) 849-7643; website: www.thyroid.org or Thyroid Foundation of America, 410 Stuart St., Boston, MA. 02116; (800) 832-8321; website: www.tsh.org.

MEDICATION
• Radioactive iodine or drugs to suppress (stop) the thyroid from producing hormones may be prescribed.
• Injections may be recommended for benign nodules to shrink them. It may require one or more injections over a few months.
• Antithyroid drugs or replacement thyroid hormone may be prescribed.

ACTIVITY—No limits, unless surgery is performed.

DIET—No special diet.

CALL YOUR DOCTOR IF

• You or a family member has symptoms of thyroid nodules or thyroid enlargement.
• New, unexplained symptoms develop. Drugs used in treatment may produce side effects.

THYROIDITIS

GENERAL INFORMATION

DEFINITION—Thyroiditis is a group of inflammatory thyroid disorders. The thyroid gland is a hormone-producing organ at the base of the neck, next to the trachea (windpipe). Types include:
• Chronic lymphocytic thyroiditis (Hashimoto's thyroiditis or autoimmune thyroiditis) is the most common type.
• Subacute granulomatous thyroiditis (DeQuervain's thyroiditis). It is less common.
• Subacute lymphocytic thyroiditis (silent thyroiditis or postpartum thyroiditis). It occurs more often in women who have recently delivered a baby.
• Acute suppurative thyroiditis (rarer type).

BODY PARTS INVOLVED—Thyroid gland.

SEX OR AGE MOST AFFECTED—Middle-aged persons of both sexes between ages 30 and 50, but more common in women.

SIGNS & SYMPTOMS
• No symptoms may occur or they may be very mild.
• Enlarged thyroid gland (goiter).
• May have trouble swallowing.
• Pain or tenderness in the thyroid (sometimes).
• Fever (sometimes).
• Underactive thyroid (hypothyroidism). It may cause fatigue, weight gain, and trouble concentrating.
• Overactive thyroid (hyperthyroidism). It is less common, and may cause weight loss and sleep problems.

CAUSES—Thyroiditis can be brought on by a number of different reasons. In the most common type, it is an immune system problem, but why this occurs is unknown. Other causes include viral or bacterial infections.

RISK INCREASES WITH
• Disorder of the body's immune system.
• Pregnancy.
• Family history of thyroid disease.
• Previous thyroid disorders.
• Various viruses, such as mumps or influenza.
• Bacterial infection of the thyroid gland (rare).

HOW TO PREVENT—No specific preventive measures.

WHAT TO EXPECT

DIAGNOSTIC MEASURES
• Your own observation of symptoms.
• Your health care provider will usually do a physical exam and ask about your symptoms.
• Medical tests include blood studies to check your thyroid function. Other tests may be done to confirm the diagnosis.

APPROPRIATE HEALTH CARE
• Treatment, if needed, is with drugs, and will depend on the type of thyroiditis.
• If symptoms are not severe, treatment may involve watchful waiting. This means monitoring thyroid function for a few months before deciding on treatment.
• Very rarely, thyroid surgery may be an option if other treatment does not improve painful symptoms.

POSSIBLE COMPLICATIONS—Permanent loss of thyroid function. This requires lifelong thyroid hormone replacement.

PROBABLE OUTCOME—Will depend on the type. The chronic type can be treated successfully with thyroid hormone therapy. It may take several weeks of therapy for symptoms to improve. Other types of thyroiditis may clear up on their own in 4 to 6 months.

HOW TO TREAT

GENERAL MEASURES
• With any type of thyroiditis, it is important to follow up with your health care provider for periodic exams.
• To learn more: American Thyroid Association, 6066 Leesburg Pike, Suite 650, Falls Church, VA 22041; (800) 849-7643; website: www.thyroid.org or Thyroid Foundation of America, 410 Stuart St., Boston, MA. 02116; (800) 832-8321; website: www.tsh.org.

MEDICATION
• Antithyroid drugs or thyroid replacement hormones, depending on the activity of your thyroid hormones.
• Beta-adrenergic blockers to suppress symptoms of an overactive thyroid may be prescribed.
• Antibiotics to treat infection, if needed.
• Cortisone drugs to decrease inflammation may rarely be prescribed.
• You may use aspirin (not for children) or ibuprofen to control mild pain.

ACTIVITY—No limits.

DIET—No special diet.

CALL YOUR DOCTOR IF

• You or a family member has symptoms of thyroiditis.
• New, unexplained symptoms develop. Drugs used in treatment may produce side effects.

TINEA CRURIS
(Jock Itch)

 GENERAL INFORMATION

DEFINITION—Fungal infection of the skin in the groin.

BODY PARTS INVOLVED—Groin and nearby skin.

SEX OR AGE MOST AFFECTED—Both sexes (more likely to occur in men than in women) and in adults more than children.

SIGNS & SYMPTOMS
• Scaling patches on the skin of the groin, thighs, and buttocks.
• Patches have well-defined edges.
• Sometimes small, pus-filled blisters appear.
• Itching of involved areas.
• Pain (if the skin also becomes infected with bacteria).

CAUSES—Infection by fungi called dermatophytes. These germs tend to grow in the darkness, warmth, and moisture of the body's groin area.

RISK INCREASES WITH
• Hot, humid weather.
• Excessive sweating.
• Tight clothing.
• Obesity, which fosters sweating.
• Friction of skin against skin from constant movement.
• Contact with infected surfaces, such as towels or benches.
• Weak immune system due to illness or drugs.
• Diabetes.
• Other fungal infection such as athlete's foot (tinea pedis).
• Military personnel or athletic team members who may have close contact to one another.
• Sharing clothing.

HOW TO PREVENT
• Dry completely after bathing. Use clean towel.
• Don't sit around in a wet bathing suit.
• Wear loose fitting, cotton underwear.
• Wear clean, dry athletic supporters and underwear for each workout.
• Don't share clothing.
• Use nonprescription tolnaftate (Tinactin) after bathing if you have had tinea cruris before. This powder can help prevent a recurrence.

 WHAT TO EXPECT

DIAGNOSTIC MEASURES
• Your own observation of symptoms.
• Your health care provider will do a physical exam of the affected area.
• Medical tests may include a microscopic exam of scraped-off scales.

APPROPRIATE HEALTH CARE—Treatment usually involves drugs applied to the skin and sometimes taken by mouth. Use them for the length of time prescribed, even if the rash goes away.

POSSIBLE COMPLICATIONS
• Recurrences are common.
• Bacterial infection in the affected area.

PROBABLE OUTCOME—Symptoms can be controlled in 2 to 4 weeks with treatment.

 HOW TO TREAT

GENERAL MEASURES
• For home care, follow the steps listed in Preventive Measures.
• If you also have an athlete's foot infection, treat both areas with equal care. Put socks on before underwear to prevent spread of germs from feet to groin.

MEDICATION
• You may use nonprescription, topical antifungal drugs for treatment and prevention.
• Other topical or oral (taken by mouth) antifungal drugs may be prescribed.

ACTIVITY—No limits.

DIET—No special diet. A weight loss diet may help improve symptoms in overweight patients.

 CALL YOUR DOCTOR IF

• You or a family member has symptoms of tinea cruris.
• Rash worsens despite treatment.
• Infection recurs after treatment.

TINEA VERSICOLOR

GENERAL INFORMATION

DEFINITION—An infection caused by a yeast type of skin fungus that changes the color of skin that it affects.

BODY PARTS INVOLVED—Skin of the chest, back, shoulders, upper arms, trunk or groin. This rarely affects the face.

SEX OR AGE MOST AFFECTED—Both sexes and is more common in teens and young adults.

SIGNS & SYMPTOMS
* Small, scaly spots (or patches) on the skin. They may appear white to pink or tan to dark. They show up differently on light skin as compared to darker skin.
* Affected skin may itch (more likely if the person gets hot).
* Spots begin small and spread. They may join together to form larger patches.
* In hot climates, a person may have the spots all year around. In other climates, they may fade during the cooler months.

CAUSES—A fungus called *Pityrosporum orbiculare*. It is present on normal skin, but it can't be seen and it normally causes no problems. Why it grows more active and causes symptoms for some people is unknown. It is not considered contagious.

RISK INCREASES WITH
* Exposure to heat and high humidity.
* Genetic predisposition.
* Malnutrition (a lack of [or too much] needed nutrients).
* Cushing's syndrome.
* Weak immune system due to illness or drugs.

HOW TO PREVENT—No specific preventive measures. Once you have had the infection, re-treatment can help stop a recurrence.

WHAT TO EXPECT

DIAGNOSTIC MEASURES
* Your own observation of symptoms.
* Your health care provider can usually diagnose the disorder by an exam of the affected skin.
* Medical tests may include a microscopic exam of scales scraped from the skin to confirm the diagnosis.

APPROPRIATE HEALTH CARE
* Numerous topical products are effective in clearing tinea versicolor.
* Your health care provider will usually recommend a method to help prevent a recurrence. Several options are available. One method is to repeat treatment every week for 3 to 4 weeks and then once a month for 3 to 4 months.

POSSIBLE COMPLICATIONS
* Recurrence is common. The episodes of recurrence decline with age.
* The cosmetic appearance of the skin may cause some emotional distress, especially in young teens.

PROBABLE OUTCOME—With treatment, the patches will clear up in 1 to 2 months. There is no permanent scarring or changes in skin color.

HOW TO TREAT

GENERAL MEASURES—Self-care involves application of tropical antifungal product.

MEDICATION
* Nonprescription, antifungal, topical products such as shampoos, creams, or lotions may be recommended. These are applied to the affected areas. Use product as directed on the label.
* In some cases, drugs taken by mouth may be prescribed.

ACTIVITY—No limits. Try to avoid activities that cause excess sweating. If heavy sweating occurs, shower as soon as possible.

DIET—No special diet.

CALL YOUR DOCTOR IF

* You or a family member has symptoms of tinea versicolor.
* Infection doesn't improve despite treatment.

TINNITUS

GENERAL INFORMATION

DEFINITION—A persistent sound heard in one or both ears when there is no environmental noise. Tinnitus can be a common symptom of nearly all ear disorders, as well as other medical problems.

BODY PARTS INVOLVED—Ears.

SEX OR AGE MOST AFFECTED—Both sexes; all ages.

SIGNS & SYMPTOMS—A noise that may be a ringing, buzzing, roaring, whistling, or hissing sound, that is heard in one or both ears. The sound may be continuous, off and on, pulsing, or in time with the heartbeat.

CAUSES—There has probably been some sort of damage to the hearing system, but why this might cause tinnitus is unknown. Tinnitus does not cause deafness, nor does deafness cause tinnitus. They can both occur together in some patients.

RISK INCREASES WITH
* Hearing loss.
* Earache or ear infection.
* Labyrinthitis.
* Meniere disease.
* Otitis media or externa.
* Otosclerosis.
* Ototoxicity.
* Earwax blockage.
* Aneurysm or tumor in the head (rare).
* Foreign body in the ear.
* Certain drugs (antibiotics, diuretics, and others).
* High or low blood pressure.
* Head trauma.
* Anemia.
* Hypothyroidism or hyperthyroidism.
* Allergies.
* Exposure to excessively loud noise, either once or over a period of time.

PREVENTIVE MEASURES—No specific prevention known. Avoid the risk factors where possible.

WHAT TO EXPECT

DIAGNOSTIC MEASURES
* Your own observation of symptoms.
* Your health care provider may do a physical exam and an ear exam. Questions will be asked about your symptoms.
* Medical tests may be done to check for an underlying disorder.

APPROPRIATE HEALTH CARE
* If tinnitus is ongoing, the treatment is basically finding methods that help you to cope with the constant noise. Try one method for a time to see if it helps. Sometimes, a combination of different methods will work.
* Electrical stimulation with cochlear implant may help tinnitus, but it is usually used only for severe deafness.
* Tinnitus retraining therapy (TRT) may help. It combines counseling with sound therapy.

POSSIBLE COMPLICATIONS—There are usually no medical complications. Emotional problems may develop due to feelings of distress for those who find the noise very difficult to live with.

PROBABLE OUTCOME—Treatment of an underlying disorder may help. Often there is no cure, and learning to cope is the only therapy. Some people tolerate the condition much better than others. Research is ongoing to find the cause and effective treatment.

HOW TO TREAT

GENERAL MEASURES
* Try to ignore the sound by directing your attention to other things and activities. Counseling or biofeedback training may help you learn to do this technique.
* Play music in the background during the day and while falling asleep.
* Learn techniques to control stress in your life. This helps some people with tinnitus.
* Quit smoking. Find a way to stop that works.
* A hearing aid for any associated deafness may help mask tinnitus.
* Wear a tinnitus suppressor or masker. This is a device that fits in the ear like a hearing aid, and presents a more pleasant sound.
* Dental treatment may be recommended.
* To learn more: American Tinnitus Association, P.O. Box 5, Portland, OR 97207; (800) 634-8978; website: www.ata.org.

MEDICATION—There are no drugs for tinnitus. Drugs normally prescribed for other conditions may help tinnitus in some people.

ACTIVITY—No limits.

DIET—No special diet.

CALL YOUR DOCTOR IF

* You or a family member has symptoms of tinnitus.
* Feelings of distress about tinnitus worsen.

TOENAIL, INGROWN

GENERAL INFORMATION

DEFINITION—A common problem in which one or both edges of a nail grows into the flesh of a toe, usually the great (big) toe. This can lead to infection and inflammation.

BODY PARTS INVOLVED—Toes.

SEX OR AGE MOST AFFECTED—Both sexes; most common in adolescents and adults.

SIGNS & SYMPTOMS—Pain, tenderness, redness, swelling, and heat in the toe where the sharp nail-edge pierces the nearby fold of tissue. Once tissue around the nail becomes red and sore, infection often develops.

CAUSES—An ingrown toenail is likely to occur with one of the following conditions:
* The nail is more curved than normal.
* The toenail is clipped back too far, allowing tissue to grow up over it.
* Shoes fit poorly, forcing the toe of the shoe against the nail and surrounding tissue.
* Injury to the nail, or infection of the nail.
* Sports activities that requires sudden stops ("toe jamming").

RISK INCREASES WITH—Any of the causes listed.

HOW TO PREVENT
* Wear roomy, well-fitting shoes and socks.
* Carefully cut toenails straight across, and not too short.
* People with diabetes or blood vessel disease have poor healing abilities. Be very careful in trimming your toenails. Foot injury is a risk with these disorders because of changes in blood flow to the feet.
* If you often handle heavy objects in your work, consider wearing work shoes with steel toe boxes.
* Keep feet clean and dry.

WHAT TO EXPECT

DIAGNOSTIC MEASURES
* Your own observation of symptoms.
* See your health care provider if home care does not help. Diagnosis is confirmed by an exam of the affected toe.

APPROPRIATE HEALTH CARE
* If there is an infection, drugs usually relieve symptoms within 1 week.
* If an ingrown toenail occurs often, then surgery is often the best treatment. The type of surgery will depend on how severe the problem is. It may involve just removing overgrown skin tissue, removing a portion of the toenail, or complete removal of the toenail.

POSSIBLE COMPLICATIONS—An ingrown toenail may become very painful, red, and swollen with pus if treatment for infection is delayed too long. Sometimes, a bloody growth called proud flesh builds up on the side of the nail.

PROBABLE OUTCOME—Curable with treatment.

HOW TO TREAT

GENERAL MEASURES—The following home treatment may help prevent the need for surgery:
* Soak the toe for 20 minutes twice a day in a gallon of warm water. You may add either 2 tablespoons of Epsom salts or 2 tablespoons of a mild detergent.
* Lift the nail corners gently, and wedge a very small piece of cotton under the ingrown nail edges. This will lift the nail slightly so it can grow past the skin tissue it is digging into. Replace the cotton daily. Do not cut a "V" in the middle of the nail. This is not helpful.
* There are certain products you can buy that may soften the nail and the skin around it, which can help relieve the pain. Follow the directions carefully. These products should not be used if you have diabetes or a blood vessel problem.

MEDICATION
* Antibiotic ointment may be prescribed to treat any infection.
* You may use ibuprofen or acetaminophen for pain.

ACTIVITY
* Resume your normal activities as soon as symptoms improve. You may need to wear sandals or a shoe with the toe cut out until the toe heals.
* If you have surgery, your health care provider will instruct you about aftercare, such as keeping the foot propped up as much as possible.

DIET—No special diet.

CALL YOUR DOCTOR IF

* You have symptoms of an ingrown toenail that persist despite self-treatment.
* The following occur during treatment or after surgery:
  - Fever.
  - Increased pain.
  - Signs of infection (pain, redness, heat, swelling, or tenderness) in the toe.
  - Red streaks going up the foot or ankle.

TONGUE INFLAMMATION
(Glossitis)

GENERAL INFORMATION

DEFINITION—Acute or chronic inflammation of the tongue from a variety of causes. This is sometimes contagious, but not cancerous.

BODY PARTS INVOLVED—Tongue and adjacent parts of the mouth.

SEX OR AGE MOST AFFECTED—Both sexes; all ages.

SIGNS & SYMPTOMS—Any of the following:
* Bright red, swollen tongue.
* Tongue looks and feels smooth.
* Tongue may be sore and tender.
* Hairy-looking tongue, sometimes with a black surface.
* A tongue with a red tip and edges.

CAUSES
* Bacterial or viral (including herpes) infections.
* Burns.
* Injury from jagged teeth, ill-fitting dentures, mouth-breathing, or repeated biting during seizures.
* Excessive use of alcohol, tobacco, hot food or spices.
* Poor dental health.
* Allergy to toothpaste, mouthwash (especially mouthwash containing peroxide), candy, dye, or material used in dental work.
* Lack of B vitamins, resulting in B-12-deficiency anemia, pellagra, or iron-deficiency anemia.
* Adverse reaction to drugs.

RISK INCREASES WITH
* Poor nutrition, especially vitamin deficiencies.
* Smoking.
* Chemical or environmental exposure to irritating or corrosive chemicals.
* Alcoholism.
* Anxiety or depression.
* Diabetes.

HOW TO PREVENT
* Practice good oral hygiene. Brush teeth and tongue at least twice a day, and floss teeth daily. Obtain regular dental checkups.
* Don't smoke.
* Prevent tongue injury by wearing protective headgear for contact sports or cycling.

WHAT TO EXPECT

DIAGNOSTIC MEASURES
* Your own observation of symptoms.
* Your health care provider will do an exam of the mouth and tongue.
* Medical tests may include blood studies to check for any underlying disorder.

APPROPRIATE HEALTH CARE—Treatment will be directed at the underlying cause along with self-help measures.

POSSIBLE COMPLICATIONS
* Tongue inflammation can become chronic if not adequately treated.
* Tongue may become swollen and block the airway.

PROBABLE OUTCOME—Usually curable in 2 weeks with treatment.

HOW TO TREAT

GENERAL MEASURES
* Observe if there is an association between eating specific foods and tongue symptoms. Irritating foods may include chocolate, citrus, acidic foods (vinegar, pickles), salted nuts, or potato chips.
* Rinse mouth 3 or more times a day with a salt solution (mix one-half teaspoon of salt in one cup of warm water).
* If tongue symptoms are caused by teeth or denture problems, consult your dentist. The problem won't heal until the cause is eliminated.

MEDICATION
* For minor pain, you may use nonprescription drugs, such as anesthetic mouthwashes or acetaminophen.
* For infection and pain, antibiotics or topical anesthetics may be prescribed.

ACTIVITY—No limits.

DIET
* No special diet, except to avoid foods that may cause the symptoms.
* Drink as many fluids and eat as well-balanced a diet as possible while healing.
* To reduce pain, sip liquids through straws. Foods or fluids that cause the least pain are milk, liquid gelatin, yogurt, ice cream, and custard.

CALL YOUR DOCTOR IF

* You or a family member has symptoms of tongue inflammation.
* Symptoms don't improve in 3 days despite treatment.
* Pain gets worse and isn't relieved by treatment.
* Tongue swells and interferes with swallowing.

TONSILLITIS

GENERAL INFORMATION

DEFINITION—Tonsils that are inflamed (red, sore, and swollen). The tonsils are located at the back of the throat on each side. They are small at birth, enlarge during childhood, and become smaller during the teen years. Tonsils usually help prevent infections in the nose, mouth, and throat from spreading to other places in the body. However, they themselves can become infected. Tonsillitis can be spread from person to person.

BODY PARTS INVOLVED—Tonsils; throat.

SEX OR AGE MOST AFFECTED—Both sexes and all ages, but most common in children between ages 5 and 10.

SIGNS & SYMPTOMS
- Sore throat and pain when you swallow.
- Tonsils are redder than normal.
- Throat may have white or yellow patches.
- Swollen glands on either side of the jaw.
- Fever.
- Headache.
- Ear pain.
- A very young child may not want to eat.

CAUSES—Usually a bacterial (often *streptococcus*, or "strep" as it is called) or a virus infection.

RISK INCREASES WITH
- Young children.
- Daycare centers (for both children and teachers).
- Living, working, or being in crowded places.
- Smoking.
- Having a chronic illness, such as diabetes.

HOW TO PREVENT—None specific. Wash hands often to help prevent spread of any germs.

WHAT TO EXPECT

DIAGNOSTIC MEASURES
- Your own observation of symptoms.
- Your health care provider will examine your head, neck, and throat.
- Medical tests may include a rapid strep test and a throat culture (to find which germ is the cause). Family members may also need a strep test. A person may carry the strep germ, but not have any symptoms.

APPROPRIATE HEALTH CARE
- Treatment usually involves drug therapy and self-care. Surgery may be recommended.
- If surgery to remove the tonsils is needed, your health care provider will discuss the details. It is usually done on an outpatient basis. (See Tonsil & Adenoid Removal in Surgery section.)

POSSIBLE COMPLICATIONS
- Abscess (an infected sore on the tonsils).
- Chronic tonsillitis. It can cause ear infection and enlarged tonsils. This may lead to breathing problems and snoring.
- Rheumatic fever may occur if the cause is strep and it is not treated, or if treatment is stopped too soon.

PROBABLE OUTCOME—Symptoms generally begin to improve in 2 to 3 days. Treatment will take longer to ensure that germs are gone. If tonsillitis is severe and occurs often, your health care provider may suggest surgery (tonsillectomy) to remove the tonsils.

HOW TO TREAT

GENERAL MEASURES
- To relieve the sore throat, gargle frequently with warm or cold double-strength tea or warm salt water (mix one-half teaspoon of salt in one cup of water).
- Suck on hard candy such as lemon drops, to increase moisture in the mouth.

MEDICATION
- If the cause is strep, take prescribed antibiotic (usually penicillin) for at least 10 days, or as directed.
- To relieve pain, you may use acetaminophen. Don't give aspirin to children under age 18.

ACTIVITY
- Stay away from others until fever, pain, and other symptoms disappear.
- Bed rest if there is fever. Then return to your regular routine.

DIET—Drink plenty of fluids. While the throat is very sore, use liquids for food. This includes milk shakes, soups, and high-protein fluids (diet or instant-breakfast milk drinks).

CALL YOUR DOCTOR IF

- You or a family member has symptoms of tonsillitis. If there is any trouble with breathing, call right away.
- Symptoms worsen, or other symptoms occur during treatment.

TOOTH ABSCESS
(Periapical Abscess; Periodontal Abscess)

 GENERAL INFORMATION

DEFINITION—An abscess (pus-filled sac) around a tooth root, which is imbedded in bone of the upper or lower jaw.

BODY PARTS INVOLVED—Teeth, gums; jawbone.

SEX OR AGE MOST AFFECTED—Both sexes; all ages.

SIGNS & SYMPTOMS
• Persistent toothache or throbbing, extreme pain upon biting or chewing.
• Swelling and tenderness in the neck glands and on the side of the face.
• Earache.
• Fever.
• General ill feeling.
• Foul taste and bad breath (if the abscess opens spontaneously).

CAUSES—The pulp (nerves and blood vessels that fill the central cavity of a tooth) is invaded by bacteria, usually as a result of dental caries (tooth decay) that destroy a tooth's enamel and dentin, or when a tooth is injured. Abscess also occur from periodontal disease (bacteria invades pockets between the teeth and gums).

RISK INCREASES WITH
• Tooth decay due to plaque.
• Early childhood caries (baby bottle tooth decay).
• Gingivitis
• Infection following an injury or surgery.
• Weak immune system due to illness or drugs.

HOW TO PREVENT
• Prevent decay with brushing and flossing:
  - Use a soft-bristle toothbrush to remove plaque from the teeth's front and back surfaces, especially at the gum line.
  - Learn to use dental floss correctly. Ask your dentist or hygienist to demonstrate the technique.
• Use fluoride mouthwash, toothpaste, tablets or liquid supplement if recommended by dentist.
• Don't let an infant fall asleep with a bottle of milk, juice, or formula in the mouth.
• Reduce sugar consumption. Tooth decay increases as sugar consumption increases.

 WHAT TO EXPECT

DIAGNOSTIC MEASURES
• Your own observation of symptoms.
• Your dental care provider (dentist) will do an exam of the mouth.
• Medical tests may include x-rays of the mouth and a culture of a sample of the pus.

APPROPRIATE HEALTH CARE
• Treatment may include drug therapy, self-care, and/or surgery.
• Surgery may involve a procedure to drain the pus from the affected area. Root canal surgery may be needed to preserve the tooth. See Root Canal Treatment in the Surgery section.

POSSIBLE COMPLICATIONS
• If untreated, the abscess can erode a small channel to the gum surface where it forms a gumboil (swelling). If the gumboil bursts, it lets foul-tasting pus into the mouth. The abscess can also erode into the jawbone and produce an infection in the bone itself (osteomyelitis).
• Loss of the tooth.
• Spread of infection through the bloodstream to other body parts.

PROBABLE OUTCOME—With treatment and follow up care, the outlook is good.

 HOW TO TREAT

GENERAL MEASURES
• Rinse your mouth with warm salt water (mix one-half teaspoon of salt in one cup of water). Repeat each hour or as often as feels good.
• Don't chew on the affected side of your mouth for at least 2 days.
• Follow medical instructions for home care after any dental surgery.

MEDICATION
• For minor pain, you may use nonprescription drugs such as acetaminophen.
• Antibiotics for infection or stronger pain relievers may be prescribed.

ACTIVITY—Normally no limits. Activities level may depend on your symptoms.

DIET—A liquid or soft diet may be necessary for 1 or 2 days until pain subsides.

 CALL YOUR DENTIST IF

• You or a family member has symptoms of a tooth abscess.
• The following occurs during treatment:: fever of 101°F (38.3°C) or higher or pain becomes severe.
• New, unexplained symptoms develop. Drugs used in treatment may produce side effects.

TOOTH DECAY
(Caries; Dental Decay; Cavities)

GENERAL INFORMATION

DEFINITION—Disintegration of tooth enamel, allowing injury to the dentin (layer below the enamel) and eventual involvement of the pulp (the layer below the dentin), which contains nerves and blood vessels. Tooth decay (also called caries) and the common cold are the most common human disorders.

BODY PARTS INVOLVED—Teeth.

SEX OR AGE MOST AFFECTED—Both sexes; all ages.

SIGNS & SYMPTOMS
* Tooth sensitivity to heat and cold.
* Tooth discomfort after eating sugar.
* Darkening on or between the teeth (cavity) when the decay has progressed enough to be seen. The most common tooth-cavity sites are the gum line, biting surfaces and surfaces between adjacent teeth.
* Unpleasant taste in the mouth and bad breath because of stagnant food and bacteria trapped in the cavity.
* Persistent tooth pain (in the final stages of decay when the pulp becomes inflamed).

CAUSES—Cavities are caused by acid destruction of tooth material. Acid is produced by bacteria in the mouth. The bacteria feed on food debris—usually sugar—and produce the acid that dissolves tooth material.
The combination of sugars from food debris, bacteria and chemicals in the saliva form a substance called plaque. Plaque becomes a localized site of acid production, which forms continuously at the neck of each tooth. This plaque must be thoroughly cleaned away at the gum line daily or it fosters tooth decay.

RISK INCREASES WITH
* Poor nutrition and improper diet.
* Poor dental hygiene.

HOW TO PREVENT
* Brush and floss teeth regularly.
* Consult your dentist about using fluoride mouthwash, liquid, tablets or having fluoride treatments once or twice a year.
* Drinking fluoridated water or taking fluoride supplements during pregnancy has not proven to protect the unborn child's teeth.
* Sealants may help prevent enamel erosion.

WHAT TO EXPECT

DIAGNOSTIC MEASURES
* Your own observation of symptoms.
* Your dental care provider (dentist) will do an exam of the teeth. The decayed area feels soft when the dentist probes it with a sharp instrument.
* X-rays of the teeth and mouth are usually done.

APPROPRIATE HEALTH CARE—Dentist's treatment to remove all decay in the tooth and replace it with a restorative material (filling). The filling prevents further decay.

POSSIBLE COMPLICATIONS
* Abscess around a decayed tooth.
* Death of the tooth, caused by destruction of the tooth pulp that contains the tooth's nerve and blood supply.

PROBABLE OUTCOME—Usually curable with dental treatment.

HOW TO TREAT

GENERAL MEASURES—No specific instructions.

MEDICATION
* For minor pain, you may use nonprescription drugs such as acetaminophen.
* Your dentist may prescribe stronger pain relievers or fluoride supplements.

ACTIVITY—No limits.

DIET—For 48 hours after your dentist fills the decayed tooth, don't put pressure on the tooth, as by eating apples, hard candy, raw vegetables or chewing on ice. Avoid very hot or cold foods. The tooth remains sensitive for 48 hours to 10 days after a cavity has been filled.

CALL YOUR DENTIST IF

* You or a family member has symptoms of tooth decay.
* You develop fever, increased pain that is not relieved by nonprescription drugs, or discomfort with hot or cold food that persists longer than 2 weeks after the filling procedure.

TOOTH GRINDING
(Bruxism)

GENERAL INFORMATION

DEFINITION—The habit of grinding or clenching the teeth. Bruxism is the medical term for the problem. Tooth grinding is often done while asleep, but grinding or tapping teeth during the day is also common. Continual tooth grinding may erode gums and supporting bones in the mouth.

BODY PARTS INVOLVED—Teeth; gums; temporomandibular joints.

SEX OR AGE MOST AFFECTED—Both sexes; all ages.

SIGNS & SYMPTOMS
* Pain in the jaw muscles. Earaches may occur also.
* Clenching of the jaw, or clicking noises in the jaw.
* Annoying, tooth grinding noises at night. These may be loud enough to awaken others.
* Teeth may become loose and more sensitive to cold and heat.
* Damage to teeth, supporting gums, and bone (a dentist will notice the changes in a dental exam).
* Headaches.
* Daytime sleepiness.

CAUSES
* There is no one specific cause. Anxiety, tension, and stress appear to play a role.
* Unconscious attempt to correct an abnormal "bite."
* Tooth grinding occurs in children. They may grind their teeth when they have a cold, ear ache, allergies, or other problems. The children usually outgrow the habit, and it typically causes no damage to the teeth.

RISK INCREASES WITH
* One study found that it occurs more often in people who drink alcohol at bedtime, drink more than 6 cups of coffee a day, smoked cigarettes, or suffered from depression and/or anxiety.
* Suppressed anger may be a risk factor.
* Some antidepressant or antipsychotic drugs may increase the risk.

HOW TO PREVENT—Avoid stressful situations if possible.

WHAT TO EXPECT

DIAGNOSTIC MEASURES
* Your own observation of symptoms.
* See your dentist if self-help measures aren't working. Your dentist will examine your teeth and the jaw areas of your face. Different treatment options will be discussed.

APPROPRIATE HEALTH CARE
* Dental work can help resolve certain problems such as an abnormal bite, crooked or missing teeth.
* A night guard may be prescribed. This is a custom-made plastic device worn at night to stop upper and lower teeth from coming together.
* Your dentist may suggest a sound alarm device. It is worn at night and sounds an alarm to wake you when it senses jaw movements.
* Biofeedback training (relaxation exercises) or counseling to learn ways to cope more effectively with stress may be needed.
* Physical therapy, hypnosis therapy, or discontinuing drugs that are a risk factor may help some patients.

POSSIBLE COMPLICATIONS
* Without treatment, teeth, bones, and gums may erode or crack from the pressure of grinding.
* Problems with the temporomandibular joint. This is the hinge-like area where your upper jaw connects to the lower jaw.
* Continued problems with disrupted sleep.

PROBABLE OUTCOME—Treatment can help relieve the symptoms and limit any further damage to the teeth or other complications.

HOW TO TREAT

GENERAL MEASURES—Self-treatment options may sometimes help.
* Cut down on alcohol and caffeine.
* Try taking a warm bath before bedtime.
* Use a warm washcloth to apply heat to the jaw area.
* Decrease the stress in your life, where possible.
* Have your spouse wake you at night when you grind your teeth. Then get up and do some simple activity for about 10 minutes before you go back to sleep.

MEDICATION—Your health care provider or dentist may prescribe drugs for a short period for certain problems. These include muscle relaxants or mild sleeping aids.

ACTIVITY—No limits.

DIET—No special diet.

CALL YOUR DENTIST IF

* You or a family member grinds teeth at night. It is also a good idea to call your dentist.
* Once treatment begins, call your dentist if you have new symptoms or if other symptoms become worse.

TORTICOLLIS
(Wryneck)

GENERAL INFORMATION

DEFINITION—A problem of the neck muscles that causes a twisted head movement. Torticollis is a type of movement disorder (dystonia). It may be acquired or congenital.

BODY PARTS INVOLVED—Brain and central nervous system; muscular system.

SEX OR AGE MOST AFFECTED—Adults ages 30 to 60 (women more than men). Congenital muscle torticollis affects newborns.

SIGNS & SYMPTOMS
• Symptoms may begin slowly and progress over time or develop suddenly.
• Head turns (or tilts) toward one shoulder while the chin turns toward the opposite shoulder. The head may be pulled forward or backward.
• The head may not move from the abnormal position (tonic), may have jerky head movements (clonic), or may have both types.
• Neck muscles are tense and tender.
• May be pain in the neck, back, or shoulder.
• In a newborn, a lump may be felt in the neck muscle.

CAUSES
• In newborns, the exact cause is unknown. It may be due to a muscle injury prior to, during, or after birth. There are other possible causes. It sometimes occurs along with a hip dislocation.
• In acquired cases, the nerves and muscles involved are affected by various causes. Often, no cause is found. This is called idiopathic spasmodic torticollis.

RISK INCREASES WITH
Newborn:
• Birth defect.
• Injury to neck muscles or vertebrae (spinal bones) at birth or later.
• Breech delivery of newborn.
• Large baby.
Others:
• Family history of torticollis.
• Cervical spine problems (injury, fractures, scar tissue, tumor, infections, ligament problems, and others).
• Inflammatory problem (myositis and others).
• Certain prescribed drugs.
• Some drugs of abuse.
• Infection in tissues around neck muscles.

HOW TO PREVENT—No specific measures.

WHAT TO EXPECT

DIAGNOSTIC MEASURES
• Your own observation of symptoms.

• Your health care provider will do a physical exam of the affected area and ask questions about your symptoms and activities.
• Medical tests may include x-rays, CT, MRI, and studies of muscle movements.

APPROPRIATE HEALTH CARE
• Congenital torticollis is initially treated with physical therapy, including daily passive therapy for at least a year. If therapy is not successful, then surgery to lengthen neck muscles is performed.
• For other forms of torticollis, drug therapies may help, along with physical therapy and massages.
• If a drug is causing the problem, it should be stopped.
• A neck brace or collar may be recommended.
• Ultrasound therapy may be recommended.
• Rarely, a surgical procedure to denervate (cut the nerves) in the neck muscles may be recommended.

POSSIBLE COMPLICATIONS—Condition becomes chronic.

PROBABLE OUTCOME
• Congenital torticollis can usually be corrected with muscle-stretching exercises or surgery.
• Acquired form may improve with treatment of underlying disorder. It may progress in some patients. Treatment may help the symptoms. Remission can sometimes occur.

HOW TO TREAT

GENERAL MEASURES
• Relieve pain from neck spasms with heat or massage. Take hot showers or use warm, moist compresses, heating ointments, or heating pad.
• Stress may worsen symptoms. Learn stress-reduction techniques, including biofeedback.
• To learn more: National Spasmodic Torticollis Association, 9920 Talbot Ave., Suite 233, Fountain Valley, CA 92708; (800) 487-8385; website: www.torticollis.org.

MEDICATION
• Muscle relaxants, anticholinergics, benzodiazepines, and others may be prescribed. They may be taken by mouth or injected.
• Injections of botulinum toxin type A into the neck muscles may be prescribed.

ACTIVITY—As tolerated.

DIET—No special diet.

CALL YOUR DOCTOR IF

• You or a family member has symptoms of torticollis.
• Symptoms don't improve with treatment.

TOXIC SHOCK SYNDROME (TSS)

 GENERAL INFORMATION

DEFINITION—A rare, bacteria infection that can be life-threatening. It is not contagious.

BODY PARTS INVOLVED—Almost all organ systems in the body.

SEX OR AGE MOST AFFECTED—It has been associated with tampon use in healthy, menstruating women, but can occur in both sexes and all ages.

SIGNS & SYMPTOMS
* Sudden, high fever in a previously healthy person.
* Vomiting and watery diarrhea.
* Rash that resembles sunburn.
* Low blood pressure.
* Excessive thirst.
* Rapid pulse.
* Feeling of impending doom.
* Mental changes, such as confusion.
* Extreme fatigue and weakness.
* Headache.
* Sore throat.

CAUSES—Bacteria (*staphylococcus aureus* or *streptococcus pyogenes*) produces toxins that enter the bloodstream, causing sudden symptoms. Most serious cases have come from women using tampons. Toxic shock syndrome can also arise from wounds or infections in the throat, skin, lungs, or bone.

RISK INCREASES WITH
* Prolonged use of superabsorbent tampons during menstrual periods.
* Bacterial infections.
* Postpartum women.
* Postoperative patients, particularly after nasal surgery.
* Surgical wound infections.
* Diabetes
* HIV.
* Viral infection (influenza A or varicella).
* Chronic heart or lung disease.

HOW TO PREVENT—It can't always be prevented. Reduce risk factors where possible.
* Avoid tampons or alternate them with sanitary napkins. Use lowest absorbency tampon (that handles your menstrual flow) and change tampons frequently.
* Wash hands often to prevent spread of any germs.
* Get medical care for infected wounds.

 WHAT TO EXPECT

DIAGNOSTIC MEASURES
* Your own observation of symptoms.
* Your health care provider will do a physical exam and ask questions about tampon use and your medical history.
* A variety of medical tests will be done to confirm the diagnosis and check for any complications.

APPROPRIATE HEALTH CARE
* Immediate hospital care is required to give intravenous (IV) fluids, antibiotics, and electrolytes to correct fluid and electrolyte loss and dehydration. Treatment is provided for kidney or heart problems and to provide mechanical breathing support, if needed.
* Surgery may be required in some cases.

POSSIBLE COMPLICATIONS
* Severe shock.
* Kidney failure.
* Congestive heart failure.
* Respiratory distress.
* Loss of hair and nails.
* Recurrence of TSS.
* Mortality may be high in severe cases.

PROBABLE OUTCOME—With early diagnosis and prompt hospital treatment most patients recover. Some cases are fatal. Skin of the palms and soles often peels during recovery.

 HOW TO TREAT

GENERAL MEASURES—Close follow up medical care is important as the disorder can recur.

MEDICATION
* Antibiotics, usually given through a vein (IV), for infection.
* Intravenous fluids and electrolytes are often required for treatment.

ACTIVITY—Start to resume your normal activities as symptoms improve.

DIET—No special diet after recovery. Intravenous nourishment is usually needed during time in the hospital.

 CALL YOUR DOCTOR IF

* You or a family member has symptoms of toxic shock syndrome. Call immediately! Shock develops rapidly.
* New, unexplained symptoms develop. Drugs used in treatment may produce side effects.

TOXOPLASMOSIS

 GENERAL INFORMATION

DEFINITION—An infection in humans and animals caused by a tiny parasite, *Toxoplasma gondii*. It can live up to a year in water or moist soil. The parasite can infect most types of animals, but cats are the most often infected. Humans can get the infection in several different ways.

BODY PARTS INVOLVED—Nerves, heart, gastrointestinal, skin.

SEX OR AGE MOST AFFECTED—Both sexes: all ages.

SIGNS & SYMPTOMS
• No symptoms usually (80% to 90% of patients).
• Fever, sore throat, or fatigue.
• Swollen lymph glands.
• Muscle aches.
• Rash (sometimes).
• Inflammation (redness and soreness) of the retina (retinitis).

CAUSES
• People can get a toxoplasmosis infection by eating foods or drinking water that contain the germs. Infection can occur if you touch something, such as infected cat litter, with your hands then accidentally touch your mouth or eyes.
• Pregnant women who get the infection can transmit it to their offspring.
• Blood transfusion or organ transplantation (rare).

RISK INCREASES WITH
• Eating raw or partially-cooked meat (e.g., pork, lamb, beef, or venison). Eating raw fruits or vegetables grown in infected soil. Handling raw meats, and then touching your mouth.
• Infected cats (who usually have no symptoms). They pass germs in their stools (feces) into litter boxes, the soil in gardens, or in a child's sand box. The germs get on a person's hands when they change litter or garden. The hands then accidentally touch the mouth or eyes. Children who eat the sand or soil can become infected.
• Weak immune system due to illness or drugs.

HOW TO PREVENT
• Cook meat thoroughly. Carefully wash any surface that raw meat has touched, including your hands. Wash raw fruits and vegetables before eating them.
• Persons with weak immune systems and pregnant women should avoid contact with cat feces. If you do change cat litter or garden, be sure to wear gloves.
• Change cat litter boxes daily. Feed indoor cats only canned, dry or cooked meat (no raw meat).
• Protect children's play areas, including sand boxes, from cat and dog feces.

 WHAT TO EXPECT

DIAGNOSTIC MEASURES
• Your health care provider may do a physical exam and ask questions about your symptoms and activities.
• A blood test is needed to confirm the diagnosis.

APPROPRIATE HEALTH CARE
• Treatment is usually not needed for a healthy person with no symptoms or if their symptoms are mild.
• For an infected pregnant female, your obstetric provider will discuss the treatment available, the risks involved, and the expected outcomes.
• For a person with a weakened immune system, treatment is usually with drugs.
• Infected newborns (with or without symptoms) are usually treated with drugs to help prevent complications that may occur as they get older.
• If drugs are prescribed, your health care provider will do frequent blood tests to monitor for side effects.

POSSIBLE COMPLICATIONS
• Complications are rare. Inflammation may occur in the eyes (retinitis), the brain (encephalitis), or heart (myocarditis). People with weak immune systems are more likely to have complications.
• Pregnant women may have a miscarriage or stillbirth.
• Serious health problems or death may result for newborns who get infection from the mother.

PROBABLE OUTCOME—The majority of infected persons have no symptoms. Those with mild symptoms recover on their own.

 HOW TO TREAT

GENERAL MEASURES—None specific.

MEDICATION
• Pyrimethamine and sulfadiazine are the drugs most often prescribed to treat toxoplasmosis. These or other drugs may be prescribed for a pregnant woman.
• Corticosteroids, if necessary, for inflammation.
• Other drugs are currently being tested.

ACTIVITY—usually no limits.

DIET—No special diet.

 CALL YOUR DOCTOR IF

• You or your child has symptoms of toxoplasmosis.
• Symptoms don't improve after diagnosis and treatment, or drugs cause any side effects.

TRANSIENT ISCHEMIC ATTACK (TIA)

GENERAL INFORMATION

DEFINITION—A type of stroke that lasts only a few minutes. They are sometimes called "mini strokes." The term transient is used to describe a condition that lasts a short time. Ischemic describes an inadequate blood flow.

BODY PARTS INVOLVED—Blood vessels to the brain and the part of the brain supplied by the affected blood vessels.

SEX OR AGE MOST AFFECTED—Both sexes and usually adults over age 40.

SIGNS & SYMPTOMS
• Symptoms are brief. Most last less than 5 minutes. A few may last an hour and rarely, up to 24 hours.
• Loss of muscle function on one side of the body.
• Headache.
• Dizziness.
• Tingling in the arms and legs.
• Numbness.
• Vision disturbance or temporary blindness in one eye.
• Confusion.
• Faintness without loss of consciousness.
• Slurred speech or inability to speak.

CAUSES—TIAs happen when blood flow to a part of the brain is reduced for a short period. The reduced blood flow may be due to a small blood clot in an artery. It may be caused by a spasm of a brain artery causing it to narrow. TIAs normally do not cause lasting injury to the brain such as a stroke does.

RISK INCREASES WITH
• Aging, males or African Americans.
• Personal or family history of high blood pressure, atherosclerosis (hardening of the arteries), or stroke.
• Smoking or excess alcohol use.
• Diabetes, heart disease, or carotid artery disease.
• High cholesterol levels or high homocysteine levels.
• Obesity.
• Sedentary lifestyle (being physically inactive).

HOW TO PREVENT
• Exercise daily. Maintain a healthy weight. Eat a healthy diet.
• Don't smoke or use alcohol to excess.
• Have your blood pressure checked regularly. If it is high, get medical advice for treatment to reduce it.
• Daily aspirin may help. Ask your health care provider.

WHAT TO EXPECT

DIAGNOSTIC MEASURES
• Your own observation of symptoms.
• Your health care provider will do a physical exam and ask questions about your symptoms and activities.
• Medical tests may include studies to check your heart, brain and blood vessel function.

APPROPRIATE HEALTH CARE
• Emergency hospital care may be needed.
• Treatment may include drugs, taking control of risk factors (diabetes, high blood pressure, heart disease, and others), and lifestyle changes.
• Surgery (endarterectomy) may be needed to remove plaques (fatty deposits) from carotid arteries in the neck.
• Heart valve-replacement surgery may be needed.

POSSIBLE COMPLICATIONS—Stroke. Without treatment, over 30% of persons who have TIAs have strokes within 5 years.

PROBABLE OUTCOME
• Normally no lasting effects (such as weakness on one side) from a TIA. Treatment of TIAs can help reduce your risk factors for stroke.
• TIAs often recur. Symptoms of each attack may be similar or different from others.

HOW TO TREAT

GENERAL MEASURES
• Stop smoking and/or alcohol use. Get counseling, join a support group, or find other methods to help you quit.
• To learn more: American Stroke Association, 7272 Greenville Ave., Dallas, TX 75231; (888) 478-7653; website: www.strokeassociation.org.

MEDICATION—Anticoagulants (blood thinners) may be prescribed to decrease the risk of blood clots. Aspirin or other drugs may be prescribed to decrease the risk of future stroke.

ACTIVITY
• If you have frequent TIAs, you may be advised to avoid or limit certain activities that could risk injury to you or others.
• Exercise daily or as advised.

DIET—Eat a well-balanced diet that is low in salt and fat. Include fresh fruits, vegetables, and fiber. Begin a weight loss diet if overweight.

☎ CALL YOUR DOCTOR IF

• You or a family member has symptoms of a TIA. Seek emergency help.
• Other symptoms occur after treatment begins.

TRANSIENT SYNOVITIS OF THE HIP
(Toxic Synovitis)

GENERAL INFORMATION

DEFINITION—An inflammation (swelling and pain) of the tissues around the hip joint. It usually affects one hip, not both, and is a common cause of sudden hip pain in young children. Transient is used to describe a condition that lasts a short time. Synovitis describes an inflamed joint in the body.

BODY PARTS INVOLVED—Hip and legs.

SEX OR AGE MOST AFFECTED—It occurs more often in children ages 3 to 10, and most are boys. It can occur in infants and adults.

SIGNS & SYMPTOMS
- Mild or more severe pain in the hip. It may start quickly or come on slowly.
- Some children may have pain in the inner thigh or knee area.
- Difficulty walking or standing.
- Walking with a limp.
- Hip is tender to the touch.
- Mild fever less than 101°F (38.3°C) may occur.

CAUSES—The exact cause is unknown. A virus, an allergic reaction, a minor injury, drug or vaccine reaction may be involved.

RISK INCREASES WITH—Unknown.

HOW TO PREVENT—None known.

WHAT TO EXPECT

DIAGNOSTIC MEASURES
- Your own or child's observation of symptoms.
- Your child's health care provider will do a physical exam with careful attention to the painful hip area.
- Medical tests may include blood studies, x-rays, and other tests. These are done to confirm the diagnosis and make sure that there is not another problem involved. The main concern is a possibility of septic arthritis (a bacterial inflammation of a joint).

APPROPRIATE HEALTH CARE
- The main treatment is rest at home with drug therapy for pain if needed.
- Rarely, traction (at home or in the hospital) may be recommended.

POSSIBLE COMPLICATIONS—Complications are rare, but may involve other problems with hip or thigh-bones.

PROBABLE OUTCOME
- The pain may start to improve within 24 to 48 hours, and is usually gone completely within 2 weeks. Some children may have minor pain for several weeks.
- A few children may get the disorder again. If it does recur, it is usually within 6 months.

HOW TO TREAT

GENERAL MEASURES
- Use heat and massage to help ease the symptoms.
- Check your child's temperature daily to see if high fever develops.

MEDICATION—Naproxen or ibuprofen may be prescribed for treating pain and inflammation.

ACTIVITY—Limit activities until the pain symptoms are gone.

DIET—No special diet.

CALL YOUR DOCTOR IF

- Your child has symptoms of transient synovitis of the hip.
- After diagnosis, your child develops a high fever, other symptoms get worse, or symptoms don't improve within 10 days.

TRENCH MOUTH
(Necrotizing Ulcerative Gingivitis; Vincent's Disease)

 GENERAL INFORMATION

DEFINITION—A severe infection of gum tissue between the teeth. It is not contagious or cancerous.

BODY PARTS INVOLVED—Gums. If untreated, trench mouth can spread to: lymph glands in the neck; tonsils; vocal cords; bronchial tubes; rectum; or vagina.

SEX OR AGE MOST AFFECTED—Both sexes and all ages, but most common in ages 15 to 35.

SIGNS & SYMPTOMS
* Painful gums.
* Gums that bleed when pressed.
* Excess saliva.
* Bad breath.
* Ulcers (sores) covered with gray membrane on the gums.
* Swallowing with difficulty.
* Speaking difficulty.

CAUSES—Bacterial or other infection of the gums.

RISK INCREASES WITH
* Poor nutrition.
* Weak immune system due to illness or drugs.
* Smoking.
* Stress.
* Poor oral hygiene. Tartar, plaque, or food debris between teeth.

HOW TO PREVENT
* Maintain good oral hygiene.
 - To brush teeth: Scrub clear, sticky plaque off teeth daily with a soft toothbrush. Place the brush at the gum line and gently rotate, pointing bristles toward the gum. Brush one section of teeth at a time. Then brush tongue. A soft brush is less likely to damage teeth and gums than a hard brush.
 - To floss: Use waxed or unwaxed dental floss according to instructions on the package label or your dentist's instructions.
* Eat a well-balanced diet.
* Don't smoke.

 WHAT TO EXPECT

DIAGNOSTIC MEASURES
* Your own observation of symptoms.
* Your dental care provider or health care provider will do an exam of the gums.
* Dental x-rays or facial x-rays may be done.

APPROPRIATE HEALTH CARE
* Removal of dead gum tissue may be done as a treatment.
* Tooth cleaning (called scaling and root planing) is usually recommended. This type of cleaning removes plaque and tartar below the gumline.

POSSIBLE COMPLICATIONS
* Surgery may be needed if gums are extensively damaged.
* Infection may spread to other areas of the face (cheeks, lips, and jawbone) and cause tissue damage.

PROBABLE OUTCOME—Usually curable in two weeks with treatment. Frequent dental checkups, up to once a month, after treatment.

 HOW TO TREAT

GENERAL MEASURES
* Rinse your mouth with warm salt water a few times a day. Use one-half teaspoon of salt in one cup of water.
* Follow steps listed in Preventive Measures on how to brush and floss your teeth.
* Don't smoke. Find a way to quit that works.
* Find ways to help control stress in your life.
* Avoid any gum irritation until gums heal completely.

MEDICATION
* Antibiotics may be prescribed for infection.
* You may use nonprescription drugs, such as acetaminophen, for minor pain.

ACTIVITY—usually, no limits.

DIET
* A liquid or soft diet may be necessary for one to two days because of gum tenderness. When pain subsides, eat a normal, healthy diet. Avoid spicy or hot (temperature) food.
* Drink plenty of fluids each day.

 CALL YOUR DOCTOR IF

* Or call your dentist if you or a family member has symptoms of trench mouth.
* One or more of the following occur during treatment:
 - Fever.
 - Swelling of neck or face.
 - Swallowing difficulty.
 - Inability to eat.

TRICHINOSIS

GENERAL INFORMATION

DEFINITION—Infection caused by larvae of parasites that live in the intestines of pigs (rarely meat of bears and some marine animals). People may be infected and never have symptoms. The infection affects different places in the body:
• Gastrointestinal tract (where larvae enter).
• Lymphatic system and bloodstream (through which they are transported).
• Large muscles of the body. The diaphragm (large muscle used in breathing that separates the chest from the abdomen), arms and legs (in which the larvae become embedded).

BODY PARTS INVOLVED—Gastrointestinal, lymphatic system and bloodstream, large muscles of the body, and arms and legs.

SEX OR AGE MOST AFFECTED—Both sexes; all ages.

SIGNS & SYMPTOMS
Early stages (usually begin in 7 to 10 days):
• Appetite loss, nausea, vomiting, diarrhea and stomach cramps.
Later stages:
• Puffy eyelids and face.
• Muscle pain.
• Headache.
• Itching, burning skin.
• Sweating.
• High fever (102°F to 104°F or 38.9°C to 40°C).
Late stages:
• Symptoms decrease, but some muscle tissues remain permanently infected with microscopic cysts. In rare cases, these cause heart and central nervous system disorders.

CAUSES—Infection with a parasite, *Trichinella spiralis*. It is transmitted to humans when they eat infected animals. Thorough cooking kills the parasite and makes infected meat safe to eat. The parasites pass from animal to animal in contaminated food (usually raw garbage).

RISK INCREASES WITH
• Eating improperly cooked or raw pork.
• Weak immune system due to illness or drugs.

HOW TO PREVENT—Don't eat raw or undercooked pork meats (including ready-to-eat pork sausage). Cook all meats thoroughly.

WHAT TO EXPECT

DIAGNOSTIC MEASURES
• Your own observation of symptoms.
• Your health care provider will usually do a physical exam and ask about your symptoms and diet.

• Medical tests including blood studies, and a muscle biopsy may be done to confirm the diagnosis. With a biopsy, a small amount of muscle tissue is removed for viewing under a microscope.

APPROPRIATE HEALTH CARE
• Treatment usually includes drug therapy for pain and fever and rest at home. Antiworm drugs may help in some cases.
• Hospital care for severe cases. Breathing support and intravenous (IV) fluids may be needed.

POSSIBLE COMPLICATIONS—Overwhelming infection, which can lead to:
• Heart and lung complications.
• Central nervous system problems.
• Kidney damage.
• Vision or hearing disorders.
• Some deaths have been reported.

PROBABLE OUTCOME—Usually curable in 5-6 weeks in most persons with rest and treatment and, in severe cases, hospital care.

HOW TO TREAT

GENERAL MEASURES—Follow medical advice for care at home.

MEDICATION
• Anthelmintic (antiworm) drugs to kill the parasites may be prescribed. They can help if larvae are in the intestinal tract. They will not help help if the muscles are infected.
• Corticosteroids for patients with severe symptoms or with central nervous system involvement.
• You may take nonprescription drugs, such as acetaminophen, to reduce fever and discomfort.

ACTIVITY—Rest in bed until symptoms improve. While confined to bed, move legs often to reduce the likelihood of deep-vein blood clots. Resume normal activities gradually.

DIET—No special diet. Drink plenty of fluids.

CALL YOUR DOCTOR IF

• You or a family member has symptoms of trichinosis.
• New, unexplained symptoms develop. Drugs used in treatment may produce side effects, especially nausea, vomiting, skin rash or fever.

TRICHOMONIASIS

 GENERAL INFORMATION

DEFINITION—Trichomoniasis is a sexually transmitted disease (STD).

BODY PARTS INVOLVED—Reproductive system.

SEX OR AGE MOST AFFECTED—It affects both sexes, but is more common in women. It usually affects sexually active adolescents and adults.

SIGNS & SYMPTOMS
* Women:
- Discomfort varies greatly from woman to woman and from time to time in the same woman.
- Foul-smelling, frothy vaginal discharge that is most apparent several days after a menstrual period.
- Vaginal itching and pain.
- Pain with intercourse.
- Redness of the vaginal lips (labia) and vulva.
- Painful and frequent urination.
* Men:
- Infected men usually have no symptoms.
- Rarely may have painful urination and a pale white discharge from the penis.

CAUSES—Infection from a tiny parasite, *Trichomonas vaginalis*. The infection is spread from person to person during sexual intercourse. Symptoms may start 5 to 28 days after being exposed. The parasite may also live in the body for years without producing symptoms. Since it thrives in both men and women, both sexual partners must receive treatment.

RISK INCREASES WITH
* Having multiple sexual partners.
* Having sex with someone who has, or had, multiple sexual partners.
* Engaging in unsafe sex.
* On very rare occasions, the infection can be spread by sharing moist towels, washcloths or possibly from hot tubs.

HOW TO PREVENT
* Use latex (rubber) condoms during sexual intercourse.
* Limit your sexual partners or practice abstinence. The more sex partners you have, the greater your risk of any sexual transmitted disease.

 WHAT TO EXPECT

DIAGNOSTIC MEASURES
* Your own observation of symptoms.
* Your health care provider will do a physical exam and a pelvic exam in women.

* Medical tests may include Pap smear, and studies of vaginal discharge and urine. Tests to check for other STDs are often done.

APPROPRIATE HEALTH CARE—Treatment is with drug therapy. Your sexual partner(s) must be treated at the same time. This will prevent you from getting reinfected.

POSSIBLE COMPLICATIONS—If the infection is untreated, it can lead to other problems. Women may be more at risk for HIV infection (if exposed). If pregnant, it may cause early delivery and low birth weight baby. In men, prostate, bladder or urethra problems may occur.

PROBABLE OUTCOME—Can be cured with treatment.

 HOW TO TREAT

GENERAL MEASURES
* Don't douche unless prescribed for you.
* Wear cotton underpants or pantyhose with a cotton crotch.
* Take showers instead of tub baths.
* If urinating causes burning, urinate through a tubular device, such as a toilet-paper roll or plastic cup with the bottom cut out. Pour a cup of warm water over the genital area while you urinate.
* Don't sit around in wet clothing, especially in a wet bathing suit.
* To learn more: Centers for Disease Control & Prevention (CDC) National STD Hotline (800) 227-8922; website: www.cdc.gov/std.

MEDICATION
* Metronidazole (Flagyl) taken for 1-14 days is usually prescribed for you and your sexual partner. Follow directions carefully. Don't drink alcohol when you take this drug. If combined, they interact and cause a reaction with nausea, vomiting, sweating, weakness and other symptoms.
* Drugs for possible other sexually transmitted diseases may be prescribed.

ACTIVITY—Avoid sexual activity until treatment is complete. Allow about 10 days for recovery.

DIET—No special diet, except for avoiding alcohol.

 CALL YOUR DOCTOR IF

* You or a family member has symptoms of trichomoniasis.
* Symptoms get worse despite treatment.
* Unusual vaginal bleeding or swelling develops.

TRIGEMINAL NEURALGIA
(Tic Douloureux)

 GENERAL INFORMATION

DEFINITION—A condition involving the 5th cranial (trigeminal) nerve that causes episodes of severe facial pain.

BODY PARTS INVOLVED—Nerve branches from the trigeminal or 5th cranial nerve (nerve from the brain that supplies sensation to the face, scalp, teeth, mouth and nose).

SEX OR AGE MOST AFFECTED—The condition is more common in adults over age 40. Women are affected more than men.

SIGNS & SYMPTOMS
* Attacks of severe facial pain, described as "jabbing" or "searing" or like an electrical shock. These attacks (or bouts) of pain usually last for seconds, or sometimes for 1 to 2 minutes. A dull ache may be felt between bouts, or there may be little or no discomfort.
* Facial spasm (or tic) often occurs at the same time as pain.
* Only one side of the face is usually affected, but it may occur at different times on both sides.
* Pain is often triggered by touching or stroking the face, brushing teeth, shaving, exposure to wind, or chewing.
* Attacks may occur several times a day. They may disappear for weeks or months.
* A less common form, called atypical trigeminal neuralgia, may cause less-intense symptoms.

CAUSES—The exact cause is unknown (often called idiopathic). It may involve a nerve or blood vessel problem such as injury, irritation, inflammation, or disease.

RISK INCREASES WITH—Multiple sclerosis.

HOW TO PREVENT—No specific preventive measures.

 WHAT TO EXPECT

DIAGNOSTIC MEASURES
* Your own observation of symptoms.
* Your health care provider will do a physical exam of the affected facial area and ask about your symptoms and activities. This is usually sufficient for diagnosis.
* Medical tests may be done to check for other problems.

APPROPRIATE HEALTH CARE
* Most patients obtain pain relief with drug therapy. However, as time goes by, the drugs may become ineffective in some patients and the pain then "breaks through."
* Alternate type of treatments have been used by some, but they are not always effective. These include acupuncture, herbal remedies, chiropractic care, electrical stimulation, hypnosis, myotherapy (muscle release), and others.
* Surgery may be effective when drugs don't help. The different procedures available will be explained to you.

POSSIBLE COMPLICATIONS—Interference with normal activities due to severe pain episodes.

PROBABLE OUTCOME—Symptom relief is usually possible with treatment. Sometimes surgery may be required. A patient may experience pain-free intervals (lasting from months to years), and then the pain returns exactly as before.

 HOW TO TREAT

GENERAL MEASURES
* Maintain good oral health with dental checkups at least twice a year.
* Learn to control stress. It may trigger or worsen pain.
* To learn more: Facial Neuralgia Resources, website: www.facial-neuralgia.org or Trigeminal Neuralgia Association, 2801 South Archer Rd., Suite C, Gainesville, GA 32608; (352) 376-9955 (not toll free); website: www.tna-support.org.

MEDICATION
* Anticonvulsant (antiseizure) drugs are often prescribed to help relieve the pain.
* Other drugs including antidepressants, muscle relaxants, or antispasmodics may be helpful in some cases. Ordinary pain relievers are not helpful for this disorder.
* Products applied to the skin may help some patients. These include capsaicin (Zostrix) or lidocaine. Get medical approval before using.
* Experimental drugs are being researched.

ACTIVITY—No limits. Avoid blasts of hot or cold air.

DIET—No special diet.

 CALL YOUR DOCTOR IF

* You or a family member has symptoms of trigeminal neuralgia.
* New, unexplained symptoms develop. Drugs used in treatment may produce side effects.

TUBERCULOSIS (TB)

 GENERAL INFORMATION

DEFINITION—A chronic bacterial infection that mainly involves the lungs. Tuberculosis (TB) is occurring more often due to AIDS, poverty, homelessness, abuse of alcohol and other drugs, and failure of infected persons to take the prescribed drugs.

BODY PARTS INVOLVED—Lungs primarily, but may spread to other organs. Childhood tuberculosis is usually confined to the middle of the lungs, but it may spread to cause meningitis. Tuberculosis in adults usually affects the top of the lungs.

SEX OR AGE MOST AFFECTED—Both sexes; all ages.

SIGNS & SYMPTOMS
Early stages:
• No symptoms (often).
• Flu-like symptoms.
Middle stages:
• Low fever.
• Weight loss.
• Chronic fatigue.
• Heavy sweating, especially at night.
Later stages:
• Cough, with sputum that over time becomes bloody, yellow, thick, or gray.
• Chest pain and/or shortness of breath.
• Reddish or cloudy urine (sometimes).

CAUSES—Infection by the germ, *Mycobacterium tuberculosis*. Germs are transmitted in the air from one person to another. Many persons are infected with TB that is inactive and there are no symptoms (called latent TB infection or LTBI). About 1 in 10 of these people will eventually develop active TB.

RISK INCREASES WITH
• Adults over 60 (decline in health from aging).
• Newborns and infants.
• Chronic illness that affects immune system.
• Use of cortisone or drugs that suppress the immune system. These may cause inactive TB to become active.
• Crowded or unclean living conditions.
• Alcohol and drug abuse.
• Homeless people.
• Living in, or coming from, third world countries.

HOW TO PREVENT
• Preventive treatment for several months with isoniazid (INH) if tuberculin skin test is positive.
• Treating latent TB to prevent active TB.
• A vaccine called BCG is used in countries where TB is very common. It is less often used in the United States.

 WHAT TO EXPECT

DIAGNOSTIC MEASURES
• Your health care provider will do a physical exam and ask about your symptoms.
• Medical tests may include TB skin test, blood studies, sputum study, and chest x-ray.

APPROPRIATE HEALTH CARE
• Treatment is with drugs. It is important to take the drugs as prescribed to be sure the infection is cured. People may stop the drugs once they feel better, but the infection is still active. If this happens, the patient can spread the infection to others. In addition, this allows the TB bacteria to "outwit" the TB drugs and soon those drugs become ineffective.
• A TB infection that becomes resistant to drugs is termed multidrug-resistant TB (MDR-TB). Stronger TB drugs have to be used which have serious side effects. MDR-TB is more difficult to cure, and it can be fatal.
• It may be necessary to isolate (separate from other persons) or have hospital care.

POSSIBLE COMPLICATIONS
• Lung abscess, chronic obstructive pulmonary disease, bronchiectasis, or respiratory failure.
• Infection to brain, bone, spine, and kidneys.
• Without treatment, TB can be fatal.

PROBABLE OUTCOME—Usually curable with treatment.

 HOW TO TREAT

GENERAL MEASURES
• While infectious, use tissue to cover mouth when coughing, sleep in a separate bed, keep away from others; don't go to work or school.
• Have regular follow-up visits with your health care provider to see if treatment is working.
• To learn more: Centers for Disease Control & Prevention (CDC), 1600 Clifton Rd., NE, Mailstop E-10, Atlanta, GA 30333; website: www.cdc.gov/nchstp/tb.

MEDICATION—Antitubercular drugs, usually for 6 to 12 months. Several types are given at the same time to avoid bacterial resistance to the drugs. Patients are probably not infectious after 10 days to 2 weeks of treatment. MDR-TB may need treatment for up to two years.

ACTIVITY—Extra rest until symptoms improve. You may need to restrict activities for 6 months.

DIET—No special diet.

CALL YOUR DOCTOR IF

• You or a family member has symptoms of TB.
• Symptoms persist or worsen despite treatment or new symptoms develop.

TYPHOID FEVER

GENERAL INFORMATION

DEFINITION—A bacterial infection of the gastrointestinal tract. In the United States, people affected have usually been traveling internationally.

BODY PARTS INVOLVED—Gastrointestinal tract; skin; central nervous system.

SEX OR AGE MOST AFFECTED—Both sexes; all ages. Infants and persons over 60 usually have the severest cases.

SIGNS & SYMPTOMS
• Fever, headache, fatigue.
• Constipation and dry cough. Diarrhea is less common.
• Bloated abdomen with some discomfort.
• Confusion and feeling listless.
• Rash (rose spots) on the front of the body.
• Eye symptoms, such as vision changes (sometimes).
• Later symptoms may include foul smelling diarrhea, weight loss, weakness, slow pulse, rapid breathing, delirium, and others.

CAUSES—Infection with *Salmonella typhi*, a type of bacteria. The infection is spread by persons who are ill with the infection, or carriers who have been ill and recovered, but still carry the germs. You can become ill if you eat food or drink beverages prepared by one of these persons. Also, the germs may get into sewage and contaminate water that is used for drinking or washing foods. Shellfish from contaminated water or canned meat prepared improperly can cause outbreaks of the infection. Symptoms may appear 10 to 20 days after exposure.

RISK INCREASES WITH
• Travel to developing countries.
• Weak immune system due to illness or drugs.

HOW TO PREVENT
• For travel to countries where typhoid is present, consider typhoid vaccine (injection or oral form). It is not 100% protective, so take precautions with food and water. During travel, avoid tap water, salad and raw vegetables, unpeeled fruits, and dairy products. Follow the advice "boil it, cook it, peel it, or forget it."
• Wash your hands after using the bathroom and before handling food.

WHAT TO EXPECT

DIAGNOSTIC MEASURES
• Your own observation of symptoms.
• Your health care provider will do a physical exam and ask about your symptoms and recent travel.
• Medical tests are usually done to confirm the diagnosis.

APPROPRIATE HEALTH CARE
• Hospital care is needed for severe cases; others can be cared for at home. Follow any special instructions provided for preventing infection from being spread to other persons.
• People in certain types of jobs, such as food handlers, health care, or child care workers, will need to be tested for the germs before they can resume their usual work. They usually need three negative tests.
• Surgery may be needed in severe cases if complications occur, such as bleeding or an abscess.

POSSIBLE COMPLICATIONS
• Perforation of the intestines.
• Gastrointestinal hemorrhage or abscess.
• Pneumonia.
• Bone infection.
• Congestive heart failure.
• Without treatment, it can be fatal.

PROBABLE OUTCOME—Usually curable in 2 to 3 weeks with treatment. Relapse may occur in 10-20% of patients. Treatment is repeated.

HOW TO TREAT

GENERAL MEASURES
• Use a heating pad or warm compress to relieve abdominal cramps.
• Wash hands carefully and often.

MEDICATION
• Antibiotics will be prescribed. They may be given by injection or taken by mouth.
• For severe cases, steroids will be prescribed in addition to antibiotics.
• Eye symptoms may require eye drops or ointments.

ACTIVITY—Bed rest is necessary until all symptoms have been gone at least 3 days. The legs should be moved often in bed to prevent deep-vein blood clots from forming.

DIET—Diet will be determined by the symptoms.

CALL YOUR DOCTOR IF

• You or a family member has symptoms of typhoid fever.
• New symptoms develop or other symptoms become worse, despite treatment.

ULCER, PEPTIC
(Duodenal Ulcer; Gastric Ulcer)

GENERAL INFORMATION

DEFINITION—An ulcer is a lesion (sore) in the gastrointestinal tract. Ulcers that form in the upper part of the small intestine are duodenal ulcers. They are the most common type. Ulcers that form in the stomach are called gastric ulcers. They are less common.

BODY PARTS INVOLVED—Gastrointestinal tract.

SEX OR AGE MOST AFFECTED—Both sexes; all ages, but most common in adults.

SIGNS & SYMPTOMS
• Pain in the upper abdomen, or sometimes, the lower chest. It may be a burning, boring, or gnawing feeling that lasts 30 minutes to 3 hours. It may be worse before or after eating. It often awakens a person during the night. The pain may come and go. Weeks of off and on pain may alternate with short, pain-free periods.
• Pain is temporarily relieved with use of antacids.
• Appetite loss and weight loss. With duodenal, it may be weight gain, as person eats more to ease discomfort.
• Vomiting (sometimes may contain blood).
• Blood in the stool.

CAUSES
• Almost all ulcers are caused by either an infection with *Helicobacter pylori* bacteria or nonsteroidal anti-inflammatory drugs. *Helicobacter pylori* bacteria is present in many healthy people. Why it causes ulcers in some is unknown.
• Ulcers are not caused by stress, or anxiety or eating spicy foods, although they may aggravate existing ulcers.

RISK INCREASES WITH
• Family history of ulcers.
• Elderly.
• Smoking.
• Excess alcohol use (possibly).
• Use of nonsteroidal anti-inflammatory drugs (e.g., aspirin).
• Type-O blood (for duodenal ulcers).

HOW TO PREVENT—None specific. Avoid those risk factors that you can control.

WHAT TO EXPECT

DIAGNOSTIC MEASURES
• Your own observation of symptoms.
• Your health care provider will do a physical exam and ask about your symptoms and activities.
• Medical tests may include blood studies, gastrointestinal tract studies, and a test to check for *Helicobacter pylori*.

APPROPRIATE HEALTH CARE
• Treatment is with drug therapy and, life-style changes (if needed).
• Hospital care may be needed for complications such as bleeding ulcer or severe perforation or obstruction.
• Surgery for some patients for complications or if drug treatment is not effective.

POSSIBLE COMPLICATIONS
• Perforation. This is an erosion of the ulcer through the intestinal wall. It can cause infection or bleeding into the abdomen.
• Bleeding into the intestine.
• Anemia from blood loss.
• Duodenal ulcers are almost always benign, while gastric ulcers may rarely become malignant.
• Intestinal obstruction.

PROBABLE OUTCOME—Usually curable with treatment, but relapses can occur.

HOW TO TREAT

GENERAL MEASURES
• Quit smoking. Find a way to stop that works.
• If you drink alcohol heavily, stop or cut down.
• If stress is a problem, learn ways to cope.
• To learn more: National Digestive Diseases Information Clearinghouse, 2 Information Way, Bethesda, MD 20892, (800) 891-5389; website: www.digestive.niddk.nih.gov.

MEDICATION—You may be prescribed:
• Antibiotics to treat the *Helicobacter pylori* infection.
• Antacids to neutralize excess stomach acid.
• H-2 blockers or proton pump inhibitors to reduce stomach acid. Long-term therapy may be required for some patients.
• Drugs to coat and protect the lining of the stomach and the duodenum.

ACTIVITY—No limits.

DIET
• Eat small, healthy meals on a regular scheduled.
• Avoid foods that bring on pain.

CALL YOUR DOCTOR IF

• You or a family member has symptoms of an ulcer.
• Vomiting occurs that is bloody or looks like coffee grounds, or stool is bloody, black, or tarry-looking.
• You feel weak, tired, have pale skin, or back pain.

URETHRITIS

GENERAL INFORMATION

DEFINITION—Inflammation or infection of the urethra. The urethra is the tube that carries urine out of the bladder when you urinate. In women, it is about an inch long. In men, it is the full length of the penis.

BODY PARTS INVOLVED—Urethra; bladder (sometimes).

SEX OR AGE MOST AFFECTED—It can affect all ages and both sexes. In women, it often occurs along with a bladder infection or inflammation (cystitis).

SIGNS & SYMPTOMS
* Painful (may be severe) or burning urination.
* Discharge that may be cloudy, yellow-green mucus, or may be watery and white.
* Genital itching.
* Frequent urge to urinate, even when there is not much urine in the bladder.
* Men may have no symptoms.

CAUSES
* An infection that is spread by a sexual transmitted disease (STD). Most common causes are gonorrhea and chlamydia. Less often, herpes virus, human papilloma virus (HPV), trichomoniasis, and other infections are the cause. Non-specific urethritis (NSU) is the term used when there is infection present, but the cause is unknown.
* Lower estrogen levels in postmenopausal women.
* Yeast infection in women.
* Other causes could be from an injury or surgery, or from a chemical such as an antiseptic. Bubble bath or bath oils have been known to cause urethritis. This type of urethritis can not be spread to anyone else.

RISK INCREASES WITH
* Bacterial infection that spreads and enters the urethra from the skin around the genitals and anal area.
* Contact with an infected sexual partner.
* Use of a urinary catheter (tube used to remove urine).
* Multiple sexual partners.
* High-risk sexual behavior.
* Current or previous sexually transmitted disease.
* Loss of estrogen in postmenopausal women.

HOW TO PREVENT
* Practicing safer sexual behaviors. This includes having only one sexual partner and using rubber (latex) condoms to help protect against infections.
* Keep genital area clean and dry. Be sure sexual partner is clean.
* Avoid irritants and chemicals that cause redness, burning, or itching in the genital area.

WHAT TO EXPECT

DIAGNOSTIC MEASURES
* Your own observation of symptoms.
* Your health care provider will usually do an exam of the genital area.
* Medical tests may include blood studies and a culture of urine and any discharge.

APPROPRIATE HEALTH CARE
* Treatment will depend on the cause.
* Drugs may be prescribed. If infection is present, your sexual partner(s) will sometimes need treatment also.
* If the cause is trauma or chemical irritants, avoid the source of injury or irritant.

POSSIBLE COMPLICATIONS
* Complications are rare, unless it is not treated, or treatment is not adequate.
* In women, urinary tract infections, pelvic inflammatory disease (PID), or infertility may occur. There is also a risk of complications in pregnancy and in a newborn.
* In men, urinary tract infections or prostatitis (prostate infection) may occur.

PROBABLE OUTCOME—Proper treatment usually brings complete recovery.

HOW TO TREAT

GENERAL MEASURES
* To relieve pain, take sitz baths. Sit in a tub of warm water for 15 minutes at least twice a day.
* Keep the area around the genitals clean. Use unscented, plain soap.

MEDICATION
* Antibiotics for infection will usually be prescribed. Finish the complete dose, even if symptoms clear up.
* In cases of severe pain, phenazopyridine (Pyridium) may be prescribed. Pyridium produces bright orange (tea) colored urine.
* In menopausal women, estrogen applied to the vaginal area, or taken by mouth may be helpful.

ACTIVITY—Avoid sexual intercourse until you have been free of symptoms for 2 weeks. Otherwise, no limits.

DIET
* Drink plenty of fluids every day.
* Drink cranberry juice to acidify urine. Some drugs are more effective with acid urine.

CALL YOUR DOCTOR IF

* You or a family member has symptoms of urethritis.
* Symptoms recur after treatment.

UTERINE BLEEDING, DYSFUNCTIONAL
(Premenopausal Abnormal Uterine Bleeding)

 GENERAL INFORMATION

DEFINITION—Bleeding that is abnormal, irregular, and not part of a normal period. There is no tumor, infection, or pregnancy involved.

BODY PARTS INVOLVED—Uterus; vagina.

SEX OR AGE MOST AFFECTED—Women over age 40 and in those under age 20.

SIGNS & SYMPTOMS
• Bleeding between periods. Flow may be light or heavy, prolonged, and may contain clots.
• Periods last for 7 to 14 or even 18 days, and/or have spotting between periods.

CAUSES—The normal menstrual cycle depends on a balance of estrogen and progesterone. Bleeding problems occur if they get out of balance. There is too much estrogen or not enough progesterone. This happens most often due to anovulation (failure of the ovaries to produce or release eggs). Anovulation is more likely to occur in women who are close to menopause and young girls whose menstrual cycles have just started.

RISK INCREASES WITH
• Women over age 40 and under age 20.
• Polycystic ovary syndrome (cysts on the ovaries).
• Obesity.
• Athletes.
• Emotional stress.
• Eating disorders.

HOW TO PREVENT—No specific preventive measures.

 WHAT TO EXPECT

DIAGNOSTIC MEASURES
• Your own observation of symptoms.
• Your health care provider will usually do a physical exam and a pelvic exam. Questions will be asked about your symptoms and activities. Dysfunctional uterine bleeding is diagnosed after other causes of abnormal uterine bleeding have been ruled out. These include diseases, drugs, pregnancy, eating disorders, gynecological infections, polyps or other growths, or tumors.
• Medical tests are needed to help confirm the diagnosis. These will be explained to you.

APPROPRIATE HEALTH CARE
• Goals of treatment are to return periods to a normal cycle or stop the bleeding altogether. Treatment will depend on a woman's age, other medical conditions, and the severity of the bleeding.

• If bleeding is severe, a hospital stay may be needed to bring it under control.
• Treatment will be given for anemia if it exists.
• If symptoms are not severe, treatment may involve watchful waiting. This means monitoring the bleeding for a few months before treating it.
• Hormone therapy is usually the first treatment step, particularly in younger women.
• If hormones do not help the bleeding, surgery may be needed. Your health care provider will discuss options, benefits, and risks. Together, you'll decide on treatment.
  - Dilation and curettage (D & C) may be the recommended procedure.
  - Other surgery options include endometrial ablation (destruction or removal of the uterine lining), or hysterectomy. These procedures mean a woman can no longer become pregnant. They may be used for women who are close to menopause.

POSSIBLE COMPLICATIONS
• Anemia due to excessive bleeding.
• Cancer (rare).
• Infertility from lack of ovulation.

PROBABLE OUTCOME—Outcome will depend on the woman's medical condition, age, the severity of the problem, and treatment.

 HOW TO TREAT

GENERAL MEASURES—To learn more: National Women's Health Information Center (800) 994-9662; website: www.4women.gov.

MEDICATION
• Hormone therapy may be prescribed. This includes birth control pills, hormone-replacement therapy, or progesterone.
• Iron supplements may be needed for anemia.

ACTIVITY—No limits.

DIET—With anemia, an iron-rich diet may be recommended.

 CALL YOUR DOCTOR IF

• You or a family member has abnormal uterine bleeding.
• The following occur during treatment:
  - Bleeding becomes heavy (filling a pad or tampon more often than once an hour).
  - Signs of infection develop, such as fever, a general ill feeling, headache, dizziness, or muscle aches.
• New, unexplained symptoms develop. Drugs used in treatment may produce side effects.

UTERINE CANCER
(Endometrial Carcinoma; Uterine Sarcoma)

 GENERAL INFORMATION

DEFINITION—Cancer of the endometrium (lining of the uterus). It is the most common female pelvic cancer in the United States. Sarcoma is a less common type of uterine cancer. It involves the muscles and/or other supporting tissues of the uterus.

BODY PARTS INVOLVED—Uterus.

SEX OR AGE MOST AFFECTED—It usually affects postmenopausal women ages 50 to 60 and older.

SIGNS & SYMPTOMS
• Bleeding or spotting, often after sexual intercourse. This usually happens after menstrual periods have stopped for 12 months or more. A watery or blood-streaked vaginal discharge may occur before bleeding or spotting.
• Cramps (sometimes).
• Pain or mass in the pelvic area.
• Weight loss.

CAUSES—Exact cause is unknown. Increased estrogen levels are thought to play a role.

RISK INCREASES WITH
• Diabetes.
• Obesity.
• Women who have never given birth to a child.
• High blood pressure.
• Use of estrogen without also using progesterone.
• History of breast, ovarian or colon cancer.
• Family history of endometrial cancer.
• Use of the drug tamoxifen.
• History of uterine polyps, menstrual cycles without ovulation, or other signs of hormone imbalance.
• Delayed menopause (after age 52).
• Previous pelvic radiation therapy.

HOW TO PREVENT
• There are no specific preventive measures.
• Pelvic exams every 6 to 12 months may aid in early detection when treatment is more effective. Exams are very important for women with risk factors.
• Obtain medical care for any bleeding or spotting after menopause.
• Control diabetes or high blood pressure, and maintain ideal body weight.

 WHAT TO EXPECT

DIAGNOSTIC MEASURES
• Your own observation of symptoms, especially abnormal bleeding.
• Your health care provider will do a physical exam and a pelvic exam. Medical tests are

done, first to diagnose the cancer, and then to find out if it has spread to other body organs (staging). Tests will be explained to you. They may include blood tests, Pap smear, liver function tests, chest x-ray, CT scan, mammogram, barium enema, MRI, vaginal ultrasound, endometrial biopsy, and/or dilatation and curettage (D & C).

APPROPRIATE HEALTH CARE
• Treatment will depend on the extent of the disease, your health and your preferences. It may involve one or more of the following: Surgery, radiation, hormone therapy, and chemotherapy (anticancer drugs).
• In some cases, other disorders, such as diabetes, high blood pressure, or anemia must be brought under control before the cancer can be treated.
• Surgery treatment may include removing the uterus and, usually, ovaries and fallopian tubes.
• Counseling may help you cope with cancer.

POSSIBLE COMPLICATIONS
• If bleeding is not treated, anemia may occur.
• Spread of cancer to other organs. This can be fatal.
• Treatment is not effective, or cancer recurs.

PROBABLE OUTCOME—With early diagnosis and treatment, 90% of patients survive at least 5 years. Older patients and delayed diagnosis have a poorer outcome.

 HOW TO TREAT

GENERAL MEASURES—To learn more: American Cancer Society, (800) ACS-2345; website: www.cancer.org or National Cancer Institute, (800) 4-CANCER; website: www.nci.nih.gov.

MEDICATION
• Chemotherapy or hormone therapy may be prescribed.
• Antibiotic therapy, if needed for infection.

ACTIVITY—Resume normal activities, including sexual activity, when you recover from treatment.

DIET—Eat a healthy diet, even if you lose your appetite from radiation or drug therapy.

 CALL YOUR DOCTOR IF

• You or a family member has symptoms of cancer of the uterus.
• After surgery, you have more bleeding or signs of infection, such as fever, muscle aches, and headache.
• Drugs used in treatment produce side effects.

ILLNESS & DISORDERS

UTERINE FIBROIDS
(Myomas; Leiomyomas)

 GENERAL INFORMATION

DEFINITION—An abnormal growth of cells in the muscular wall (myometrium) of the uterus. The term *fibroid* is misleading. The cells are not fibrous. They are composed of abnormal muscle cells. Uterine fibroids are common, and almost always benign (not cancerous). Fibroid size can be very tiny to the size of a cantaloupe or larger. Rarely, fibroids can involve the cervix. Major types of fibroids include:
- Subserous, which appear on the outside of the uterus.
- Intramural, which are confined to the wall of the uterus.
- Submucous, which appear inside the uterus.
- Pedunculated myomas, which are attached to the uterine wall by stalks.

BODY PARTS INVOLVED—Uterus.

SEX OR AGE MOST AFFECTED—20-40% of women over 35.

SIGNS & SYMPTOMS
- Often, no symptoms occur. The fibroids may be diagnosed during a pelvic exam.
- Menstruation is more frequent, with (possibly) heavy bleeding, and (sometimes) passing clots.
- Bleeding between periods.
- Feelings of pressure on the bladder, rectum, or spine.
- Anemia (weakness, fatigue and paleness).
- Increased vaginal discharge (rare).
- Painful sexual intercourse, or bleeding after intercourse (rare).

CAUSES—Exact cause is unknown. It may involve excess estrogen in the body.

RISK INCREASES WITH
- Use of certain oral contraceptives and estrogen replacement therapy, as these stimulate fibroid growth.
- Genetic factors. They occur more often in African American women.
- Family history of fibroids.
- Diet high in fat and/or obesity may be a risk.

HOW TO PREVENT—Cannot be prevented at present. Routine pelvic exams can help with early diagnosis and treatment.

 WHAT TO EXPECT

DIAGNOSTIC MEASURES
- Your health care provider will do a physical exam and a pelvic exam.
- Medical tests may include blood studies and an ultrasound. Specialized tests (laparoscopy, hysterosalpingogram, hysteroscopy, or biopsy) may be done to verify the type of fibroid.

APPROPRIATE HEALTH CARE
- Treatment will vary depending on symptoms and diagnostic tests, location and size of the fibroids, health status, and desire for pregnancy.
- No treatment may be needed if symptoms are mild (follow up exam every 3 to 12 months).
- Hormone therapy (suppress natural estrogen) may be the first treatment or before surgery.
- Surgery may be recommended. Hysterectomy is surgery to remove the uterus. Myomectomy removes the fibroids. Laparoscopy technique can be used.
- Uterine fibroid embolization (UFE), also called uterine artery embolization (UAE), is a nonsurgical procedure. It treats fibroids by cutting off their blood flow.
- Radiofrequency ablation (RFA) or myomacoagulation (called myolysis) uses electric current to treat fibroids.
- Cryomyolysis uses a probe to freeze fibroids.
- Ultrasound with an MRI uses soundwaves to heat and destroy fibroid tissue.

POSSIBLE COMPLICATIONS
- Heavy bleeding and anemia.
- Complications may occur in a pregnancy.
- Fibroids may return after some treatments.
- Fibroids may affect fertility.
- Fibroids become cancerous (about 1 in 1000).

PROBABLE OUTCOME
- Treatment is usually not needed when there are no symptoms or the symptoms are mild.
- Drugs can help relieve some symptoms, but will not cure fibroids. Fibroids can be removed or destroyed with several different methods.
- Fibroid size may decrease after menopause.

 HOW TO TREAT

GENERAL MEASURES—Be sure you understand all of your treatment options.

MEDICATION
- A combination of nonsteroidal anti-inflammatories, birth control pills, or progestins may be prescribed.
- Iron may be prescribed for anemia.
- A gonadotropin-releasing hormone may be prescribed. It will induce an abrupt, artificial menopause that stops the bleeding and reduces size of the fibroid.

ACTIVITY—No limits usually (may depend on treatment).

DIET—No special diet.

 CALL YOUR DOCTOR IF

You or a family member has symptoms of fibroids.

UTERINE PROLAPSE

GENERAL INFORMATION

DEFINITION—A uterus that has fallen or dropped from its normal location. This causes it to bulge into or beyond the vagina. Other types of genital prolapse may also occur:
- Cystocele (part of bladder bulges into the vagina).
- Enterocele (small bowel bulges into the vagina).
- Rectocele (rectum bulges into the vagina).

BODY PARTS INVOLVED—Uterus; ligaments that suspend the uterus; vagina.

SEX OR AGE MOST AFFECTED—Women over age 40.

SIGNS & SYMPTOMS
- A lump in front or back of the vagina, or a lump that extends outside of the vagina.
- Vague discomfort or pressure in the pelvic region.
- Backache that gets worse with lifting.
- Frequent and painful urination.
- Stress incontinence (urine leakage when laughing, sneezing, or coughing) may occur.
- Problem in moving bowels.
- Pain with sexual intercourse.

CAUSES—Prolapse occurs when muscles and ligaments of the pelvic floor become overstretched and weak.

RISK INCREASES WITH
- Being overweight.
- Having one or more vaginal births.
- Obstetrical trauma and lacerations sustained during labor and delivery.
- Normal aging and decreased estrogen.
- Strain on the supportive muscles such as from chronic cough or chronic constipation.
- Work or other activities requiring heavy lifting.
- Tumors (rare).

HOW TO PREVENT
- May not be able to prevent, but can reduce the risk.
- Maintain a healthy body weight.
- Practice pelvic floor exercises during pregnancy and after childbirth.
- Exercise on a regular basis to maintain muscle strength.
- Avoid constipation.
- Consider estrogen therapy after menopause.

WHAT TO EXPECT

DIAGNOSTIC MEASURES
- Your own observation of symptoms.
- Your health care provider can usually diagnose the prolapse with a pelvic exam.
- Medical tests may be done to check for other pelvic disorders or complications.

APPROPRIATE HEALTH CARE
- Treatment options depend on the severity of the prolapse. Other factors to consider are the patient's age, if pregnancy is still desired, and other pelvic disorders.
- Patients with mild symptoms can usually be treated without surgery. This may include an exercise program (e.g., Kegel), hormone therapy, or use of a pessary (support device).
- A pessary is small device inserted into the vagina to help maintain the uterus in a normal position. They come in different shapes, and are individually fitted.
- Surgery may be needed for severe prolapse. Several methods are available and it can be performed to save the uterus if desired. Your options will be discussed.

POSSIBLE COMPLICATIONS
- The cervix may become irritated and sore.
- Higher risk of infection or injury to pelvic organs.
- Hemorrhoids from straining due to constipation.
- Problems with bladder, bowel, or sexual functions.
- Prolapse may recur.

PROBABLE OUTCOME—Mild prolapse usually responds to conservative treatment. A more severe prolapse can be helped with surgery.

HOW TO TREAT

GENERAL MEASURES
- Avoid wearing tight girdles or clothing that increases intra-abdominal pressure.
- Get treatment for a chronic coughing problem.
- Quit smoking. Find a plan that works for you.
- Kegel exercises. Learn to recognize, control, and develop pelvic muscles. They are the ones you use to interrupt urination in mid-stream.
- To learn more: National Women's Health Information Center (800) 994-9662; website: www.4women.gov.

MEDICATION
- Estrogen (cream or pills) may be prescribed to improve blood flow to pelvic muscles.
- Stool softeners may be used for constipation.

ACTIVITY
- Avoid heavy lifting.
- After any surgery, follow medical advice.

DIET
- Keep your weight under control.
- High fiber diet helps prevent constipation.

CALL YOUR DOCTOR IF

- You or a family member has symptoms of uterine prolapse.
- Symptoms don't improve, despite treatment.

VAGINA OR VULVA CANCER

GENERAL INFORMATION

DEFINITION—A rare type of cancer that involves the growth of malignant cells in the vagina or on the vulva. The vagina is the opening to the birth canal. The vulva is the whole area surrounding the vagina and extending to the thighs including the clitoris and vaginal lips.

BODY PARTS INVOLVED—Vagina; vulva.

SEX OR AGE MOST AFFECTED—It occurs mostly in women over age 50. One type (rhabdomyosarcoma) occurs in children.

SIGNS & SYMPTOMS
• Vulvar itching.
• Abnormal vaginal bleeding.
• Discomfort or bleeding with intercourse.
• Small or large, firm, painless sores on the vulva that may bleed easily.
• Changes in skin color.

CAUSES—For unknown reasons, abnormal cells begin to develop and grow out of control. These abnormal cells may be benign (not cancer), precancer, or cancer cells. Certain risk factors have been identified.

RISK INCREASES WITH
• Women over age 60.
• Being born between 1938 and 1971 to a mother who took DES to control spotting or bleeding in pregnancy. DES is diethylstilbestrol, a drug prescribed up to 1971.
• Family history of cancer of reproductive organs.
• Human papillomavirus (HPV), the cause of genital warts.
• Smoking.
• Multiple sex partners.
• A history of sexually transmitted diseases.
• Other cancer.

HOW TO PREVENT
• No specific preventive measures. Have a yearly pelvic exam and Pap smear to detect possible problems early.
• Become familiar with the appearance of your genitals. Use a mirror and examine once a month. Darker spots around the labia are generally not vaginal or vulvar cancer. They may be a sign of melanoma, a skin cancer. Seek medical care for any dark skin change.

WHAT TO EXPECT

DIAGNOSTIC MEASURES
• Your own observation of symptoms.
• Your health care provider will do a physical exam and a pelvic exam and ask questions about your symptoms.

• Medical tests will be done to diagnose cancer and to check if it has spread to other parts of the body (called staging).

APPROPRIATE HEALTH CARE
• Treatment options include surgery, radiation, and (sometimes) chemotherapy. It depends on the location and stage of the cancer, and the age and physical health of the patient. Precancer conditions may be treated.
• Surgery involves leaving normal skin while removing the cancer. Different options are used depending on the cancer stage. All or part of the vagina and vulva may be removed. Lymph node removal may be needed if cancer has spread.
• Laser therapy may be used for treatment of some vulvar cancer.
• Radiation treatment (sometimes). External radiation shrinks the primary tumor. Internal radiation (implants) affects cancer that has spread to nearby tissues.

POSSIBLE COMPLICATIONS—Spread to other places in the body. Common sites of spread are lymph nodes in the groin, wall of the pelvis, bladder, rectum, bone, lungs, or liver. This could be fatal.

PROBABLE OUTCOME—Early diagnosis and treatment offer a good chance for complete recovery. Symptoms can be relieved or controlled during treatment.

HOW TO TREAT

GENERAL MEASURES—To learn more: American Cancer Society, (800) ACS-2345; website: www.cancer.org or National Cancer Institute, (800) 4-CANCER; website: www.nci.nih.gov.

MEDICATION
• Anticancer (chemotherapy) drugs may be given by pill, through a vein, or applied topically.
• Pain relievers (if needed) may be prescribed.
• Use stool softener (if needed) to prevent constipation.

ACTIVITY
• After surgery, resume your normal activities gradually, allowing 6 weeks for full recovery.
• Sexual relations may be resumed when healing is complete or as advised by your health care provider.

DIET—No special diet.

CALL YOUR DOCTOR IF

• You or a family member has symptoms of cancer of the vagina or vulva.
• After treatment, signs of infection, such as pain, fever, swelling, or excessive vaginal bleeding occur.

VAGINISMUS

GENERAL INFORMATION

DEFINITION—Vaginismus involves spasms (clenching up) of the pelvic muscles. This may prevent sexual intercourse. Types:
• *Primary vaginismus*—a woman has never been able to have sexual intercourse.
• *Secondary vaginismus*—a woman has had intercourse at one time, but is no longer able to because of the spasms.

BODY PARTS INVOLVED—Pelvic muscles.

SEX OR AGE MOST AFFECTED—Females after puberty.

SIGNS & SYMPTOMS
• Muscle spasms around the vagina and rectum. They may be quite painful.
• The vagina closes so tightly that the penis cannot penetrate for sexual intercourse. It also prevents inserting any object into the vagina, such as a tampon, diaphragm, or speculum (used for pelvic exam).

CAUSES—It may be caused by physical or mental (emotional) factors, or a combination of the two.

RISK INCREASES WITH
• An unconscious desire to prevent penile penetration. This may be due to fear of pain, anxiety, hostility, anger, or a distaste for sex.
• Being brought up to think that sex is a sin or dirty.
• Previous sexual trauma (incest, rape, sexual abuse).
• The first sexual experience for a woman.
• A sexual partner who is not sensitive; insufficient or unskillful foreplay.
• Emotional stress.
• Infections, allergic reactions, or a rigid, intact hymen.
• Surgical or postdelivery scarring.
• Endometriosis (a gynecological condition).

HOW TO PREVENT—Pelvic exam by a health care provider and counseling prior to beginning of sexual activity.

WHAT TO EXPECT

DIAGNOSTIC MEASURES
• Your own observation of symptoms.
• You health care provider will do a physical exam and a pelvic exam if possible. Sedation may be needed for a complete exam. A sexual history is important. This will include early childhood experiences, family attitudes toward sex, previous and current sexual responses. Contraceptive practices, reproductive goals, feelings about your sexual partner, and specifics about the pain you experience will be discussed.

APPROPRIATE HEALTH CARE
• Treatment will be given for any medical problems. This is often followed by therapy to help with emotional problems, and to reduce the muscle spasms.
• One therapy involves dilating (widening) the vaginal opening gently and gradually with rubber or glass dilators. Treatments may be started at the medical office and then practiced at home.
• Prior to dilation therapy or attempted intercourse, sit in a tub of warm water for 10 to 15 minutes. Baths often relax muscles and relieve discomfort.
• Kegel exercises to control the pelvic muscles may be helpful. You will be instructed on how to do them.
• Counseling is helpful for many patients and their partners. It can help resolve any conflicts and concerns in your life, and to better communicate with your partner.

POSSIBLE COMPLICATIONS—Emotional problems caused by guilt, anxiety, loss of self-esteem, and feeling inadequate. Relationship problems with your sexual partner.

PROBABLE OUTCOME—Medical treatment and counseling can help. Treating the underlying cause may clear up the condition.

HOW TO TREAT

GENERAL MEASURES—You and your partner may try other sexual activities. This can include massage, oral sex, or masturbation.

MEDICATION
• Anti-anxiety drugs or muscle relaxants may be prescribed for a short period of time.
• Before attempting intercourse, you and your partner should use a lubricant, such as K-Y Lubricating Jelly.

ACTIVITY—No limits.

DIET—No special diet.

CALL YOUR DOCTOR IF

• You or a family member has symptoms of vaginismus.
• Symptoms don't improve after 3 weeks, despite treatment. Symptoms recur after treatment.

VAGINITIS
(Vulvovaginitis; Vaginitis, Atrophic)

GENERAL INFORMATION

DEFINITION—Vaginitis is an inflammation of the vagina. Types of vaginitis include:
• *Infectious:* this is the most common type and is usually caused by a bacterial infection. It may also be due to a yeast or parasitic infection.
• *Noninfectious:* may be caused by vaginal dryness (atrophic), allergic reaction, or chemical irritation.

BODY PARTS INVOLVED—Vagina; urethra; bladder; skin around the genitals.

SEX OR AGE MOST AFFECTED—Female adolescents and adults. It most often occurs during the reproductive years.

SIGNS & SYMPTOMS
• The vagina normally has a thin, whitish or clear discharge which may change to:
  - Texture (thick, thin, or curd-like).
  - Color (white, gray, or yellowish).
  - Odor (fishy smell).
  - Amount (heavy or light).
• Itching, burning, irritation, redness, swelling, and possibly pain in the vagina or vulva (external genitals).
• Vaginal dryness (due to atrophy).
• Pain with sexual intercourse.
• Pain and burning when urinating.
• Symptoms may vary with the menstrual cycle.

CAUSES
• Infectious vaginitis causes include: bacterial vaginosis (most common cause), vulvovaginal candidiasis (a yeast infection), or trichomoniasis (a parasitic infection).
• Noninfectious causes include a decrease of natural estrogen (at menopause), an irritant (such as clothes that rub), or an allergic reaction (such as a spermicide).

RISK INCREASES WITH
• Use of antibiotic drugs.
• Use of spermicide or intrauterine device (IUD).
• Sexual intercourse.
• Having multiple sex partners.
• Douching.
• Change in hormone levels (pregnancy, breast-feeding, menopause, or birth-control pills).

HOW TO PREVENT
• Wear underwear and pantyhose with a cotton crotch. Avoid wearing clothing that is overly tight, such as jeans.
• Keep genitals clean and dry. Don't douche.
• Don't sit around in a wet bathing suit.
• Avoid perfumed or deodorant soap, detergents, fabric softeners, bubble baths, powder, and vaginal sprays.
• Always wipe away from the vagina—front to back—after bowel movements.
• Use a latex condom for sexual intercourse unless you and your partner are monogamous (having one mate).

WHAT TO EXPECT

DIAGNOSTIC MEASURES
• Your own observation of symptoms.
• Your health care provider will usually do a physical exam and a pelvic exam.
• Tests may be done of the vaginal discharge.

APPROPRIATE HEALTH CARE
• Treatment will depend on the cause of the vaginitis. Drugs are usually prescribed for infections and sometimes for vaginal dryness or irritation. Your sexual partner needs treatment if trichomoniasis is the cause.
• If the vaginitis is due to an irritant or allergic reaction, stop using the offending product.

POSSIBLE COMPLICATIONS
• Vaginitis may recur after treatment.
• Without treatment, it can lead to serious medical problems, be a risk factor for sexually transmitted diseases, or cause pregnancy complications.

PROBABLE OUTCOME—With treatment, symptoms usually clear up in 3 to 4 days.

HOW TO TREAT

GENERAL MEASURES
• Don't assume you have a yeast infection and use antifungal drugs to self-treat without a diagnosis. Those drugs won't help other types of infection. In addition, a vaginal infection should not be self-treated with herbal remedies, douches, or deodorant sprays.
• To learn more: National Women's Health Information Center (800) 994-9662; website: www.4women.gov.

MEDICATION
• An antibiotic, antifungal, or antiparasitic drug may be prescribed. Take the entire drug course.
• For vaginal dryness, estrogen creams or oral tablets may be recommended.
• For vaginal irritation, steroid or hormone creams may be prescribed.

ACTIVITY—Avoid sex intercourse during treatment.

DIET—No special diet.

CALL YOUR DOCTOR IF

• You or a family member has symptoms of vaginitis.
• Symptoms recur following treatment.

VAGINOSIS, BACTERIAL
(Vaginosis, *Gardnerella*; Vaginitis, Nonspecific)

 GENERAL INFORMATION

DEFINITION—Vaginosis is an infection of the vagina. Bacterial vaginosis (BV) means that bacteria are the cause of the infection. It is not thought to be a sexually transmitted disease (STD), but sexual activity has been linked to this infection. It may cause vaginitis that has symptoms of soreness, itching, and irritation.

BODY PARTS INVOLVED—Vagina and adjacent skin.

SEX OR AGE MOST AFFECTED—Females of all ages (most often in the childbearing years).

SIGNS & SYMPTOMS
• About 50% of women have no symptoms.
• Vaginal discharge that may have an unpleasant odor (referred to as a "fishy" smell). The color and amount of discharge varies from woman to woman.

CAUSES—Normally, there are a number of harmless bacteria in the vagina. They may help protect against other infections such as yeast infection. These harmless bacteria sometimes get out of balance and undesirable bacteria are able to grow. Why this occurs is unknown. Undesirable bacteria types are *Gardnerella vaginalis, Mycoplasma hominis,* and *Mobiluncus species.*

RISK INCREASES WITH
• Intrauterine contraceptive device (IUD).
• Smokers.
• Early age at first intercourse.
• Higher number of lifetime sexual partners.
• New sexual partner, or increase in number of sexual partners in the month before diagnosis.
• Recent use of antibiotic drugs.

HOW TO PREVENT
• There are no specific preventive measures. The following general measures may help to prevent bacterial vaginosis or other vaginal disorders.
• Use condoms with new sexual partners to help protect against infections, possibly bacterial vaginosis.
• Keep the genital area clean and dry. Use plain unscented soap. Be sure sexual partner is clean. Avoid vaginal douching.
• Take showers rather than tub baths. If you take a bath, don't add oils or bubble bath to the water.
• Wear cotton underwear or pantyhose with a cotton crotch.
• Don't sit around in wet clothes, such as a bathing suit.
• After going to the bathroom, wipe from front to back (vagina to anus).
• Change tampons or sanitary pads frequently.

 WHAT TO EXPECT

DIAGNOSTIC MEASURES
• Your health care provider will do a physical exam including a pelvic exam. Because some women have no symptoms of the infection, it may be diagnosed on a routine exam.
• Medical tests may include studies of vaginal discharge and a Pap smear.

APPROPRIATE HEALTH CARE
• Treatment is usually recommended for women who have symptoms and women who will be having surgical procedures.
• For pregnant women with the infection, your obstetric provider will discuss the diagnosis, risks, and treatment recommendations.

POSSIBLE COMPLICATIONS
• Recurrence is common, but it can be retreated.
• Infection with another vaginal disorder.
• Increased risk of infection with uterine surgery.
• May have problems with pregnancy and delivery.

PROBABLE OUTCOME—Mild cases may get better without treatment. Treatment can relieve symptoms in other cases.

 HOW TO TREAT

GENERAL MEASURES
• If you smoke, find a way to quit that works.
• Testing and treating male sexual partners is usually not needed.
• Douches or deodorant sprays that mask vaginal odor should not be used to treat BV. They may eliminate the odor, but they will not cure the condition.
• To learn more: National Women's Health Information Center (800) 994-9662; website: www.4women.gov.

MEDICATION—Metronidazole (Flagyl) or clindamycin (Cleocin) are often prescribed for treatment of bacterial vaginosis. They are available in both an oral and topical form.

ACTIVITY—No limits.

DIET—No special diet.

 CALL YOUR DOCTOR IF

• You or a family member has a vaginal discharge.
• Symptoms persist longer than 1 week or worsen, despite treatment.
• Vaginal bleeding or swelling develops.

VARICOCELE

GENERAL INFORMATION

DEFINITION—A varicocele is a tangled network of blood vessels, or varicose veins, in the testicles. Varicocele occurs more often in the left testicle than the right, and, less often, in both. They can take up to 20 years to grow large enough to be noticeable. It is a common condition (occurs in about 15% of men).

BODY PARTS INVOLVED—Vagina and adjacent skin.

SEX OR AGE MOST AFFECTED—Males (often in their 20s or 30s).

SIGNS & SYMPTOMS
* In most cases, there are no symptoms. They may be diagnosed during a routine physical exam.
* Ache in the testicle. Sometimes they cause pain.
* Feeling of heaviness or dragging in the scrotum (the pouch of skin that contains the testicles).
* Atrophy (shrinkage) of the testicle.
* Enlarged veins can be felt (like feeling a "bag of worms"), and can make the testicle look lumpy.

CAUSES
* Normally, blood in the testicles travels through a series of small veins into a large vein that goes up through the abdomen. A series of one-way valves in the veins prevents the reverse flow of blood back to the testicles. Sometimes, these one-way valves become damaged or defective. This causes the blood to flow backward. This reverse flow of blood stretches and enlarges the tiny veins around the testicle to cause a varicocele.
* Because of the varicocele, the blood does not cool as it does in a normal vein. The increased temperature of the blood raises the temperature of the testicles. This is believed to contribute to infertility, as heat can damage or destroy sperm. The raised temperature may also block production of new, healthy sperm.

RISK INCREASES WITH—Men in their 20s or 30s.

HOW TO PREVENT—No known preventive measures.

WHAT TO EXPECT

DIAGNOSTIC MEASURES
* Your health care provider will do an exam of the genital area. Varicoceles may be seen with the naked eye or by palpating (feeling) the area while a patient is standing up.
* Small varicoceles may be diagnosed with ultrasound or other medical tests.

APPROPRIATE HEALTH CARE
* No treatment may be needed if there are no symptoms or the symptoms are mild and infertility is not an issue. Wear an athletic supporter or a pair of snug-fitting underwear to provide the scrotum with support.
* Surgery or other treatment may be recommended if the varicocele causes pain, atrophy, or infertility.
* Most varicoceles can be corrected through a surgical procedure called varicocelectomy (tying off the affected spermatic veins). It is usually performed under general or local anesthesia as an outpatient.
* Laparoscopy may be an option. It involves the insertion of a thin, lighted tube (called a laparoscope) through a small incision (cut) in the abdomen to locate and tie off the varicocele.
* A nonsurgical alternative called varicocele embolization may be recommended. A small catheter (tube) is inserted into the groin. Substances that will block the flow of blood are inserted through the catheter. The affected veins are sealed off, causing the blood flow to return to its normal path.

POSSIBLE COMPLICATIONS
* Low sperm count.
* Male infertility.
* Varicocele may recur after treatment.
* Some patients develop a condition called hydrocele. This is a fluid-filled cyst that forms around the testicle. Minor surgery is used to correct the problem.

PROBABLE OUTCOME
* Successful treatment can reduce the swelling and discomfort of varicoceles that cause symptoms.
* Treatment may help with infertility. It takes about 90 days for a sufficient quantity of new sperm to be produced to permit fertilization. Semen study is usually done at 3 and 6 months after treatment.

HOW TO TREAT

GENERAL MEASURES—None specific.

MEDICATION—Drugs are normally not needed.

ACTIVITY—No limits.

DIET—No special diet.

CALL YOUR DOCTOR IF

* You or a family member has symptoms of a varicocele.
* Varicocele symptoms recur after treatment.

VARICOSE VEINS

GENERAL INFORMATION

DEFINITION—Veins, usually in the legs, which become permanently enlarged and often twisted. Varicose veins can involve superficial veins, deep veins, and veins that connect superficial and deep veins.

BODY PARTS INVOLVED—Veins in the legs, including superficial veins, deep veins and veins that connect superficial and deep veins. Veins in the vaginal lips during pregnancy and those around the anus (hemorrhoids) also may become varicose.

SEX OR AGE MOST AFFECTED—Adults of both sexes.

SIGNS & SYMPTOMS
* Enlarged, bulging, ropelike, bluish veins that are visible under the skin. They appear most often in the back of the calf or on the inside of the leg from the ankle to the groin.
* Vague discomfort and aching, or pain in the legs, especially after standing.
* Fatigue.

CAUSES—The veins of the legs contain one-way valves every few inches to help blood return against gravity to the heart. If the valves leak, blood pressure in the veins prevents blood from draining properly. Valves may fail because of previous vein disease, such as thrombophlebitis; prolonged standing; or pressure on veins in the pelvis from pregnancy, tumors, or fluid in the abdomen.

RISK INCREASES WITH
* Increasing age.
* Being overweight.
* Straining. This may be from constipation, a chronic cough, prostate problems, or urinary retention.
* Family history of varicose veins.
* Work that requires prolonged sitting or standing.
* Pregnancy or menstruation.
* Injury or prior surgery on the legs.

HOW TO PREVENT
* Exercise regularly (walking, swimming, or bicycling) to keep circulation healthy.
* Don't sit or stand for long periods. Move around.

WHAT TO EXPECT

DIAGNOSTIC MEASURES
* Your own observation of symptoms.
* Your health care provider will do a physical exam of the affected veins and ask about your symptoms.
* Medical tests may include ultrasound and other studies.

APPROPRIATE HEALTH CARE
* Simple self-care methods may be recommended.
* Surgery and other treatment methods may be done for pain, recurrent phlebitis (inflamed veins), skin changes, or for cosmetic reasons.
* Veins can be sealed off by using sclerotherapy (injections), laser, intense-pulsed light therapy, or radio-frequency ablation. Veins can also be removed with surgery. Your health care provider will discuss your options, the risks, and benefits of each one with you.
* Spider veins (idiopathic telangiectases) are small superficial veins. They may be treated with a laser or with injections.

POSSIBLE COMPLICATIONS
* Ulcer near the ankle (stasis dermatitis) caused by poor blood flow to the skin. This may be slow to heal.
* Deep-vein blood clot.
* Venous insufficiency. Blood does not completely return to the heart.
* Varicose veins may return after treatment.

PROBABLE OUTCOME—Self-care steps may help symptoms. Medical treatment has a high success rate.

HOW TO TREAT

GENERAL MEASURES
* Take frequent rest periods with legs elevated.
* Use lightweight, elastic compression hosiery. Put them on before getting out of bed.
* Don't wear girdles or other tight clothing.
* Avoid long periods of sitting or standing. Take breaks and walk around.
* Wear comfortable shoes and avoid high heels.
* Cross legs at ankles and not at the knees.

MEDICATION
* A chemical may be injected (sclerotherapy) into small varicose veins to make them collapse and disappear over time Other veins will take over blood flow.
* Drugs for pain may be prescribed following surgery.

ACTIVITY
* Walking and being active after any treatment is important to help promote healing.
* Compression hose will usually need to be worn for a period of time after any form of treatment.

DIET
* Eat healthy. Avoid alcohol.
* Consider a weight-loss diet, if overweight.

CALL YOUR DOCTOR IF

* You or a family member has varicose veins.
* After diagnosis, the veins cause problems.

VITAMIN DEFICIENCIES

GENERAL INFORMATION

DEFINITION—Insufficient intake or absorption of a vitamin. This deficiency is rare in the U.S. and is usually due to failure of the intestine to absorb enough of the vitamin.

BODY PARTS INVOLVED—Total body tissues.

SEX OR AGE MOST AFFECTED—Both sexes; all ages.

SIGNS & SYMPTOMS
• **Vitamin A**—Night blindness, dry eyes, rough skin, loss of appetite, diarrhea, anemia.
• **Vitamin B1**—Loss of sensation in the legs, weakness, congestive heart failure, lack of urinary control, psychosis, abdominal pain.
• **Vitamin B2**—Cracked lips, pallor, sore tongue.
• **Vitamin B3 (Niacin)**—Fatigue and weakness, poor appetite, sore mouth and tongue, indigestion, nausea, vomiting, diarrhea.
• **Vitamin B6**—Dermatitis, sore mouth and tongue, abdominal pain, vomiting, diarrhea.
• **Vitamin B12**—Weakness, sore tongue, nausea, bleeding gums, numbness in hands and feet, jaundice, headache, poor memory, depression.
• **Vitamin C**—Tender legs, bleeding and bruising under the skin, anemia, bleeding gums, loss of teeth, rough skin, increased susceptibility to infection, weakness and fatigue.
• **Vitamin D**—Restlessness, poor sleep habits, profuse sweating, bowed legs in infants, delayed walking in infants, bone pain, muscle weakness.
• **Vitamin E**—Muscle weakness, swelling of the ankles, abdomen and face in infants, anemia in premature infants.
• **Vitamin K**—Unusual bleeding or bruising.

CAUSES
• Inadequate diet.
• Impaired absorption from disease or drug use.

RISK INCREASES WITH
• Fad diets.
• Use of several medications.
• Alcohol or drug (including laxative) abuse.
• Malabsorption; disease; pregnancy.
• Poverty; very young or very old.
• Intestinal parasites; gastrointestinal surgery.

HOW TO PREVENT
• Proper diet.
• Supplemental vitamins if needed.

WHAT TO EXPECT

DIAGNOSTIC MEASURES
• Your own observation of symptoms.
• Your health care provider will do a physical exam.

• Medical tests may include blood and urine studies, x-rays of bones, and others.

APPROPRIATE HEALTH CARE
• Treatment will involve correction of the underlying cause.
• Hospital care may be required for severe malnutrition or alcoholism.

POSSIBLE COMPLICATIONS
• Vision problems; infections, death, if untreated (Vitamin A deficiency).
• Brain, nerve damage; heart disease (Vitamin B deficiency).
• Bone dislocations, osteopenia, osteoporosis, fractures (Vitamin C & D deficiency). Difficult or impossible vaginal childbirth in women with flattened pelvic bones. Cesarean section is usually required (Vitamin D deficiency).
• Chronic anemia (Vitamin E deficiency).
• Severe or fatal hemorrhage (Vitamin K deficiency).

PROBABLE OUTCOME—Usually curable with vitamin supplementation.

HOW TO TREAT

GENERAL MEASURES—No specific instructions.

MEDICATION—You may be prescribed vitamin supplements depending on the type of deficiency. Don't take more than the prescribed amount.

ACTIVITY
• Exercise daily if possible. Avoid excessive bed rest.
• Don't drive at night if you have vision problems.
• Handle children carefully to avoid bone or joint injury until deficiency is corrected.

DIET—Eat a well balanced diet that includes foods rich in vitamins. Take prenatal vitamins if you are pregnant. Provide your infant with vitamin supplements or vitamin fortified formula.

CALL YOUR DOCTOR IF

• You or a family member has symptoms of vitamin deficiency.
• Symptoms don't improve in 3 weeks, despite treatment.
• Unexplained bleeding or bruising develops.
• Pain or suspected fracture occurs following an injury, even a minor injury.

VITILIGO

GENERAL INFORMATION

DEFINITION—Loss of skin pigment (color) that results in white patches. This condition can affect persons of any race or ethnic group.

BODY PARTS INVOLVED—It affects skin on the hands, face and lips, arms, armpits, legs, and sometimes, the genitals.

SEX OR AGE MOST AFFECTED—Both sexes. It is more common in late childhood (9 to 12 years) to mid-adulthood.

SIGNS & SYMPTOMS
• Patches of different skin color.
• They are flat, usually white, and can't be felt with the fingers. Skin texture does not change.
• They don't hurt or itch.
• They spread to form very large, irregularly shaped areas without pigment.
• The amount of skin affected differs in each person. Some may have small areas, while others may gradually lose pigment over their entire body.
• Hair color may turn gray prematurely.

CAUSES—Exact cause is unknown, but it is probably partly an autoimmune disorder. The immune system by mistake attacks the body itself. With vitiligo, it attacks the pigment-producing cells (melanocytes), and they become weak or die resulting in a lack of pigment production. Genetics may be involved since it runs in families.

RISK INCREASES WITH
• Family history of vitiligo.
• Exposure to some chemicals, such as phenol. It is used in photography, and is also found in some hair color products, household stains, and other products.
• Hyperthyroidism (overactive thyroid) and hypothyroidism (underactive thyroid).
• Autoimmune disorders.

HOW TO PREVENT—Cannot be prevented at present.

WHAT TO EXPECT

DIAGNOSTIC MEASURES
• Your own observation of symptoms.
• Your health care provider can diagnose the disorder with an exam of the affected skin.
• Medical tests may be done to check for disorders such as a thyroid problem.

APPROPRIATE HEALTH CARE
• Treatment is sometimes not needed. The disorder is benign and often more of a cosmetic concern.
• Counseling may be helpful for patients if the disorder is causing emotional problems.

• If treatment is desired, your health care provider will discuss several options. Treatment with drugs can involve repigmenting the skin or removing the remaining pigment. Surgery involving skin grafts or tattooing the affected skin are options for some patients.

POSSIBLE COMPLICATIONS
• The disorder may never disappear completely, causing permanent white skin areas.
• Emotional problems may occur.

PROBABLE OUTCOME
• Treatment can be prolonged and often unsatisfactory. Complete and permanent repigmentation rarely occurs. It is impossible to predict how much improvement will occur with treatment. Younger individuals (under 30) and those who obtain treatment early usually respond best. Allow 1 year to evaluate results.
• Research is ongoing to look for the causes and find new, effective forms of treatment.

HOW TO TREAT

GENERAL MEASURES
• Some patients with limited disease may choose to use a make-up product. Cover the affected skin with opaque makeup, self-tanning products, or dyes to make it less noticeable.
• Some sun exposure may help improve skin color. Ask your health care provider. If advised, use sunscreen (with SPF of 15 or higher) to avoid sunburn.
• To learn more: National Vitiligo Foundation, 611 S. Fleishel Ave., Tyler, TX 75701; (903) 531-0074 (not toll free); website: www.nvfi.org.

MEDICATION
• Steroid creams may be prescribed to help repigment small areas.
• Psoralen drugs used with exposure to ultraviolet A (UVA) may be prescribed. It is called PUVA. This stimulates pigmentation. It helps some, but not all patients. Adverse effects of these drugs are frequent.
• Monobenzyl ether of hydroquinone may be prescribed for depigmentation. It can permanently remove pigment so that skin color is uniform. It takes about 6 months to a year. Success rate is about 75%.
• Other drugs may be prescribed.

ACTIVITY—No limits.

DIET—No special diet.

CALL YOUR DOCTOR IF

You or a family member has symptoms of vitiligo.

VOCAL-CORD NODULES
("Singer's Nodes")

 GENERAL INFORMATION

DEFINITION—Noncancerous growths of tissue on the vocal cords.

BODY PARTS INVOLVED—Larynx (voicebox).

SEX OR AGE MOST AFFECTED—The condition can be common in children and occurs in women more than men.

SIGNS & SYMPTOMS
* Persistent hoarseness without pain.
* Breathy or scratchy voice.
* Singers may notice they have a voice alteration.

CAUSES—The vocal cords are located in the voice box (larynx) in the middle of the throat. They are made up of two fibrous bands that vibrate to produce sound. The bands are covered with skin-like tissue. This tissue becomes thickened when the vocal cords are used a lot. A part of the thickened tissue can grow and produce nodules. They appear as red, swollen bumps and may be the size of a pinhead up to a small pea. When nodules occur, the vocal cords cannot close completely. This causes the voice to sound hoarse.

RISK INCREASES WITH
* Continued overuse of the voice by singing, shouting, yelling, lecturing, or other forms of talking too loudly or too much.
* Excessive coughing or throat clearing.
* Using the voice incorrectly.
* People who use the voice a lot such as singers, teachers, ministers, auctioneers, cheerleaders, aerobic instructors, and others.
* Smoking or exposure to smoke.
* Chronic infection caused by allergies or irritants.
* Reflux (stomach acid backs up into throat).

HOW TO PREVENT
* Take voice or speech lessons to learn proper techniques for speaking or singing.
* Don't smoke. Avoid being around smokers.
* Drink plenty of fluids.
* Try not to use the voice too long or too loudly.
* Rest your voice for a while when it appears to have been overused.

 WHAT TO EXPECT

DIAGNOSTIC MEASURES
* Your own observation of symptoms.
* Your health care provider will do a physical exam of the throat and vocal cords.
* Medical tests may include a biopsy of the nodule to rule out cancer. A biopsy involves removing a small piece of tissue for viewing under a microscope.

APPROPRIATE HEALTH CARE
* Treatment often involves voice therapy (voice behavior). This may include voice rest (using your voice less, controlling the loudness and not talking much for a few days). Therapy includes behavior training on healthy use of the voice and proper voice techniques. Therapy may take 1 to 2 sessions a week for 5 to 6 weeks.
* Surgery (rarely) to remove nodules may be needed if voice therapy is not effective. Surgery is usually not done in children under age 12.

POSSIBLE COMPLICATIONS
* Without treatment, permanent hoarseness or voice change may occur.
* Nodules may regrow after treatment if voice continues to be overused.

PROBABLE OUTCOME—Almost always curable with voice therapy treatment or surgery.

 HOW TO TREAT

GENERAL MEASURES—Don't smoke, and avoid smoky environments.

MEDICATION—Drugs are usually not needed for this disorder.

ACTIVITY—No limits except those for voice usage.

DIET—No special diet.

 CALL YOUR DOCTOR IF

* You or a family member is hoarse for more than 2 weeks.
* Symptoms recur after treatment.

VULVOVAGINITIS BEFORE PUBERTY

 GENERAL INFORMATION

DEFINITION—Infection or inflammation (redness and soreness) of the vagina or vulva before a young girl reaches puberty. Before puberty, the skin around the vaginal area can be very sensitive, and it can easily become red and inflamed.

BODY PARTS INVOLVED—Vagina; cervix; vulva (vaginal lips); skin around the genitals.

SEX OR AGE MOST AFFECTED—Female infants and children.

SIGNS & SYMPTOMS
• Redness, pain, and itching around the genital area.
• Vaginal discharge. It may or may not have an odor.
• Pain with urination.
• Bleeding from the affected area (sometimes).

CAUSES
• Infections caused by bacteria, parasites (including pinworms), yeast-like fungi, or viruses.
• Allergies to synthetic fabrics, soap, or other items in contact with the genitals.
• Scratches, abrasions or genital injury from foreign body in the vagina (this could be some toilet paper).
• Genital injury from sexual abuse.
• Irritation from bubble bath or oils put in bath water.

RISK INCREASES WITH
• Poor hygiene such as infrequent bathing, not wiping, or wiping incorrectly after urinating.
• Diabetes.
• Trauma or injury to the vaginal area.
• Overweight.
• Wearing tight clothing (leotards, jeans, underwear, or bathing suits).

HOW TO PREVENT
• Teach the child to wipe from the vagina toward the anus after bowel movements.
• Don't let the child sit around in wet clothing, especially a wet bathing suit. Avoid tight clothing.
• Have the child bathe or shower frequently.
• Don't use scented soap or bubble baths, dyed or perfumed toilet tissue.
• Provide the child with cotton underpants or nylon underpants with a cotton crotch.
• Teach your child to resist and report any attempted sexual contact by anyone.
• Don't wash your child's hair in the bath. Shampoo the hair over a sink instead. If you do it in the bath, wash it at the end of the bath. Be sure to rinse off any shampoo that may have gotten on the genital area.
• Use a bland ointment for protection of the skin.

 WHAT TO EXPECT

DIAGNOSTIC MEASURES
• Your own observation of symptoms.
• Your child's health care provider will usually do a physical exam, including a gentle exam of the genital area.
• Medical tests may include blood studies and a culture of any vaginal discharge.

APPROPRIATE HEALTH CARE
• Treatment will depend on the cause. Drug therapy may be needed for an infection.
• Treatment may involve removing any foreign object in the vagina.
• Stop the use of any product that may cause irritation or allergy, such as soap or bubble bath.
• Your child's health care provider will discuss any possibility of child abuse with you.

POSSIBLE COMPLICATIONS—Symptoms may persist or other skin infections may develop. Rarely, an infection may worsen.

PROBABLE OUTCOME—Symptoms often clear up by using preventive measures. In cases of infection, drugs will provide a cure.

 HOW TO TREAT

GENERAL MEASURES
• Follow steps in Preventive Measures.
• Prevent urine from stinging inflamed skin: The child may urinate while in the shower. Urinate through a toilet-paper roll or plastic cup with the bottom cut out. Pour a cup of warm water over the genital area while urinating.
• Taking sitz baths (warm water baths) in clear water 2 to 4 times a day may help relieve symptoms.

MEDICATION
• Nonprescription topical ointments, or 0.5% or 1% hydrocortisone cream, 3 to 4 times a day may be recommended to relieve burning and itching.
• Drugs for infection (including antibiotics, antifungal, or antiparasitic drugs) may be prescribed.

ACTIVITY—No limits.

DIET—No special diet.

 CALL YOUR DOCTOR IF

• Your child has symptoms of vulvovaginitis.
• Symptoms don't improve in 7 to 10 days or symptoms worsen, despite treatment.
• You suspect your child has been sexually abused.

ILLNESS & DISORDERS

VULVOVAGINAL CANDIDIASIS
(Vaginal Yeast Infection)

 GENERAL INFORMATION

DEFINITION—Vulvovaginal candidiasis is an infection of the vagina and vulva (external genitals).

BODY PARTS INVOLVED—Vagina; cervix; vulva (vaginal lips); skin around the genitals.

SEX OR AGE MOST AFFECTED—It can affect women of all ages but occurs most often in the childbearing years. Men may have candidiasis infection with no symptoms.

SIGNS & SYMPTOMS
* The symptoms vary among women and from time to time, in the same woman.
* White, "curdy" vaginal discharge (resembles lumps of cottage cheese). Odor may be unpleasant, but not foul.
* Swollen, red, tender, itching vaginal lips (labia) and surrounding skin.
* Burning during urination.
* Change in vaginal color from pale pink to red.
* Pain during sexual intercourse (dyspareunia).

CAUSES—Most often, the cause is a yeast-like fungus called *Candida albicans*. Healthy women have this yeast in their vagina (and the mouth and intestines). If the normal conditions of the vagina change, the yeast can overgrow and cause infection. Rarely, *Candida* may be passed from person to person, by sexual intercourse.

RISK INCREASES WITH
* Pregnancy.
* Diabetes.
* Drugs (antibiotics, corticosteroids, birth control pills).
* Weak immune system from drugs or disease.
* Recent illness, poor diet, or lack of sleep.

HOW TO PREVENT
* There are no specific preventive measures. The following steps may help to prevent vaginal disorders.
* Use condoms with new sexual partners to help protect against some infections.
* Keep the genital area clean and dry. Use plain unscented soap. Be sure sexual partner is clean. Avoid vaginal douching.
* Take showers rather than tub baths. If you take a bath, don't add oils or bubble bath to the water.
* Wear cotton underwear or pantyhose with a cotton crotch. Avoid tight jeans, pants, or pantyhose.
* Don't sit around in wet clothes, such as bathing suits.
* After going to the bathroom, wipe from front to back (vagina to anus).
* Change tampons or sanitary pads frequently.
* Take antibiotics only when prescribed for you.

 WHAT TO EXPECT

DIAGNOSTIC MEASURES
* Your own observation of symptoms.
* Your health care provider will usually do a physical exam and a pelvic exam and ask questions about your symptoms.
* Tests of the vaginal discharge may be done.

APPROPRIATE HEALTH CARE—Drug therapy is usually recommended.

POSSIBLE COMPLICATIONS
* Vaginitis (soreness, itching, and irritation).
* Some women may develop recurrent vulvovaginal candidiasis (RVVC). This is when four or more episodes of vulvovaginal candidiasis have occurred in one year.

PROBABLE OUTCOME—Symptoms will normally clear up with treatment.

 HOW TO TREAT

GENERAL MEASURES
* Don't assume you have a yeast infection and use antifungal (yeast) drugs without diagnosis. A vaginal infection should not be treated with douches, deodorant sprays, or herbal remedies.
* If urinating causes burning, urinate through a tubular device, such as a toilet-paper roll or plastic cup with the bottom cut out, or pour cup of warm water over the area while you urinate.

MEDICATION
* Antifungal drugs, either in vaginal creams or suppositories or in oral form, may be recommended. Some nonprescription examples are miconazole nitrate (Monistat-7) and clotrimazole (Gyne-Lotrimin, Mycelex-7, and FemCare). Follow the instructions on the product. If you have tried one of these drugs and it has not worked for you, your health care provider may prescribe a prescription-only drug.
* Recurrent vulvovaginal candidiasis treatment usually involves two weeks of intensive antifungal drugs, then up to six months of a lower "maintenance" dose.

ACTIVITY—Delay sexual relations until symptoms clear up.

DIET—Some women find that eating yogurt or a low sugar diet can help in preventing or treating yeast infections.

📞 **CALL YOUR DOCTOR IF**

* You or a family member has symptoms of vulvovaginal candidiasis.
* Symptoms get worse or recur after treatment.

WARTS
(Verruca Vulgaris; Plantar Warts)

GENERAL INFORMATION

DEFINITION—Skin growths caused by a virus in the outer skin layer. Warts are not cancerous. They are mildly contagious from person to person and from one area to another on the same person. Note: this information does not discuss genital warts.

BODY PARTS INVOLVED—Skin anywhere, but most likely on the fingers, hands and arms.

SEX OR AGE MOST AFFECTED—Both sexes; most common in children and young adults between ages 1 and 30, but occur at any age.

SIGNS & SYMPTOMS—A small, raised bump on the skin with the following features:
* Warts begin very small and grow larger.
* Warts have a rough surface and clearly defined borders. They are usually the same color as the skin, but sometimes darker.
* Warts often appear in clusters around a "mother wart."
* If you cut into the wart surface, it contains small black dots or bleeding points.
* Warts are painless and typically don't itch.
* Plantar warts appear on the soles of the feet.

CAUSES—Infection of the outer skin layer (epidermis) by the human papillomavirus (HPV) family. The virus causes some cells to grow more rapidly than normal. Warts are very common.

RISK INCREASES WITH
* Use of public showers.
* Skin injury.
* Weak immune system due to drugs or illness.

HOW TO PREVENT
* There is no sure way to prevent warts. Reduce risk by wearing thong sandals in public locker rooms, swimming pools, or showers. Don't share towels.
* To keep from spreading warts, don't scratch them. Warts spread readily to small cuts and scratches.

WHAT TO EXPECT

DIAGNOSTIC MEASURES
* Your own observation of symptoms.
* Health care provider exam if needed.

APPROPRIATE HEALTH CARE
* There are a variety of nonprescription products and home (or folk) remedies for warts. Family members or friends may recommend trying different treatments.

* Your health care provider has other options for treatment. These can be done during an office visit. Some treatments may be somewhat painful, so be sure to discuss the risks and benefits. Options:
    - Cryotherapy (freezing) with liquid nitrogen. Freezing causes a blister to form that heals in about a week. More than one treatment may be needed for complete wart removal.
    - Electrosurgery (using heat). This treatment is often done in one office visit. An electric needle is used to cut away the wart or destroy it.
    - Surgery with a knife (scalpel) or laser.
    - Injection of a drug into the wart.

POSSIBLE COMPLICATIONS
* Spread to other places in the body.
* Scars where warts were removed.
* Recurrence of warts after treatment.

PROBABLE OUTCOME—There is no one specific treatment for warts that works for everybody. Some warts go away on their own, others are cured with nonprescription drugs. Some may require medical care that could include surgery. There are also many "home remedies" that may work for some people. Nonsurgical treatment for warts may take some time, so be patient.

HOW TO TREAT

GENERAL MEASURES—Follow instructions from your health care provider for home care after any medical treatment.

MEDICATION
* There are nonprescription drugs for treatment of warts. Most are applied to skin daily for several weeks. Also available is a freezing aerosol product. Follow the instructions provided with any product that you buy.
* Your health care provider may prescribe stronger drugs or injections for removing the warts.

ACTIVITY—No limits.

DIET—No special diet.

CALL YOUR DOCTOR IF

* You or your child has warts that cause concern or warts appear on the face or genital area.
* Self-treatment for warts has not worked.
* After treatment, the treated skin becomes hot, red, and painful.
* Warts don't disappear completely after treatment.
* Other warts appear after treatment.

WARTS, GENITAL
(Condylomata Acuminata; Venereal Warts)

 GENERAL INFORMATION

DEFINITION—Warts that grow in the genital area. They are not the same warts commonly found on hands or feet.

BODY PARTS INVOLVED—Urethra; genitals; rectum.

SEX OR AGE MOST AFFECTED—Both sexes of sexually active young people and adults. Women are affected more often than men.

SIGNS & SYMPTOMS
• Warts appear on moist surfaces of the genital area. They are thin, flexible, solid raised areas of the skin, growing in stalks or clusters. They are taller than they are wide. They may be tiny or grow in larger clusters. Small warts usually cause no symptoms.
• In women, they may be on the inside and outside of the vagina, on the cervix, or around the anus.
• Men may have warts on the tip or shaft of the penis or around the anus.
• They don't hurt or itch.
• Women may have a vaginal discharge.

CAUSES
• Genital warts are caused by certain types of the human papillomavirus (HPV). More than 100 types of HPV have been identified and most are harmless. About 30 types are spread through sexual contact.
• Genital warts spread very easily from one person to another. They are spread through genital, anal, or oral sex with an infected person. They have an incubation period of 1 to 6 months. Genital warts are considered a sexually transmitted disease (STD). Some types of HPV that cause genital warts can also cause, or be a risk factor for, genital cancers.

RISK INCREASES WITH
• Other venereal disease.
• Multiple sexual partners.
• Smoking.
• Early age for first sexual intercourse.
• Use of oral contraceptives.

HOW TO PREVENT
• Men and women need to avoid sexual activity with a person who has visible genital warts.
• Use rubber (latex) condoms during sexual intercourse to reduce the risk of genital warts.

 WHAT TO EXPECT

DIAGNOSTIC MEASURES
• Your own observation of symptoms.
• Your health care provider will do a physical exam including a pelvic exam. Vinegar (acetic acid) may be applied to the skin area to better see any warts. A special magnifying instrument may be used to view the affected area.
• Medical tests may include a Pap smear. If it shows abnormal cells, further follow up testing will be done.

APPROPRIATE HEALTH CARE
• Treatment will be determined by size and location of the warts.
• Some warts may be treated with drugs that are applied to the skin.
• Other warts may be frozen (cryotherapy), burned (electrocautery), or removed with laser treatment.
• Warts that are large and have not responded to other treatment may need to be surgically removed.
• Pregnant women with genital warts will be examined by their obstetric providers. The possible problems for mother and for the baby and options for treatment will be discussed.

POSSIBLE COMPLICATIONS
• HPV can increase the risk for certain cancers.
• Problems in pregnant woman and newborn.

PROBABLE OUTCOME—Small warts often disappear on their own. Because the virus is a risk factor for genital cancer, get medical care. Treatment can get rid of the warts, but the virus stays in the body. Recurrence of warts after treatment is common. Most HPV infections do not progress to cancer.

 HOW TO TREAT

GENERAL MEASURES
• Follow your health care provider's advice about home care after treatment.
• Don't pick, squeeze, or scratch the warts. You can spread them to other places in your body.

MEDICATION—There are several types of drugs that can be used on the warts. Some are applied at a medical office and others can be used at home. Your health care provider will discuss the options, the risks, and benefits of each type. Follow instructions carefully if you decide on home treatment.

ACTIVITY—No limits, except to avoid sexual relations until warts are completely gone.

DIET—No special diet.

 CALL YOUR DOCTOR IF

• You or a family member has symptoms of genital warts.
• The treated area becomes infected (red, swollen, painful, or tender).
• Warts return after treatment.

WEST NILE VIRUS

 ## GENERAL INFORMATION

DEFINITION—A virus that can cause a mild or, less often, a serious disease in humans. Outbreaks often occur in the summer and continue into the fall, but can happen year round. Most people who are infected will not show any symptoms. About 20% will have mild symptoms typically lasting a few days. This is called West Nile fever. A few (1 in 150 infected persons) will develop severe disease.

BODY PARTS INVOLVED—Whole body.

SEX OR AGE MOST AFFECTED—Both sexes; all ages.

SIGNS & SYMPTOMS
• Mild symptoms:
- Fever.
- Headache.
- Body aches.
- Nausea and vomiting.
- Swollen lymph glands.
- Skin rash on the chest, stomach, and back.
• Severe symptoms can include high fever, headache, neck stiffness, stupor, disorientation, coma, tremors, convulsions, muscle weakness, vision loss, numbness, and paralysis.

CAUSES—Bite of an infected mosquito. Mosquitoes are carriers that become infected when they feed on infected birds. Infected mosquitoes can then spread the infection to humans and other animals when they bite. In a very few cases, it has spread through blood transfusions, organ transplants, breastfeeding, and during pregnancy from mother to baby. It is not spread through casual contact such as touching or kissing a person with the virus. People may develop symptoms between 3 and 14 days after they are bitten by an infected mosquito.

RISK INCREASES WITH
• People who spend a lot of time outdoors.
• Having mosquitoes in or around the home.
• People with chronic disease, weak immune system, or the elderly are more likely to develop severe illness.

HOW TO PREVENT
• When outdoors, use mosquito repellent containing DEET, picaridin, or oil of lemon eucalyptus on the skin. Wear protective, light-colored clothing. Spray clothing with DEET or permethrin products.
• Put screens on windows and doors. Drain standing water from buckets, flower pots, and other items.
• Don't handle dead birds. Call local health department.
• Mosquito control programs in communities can help.
• Vaccines for the virus are being researched.

 ## WHAT TO EXPECT

DIAGNOSTIC MEASURES
• See your health care provider if you have any concern about the symptoms. A physical exam may be done and questions asked about your symptoms and activities.
• A blood test may be done if needed to confirm diagnosis.

APPROPRIATE HEALTH CARE
• Most people will not seek or need medical care. Mild symptoms are similar to other virus infections that people usually treat themselves.
• No treatment is available to cure the infection. Drugs may help relieve symptoms such as fever or headache.
• Severe symptoms require hospital care. Treatment can include fluids given through a vein (IV), breathing support (sometimes with a machine), and steps to prevent more complications.

POSSIBLE COMPLICATIONS
• Encephalitis (inflammation of the brain).
• Meningitis (inflammation of the brain's lining).
• Meningoencephalitis (both of the above).
• Permanent brain damage or muscle weakness, or death (rare).

PROBABLE OUTCOME—Mild symptoms clear up without treatment. In severe cases, most patients recover with hospital care, but the illness may be fatal.

 ## HOW TO TREAT

GENERAL MEASURES
• Follow instructions from your health care provider for home care after any medical treatment.
• To learn more: Centers for Disease Control and Prevention, (888) 246-2675; website: www.cdc.gov, or call your local health department.

MEDICATION—You may use nonprescription drugs for mild symptoms such as fever, pain, or headache remedies. Antibiotics do not help virus infections. Research continues for new antiviral drugs for prevention and treatment.

ACTIVITY—No limits (with mild symptoms).

DIET—No special diet.

 ## CALL YOUR DOCTOR IF

• You or a family member has symptoms of West Nile virus infection that you are concerned about.
• Symptoms are severe, get emergency care.

ILLNESS & DISORDERS

WHIPLASH
(Cervical Sprain or Strain)

 GENERAL INFORMATION

DEFINITION—Injury to the neck caused when it is whipped forcefully backward and then forward, usually in an accident.

BODY PARTS INVOLVED—Muscles, tendons, ligaments, disks, and nerves in the neck.

SEX OR AGE MOST AFFECTED—Both sexes (women more than men); all ages.

SIGNS & SYMPTOMS
* Pain in the front and back of the neck either immediately following or up to 24 hours after injury.
* Stiffness in the neck. Difficult to move neck around.
* Pain may go into the shoulder or arm.
* Headache.

CAUSES—Injury, usually from a motor-vehicle accident or contact sports. It may also be caused by being punched or hit by a falling object, or rarely, in cases of child abuse.

RISK INCREASES WITH
* Situations that make accidents more likely, such as:
  - Driving in rainy, icy, or snowy weather.
  - "Tail-gating" or other poor driving habits.
  - Driving after excess alcohol use or use of mind-altering drugs.
* Previous neck injury.
* People who have bone or joint disease.

HOW TO PREVENT
* Use seatbelts and the padded headrests in your motor vehicle. These have decreased the frequency and severity of auto whiplash injuries. Drive carefully and defensively. Don't drink alcohol and drive.
* Use proper head gear for contact sports.

 WHAT TO EXPECT

DIAGNOSTIC MEASURES
* Your own observation of symptoms.
* Your health care provider will do a physical exam of the head and neck and ask questions about your symptoms and the cause of injury.
* An x-ray, CT, or MRI (see Glossary for all) may be done to rule out injury to the spine.

APPROPRIATE HEALTH CARE
* Treatment will depend on the extent of injury. Steps may include drugs and/or injections, physical therapy, exercises, massage, chiropractor care, heat or ice, wearing a neck collar, ultrasound, or traction. You and your health care provider can discuss a treatment plan for your individual needs.
* Surgery to remove injured spinal disk (rare).

POSSIBLE COMPLICATIONS
* Temporary numbness and weakness in the arms, if nerve roots are injured. This may persist until recovery.
* A few may have symptoms for a year, while others may have some symptoms even after two years. It may affect quality of life for a person. Depression may occur.

PROBABLE OUTCOME—The injury is usually not serious and permanent damage is rare. Most people recover in a few weeks to 3 months.

 HOW TO TREAT

GENERAL MEASURES
* Apply ice packs (over a towel) to the injured area for 10 to 20 minutes each hour during the first 24 hours.
* After 24 hours, use ice packs or heat to relieve pain. Heat may include warm showers twice a day, in which the water beats on your neck and shoulders for 10 to 20 minutes. Between showers, apply warm soaks to the neck several times a day for 10 to 15 minutes.

MEDICATION
* Pain relievers or muscle relaxants may be prescribed.
* You may use ibuprofen or acetaminophen for minor pain.

ACTIVITY—People who stay active and exercise the neck muscles as directed appear to recover more quickly. Resume routine activities and work as soon as possible. Some adjustments at your job may be needed for a short time.

DIET—No special diet. Avoid alcohol.

 CALL YOUR DOCTOR IF

* You or a family member has a neck injury. Seek emergency care if you feel symptoms are more severe.
* Pain, numbness, tingling, or weakness develops in the arm or face. This may require emergency help.
* Symptoms continue after treatment.

WHOOPING COUGH
(Pertussis)

GENERAL INFORMATION

DEFINITION—A serious, contagious infection of the nose, throat, and lungs. Pertussis is the medical name for whooping cough. Use of a vaccine has greatly reduced the occurrence of the disease.

BODY PARTS INVOLVED—Bronchial tubes; larynx; lungs.

SEX OR AGE MOST AFFECTED—All ages, but most common in children.

SIGNS & SYMPTOMS
Early stages:
* Runny nose.
* Dry cough that leads to a cough with thick sputum.
* Slight fever.
Late stages:
* Severe, ongoing coughing bouts that last up to 1 minute. The face turns red or blue from lack of oxygen while coughing. At the end of each coughing effort, the person gasps for breath with a "whooping" sound.
* Vomiting and diarrhea.
* Little or no fever.

CAUSES—*Bordetella pertussis* bacteria. Germs are spread by contact with an infected person, breathing in germs in the air, or touching an object with germs on it. The time from being exposed to the germs to having symptoms is about 7 to 10 days, and not more than 21 days.

RISK INCREASES WITH
* Children who have not been immunized or have not completed the whole series of vaccine shots needed.
* The vaccine protection fades as children get older. Teens and adults can easily get the infection if exposed.
* A person who does not know they have the infection may spread the germs. This can happen during the first 21 days of their cough.

HOW TO PREVENT
* Pertussis vaccine started in infancy.
* Adult forms of the vaccine are being tested.
* Keep infants away from anyone with a cough illness.

WHAT TO EXPECT

DIAGNOSTIC MEASURES
* Your own observation of symptoms.
* Your health care provider will do a physical exam. The diagnosis can be made based on the symptoms and knowing about contact with an infected person.
* Medical tests are usually done to confirm the diagnosis.

APPROPRIATE HEALTH CARE
* Treatment depends on how severe the symptoms are.
* Severely ill infants will need hospital care.
* Children can usually be treated at home. They should get extra rest, drink plenty of fluids, take any prescribed drugs, and be watched for any complications.

POSSIBLE COMPLICATIONS
* Children under age one are at high risk for complications. They are less likely in older children and adults.
* Complications include severe ear infection, nose-bleeds, dehydration, pneumonia, convulsions, and in rare cases, brain damage and death.

PROBABLE OUTCOME—Usually curable in about 6 weeks with treatment (may range from 3 weeks to 3 months). The usual course of illness is: 2 weeks with the cough; 2 weeks with bouts of the "whooping" cough; and 2 weeks for recovery. Some persistent coughs may continue for months.

HOW TO TREAT

GENERAL MEASURES—Keep an ill person at home and away from others when possible.

MEDICATION
* An antibiotic, most often erythromycin, is usually prescribed. If started early in the infection, it helps improve symptoms. It also reduces the risk of spreading germs.
* Close contacts of an infected person are usually prescribed antibiotics to help prevent the infection (even if they have had the vaccine).

ACTIVITY
* Keep the child in bed or resting until the fever disappears. Normal activity should be resumed slowly, according to strength.
* Return to daycare, school, or work is permitted after taking antibiotics for five days. Without antibiotics, it will be 3 to 4 weeks after the start of symptoms.

DIET
* Drink extra fluids, such as fruit juice, tea, carbonated drinks, and clear soups.
* No special diet. Small, frequent meals may decrease vomiting.

CALL YOUR DOCTOR IF

* You or a family member has symptoms of whooping cough or has been exposed to anyone with it.
* Your child's coughing is severe.
* Vomiting persists more than 1 or 2 days.
* You are concerned about any symptoms.

WILMS' TUMOR
(Nephroblastoma)

 GENERAL INFORMATION

DEFINITION—A malignant, mixed tumor (one that contains several cell types) of the kidneys. Only one kidney is affected in 90% of cases. The kidneys are a pair of organs that are shaped like kidney beans. They are located on either side of the backbone. Kidneys filter and clean the blood in the body and make urine.

BODY PARTS INVOLVED—Kidneys.

SEX OR AGE MOST AFFECTED—It usually affects children of both sexes under age 7, with a peak incidence between ages 3 and 4. Very rarely, it may not appear until teen years or adulthood.

SIGNS & SYMPTOMS
• Enlarged abdomen. A large, firm, smooth tumor can usually be felt within the abdominal wall.
• Blood in the urine (urine may appear cloudy).
• Abdominal pain (sometimes).
• Repeated vomiting.
• Fever.
• Weight loss.
• High blood pressure (this may have no symptoms).

CAUSES—Exact cause is unknown. It often occurs along with other congenital (being born with) abnormalities. These include urinary-tract problems, absence of iris in the eyes (aniridia), and enlargement of one side of the body.

RISK INCREASES WITH
• Congenital abnormalities.
• African Americans are more often affected.
• Girls (are more often affected than boys).

HOW TO PREVENT—Cannot be prevented at present.

 WHAT TO EXPECT

DIAGNOSTIC MEASURES
• Your own observation of symptoms.
• Your child's health care provider will do a physical exam.
• Different medical tests are done to verify the diagnosis and to determine if the cancer has spread to other places in the body (called staging).

APPROPRIATE HEALTH CARE
• The treatment plan will be determined by the stage of the cancer, the type of cancer cells, the size of the tumor, and your child's age and health status. Your child's health care provider will discuss all aspects of treatment with you.

• Surgery is usually needed for treatment. It may involve removal of the tumor and the whole affected kidney or less often, a portion of the kidney. Body tissue around the kidney and lymph nodes may need to be removed.
• Chemotherapy (anticancer drugs) may be done before and/or after surgery. Radiation may be done for certain stages of the tumor.

POSSIBLE COMPLICATIONS
• Cancer may recur after treatment.
• Tumor may spread to lungs, bones, liver, or brain, if untreated.
• Adverse reactions, including hair loss, from radiation treatment and chemotherapy.
• Surgery procedures may have complications.
• Kidney function problems.
• Chemotherapy and radiation treatment are risk factors for developing other types of cancer.

PROBABLE OUTCOME—With appropriate treatment, the outlook is good. In most cases, Wilms' tumor is curable with surgery, radiation treatment, and chemotherapy (anticancer) drugs. Long-term follow-up care is needed to watch for any late effects of treatment.

 HOW TO TREAT

GENERAL MEASURES—To learn more: American Cancer Society, (800) ACS-2345; website: www.cancer.org or National Cancer Institute, (800) 4-CANCER; website: www.nci.nih.gov.

MEDICATION—Your child may be prescribed anticancer drugs, antinausea drugs, pain relievers, antibiotics (if infection occurs), and stool softeners to prevent constipation following surgery.

ACTIVITY—An active lifestyle is possible with one kidney. Sports activities that carry a risk of kidney injury (e.g., hockey or boxing) should be avoided.

DIET—No special diet.

 CALL YOUR DOCTOR IF

• Your child has symptoms of Wilms' tumor.
• The following occur during treatment:
  - Vomiting, abdominal pain or constipation.
  - Shortness of breath.
  - Swelling in feet or ankles.
• New, unexplained symptoms develop. Drugs used in treatment may cause side effects.

WILSON DISEASE

GENERAL INFORMATION

DEFINITION—An inherited disorder in which excessive amounts of copper accumulate in the body. Although the accumulation of copper begins at birth, symptoms of the disorder appear later in life, between the ages of 6 and 40. The liver of a person who has Wilson disease does not release copper into bile as it should. Bile is a liquid produced by the liver that helps with digestion. As the intestines absorb copper from food, the copper builds up in the liver and injures liver tissue. Eventually, the damage causes the liver to release the copper into the bloodstream, which carries the copper throughout the body. The copper buildup leads to damage in the kidneys, brain, and eyes.

BODY PARTS INVOLVED—The liver, blood, central nervous system, urinary system and/or musculoskeletal system.

SEX OR AGE MOST AFFECTED—Both sexes, all ages.

SIGNS & SYMPTOMS
• Jaundice (yellowing of the eyes and skin).
• Vomiting blood.
• Speech and language problems.
• Tremors in the arms and hands.
• Rigid muscles.
• Difficulty in walking and swallowing.
• Menstrual problems, infertility or miscarriage.
• Abnormal eye movements.
• Mental, behavior and/or personality changes.
• Many signs may be detected by a doctor. The Kayser-Fleischer ring—a rusty brown ring around the cornea of the eye that can be seen only through an eye exam. Others signs include swelling of the liver and spleen; fluid buildup in the lining of the abdomen; anemia; low platelet and white blood cell count in the blood; high levels of amino acids, protein, uric acid, and carbohydrates in urine; and softening of bones.

CAUSES—Both parents must carry the gene that each passes to the affected child. A person with one abnormal gene is a carrier.

RISK INCREASES WITH—Family history of Wilson disease (but most patients have no family history).

HOW TO PREVENT—There are no known preventive measures. Genetic testing may be helpful in diagnosing a patient's relatives.

WHAT TO EXPECT

DIAGNOSTIC MEASURES
• Your own observation of symptoms.
• Your health care provider will do a physical exam. It is usually diagnosed through tests that measure the amount of copper in the blood,

urine, and liver. An eye exam would detect the Kayser-Fleischer ring.
• Other tests may include x-ray, MRI, CT, liver biopsy and genetic testing.

APPROPRIATE HEALTH CARE
• Treatment generally consists of anti-copper agents to remove excess copper from the body and to prevent it from reaccumulating.
• Other symptoms will be treated as needed.
• In rare cases in which there is severe liver disease, a liver transplant may be needed.

POSSIBLE COMPLICATIONS
• The primary consequence for approximately 40% of patients is liver disease. The onset of liver disease is usually at age 8-16 years.
• Damage to the nervous system and disabling symptoms.
• Without proper treatment, Wilson disease is generally fatal, usually by the age of 30.

PROBABLE OUTCOME—Lifelong treatment is required. If treatment is begun early enough, symptomatic recovery is usually complete, and a life of normal length and quality can be expected.

HOW TO TREAT

GENERAL MEASURES
• Follow medical advice for home care after diagnosis.
• To learn more: Wilson's Disease Association, 1802 Brookside Dr., Wooster, OH 44691; (800) 399-0266; website: www.wilsonsdisease.org.

MEDICATION
• Drug therapy may include trientine, D-penicillamine or tetrathiomolydate (undergoing study). Zinc for maintenance therapy stops the intestines from absorbing copper and promotes copper excretion.
• Other drugs as needed for complications.
• Patients may also need to take vitamin B6.

ACTIVITY
• Activities may be limited until symptoms improve. Return to normal activities gradually.
• Exercise or physical therapy may help improve some muscular symptoms.

DIET—A low copper diet may be prescribed. Avoid foods that are high in copper. These include shellfish, liver, mushrooms, broccoli, chocolate, nuts, dried fruit, and liver.

CALL YOUR DOCTOR IF

• You or a family member has symptoms of Wilson disease.
• Symptoms worsen despite treatment.
• Drugs used in treatment cause unexpected side effects.

ZINC DEFICIENCY

GENERAL INFORMATION

DEFINITION—Inadequate amounts of zinc in body cells. This affects the function of the testicles, liver, and muscles, and affects the structure of bones, teeth, hair, and skin. Zinc is a vital part of many enzymes that aid chemical reactions needed for normal body function. This includes immune function and skin healing.

BODY PARTS INVOLVED—All body cells.

SEX OR AGE MOST AFFECTED—Both sexes; all ages.

SIGNS & SYMPTOMS
- Poor appetite.
- Poor growth.
- Sensations of unpleasant tastes and odors, and decreased senses of taste and smell.
- Decreased sex drive.
- Darkening of the skin all over the body.
- Sparse hair growth.
- Deformed nails.

CAUSES
- Zinc intake is not adequate.
- Zinc is poorly absorbed in the body.
- Increased losses of zinc from the body.
- Increased need for zinc by the body (such as in ages 14-16).

RISK INCREASES WITH
- Alcoholism. Alcohol increases the loss of zinc.
- Excessive intake of substances that bind zinc and prevent its absorption from the gastrointestinal tract. These include calcium, vitamin D, high fiber-diet, and phytate enzyme (found in whole-meal bread).
- Surgical removal of any part of the gastrointestinal tract, especially the stomach.
- Parasitic infection in the gastrointestinal tract.
- Excessive milk drinking in preschool children.
- Use of cortisone drugs increases zinc excretion.
- Pregnancy.
- Taking diuretic drugs.
- Diabetes, kidney disease, or cirrhosis.
- Burns or major trauma.
- Diet that is lacking in meat, liver, eggs, or seafood.
- Longterm intravenous feeding.
- Acrodermatitis enteropathica, a rare hereditary disorder in which zinc cannot be absorbed.

HOW TO PREVENT
- Adults should not drink or eat more than the recommended amounts of milk, other dairy products, or whole-meal bread. Keep calcium intake at 1500 mg or less daily.
- Don't take large doses of vitamin D supplements without medical approval.
- Take zinc supplements if you have had gastrointestinal surgery.
- Obtain medical care for any parasite infections.
- Don't drink more than 1 or 2 alcoholic drinks, if any, a day.

WHAT TO EXPECT

DIAGNOSTIC MEASURES
- Your own observation of symptoms.
- Your health care provider may do a physical exam and ask questions about your symptoms, your activities, diet, and alcohol use.
- Medical tests may include blood studies to determine zinc levels and other tests to determine any underlying disorder.

APPROPRIATE HEALTH CARE—Treatment usually consists of correcting the cause and the use of zinc supplements.

POSSIBLE COMPLICATIONS
- Iron-deficiency anemia. Zinc is necessary for iron absorption.
- Poor wound healing.
- Liver and spleen enlargement.
- Excess zinc replacement or overdose may interfere with the body's manufacture of necessary enzymes.

PROBABLE OUTCOME—Usually curable in 2 months with zinc supplements and removal or treatment of the underlying causes.

HOW TO TREAT

GENERAL MEASURES—Follow medical instructions. Compliance with your medical treatment plan is essential for the best outcome.

MEDICATION
- Zinc supplements will be prescribed. Take with milk or meals to prevent stomach upset.
- Drugs may be prescribed for an underlying disorder that is diagnosed.

ACTIVITY—No limits.

DIET—Eat foods high in zinc such as red meat. Avoid excessive intake of whole-meal bread (if advised).

CALL YOUR DOCTOR IF

- You or a family member has symptoms of zinc deficiency.
- Symptoms recur after treatment.

Surgeries

ABDOMINAL AORTIC ANEURYSM REPAIR

GENERAL INFORMATION

DEFINITION—An aneurysm is a weakened, dilated (widened) segment of an artery. The surgery replaces a segment of the dilated aorta in the abdomen with graft material to strengthen the wall.

BODY PARTS INVOLVED—Abdominal cavity, aorta, and sometimes the iliac arteries.

REASONS FOR SURGERY—To prevent a rupture of the abdominal aortic aneurysm which usually results in massive hemorrhage and death.

SURGICAL RISK INCREASES WITH
* Age.
* Diabetes.
* Poor kidney function.
* High blood pressure.
* Poor nutrition.
* Chronic lung disease.

WHAT TO EXPECT

WHO OPERATES—General surgeon, vascular surgeon, cardiothoracic surgeon.

WHERE PERFORMED—Hospital.

DIAGNOSTIC TESTS
* Before surgery: Blood tests, chest x-ray, CT scan, EKG (see Glossary for these two terms).
* After surgery: Blood tests.

ANESTHESIA—General anesthesia.

DESCRIPTION OF OPERATION
* The abdomen is opened through a long vertical midline incision from the ribcage to the pubis.
* The bowels are mobilized and pulled off to the side to expose the aneurysm.
* Control of blood flow in the aorta is obtained above and below the aneurysm with clamps.
* The aneurysm is opened and inspected. A graft is sewn to the upper end just below the arteries to the kidneys and to the lower end just above the split going to the legs. Sometimes the graft must be sewn to the individual leg arteries if the aneurysm extends too close to or beyond the split. The walls of the original aorta are sewn over the graft.
* The wound is closed once all bleeding is controlled.
* Infrequently the aneurysm is resected and removed.
* Another option for repair may be placement of an endovascular graft inside the intact aneurysm. This can be done with a nonsurgical technique.

POSSIBLE COMPLICATIONS
* Bleeding from the graft site.
* Kidney failure.
* Poor circulation to the intestines which can lead to gangrene.
* Poor circulation to the lower extremities.
* Incisional hernia.

AVERAGE HOSPITAL STAY—Usually 5-10 days with the first day or two in the intensive care unit.

PROBABLE OUTCOME—Expect full recovery in 8-12 weeks with no recurrence of the aneurysm. Older patients may take many months (or years) to regain strength.

POSTOPERATIVE CARE

GENERAL MEASURES
* Hard ridges will form along the incisions. As they heal, the ridges will gradually recede.
* Use heat on the incision to help relieve incisional pain.
* Shower as usual. You may wash the incisions gently with mild soap. After showering, replace any dressings with a new dry dressing.
* Wear compression stockings when up for the first few weeks after surgery.

MEDICATION
* Your doctor may prescribe pain relievers. Use only as much as you need to be comfortable.
* You may use nonprescription pain relievers such as acetaminophen for minor pain. Ask your doctor if it is okay to take ibuprofen or aspirin.

ACTIVITY
* Start ambulating (walking) as soon as you are home. Take frequent naps as needed during the day when tired. Avoid strenuous activity for 6 to 8 weeks.
* You may swim once all sutures are out.
* Resume sexual relations when comfortable and when advised by your surgeon.

DIET—No special diet.

CALL YOUR DOCTOR IF

* Pain, swelling, redness, drainage or bleeding increases in the surgical area.
* You develop signs of infection, including headache, muscle aches, dizziness fever, or a general ill feeling.
* You develop nausea and vomiting.
* You have prolonged constipation.
* Legs are cold, numb, or painful.
* New unexplained symptoms develop.

ABDOMINAL AORTIC ANEURYSM REPAIR

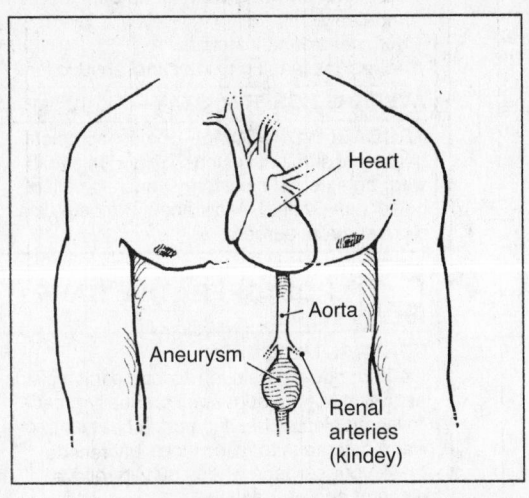

Most aortic aneurysms occur between the venal arteries and the bifurcation (split) which goes to the legs.

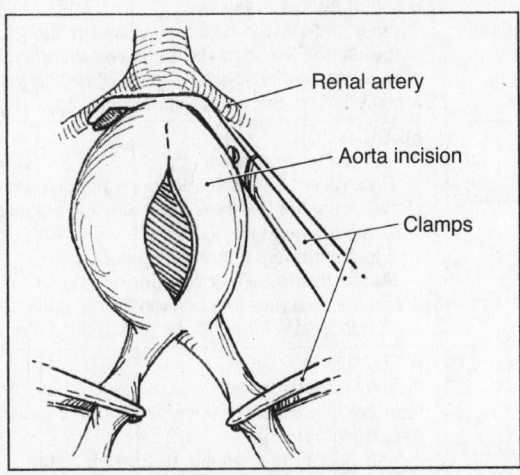

The aorta is clamped above and below the aneurysm and opened.

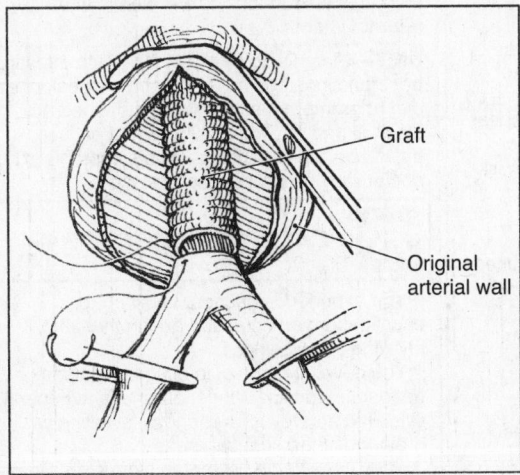

The graft is sewn inside the aorta and the wall of the aneurysm is closed over the graft.

ABDOMINOPERINEAL RESECTION

 GENERAL INFORMATION

DEFINITION—Removal of cancerous cells in the rectum and anus through an incision in the lower abdomen and the perineum. Enough of the anus and rectum are removed so that the intestines cannot be reconnected. A colostomy (see Colostomy in Surgery section) is performed at the same time so that digestive function is not disrupted.

BODY PARTS INVOLVED—Rectum; anus; sigmoid colon; perineum; abdomen.

REASONS FOR SURGERY—Cancer of the rectum or anus.

SURGICAL RISK INCREASES WITH
• Adults over 60.
• Diabetes.
• Obesity; smoking.
• Poor nutrition.
• Recent illness.
• Alcoholism or other chronic illness.
• Use of some prescription and nonprescription drugs. Inform your doctor of any drugs, medications, or vitamin and herb supplements you are using or have used in the last month.

 WHAT TO EXPECT

WHO OPERATES—Proctologist, general surgeon or colon and rectal surgeon.

WHERE PERFORMED—Hospital.

DIAGNOSTIC TESTS
• Before surgery: Colonoscopy; sigmoidoscopy; barium enema; ultrasound; CT scan (see Glossary for these terms); blood and urine studies.
• After surgery: Laboratory examination of removed tissue; blood studies.

ANESTHESIA—General anesthesia by injection and inhalation with an airway tube placed in the windpipe.

DESCRIPTION OF OPERATION
• An incision is made in the abdomen. The abdominal muscles are divided and the peritoneal cavity is entered. The sigmoid colon is located, isolated and divided. The closer bowel portion is brought to the skin surface for a colostomy.
• The colostomy bag is fitted and placed in position.
• The farther bowel portion is closed and placed deep in the pelvis.
• Incisions are made in the perineum.
• The rectum, anus and end of the bowel (intestine) are isolated and cut free of connective tissue.
• Tubes are left in to allow drainage.
• The skin edges of both incisions are closed with sutures or clips, which usually can be removed in 7 to 10 days after surgery.

POSSIBLE COMPLICATIONS
• Excessive bleeding.
• Hernia around colostomy or surgery incision.
• Impotence.
• Surgical-wound infection.
• Adhesions leading to intestinal obstruction.

AVERAGE HOSPITAL STAY—7 to 10 days.

PROBABLE OUTCOME—Expect complete healing of surgical wounds. You will need to wear an external colostomy pouch to collect bowel movements. Allow about 3 months for recovery from surgery.

 POSTOPERATIVE CARE

GENERAL MEASURES
• A hard ridge should form along each incision. As they heal, the ridges will gradually recede.
• Use an electric heating pad, a heat lamp or a warm compress to relieve incisional pain.
• Ask your surgeon when you may begin to bathe or shower as usual.
• Move and elevate legs often while in bed to decrease the likelihood of deep-vein blood clots.
• An enterostomy specialist (see Glossary) will teach you how to care for your colostomy.

MEDICATION
• Your doctor may prescribe:
  - Pain relievers. Don't take prescription pain medication longer than 4 to 7 days. Use only as much as you need.
  - Stool softeners to prevent constipation.
  - Antibiotics to fight or prevent infection.
• You may use nonprescription drugs, such as acetaminophen, for minor pain. Avoid aspirin.

ACTIVITY
• To help recovery and aid your well-being, resume daily activities, including work, as soon as possible.
• Avoid vigorous exercise for 6 weeks after surgery. Resume driving 2-3 weeks after returning home.

DIET—Clear liquid diet until the gastrointestinal tract functions again. Then eat a well-balanced diet to promote healing. Avoid caffeine and alcohol, and any food or spice that causes painful or unpleasant digestive symptoms. Your doctor may prescribe a special diet.

 CALL YOUR DOCTOR IF

• You experience nausea, vomiting, or constipation; or increased abdominal pain, swelling or bleeding.
• You develop signs of infection, including headache, muscle aches, dizziness, a general ill feeling and fever; or redness, swelling or drainage in the surgical areas.
• New, unexplained symptoms develop. Drugs used in treatment may produce side effects.

ABDOMINOPERINEAL RESECTION

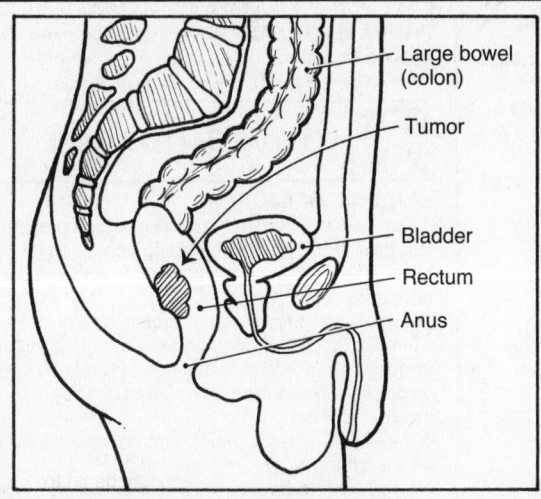

Large bowel (colon)

Tumor

Bladder

Rectum

Anus

An illustration of the appearance and anatomical relationships of the large bowel with representation of a rectal tumor.

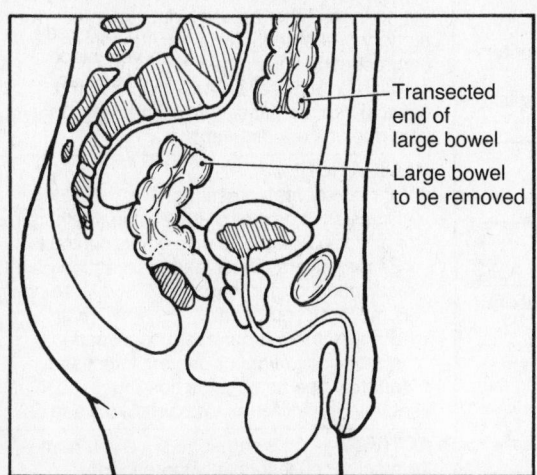

Transected end of large bowel

Large bowel to be removed

The large bowel is transected above the tumor. The distal segment is closed prior to removal.

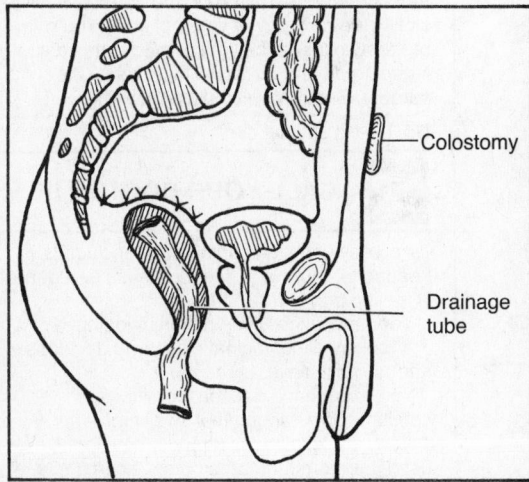

Colostomy

Drainage tube

Tumor removed, along with rectum, large bowel and anus.
• Drainage tube left in place to be removed after healing.
The proximal transected end of large bowel is brought out through the abdominal wall and skin to form a colostomy.

SURGERIES

ABORTION
(Suction Curettage)

GENERAL INFORMATION

DEFINITION—Removal of a fetus and accompanying tissue from the uterus. It can be used to terminate a pregnancy, or to remove a fetus that has died in utero, and is usually performed in pregnancies of 12 weeks duration or less.

BODY PARTS INVOLVED—Uterus; placenta; vagina (route for surgery).

REASONS FOR SURGERY
* Missed or incomplete miscarriage.
* Elective termination of pregnancy. The patient should receive competent counseling before making this decision.

SURGICAL RISK INCREASES WITH
* Obesity.
* Smoking.
* Poor nutrition.
* Recent or chronic illness.
* Use of some prescription and nonprescription drugs. Inform your doctor of any drugs, medications, or vitamin and herb supplements you are using or have used in the last month.

WHAT TO EXPECT

WHO OPERATES—General surgeon or obstetrician-gynecologist.

WHERE PERFORMED—Hospital or outpatient surgical facility.

DIAGNOSTIC TESTS
* Before surgery: Pregnancy test; psychological counseling and testing; blood and urine studies.
* After surgery: Laboratory examination of removed tissue.

ANESTHESIA—Local anesthesia by injection; sometimes accompanied by sedation.

DESCRIPTION OF OPERATION
* The opening of the cervix is dilated by the use of instruments or laminaria (see Glossary).
* A small plastic tube is passed through the vagina and cervix into the uterus. The tube is connected to a suction apparatus.
* Gentle suction through the tube removes the uterine contents. You may feel cramps in the lower abdomen, nausea, sweating and faintness.
* The tube is removed, and the lining of the uterus is scraped with a curette to be sure all the placental tissue is removed.

POSSIBLE COMPLICATIONS
* Excessive bleeding.
* Perforation or infection of the uterus.
* Potential psychological problems.

AVERAGE HOSPITAL STAY—None.

PROBABLE OUTCOME—Expect complete healing without complications. Allow several days to one week for recovery from surgery.

POSTOPERATIVE CARE

GENERAL MEASURES
* Use sanitary pads for bleeding, which may last for several days. If bleeding continues for more than 14 days after surgery, you may use tampons.
* If you have pain, place a heating pad or hot-water bottle on the abdomen or back. Hot baths frequently aid muscle relaxation and relieve discomfort. Repeat baths as often as they provide comfort.
* Avoid sexual relations and do not douche for 2 weeks after surgery.
* If you wish to take birth-control pills, begin taking them either on the night you return from surgery or the next day; a backup form of contraception should be used for the first month. If you prefer an IUD, diaphragm or cervical cap, the fitting can be made during your next doctor's appointment.

MEDICATION
* Your doctor may prescribe:
  - Drugs such as methylergonovine (Methergine) or oxytocin (Pitocin) to help uterus contract.
  - Pain relievers. Don't take prescription pain medication longer than 4 to 7 days. Use only as much as you need.
  - Stool softeners to prevent constipation.
  - Antibiotics to fight or prevent infection.
* You may use nonprescription drugs, such as acetaminophen, for minor pain. Avoid aspirin.

ACTIVITY—Have someone drive you home from surgery. Rest quietly there for the remainder of the day. Resume normal activities slowly the next day, if you feel able. You will probably experience light or moderate vaginal bleeding on and off for 10 to 14 days after surgery. Bed rest will reduce bleeding.

DIET—No special diet.

CALL YOUR DOCTOR IF

* You develop signs of infection, including headache, muscle aches, dizziness or a general ill feeling and fever.
* You have excessive vaginal bleeding.
* A foul smelling vaginal discharge develops after several days.
* You experience nausea, vomiting, constipation or abdominal swelling.
* New, unexplained symptoms develop. Drugs used in treatment may produce side effects.

ABORTION
(Suction Curettage)

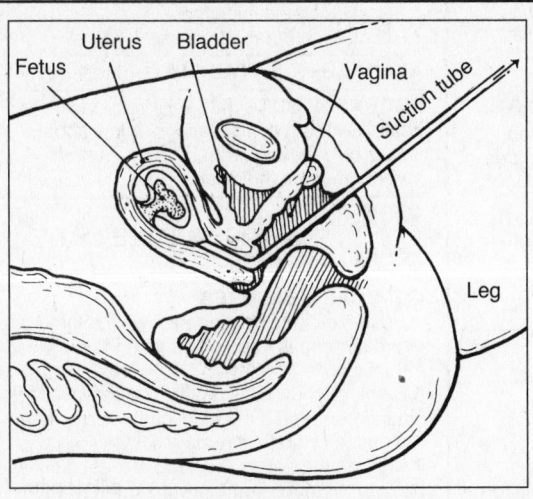

Uterus Bladder

Fetus

Vagina

Suction tube

Leg

A side view of an adult female showing a small fetus within the uterus (womb).
 • Suction tube in place. One end of the the tube is attached to the suction machine and the other end is passed through the vagina and cervix into the uterus.

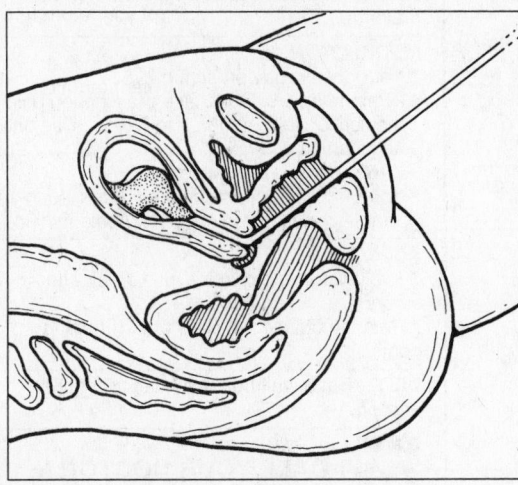

Gentle suction through the tube removes the fetus and placenta.

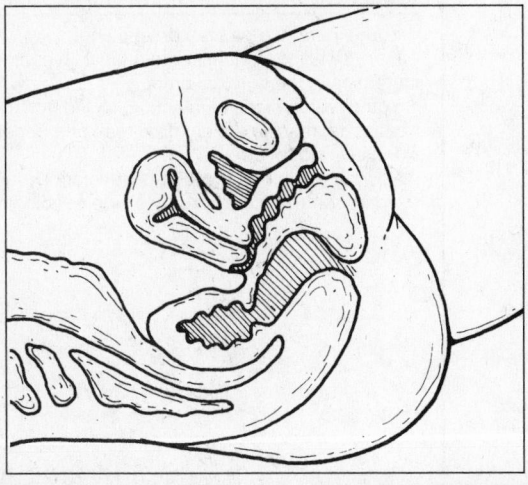

Suction tube removed. Uterus is now empty. Pregnancy terminated.

SURGERIES

ABSCESS DRAINAGE SUPERFICIAL

GENERAL INFORMATION

DEFINITION—To open and drain an abscess.

BODY PARTS INVOLVED—Abscesses may occur anywhere in the body. The most common areas include: female breast during lactation; armpit; anal area; groin; vaginal lips; face; area around the tonsils; scrotum; back; and arms, legs, hands and feet.

REASONS FOR SURGERY—Treatment of infections. If an abscess breaks open and drains spontaneously, surgery is often still required to assure complete drainage.

SURGICAL RISK INCREASES WITH
- Obesity.
- Smoking.
- Poor nutrition.
- Diabetes.
- Recent or chronic illness.
- Use of some prescription and nonprescription drugs. Inform your doctor of any drugs, medications, or vitamin and herb supplements you are using or have used in the last month.

WHAT TO EXPECT

WHO OPERATES—Family doctor or general surgeon.

WHERE PERFORMED—Doctor's office, outpatient surgical facility, hospital or emergency room.

DIAGNOSTIC TESTS
- Before surgery: Blood and urine studies (sometimes).
- After surgery: Laboratory examination of removed pus (sometimes).

ANESTHESIA
- Local anesthesia by injection.
- General anesthesia by injection and inhalation.

DESCRIPTION OF OPERATION
- An incision is made over the abscess.
- The incision is spread apart, and a sterile-gloved finger or instrument is inserted inside the abscess to break up small pockets. The pus is drained and the cavity is irrigated.
- Gauze is packed into the space left by the abscess. Sometimes a soft rubber drain may be left in the incision; either method allows the cavity to heal from the bottom outward. The drain is usually removed 24 to 48 hours after surgery.
- The skin is left open to prevent recurrence of the abscess.
- A gauze dressing is applied over the wound.

POSSIBLE COMPLICATIONS
- Excessive bleeding.
- Surgical-wound infection.
- Recurrence of the abscess.

AVERAGE HOSPITAL STAY—0 to 1 day.

PROBABLE OUTCOME—Expect complete healing without complications. Allow about 2 weeks for recovery from surgery. Further surgery may be indicated.

POSTOPERATIVE CARE

GENERAL MEASURES
- Use an electric heating pad, a heat lamp or a warm compress to relieve pain and help clear the infection.
- Bathe or shower as usual. You may wash the wound gently with mild, unscented soap after the gauze or drain is removed.
- Change the gauze dressing at least daily after bathing, or more frequently if saturated with drainage.

MEDICATION
- Your doctor may prescribe:
  - Pain relievers. Don't take prescription pain medication longer than 4 to 7 days. Use only as much as you need.
  - Antibiotics to fight infection.
- You may use nonprescription drugs, such as acetaminophen, for minor pain. Avoid aspirin.

ACTIVITY
- Avoid vigorous exercise for 1 week after surgery.
- Resume driving 1-2 days after returning home.

DIET—Eat a well-balanced diet to promote healing.

CALL YOUR DOCTOR IF

- You experience nausea or vomiting.
- Pain, swelling, redness, drainage or bleeding increases in the surgical area.
- You develop signs of infection, including headache, muscle aches, dizziness or a general ill feeling and fever.
- New, unexplained symptoms develop. Drugs used in treatment may produce side effects.

ABSCESS DRAINAGE SUPERFICIAL

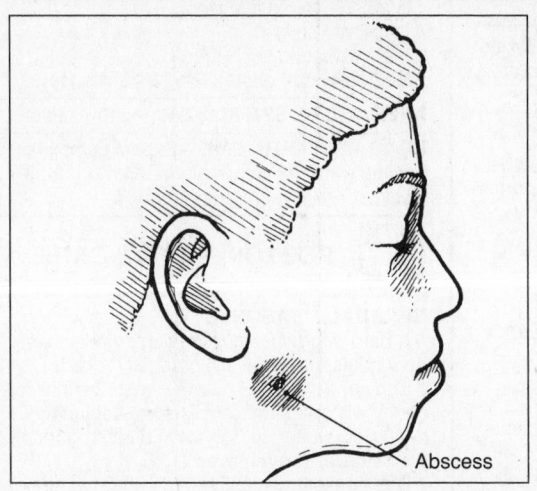

A side view of an adolescent male face showing an abscess.

Abscess

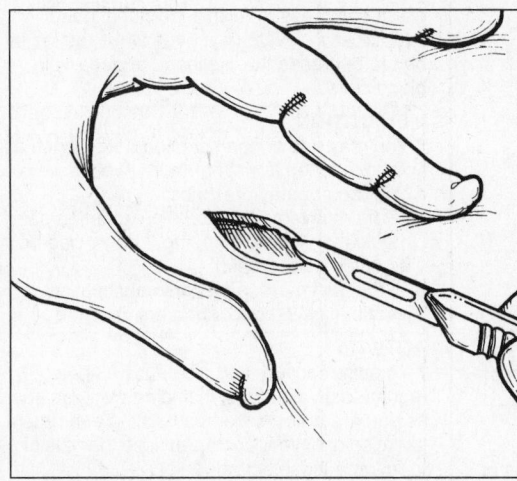

Abscess is incised, the incision spread apart, and finger inserted into abscess cavity to break up small pockets.

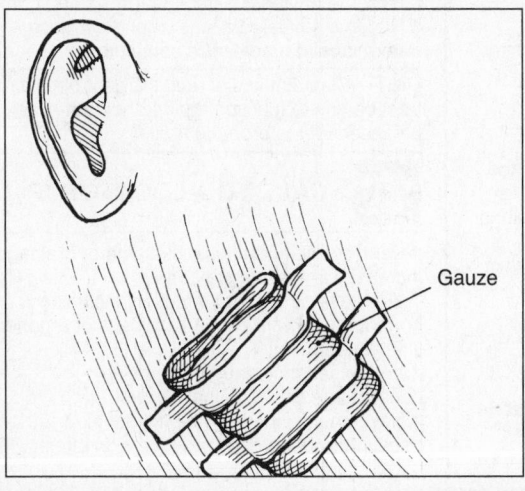

Gauze inserted into space left by the abscess. This provides a drain that allows the abscess cavity to heal from the bottom outward.

Gauze

ADHESIONS, SEPARATION OF (LYSIS OF)

GENERAL INFORMATION

DEFINITION—Separation of adhesions, fibrous bands of tissue that cause parts of the abdomen and pelvis to cling together abnormally.

BODY PARTS INVOLVED—Abdominal or pelvic organs.

REASONS FOR SURGERY—Relief of a partial or complete intestinal obstruction caused by adhesions. Adhesions usually result from:
* Previous abdominal surgery.
* Congenital defects.
* Pelvic inflammatory disease.
* Endometriosis.
* Ruptured ectopic pregnancy.
* Radiation treatment for cancers in the abdomen or pelvis.
* Any ruptured organ that has caused infection and scarring.

SURGICAL RISK INCREASES WITH
* Adults over 60; obesity; smoking.
* Excess alcohol consumption.
* Poor nutrition.
* Multiple previous surgeries.
* Diabetes.
* Recent or chronic illness.
* Use of some prescription and nonprescription drugs. Inform your doctor of any drugs, medications, or vitamin and herb supplements you are using or have used in the last month.

WHAT TO EXPECT

WHO OPERATES—General surgeon.

WHERE PERFORMED—Hospital.

DIAGNOSTIC TESTS
* Before surgery: Blood and urine studies; abdominal x-rays; sometimes, barium enema or small bowel series (see Glossary).
* After surgery: Blood studies.

ANESTHESIA—General anesthesia by injection and inhalation with an airway tube placed in the windpipe.

DESCRIPTION OF OPERATION
* An incision is made in the abdomen over the obstruction.
* The obstruction is isolated and the adhesions are divided carefully.
* The bowel is examined for strangulation (lost blood supply). Any strangulated portion is removed, and the normal ends are joined.
* The abdominal contents are then inspected for undetected disease. Other surgeries may be performed at this time.
* The abdominal contents are replaced. Muscle layers are closed with sutures, and skin is closed with sutures or clips, which can usually be removed in 1 week.

POSSIBLE COMPLICATIONS
* Excessive bleeding; blood clots.
* Surgical-wound infection.
* Incisional hernia.
* Inadvertent bowel injury.
* Recurrence of obstruction (25% chance).

AVERAGE HOSPITAL STAY—5 to 7 days.

PROBABLE OUTCOME—Expect complete healing without complications. Allow about 6 weeks for recovery from surgery.

POSTOPERATIVE CARE

GENERAL MEASURES
* A hard ridge should form along the incision. As it heals, the ridge will gradually recede.
* Shower as usual. You may wash the incision gently with mild, unscented soap beginning 24 to 48 hours after surgery. Avoid bathing until your sutures are removed.
* Use an electric heating pad, a heat lamp or a warm compress to relieve incisional pain.
* Move and elevate legs often while resting in bed to decrease the likelihood of deep-vein blood clots.

MEDICATION
* You may use nonprescription drugs, such as acetaminophen, for minor pain. Avoid aspirin.
* Your doctor may prescribe:
  - Pain relievers. Don't take prescription pain medication longer than 4 to 7 days. Use only as much as you need.
  - Stool softeners to prevent constipation.
  - Antibiotics to fight or prevent infection.

ACTIVITY
* To help recovery and aid your well-being, resume daily activities, including work, as soon as you are able. Avoid heavy lifting and heavy exercise until your doctor advises that it is okay to resume these activities.
* Resume driving 3 weeks after returning home.
* Resume sexual relations when your doctor determines that healing is complete.

DIET—Clear liquid diet until the gastrointestinal tract begins to function again. Then eat a well-balanced diet to promote healing.

CALL YOUR DOCTOR IF

* Pain, swelling, redness, bleeding or drainage increases in the surgical area.
* You develop signs of infection, including headache, muscle aches, dizziness or a general ill feeling and fever.
* You experience nausea, vomiting, constipation or abdominal swelling.
* New, unexplained symptoms develop. Drugs used in treatment may produce side effects.

ADHESIONS, SEPARATION OF (LYSIS OF)

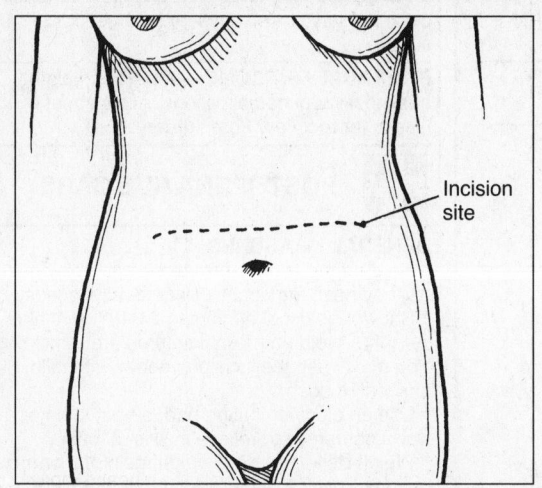

An illustration of the surgical site to enter the abdomen.

Incision site

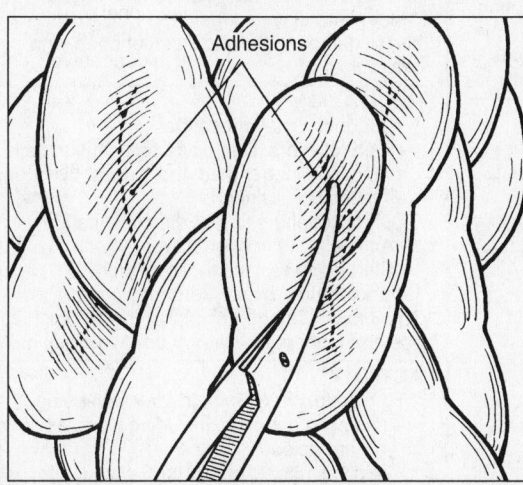

The adhesion causes the small bowel to be obstructed. Here a surgical instrument cuts the adhesions free.

Adhesions

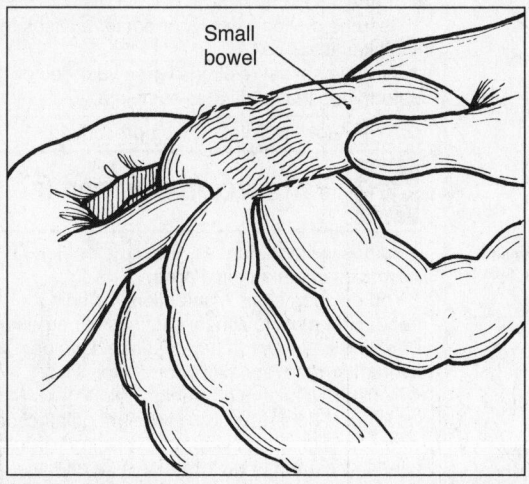

The bowel is manually inspected for other disease.

Small bowel

SURGERIES

ADRENAL GLAND REMOVAL
(Adrenalectomy)

GENERAL INFORMATION

DEFINITION—Removal of one or both of the adrenal glands.

BODY PARTS INVOLVED—Adrenal glands.

REASONS FOR SURGERY
- Cushing's syndrome.
- Pheochromocytoma (a tumor).
- Other adrenal gland tumors.

SURGICAL RISK INCREASES WITH
- Adults over 60.
- Obesity.
- Smoking.
- Stress.
- Poor nutrition.
- Diabetes.
- Recent illness.
- Alcoholism or other chronic illness.
- Use of some prescription and nonprescription drugs. Inform your doctor of any drugs, medications, or vitamin and herb supplements you are using or have used in the last month.

WHAT TO EXPECT

WHO OPERATES—General surgeon.

WHERE PERFORMED—Hospital.

DIAGNOSTIC TESTS
- Before surgery: Blood and urine studies; x-rays of kidneys; CT scan (see Glossary) of adrenal area.
- After surgery: Blood studies; laboratory examination of removed tissue.

ANESTHESIA—General anesthesia by injection and inhalation with an airway tube placed in the windpipe.

DESCRIPTION OF OPERATION
- The adrenal glands can frequently be removed using Laparoscopy (see in Surgery section), rather than open surgery.
- When open surgery is required, the incision may be in the abdomen or the flank (on the back, near the kidneys).
- The adrenal glands are located, isolated, cut free and removed. Tubes are left in to allow drainage.
- The skin incisions are closed with sutures or clips, which usually can be removed about 1 week after surgery.

POSSIBLE COMPLICATIONS
- Excessive bleeding.
- Surgical-wound infection.
- Adrenal-hormone shortage.
- Fluid retention.
- Increased risk of life-threatening infections.

AVERAGE HOSPITAL STAY—5 to 7 days for open surgery; 1 to 2 days for laparoscopic surgery.

PROBABLE OUTCOME—Expect complete healing without complications. Allow about 6 weeks for recovery from surgery.

POSTOPERATIVE CARE

GENERAL MEASURES
- Hard ridges should form along the incisions. As they heal, the ridges will gradually recede.
- Shower as usual beginning 24-48 hours after surgery. Avoid baths until sutures are removed. You may wash the incisions gently with mild, unscented soap.
- Use an electric heating pad, a heat lamp or a warm compress to relieve incisional pain.
- Weigh daily. Report a weight gain of 2 or more pounds in any 24-hour period to your doctor.
- Move and elevate legs often while resting in bed to decrease the likelihood of deep-vein blood clots.

MEDICATION
- Your doctor may prescribe:
  - Pain relievers. Don't take prescription pain medication longer than 4 to 7 days. Use only as much as you need.
  - Stool softeners to prevent constipation.
  - Antibiotics to fight or prevent infection.
  - Steroids to replace those formerly manufactured by the adrenal glands.
- You may use nonprescription drugs, such as acetaminophen, for minor pain. Avoid aspirin.

ACTIVITY
- To help recovery and aid your well-being, resume daily activities, including work, as soon as you are able.
- Avoid vigorous exercise for 6 weeks after surgery.
- Resume driving when your doctor advises that it is okay to do so.
- Resume sexual relations when your doctor determines that healing is complete.

DIET—A low-salt diet may be prescribed.

CALL YOUR DOCTOR IF

- Pain, swelling, redness, drainage or bleeding increases in the surgical area.
- You develop signs of infection, including headache, muscle aches, dizziness or a general ill feeling and fever. If any of these develop, even after recovery, call your doctor.
- Nausea, vomiting, dizziness, fatigue, weakness, fluid retention, or weight gain occurs.
- New unexplained symptoms develop. Drugs used in treatment may produce side effects.

ADRENAL GLAND REMOVAL
(Adrenalectomy)

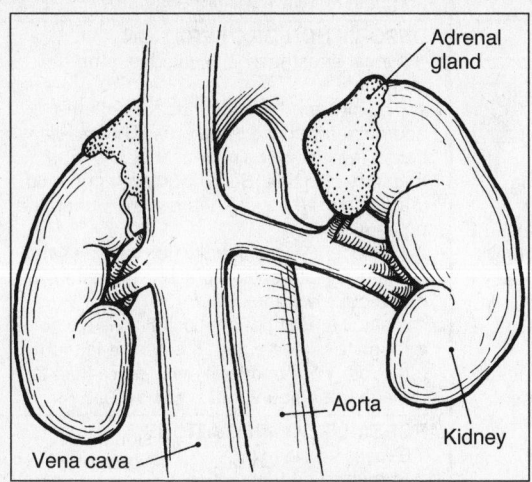

An illustration of the adrenal glands.

Adrenal
gland

Aorta

Kidney

Vena cava

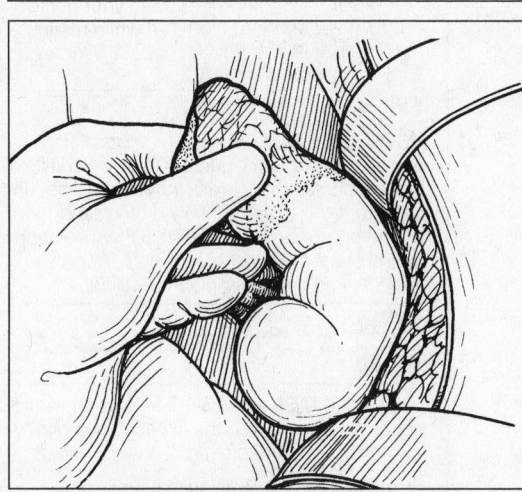

The adrenal gland is freed from the kidney on the left side of the patient.

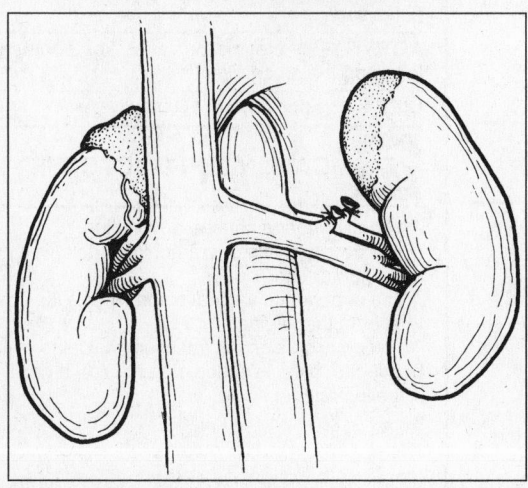

Adrenal glands removed.

AMNIOCENTESIS

GENERAL INFORMATION

DEFINITION—Removal of fluid from the amniotic sac during pregnancy.

BODY PARTS INVOLVED—Uterus; amniotic sac.

REASONS FOR SURGERY—Laboratory examination of amniotic fluid helps diagnose abnormalities of the unborn child. Although genetic testing may be done as early as the 11th week of pregnancy, the best time is usually between the 14th and 20th weeks of pregnancy. There is ample fluid, time to treat certain problems before the baby is born, and enough time exists to terminate the pregnancy if necessary. Amniocentesis may also be done in the third trimester to assess fetal development. Amniocentesis is often done for one or more of the following reasons:
* Mother is over 35 years old.
* Either parent has a chromosome abnormality.
* Mother has previously had a child with a chromosome abnormality, such as Down syndrome.
* Patient had abnormal results from a blood screening test, such as maternal serum alpha-fetoprotein (MSAFP or AFP) test.
* Mother produces antibodies, most commonly to the fetal blood cells, that can cause the unborn child to be very anemic. The amniotic fluid is tested for a chemical (bilirubin) that serves as a marker for fetal anemia.
* To evaluate pregnancy for infection.
* To remove excess amniotic fluid; most commonly in twins when one baby has too much amniotic fluid and the other has too little.
* Mother carries a sex-linked abnormality, and the unborn child's sex must be determined.
* To evaluate fetal lung maturity.
* Unborn child's maturity or other conditions must be determined late in pregnancy.

SURGICAL RISK INCREASES WITH
* Obesity.
* Previous abdominal surgery.
* Previous infection in pelvic organs.

WHAT TO EXPECT

WHO OPERATES—Obstetrician-gynecologist or family doctor.

WHERE PERFORMED—Outpatient surgical facility or hospital.

DIAGNOSTIC TESTS
* Before surgery: Blood and urine studies.
* During surgery: Ultrasonography (see Glossary).
* After surgery: Laboratory examination of the amniotic fluid.

ANESTHESIA—Local anesthesia by injection. To ensure the unborn child's safety, sedatives and pain relievers will not be used.

DESCRIPTION OF OPERATION
* A local anesthetic is injected into the abdomen.
* A hollow needle is inserted through the abdominal wall into the uterus. The needle will cause temporary pain, but should not hurt more than any injection. Some women report mild cramping, or a feeling of pressure, during the procedure.
* Amniocentesis is usually performed using continuous ultrasound to allow a constant view of the needle's path.
* A small amount of amniotic fluid is suctioned through the needle, and the needle is then removed. Your body will make more fluid to replace the amount that is removed.

POSSIBLE COMPLICATIONS
* Excessive bleeding.
* Surgical-wound infection.
* Unwanted abortion triggered by procedure in 1 out of 150 to 200 cases.
* Injury to the fetus (rare).

AVERAGE HOSPITAL STAY—None.

PROBABLE OUTCOME—More than 95% of amniocentesis tests indicate no abnormalities. Some couples at high risk want the procedure done to reduce their anxiety during pregnancy. However, normal amniocentesis results cannot guarantee a child without defects. At present, there are no tests for all abnormalities.

POSTOPERATIVE CARE

GENERAL MEASURES—Bathe or shower as usual. You may wash the injection site gently with mild, unscented soap.

MEDICATION—Medicine is usually not necessary.

ACTIVITY—No restrictions after 2 or 3 hours following the procedure.

DIET—No special diet.

CALL YOUR DOCTOR IF

* You experience nausea or vomiting.
* You develop pain or cramping in the lower abdomen or shoulder.
* You experience vaginal bleeding or a loss of fluid from the vagina.
* You develop signs of infection, including headache, muscle aches, dizziness or a general ill feeling and fever.

AMNIOCENTESIS

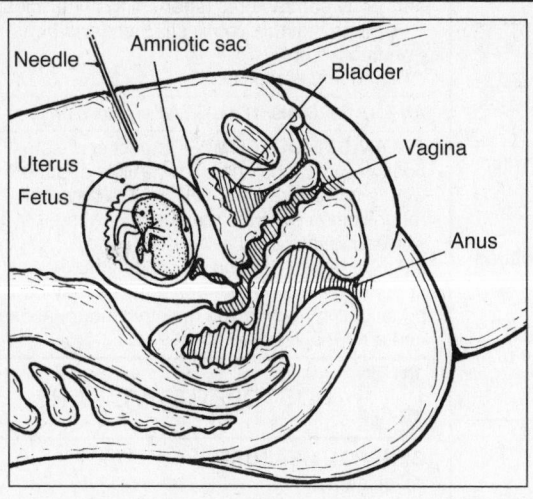

Needle
Amniotic sac
Bladder
Uterus
Fetus
Vagina
Anus

An illustration of the structures near any amniocentesis procedure.
 • Hollow needle inserted through the skin and abdominal wall.

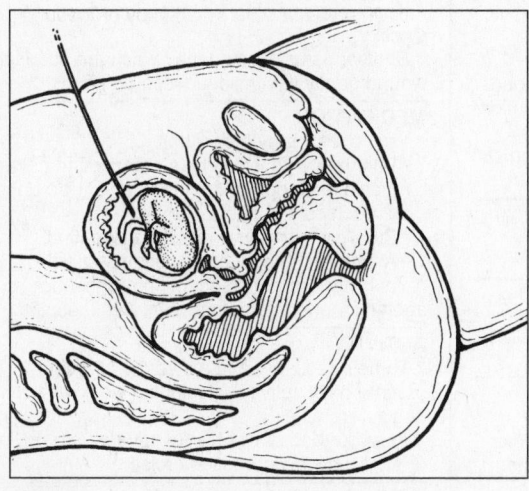

Hollow needle penetrates the cavity of the uterus.

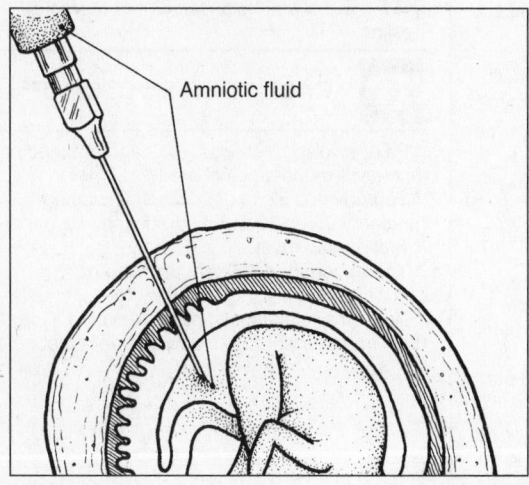

Amniotic fluid

Amniotic fluid suctioned through the needle and collected for study.

AMPUTATION

GENERAL INFORMATION

DEFINITION—Removal of a limb or appendage.

BODY PARTS INVOLVED—Arms, legs, hands, feet; fingers, or toes.

REASONS FOR SURGERY—Performed when blood circulation to a part of the body is irreversibly interrupted, usually caused by one of the following:
- Injury to blood vessels that cannot be repaired or reconstructed.
- Hardening or obstructions of the arteries.
- Impaired blood circulation due to diabetes.
- Buerger's disease, Raynaud's phenomena.
- Severe infection with gangrene.
- Severe frostbite.

SURGICAL RISK INCREASES WITH
- Adults over 60.
- Smoking; obesity; stress; poor nutrition.
- Excess alcohol consumption.
- Coronary artery disease.
- Diabetes.
- Disease that increases coagulability of blood.
- Use of some prescription and nonprescription drugs. Inform your doctor of any drugs, medications, or vitamin and herb supplements you are using or have used in the last month.

WHAT TO EXPECT

WHO OPERATES—General surgeon, vascular surgeon, or orthopedic surgeon.

WHERE PERFORMED—Hospital.

DIAGNOSTIC TESTS
- Before surgery: Blood and urine studies; x-rays of part to be amputated; arterial doppler studies or arteriography (see Glossary for both).
- After surgery: Blood studies.

ANESTHESIA—General anesthesia by injection and inhalation with an airway tube placed in the windpipe or spinal anesthesia.

DESCRIPTION OF OPERATION
- An incision is made around the part to be amputated.
- Tissue, muscles, blood vessels, nerves and bone are severed.
- The bone is filed smooth, and the bone end is covered with connective tissue. Frequently tubes are left in the wound to allow drainage.
- Muscles are closed with large sutures. The skin is closed with fine sutures, which are left in place for 2 to 4 weeks after surgery.
- A snug bandage is often wrapped around the affected area of the body, and may be left in place for several days following surgery.
- In some cases, an immediate, temporary prosthesis (artificial limb) is fitted.

POSSIBLE COMPLICATIONS
- Excessive bleeding, surgical-wound infection or muscle contractures (shortening of muscles).
- Feelings that the limb is still there and hurts ("phantom limb").
- Pulmonary embolism.

AVERAGE HOSPITAL STAY—2 to 7 days.

PROBABLE OUTCOME—Expect complete healing without complications. Allow about 6 weeks for recovery from surgery. A physical rehabilitation program may be frustrating, but it will lead to improved self-esteem and independence. Depending on the limb or appendage amputated, a prosthesis may be beneficial in helping you maintain independence and a normal lifestyle.

POSTOPERATIVE CARE

GENERAL MEASURES
- Don't smoke.
- Keep stump slightly elevated to reduce swelling.
- Shower as usual. You may wash the surgical wound gently with mild, unscented soap.

MEDICATION
- Your doctor may prescribe:
  - Pain relievers. Don't take prescription pain medication longer than 4 to 7 days. Use only as much as you need.
  - Stool softeners to prevent constipation.
  - Antibiotics to fight or prevent infection.
- You may use nonprescription drugs, such as acetaminophen, for minor pain. Avoid aspirin.

ACTIVITY
- To help recovery and aid your well-being, resume daily activities, including work, as soon as you are able.
- Ask your doctor when you may resume driving or engaging in vigorous exercise.

DIET—Eat a well-balanced diet to promote healing.

CALL YOUR DOCTOR IF

- Pain, swelling, redness, drainage or bleeding increases in the surgical area.
- You develop signs of infection, including headache, muscle aches, dizziness or a general ill feeling and fever.
- You experience nausea, vomiting or constipation.
- New, unexplained symptoms develop. Drugs used in treatment may produce side effects.

AMPUTATION

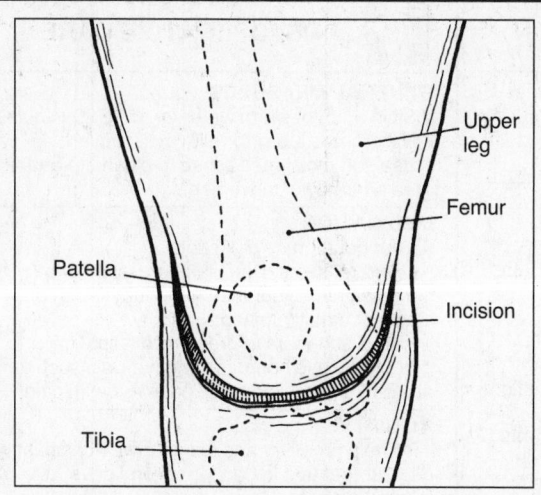

An illustration of a lower leg amputation.

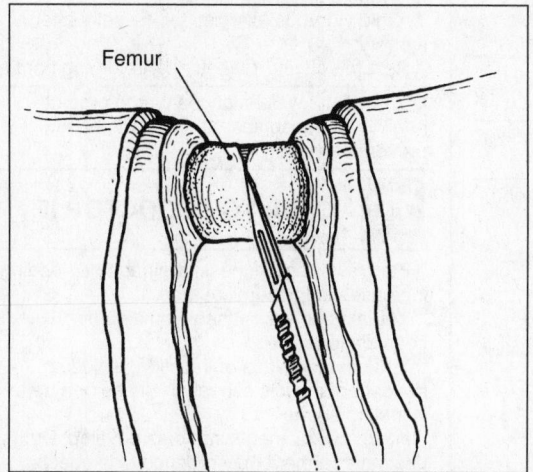

Skin, connective tissue, muscles, blood vessels, nerves, and bone are severed.

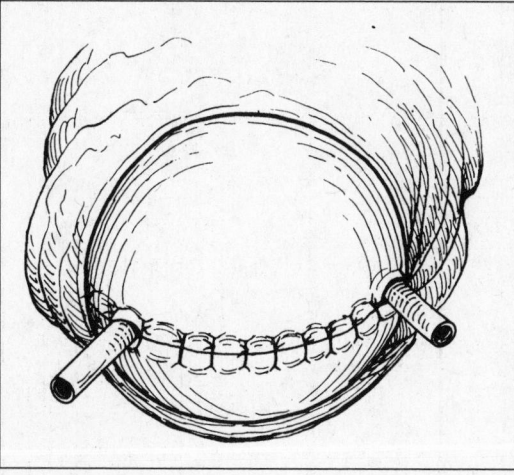

Bone end filed smooth and covered with connective tissue.
- Muscles closed with large sutures, skin closed with fine sutures.
- Drains remain in place.

ANAL FISSURE REMOVAL & ANAL SPHINCTEROTOMY

GENERAL INFORMATION

DEFINITION—Removal of an anal fissure, a crack or tear in the membrane that lines the anus, and incision of the muscular anal sphincter.

BODY PARTS INVOLVED—Anus and lining membrane; anal muscles (sphincter).

REASONS FOR SURGERY—Relief of pain.

SURGICAL RISK INCREASES WITH
* Obesity; smoking.
* Recent or chronic illness.
* Diabetes.
* Use of some prescription and nonprescription drugs. Inform your doctor of any drugs, medications, or vitamin and herb supplements you are using or have used in the last month.

WHAT TO EXPECT

WHO OPERATES—General surgeon or proctologist.

WHERE PERFORMED—Hospital or outpatient surgical facility.

DIAGNOSTIC TESTS—Before surgery: Blood and urine studies; anoscopy; sigmoidoscopy (see Glossary for both).

ANESTHESIA
* Local anesthesia by injection.
* Spinal anesthesia by injection.
* General anesthesia by injection and inhalation with an airway tube placed in the windpipe.

DESCRIPTION OF OPERATION
* Sometimes dilatation (see Glossary) of the sphincter muscles is sufficient to treat the problem.
* In other cases, one of the outer sphincter muscles is cut to prevent recurrence.
* Rarely, the fissure is cut from the surrounding tissue and removed.
* Bleeding vessels are tied or closed with electrocauterization.
* The surgical area may be left open to hasten healing. Bandages are applied.

POSSIBLE COMPLICATIONS
* Excessive bleeding or pain.
* Surgical-wound infection.
* Inability to control bowel movements until healing is complete.
* Incontinence.

AVERAGE HOSPITAL STAY—0 to 1 day.

PROBABLE OUTCOME—Expect complete healing without complications. Allow about 3 weeks for recovery from surgery.

POSTOPERATIVE CARE

GENERAL MEASURES
* Sit in a tub of warm water for 15 to 20 minutes several times a day to relieve discomfort.
* Use soft moistened tissue to clean the anal area after bowel movements.

MEDICATION
* Your doctor may prescribe:
  - Pain relievers. Don't take prescription pain medication longer than 4 to 7 days. Use only as much as you need.
  - Stool softeners to prevent constipation.
* You may use nonprescription drugs, such as acetaminophen, for minor pain. Avoid aspirin.

ACTIVITY
* To help recovery and aid your well-being, stay off your feet and in bed for several days following surgery.
* Avoid vigorous exercise for 4 weeks after surgery.
* Resume driving 1 week after returning home.

DIET—Eat a well-balanced diet to promote healing. Increase fiber and fluid intake to prevent constipation.

CALL YOUR DOCTOR IF

* Pain, swelling, redness, drainage or bleeding increases in the surgical area.
* You experience nausea, vomiting or constipation.
* You develop signs of infection, including headache, muscle aches, dizziness or a general ill feeling and fever.
* New, unexplained symptoms develop. Drugs used in treatment may produce side effects.

ANAL FISSURE REMOVAL & ANAL SPHINCTEROTOMY

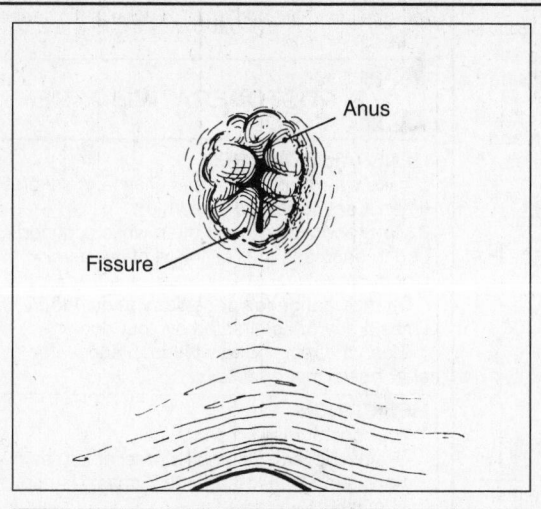

An illustration of an anal fissure. This view places the patient lying on back with legs extended.

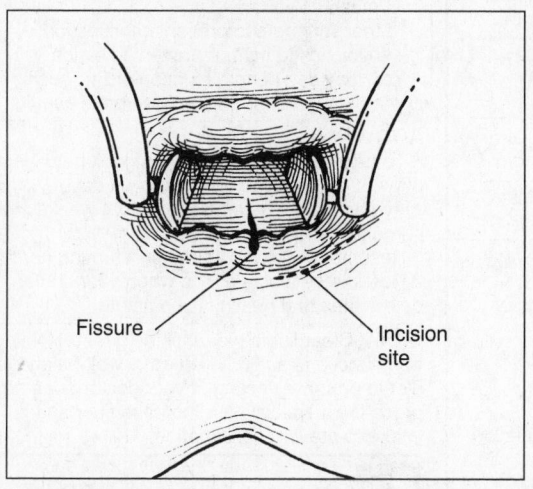

Sphincter muscle is expanded with special instrument. The incision site is indicated above the sphincter muscle.

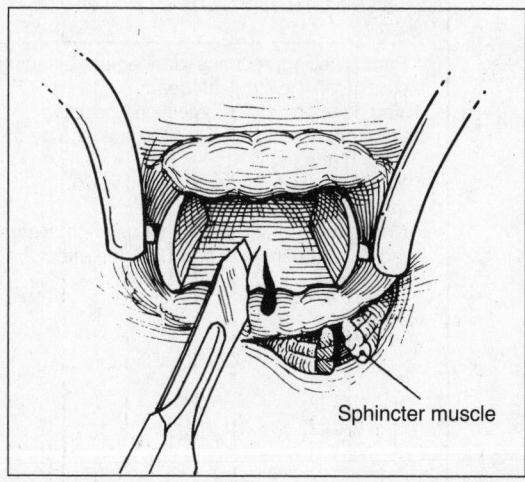

Fissure cut free from surrounding tissue and removed. Sphincter muscle has been cut.

SURGERIES

ANAL FISTULA REPAIR

GENERAL INFORMATION

DEFINITION—Opening or removal of an anal fistula, an abnormal tract extending from inside the rectum to the skin outside of the anus.

BODY PARTS INVOLVED—Rectum; skin and underlying tissue around the rectum and anus.

REASONS FOR SURGERY
* Repeated abscesses in the anal and rectal areas.
* Chronic drainage from a fistula.

SURGICAL RISK INCREASES WITH
* Diabetes.
* Poor nutrition.
* Recent or chronic illness.
* Obesity.
* Smoking.
* Use of some prescription and nonprescription drugs. Inform your doctor of any drugs, medications, or vitamin and herb supplements you are using or have used in the last month.

WHAT TO EXPECT

WHO OPERATES—General surgeon or proctologist.

WHERE PERFORMED—Outpatient surgical facility or hospital.

DIAGNOSTIC TESTS—Before surgery: x-rays of lower gastrointestinal tract; colonoscopy, anoscopy or sigmoidoscopy (see Glossary for all 3).

ANESTHESIA
* Local anesthesia by injection.
* Spinal anesthesia by injection.
* General anesthesia by injection and inhalation with an airway tube placed in the windpipe.

DESCRIPTION OF OPERATION
* Abscesses are drained, if necessary.
* The fistula is located with a delicate probe, and the skin and tissue over the fistula is opened.
* The surgical wound is left open to heal from inside out.
* Occasionally, the internal opening of the fistula may be located very high inside the rectum. In this case, it may be necessary to perform the operation in two stages a few weeks apart.

POSSIBLE COMPLICATIONS
* Excessive bleeding.
* Surgical-wound infection.
* Slow healing or recurrence.
* Incontinence.

AVERAGE HOSPITAL STAY—0 to 3 Days.

PROBABLE OUTCOME—Expect complete healing without complications in 4 to 5 weeks for small fistulas, and up to 16 weeks for deeper ones.

POSTOPERATIVE CARE

GENERAL MEASURES
* Take warm sitz baths (see Glossary) several times a day to relieve discomfort.
* Move and elevate legs often while confined to bed to decrease the likelihood of deep-vein blood clots.
* Change bandages or sanitary pads 4 to 5 times a day or as directed by your doctor.
* Clean the rectal area with soap and water after bowel movements.

MEDICATION
* Your doctor may prescribe:
  - Pain relievers. Don't take prescription pain medication longer than 4 to 7 days. Use only as much as you need.
  - Stool softeners to prevent constipation.
  - Antibiotics to fight or prevent infection.
* You may use nonprescription drugs, such as acetaminophen, for minor pain. Avoid aspirin.

ACTIVITY
* To help recovery and aid your well-being, stay off your feet and in bed for several days.
* Avoid vigorous exercise for 3 to 4 weeks after surgery.
* Resume driving 1 week after returning home.
* Resume sexual relations when your doctor determines that healing is complete.

DIET—Clear liquid diet until the gastrointestinal tract functions again. Then eat a well-balanced diet to promote healing, if your doctor does not prescribe a special diet. Increase fiber and fluid intake to prevent constipation.

CALL YOUR DOCTOR IF

* Pain, swelling, redness, drainage or bleeding increases in the surgical area.
* You develop signs of infection, including headache, muscle aches, dizziness or a general ill feeling and fever.
* You experience nausea, vomiting or constipation.
* New, unexplained symptoms develop. Drugs used in treatment may produce side effects.

ANAL FISTULA REPAIR

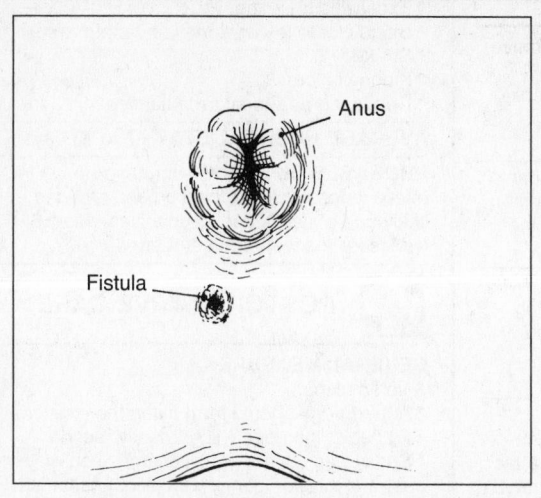

An illustration of an anal fissure. The opening of the tract that appears on the skin may occur in various places in the area surrounding the anus.

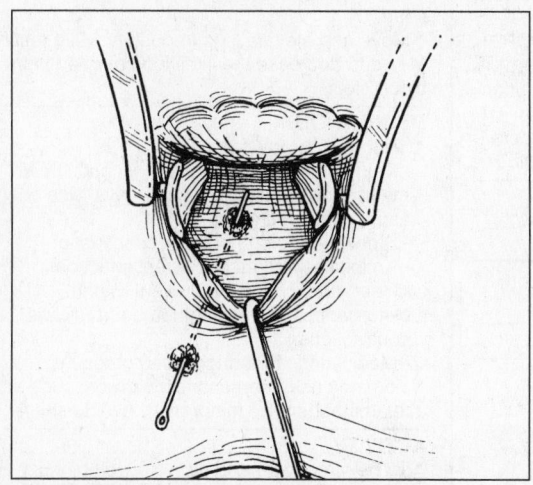

Anus retracted to expose the fistula tract. A probe is inserted to locate the inner opening of the fistula.

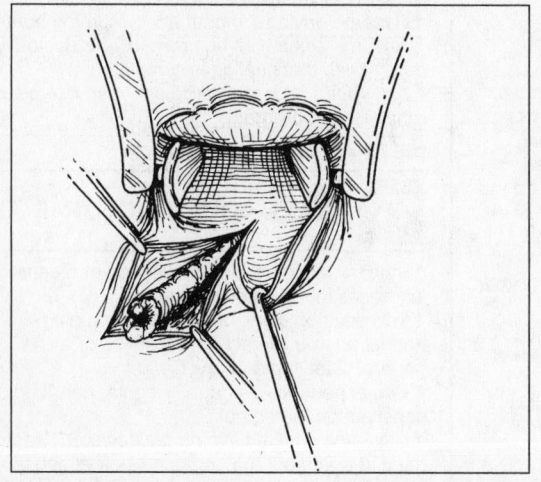

Fistula is opened and the surgical wound is then left open to allow healing from inside out.

ANEURYSM REPAIR

GENERAL INFORMATION

DEFINITION—A surgical procedure to remove an aneurysm (a swelling, dilatation or ballooning of a blood vessel due to weakening that is caused by disease, injury or a congenital defect in the artery wall).

BODY PARTS INVOLVED—Aneurysms can form anywhere in the body. The most common sites are the aorta, the arteries supplying the brain, and the heart.

REASONS FOR SURGERY
* Prevent rupture and uncontrolled bleeding
* Pressure of an aneurysm on surrounding structures.
* Reduce risk of blood clots.

SURGICAL RISK INCREASES WITH
* Obesity; smoking.
* Recent or chronic illness such as heart attack, high blood pressure, thyroid disease, diabetes, or kidney disease.
* Chronic obstructive pulmonary disease (COPD).
* Chronic congestive heart failure (advanced).
* Use of some prescription and nonprescription drugs. Inform your doctor of any drugs, medications, or vitamin and herb supplements you are using or have used in the last month.

WHAT TO EXPECT

WHO OPERATES—Cardiovascular surgeon, vascular surgeon, or neurosurgeon.

WHERE PERFORMED—Hospital.

DIAGNOSTIC TESTS
* Before surgery: Blood studies; chest x-ray; cardiac catheterization; ECG; sonogram; CT scan; arteriogram (see Glossary for all).
* After surgery: ECG; chest x-ray.

ANESTHESIA—General anesthesia by injection and inhalation with an airway tube placed in the windpipe.

DESCRIPTION OF OPERATION—Surgery for an aneurysm on the heart is described here:
* The patient is connected to the heart-lung equipment to allow the heart to be stopped temporarily so surgery can be performed on the diseased tissue.
* The heart is made to stop by cooling and weak electrical shock.
* The aneurysm is removed along with a border of normal heart tissue.
* The edges of the heart are sewn together. A graft may be sewn into place between the two cut edges.
* The heart is warmed, then the heartbeat is restored by a weak electrical shock.
Note: Coronary artery bypass surgery is frequently performed at the same time.

POSSIBLE COMPLICATIONS
* Surgical wound infection.
* Excessive bleeding.
* Blood clot to leg or kidney and other areas.
* Stroke.
* Kidney failure.
* Continued heartbeat irregularities.

AVERAGE HOSPITAL STAY—7 to 10 days.

PROBABLE OUTCOME—Improved effectiveness of heart function and reduced likelihood of heartbeat irregularities. Allow 6 weeks for recovery from surgery.

POSTOPERATIVE CARE

GENERAL MEASURES
* No smoking.
* A hard ridge should form along the incision. As it heals, the ridge will gradually recede.
* Shower as usual after discharge. You may wash the incision gently with mild, unscented soap.
* Move and elevate legs frequently while resting in bed to decrease the likelihood of deep-vein blood clots.

MEDICATION
* Your doctor may prescribe:
  - Pain relievers. Don't take prescription pain medication longer than 4 to 7 days. Use only as much as you need.
  - Stool softeners to prevent constipation.
  - Antibiotics to fight or prevent infection.
  - Heart medications to prevent rhythm disturbances and strengthen heart muscle contractions.
  - Medications to reduce blood pressure.
* You may use nonprescription drugs, such as acetaminophen, for minor pain. Avoid aspirin.

ACTIVITY
* To help recovery and aid your well-being, resume daily activities as soon as possible.
* Resume driving 1 month after returning home.
* Resume sexual relations when your doctor determines that healing is complete.
* Ask your doctor for advice about an exercise rehabilitation program.

DIET—As directed by your doctor.

CALL YOUR DOCTOR IF

* Pain, swelling, redness, drainage or bleeding increases in the surgical area.
* You develop signs of infection, including headache, muscle aches, dizziness or a general ill feeling and fever.
* You experience a cough, irregular heartbeat, constipation, or leg pain.
* New, unexplained symptoms develop. Drugs used in treatment may produce side effects.

ANEURYSM REPAIR

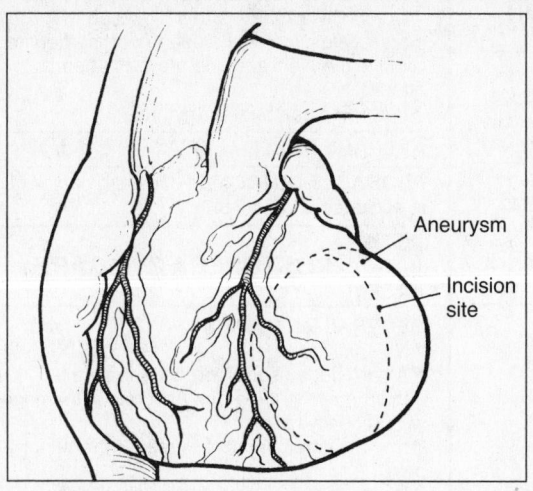

An illustration of the heart as seen after the chest wall has been opened showing the ballooning out of the left ventricle representing the aneurysm as well as the proposed incision site.

Aneurysm

Incision site

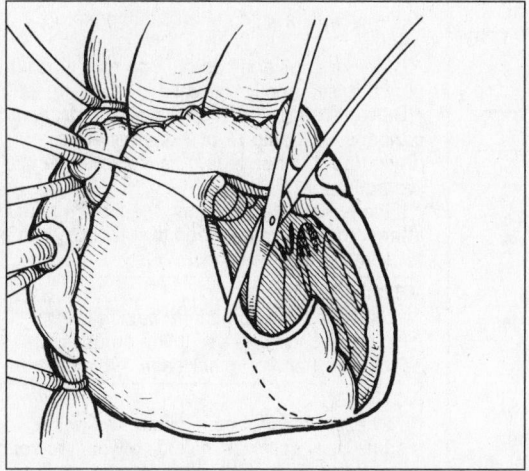

The aneurysm is incised and any blood clot inside is removed. The weakened scarred area is excised and the remaining heart muscle closed in layers.

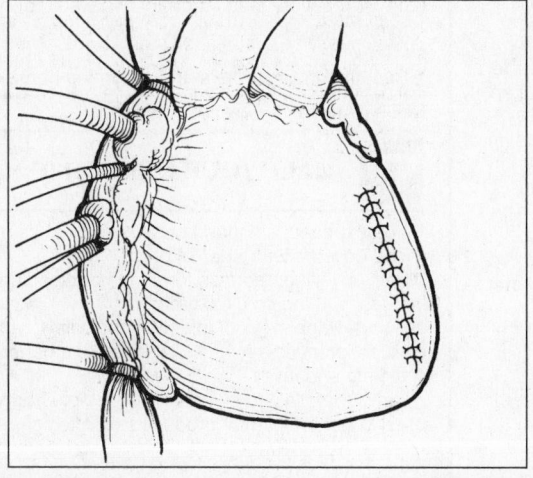

The appearance of the heart after the aneurysm has been excised and the remaining heart muscle closed with the sutures.

SURGERIES

ANGIOPLASTY, CORONARY
(Percutaneous Transluminal Coronary Angioplasty)

 GENERAL INFORMATION

DEFINITION—A non-surgical shaping or alteration of blood vessels. In this procedure, a catheter with an inflatable balloon is inserted into a blocked or partially blocked coronary artery.

BODY PARTS INVOLVED—Coronary arteries (the blood vessels that supply nourishment to the heart muscle).

REASONS FOR SURGERY—To open a block or partial block of a coronary artery.

SURGICAL RISK INCREASES WITH
• Obesity; smoking.
• Excess alcohol consumption.
• Angina (for more than 1 year).
• Calcification of blood vessels.
• Use of some prescription and nonprescription drugs. Inform your doctor of any drugs, medications, or vitamin and herb supplements you are using or have used in the last month.

 WHAT TO EXPECT

WHO OPERATES—Cardiologist.

WHERE PERFORMED—Hospital.

DIAGNOSTIC TESTS
• Before surgery: Heart catheterization with x-ray and fluoroscopic examinations (see Glossary).
• During surgery: X-rays after injection of dye through the catheter into various parts of the heart.

ANESTHESIA—Local, with sedation.

DESCRIPTION OF OPERATION
• The cardiac balloon catheter is inserted into an artery in the arm or leg. Fluoroscopy (see Glossary) provides guidance for the catheter to pass through the artery to the heart.
• Blood-pressure readings are taken, and the heart's ability to pump blood is tested.
• The catheter is guided into the coronary-artery system. Fluoroscopy allows identification of any disease in the coronary arteries.
• The catheter is passed through the occlusion, the balloon is inflated, and the occlusion is compressed, allowing blood to flow through once again.
• Stents may be placed to keep the artery open.
• When all examinations have been completed, the catheter balloon is withdrawn, and the artery is compressed until bleeding stops.

POSSIBLE COMPLICATIONS
• Break or rupture in the dilated artery lining.
• Dislodged plaque that blocks the artery further downstream.
• Coronary spasm.

• Reaction to the dye used in x-ray studies.
• Complete coronary artery blockage which necessitates immediate open-heart surgery to remove the blockage and prevent a heart attack.
• Irregular heart beat (arrhythmia).

AVERAGE HOSPITAL STAY—0 to 1 day.

PROBABLE OUTCOME—Opening of blockage in occluded coronary artery.

 POSTOPERATIVE CARE

GENERAL MEASURES
• No smoking.
• A hard ridge usually forms beneath the puncture site in the groin. As it heals, the ridge will gradually recede.
• Use a warm compress to relieve incisional pain.
• Discoloration under the skin where the catheter was inserted should disappear in 2 weeks.
• Bathe or shower as usual. You may wash the puncture site gently with mild, unscented soap.
• Between showers, keep the wound dry with a bandage for the first 2 or 3 days after the procedure. If a bandage gets wet, change it promptly.
• If the wound bleeds during the first 24 hours after surgery, press a clean tissue or cloth to it for 10 to 15 minutes continuously.

MEDICATION
• Your doctor may prescribe pain relievers.
• You may use nonprescription drugs, such as acetaminophen, for minor pain. Avoid aspirin.

ACTIVITY
• To help recovery and aid your well-being, resume daily activities, including work, as soon as possible. This procedure requires much less time for recovery than coronary bypass surgery.
• Avoid vigorous exercise for 2 weeks after surgery.
• Resume driving 2 days after returning home.

DIET—As directed by your doctor.

 CALL YOUR DOCTOR IF

• You experience sudden or severe chest pain.
• You develop shortness of breath.
• Pain, swelling, redness, drainage or bleeding increases in the surgical area.
• You develop signs of infection, including headache, muscle aches, dizziness or a general ill feeling and fever.
• New, unexplained symptoms develop. Drugs used in treatment may produce side effects.

ANGIOPLASTY, CORONARY
(Percutaneous Transluminal Coronary Angioplasty)

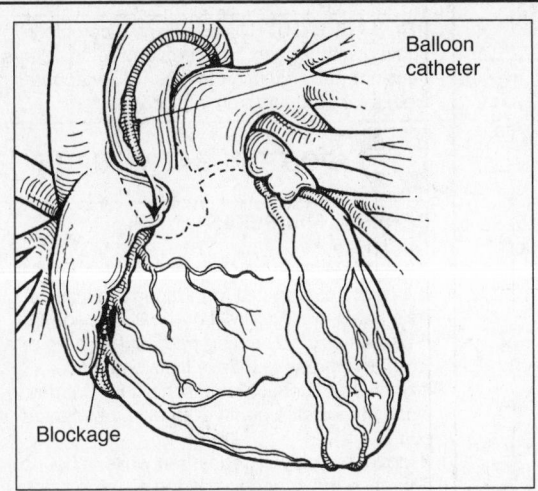

Balloon catheter

Blockage

An illustration of the cardiac balloon catheter about to enter the right coronary artery.

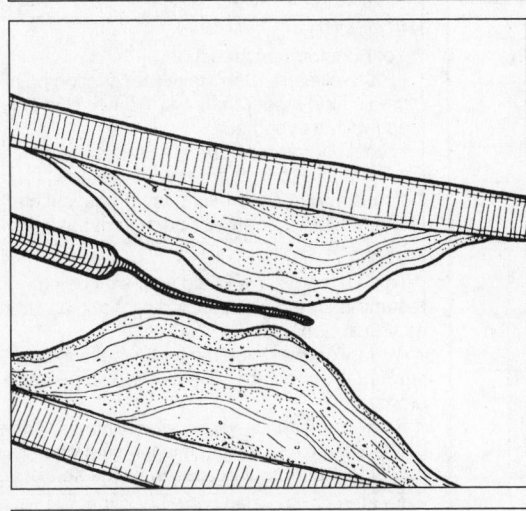

Fluoroscopy allows identification of any disease in the coronary arteries and the catheter is passed through the occlusion.

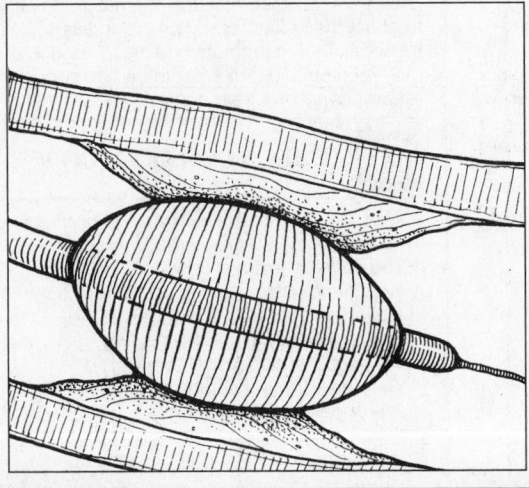

Then the balloon is inflated, the plaque is broken, and the occlusion is dilated allowing blood to flow freely once again. After all examinations have been completed, the catheter balloon is withdrawn.

AORTO-ILIAC BYPASS GRAFT
(Aortoiliofemoral Reconstruction)

 GENERAL INFORMATION

DEFINITION—Placement of an artificial graft to bypass a blood clot or narrowing in the arteries that supply blood to the abdomen, genital area and legs.

BODY PARTS INVOLVED—Aorta; iliac arteries.

REASONS FOR SURGERY—Restoration of normal blood circulation in the legs.

SURGICAL RISK INCREASES WITH
* Alcoholism; obesity; smoking.
* Diabetes; coronary artery disease; or atherosclerosis.
* Use of some prescription and nonprescription drugs. Inform your doctor of any drugs, medications, or vitamin and herb supplements you are using or have used in the last month.

 WHAT TO EXPECT

WHO OPERATES—General surgeon or vascular surgeon.

WHERE PERFORMED—Hospital.

DIAGNOSTIC TESTS
* Before surgery: Blood and urine studies; ultrasound; arteriograms (see Glossary for both).
* After surgery: Blood studies.

ANESTHESIA—General anesthesia by injection and inhalation with an airway tube placed in the windpipe.

DESCRIPTION OF OPERATION
* An incision is made in the abdomen.
* The abdominal muscles are separated to expose the abdominal organs, which are inspected for undetected disease. (Other surgeries may be performed at this time.)
* The aorta and iliac arteries are located and clamped to isolate the obstruction.
* An artificial graft is selected and fitted in place. One end attaches to the aorta and the other two ends to the iliac arteries.
* The graft is sewn in place and the clamps are released. Blood can now circulate freely.
* The muscles of the abdomen are closed in layers. The skin is closed with sutures or clips, which usually can be removed about 1 week after surgery.

POSSIBLE COMPLICATIONS
* Excessive bleeding.
* Surgical-wound infection; graft infection.
* Incisional hernia.
* Inadvertent injury to the ureter.
* Impotence.
* Occlusion of arteries beyond the grafted vessels.

AVERAGE HOSPITAL STAY—5 to 7 days.

PROBABLE OUTCOME—Expect complete healing without complications and restoration of near-normal circulation to legs. Allow about 6 weeks for recovery from surgery.

 POSTOPERATIVE CARE

GENERAL MEASURES
* Don't smoke.
* Keep feet clean and dry.
* A hard ridge should form along the incision. As it heals, the ridge will gradually recede.
* Use an electric heating pad, a heat lamp or a warm compress to relieve incisional pain.
* Shower as usual after discharge. You may wash the incision gently with mild, unscented soap.
* Move and elevate legs often while in bed to decrease the chance of deep-vein blood clots.

MEDICATION
* Your doctor may prescribe:
  - Pain relievers. Don't take prescription pain medication longer than 4 to 7 days. Use only as much as you need.
  - Stool softeners to prevent constipation.
  - Antibiotics to fight or prevent infection.
* You may use nonprescription drugs, such as acetaminophen, for minor pain. Avoid aspirin.

ACTIVITY
* To help recovery and aid your well-being, resume daily activities, including work, as soon as you are able.
* Avoid vigorous exercise for 6 weeks after surgery. Your doctor will prescribe an exercise program.
* Resume driving 5 weeks after returning home.
* Resume sexual relations when your doctor has determined that healing is complete.

DIET—Clear liquid diet until the gastrointestinal tract begins to function again. Then eat a well-balanced diet to promote healing. Your doctor may recommend a diet low in fat and sodium (see Appendix for both diets).

 CALL YOUR DOCTOR IF

* Pain, swelling, redness, drainage or bleeding increases in the surgical area.
* You develop signs of infection, including headache, muscle aches, dizziness or a general ill feeling and fever.
* You experience nausea, vomiting, constipation or abdominal swelling.
* Your legs or feet become cold, discolored, numb or painful.
* New, unexplained symptoms develop. Drugs used in treatment may produce side effects.

AORTO-ILIAC BYPASS GRAFT
(Aortoiliofemoral Reconstruction)

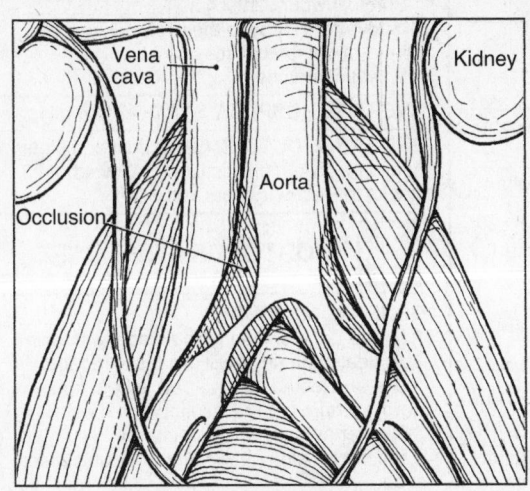

An illustration of the aorta, iliac arteries, and the occlusions to be bypassed.

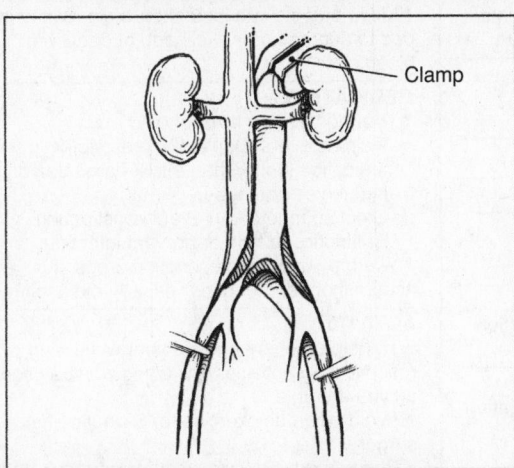

The aorta and iliac arteries are clamped to isolate the obstruction.

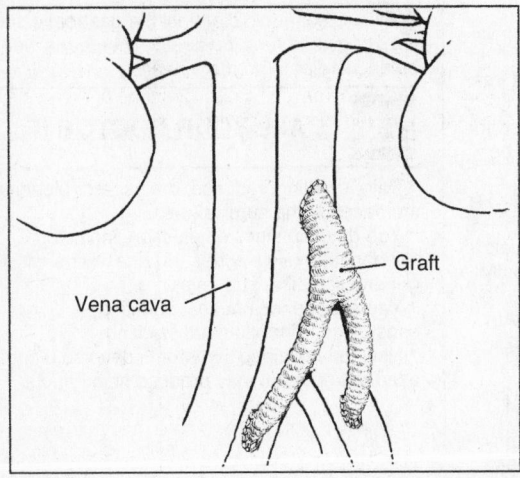

Polyester graft fitted in place. The upper end fits the aorta and the two lower ends fit the iliac arteries.
 • After the graft is in place, the clamps are released. Blood can now again circulate freely.

SURGERIES

APPENDECTOMY

GENERAL INFORMATION

DEFINITION—Removal of the appendix, an outgrowth of tissue from the cecum, the first part of the large intestine.

BODY PARTS INVOLVED—Appendix; cecum; peritoneum.

REASONS FOR SURGERY—Treatment of an infected appendix. Signs and symptoms of infection can include:
- Abdominal pain; nausea; vomiting.
- Loss of appetite.
- Tenderness in the right lower abdomen.
- Low-grade fever.
- Elevated white blood-cell count.

SURGICAL RISK INCREASES WITH
- Alcoholism; obesity; smoking.
- Chronic heart, lung, liver or kidney disease.
- Use of some prescription and nonprescription drugs. Inform your doctor of any drugs, medications, or vitamin and herb supplements you are using or have used in the last month.

WHAT TO EXPECT

WHO OPERATES—General surgeon.

WHERE PERFORMED—Hospital.

DIAGNOSTIC TESTS
- Before surgery: Blood and urine studies, x-rays of abdomen, ultrasound and CT scan (see Glossary).
- After surgery: Blood studies and examination of removed tissue.

ANESTHESIA
- General anesthesia by injection and inhalation with an airway tube placed in the windpipe.
- Spinal anesthesia by injection.

DESCRIPTION OF OPERATION
- An incision is made in the lower abdomen.
- The abdominal muscles and organs are separated and the appendix is isolated, cut free and removed.
- The area around the appendix is inspected for undetected diseases. Other surgeries may be performed at this time.
- Any fluid or pus from the infected appendix is suctioned away.
- Sometimes, a drain is placed in the area left by the removed appendix. The drain is usually removed 2 to 3 days following surgery.
- The abdominal cavity is closed, and the skin is closed with sutures, which usually can be removed 1 week after surgery.
- Alternatively, surgery may be performed using a laparoscope (see Glossary). In this case, several small incisions would be made in the abdomen to facilitate viewing and removal of the appendix.

POSSIBLE COMPLICATIONS
- Excessive bleeding.
- Surgical-wound infection.
- Inadvertent injury to the ureter.
- Intra-abdominal abscess.
- Bowel obstruction.

AVERAGE HOSPITAL STAY—2 to 4 days.

PROBABLE OUTCOME—Expect complete healing without complications. Allow about 3 weeks for recovery from surgery.

POSTOPERATIVE CARE

GENERAL MEASURES
- A hard ridge should form along the incision. As it heals, the ridge will gradually recede.
- Use an electric heating pad, a heat lamp or a warm compress to relieve incisional pain.
- Shower as usual after discharge. You may wash the incision gently with mild, unscented soap.
- Move and elevate legs often while resting in bed to decrease the likelihood of deep-vein blood clots.

MEDICATION
- Your doctor may prescribe:
  - Pain relievers. Don't take prescription pain medication longer than 4 to 7 days. Use only as much as you need.
  - Stool softeners to prevent constipation.
  - Antibiotics to fight or prevent infection.
- You may use nonprescription drugs, such as acetaminophen, for minor pain. Avoid aspirin.

ACTIVITY
- To help recovery and aid your well-being, resume daily activities, including work, as soon as you are able.
- Avoid vigorous exercise for 6 weeks after surgery.
- Resume driving 2 weeks after returning home.

DIET—Clear liquid diet until the gastrointestinal tract begins to function again. Then eat a well-balanced diet to promote healing.

CALL YOUR DOCTOR IF

- Pain, swelling, redness, drainage or bleeding increases in the surgical area.
- You develop signs of infection, including headache, muscle aches, dizziness or a general ill feeling and fever.
- You experience nausea, vomiting, constipation or abdominal swelling.
- New, unexplained symptoms develop. Drugs used in treatment may produce side effects.

APPENDECTOMY

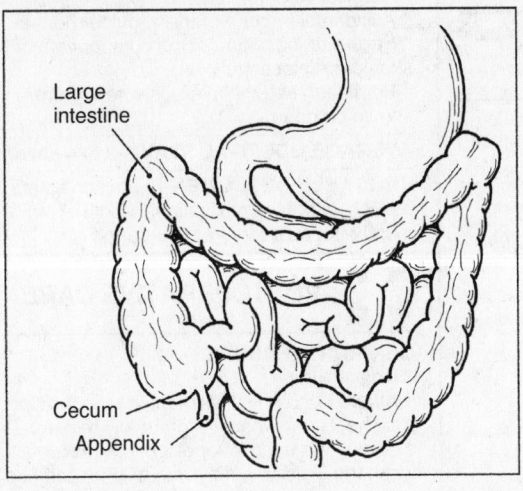

An illustration of the vermiform appendix attached to the cecum (the first part of the large intestine).

Large intestine

Cecum

Appendix

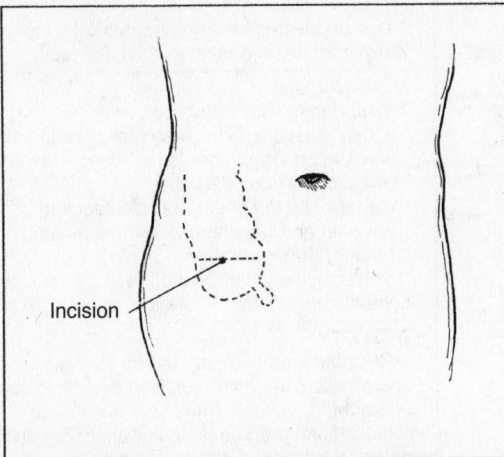

The incision is usually made at a point approximately 2/3 the distance between the navel and the point of the hip.

Incision

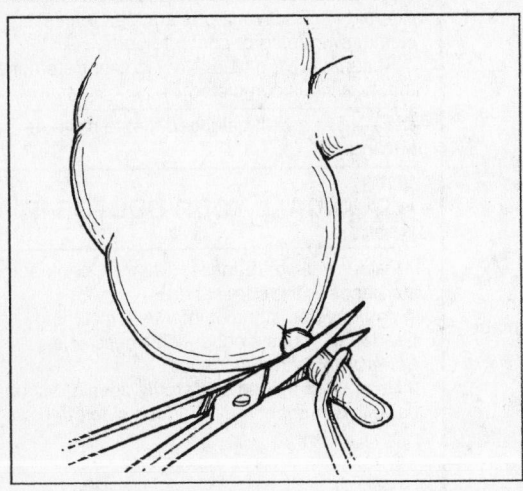

Appendix isolated, cut free and removed. The stump is then cauterized and sterilized to prevent infection.

SURGERIES

ARTHROPLASTY, SHOULDER

GENERAL INFORMATION

DEFINITION—Surgical replacement and repair of an injured or diseased shoulder to re-establish a movable joint.

BODY PARTS INVOLVED—Shoulder joint; muscles, ligaments, bones, cartilage and bursa forming the shoulder joint.

REASONS FOR SURGERY—Diseased or injured shoulder causing chronic pain or disability impairing the quality of life. Disorders treated include rheumatoid arthritis, osteoarthritis, rotator cuff arthropathy, avascular necrosis, congenital defects, old trauma and failed shoulder prosthesis.

SURGICAL RISK INCREASES WITH
- Obesity; smoking.
- Excess alcohol consumption.
- Recent or chronic illness.
- Diabetes.
- Use of some prescription and nonprescription drugs. Inform your doctor of any drugs, medications, or vitamin and herb supplements you are using or have used in the last month.

WHAT TO EXPECT

WHO OPERATES—Orthopedic surgeon.

WHERE PERFORMED—Hospital.

DIAGNOSTIC TESTS
- Before surgery: X-rays of joint; CT scan or MRI (see Glossary for both); joint aspiration (to check for active infection); blood and urine studies.
- During surgery: X-rays.
- After surgery: X-rays, blood tests, and examination of tissue removed.

ANESTHESIA—General anesthesia by injection and inhalation with an airway tube placed in the windpipe.

DESCRIPTION OF OPERATION
- An incision is made into the affected shoulder.
- The surgeon will do any repair work necessary; there may be a need to remove tissue fragments, reattach tendons to bones and muscles, stitch or staple torn tissue.
- A total shoulder replacement may be necessary for severe shoulder disability. One type is designed to maintain and reproduce the normal anatomy of the shoulder joint. Another type may be used if there is rotator cuff damage that cannot be repaired.
- The incision is closed with stitches and bandaged. The shoulder is immobilized in a sling, splint or cast that is left on for 2 to 3 weeks.

POSSIBLE COMPLICATIONS
- Excessive bleeding; blood clots.
- Surgical-wound infection.
- Accidental fracture of the shoulder bones.
- Failure or loosening of the components of the shoulder replacement.
- Formation of bone in areas where there should be none.

AVERAGE HOSPITAL STAY—2 to 4 days.

PROBABLE OUTCOME—Expect complete healing without complications. Allow about 6 months for recovery from surgery.

POSTOPERATIVE CARE

GENERAL MEASURES
- No smoking.
- A hard ridge should form along the incision. As it heals, the ridge will gradually recede.
- Shower as usual after discharge. You may wash the incision gently with mild, unscented soap.
- Use an electric heating pad, a heat lamp or a warm compress to relieve incisional pain.

MEDICATION
- Your doctor may prescribe:
  - Pain relievers. Don't take prescription pain medication longer than 4 to 7 days. Use only as much as you need.
  - Antibiotics to fight or prevent infection. If you have an artificial shoulder joint, use antibiotics before future dental work.
- You may use nonprescription drugs, such as acetaminophen, for minor pain. Avoid aspirin.

ACTIVITY
- As prescribed and directed by your surgeon and physical therapist. Passive exercises can begin 3-6 days after surgery. A sustained rehabilitation program is important to regain as much shoulder mobility as possible.
- Avoid very active sports such as tennis, skiing, swimming or contact sports.
- Resume driving when your doctor determines that healing is complete.

DIET—Eat a well-balanced diet to promote healing.

CALL YOUR DOCTOR IF

- Pain, swelling, redness, drainage or bleeding increases in the surgical area.
- You develop signs of infection, including headache, muscle aches, dizziness or a general ill feeling and fever.
- New, unexplained symptoms develop. Drugs used in treatment may produce side effects.

ARTHROPLASTY, SHOULDER

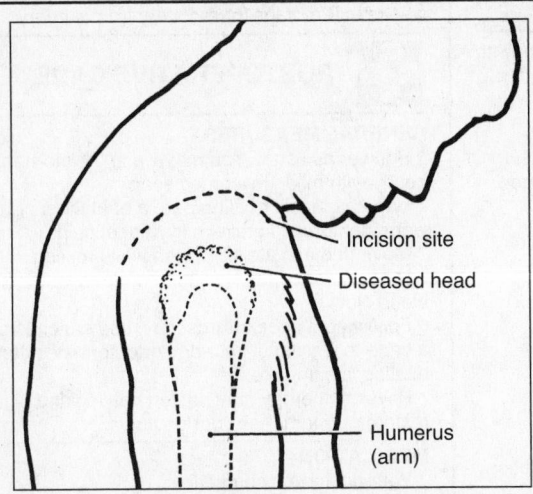

Shoulder is prepared for incision.

Incision site

Diseased head

Humerus
(arm)

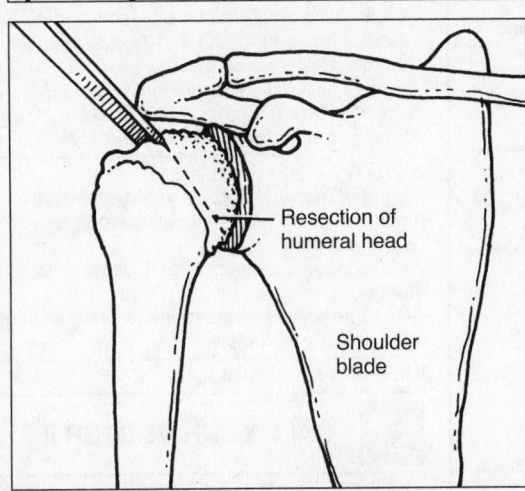

After the humeral head has been surgically exposed, the diseased surface is removed.

Resection of
humeral head

Shoulder
blade

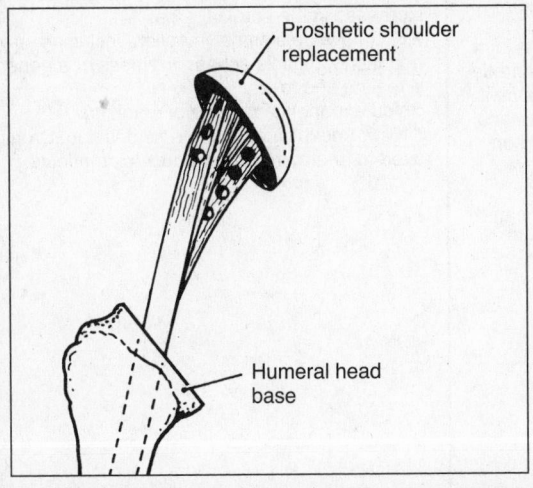

Prosthetic shoulder
replacement

A prosthetic device is inserted into the humeral base. Cement is used to adhere device to the bone. Shoulder is closed and immobilized for a period of time (not illustrated).

Humeral head
base

ARTHROSCOPY

GENERAL INFORMATION

DEFINITION—Visual examination of a joint with an arthroscope, a fiber-optic instrument with a lighted tip (with or without repair of damaged tissue).

BODY PARTS INVOLVED—Joint, usually in the knee, but often performed in the shoulder.

REASONS FOR SURGERY
* Diagnosis of disease or injury inside a joint.
* Removal of bone or cartilage or repair of tendons or ligaments.

SURGICAL RISK INCREASES WITH
* Adults over 60.
* Obesity; smoking.
* Poor nutrition.
* Recent or chronic illness.
* Diabetes.
* Use of some prescription and nonprescription drugs. Inform your doctor of any drugs, medications, or vitamin and herb supplements you are using or have used in the last month.

WHAT TO EXPECT

WHO OPERATES—Orthopedist.

WHERE PERFORMED—Hospital or outpatient surgical facility.

DIAGNOSTIC TESTS
* Before surgery: Blood and urine studies; x-rays of joint.
* After surgery: Blood studies; x-rays; examination of removed fluid or tissue.

ANESTHESIA
* Local anesthesia by injection.
* Spinal anesthesia by injection.
* General anesthesia by injection and inhalation with an airway tube placed in the windpipe.

DESCRIPTION OF OPERATION
* A small incision is made at the side of the joint to be examined (several openings may be made for a complete examination). The arthroscope is inserted into the joint. Diagnostic and/or surgical procedures are then performed, depending on the problem.
* The arthroscope is removed. The skin is closed with sutures or clips, which usually can be removed about 7 to 10 days after surgery.

POSSIBLE COMPLICATIONS
* Bleeding into joint.
* Surgical-wound infection.
* Slow healing.

AVERAGE HOSPITAL STAY—0 to 1 day.

PROBABLE OUTCOME—Expect complete healing without complications. Allow about 6 weeks to 3 months for recovery from surgery.

POSTOPERATIVE CARE

GENERAL MEASURES
* Shower as usual. You may wash the incision gently with mild, unscented soap.
* Use an electric heating pad, a heat lamp or a warm compress to relieve incisional pain.
* Move and elevate legs often while resting in bed to decrease the likelihood of deep-vein blood clots.
* Following a knee arthroscopy, use crutches or a cane to walk until your doctor determines that healing is complete.
* Physical therapy may hasten healing and restore strength. Ask your doctor.

MEDICATION
* Your doctor may prescribe:
  - Pain relievers. Don't take prescription pain medication longer than 4 to 7 days. Use only as much as you need.
  - Antibiotics to fight or prevent infection.
* You may use nonprescription drugs, such as acetaminophen, for minor pain. Avoid aspirin.

ACTIVITY
* To help recovery and aid your well-being, resume daily activities, including work, as soon as you are able.
* Avoid vigorous exercise for 6 weeks after surgery.
* Resume driving when your doctor determines that healing is complete.

DIET—No special diet.

CALL YOUR DOCTOR IF

* Pain, swelling, redness, drainage or bleeding increases in the surgical area.
* You develop signs of infection, including headache, muscle aches, dizziness or a general ill feeling and fever.
* You experience nausea or vomiting.
* New, unexplained symptoms develop. Drugs used in treatment may produce side effects.

ARTHROSCOPY

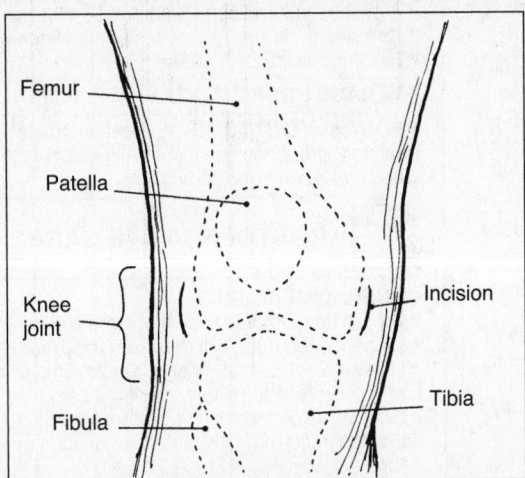

Femur

Patella

Knee
joint

Fibula

Incision

Tibia

An illustration of the knee joint area
frequently examined by arthroscopy.

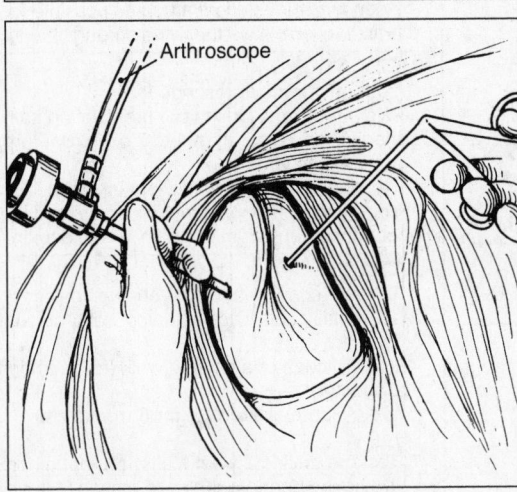

Arthroscope

After an incision is made at the side
of the joint to be examined, the
arthroscope is inserted into the joint.
 • The operator inspects the joint
   and performs whatever surgical
   procedures are indicated.

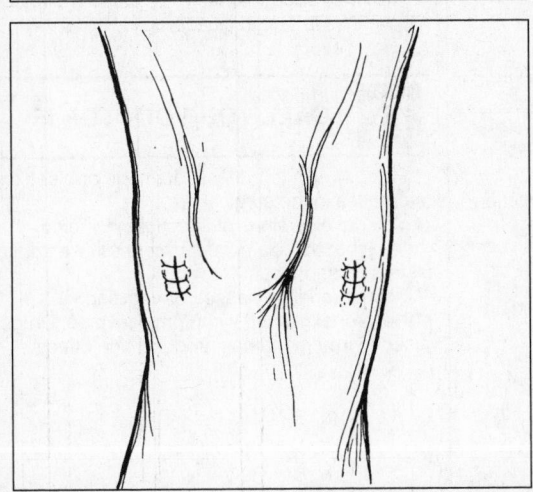

After the arthroscope is removed, the
small incisions in the skin are closed.

BAKER'S CYST REMOVAL

GENERAL INFORMATION

DEFINITION—Removal of Baker's cyst, a benign cystic tumor on the back of the knee joint. The cyst consists of accumulated fluid that protrudes between two groups of muscles behind the knee. Baker's cyst may result from injury or from diseases, such as arthritis, gout or inflammation of the membrane lining the knee joint.

BODY PARTS INVOLVED—Space behind the knee joint on either or both sides of the knee.

REASONS FOR SURGERY—If the cyst has resulted from disease, it may disappear after successful treatment of the underlying disease. Often, local steroid injections are successful in treating a Baker's cyst. Otherwise, the cyst is removed when it becomes painful or unsightly. In children, the cyst is usually left to heal by itself, and is not removed unless it presses on nerves or blood vessels.

SURGICAL RISK INCREASES WITH
* Obesity; smoking.
* Poor nutrition.
* Recent or chronic illness.
* Diabetes.
* Use of some prescription and nonprescription drugs. Inform your doctor of any drugs, medications, or vitamin and herb supplements you are using or have used in the last month.

WHAT TO EXPECT

WHO OPERATES—General surgeon or orthopedist.

WHERE PERFORMED—Outpatient surgical facility or hospital.

DIAGNOSTIC TESTS
* Before surgery: Blood and urine studies; x-rays of both knees; ultrasound; venography; arthrograms (see Glossary for all).
* After surgery: Blood studies; examination of tissue removed.

ANESTHESIA
* Local anesthesia by injection.
* Spinal anesthesia by injection.
* General anesthesia by injection and inhalation with an airway tube placed in the windpipe.

DESCRIPTION OF OPERATION
* An incision is made over the cyst.
* The cyst is located, cut free from surrounding tissue and removed.
* A synthetic patch is sometimes sutured in place to cover the defect left from removal of the cyst.
* The skin is closed with fine sutures, which usually can be removed about 2 weeks after surgery.

POSSIBLE COMPLICATIONS
* Excessive bleeding.
* Surgical-wound infection.
* Slow healing and continued pain.
* Damage to nerves or arteries behind knee.
* Recurrence (rare).

AVERAGE HOSPITAL STAY—0 to 1 day.

PROBABLE OUTCOME—Expect complete healing without complications. Allow about 4 weeks for recovery from surgery.

POSTOPERATIVE CARE

GENERAL MEASURES
* A hard ridge should form along the incision. As it heals, the ridge will gradually recede.
* Use an electric heating pad, a heat lamp or a warm compress to relieve incisional pain.
* Shower as usual after discharge. You may wash the incision gently with mild, unscented soap.
* Keep legs elevated as much as possible for the first several days following surgery.

MEDICATION
* Your doctor may prescribe:
  - Pain relievers. Don't take prescription pain medication longer than 4 to 7 days. Use only as much as you need.
  - Antibiotics to fight or prevent infection.
* You may use nonprescription drugs, such as acetaminophen, for minor pain. Avoid aspirin.

ACTIVITY
* To help recovery and aid your well-being, resume daily activities, including work, as soon as you are able.
* Use crutches or a cane to walk (as directed by your doctor).
* Avoid vigorous exercise for 6 weeks after surgery.
* Resume driving 2 weeks after returning home if you have adequate range-of-motion in knee.

DIET—Eat a well-balanced diet to promote healing.

CALL YOUR DOCTOR IF

* Pain, swelling, redness, drainage or bleeding increases in the surgical area.
* You develop signs of infection, including headache, muscle aches, dizziness or a general ill feeling and fever.
* You experience nausea or vomiting.
* New, unexplained symptoms develop. Drugs used in treatment may produce side effects.

BAKER'S CYST REMOVAL

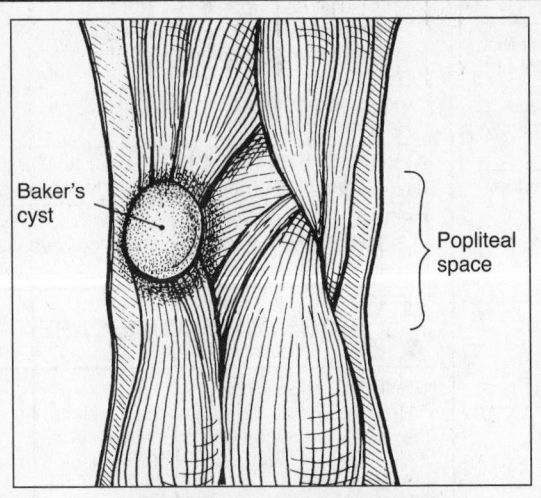

An illustration of a Baker's cyst located in the popliteal space behind the knee joint.

Baker's cyst

Popliteal space

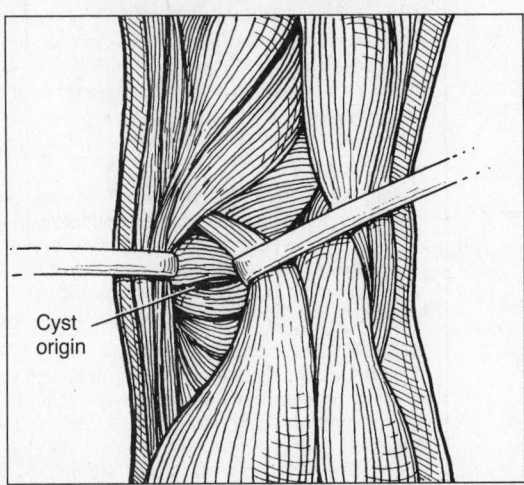

Muscles pulled apart to expose the area where the cyst begins.

Cyst origin

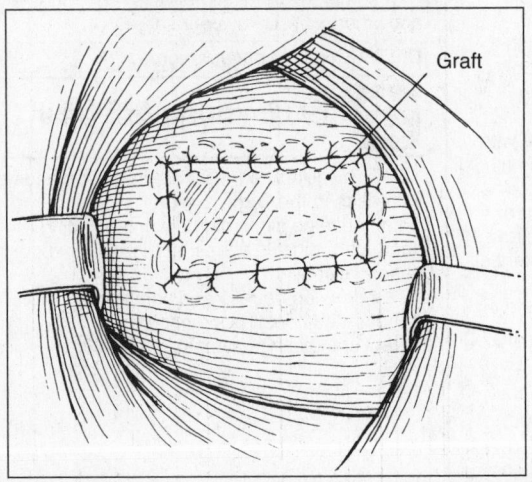

Synthetic patch sutured in place to cover the defect left after surgical removal of the cyst.

Graft

BARIATRIC SURGERY (Gastric Bypass)

 ## GENERAL INFORMATION

DEFINITION—A surgical procedure to limit food intake and absorption with the ultimate goal of losing weight.

BODY PARTS INVOLVED—Abdominal cavity, stomach, small intestines.

REASONS FOR SURGERY—To treat morbid obesity.

SURGICAL RISK INCREASES WITH
* Age.
* Diabetes.
* Poor kidney function.
* High blood pressure.
* Chronic lung disease.
* Degree of obesity.

 ## WHAT TO EXPECT

WHO OPERATES—General surgeon.

WHERE PERFORMED—Hospital.

DIAGNOSTIC TESTS
* Before surgery: Blood tests, chest x-ray, EKG (see Glossary).
* After surgery: Blood tests.

ANESTHESIA—General anesthesia.

DESCRIPTION OF OPERATION
* There are two main types of surgery done for weight loss—restrictive operations to limit the stomach size and bypass operations to limit the absorption of food. Sometimes a combination of the two is done.
* The most common restrictive operations involve a small upper abdominal incision. A "band-like" device is placed around the upper stomach to limit the flow of food through the stomach and into the intestines. This is usually adjustable to permit more food or less food if needed. Another method of restriction is performed using staples across the stomach with a small opening for food to pass through. These procedures can often be done using laparoscopy rather than an incision.
* The bypass procedure is often combined with making the stomach pouch smaller. The small intestine is then brought up to this shortened stomach so that only the last couple of feet of intestine is exposed to the food passing through, severely limiting absorption of potential calories.

POSSIBLE COMPLICATIONS
* Bleeding.
* Kidney failure.
* Failure of bowel connections to heal with leakage of intestinal contents.
* Blood clots.
* Incisional hernia.
* Respiratory failure.

AVERAGE HOSPITAL STAY—Usually 3-10 days (depending on the procedure done).

PROBABLE OUTCOME—Expect full recovery in 6-8 weeks with continued weight loss over 1-2 years.

 ## POSTOPERATIVE CARE

GENERAL MEASURES
* Hard ridges will form along the incisions. As they heal, the ridges will gradually recede.
* Use heat on the incision to help relieve incisional pain.
* Shower as usual. You may wash the incisions gently with mild soap. After showering, replace any dressings with a new dry dressing.
* Wear compression stockings when up for the first few weeks after surgery.
* Discuss diet with your surgeon.

MEDICATION
* Your doctor may prescribe pain relievers. Use only as much as you need to be comfortable.
* You may use nonprescription pain relievers such as acetaminophen for minor pain. Ask your doctor if it is okay to take ibuprofen or aspirin.

ACTIVITY
* Start ambulating (walking) as soon as you are home. Take frequent naps as needed during the day when tired. Avoid strenuous activity for 6 to 8 weeks.
* You may swim once all sutures are out.
* Resume sexual relations when comfortable and when advised by your surgeon.

DIET—Consult your surgeon.

 ## CALL YOUR DOCTOR IF

* Pain, swelling, redness, drainage or bleeding increases in the surgical area.
* You develop signs of infection, including headache, muscle aches, dizziness, fever, or a general ill feeling.
* You develop nausea and vomiting.
* Prolonged constipation occurs.
* New unexplained symptoms develop.

BARIATRIC SURGERY (Gastric Bypass)

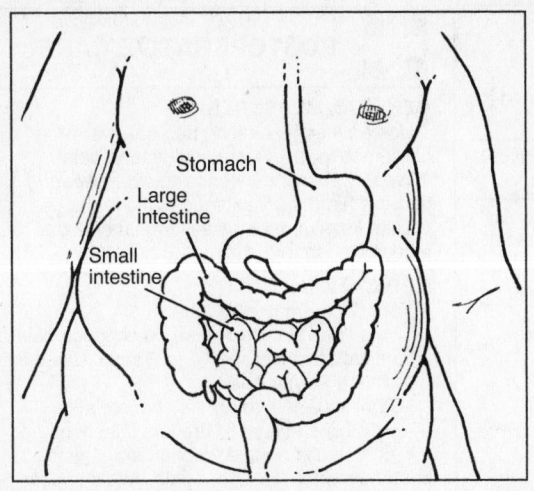

An illustration of the stomach and surrounding structures.

Stomach

Large intestine

Small intestine

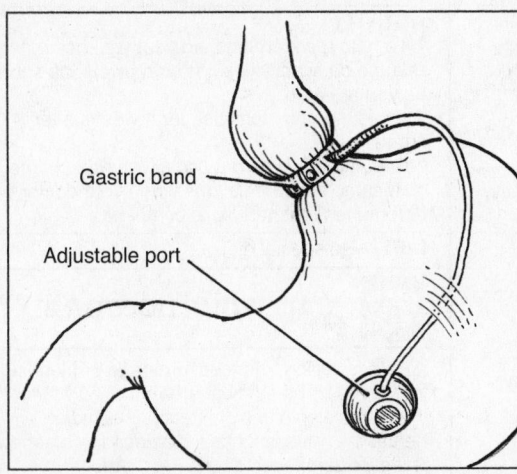

One method of restricting food passage is a mechanical banding of the upper stomach. The port is used to adjust the constriction of the band.

Gastric band

Adjustable port

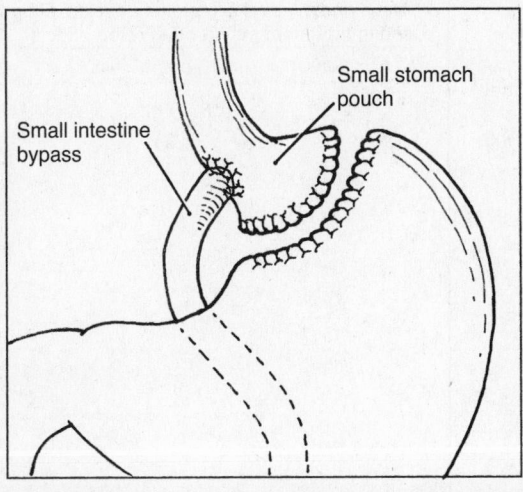

Another method is to reduce the size of the stomach pouch and reattach it to a shortened segment of the small intestine.

Small stomach pouch

Small intestine bypass

BARTHOLIN'S GLAND, ABSCESS DRAINAGE

GENERAL INFORMATION

DEFINITION—Removal of a blockage of the Bartholin's glands caused by a cyst or an abscess (on accumulation of mucus or infection). These two small glands are located in the base of the vaginal lips.

BODY PARTS INVOLVED—Bartholin's glands; lips of vagina.

REASONS FOR SURGERY—Appropriate treatment of an abscess or cyst which will result in near immediate relief of symptoms and will reduce the risk of subsequent infection.

SURGICAL RISK INCREASES WITH
* Obesity.
* Smoking.
* Poor nutrition.
* Recent illness.
* Alcoholism or chronic illness.
* Diabetes.
* Use of some prescription and nonprescription drugs. Inform your doctor of any drugs, medications, or vitamin and herb supplements you are using or have used in the last month.

WHAT TO EXPECT

WHO OPERATES—Obstetrician-gynecologist, family doctor or general surgeon.

WHERE PERFORMED—Doctor's office, outpatient surgical facility or hospital.

DIAGNOSTIC TESTS
* Before surgery: Blood and urine studies; laboratory examination of vaginal discharge.
* After surgery: Laboratory examination of pus or secretions from opened glands.

ANESTHESIA
* Local anesthesia by injection.
* Regional anesthesia by injection.
* General anesthesia; usually by inhalation.

DESCRIPTION OF OPERATION
* A small incision is made in the labia over the area of the abscess. A catheter is placed through the incision, and is allowed to drain into the vagina. The catheter is left in place for approximately 2 weeks.
* The alternate method is marsupialization. In this procedure, the edges of the glands are opened and the linings are folded back and sewn open. This forms a small pouch that drains easily. Sutures that will be absorbed by the body are used to form the pouch.

POSSIBLE COMPLICATIONS
* Excessive bleeding.
* Surgical-wound infection.

AVERAGE HOSPITAL STAY—0 to 1 day.

PROBABLE OUTCOME—Expect complete healing without complications. Allow about 2 weeks for recovery from surgery.

POSTOPERATIVE CARE

GENERAL MEASURES
* Use an electric heating pad or a warm compress to relieve surgical-wound pain.
* Wear cotton underwear and avoid wearing tight clothing, such as snug-fitting jeans.
* Take lukewarm baths several times a day to relieve discomfort.

MEDICATION
* Your doctor may prescribe:
  - Pain relievers. Don't take prescription pain medication longer than 4 to 7 days. Use only as much as you need.
  - Stool softeners to prevent constipation.
  - Antibiotics to fight or prevent infection.
* You may use nonprescription drugs, such as acetaminophen, for minor pain. Avoid aspirin.

ACTIVITY
* To help recovery and aid your well-being, resume daily activities, including work, as soon as you are able.
* Avoid vigorous exercise for 4 weeks after surgery.
* Resume driving 4 days after returning home.
* Resume sexual relations when your doctor determines that healing is complete.

DIET—No special diet.

CALL YOUR DOCTOR IF

* Pain, swelling, redness, drainage or bleeding increases in the surgical area.
* You develop signs of infection, including headache, muscle aches, dizziness or a general ill feeling and fever.
* New, unexplained symptoms develop. Drugs used in treatment may produce side effects.

BARTHOLIN'S GLAND, ABSCESS DRAINAGE

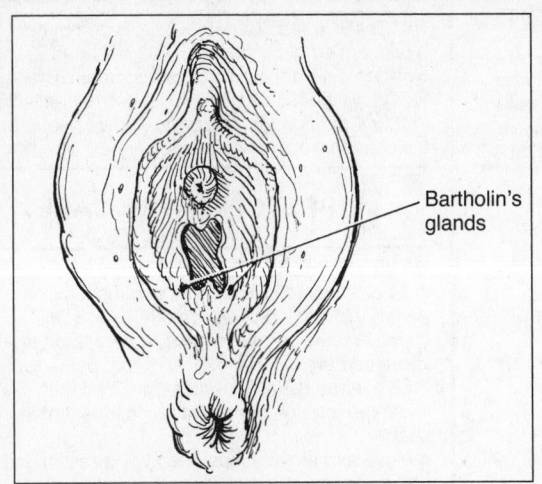

An illustration showing the normal appearance of the Bartholin's glands, which are two small glands located at the base of the vaginal lips.

Bartholin's glands

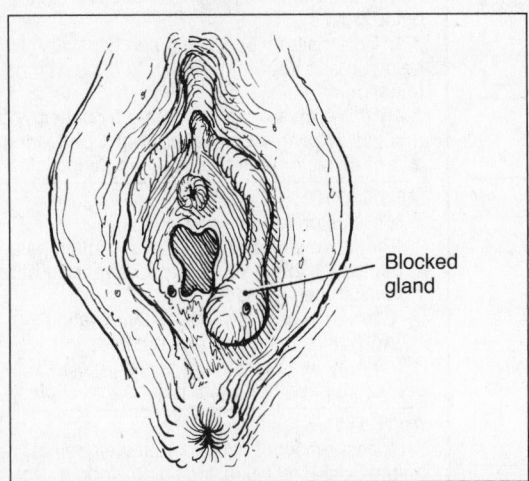

The appearance of a Bartholin's gland which is blocked because of a cyst or abscess.

Blocked gland

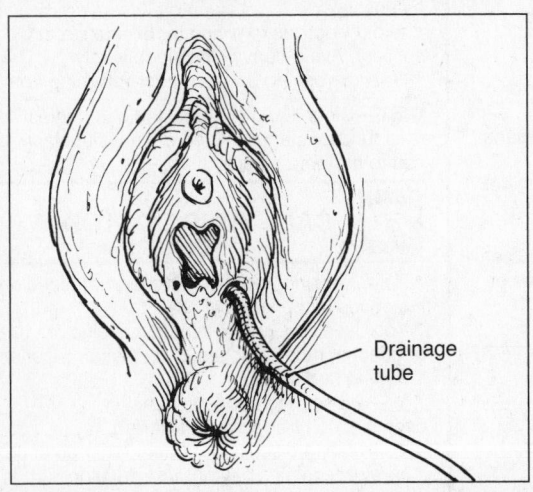

A small incision has been placed in the labia over the area of the abscess. A catheter has been placed in the incision and is allowed to drain into the vagina.

Drainage tube

BLADDER (URINARY) REMOVAL (Cystectomy)

GENERAL INFORMATION

DEFINITION—Removal of the urinary bladder and adjacent tissues and organs, and diversion of the urinary stream. This involves an artificial opening, which is called an "ostomy" or "stoma."

BODY PARTS INVOLVED
• Males: Bladder; prostate; urethra; ureters; seminal vesicles; small intestine.
• Females: Urinary bladder; urethra; ureters; cervix; vagina; small intestine.

REASONS FOR SURGERY—Cancer of the bladder.

SURGICAL RISK INCREASES WITH
• Poor nutrition.
• Obesity.
• Repeated surgeries on the bladder.
• Diabetes.
• Use of some prescription and nonprescription drugs. Inform your doctor of any drugs, medications, or vitamin and herb supplements you are using or have used in the last month.

WHAT TO EXPECT

WHO OPERATES—Urologist.

WHERE PERFORMED—Hospital.

DIAGNOSTIC TESTS
• Before surgery: Blood and urine studies; x-rays of kidneys and chest; ultrasound; CT scan; cystoscopy (see Glossary for all).
• During surgery: Cystoscopy (see Glossary).

ANESTHESIA—General anesthesia by injection and inhalation with an airway tube placed in the windpipe.

DESCRIPTION OF OPERATION
• An incision is made in the abdomen. The muscles are separated and the abdominal cavity is entered.
• The blood supply and the ureters are cut and tied.
• The bladder and adjacent tissues and organs are cut free and removed.
• The ureters are diverted through an intestinal pouch (called an ileal conduit) to an opening made in the skin (the stoma).
• The muscles are replaced and sewn together with sutures. The skin is closed with sutures or clips, which usually can be removed about 1 week after surgery.

POSSIBLE COMPLICATIONS
• Excessive bleeding; blood clots.
• Incisional hernia or infection.
• Impotence in males.
• Recurring urinary tract infections.
• Obstruction of the ureter; leakage of urine.

AVERAGE HOSPITAL STAY— 7 to 10 days.

PROBABLE OUTCOME—Expect complete healing of surgical wounds. You will need to wear an external pouch to collect urine. The stoma will heal and shrink to its permanent size in 2 to 4 months after surgery. Allow about 6 to 8 weeks for recovery from surgery.

POSTOPERATIVE CARE

GENERAL MEASURES
• A hard ridge should form along the incision. As it heals, the ridge will gradually recede.
• Use an electric heating pad, a heat lamp or a warm compress to relieve incisional pain.
• Shower as usual aer discharge. You may wash the incision gently with mild, unscented soap.
• Move and elevate legs often while resting in bed to decrease the likelihood of deep-vein blood clots.
• An enterostomy specialist (see Glossary) will help you and your family learn to cope with new urination habits.
• Dry the area around the stoma by patting, not rubbing. Apply gauze soaked with 1 part vinegar to 3 parts water over the stoma to keep it clean.

MEDICATION
• Your doctor may prescribe:
  - Pain relievers. Don't take prescription pain medication longer than 4 to 7 days. Use only as much as you need.
  - Stool softeners to prevent constipation.
  - Antibiotics to fight or prevent infection.
• You may use nonprescription drugs, such as acetaminophen, for minor pain. Avoid aspirin.

ACTIVITY
• To help recovery and aid your well-being, resume daily activities, including work, as soon as possible.
• Avoid vigorous exercise for 6 weeks after surgery. Avoid heavy lifting indefinitely.
• Resume driving 3 weeks after returning home.

DIET—Clear liquid diet until the gastrointestinal tract functions again. Then eat a well-balanced diet to promote healing.

CALL YOUR DOCTOR IF

• Pain, swelling, redness, drainage or bleeding increases in the surgical area.
• You develop signs of infection, including headache, muscle aches, dizziness or a general ill feeling and fever.
• You experience nausea, vomiting, constipation or abdominal swelling.
• You wish to discuss treatment for impotence.
• New, unexplained symptoms develop. Drugs used in treatment may produce side effects.

BLADDER (URINARY) REMOVAL
(Cystectomy)

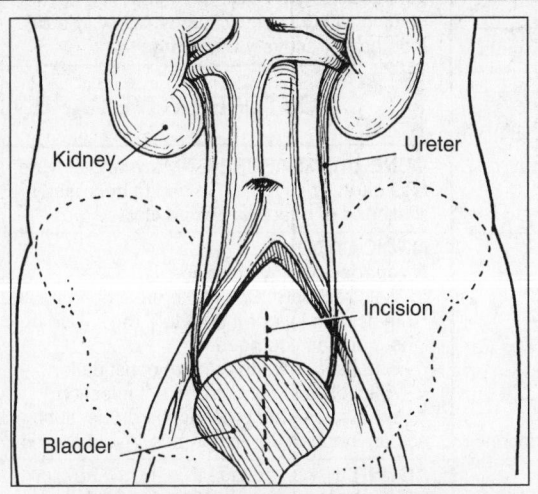

An illustration of the bladder and other parts of the urinary tract.

Kidney

Ureter

Incision

Bladder

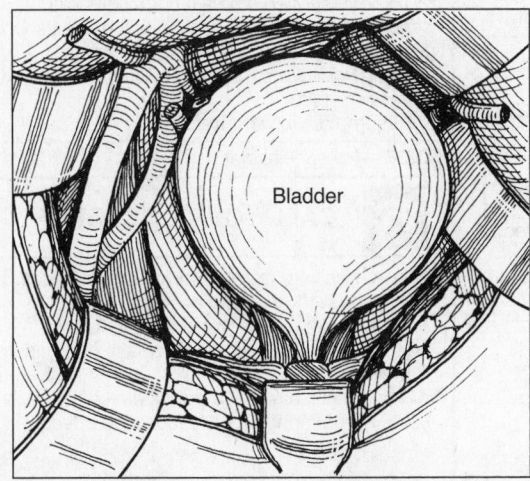

Bladder

The bladder and adjacent tissues and organs are cut free and removed.
- The ureters are divided and an intestinal pouch is created by isolating a small/short segment of small bowel (ileum).

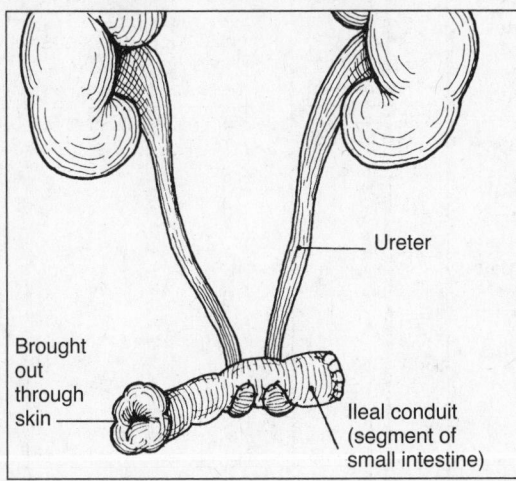

After the bladder has been removed, the ureters are connected to an ileal conduit to drain the kidneys.

Ureter

Brought out through skin

Ileal conduit (segment of small intestine)

SURGERIES

BONE GRAFT

GENERAL INFORMATION

DEFINITION—Filling space between fragments of a broken bone.

BODY PARTS INVOLVED—Bone.

REASONS FOR SURGERY
* Joining of two or more parts of a bone that have broken and not grown back together.
* Fusion of the spine after injury or surgery.

SURGICAL RISK INCREASES WITH
* Adults over 60.
* Obesity.
* Smoking.
* Poor nutrition.
* Diabetes.
* Rheumatoid arthritis.
* Recent or chronic illness.
* Use of some prescription and nonprescription drugs. Inform your doctor of any drugs, medications, or vitamin and herb supplements you are using or have used in the last month.

WHAT TO EXPECT

WHO OPERATES—Orthopedist.

WHERE PERFORMED—Hospital.

DIAGNOSTIC TESTS
* Before surgery: X-rays of area to be grafted; blood and urine studies.
* After surgery: Blood studies; x-rays of grafted area.

ANESTHESIA—General anesthesia by injection and inhalation with an airway tube placed in the windpipe.

DESCRIPTION OF OPERATION
* If bone for the graft is to be an autograft (taken from the patient), it is usually removed from the top of the hip bone, the spine, or the ribs. Otherwise, bone is obtained from a bone bank (see Glossary).
* An incision is made over the affected bone. The bone is located and isolated.
* The bone to be grafted is shaped to fit the affected area. The bone is held in place with wire or screws.
* The skin is closed with sutures or clips, which usually can be removed about 1 week after surgery.
* A splint or plaster cast keeps the affected part rigid and promotes healing (sometimes).

POSSIBLE COMPLICATIONS
* Excessive bleeding.
* Surgical-wound infection.
* Rejection of transplanted bone.
* Continued non-healing.

AVERAGE HOSPITAL STAY—7 to 10 days.

PROBABLE OUTCOME—Expect complete healing without complications. Allow about 3 months for recovery from surgery.

POSTOPERATIVE CARE

GENERAL MEASURES—Move and elevate legs often while resting in bed to decrease the likelihood of deep-vein blood clots.

MEDICATION
* Your doctor may prescribe:
  - Pain relievers. Don't take prescription pain medication longer than 4 to 7 days. Use only as much as you need.
  - Stool softeners to prevent constipation.
  - Antibiotics to fight or prevent infection.
* You may use nonprescription drugs, such as acetaminophen, for minor pain. Avoid aspirin.

ACTIVITY
* To help recovery and aid your well-being, resume daily activities, including work, as soon as your doctor advises that you are able.
* Avoid vigorous exercise for 3 months after surgery.
* Resume driving when able.

DIET—No special diet.

CALL YOUR DOCTOR IF

* Pain, swelling, redness, drainage or bleeding increases in the surgical area.
* You develop signs of infection, including headache, muscle aches, dizziness or a general ill feeling and fever.
* New, unexplained symptoms develop. Drugs used in treatment may produce side effects.

BONE GRAFT

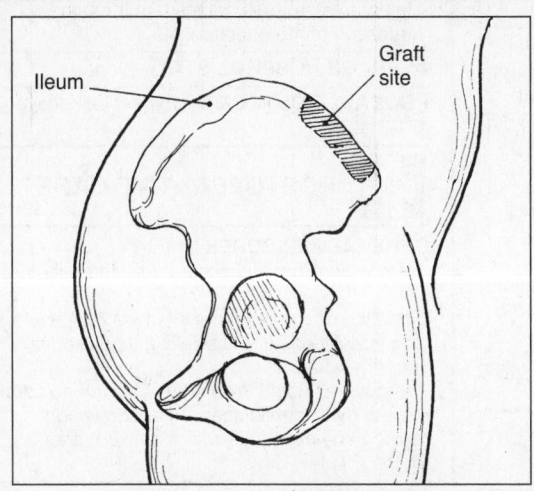

Ileum

Graft site

An illustration of a frequent bone graft site. In this case, located on the crest of the ileum (hip bone).
(These illustrations are used as examples. The principles and techniques are similar for bone grafts in other locations.)

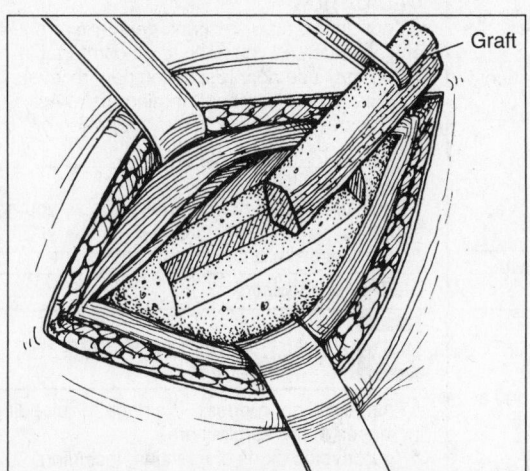

Graft

After muscles and covering tissues are separated, the segment of bone is removed from its normal site.

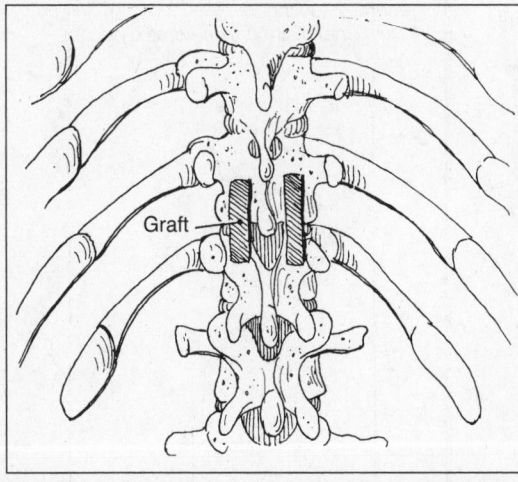

Graft

The bone graft is transplanted to another part of the body (in this example, the spine) where it will provide stabilization.

BONE MARROW ASPIRATION & BIOPSY

 GENERAL INFORMATION

DEFINITION—Drawing tissue and cells from the marrow of one of the large bones in order to study the number and types of cells present.

BODY PARTS INVOLVED—Usually pelvis bone, sometimes sternum or leg bone.

REASONS FOR SURGERY—To determine if there are abnormal cells, such as tumor cells, or to see if there are adequate numbers of the cells which make up the various blood components. The two most common indications are to look for cancer cells like leukemias or to try to determine a cause for anemia..

SURGICAL RISK INCREASES WITH—Clotting disorders.

 WHAT TO EXPECT

WHO OPERATES—Hematologist-oncologist or internist.

WHERE PERFORMED—Hospital or outpatient facility or physician's office.

DIAGNOSTIC TESTS
• Before procedure: None other than those to work up underlying disease process.
• After procedure: Laboratory study of removed tissue and cells.

ANESTHESIA—Local anaesthesia, local with sedation, or general anaesthesia

DESCRIPTION OF OPERATION
• The biopsy/aspiration is usually performed in the posterior portion of the pelvis bone.
• A local anesthetic is injected over the site and a large bore needle is pushed down against the outer cortex of the bone. The needle is then pushed through the outer bone and enters the marrow space. A syringe is used to aspirate tissue and cells from the marrow and the needle is withdrawn.
• There is frequently sharp pain elicited by the aspiration of cells. No sutures are required.

POSSIBLE COMPLICATIONS
• Bleeding from the puncture site.
• Injury to structures adjacent to the bone.
• Infection of the puncture site.

AVERAGE HOSPITAL STAY—None.

PROBABLE OUTCOME—Expect full recovery in 1-2 days.

 POSTOPERATIVE CARE

GENERAL MEASURES
• Slight swelling may occur under the puncture site
• Use ice on the puncture site for 12-24 hours to minimize bleeding and swelling if advised by your physician.
• Shower as usual. You may wash the puncture site gently with mild soap. After showering, replace any dressings with a new dry dressing for the first few days.

MEDICATION
• Your doctor may prescribe pain relievers. Use only as much as you need to be comfortable.
• You may use nonprescription pain relievers such as acetaminophen for minor pain. Ask your doctor if it is okay to take ibuprofen or aspirin.

ACTIVITY
• Start ambulating (walking) as soon as you are home.
• You may swim once all sutures are out.

DIET—No special diet.

 CALL YOUR DOCTOR IF

• Pain, swelling, redness, drainage, or bleeding increases in the surgical area.
• You develop signs of infection, including headache, muscle aches, dizziness, fever, or a general ill feeling.
• New unexplained symptoms develop.

BONE MARROW ASPIRATION & BIOPSY

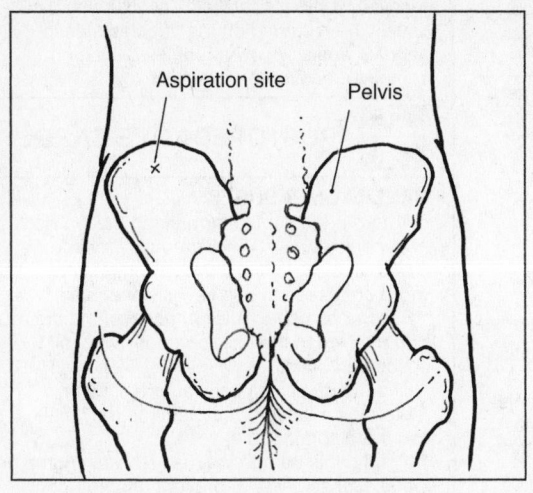

A site is chosen on the posterior and lateral portion of the pelvis bone.

Aspiration site   Pelvis

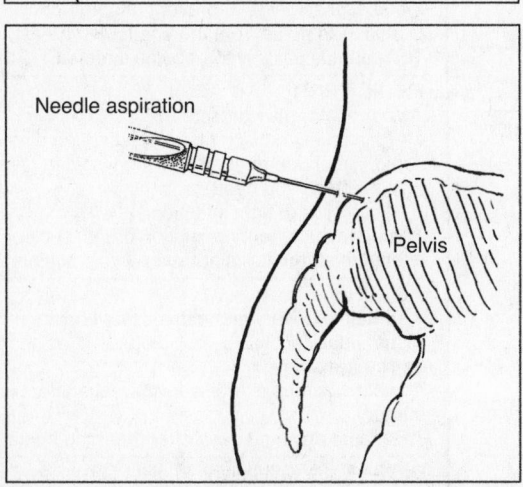

A needle is inserted through the skin and pushed through the outer layer of the bone.

Needle aspiration

Pelvis

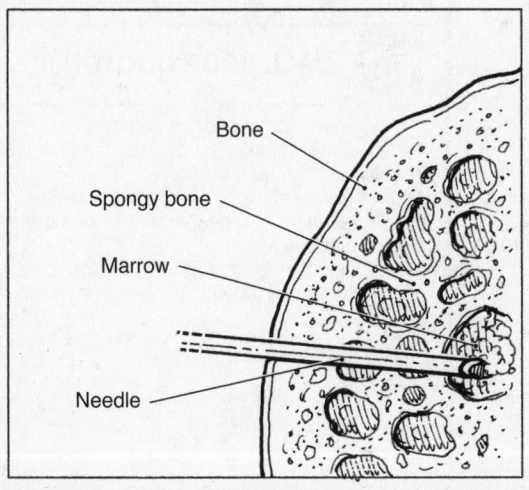

Cells and fluid are aspirated from the soft marrow of the pelvic bone.

Bone

Spongy bone

Marrow

Needle

BREAST ABSCESS DRAINAGE

 GENERAL INFORMATION

DEFINITION—To open and drain an abscess in the female breast.

BODY PARTS INVOLVED—Lactating breast; nipple; lactiferous ducts.

REASONS FOR SURGERY—Relief of pain and prevention of the spread of infection.

SURGICAL RISK INCREASES WITH
- Obesity.
- Smoking.
- Poor nutrition.
- Recent or chronic illness.
- Diabetes.
- Use of some prescription and nonprescription drugs. Inform your doctor of any drugs, medications, or vitamin and herb supplements you are using or have used in the last month.

 WHAT TO EXPECT

WHO OPERATES—General surgeon or obstetrician-gynecologist.

WHERE PERFORMED—Hospital, emergency room, doctor's office or outpatient surgical facility.

DIAGNOSTIC TESTS
- Before surgery: Blood and urine studies; ultrasound; mammogram; aspiration (see Glossary for all).
- After surgery: Laboratory examination of removed pus.

ANESTHESIA
- Local anesthesia by injection.
- General anesthesia by injection and inhalation with an airway tube placed in the windpipe.

DESCRIPTION OF OPERATION
- An incision is made in the breast over the abscess. The incision is deepened and pus is removed.
- An instrument is forced into the abscess. Pockets of pus are broken up by the surgeon's finger. The opening is enlarged and the area is irrigated with a salt solution.
- Gauze packing is inserted to allow drainage. A small, plastic tube may be placed in the incision to collect additional pus and allow drainage. The drain or gauze packing is usually removed 3 to 5 days following surgery.

POSSIBLE COMPLICATIONS
- Excessive bleeding.
- Surgical-wound infection.
- Slow healing.
- Breast engorgement, if breast is not emptied regularly of milk. Leakage of milk through incision
- Recurrence of abscess.

AVERAGE HOSPITAL STAY—0 to 2 days.

PROBABLE OUTCOME—Expect complete recovery without complications. Nursing can usually be resumed on the affected side in about 2 weeks. Allow about 3 weeks for complete recovery from surgery.

 POSTOPERATIVE CARE

GENERAL MEASURES
- A hard ridge should form along the incision. As it heals, the ridge will gradually recede.
- Use an electric heating pad, a heat lamp or a warm compress to relieve incisional pain.
- Shower as usual. After removal of the drain, You may wash the incision gently with mild, unscented soap.
- Change dressings daily after a shower.
- Wearing a loose bra at bedtime may make you more comfortable.
- If you continue nursing, use a breast pump on the abscessed side to prevent engorgement. Continue to nurse from the unaffected breast. The infant is unlikely to become infected.

MEDICATION
- Your doctor may prescribe:
  - Pain relievers. Don't take prescription pain medication longer than 4 to 7 days. Use only as much as you need.
  - Antibiotics to fight infection.
- You may use nonprescription drugs, such as acetaminophen, for minor pain. Avoid aspirin.

ACTIVITY
- To help recovery and aid your well-being, resume daily activities, including work, as soon as you are able.
- Avoid vigorous exercise for 3 weeks after surgery.
- Resume driving 2 days after returning home.

DIET—Eat a well-balanced diet to promote healing. Drink at least 8 glasses of water daily.

 CALL YOUR DOCTOR IF

- You experience nausea or vomiting.
- Pain, swelling, redness, drainage or bleeding increases in the surgical area.
- You develop signs of infection, including headache, muscle aches, dizziness or a general ill feeling and fever.
- New, unexplained symptoms develop. Drugs used in treatment may produce side effects.

BREAST ABSCESS DRAINAGE

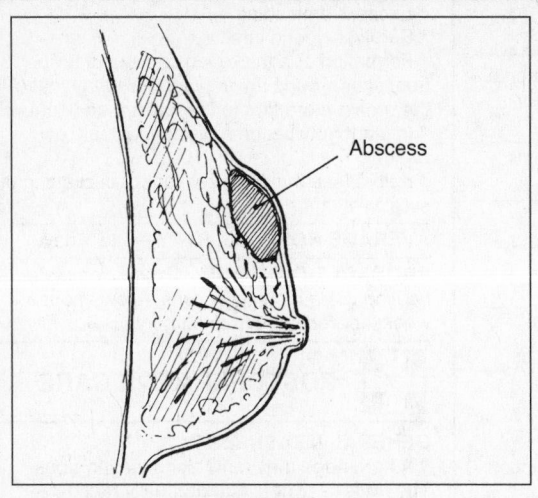

A side illustration of a breast abscess that has become red, warm and fluctuant.

Abscess

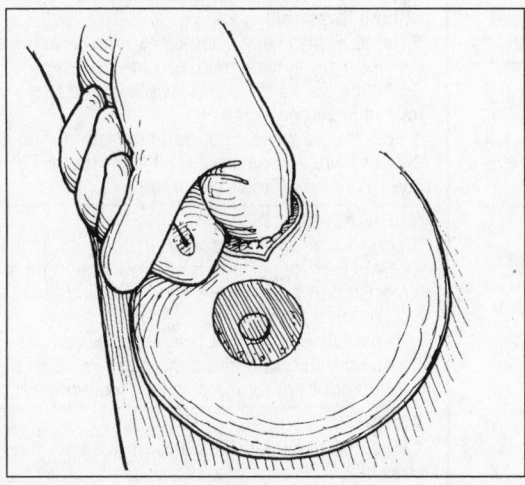

The incision is made into the abscess cavity, a pocket is created, the incision is deepened and pus is removed. An instrument having been forced into the abscess, pockets of pus are now broken up by the surgeon's finger. The opening is enlarged and the area is irrigated with a salt solution. Gauze packing is inserted for drainage.

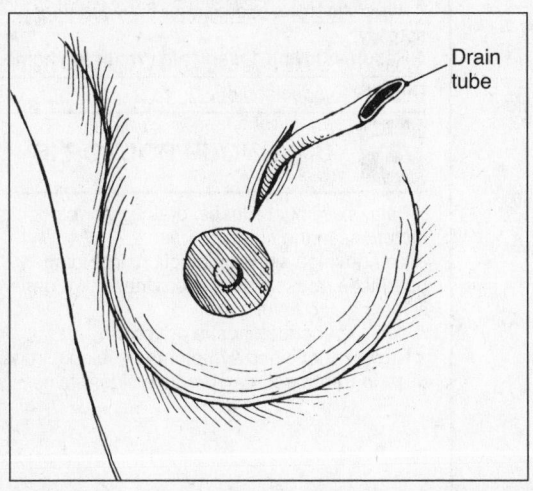

Drain tube

A small, plastic drain may be placed in the incision to collect additional pus and allow drainage. The drain or gauze packing remains in place for several days and is then removed.

SURGERIES

BREAST AUGMENTATION
(Augmentation Mammoplasty)

 GENERAL INFORMATION

DEFINITION—Implantation of artificial material inside the female breasts to enlarge them or give them a different shape.

BODY PARTS INVOLVED—Female breasts; underlying muscles.

REASONS FOR SURGERY
• Enlargement of the breasts in patients who have less breast tissue than they desire.
• Correction of asymmetry of the breasts.

SURGICAL RISK INCREASES WITH
• Smoking.
• Obesity.
• Excess alcohol consumption.
• Recent or chronic illness.
• Diabetes.
• Use of some prescription and nonprescription drugs. Inform your doctor of any drugs, medications, or vitamin and herb supplements you are using or have used in the last month.

 WHAT TO EXPECT

WHO OPERATES—Plastic and reconstructive surgeon.

WHERE PERFORMED—Hospital; doctor's office; or outpatient surgical facility.

DIAGNOSTIC TESTS
• Before surgery: Blood studies; mammogram (see Glossary).
• After surgery: Usually none.

ANESTHESIA
• General anesthesia by injection and inhalation.
• Local anesthesia with sedation.

DESCRIPTION OF OPERATION
• Incisions may be made under the breast, through the nipple or in the armpit.
• The breast tissue is brought forward by raising muscles from below the breast or the muscles next to the chest wall.
• A pocket is created, and the implant (a mammary prosthesis filled with saline) is inserted. The procedures are usually repeated on the other breast.
• The skin is closed with sutures or clips, which usually can be removed about 1 week after surgery. A light bandage is applied.
• Occasionally, a drain may be left in place for several days to promote healing.
• A bra or elastic bandage is fitted to give support and to reduce possible bleeding.

POSSIBLE COMPLICATIONS
• Excessive bleeding.
• Surgical-wound infection.
• Formation of a thickened capsule of tissue from scar around the implant. This may make the breast more firm to the touch than usual.
• Implant may become dislodged, leak, or rupture.
• Keloid (see in Illness section) or thickening of surgical scars.

AVERAGE HOSPITAL STAY—0 to 1 day.

PROBABLE OUTCOME—Expect complete healing without complications. Allow about 2 weeks for recovery from surgery.

 POSTOPERATIVE CARE

GENERAL MEASURES
• A hard ridge may form along the incisions. The ridges will heal and gradually recede without treatment.
• Bathe or shower as usual. You may wash the incisions gently with mild, unscented soap.
• Use ice packs to reduce swelling and to relieve incisional pain.
• You should wear a support bra both during the day and while you sleep, until your doctor determines that healing is complete.

MEDICATION
• Your doctor may prescribe:
  - Pain relievers. Don't take prescription pain medication longer than 4 to 7 days. Use only as much as you need.
  - Antibiotics to fight or prevent infection.
• You may use nonprescription drugs, such as acetaminophen, for minor pain. Avoid aspirin.

ACTIVITY
• Resume daily activities and work as soon as possible.
• Avoid vigorous exercise for 6 weeks after surgery.
• Resume driving 1 week after returning home.

DIET—No special diet.

 CALL YOUR DOCTOR IF

• Pain, swelling, redness, drainage or bleeding increases in the surgical area.
• You develop signs of infection, including headache, muscle aches, dizziness or a general ill feeling and fever.
• You experience nausea or vomiting.
• New, unexplained symptoms develop. Drugs used in treatment may produce side effects.

BREAST AUGMENTATION
(Augmentation Mammoplasty)

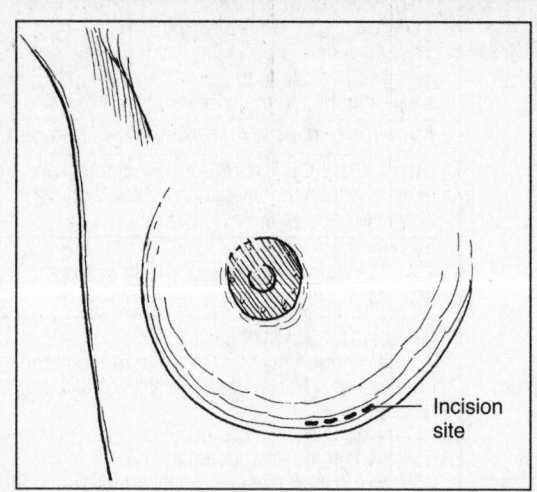

Incision site

Incisions for the implant may be made under the breast, through the nipple or in the armpit. In this example, it is under the breast line in the chest wall skin.

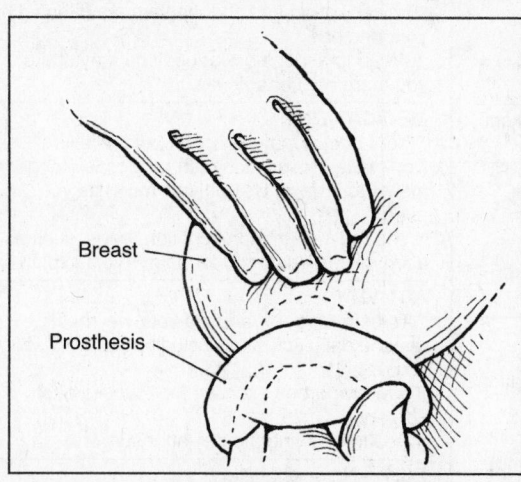

Breast

Prosthesis

After the pocket is created, a prosthesis is inserted. The procedure is usually repeated on the other breast.

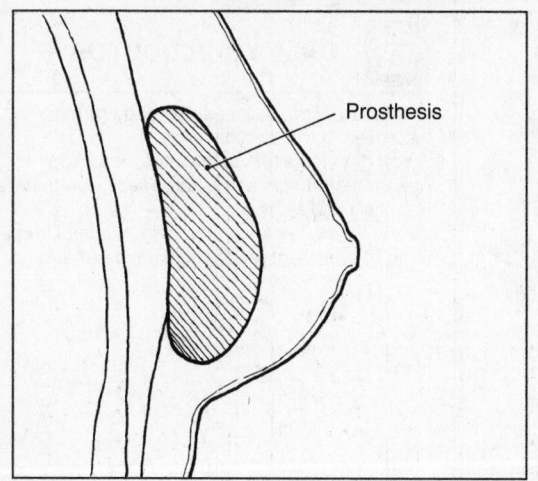

Prosthesis

Skin is closed with sutures that absorb or that can be removed about 1 week after surgery. A light bandage is usually all that is necessary for a dressing following surgery.

SURGERIES

BREAST BIOPSY BY EXCISION

GENERAL INFORMATION

DEFINITION—Removal of suspected abnormal tissue from the breast.

BODY PARTS INVOLVED—Female breast; male breast (rare).

REASONS FOR SURGERY—Clinical or mammographic signs or symptoms that may indicate breast cancer.

SURGICAL RISK INCREASES WITH
* Obesity.
* Smoking.
* Poor nutrition.
* Recent or chronic illness.
* Diabetes.
* Use of some prescription and nonprescription drugs. Inform your doctor of any drugs, medications, or vitamin and herb supplements you are using or have used in the last month.

WHAT TO EXPECT

WHO OPERATES—General surgeon.

WHERE PERFORMED—Hospital or outpatient surgical facility.

DIAGNOSTIC TESTS
* Before surgery: Blood and urine studies; mammogram; ultrasound (see Glossary for both).
* After surgery: Laboratory examination of removed tissue.

ANESTHESIA
* Local anesthesia often with sedation.
* General anesthesia by injection and inhalation with an airway tube placed in the windpipe.

DESCRIPTION OF OPERATION
* A special wire (the size of a thin guitar string) with a hooked tip may be inserted into the breast to localize the abnormality.
* An incision is made over the tissue to be removed. It is often possible to make a very cosmetic incision by cutting at the edge of the areola.
* The suspect tissue is cut free of the surrounding breast tissue and removed.
* Bleeding is controlled with ties or electrocautery.
* The skin is closed with sutures, which usually can be removed about 1 week after surgery.
* The removed tissue is sent to the pathology laboratory for microscopic examination.

POSSIBLE COMPLICATIONS
* Excessive bleeding.
* Surgical-wound infection.
* Unsightly scar on breast (rare).
* In cases of a large biopsy, or if the tissue removed is close to the skin, there may be some changes to the contour of the breast.

AVERAGE HOSPITAL STAY—Usually none.

PROBABLE OUTCOME—Expect complete healing without complications. Allow about 2 weeks for recovery from surgery.

POSTOPERATIVE CARE

GENERAL MEASURES
* A hard ridge may form along or beneath the incision. As it heals, the ridge will gradually recede.
* Shower as usual. You may wash the incision gently with mild, unscented soap.
* Wear a supportive bra. Apply bandages to the surgical wound and change them as directed by your doctor.
* Wearing a loose bra at bedtime may make you more comfortable.

MEDICATION
* Your doctor may prescribe pain relievers. Don't take prescription pain medication longer than 4 to 7 days. Use only as much as you need.
* You may use nonprescription drugs, such as acetaminophen, for minor pain. Avoid aspirin.

ACTIVITY
* To help recovery and aid your well-being, resume daily activities, including work, as soon as possible.
* Avoid vigorous exercise for 2 weeks after surgery.
* Resume driving the day after surgery.

DIET—No special diet.

CALL YOUR DOCTOR IF

* Pain, swelling, redness, drainage or bleeding increases in the surgical area.
* You develop signs of infection, including headache, muscle aches, dizziness or a general ill feeling and fever.
* New, unexplained symptoms develop. Drugs used in treatment may produce side effects.

BREAST BIOPSY BY EXCISION

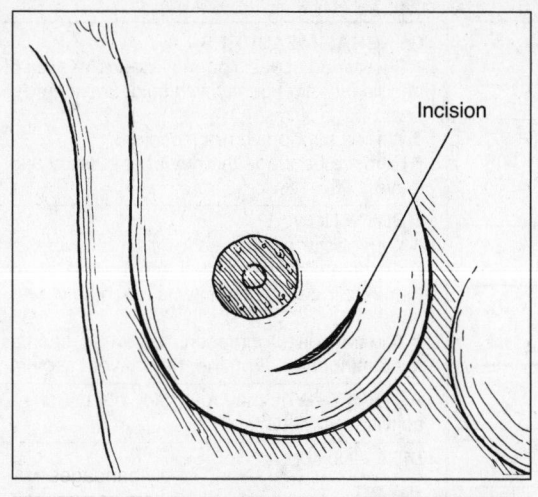

Incision

An illustration of a typical incision over the site of suspected abnormal breast tissue.

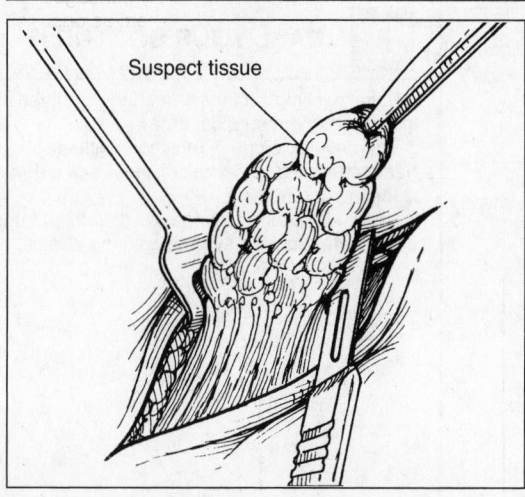

Suspect tissue

The suspect tissue is cut free of the surrounding breast tissue and removed.

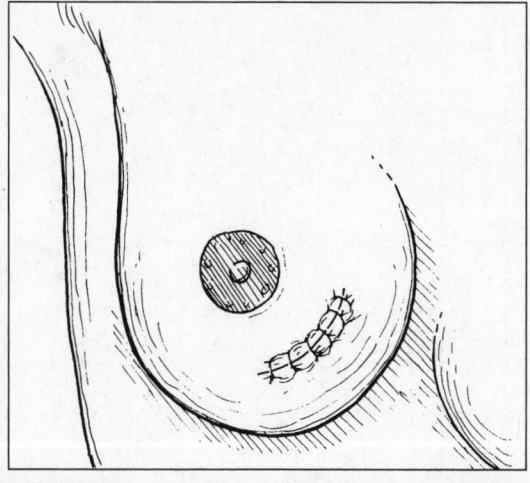

Appearance of the breast after closure of the skin, following tissue removal.

SURGERIES

BREAST BIOPSY BY NEEDLE ASPIRATION

 GENERAL INFORMATION

DEFINITION—Removal of fluid or tissue from the breasts.

BODY PARTS INVOLVED—Breast.

REASONS FOR SURGERY—Diagnosis of a thickening or lump. Needle biopsy is often the best first step for diagnosis of a lump in the breast.

SURGICAL RISK INCREASES WITH—Bleeding disorders.

 WHAT TO EXPECT

WHO OPERATES—Family doctor or general surgeon.

WHERE PERFORMED—Hospital, doctor's office or outpatient surgical facility.

DIAGNOSTIC TESTS
• Before surgery: Medical history and physical examination; ultrasound; mammogram (see Glossary for both).
• After surgery: Laboratory examination of removed fluid or tissue.

ANESTHESIA—Local anesthesia by injection (sometimes). Often, no anesthetic is necessary.

DESCRIPTION OF OPERATION
• A small, hollow needle is inserted into the thickening or lump.
• If the thickening or lump is a cyst, fluid usually can be removed and the cyst will shrink or disappear. This is often considered both therapeutic and diagnostic.
• In some cases, the removed fluid is sent to the laboratory to be examined for abnormal cells.
• If a solid tumor is detected, the tissue is recovered by passing the needle through the suspicious tissue several times, while using a syringe to aspirate as large a sample of cells as possible. The tissue is sent to the laboratory for microscopic examination.
• The needle is withdrawn and pressure is exerted on the site of the biopsy; a bandage is then applied.

POSSIBLE COMPLICATIONS
• Infection in surgical area (rare).
• Collection of blood (hematoma) under the skin where needle was inserted.

AVERAGE HOSPITAL STAY—Outpatient.

PROBABLE OUTCOME—Expect complete healing without complications. No recovery time is required.

 POSTOPERATIVE CARE

GENERAL MEASURES
• Shower as usual. You may wash the area of needle insertion gently with mild, unscented soap.
• Wear a supportive bra if desired.
• Remove bandage the day after surgery and leave it off.

MEDICATION
• Your doctor may prescribe pain relievers. Don't take prescription pain medication longer than 4 to 7 days. Use only as much as you need.
• You may use nonprescription drugs, such as acetaminophen, for minor pain. Avoid aspirin.

ACTIVITY—You may return to your usual activities immediately.

DIET—No special diet.

 CALL YOUR DOCTOR IF

• Pain, swelling, redness, drainage or bleeding increases in the surgical area.
• You develop signs of infection, including headache, muscle aches, dizziness or a general ill feeling and fever.
• New, unexplained symptoms develop. Drugs used in treatment may produce side effects.

BREAST BIOPSY BY NEEDLE ASPIRATION

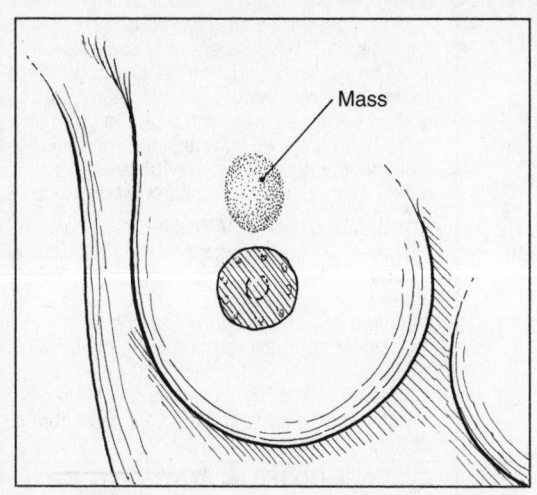

An illustration of a typical mass within the breast.

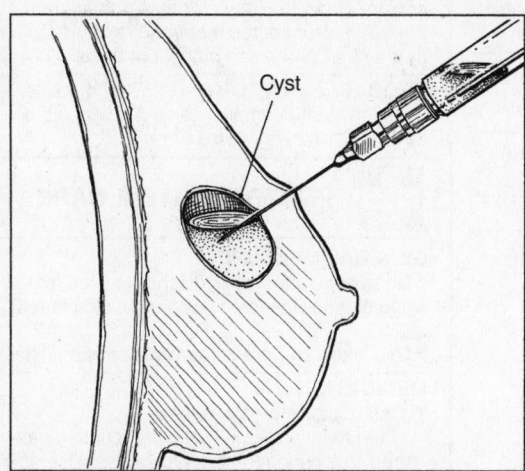

A small, hollow needle is inserted into the thickening or lump. Fluid is aspirated if the lump is a cyst.

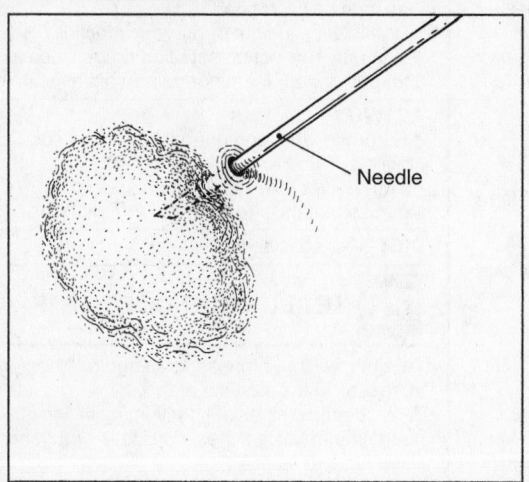

If a solid tumor is detected, tissue is aspirated through the needle and a laboratory examination is done to determine whether the tissue is benign or malignant.

SURGERIES

BREAST RECONSTRUCTION

GENERAL INFORMATION

DEFINITION—Rebuilding the female breast after mastectomy; using an implant or other body tissue.

BODY PARTS INVOLVED—Breasts; chest wall muscles; abdominal wall or back.

REASONS FOR SURGERY—Reconstruction of the breast following a mastectomy for breast cancer is usually done for psychological and cosmetic reasons. It also helps to reestablish symmetry. In most states, health insurance is required to cover reconstruction.

SURGICAL RISK INCREASES WITH
• Obesity; smoking.
• Excess alcohol consumption.
• Recent or chronic illness;diabetes.
• Previous radiation to the breast.
• Use of some prescription and nonprescription drugs. Inform your doctor of any drugs, medications, or vitamin and herb supplements you are using or have used in the last month.

WHAT TO EXPECT

WHO OPERATES—Plastic surgeon; general surgeon or oncology surgeon (sometimes).

WHERE PERFORMED—Hospital.

DIAGNOSTIC TESTS
• Before surgery: As required for the mastectomy procedure.
• After surgery: As required for follow up of cancer therapy or monitoring.

ANESTHESIA—General anesthesia by injection and inhalation, with an airway tube placed in the windpipe.

DESCRIPTION OF OPERATION—Several options are available and additional methods are undergoing development. You and your surgeon should have a clear understanding of what is to be done during surgery, but the surgeon will need some leeway in case unexpected problems occur.
• Expander/implant reconstruction is the most common. It consists of placement of an expander (empty or partially filled plastic shell) under the muscle either at the time of mastectomy or after the mastectomy surgery has healed. The expander is slowly inflated with saline over 2 to 3 months and eventually replaced by a permanent implant filled with saline. The opposite breast may need a reduction or "lift" to achieve symmetry.
• Autologous graft is a more complex reconstruction which can achieve a superior cosmetic result without the need for any "foreign" implant. Tissue is moved to the chest wall from the lower abdomen or back to

reconstruct the breast. This can also be done at the time of the mastectomy or as a delayed procedure.
• The nipple-areola area can also be reconstructed. This is generally done after the initial breast reconstruction healing is complete so that the positioning is correct. Skin may be grafted from the inner thigh near the groin or color may be added by tattooing. For some patients, the nipple area may be preserved during mastectomy and used in reconstruction.

POSSIBLE COMPLICATIONS
• Excessive bleeding; surgical-wound infection.
• Accumulation of blood (hematoma) or fluid under the surgical area.
• Limited shoulder motion.
• Capsular contracture (hardening of the implant).
• Abdominal wall hernia (with autologous graft).
• Failure of the implant due to slippage, rupture, infection or scarring.

AVERAGE HOSPITAL STAY—1 to 2 days for implant and 4 to 6 days for autologous graft. Follow up procedures may require shorter times or may be done on an outpatient basis.

PROBABLE OUTCOME—Expect complete healing without complications. Allow about 6 weeks for recovery from surgery.

POSTOPERATIVE CARE

GENERAL MEASURES
• Shower as usual after discharge. You may wash the incision gently with mild, unscented soap.
• Use warm compress to relieve incisional pain.

MEDICATION
• Your doctor may prescribe:
  - Pain relievers. Don't take prescription pain medication longer than 4 to 7 days. Use only as much as you need.
  - Antibiotics to fight or prevent infection.
• You may use nonprescription drugs, such as acetaminophen, for minor pain.Avoid aspirin.

ACTIVITY
• Return to work and normal activity as soon as possible.
• Your doctor may recommend special exercises to aid in recovery of arm mobility.

DIET—No special diet.

CALL YOUR DOCTOR IF

• Pain, swelling, redness, drainage or bleeding increases in the surgical area.
• You develop signs of infection, including headache, muscle aches, dizziness or a general ill feeling and fever.

BREAST RECONSTRUCTION

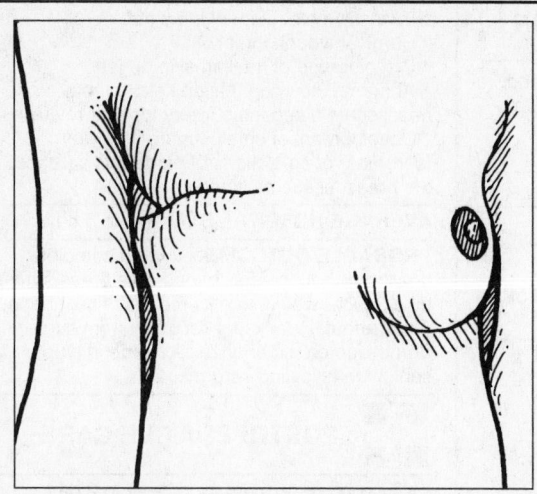

Illustration shows the appearance of right breast after mastectomy.

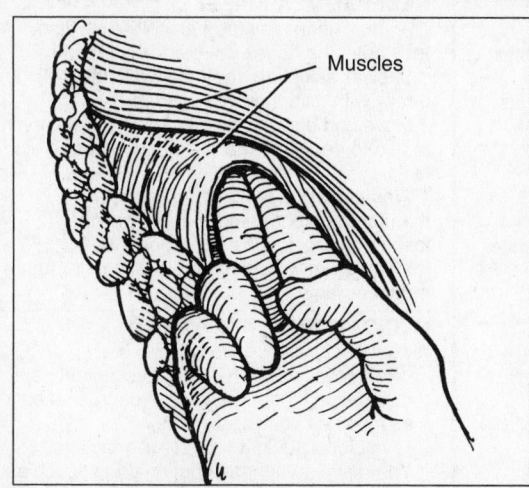

Muscles

A pocket is prepared for an implant.

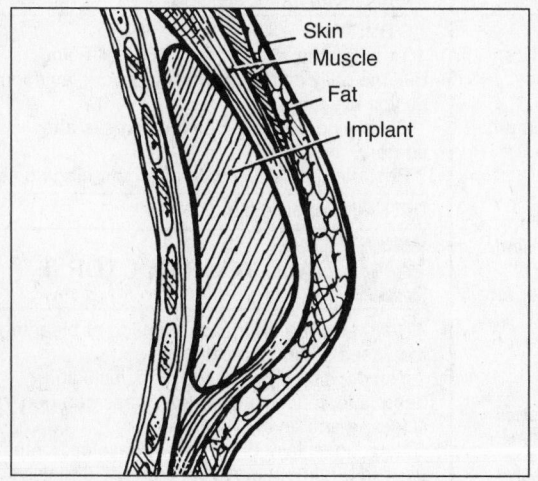

Skin
Muscle
Fat
Implant

Side view of the breast showing the implant in position.

BREAST REDUCTION
(Reduction Mammoplasty)

GENERAL INFORMATION

DEFINITION—Removal of excess tissue and overlying skin from the female breasts. Usually this surgery also includes reconstruction of breast shape.

BODY PARTS INVOLVED—Breasts.

REASONS FOR SURGERY
* Reduction of overly large breasts to improve appearance and/or emotional well-being.
* Relief of back and neck pain from weight of overly large breasts.
* Reconstruction of a breast to match a surgical change made in the other breast.

SURGICAL RISK INCREASES WITH
* Obesity.
* Smoking.
* Excess alcohol consumption.
* Diabetes.
* Poor nutrition.
* Use of some prescription and nonprescription drugs. Inform your doctor of any drugs, medications, or vitamin and herb supplements you are using or have used in the last month.

WHAT TO EXPECT

WHO OPERATES—Plastic and reconstructive surgeon.

WHERE PERFORMED—Hospital.

DIAGNOSTIC TESTS
* Before surgery: Blood and urine studies; mammogram (see Glossary).
* After surgery: Blood studies.

ANESTHESIA—General anesthesia by injection and inhalation with an airway tube placed in the windpipe.

DESCRIPTION OF OPERATION
* The breast is marked where the skin will be removed and where the nipple will be after tissue is removed.
* The skin between the new nipple location and the natural nipple location is incised and removed. The nipple stays attached to underlying tissue.
* Another incision is made below the nipple. Excess tissue is removed through this incision.
* The removed tissue is sent to a pathology laboratory to be examined and analyzed for any early signs of breast cancer.
* Drains are sometimes left in place to prevent fluid or blood from accumulating under the sutures.
* The skin is closed with fine sutures, which usually can be removed about 10 to 14 days after surgery.

POSSIBLE COMPLICATIONS
* Excessive bleeding; blood clots.
* Surgical-wound infection.
* Discoloration of healing skin edges.
* Abnormal scarring (called keloids) may necessitate a second surgery for scar revision.
* Development of small, tumor-like cysts (seromas) or collections of blood and serum in the breast tissue as it heals.

AVERAGE HOSPITAL STAY—4 to 5 days.

PROBABLE OUTCOME—Expect complete healing without complications. The breasts may take 3 to 12 weeks to assume their final shape. Allow about 4 weeks for recovery from surgery. Some women experience a change in nipple sensation following surgery.

POSTOPERATIVE CARE

GENERAL MEASURES
* A small ridge may form along the incisions. As they heal, the ridges will gradually recede.
* Shower as usual. You may wash the incision gently with mild, unscented soap.
* Move and elevate your legs often while resting in bed to decrease the likelihood of deep-vein clots.
* Women over age 30 should have a mammogram both before and 6 months following surgery. The postoperative mammogram will serve as a baseline for future mammograms.

MEDICATION
* Your doctor may prescribe:
  - Pain relievers. Don't take prescription pain medication longer than 4 to 7 days. Use only as much as you need.
  - Antibiotics to fight or prevent infection.
* You may use nonprescription drugs, such as acetaminophen, for minor pain. Avoid aspirin.

ACTIVITY
* To help recovery and aid your well-being, resume daily activities, including work, as soon as you are able.
* Avoid vigorous exercise for 6 weeks after surgery.
* Resume driving 1 month after returning home.

DIET—No special diet.

CALL YOUR DOCTOR IF

* Pain, swelling, redness, drainage or bleeding increases in the surgical area.
* You develop signs of infection, including headache, muscle aches, dizziness or a general ill feeling and fever.
* New, unexplained symptoms develop. Drugs used in treatment may produce side effects.

BREAST REDUCTION
(Reduction Mammoplasty)

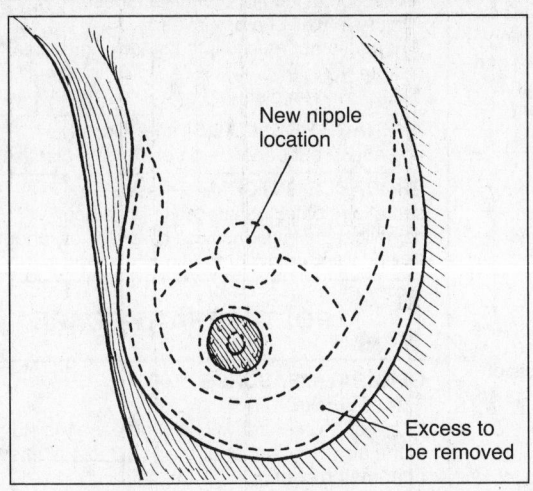

New nipple location

Excess to be removed

An illustration showing markings on the breast where skin will be removed and the nipple will be placed after the reduction procedure.

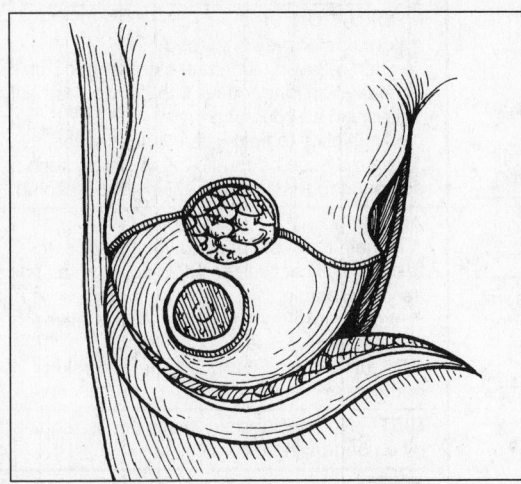

Skin between the new nipple location and the natural nipple location is incised and removed. The nipple stays attached to the underlying tissue.

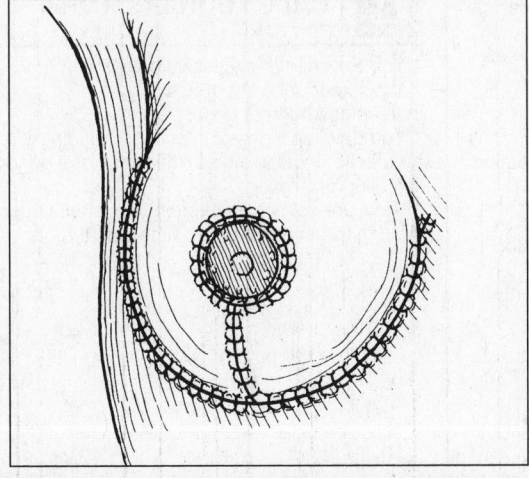

Another incision is made below the nipple. Excess tissue is removed, drains are left in place to prevent collection of fluid, and skin is closed with fine sutures. Sutures are usually removed about 10 to 14 days after surgery.

SURGERIES

BRONCHOSCOPY

GENERAL INFORMATION

DEFINITION—Visual examination of the lining of the bronchial tubes and removal of tissue and secretions. The procedure is performed with a flexible bronchoscope, an optical instrument with a lighted tip.

BODY PARTS INVOLVED—Windpipe (trachea); larynx; bronchial tree.

REASONS FOR SURGERY
* Suspected cancer in the bronchial tubes.
* Foreign matter that has been inhaled accidentally.
* Bleeding in the bronchial tubes.
* X-ray studies (bronchograms) to diagnose diseases of the lung, such as bronchiectasis or emphysema.

SURGICAL RISK INCREASES WITH
* Obesity.
* Smoking.
* Recent or chronic illness, especially chronic lung disease.
* Diabetes.
* Alcoholism.
* Use of some prescription and nonprescription drugs. Inform your doctor of any drugs, medications, or vitamin and herb supplements you are using or have used in the last month.

WHAT TO EXPECT

WHO OPERATES—Thoracic surgeon, general surgeon, pulmonary specialist or ear, nose and throat specialist.

WHERE PERFORMED—Hospital or outpatient surgical facility.

DIAGNOSTIC TESTS
* Before surgery: Blood and urine studies; x-rays of chest; CT scan (see Glossary).
* During surgery: Bronchogram (see Glossary).
* After surgery: Laboratory examination of removed tissue and secretions; x-rays to check for complications.

ANESTHESIA
* Local anesthesia with sedation.
* General anesthesia by injection and inhalation with an airway tube placed in the windpipe.

DESCRIPTION OF OPERATION
* The bronchoscope is inserted in the mouth, past the back of the tongue, into the main bronchial tube and its branches. Supplemental oxygen is supplied during the procedure.
* Foreign matter is removed, if necessary. Tissue is gathered and secretions are collected.
* The bronchoscope is removed.

POSSIBLE COMPLICATIONS
* Excessive bleeding.
* Infection in lung or bronchial tubes.
* Injury to wall of a bronchus.
* Aspiration of mucus into the lower bronchial tissues.
* Heart rhythm disturbances.

AVERAGE HOSPITAL STAY—Usually outpatient, but depends on underlying disease.

PROBABLE OUTCOME—Tissue and secretions obtained successfully without complications in virtually all cases. Allow about 24 hours for recovery from the procedure.

POSTOPERATIVE CARE

GENERAL MEASURES
* Don't smoke.
* Use of a vaporizer will help increase moisture in the air you breathe for the first 3 to 4 nights after the procedure.

MEDICATION
* Your doctor may prescribe:
  - Pain relievers. Don't take prescription pain medication longer than 4 to 7 days. Use only as much as you need.
  - Antibiotics to fight or prevent infection.
* You may use nonprescription drugs, such as acetaminophen, for minor pain. Avoid aspirin.

ACTIVITY
* To help recovery and aid your well-being, resume daily activities, including work, as soon as you are able.
* Avoid vigorous exercise for 7 days after the procedure.
* Resume driving 24 hours after returning home.

DIET—No special diet (unless one is required by an underlying disorder).

CALL YOUR DOCTOR IF

* You experience excessive bleeding.
* You experience shortness of breath, increasing cough or chest pain.
* You develop signs of infection, including headache, muscle aches, dizziness or a general ill feeling and fever.
* New, unexplained symptoms develop. Drugs used in treatment may produce side effects.

BRONCHOSCOPY

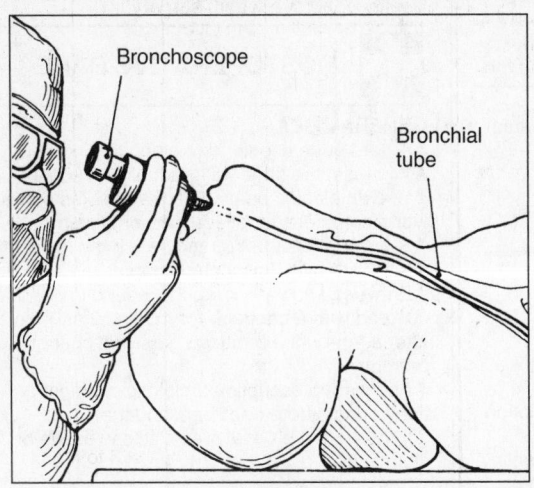

An illustration of the bronchoscope inserted into the mouth past the tongue and into the main bronchial tube and its branches.

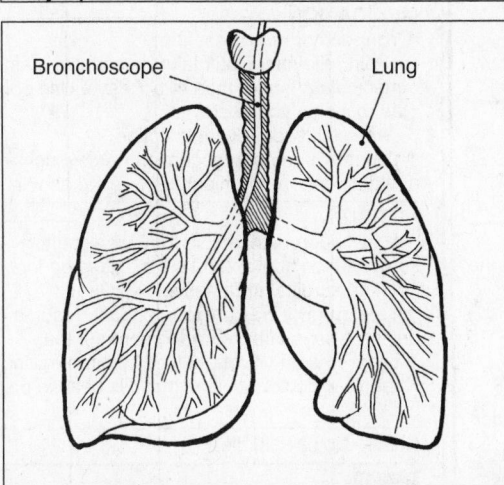

The flexible bronchoscope can be passed into either of the main stem bronchial branches.
• Foreign matter is removed by suction. If necessary, tissue is gathered and secretions are collected to be studied microscopically.

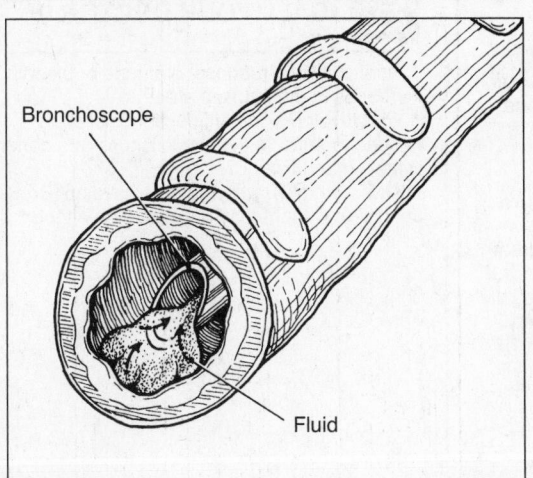

Fluid being suctioned from the bronchoscope while still in place.

BUNION REMOVAL

GENERAL INFORMATION

DEFINITION—Removal of a bunion, a bony and fibrous outgrowth at the base of the big toe.

BODY PARTS INVOLVED—Foot; joint between the metatarsal bone and big toe; fluid sac that surrounds the joint.

REASONS FOR SURGERY
* Relief of pain.
* Correction of deformity.

SURGICAL RISK INCREASES WITH
* Poor nutrition.
* Recent illness.
* Alcoholism or chronic illness.
* Diabetes.
* Vascular disease.
* Use of some prescription and nonprescription drugs. Inform your doctor of any drugs, medications, or vitamin and herb supplements you are using or have used in the last month.

WHAT TO EXPECT

WHO OPERATES—General surgeon, orthopedist or podiatrist.

WHERE PERFORMED—Doctor's office, outpatient surgical facility or hospital.

DIAGNOSTIC TESTS
* Before surgery: X-rays of foot; blood and urine studies.
* After surgery: X-rays of foot.

ANESTHESIA
* Local anesthesia by injection.
* Spinal anesthesia by injection.
* General anesthesia by injection and inhalation with an airway tube placed in the windpipe.

DESCRIPTION OF OPERATION
* An incision is made over the bunion.
* The capsule of the joint connecting the metatarsal bone and the big toe is opened.
* A section from the metatarsal bone is cut or filed away and removed. Another small bone (the sesamoid bone) attached to a tendon is removed also.
* Tendons attached to the base of the metatarsal and toe bones are cut. This allows the bones to straighten when healed.
* A pin (metal rod) may be placed in the great toe.
* The skin is closed with sutures, which usually can be removed about 10 days after surgery.

POSSIBLE COMPLICATIONS
* Excessive bleeding.
* Surgical-wound infection.
* Slow healing.

AVERAGE HOSPITAL STAY—0 to 1 day.

PROBABLE OUTCOME—Expect complete healing without complications. Allow about 6 weeks for recovery from surgery.

POSTOPERATIVE CARE

GENERAL MEASURES
* A hard ridge should form along the incision. As it heals, the ridge will gradually recede.
* Use an electric heating pad, a heat lamp or a warm compress to relieve incisional pain.
* Shower as usual. You may wash the incision gently with mild, unscented soap.
* Between showers, keep the wound dry and covered with a bandage for the first 2 or 3 days after surgery. If a bandage gets wet, change it promptly.
* Apply nonprescription antibiotic ointment to the wound before applying bandages.
* If the wound bleeds, press a clean tissue or cloth to it.

MEDICATION
* Your doctor may prescribe:
  - Pain relievers. Don't take prescription pain medication longer than 4 to 7 days. Use only as much as you need.
  - Antibiotics to prevent infection.
* You may use nonprescription drugs, such as acetaminophen, for minor pain. Avoid aspirin.

ACTIVITY
* Avoid vigorous exercise for 6 weeks after surgery. Don't put weight on the affected foot until the surgical area heals.
* If the surgery was on your left foot, resume driving 4 days after returning home. If the surgery was on your right foot, resume driving when your doctor advises that it is okay to do so.

DIET—No special diet.

CALL YOUR DOCTOR IF

* Pain, swelling, redness, drainage or bleeding increases in the surgical area.
* You develop signs of infection, including headache, muscle aches, dizziness or a general ill feeling and fever.
* New, unexplained symptoms develop. Drugs used in treatment may produce side effects.

BUNION REMOVAL

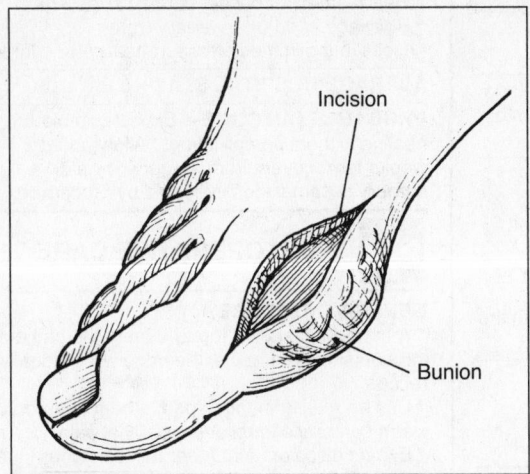

An illustration of a typical bunion. An incision is made over the bunion.

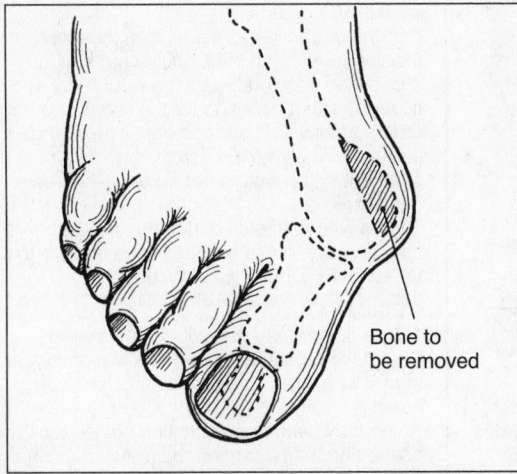

Overgrown section from the metatarsal bone is cut or filed away and removed.

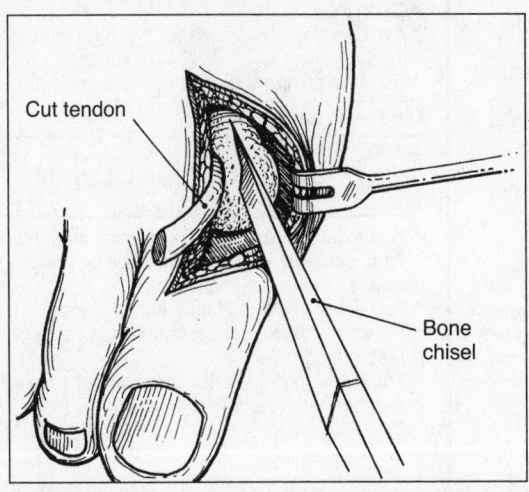

Tendons attached to the base of the metatarsal bone and toe bones are cut to allow bones to straighten when healed.

SURGERIES

CARDIAC CATHETERIZATION & ANGIOGRAMS

GENERAL INFORMATION

DEFINITION—Diagnostic procedures to examine functions of the heart.

BODY PARTS INVOLVED—Heart muscle and valves; coronary arteries; large artery in arm or leg.

REASONS FOR SURGERY
* Evaluation of chest pain.
* Diagnosis of a congenital heart defect and valvular-heart disease.
* Measurement of the heart muscle's ability to pump blood.
* Identification of narrowing or obstruction in the coronary arteries.

SURGICAL RISK INCREASES WITH
* Stress; obesity; smoking.
* Recent or chronic illness.
* Alcoholism.

WHAT TO EXPECT

WHO OPERATES—Cardiologist.

WHERE PERFORMED—Hospital.

DIAGNOSTIC TESTS
* Before surgery: Blood and urine studies; ECG (see Glossary); chest x-ray.
* During surgery: Intracardiac pressures; cardiac output; cinematography; fluoroscopy; ECG (see Glossary for all).
* After surgery: ECG; blood studies.

ANESTHESIA—Local anesthesia by injection; usually accompanied by sedation.

DESCRIPTION OF OPERATION
* The cardiac catheter is inserted into an artery in the patient's arm or leg. Fluoroscopy provides guidance for the catheter to pass through the artery to the heart.
* Blood-pressure readings are taken, and the heart's ability to pump blood is tested.
* The catheter is guided into the coronary-artery system. Dye is injected through the catheter and into the coronary arteries. Multiple images will be taken to allow identification of any disease in the coronary arteries.
* When all examinations have been completed, the catheter is withdrawn, and the artery into which it was inserted is compressed until bleeding stops. If an arm artery was used, it may need to be repaired. A tight bandage is placed over the entry site for the catheter, and you will be expected to keep that area of your body flat for approximately 6 hours.

POSSIBLE COMPLICATIONS
* Excessive bleeding; blood clot in an artery.
* Reaction to dye (allergy).
* Surgical-wound infection.

* Development of hematomas (collections of blood) where skin was pierced to enter artery.
* Heartbeat disturbance; cardiac arrest (rare).
* Blockage of coronary artery (rare) necessitating immediate open-heart procedure.

AVERAGE HOSPITAL STAY—0 to 1 day.

PROBABLE OUTCOME—Expect complete healing without complications. Allow about 2 weeks for recovery from surgery. Urgent surgery is sometimes indicated by procedure.

POSTOPERATIVE CARE

GENERAL MEASURES
* A hard ridge should form beneath the catheter incision site. As it heals, the ridge will gradually recede.
* Use an electric heating pad, a heat lamp or a warm compress to relieve incisional pain.
* Expect discoloration under the skin where the catheter was inserted. It should disappear in 2 weeks.
* Bathe or shower as usual. You may wash the incision gently with mild, unscented soap.
* Between showers, keep the wound dry and covered with a bandage for the first 2 or 3 days after surgery. If a bandage gets wet, change it promptly. Apply nonprescription antibiotic ointment to the wound before applying new bandages.
* If the wound bleeds during the first 24 hours after surgery, press a clean tissue or cloth to it for 10 to 15 minutes continuously.

MEDICATION
* Your doctor may prescribe pain relievers. Don't take prescription pain medication longer than 4 to 7 days. Use only as much as you need.
* You may use nonprescription drugs, such as acetaminophen, for minor pain. Avoid aspirin.

ACTIVITY
* Avoid vigorous exercise for 2 weeks after surgery.
* Resume driving 2 days after returning home.

DIET—No special diet.

CALL YOUR DOCTOR IF

* You experience sudden or severe chest pain.
* Pain, swelling, redness, drainage or bleeding increases in the surgical area.
* You develop signs of infection, including headache, muscle aches, dizziness or a general ill feeling and fever.
* You develop decreased sensation or pain in the limb where artery was entered.

CARDIAC CATHETERIZATION & ANGIOGRAMS

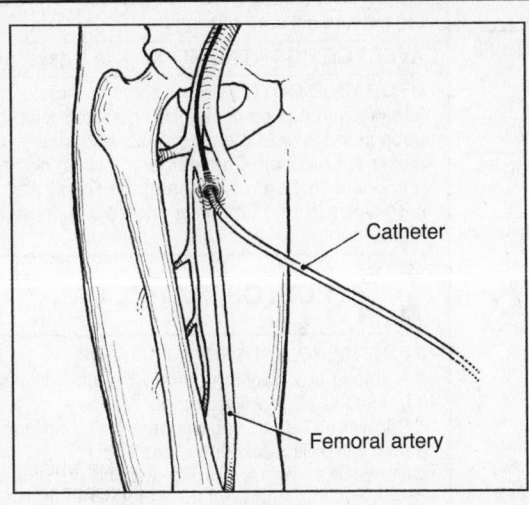

An illustration of a typical location for catheter insertion in the large artery of the leg. The catheter may also be placed in a large vessel in the arm.
- When the catheter is in place, accurate blood pressure measurements may be made continuously.

Catheter

Femoral artery

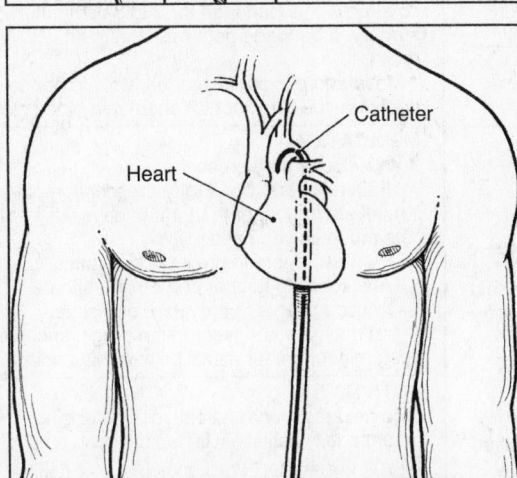

The catheter is guided into the coronary artery system. Pressure readings are made in various chambers of the heart and great blood vessels for later interpretation.

Catheter

Heart

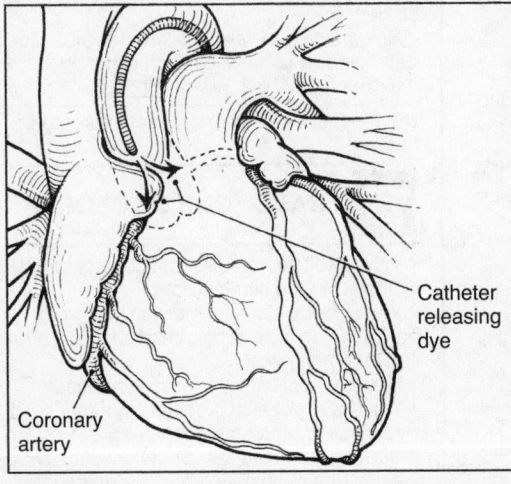

Dye is injected through the catheter to fill the coronary arteries to accurately locate any narrowing or obstructions in the coronary artery system.
- When all examinations have been completed, the catheter is withdrawn and the artery it was inserted into is compressed until bleeding stops.

Catheter releasing dye

Coronary artery

SURGERIES

CAROTID ARTERY ENDARTERECTOMY

 GENERAL INFORMATION

DEFINITION—Removal of obstruction in carotid (neck) artery usually due to hardening of arteries (arteriosclerosis).

BODY PARTS INVOLVED—Carotid arteries.

REASONS FOR SURGERY—Prevention of stroke and transient ischemic attacks (see Glossary).

SURGICAL RISK INCREASES WITH
* Adults over 80.
* Obesity; smoking.
* Poor nutrition.
* Excess alcohol consumption.
* Recent or chronic illness.
* Atherosclerosis; coronary artery disease.
* Diabetes.
* Use of some prescription and nonprescription drugs. Inform your doctor of any drugs, medications, or vitamin and herb supplements you are using or have used in the last month.

 WHAT TO EXPECT

WHO OPERATES—General surgeon, neurosurgeon, cardiovascular surgeon, or peripheral vascular surgeon.

WHERE PERFORMED—Hospital.

DIAGNOSTIC TESTS
* Before surgery: Blood and urine studies; chest x-ray; ECG; arteriograms; CT scan of head (see Glossary for all).
* After surgery: Blood studies.

ANESTHESIA
* Local anesthetic by injection and sedation.
* General anesthesia by injection and inhalation with an airway tube placed in the windpipe.

DESCRIPTION OF OPERATION
* An incision is made in the neck over the obstruction.
* The obstructed area is isolated. A tube is often placed in the carotid artery and is used to circulate blood around the obstruction while the blockage is being cleared.
* A small incision is made in the artery over the obstruction which is scraped away. The opened area is sometimes patched with a graft fashioned from a vein from another part of the body or a cloth-like material.
* The temporary bypass tube is removed as the artery is closed.
* The skin is closed with sutures or clips, which usually can be removed in 2 weeks.
* A drain is frequently left in for 24 hours.

POSSIBLE COMPLICATIONS
* Excessive bleeding; hematoma (blood clot).
* Surgical-wound infection.
* Stroke; heart problems; pneumonia.
* Inadvertent injury to a branch of the nerves to the face, vocal cord or tongue.

AVERAGE HOSPITAL STAY—2 to 3 days.

PROBABLE OUTCOME—Expect complete healing without complications and restoration of good blood flow to the brain. Allow about 2 weeks for recovery from surgery. Expect some numbness in your neck area at the site of the surgical incision; numbness should disappear in 3 to 4 months.

 POSTOPERATIVE CARE

GENERAL MEASURES
* A small ridge may form along the incision. As it heals, the ridge will gradually recede.
* Shower as usual. You may wash the incision gently with mild, unscented soap.
* Between showers, keep the wound dry and covered with a bandage for 2 to 3 days after surgery. If bandage gets wet, change it promptly.
* Move and elevate legs often while in bed to decrease the likelihood of deep-vein blood clots.

MEDICATION
* Your doctor may prescribe:
  - Pain relievers. Don't take prescription pain relievers for longer than 4 to 7 days. Use only as much as you need.
  - Stool softeners to prevent constipation.
  - Antibiotics to fight or prevent infection.
  - Anticoagulants to prevent blood clots.
* You may use nonprescription drugs, such as acetaminophen, for minor pain. Avoid aspirin.

ACTIVITY
* To help recovery and aid your well-being, resume daily activities, including work, as soon as you are able.
* Avoid vigorous exercise for 6 weeks after surgery.
* Resume sexual relations when your doctor determines that healing is complete.
* Resume driving 3 weeks after returning home.

DIET—Eat a well-balanced diet to promote healing.

 CALL YOUR DOCTOR IF

* Pain, swelling, redness, drainage or bleeding increases in the surgical area.
* You develop signs of infection, including headache, muscle aches, dizziness or a general ill feeling and fever.
* Nausea, vomiting or constipation occurs.
* You develop visual problems, numbness, weakness or problems with speech.
* New, unexplained symptoms develop. Drugs used in treatment may produce side effects.

CAROTID ARTERY ENDARTERECTOMY

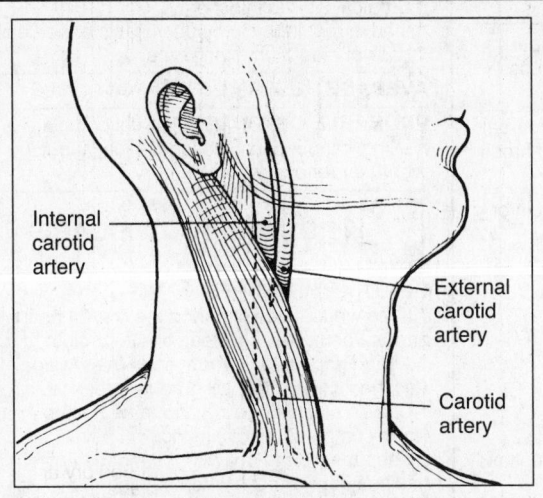

Illustration shows the anatomical locations of the carotid artery, external carotid artery and internal carotid artery.

Internal carotid artery

External carotid artery

Carotid artery

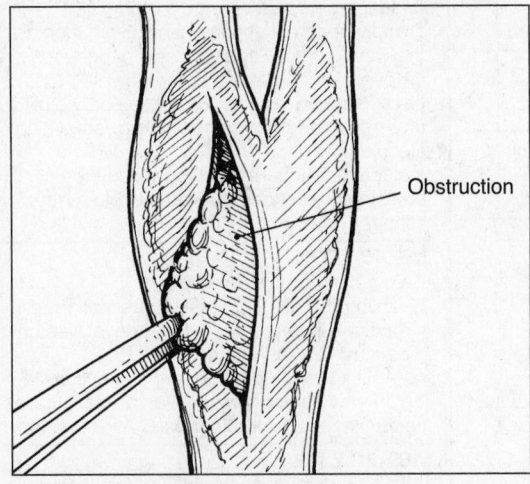

The arterial debris causing the obstruction (which was located by previous special studies) is removed.

Obstruction

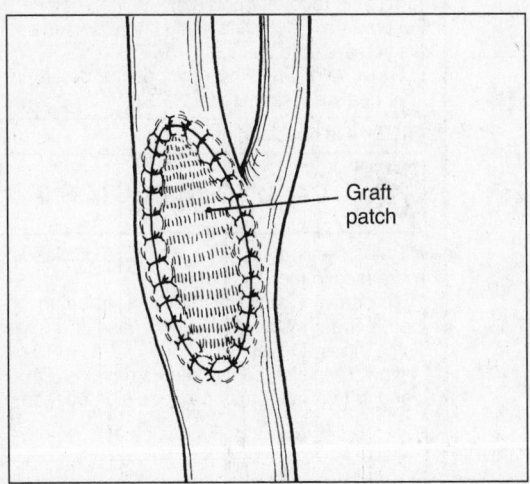

A patch is grafted in place to close the artery that has been cleared of obstruction.

Graft patch

CARPAL-TUNNEL SYNDROME REPAIR

 GENERAL INFORMATION

DEFINITION—Cutting the transverse carpal ligament, the fibrous tissue extending across the wrist.

BODY PARTS INVOLVED—Transverse carpal ligament; median nerve and surrounding fibrous tissue; wrist joint.

REASONS FOR SURGERY—Relief of pain or numbness caused by compression of the median nerve.

SURGICAL RISK INCREASES WITH
- Obesity.
- Smoking.
- Poor nutrition.
- Recent or chronic illness.
- Alcoholism.
- Diabetes.
- Use of some prescription and nonprescription drugs. Inform your doctor of any drugs, medications, or vitamin and herb supplements you are using or have used in the last month.

 WHAT TO EXPECT

WHO OPERATES—Hand surgeon, general surgeon, orthopedist or plastic and reconstructive surgeon.

WHERE PERFORMED—Hospital or outpatient surgical facility.

DIAGNOSTIC TESTS
- Before surgery: Blood and urine studies; x-rays of wrist; nerve-conduction tests (see Glossary).
- After surgery: Blood studies.

ANESTHESIA
- Local anesthesia by injection.
- Regional anesthesia by injection.
- General anesthesia by injection and inhalation with an airway tube placed in the windpipe.

DESCRIPTION OF OPERATION
- A tourniquet is applied above the wrist to prevent bleeding in the surgical area.
- An incision is made in the underside of the wrist.
- The transverse carpal ligament is located and cut, releasing the compressed median nerve.
- The skin is closed with fine sutures, which usually can be removed about 10 days after surgery. Absorbable stitches are not removed.
- A bandage is applied, and a splint is used to hold the wrist in position. In some instances, the stitched wound may be left uncovered.

POSSIBLE COMPLICATIONS
- Excessive bleeding.
- Surgical-wound infection.
- Inadvertent injury to blood vessels or nerves.
- Lack of relief from symptoms.

AVERAGE HOSPITAL STAY—0 to 1 day.

PROBABLE OUTCOME—Expect complete healing without complications. Allow about 1 month for recovery from surgery.

 POSTOPERATIVE CARE

GENERAL MEASURES
- If the wound bleeds during the first 24 hours after surgery, press a clean tissue or cloth to it.
- A hard ridge should form along the incision. As it heals, the ridge will gradually recede.
- Use an electric heating pad, a heat lamp or a warm compress to relieve incision pain.
- Keep the wound dry with a bandage until it has healed. Protect it when bathing. If a bandage gets wet, change it promptly.
- Apply nonprescription antibiotic ointment to the wound before applying new bandages.
- Keep the hand elevated for the first 1 to 2 days following surgery. Place one or two pillows under the hand and arm when you are sitting or sleeping.
- If your fingers are not wrapped in the dressing, try to keep them moving to reduce stiffness.

MEDICATION
- Your doctor may prescribe:
  - Pain relievers. Don't take prescription pain medication longer than 4 to 7 days. Use only as much as you need.
  - Antibiotics to fight or prevent infection.
- You may use nonprescription drugs, such as acetaminophen, for minor pain. Avoid aspirin.

ACTIVITY
- To help recovery and aid your well-being, resume daily activities, including work, as soon as you are able.
- Resume driving when your doctor determines that healing is complete.

DIET—No special diet.

 CALL YOUR DOCTOR IF

- Pain, swelling, redness, drainage or bleeding increases in the surgical area.
- You develop signs of infection, including headache, muscle aches, dizziness or a general ill feeling and fever.
- New, unexplained symptoms develop. Drugs used in treatment may produce side effects.

CARPAL-TUNNEL SYNDROME REPAIR

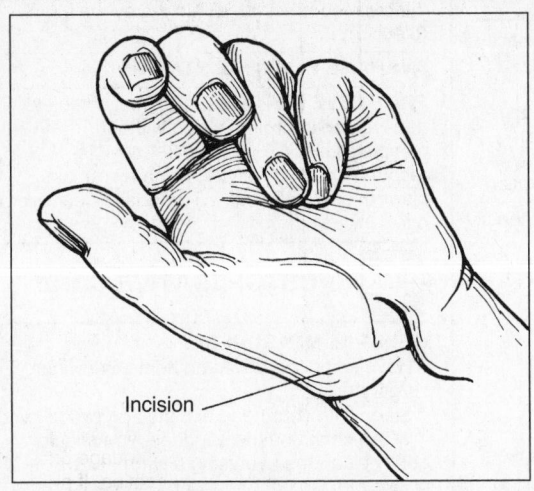

An illustration of the incision site at the wrist area where compression of the median nerve occurs.

Incision

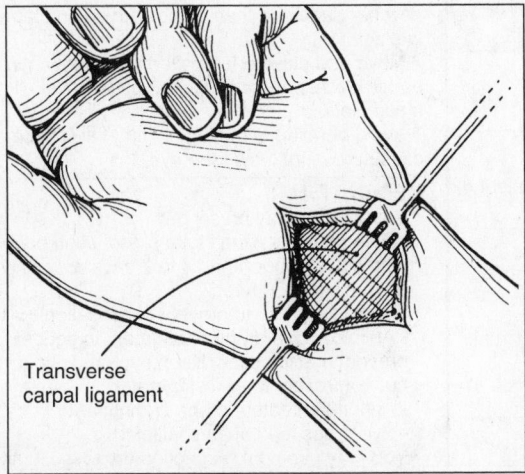

After the skin is incised, the transverse carpal ligament is exposed.

Transverse carpal ligament

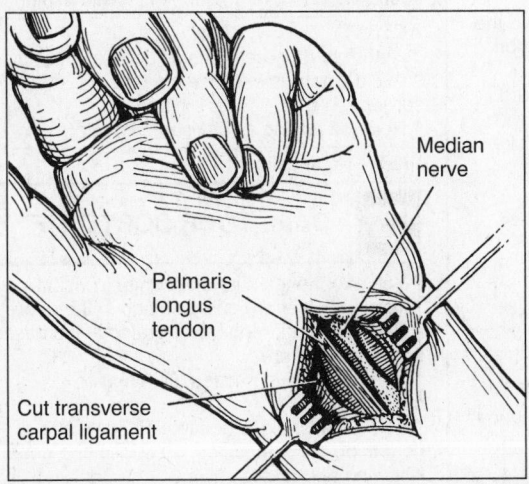

Carpal ligament is located and cut, releasing the compressed median nerve. This usually cures symptoms.

Median nerve

Palmaris longus tendon

Cut transverse carpal ligament

SURGERIES

CATARACT EXTRACTION

 GENERAL INFORMATION

DEFINITION—Removal of cataracts, an opacity or clouding of the lens of the eye. This procedure is almost always performed in conjunction with an intraocular (within the eye) lens implant. Several surgical techniques are available; the doctor will choose the one that is most appropriate to your age and eye condition.

BODY PARTS INVOLVED—Eye; cornea; lens; eyelid membrane lining.

REASONS FOR SURGERY—Restoration of normal or near-normal vision.

SURGICAL RISK INCREASES WITH
* Obesity; smoking.
* Newborns and infants.
* Recent or chronic illness.
* Diabetes.
* Use of some prescription and nonprescription drugs. Inform your doctor of any drugs, medications, or vitamin and herb supplements you are using or have used in the last month.

 WHAT TO EXPECT

WHO OPERATES—Ophthalmologist.

WHERE PERFORMED—Hospital or outpatient facility.

DIAGNOSTIC TESTS
* Before surgery: Blood and urine studies; eye examinations; ultrasound (see Glossary).
* After surgery: Eye examinations.

ANESTHESIA—Local anesthesia by injection. One injection prevents eyelid blinking and another one immobilizes the eyeball.

DESCRIPTION OF OPERATION
* A special instrument is used to hold the eyelids apart.
* A small incision is made in the cornea and the diseased lens is removed through the incision. Often, the lens is first fragmented with ultrasound and the debris is simply suctioned away.
* An artificial lens, known as an intraocular lens, is usually inserted in the eye to replace the discarded lens.
* Few or no stitches are required to close the wound.
* Pilocarpine or atropine eye-drop solutions are placed in the eye to keep the pupil open. Bandages are applied.

POSSIBLE COMPLICATIONS
* Surgical-wound infection.
* Postoperative inflammation.
* Lens capsule thickens causing hazy or cloudy vision.
* Dislocation of intraocular lens implant.

* Astigmatism.
* Retinal detachment.
* Increased pressure within the eyeball (glaucoma).

AVERAGE HOSPITAL STAY—0 to 1 day.

PROBABLE OUTCOME—Expect complete healing and improved vision without complications. Allow about 3-4 days for recovery from surgery. Vision may remain blurred for awhile, but will gradually clear over a 4 to 10 week period.

 POSTOPERATIVE CARE

GENERAL MEASURES
* Have someone drive you home following surgery.
* Sleep with your head elevated on two pillows.
* When changing the bandage, you should gently clean the eye using a warm, wet washcloth. Do not press or rub the eye. The new bandage can then be positioned and taped in place.
* Move and elevate legs often while resting in bed to decrease the likelihood of deep-vein blood clots.
* Avoid bending, straining or lying flat. These cause pressure inside the eye.

MEDICATION
* Your doctor may prescribe:
  - Pain relievers. Don't take prescription pain medication longer than 4 to 7 days. Use only as much as you need.
  - Stool softeners to prevent constipation.
  - Antibiotic eye drops or ointment to fight or prevent eye infection. Keep eye drops cold, but not frozen, in the refrigerator.
  - Anti-inflammatory drops or ointment.
  - Eye drops to keep pupil dilated.
* You may use nonprescription drugs, such as acetaminophen, for minor pain. Avoid aspirin.

ACTIVITY
* Return to daily activities as soon as possible.
* Avoid vigorous exercise for 6 weeks after surgery.
* Resume driving as advised by doctor.

DIET—No special diet.

 CALL YOUR DOCTOR IF

* You experience sudden change in vision.
* You have a sharp pain or blood in the eye.
* Pain, swelling, redness or drainage increases in the surgical area.
* You experience nausea, vomiting or constipation.
* You develop signs of infection, including headache, muscle aches, dizziness or a general ill feeling and fever.

CATARACT EXTRACTION

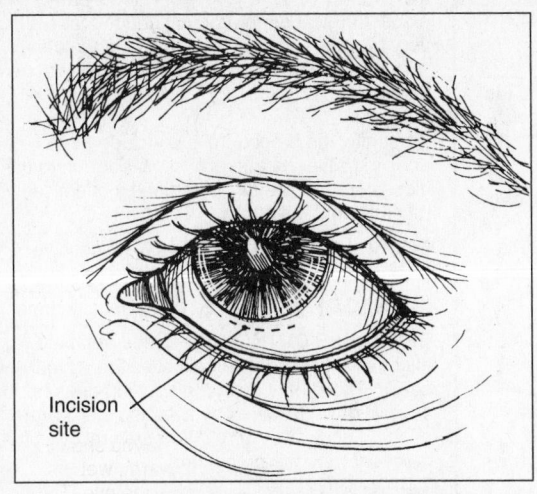

Surgical incision site below the iris.

Incision
site

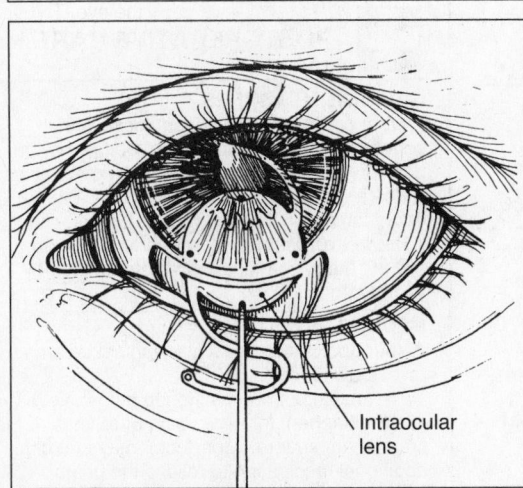

The diseased lens is removed and an intraocular lens is inserted.

Intraocular
lens

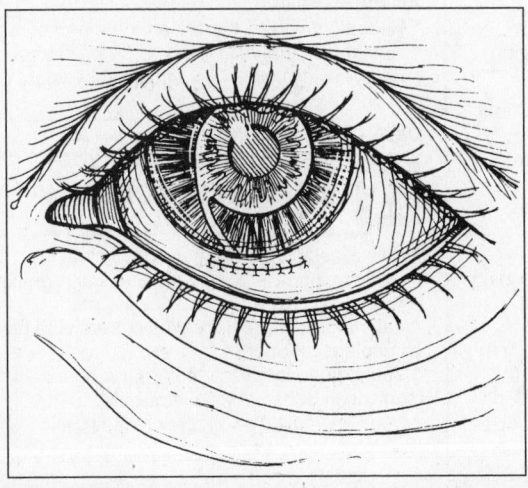

Artificial lens is in place. Incision is closed with fine sutures.

SURGERIES

CERVIX, BIOPSY OF

GENERAL INFORMATION

DEFINITION—Removal of tissue from the cervix (the lower third of the uterus).

BODY PARTS INVOLVED—Cervix; vagina (as route for surgery).

REASONS FOR SURGERY
• Investigation of diseases of the cervix. Laboratory examination of the removed tissue aids in diagnosis.
• Usually follows a visual examination or a Pap smear (see Glossary) of the cervix that revealed a possible abnormality (dysplasia).
• May be done for exploratory purposes for conditions such as infertility.
• Sometimes done as a follow-up in women who have previously been treated for early cervical cancer or dysplasia (atypical cells) of the cervix.

SURGICAL RISK INCREASES WITH
• Bleeding disorders.
• Use of drugs such as anticoagulants or aspirin.

WHAT TO EXPECT

WHO OPERATES—Obstetrician-gynecologist, family doctor or general surgeon.

WHERE PERFORMED—Doctor's office or outpatient surgical facility.

DIAGNOSTIC TESTS
• Before surgery: Pap smear (see Glossary); pelvic exam; blood and urine tests.
• During surgery: Your doctor may stain the cervix before removing any sample tissue. Areas that do not hold the stain are the most important ones to examine. The staining is harmless and painless.
• After surgery: Laboratory examination of removed tissue.

ANESTHESIA—Local anesthesia by injection.

DESCRIPTION OF OPERATION
• A speculum is inserted into the vagina to hold it open and to bring the cervix into view.
• Your physician may perform a colposcopic biopsy, in which a slender, optical instrument with a lighted tip is used to pinpoint the areas of the cervix to be biopsied.
• Another instrument is used to gather the tissue. The instrument used will vary, depending on the type of biopsy being performed. In a punch biopsy, the clinician will use a small instrument resembling a paper punch to punch out a small sample of cervical tissue; several punches may be necessary. Another common form of biopsy uses a curette (a thin, metal instrument with a spoon-shaped tip) to scrape tissue from the cervix. Still another technique

that may be used is called LEEP (loop excision electrosurgical procedure). In this procedure, a thin, hand-held wire loop, activated by an electrosurgical generator, is used to make a very precise and uniform cut across the cervix.
• The instruments are removed and the tissue is then sent to a laboratory for microscopic analysis.
• Usually, the procedure is concluded by applying silver nitrate, or a similar agent, to the biopsy sites to prevent bleeding by chemically cauterizing the wounds.

POSSIBLE COMPLICATIONS—Excessive bleeding or infection.

AVERAGE HOSPITAL STAY—Usually none.

PROBABLE OUTCOME—Tissue obtained successfully without complications in virtually all cases. There may be some spotting of blood for several days, followed by a vaginal discharge, as the biopsy sites heal. Allow several days for recovery from the procedure.

POSTOPERATIVE CARE

GENERAL MEASURES
• Wear cotton panties or pantyhose with a cotton crotch. Avoid panties made from nylon, polyester, silk or other nonventilating materials.
• Use a sanitary pad to protect your clothing. Avoid tampons, as they may lead to infection.
• Shower as usual. Use nonperfumed soap.
• Don't douche unless it is recommended by your doctor.

MEDICATION
• Your doctor may prescribe vaginal creams to relieve discomfort.
• You may use nonprescription drugs, such as acetaminophen, for minor pain or cramps. If the cramps are severe, your doctor may prescribe additional medication to relieve the pain.

ACTIVITY
• Resume driving 24 hours after the procedure.
• Resume sexual relations 1 to 2 weeks after surgery, unless otherwise specified by your doctor.

DIET—No special diet.

CALL YOUR DOCTOR IF

• You develop signs of infection, including headache, muscle aches, dizziness or a general ill feeling and fever.
• Vaginal discharge increases or begins to have an unpleasant odor.
• You experience discomfort that simple pain medication does not relieve quickly.
• Unusual vaginal swelling or bleeding develops.

CERVIX, BIOPSY OF

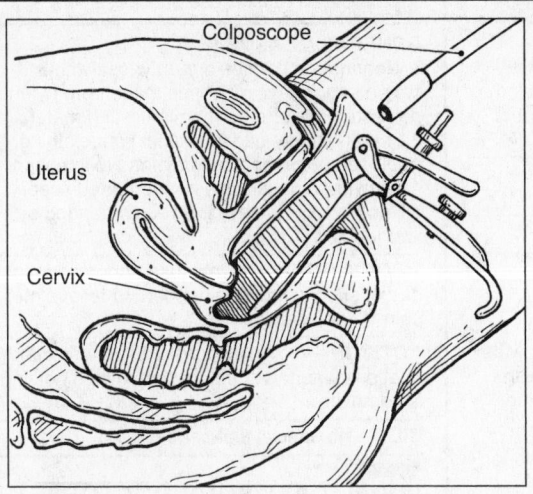

Colposcope

Uterus

Cervix

Side view of the vagina, cervix and uterus. This illustration shows a speculum inserted into the vagina to stretch it open and expose the cervix (the lower third of the uterus). A colposcope is used to pinpoint the areas to be biopsied.

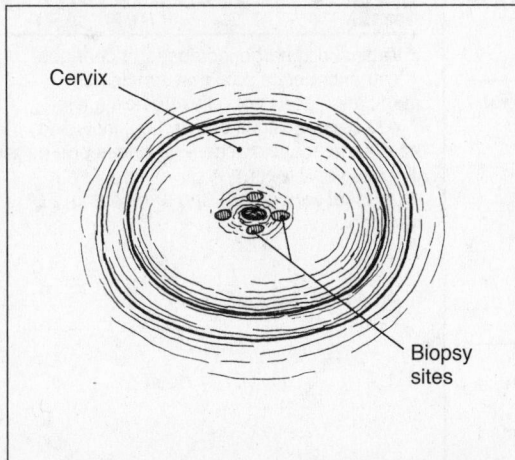

Cervix

Biopsy sites

A closer view of the cervix shows the different sites where biopsies are taken. Biopsy sites are usually chosen on the basis of the appearance of the cervix.

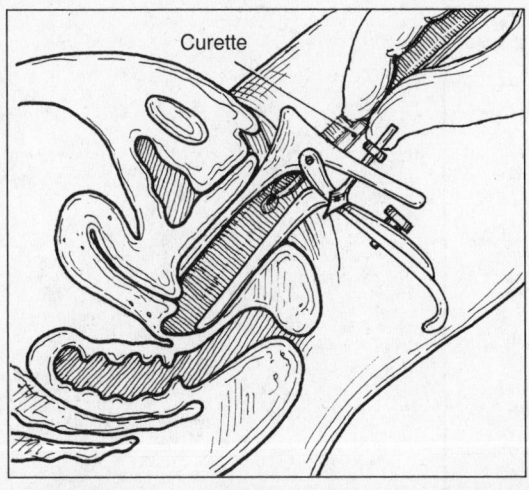

Curette

A curette is inserted and is used to remove small amounts of tissue in the suspected areas of the cervix.

CERVIX, CRYOSURGERY OF

GENERAL INFORMATION

DEFINITION—Destruction of abnormal (infected or damaged) cells in the cervix, the lower third of the uterus. An instrument called a cryosurgery probe is used to freeze abnormal cells with liquid nitrogen.

BODY PARTS INVOLVED—Cervix; vagina (as route for surgery).

REASONS FOR SURGERY
• Primary treatment of mild to moderate cervical dysplasia (abnormal cell growth).
• Sometimes used to treat severe cervical dysplasia.
• Treatment of benign (noncancerous) growths on the cervix (such as polyps) or genital warts.
• Treatment of cervicitis (inflammation of the cervix).

SURGICAL RISK INCREASES WITH—None expected.

WHAT TO EXPECT

WHO OPERATES—Obstetrician-gynecologist, family doctor or general surgeon.

WHERE PERFORMED—Doctor's office or outpatient surgical facility.

DIAGNOSTIC TESTS
• Before surgery: Pap smear (see Glossary); vaginal exam.
• After surgery: Pap smear in 2 to 3 months.

ANESTHESIA—Usually none.

DESCRIPTION OF OPERATION
• A speculum is inserted into the vagina to hold it open and to bring the cervix into view.
• The cryosurgery probe is held on the affected areas long enough to freeze and destroy abnormal cells.
• The instruments are removed. Discomfort during surgery may vary from one person to the next but should not cause much distress.

POSSIBLE COMPLICATIONS
• Surgical wound infection (rare).
• Cervical stenosis (narrowing).
• Failure of the procedure to destroy all of the cervical dysplasia, particularly with severe dysplasia.

AVERAGE HOSPITAL STAY—Usually none.

PROBABLE OUTCOME—Expect complete healing without complications. You may experience mild uterine cramping and facial flushing. Vaginal discharge is common; discharge may be profuse, foul-smelling, and last for 7 to 10 days or longer. Allow about 3 weeks for recovery from surgery.

POSTOPERATIVE CARE

GENERAL MEASURES
• Wear cotton panties or pantyhose with a cotton crotch. Avoid panties made from nylon, polyester, silk or other nonventilating materials.
• Use a sanitary pad to protect your clothing. Avoid tampons, as they may lead to infection.
• Shower as usual. Use nonperfumed soap.
• Don't douche unless it is recommended by your doctor.

MEDICATION—You may use nonprescription drugs, such as acetaminophen, to relieve minor pain. Avoid aspirin.

ACTIVITY—No restrictions. Resume sexual relations when your doctor determines healing is complete.

DIET—No special diet.

CALL YOUR DOCTOR IF

• Vaginal discharge increases or changes.
• You experience pain that simple pain medication does not relieve quickly.
• You develop signs of infection, including headache, muscle aches, dizziness or a general ill feeling and fever.
• Unusual vaginal swelling or bleeding develops.

CERVIX, CRYOSURGERY OF

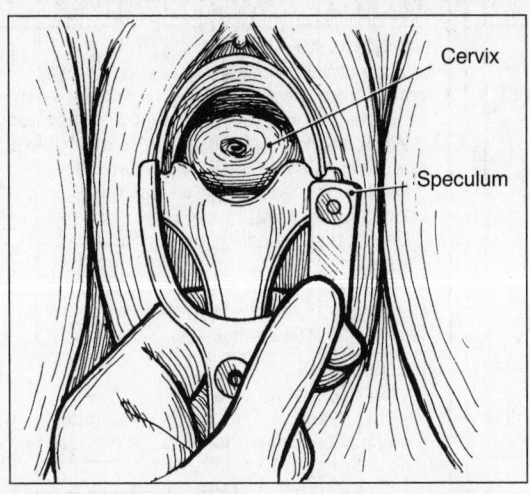

Cervix

Speculum

This view illustrates a female patient with extended legs in stirrups on an examining table to allow examination of the genital area.
  • The speculum is inserted into the vagina to stretch it open and expose the cervix.

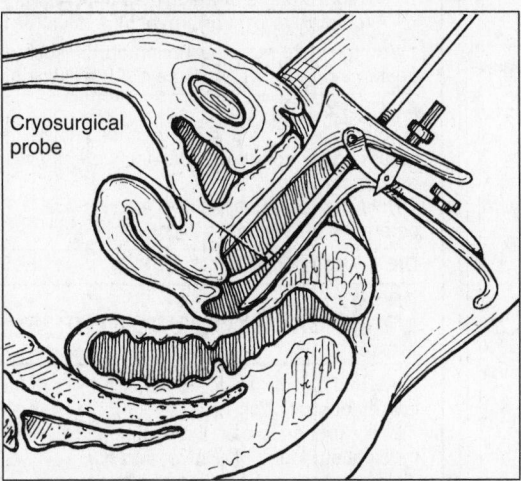

Cryosurgical probe

A side view of the pelvic structures.
  • The cryosurgery probe, which has been brought to temperatures well below zero, is held on the affected areas long enough to freeze and destroy the abnormal cervical cells.

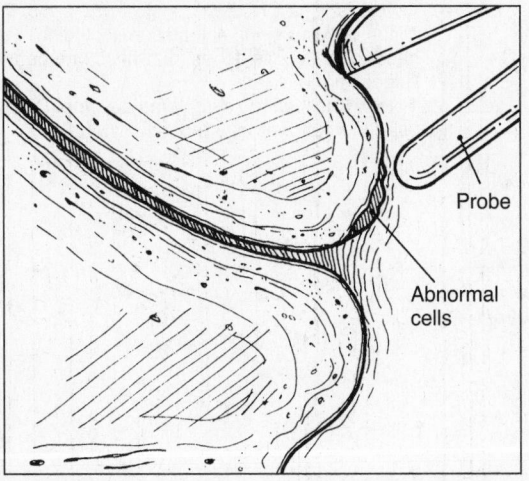

Probe

Abnormal cells

Probe removed after suspicious cells have been destroyed.

CERVIX, ELECTROCAUTERIZATION OF

 GENERAL INFORMATION

DEFINITION—Destruction of abnormal (infected or damaged) cells in the cervix, in the lower third of the uterus. An instrument called an electrocautery uses electric current to destroy the abnormal tissue.

BODY PARTS INVOLVED—Cervix; vagina (as route for surgery).

REASONS FOR SURGERY
* Presence of abnormal cells in the cervix.
* Inflammation or infection of the cervix.

SURGICAL RISK INCREASES WITH
* Diabetes.
* Use of some prescription and nonprescription drugs. Inform your doctor of any drugs, medications, or vitamin and herb supplements you are using or have used in the last month.

 WHAT TO EXPECT

WHO OPERATES—Obstetrician-gynecologist, general surgeon or family doctor.

WHERE PERFORMED—Doctor's office or outpatient surgical facility.

DIAGNOSTIC TESTS
* Before surgery: Pap smear (see Glossary); vaginal-discharge study.
* After surgery: Vaginal-discharge study; Pap smear in about 2 months.

ANESTHESIA—Usually none.

DESCRIPTION OF OPERATION
* A speculum is inserted into the vagina to hold it open and to bring the cervix into view.
* The electrocautery probe is inserted into the cervix. The flow of electric current is applied through the probe to destroy abnormal cells. You may experience some mild cramping.
* The instruments are removed. Discomfort after surgery will vary from one person to another, but any pain or cramping should be minor.

POSSIBLE COMPLICATIONS
* Surgical-wound infection.
* Inadvertent damage to normal vaginal tissue.
* Cervical stenosis (narrowing).

AVERAGE HOSPITAL STAY—None

PROBABLE OUTCOME—Healing requires up to 2 months. During this time, you will have a frequent, watery vaginal discharge. Allow about 6 weeks for recovery from surgery.

 POSTOPERATIVE CARE

GENERAL MEASURES
* Wear cotton panties or pantyhose with a cotton crotch. Avoid panties made from nylon, polyester, silk or other nonventilating materials.
* Wear a sanitary pad to protect clothing. Avoid tampons, as they may lead to infection.
* Bathe or shower as usual. Use mild, unscented soap.
* Do not douche unless prescribed by your doctor.
* Following this procedure, you should have a Pap smear (see Glossary) twice a year for 2 years, and then annually thereafter.

MEDICATION
* Your doctor may prescribe:
  - Pain relievers. Don't take prescription pain medication longer than 4 to 7 days. Use only as much as you need.
  - Vaginal creams or medicated douches.
  - Antibiotics to fight or prevent infection.
* You may use nonprescription drugs, such as acetaminophen, for minor pain. Avoid aspirin.

ACTIVITY
* To help recovery and aid your well-being, resume daily activities, including work, as soon as you are able.
* Delay sexual relations until your doctor determines that healing is complete.

DIET—No special diet.

 CALL YOUR DOCTOR IF

* Vaginal discharge increases or begins to have an unpleasant odor.
* You experience pain that simple pain medication does not relieve quickly.
* Unusual vaginal swelling or bleeding develops.
* You develop signs of infection, including headache, muscle aches, dizziness or a general ill feeling and fever.
* New, unexplained symptoms develop. Drugs used in treatment may produce side effects.

CERVIX, ELECTROCAUTERIZATION OF

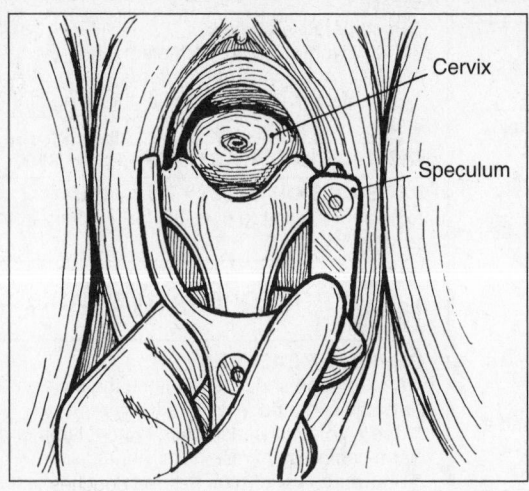

This view illustrates a female patient with extended legs in stirrups on an examining table to allow examination of the genital area.
- The speculum is inserted into the vagina to stretch it open and expose the cervix.

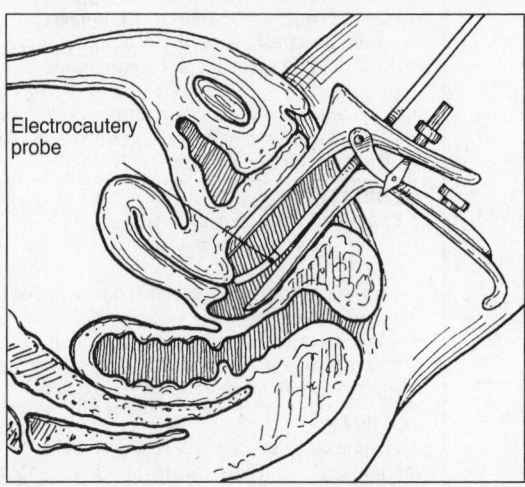

A side view of the pelvic structures showing the speculum in the vagina.
- The electrocautery probe is inserted through the speculum to reach the uterine opening in the cervical area.

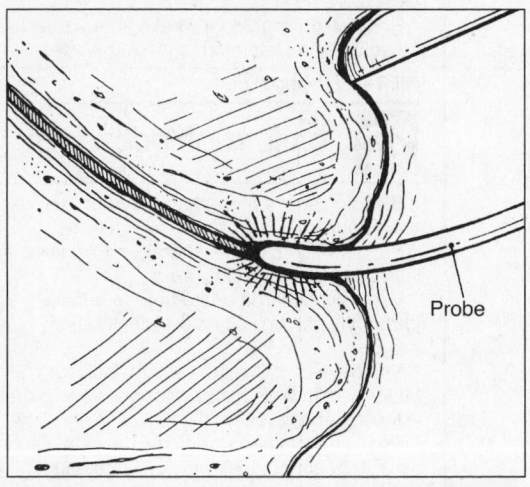

A view showing the electrocautery probe touching abnormal cervical cells. A flow of electric current is applied through the electrocautery probe to destroy the cells.

SURGERIES

CESAREAN SECTION

GENERAL INFORMATION

DEFINITION—Delivery of a baby through an incision in the mother's lower abdominal and uterine walls.

BODY PARTS INVOLVED—Uterus; abdominal wall; placenta; placental membranes; fetus.

REASONS FOR SURGERY—Danger to the mother or baby from one or more of many causes, including:
* Baby's head too large to pass through the birth canal.
* Breech presentation (see Glossary).
* Insufficient contractions of the uterus.
* Abnormal attachment of placenta.
* Severe preeclampsia (see in Illness section).
* Fetal distress.
* Failure of normal labor in a patient who had a previous cesarean section.
* Acute herpes genitalis infection.

SURGICAL RISK INCREASES WITH
* Obesity; smoking; poor nutrition.
* Excess alcohol consumption.
* Placenta previa with excessive blood loss.
* Preeclampsia or eclampsia of pregnancy (see in Illness section).
* Prior cesarean section.
* Chronic heart or lung disease.
* Use of some prescription and nonprescription drugs. Inform your doctor of any drugs, medications, or vitamin and herb supplements you are using or have used in the last month.

WHAT TO EXPECT

WHO OPERATES—Obstetrician-gynecologist.

WHERE PERFORMED—Hospital.

DIAGNOSTIC TESTS
* Before surgery: Blood and urine studies; sonogram (see Glossary).
* After surgery: Blood and urine studies.

ANESTHESIA
* Local anesthesia by injection
* Spinal anesthesia by injection.
* General anesthesia by injection and inhalation with an airway tube placed in the windpipe (sometimes).

DESCRIPTION OF OPERATION
* An incision is made in the abdomen.
* Another incision is made in the uterus.
* Baby and placenta are removed.
* The uterus is closed and the abdominal contents are replaced. Connective tissue, muscles and skin are closed. The skin is closed with sutures or clips, which usually can be removed 2 to 7 days after surgery.

POSSIBLE COMPLICATIONS
* Excessive bleeding or surgical-wound infection.
* Postoperative anemia.
* Endomyometritis (inflammation of the muscular substance of the uterus).
* Endometritis (inflammation of the lining of the uterus).

AVERAGE HOSPITAL STAY—3 to 5 days.

PROBABLE OUTCOME—No complications expected. Allow 4 to 6 weeks for recovery from surgery.

POSTOPERATIVE CARE

GENERAL MEASURES
* A hard ridge should form along the incision. As it heals, the ridge will gradually recede.
* Use an electric heating pad, a heat lamp or a warm compress to relieve incisional pain.
* Shower as usual. You may wash the incision gently with mild, unscented soap. You may resume tub baths 2 to 3 weeks after surgery.
* Don't douche unless it is recommended by your doctor.
* Move and elevate your legs often while resting in bed to improve circulation and decrease the likelihood of deep-vein clots.

MEDICATION
* Your doctor may prescribe:
  - Pain relievers. Use only as much as you need.
  - Vaginal cream, if vaginal discharge develops an unpleasant odor.
  - Antibiotics to fight or prevent infection.
* You may use nonprescription drugs, such as acetaminophen, for minor pain. Avoid aspirin.

ACTIVITY
* To help recovery and aid your well-being, resume daily activities, including work, as soon as you are able.
* Resume driving 2 to 4 weeks after surgery.
* Avoid sexual intercourse for 4 to 6 weeks.

DIET—No special diet.

CALL YOUR DOCTOR IF

* Bleeding soaks more than 1 pad or tampon each hour.
* Pain, swelling, redness, drainage or bleeding increases in the surgical area.
* Vaginal discharge or the urge to urinate frequently persists beyond 1 month after surgery.
* You develop signs of infection, including headache, muscle aches, dizziness or a general ill feeling and fever.
* New, unexplained symptoms develop. Drugs used in treatment may produce side effects.

CESAREAN SECTION

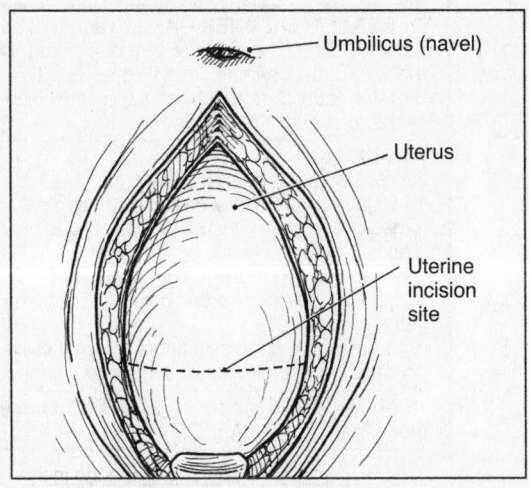

Umbilicus (navel)

Uterus

Uterine
incision
site

An illustration, looking from above, of
a patient lying flat on an operating
table.
A vertical (as illustrated) or
transverse incision is made exposing
the uterus. A transverse incision is
made in the uterus.

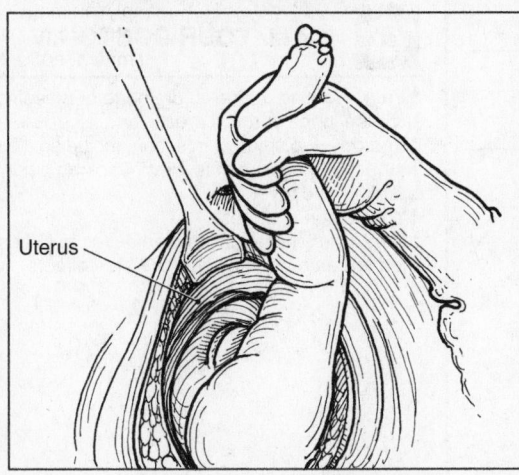

Uterus

The baby and the placenta are
removed.

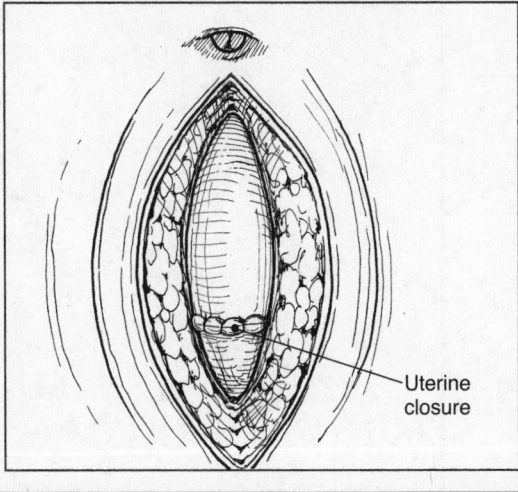

The uterus is closed, followed by
closure of connective tissue, muscles
and skin of the abdominal wall.

Uterine
closure

CHALAZION REMOVAL

 GENERAL INFORMATION

DEFINITION—Removal of a chalazion, a nontender inflammation in the cartilage of the eyelid. Chalazions are caused by a blockage in the meibomian glands (see Glossary).

BODY PARTS INVOLVED—Eyelids (upper or lower); meibomian glands.

REASONS FOR SURGERY—A chalazion is not cancerous or infectious. It is removed to improve appearance or to relieve pressure on an eyeball. Surgery is performed only after simpler treatment has failed.

SURGICAL RISK INCREASES WITH
• Diabetes.
• Use of some prescription and nonprescription drugs. Inform your doctor of any drugs, medications, or vitamin and herb supplements you are using or have used in the last month.

 WHAT TO EXPECT

WHO OPERATES—Ophthalmologist.

WHERE PERFORMED—Doctor's office or outpatient surgical facility.

DIAGNOSTIC TESTS—Complete eye examination before surgery.

ANESTHESIA—Local anesthesia by injection.

DESCRIPTION OF OPERATION
• The eyelid is turned inside out and held to expose its underside.
• The chalazion is identified.
• An incision is made on the surface of the chalazion.
• The chalazion is cut free and removed.
• The eye is bandaged.

POSSIBLE COMPLICATIONS
• Excessive bleeding.
• Surgical-wound infection.

AVERAGE HOSPITAL STAY—None.

PROBABLE OUTCOME—Expect complete healing without complications. Allow about 1 week for recovery from surgery. Chalazions may recur.

 POSTOPERATIVE CARE

GENERAL MEASURES—Apply warm (not hot) compresses to the eye to relieve discomfort. Do this for 10 to 15 minutes at a time several times daily for about 2 days after surgery. Use clean cloths, and discard them after use.

MEDICATION
• Your doctor may prescribe:
- Pain relievers. Don't take prescription pain medication longer than 4 to 7 days. Use only as much as you need.
- Antibiotic eye drops to fight or prevent infection. Keep eye drops cold, but not frozen, in the refrigerator.
• You may use nonprescription drugs, such as acetaminophen, for minor pain. Avoid aspirin.

ACTIVITY—Resume driving 2 days after the procedure.

DIET—No special diet.

 CALL YOUR DOCTOR IF

• Pain, swelling, redness, drainage or bleeding increase in the surgical area.
• You develop signs of infection, including headache, muscle aches, dizziness or a general ill feeling and fever.
• Your vision changes.
• New, unexplained symptoms develop. Drugs used in treatment may produce side effects.

CHALAZION REMOVAL

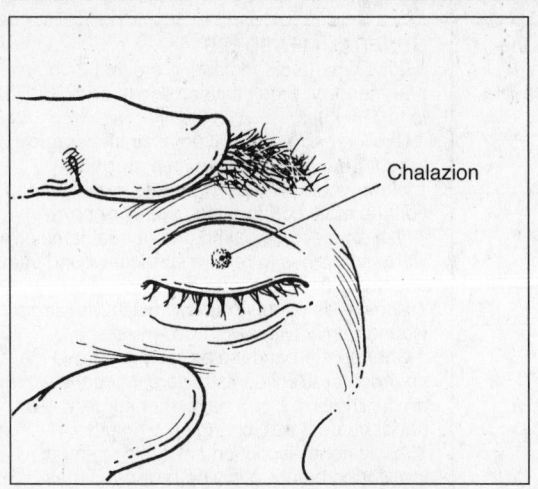

Appearance of the chalazion seen through the eyelid skin.

Chalazion

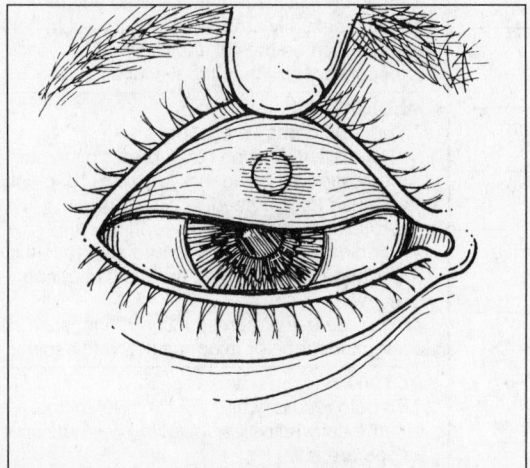

The eyelid is turned inside out and held to expose its underside. The chalazion is identified on the inverted lid.

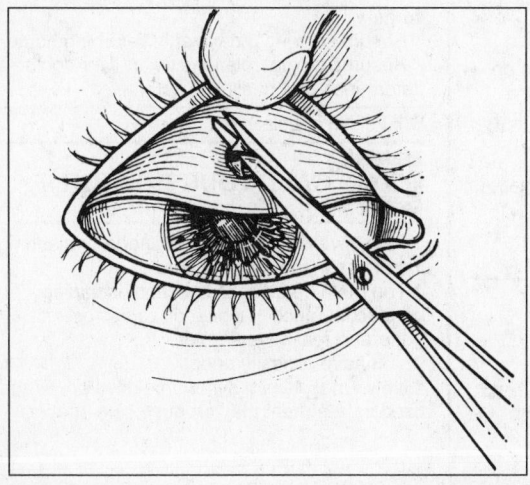

An incision made on the membranous lining of the eyelid allows the chalazion to be cut free and removed.

CIRCUMCISION

 GENERAL INFORMATION

DEFINITION—Removal of the foreskin of the penis. This section describes circumcision performed at times other than at birth or several days after birth.

BODY PARTS INVOLVED—Penis; foreskin of the penis.

REASONS FOR SURGERY
* Correction of inability to retract the foreskin completely (phimosis).
* Treatment of infection of the penis (balanitis).
* Urinary tract infection (sometimes).

SURGICAL RISK INCREASES WITH
* Poor nutrition.
* Recent or chronic illness.
* Alcoholism.
* Use of some prescription and nonprescription drugs. Inform your doctor of any drugs, medications, or vitamin and herb supplements you are using or have used in the last month.

 WHAT TO EXPECT

WHO OPERATES—Family doctor, general surgeon or urologist.

WHERE PERFORMED—Hospital or outpatient surgical facility.

DIAGNOSTIC TESTS
* Before surgery: Blood and urine studies.
* After surgery: Blood studies.

ANESTHESIA
* Local anesthesia by injection.
* General anesthesia (sometimes) by injection and inhalation with an airway tube placed in the windpipe.

DESCRIPTION OF OPERATION
* The foreskin is carefully retracted from the tip of the penis.
* A clamp is placed under the foreskin.
* The clamped foreskin is slit in two places on the top and bottom of the penis.
* The foreskin between the two slits is cut free and removed.
* The mucous membrane of the foreskin is folded back on itself and sewn to the remaining skin of the penis, usually with sutures that will be absorbed by the body.
* Petroleum jelly and a bandage are applied.

POSSIBLE COMPLICATIONS
* Excessive bleeding
* Surgical-wound infection.

AVERAGE HOSPITAL STAY—0 to 1 day.

PROBABLE OUTCOME—Expect complete healing without complications. Allow about 3 weeks for recovery from surgery.

 POSTOPERATIVE CARE

GENERAL MEASURES
* If the wound bleeds during the first 24 hours after surgery, press a clean tissue or cloth to it for 10 minutes.
* Use ice packs to relieve pain in the surgical area for the first 24 hours after surgery.
* Wear whatever type of undershorts will keep you the most comfortable (jockey or boxers).
* Use an electric heating pad, a heat lamp or a warm compress to relieve surgical-wound pain beginning 24 hours after surgery.
* Shower as usual. You may wash the surgical wound gently with mild, unscented soap.
* Change the bandage as recommended by your doctor. Between showers, keep the wound dry for the first 2 or 3 days after surgery. If a bandage gets wet, change it promptly.
* Apply nonprescription antibiotic ointment to the wound before applying new bandages.
* Avoid conditions that may cause you to become sexually aroused. Until healed, a penile erection can be painful and can put unnecessary strain on the stitches.

MEDICATION
* Your doctor may prescribe:
  - Pain relievers. Don't take prescription pain medication longer than 4 to 7 days. Use only as much as you need.
  - Antibiotics to fight or prevent infection.
  - Medications to relax you and decrease the likelihood of developing an erection during recovery.
* You may use nonprescription drugs, such as acetaminophen, for minor pain. Avoid aspirin.

ACTIVITY
* To help recovery and aid your well-being, resume daily activities, including work, as soon as you are able.
* Avoid vigorous exercise for 4 weeks after surgery.
* Resume driving 5 days after returning home.
* Resume sexual relations when your doctor determines that healing is complete.

DIET—No special diet.

 CALL YOUR DOCTOR IF

* Pain, swelling, redness, drainage or bleeding increases in the surgical area.
* You develop signs of infection, including headache, muscle aches, dizziness or a general ill feeling and fever.
* You have difficulty urinating.
* New, unexplained symptoms develop. Drugs used in treatment may produce side effects.

CIRCUMCISION

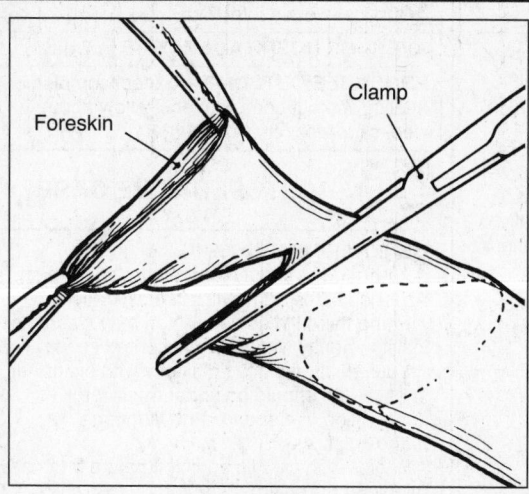

An illustration of the foreskin being carefully retracted and stretched from the tip of the penis with clamps.

Foreskin

Clamp

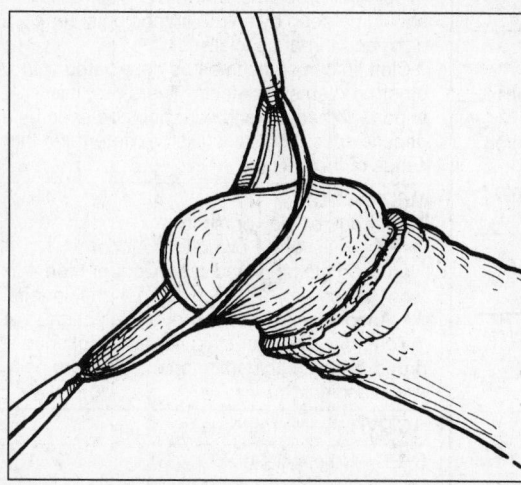

The foreskin between slits is cut free and removed.

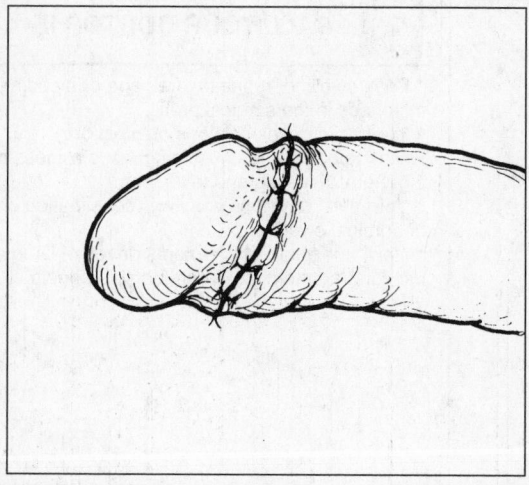

Mucus membrane of foreskin is folded back on itself and sewn to the remaining skin of the penis. Healing is rapid and sutures drop out without painful removal.

SURGERIES

CLEFT LIP REPAIR

GENERAL INFORMATION

DEFINITION—Repair of a hereditary deformity of the upper lip called a "cleft lip," in which lip, nose and palate structures do not fuse correctly prior to birth. Frequently, this defect extends to the roof of the mouth (palate) and can hamper development of normal speech. Surgery is usually performed when the patient is about 3 months old. If a cleft palate exists, it is usually repaired in a separate surgery when the patient is 12 to 18 months old.

BODY PARTS INVOLVED—Upper lip; muscles surrounding the mouth; membrane lining the mouth; roof of the mouth (palate).

REASONS FOR SURGERY
• Prevention of nursing and feeding problems that can retard normal growth.
• Rearrangement of the distorted tissues to make the lip and palate function normally and appear as normal as possible.

SURGICAL RISK INCREASES WITH
• Other congenital abnormalities.
• Poor nutrition. This often results from inability to nurse properly because of the deformity.
• Use of some prescription and nonprescription drugs. Inform your doctor of any drugs, medications, or vitamin and herb supplements you have given your child in the last month.

WHAT TO EXPECT

WHO OPERATES—Plastic and reconstructive surgeon.

WHERE PERFORMED—Hospital.

DIAGNOSTIC TESTS
• Before surgery: Blood and urine studies.
• After surgery: Blood studies.

ANESTHESIA
• Local anesthesia by injection.
• General anesthesia by a combination of injection and inhalation with an airway tube placed in the windpipe.

DESCRIPTION OF OPERATION
• The areas are marked where the lip, mouth and palate should be.
• The skin to be relocated is cut free from its underlying tissue. Bleeding is controlled with clamps, medication (epinephrine) or cautery.
• The skin flaps are adjusted to their desired position.
• The muscles and skin edges are reconstructed with fine sutures, which usually can be removed about 7 to 10 days after surgery.

POSSIBLE COMPLICATIONS
• Excessive bleeding.
• Surgical-wound infection.

AVERAGE HOSPITAL STAY—5 to 7 days.

PROBABLE OUTCOME—Expect complete healing without complications. Allow about 4 weeks for recovery from surgery.

POSTOPERATIVE CARE

GENERAL MEASURES
• A hard ridge should form along the incision. As it heals, the ridge will gradually recede.
• Bathe the child as usual. You may wash the incision gently with mild, unscented soap.
• Your child may have difficulty with his or her speech and should be under the close supervision of a speech and language pathologist.
• Babies with cleft lip and cleft palate often have middle ear problems. Therefore, your child should be seen by an otolaryngologist (ear, nose and throat specialist).
• Cleft lip can sometimes be associated with other problems or defects. Therefore, it is important that you and your baby be seen by a genetic specialist (geneticist) to determine the cause of the cleft lip.

MEDICATION
• Your doctor may prescribe:
- Pain relievers. Don't give your child prescription pain medication longer than 4 to 7 days. Use only as much as your child needs.
- Antibiotics to fight or prevent infection.
• You may give your child nonprescription drugs, such as acetaminophen, for minor pain. Avoid aspirin.

ACTIVITY—No restrictions.

DIET—No special diet.

CALL YOUR DOCTOR IF

• Pain, swelling, redness, drainage or bleeding increases in the surgical area.
• Your child develops signs of infection, including headache, muscle aches, dizziness or a general ill feeling and fever.
• Your child develops vomiting, constipation or abdominal swelling.
• New, unexplained symptoms develop. Drugs used in treatment may produce side effects.

CLEFT LIP REPAIR

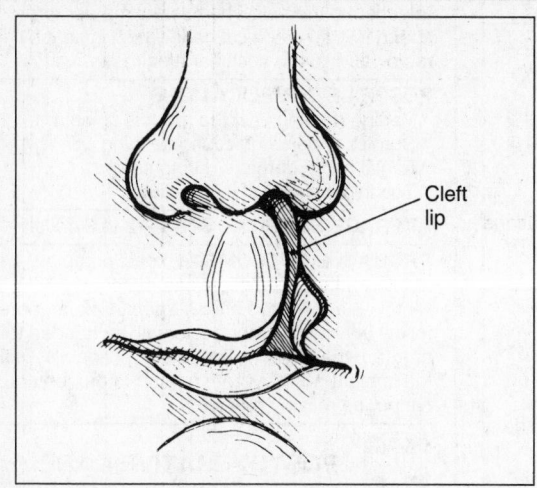

An illustration of mouth and lip skin between the lip and the nose showing the cleft lip deformity.

Cleft lip

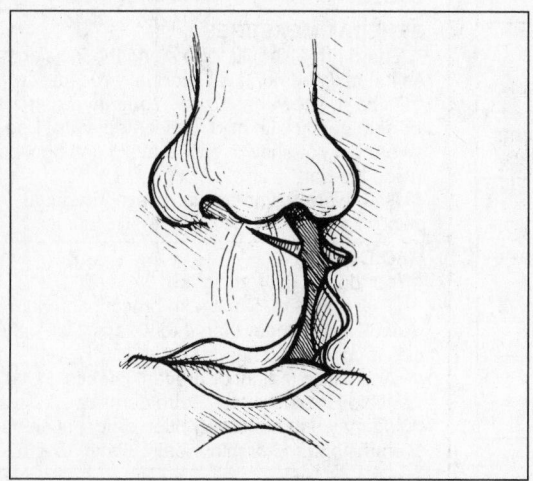

Skin to be relocated is cut free from its underlying tissue.

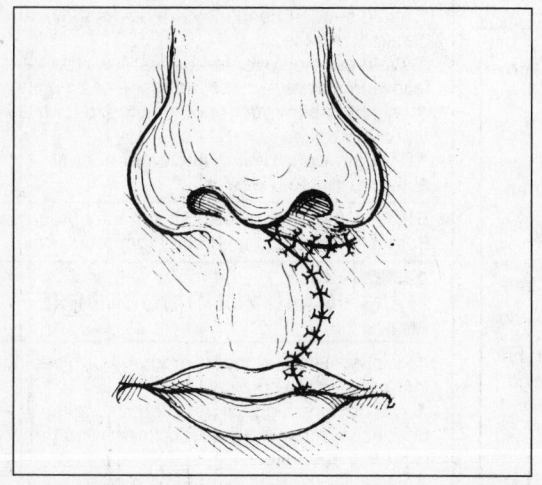

Skin flaps are adjusted to their desired new position and skin edges approximated and sewn.

SURGERIES

COCHLEAR IMPLANT

GENERAL INFORMATION

DEFINITION—Installation of a microelectronic (tiny electrodes) system designed to improve hearing in some persons with hearing impairments. A cochlear implant consists of 3 parts: a microphone, a microcomputer, and a cochlear electrode.

BODY PARTS INVOLVED—Cochlea (an organ in the inner ear that transforms sound vibrations into nerve impulses for transmission to the brain); skin behind the ear.

REASONS FOR SURGERY—Treatment for profound hearing loss. The sensitive structures within the cochlea may have been damaged by trauma, toxic effect of drugs, or infection. The auditory nerve carrying sound signals to the brain is intact, but it receives no stimulus. The implant provides signals which can be taken up by the auditory nerve. It improves, but cannot restore, normal hearing.

SURGICAL RISK INCREASES WITH
* Recent or chronic illness; diabetes.
* Use of some prescription and nonprescription drugs. Inform your doctor of any drugs, medications, or vitamin and herb supplements you are using or have used in the last month.

WHAT TO EXPECT

WHO OPERATES—Ear, nose and throat specialist (otolaryngologist).

WHERE PERFORMED—Hospital.

DIAGNOSTIC TESTS
* Before surgery: Auditory testing.
* After surgery: Auditory testing.

ANESTHESIA—General anesthesia by injection and inhalation, with an airway tube placed in the windpipe.

DESCRIPTION OF OPERATION
* An incision is made behind and slightly above the ear. A burr-type instrument is used to drill a circular hole in the bone for preparation for implanting the internal coil.
* The mastoid bone in the ear is opened to gain access for the electrodes that will be led from the internal coil into the inner ear.
* The internal coil is then positioned in the prepared site and secured with stitches.
* The electrodes are inserted deep in the inner ear.
* Once the surgical wound is healed, an external unit consisting of a stimulator with built-in microphone is provided for wearing behind the ear. It may be attached to eyeglasses or a headband or special magnets between the internal and external components.

* A microcomputer is connected to the microphone by a wire, and is worn in a pouch attached to the belt. The microcomputer turns sound into an electrical code which is sent by radio wave to the cochlear electrodes.

POSSIBLE COMPLICATIONS
* Vertigo (feeling as if the room is spinning).
* Surgical-wound infection; bleeding.
* Facial nerve damage during surgery.
* Technical failure of the implant.

AVERAGE HOSPITAL STAY—2 to 3 days.

PROBABLE OUTCOME—Expect complete healing without complications. Stitches will be removed a few days after surgery. One or more follow up visits to your doctor will be needed to program the implant. The hearing capability with the implant will vary from person to person and cannot be reliably predicted.

POSTOPERATIVE CARE

GENERAL MEASURES
* A hard ridge should form along the incision. As it heals, the ridge will gradually recede.
* Bathe or shower as usual. You may wash the incision gently with mild, unscented soap. Use an ear plug or shower cap to avoid getting water inside the ear.
* Use a warm compress to relieve incisional pain.

MEDICATION
* Your doctor may prescribe:
  - Pain relievers. Don't take prescription pain medication longer than 4 to 7 days. Use only as much as you need.
  - Antibiotics to fight or prevent infection. Use antibiotics before any future dental work.
* You may use nonprescription drugs, such as acetaminophen, for minor pain. Avoid aspirin.

ACTIVITY
* Avoid sudden head movements as they can cause dizziness.
* Avoid bending over for the first few days following surgery.
* Try not to blow your nose or sneeze for the first two weeks.
* Resume work, driving and other normal activities in 2 to 3 weeks.

DIET—While in the hospital, you may progress from a liquid diet to a soft diet to a regular diet.

CALL YOUR DOCTOR IF

* Pain, swelling, redness, drainage or bleeding increases in the surgical area.
* You develop signs of infection, including headache, muscle aches, dizziness or a general ill feeling and fever.
* New, unexplained symptoms develop.

COCHLEAR IMPLANT

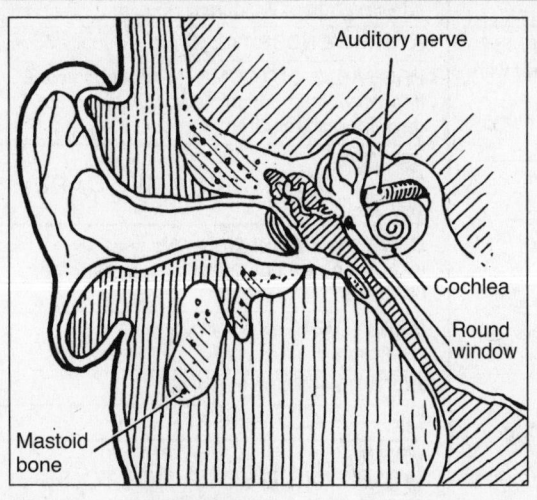

Illustration demonstrating anatomy of the ear where the implant is inserted.

Auditory nerve

Cochlea

Round window

Mastoid bone

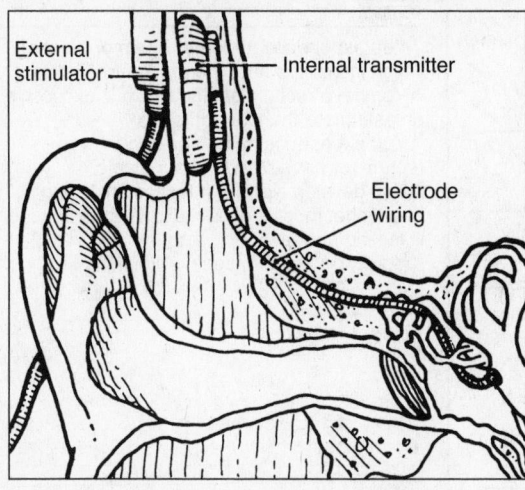

Cochlear implant devices are surgically positioned. Wiring from internal transmitter runs through the middle ear and round window into the cochlea.

External stimulator

Internal transmitter

Electrode wiring

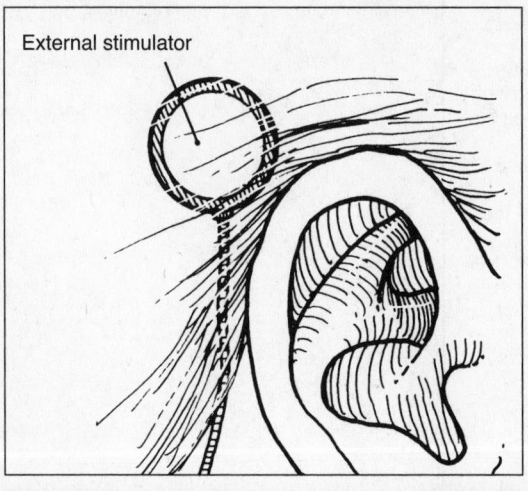

After surgery, the external stimulator is positioned. The illustration shows a wire to the power source.

External stimulator

COLONOSCOPY

GENERAL INFORMATION

DEFINITION—Visual examination of the inside of the rectum and the colon (large intestine) with a fiber-optic scope, in order to identify abnormalities and remove tissue for laboratory examination.

BODY PARTS INVOLVED—Anus; rectum; colon.

REASONS FOR SURGERY—Examination of the rectum and lower intestinal tract for disorders that may include: fissures; fistulas; narrowed sections of the intestine; unexplained blood in stools; benign or cancerous tumors; or precancerous polyps.

SURGICAL RISK INCREASES WITH
* Adults over 60.
* Obesity.
* Smoking.
* Poor nutrition.
* Recent or chronic illness.
* Use of some prescription and nonprescription drugs. Inform your doctor of any drugs, medications, or vitamin and herb supplements you are using or have used in the last month.

WHAT TO EXPECT

WHO OPERATES—General surgeon, family doctor, proctologist or gastroenterologist.

WHERE PERFORMED—Hospital, outpatient surgical facility or well-equipped doctor's office.

DIAGNOSTIC TESTS
* Before surgery: Blood and urine studies; stool examinations; x-rays of lower gastrointestinal tract.
* After surgery: Laboratory examination of removed tissue and other material.

ANESTHESIA—Intravenous sedation.

DESCRIPTION OF OPERATION
* The examination is best accomplished after thorough cleansing of large bowel with laxatives and enemas. Your physician will instruct you on how to cleanse your bowel.
* The colonoscope is lubricated, inserted into the rectum and passed into the colon.
* The colonoscope will be inserted through the full length of the large intestine.
* Affected areas are located, examined or treated. Polyps or tumors are removed for laboratory examination, and other biopsies of the colon wall may also be performed.
* Other necessary minor surgical procedures may be performed. The colonoscope is removed.

POSSIBLE COMPLICATIONS
* Excessive bleeding.
* Perforation of the colon.

AVERAGE HOSPITAL STAY—Usually none.

PROBABLE OUTCOME—Expect complete healing without complications. Allow about 4 days for recovery from surgery.

POSTOPERATIVE CARE

GENERAL MEASURES—No special instructions except those listed under other headings.

MEDICATION—Medicine is usually not necessary.

ACTIVITY—No restrictions.

DIET—No special diet.

CALL YOUR DOCTOR IF

* You experience abdominal pain or bloating which increases after the procedure.
* You have rectal bleeding which is excessive or lasts more than 24 hours.
* You experience pain or swelling in your rectum, or have blood in your stools.
* You develop signs of infection, including headache, muscle aches, dizziness or a general ill feeling and fever.
* You experience nausea or vomiting.

COLONOSCOPY

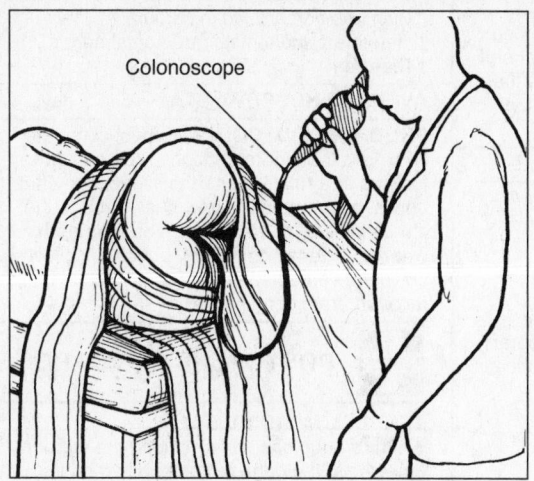

Colonoscope

An illustration of a draped patient and the colonoscope inserted into the anal opening and rectum.

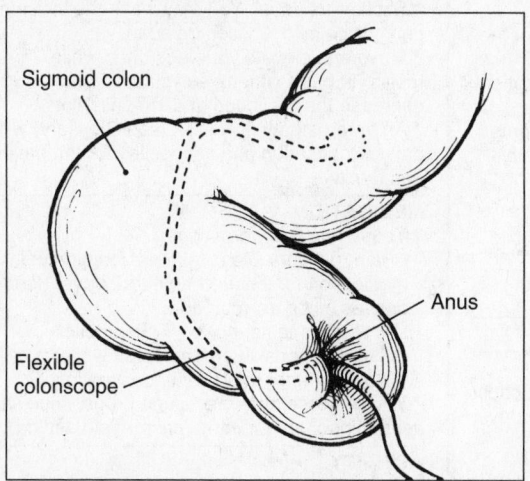

Sigmoid colon

Anus

Flexible colonscope

The colonoscope is advanced through the rectum into the sigmoid colon.

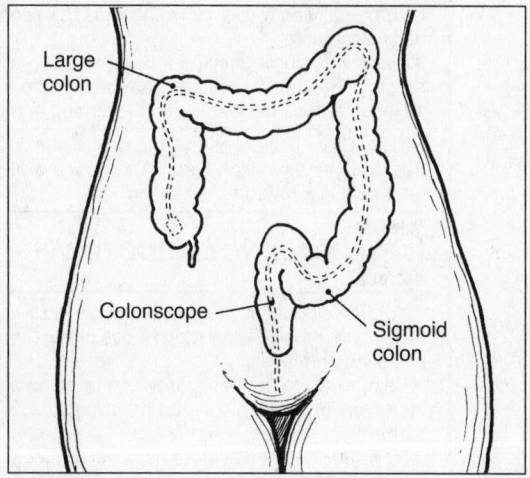

Large colon

Colonscope

Sigmoid colon

The colonoscope is inserted to the full length of the large intestine. This procedure locates possible affected areas to be examined or treated. Suspicious areas may be biopsied for microscopic examination.

SURGERIES

COLOSTOMY

GENERAL INFORMATION

DEFINITION—Creation of an artificial opening between a part of the colon (large intestine) and the surface of the body. All feces will leave the body through this opening, which is called an ostomy or stoma.

BODY PARTS INVOLVED—Large intestine.

REASONS FOR SURGERY
• Injury or infection which has caused perforation and peritonitis (see Glossary).
• Intestinal blockage, usually caused by cancer or scarring from a chronic infection.
• Colon or rectal surgery which weakens an area of the bowel and necessitates a temporary bypass of the colon until the bowel has healed.
• Anal or rectal cancer.
• Radiation therapy to colon or rectum.

SURGICAL RISK INCREASES WITH
• Obesity; poor nutrition.
• Excess alcohol consumption; smoking.
• Recent illness; diabetes; chronic illness of the heart, lungs, liver or gastrointestinal tract.
• Use of some prescription and nonprescription drugs. Inform your doctor of any drugs, medications, or vitamin and herb supplements you are using or have used in the last month.

WHAT TO EXPECT

WHO OPERATES—General surgeon; colon-rectal surgeon.

WHERE PERFORMED—Hospital.

DIAGNOSTIC TESTS
• Before surgery: Blood and urine studies; chest and gastrointestinal x-rays; ECG; colonoscopy or sigmoidoscopy (see Glossary for all).
• After surgery: Blood studies.

ANESTHESIA—General anesthesia by injection and inhalation with an airway tube placed in the windpipe.

DESCRIPTION OF OPERATION
• An incision is made in the abdomen. The abdominal muscles are separated to expose the abdominal organs, which are inspected for any undetected disease.
• The colon section that is to be opened is isolated and clamped on both sides, then cut between the clamps. The end of the colon closer to the stomach is brought out of the abdomen and clamped outside the skin. The end farther from the stomach is usually closed, but may be brought out as a separate opening (mucous fistula).
• The abdominal contents are replaced, and muscles are closed around the stoma. Skin is closed with sutures or clips, which usually can be removed in about 1 week.

POSSIBLE COMPLICATIONS
• Excessive bleeding; blood clots.
• Surgical-wound infection; incisional hernia.
• Skin irritation around the stoma.
• Hernia around the stoma (stomal hernia).
• Diarrhea.

AVERAGE HOSPITAL STAY—5 to 7 days.

PROBABLE OUTCOME—Expect complete healing without complications. You can look forward to a relatively normal life, except that bowel movements will now pass through the stoma instead of the rectum. You will need to wear an external colostomy pouch to collect bowel movements. Allow about 6 weeks for recovery from surgery.

POSTOPERATIVE CARE

GENERAL MEASURES
• A hard ridge should form along the incision. As it heals, the ridge will gradually recede.
• Shower as usual. You may wash the incision gently with mild, unscented soap.
• Move and elevate your legs often while resting in bed to improve circulation and decrease the likelihood of deep-vein clots.
• An enterostomy specialist (see Glossary) will provide education and counseling for the patient and family.

MEDICATION
• Your doctor may prescribe:
 - Pain relievers. Don't take prescription pain medication for longer than 4 to 7 days. Use only as much as you need.
 - Antibiotics to fight or prevent infection.
 - Ointment for skin around ostomy site.
 - Stool softener to prevent constipation.
• You may use nonprescription drugs, such as acetaminophen, for minor pain. Avoid aspirin.

ACTIVITY
• To help recovery and aid your well-being, resume daily activities, including work, as soon as you are able.
• Avoid vigorous exercise for 6 weeks after surgery. Resume sexual relations when able.
• Resume driving 3 weeks after returning home.

DIET—Clear liquid diet until the gastrointestinal tract begins to function again. Then eat a well-balanced diet to promote healing.

CALL YOUR DOCTOR IF

• You develop signs of infection, including headache, muscle aches, dizziness or a general ill feeling and fever.
• Pain, swelling, redness, drainage or bleeding increases in the surgical area or around the stoma.
• New, unexplained symptoms develop. Drugs in treatment may produce side effects.

COLOSTOMY

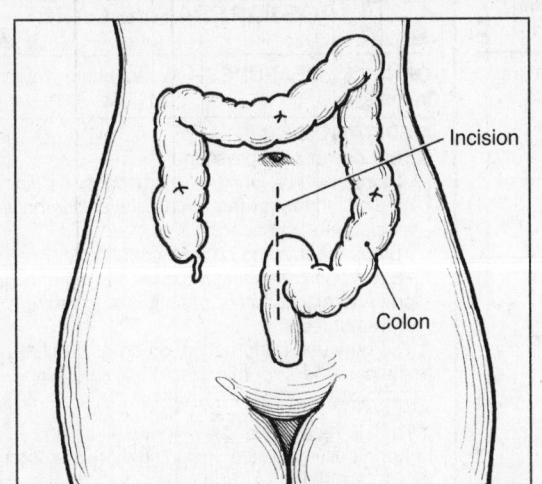

An illustration of the incision site in the abdominal wall. The "x's" mark common areas for colon transection.

Incision

Colon

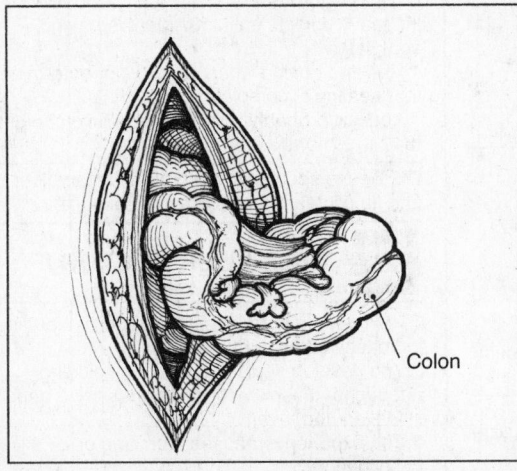

The abdominal muscle is separated to expose the abdominal organs. The colon section to be opened is isolated, clamped on both sides, then cut between the clamps.

Colon

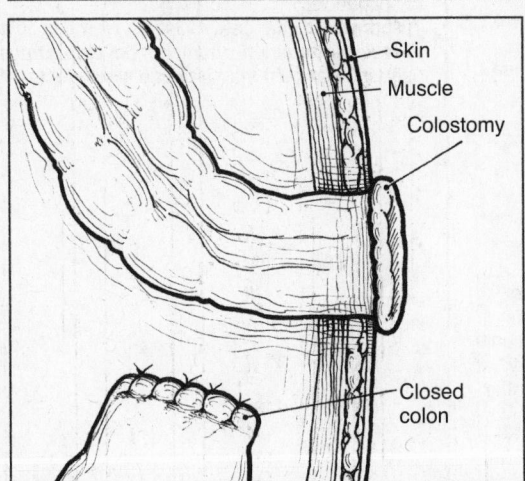

Skin

Muscle

Colostomy

Closed colon

The proximal end of the colon (closer to the stomach) is brought out of the abdomen and clamped outside the skin. The distal end (farther from the stomach) is usually closed, but may also be brought out to the skin.
  • After the operation, bowel movements will emerge through the open end of the colostomy, which has been sewn to the skin through an opening in the abdominal wall.

CORNEA TRANSPLANT
(Keratoplasty)

 ## GENERAL INFORMATION

DEFINITION—Removing a diseased or injured cornea and replacing it with a healthy cornea from a donor.

BODY PARTS INVOLVED—Cornea (the front part of the eyeball).

REASONS FOR SURGERY—Restoration of vision or prevention of blindness.

SURGICAL RISK INCREASES WITH
* Obesity.
* Smoking.
* Poor nutrition.
* Recent or chronic illness.
* Alcoholism.
* Diabetes.
* Use of some prescription and nonprescription drugs. Inform your doctor of any drugs, medications, or vitamin and herb supplements you are using or have used in the last month.

 ## WHAT TO EXPECT

WHO OPERATES—Ophthalmologist.

WHERE PERFORMED—Hospital.

DIAGNOSTIC TESTS
* Before surgery: Blood and urine studies; eye examination.
* After surgery: Eye examination.

ANESTHESIA
* Local anesthesia by injection.
* General anesthesia by injection and inhalation with an airway tube placed in the windpipe.

DESCRIPTION OF OPERATION
* The diseased or injured cornea is cut free with scissors and removed.
* The donor cornea (usually from an eye bank) is grafted into the area with tiny sutures.
* The sutures holding the transplanted cornea are removed when healing has taken place, usually about 3 to 4 weeks after surgery.

POSSIBLE COMPLICATIONS
* Surgical-wound infection.
* Rejection of transplant (rare).
* Secondary glaucoma.

AVERAGE HOSPITAL STAY—2 days.

PROBABLE OUTCOME—Expect complete healing without complications. Allow 3 to 4 weeks for recovery from surgery. Some patients can see better within a day or two of surgery; others may not gain optimum vision for months or even a year or more.

 ## POSTOPERATIVE CARE

GENERAL MEASURES—Avoid getting water in the eye.

MEDICATION
* Your doctor may prescribe:
  - Pain relievers. Don't take prescription pain medication longer than 4 to 7 days. Use only as much as you need.
  - Stool softeners to prevent constipation.
  - Eyedrops containing a topical steroid to help prevent rejection and an antibiotic to prevent or treat infection.
* You may use nonprescription drugs, such as acetaminophen, for minor pain. Avoid aspirin.

ACTIVITY
* To help recovery and aid your well-being, resume daily activities, including work, as soon as you are able.
* Avoid vigorous exercise. Don't bend over or lift heavy objects until transplant is healed completely.
* Resume driving when your doctor determines that healing is complete.
* You will probably wear an eye shield at night for 2 to 3 months.

DIET—No special diet. Increase dietary fiber and fluid intake to help prevent constipation.

 ## CALL YOUR DOCTOR IF

* Pain, swelling, redness, drainage or bleeding increases in the surgical area.
* You develop signs of infection, including headache, muscle aches, dizziness or a general ill feeling and fever.
* You experience nausea, vomiting or constipation.
* Your vision changes.
* New, unexplained symptoms develop. Drugs used in treatment may produce side effects.

CORNEA TRANSPLANT
(Keratoplasty)

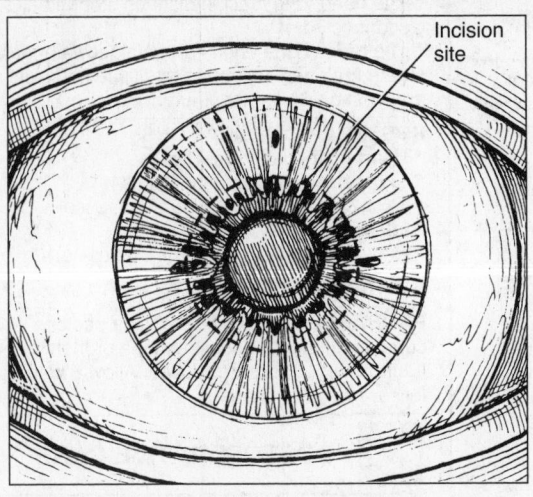

Incision site

An illustration of the incision site and cornea, which covers the pupil of the eye.

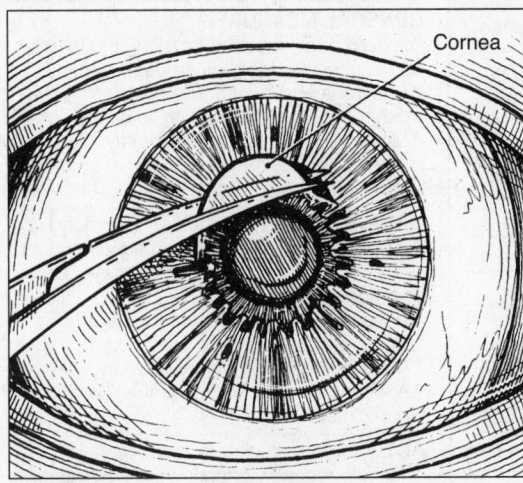

Cornea

Diseased or injured cornea is cut free with scissors and removed.

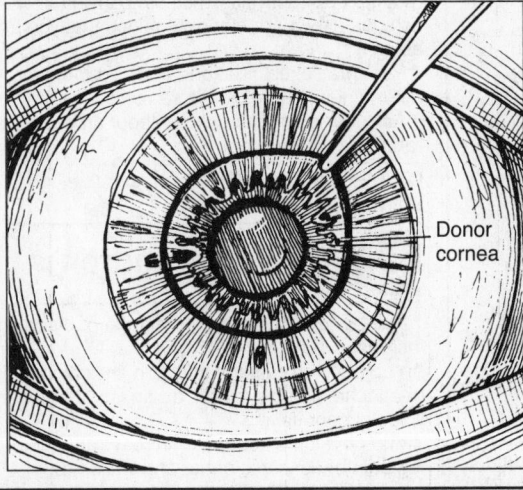

Donor cornea

The donor cornea is fastened into the area with sutures. Sutures can be removed when healing has taken place, usually about 3 to 4 weeks after surgery.

CORONARY ARTERY BYPASS GRAFT
(Heart Bypass)

 GENERAL INFORMATION

DEFINITION—Using a section of the patient's leg vein or an artery in the chest wall to bypass a partial or complete blockage in the coronary artery system.

BODY PARTS INVOLVED—Heart; coronary arteries; chest wall; large veins of legs.

REASONS FOR SURGERY
* Angina pectoris.
* Restoration of blood to the heart muscle after a heart attack.
* Prevention of a possible heart attack, if coronary arteries have narrowed.

SURGICAL RISK INCREASES WITH
* Obesity; smoking.
* Recent or chronic illness; diabetes.
* Chronic obstructive pulmonary disease (COPD); heart failure.
* Use of some prescription and nonprescription drugs. Inform your doctor of any drugs, medications, or vitamin and herb supplements you are using or have used in the last month.

 WHAT TO EXPECT

WHO OPERATES—Cardiovascular surgeon.

WHERE PERFORMED—Hospital.

DIAGNOSTIC TESTS
* Before surgery: Blood studies; chest x-ray; cardiac catheterization; ECG; sonogram (see Glossary for all).
* During surgery: ECG; angiograms (see Glossary).
* After surgery: ECG; chest x-ray; sonogram.

ANESTHESIA—General anesthesia by injection and inhalation with an airway tube placed in the windpipe.

DESCRIPTION OF OPERATION
* A section of the patient's large leg vein, or a section of the mammary artery (located in the chest), is removed and set aside to be used as the bypass vein graft.
* An incision is made through the breastbone, and the chest is spread open to expose the heart.
* The heart is stopped with a chemical solution that temporarily paralyzes the heart muscle fibers and the heart's temperature is reduced. Circulation and breathing are then performed by a heart-lung machine.
* The bypass vein graft is sutured in place to allow blood flow to resume beyond the blocked area.
* After reheating the heart, it is given a mild electric shock that causes heartbeat to resume.

* The heart-lung machine is then stopped and disconnected.
* The breastbone edges are rejoined with metal suture material, and muscles, tissue and skin are closed with lighter sutures.

POSSIBLE COMPLICATIONS
* Heart rhythm abnormalities.
* Excessive bleeding; blood clots
* Occlusion (blockage) of grafted vessels.
* Infection; kidney failure.
* New area of injury to the heart muscle; stroke.

AVERAGE HOSPITAL STAY—6-10 days.

PROBABLE OUTCOME—Angina pectoris is cured in almost all cases, and the probability of future heart attacks is reduced. Allow 6 weeks for recovery from surgery.

 POSTOPERATIVE CARE

GENERAL MEASURES
* A hard ridge should form along the incision. As it heals, the ridge will gradually recede.
* Shower as usual after discharge. You may wash the incision gently with mild soap.
* Move and elevate legs frequently while resting in bed to decrease the likelihood of deep-vein blood clots.

MEDICATION—Your doctor may prescribe:
* Pain relievers. Don't take prescription pain medication for longer than 4 to 7 days. Use only as much as you need.
* Antiarrhythmics to prevent heartbeat irregularities.
* Digitalis to strengthen the heart muscle.
* Anticoagulants to decrease the likelihood of blood clots.

ACTIVITY
* To help recovery and aid your well-being, resume daily activities, including driving or work, as soon as your doctor determines that you are able.
* Resume sexual relations when your doctor determines that healing is complete.
* Ask your doctor for advice about an exercise rehabilitation program.

DIET—Low-salt; low-fat; high-fiber (see Appendix for diets).

 CALL YOUR DOCTOR IF

* Pain, swelling, redness, drainage or bleeding increases in the surgical area.
* You develop signs of infection, including headache, muscle aches, dizziness or a general ill feeling and fever.
* You develop a cough, heartbeat irregularities, leg pain or constipation; or any other new symptoms.

CORONARY ARTERY BYPASS GRAFT
(Heart Bypass)

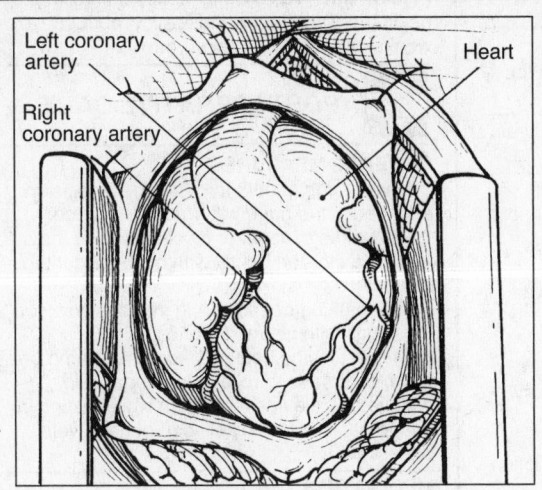

Left coronary artery

Right coronary artery

Heart

An illustration of the heart showing the coronary artery circulation.

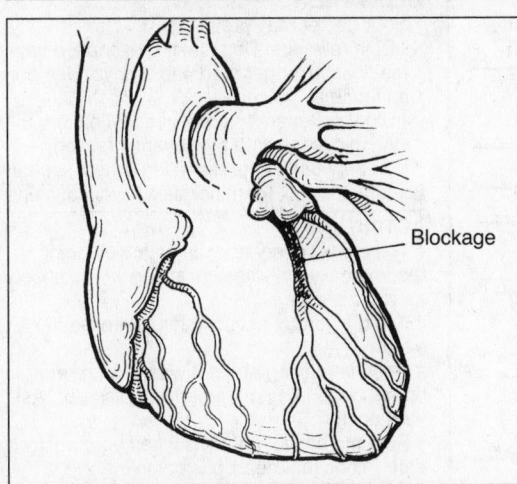

Blockage

The blocked area in this illustration is the left anterior descending coronary artery, a common site for such blockage to occur.

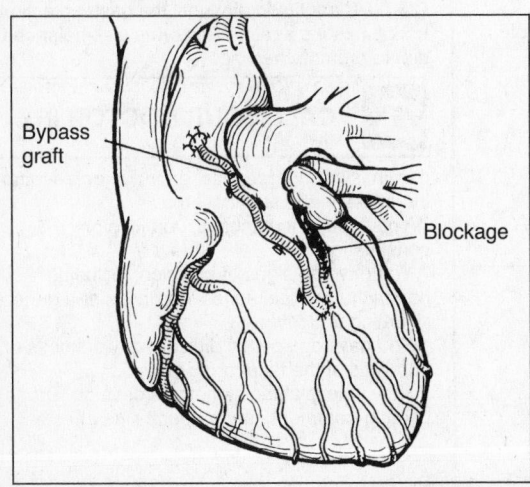

Bypass graft

Blockage

A bypass vein or artery grafted in place allows blood flow to resume beyond the blocked area and thus restore more normal circulation to some of the damaged heart muscle.

SURGERIES

CRANIOTOMY

GENERAL INFORMATION

DEFINITION—Cutting through the skull (cranium) to expose and treat disorders in the brain or associated tissues.

BODY PARTS INVOLVED—Scalp; skull; brain and membrane coverings.

REASONS FOR SURGERY
- Removal of blood clots, aneurysms or tumors.
- Repair of tears in the brain's membrane coverings.
- Drainage of a brain abscess.

SURGICAL RISK INCREASES WITH
- Smoking; excess alcohol consumption.
- Chronic illness.
- Recent illness, especially upper respiratory infection.
- Diabetes.
- Use of some prescription and nonprescription drugs. Inform your doctor of any drugs, medications, or vitamin and herb supplements you are using or have used in the last month.

WHAT TO EXPECT

WHO OPERATES—Neurosurgeon.

WHERE PERFORMED—Hospital.

DIAGNOSTIC TESTS
- Before surgery: Blood and urine studies; x-rays of skull; MRI; angiogram; EEG; ECG; CT scan (see Glossary for all).
- After surgery: EEG; x-rays of skull; blood studies; CT scan; angiogram (sometimes).

ANESTHESIA—General anesthesia by injection and inhalation with an airway tube placed in the windpipe.

DESCRIPTION OF OPERATION
- A portion of the head area is shaved. An incision is made in the scalp over the area of suspected disorder.
- A flap of bone is cut away from the skull and set aside.
- The disorder is located and treated as necessary.
- The bone flap is replaced.
- The scalp is closed with sutures or clips, which usually can be removed about 1 week after surgery.

POSSIBLE COMPLICATIONS
- Stroke; seizure.
- Excessive bleeding; blood clots.
- Surgical-wound infection.
- Brain damage.
- Swelling of the brain caused by the trauma of surgery.

PROBABLE OUTCOME—Expect complete healing of surgical wounds. Allow about 8 weeks for recovery from surgery.

POSTOPERATIVE CARE

GENERAL MEASURES
- A hard ridge should form along the incision. As it heals, the ridge will gradually recede.
- Shower as usual after discharge. You may wash the incision gently with mild, unscented soap.
- After bathing or showering, replace any wet dressings with clean, dry ones.
- Use an electric heating pad, a heat lamp or a warm compress to relieve incisional pain.
- Move and elevate legs often while resting in bed to decrease the likelihood of deep-vein blood clots.

MEDICATION
- Your doctor may prescribe:
  - Pain relievers. Don't take prescription pain medication longer than 4 to 7 days. Use only as much as you need.
  - Stool softeners to prevent constipation.
  - Antibiotics to fight or prevent infection.
- You may use nonprescription drugs, such as acetaminophen, for minor pain. Avoid aspirin.

ACTIVITY
- To help recovery and aid your well-being, resume daily activities, including work, as soon as you are able.
- Avoid vigorous exercise for 6 weeks after surgery.
- Resume driving about 3 weeks after returning home, depending on underlying disorder. Ask your doctor.
- Resume sexual relations when your doctor determines that healing is complete.

DIET—Clear liquid diet until the gastrointestinal tract functions again. Then eat a well-balanced diet to promote healing.

CALL YOUR DOCTOR IF

- Pain, swelling, redness, drainage or bleeding increases in the surgical area.
- You experience nausea, vomiting or constipation.
- You develop signs of infection, including headache, muscle aches, dizziness or a general ill feeling and fever.
- You develop speech difficulties, weakness or paralysis of the face, arms or legs.
- New, unexplained symptoms develop. Drugs used in treatment may produce side effects.

CRANIOTOMY

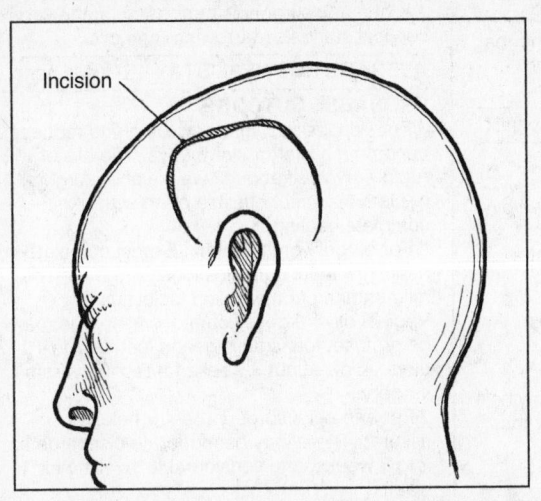

An illustration of a shaved head and a typical incision site on the scalp.

Incision

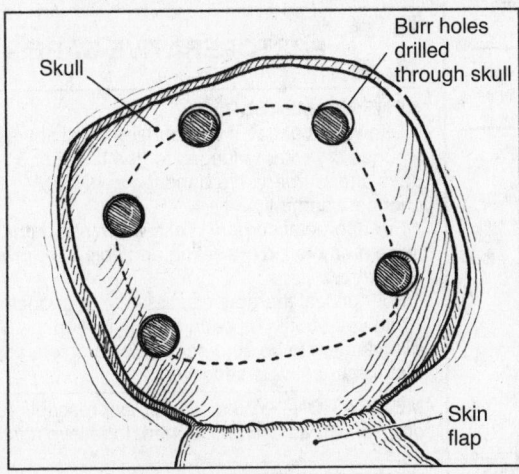

Skin over the scalp is incised, exposing the skull bone, and a flap is formed.

Burr holes drilled through skull

Skull

Skin flap

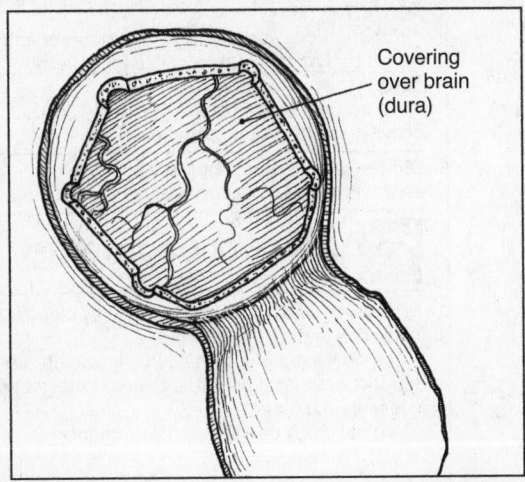

Skin and bone flap are retracted to expose the brain covering where the suspected area of pathology is located.

Covering over brain (dura)

SURGERIES

CRYOSURGERY

GENERAL INFORMATION

DEFINITION—Thermal destruction of abnormal or diseased tissue by freezing, usually with liquid nitrogen.

BODY PARTS INVOLVED—Skin; anus; cervix.

REASONS FOR SURGERY
- Removal of skin lesions such as actinic keratoses (precancerous conditions caused by the sun) and warts.
- Treatment of cervicitis (inflammation of the cervix).
- Treatment of mild to moderate cervical dysplasia (abnormal cell growth).
- Sometimes used to treat severe cervical dysplasia.
- Treatment of benign (noncancerous) growths on the cervix (such as polyps) or genital warts.
- Moderate hemorrhoids.
- Anal fissures.

SURGICAL RISK INCREASES WITH—None expected.

WHAT TO EXPECT

WHO OPERATES—Dermatologist or family doctor (to treat skin lesions); obstetrician-gynecologist (to treat cervicitis or other cervical abnormalities); or general surgeon (for hemorrhoids or fissures).

WHERE PERFORMED—Hospital, outpatient surgical facility, doctor's office or emergency room.

DIAGNOSTIC TESTS
- Before surgery: Blood and urine studies (occasionally).
- After surgery: None expected.

ANESTHESIA—Usually none. For skin lesions, the area to be treated is sometimes anesthetized with an injection of local anesthetic. A general or spinal anesthesia may be used for anorectal lesions.

DESCRIPTION OF OPERATION
- For small skin lesions, liquid nitrogen is applied to a cotton-tipped applicator. The applicator is held to the skin lesions until they are frozen and destroyed.
- For surgery on the cervix or anus, a special probe instrument is used. Liquid nitrogen circulates in the tip of this instrument causing it to become almost as cold as the liquid nitrogen itself. The instrument tip is held on the affected areas until the abnormal tissue is frozen.

POSSIBLE COMPLICATIONS
- Surgical-wound infection (rare).
- Failure of the procedure to destroy all of the abnormal tissue.

- For anorectal surgery: constipation; urinary retention; recurrence of hemorrhoids.
- When cryosurgery is performed on the cervix, cervical stenosis (narrowing) can occur.

AVERAGE HOSPITAL STAY—Usually none.

PROBABLE OUTCOME
- For skin lesions: Initial swelling and redness become a blister in 2 or 3 days. The blister will rupture by itself about 2 weeks after surgery. It will leave a scab, but little or no scar after complete healing.
- For surgery of the cervix: Expect complete healing without complications. There may be mild uterine cramping and facial flushing. Vaginal discharge is common; discharge may be profuse, foul-smelling, and last for 7 to 10 days. Allow about 3 weeks for recovery from surgery.
- For anorectal surgery (hemorrhoids or fissure): There may be moderate discharge for 2 to 3 weeks, and considerable swelling for 1 week.

POSTOPERATIVE CARE

GENERAL MEASURES
- Shower as usual. If appropriate, keep any skin wounds dry with bandages for the first 2 or 3 days after surgery. If a bandage gets wet, change it promptly.
- For anorectal surgery: Take warm sitz baths twice a day to aid in healing and help to relieve discomfort.
- For cervical therapy, discuss with your doctor when you should be seen for a follow-up examination to be sure healing is complete and that treatment was effective.

MEDICATION—You may use nonprescription drugs, such as acetaminophen, to relieve minor pain.

ACTIVITY
- For anorectal surgery: Stay off your feet and rest in bed as much as possible for several days.
- For surgery of the cervix: Avoid any sexual activity until healing is complete.

DIET—High-fiber diet or Metamucil for anorectal surgery. Otherwise, no special diet.

CALL YOUR DOCTOR IF

- Pain, swelling, redness, drainage or bleeding increases in the surgical area.
- You develop signs of infection, including headache, muscle aches, dizziness or a general ill feeling and fever.
- Vaginal discharge increases or changes.

CRYOSURGERY

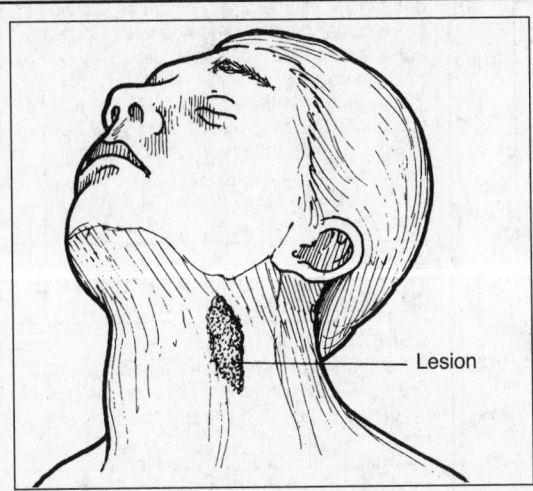

An illustration of a skin lesion on the neck to be treated with cryosurgery (very low temperature).

Lesion

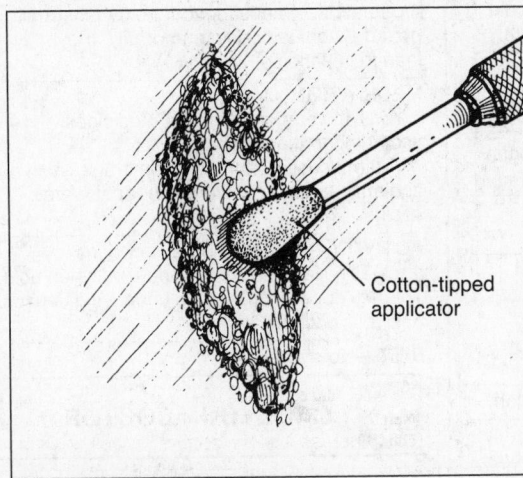

A cotton-tipped applicator that has been dipped in liquid nitrogen is held against the lesion to destroy abnormal cells.

Cotton-tipped applicator

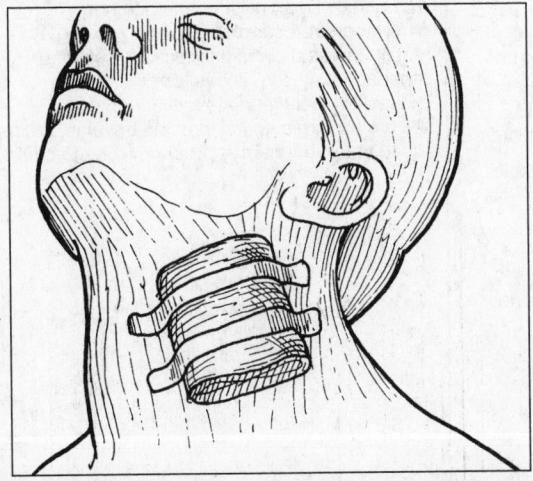

Large treated areas should be covered with bandages until healing is complete.

SURGERIES

CULDOCENTESIS

GENERAL INFORMATION

DEFINITION—Piercing the "cul-de-sac," the space deep in the vagina behind and under the cervix, in order to obtain a fluid sample for laboratory examination.

BODY PARTS INVOLVED—Vagina; lowest part of pelvis behind the uterus and cervix.

REASONS FOR SURGERY—Investigation of possible ailments in the abdomen and pelvis, including: bleeding inside the lower pelvic cavity; ruptured ectopic pregnancy; ruptured ovarian cyst; ovarian cancer; or pelvic inflammatory disease. Laboratory examination of the removed fluid aids in diagnosis.

SURGICAL RISK INCREASES WITH
- Recent or chronic illness.
- Diabetes.
- Use of some prescription and nonprescription drugs. Inform your doctor of any drugs, medications, or vitamin and herb supplements you are using or have used in the last month.

WHAT TO EXPECT

WHO OPERATES—Obstetrician-gynecologist, general surgeon or family doctor.

WHERE PERFORMED—Doctor's office; outpatient surgical facility; or hospital.

DIAGNOSTIC TESTS
- Before surgery: Pap smear; vaginal and abdominal exam; x-rays of lower abdomen.
- After surgery: Laboratory examination of removed fluid.

ANESTHESIA—Local anesthesia by injection.

DESCRIPTION OF OPERATION
- A speculum is inserted into the vagina to hold it open.
- The rear lip of the cervix is raised.
- A local anesthetic is applied to the farthest back portion of the vagina (cul-de-sac).
- The posterior wall of the vagina is penetrated with a needle and syringe.
- Fluid, if present, is aspirated. No sutures are necessary.

POSSIBLE COMPLICATIONS
- Perforation of bladder or bowel (rare).
- Excessive bleeding.
- Surgical-wound infection.

AVERAGE HOSPITAL STAY—Usually none.

PROBABLE OUTCOME
- A fluid sample is obtained successfully without complications in virtually all cases. If fluid or blood confirms other findings that suggest a serious disease or condition, you may need further surgery.
- If no fluid is obtained and there are no complications, but you still have your original symptoms, expect further observation or tests to diagnose your conditions.
- Allow about 1 week for recovery from the procedure.

POSTOPERATIVE CARE

GENERAL MEASURES
- Resume your usual activities as soon as possible, if symptoms that caused the need for surgery disappear. If symptoms recur, see your doctor.
- Continue to use your usual birth-control methods. Your periods should not be disturbed.
- Use sanitary pads for your next menstrual period. Avoid tampons temporarily; they may lead to infection.

MEDICATION
- Your doctor may prescribe medicines according to diagnosis.
- You may use nonprescription drugs, such as acetaminophen, to relieve minor pain. Avoid aspirin.

ACTIVITY—Resume normal activities gradually. Resume sexual relations when able. This will depend on various underlying causes. Ask your doctor.

DIET—No special diet.

CALL YOUR DOCTOR IF

- You experience vaginal bleeding that soaks more than 1 pad or tampon each hour.
- Symptoms recur or worsen.
- You develop signs of infection, including headache, muscle aches, dizziness, or a general ill feeling and fever.
- New, unexplained symptoms develop. Drugs used in treatment may produce side effects.

CULDOCENTESIS

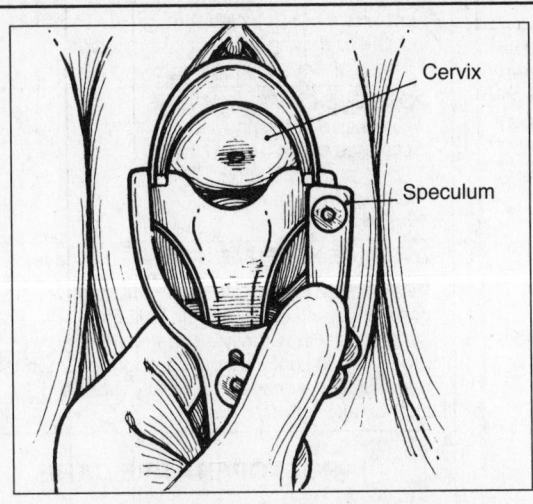

Cervix

Speculum

This view illustrates a female patient with extended legs in stirrups on an examining table to allow examination of the genital area.
   • The speculum is inserted into the vagina to stretch it open and expose the cervix.

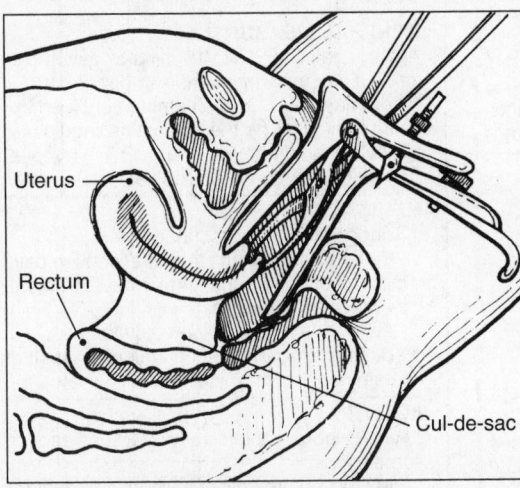

Uterus

Rectum

Cul-de-sac

Forceps grasp the rear lip of the cervix to expose the cul-de-sac (the farthest back portion of the vagina).

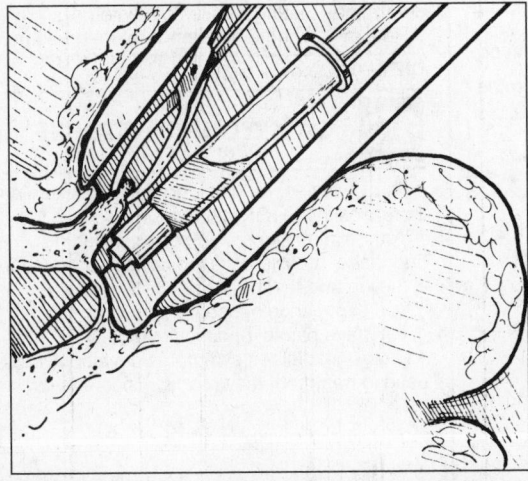

The cul-de-sac is penetrated with needle and syringe. Fluid, if present, is aspirated.

SURGERIES

CYSTOSCOPY

GENERAL INFORMATION

DEFINITION—Visual examination of the lower urinary tract and collection of a urine sample from the bladder. The examination is performed with a cystoscope, a thin fiber-optic instrument with a lighted tip.

BODY PARTS INVOLVED—Urethra; bladder; openings into the bladder.

REASONS FOR SURGERY
* Blood in the urine (hematuria).
* Inability to control urination (incontinence).
* Recurrent urinary tract infections.
* Congenital abnormalities of the urinary tract.
* Tumors of the bladder.
* Bladder or kidney stones.
* Tightening of the urethra or the ureters.

SURGICAL RISK INCREASES WITH
* Obesity.
* Smoking.
* Recent or chronic illness.
* Diabetes.
* Use of some prescription and nonprescription drugs. Inform your doctor of any drugs, medications, or vitamin and herb supplements you are using or have used in the last month.

WHAT TO EXPECT

WHO OPERATES—Urologist.

WHERE PERFORMED—Hospital, doctor's office or outpatient surgical facility.

DIAGNOSTIC TESTS
* Before surgery: Blood and urine studies; x-rays of kidneys, ureters (see Glossary) and bladder; CT scan (see Glossary).
* During surgery: Retrograde pyelograms (see Glossary).
* After surgery: Blood studies.

ANESTHESIA
* Spinal anesthesia (sometimes) by injection or injected general anesthesia.
* Local anesthesia with or without sedation.

DESCRIPTION OF OPERATION
* The patient urinates before surgery so that urine remaining in the bladder can be measured.
* The cystoscope is lubricated and inserted through the urethra into the bladder. A urine sample is collected.
* Fluid is pumped through the cystoscope to inflate the bladder, which allows visual examination of the entire bladder wall.
* Bladder or kidney stones are removed, if necessary. Tissue samples are gathered and, if necessary, lesions are treated.

* Catheters are passed through the cystoscope and guided to the openings into the ureters. A harmless dye is injected through the catheters into the ureters to perform x-ray studies.
* The cystoscope is removed.

POSSIBLE COMPLICATIONS
* Excessive bleeding.
* Damage to the urethra.
* Perforation of bladder.
* Urinary tract infection.
* Injury to the penis.

AVERAGE HOSPITAL STAY—0 to 3 days.

PROBABLE OUTCOME—Examination completed and urine sample collected successfully in virtually all cases. If the procedure is confined to inspection and manual manipulation, recovery is usually rapid and should take only 2 to 4 days.

POSTOPERATIVE CARE

GENERAL MEASURES
* Warm baths for 10 to 15 minutes several times a day may help to relieve discomfort.
* You may notice a small amount of blood in your urine following the exam; this should last no more than 24 hours.
* Drink eight 8 ounce glasses of water a day.

MEDICATION
* Your doctor may prescribe:
  - Pain relievers. Don't take prescription pain medication longer than 4 to 7 days. Use only as much as you need.
  - Antibiotics to fight or prevent infection.
* You may use nonprescription drugs, such as acetaminophen, for minor pain.

ACTIVITY
* Avoid vigorous exercise for 2 weeks after surgery.
* Resume sexual relations when your doctor determines that healing is complete.
* Resume driving 2 days after returning home.

DIET—No special diet.

CALL YOUR DOCTOR IF

* Pain, swelling, redness, drainage or bleeding increases in the surgical area.
* You develop signs of infection, including headache, muscle aches, dizziness or a general ill feeling and fever.
* You experience nausea or vomiting.
* You have painful or difficult urination.
* New, unexplained symptoms develop. Drugs used in treatment may produce side effects.

CYSTOSCOPY

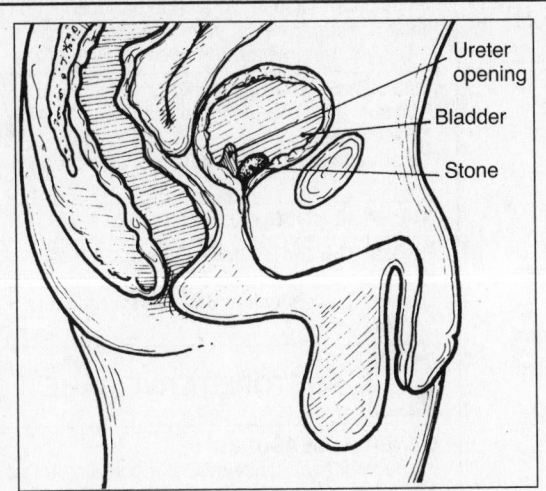

A cross-section of the male pelvis showing the urethra, bladder and openings into the bladder. A typical stone inside the bladder is illustrated.

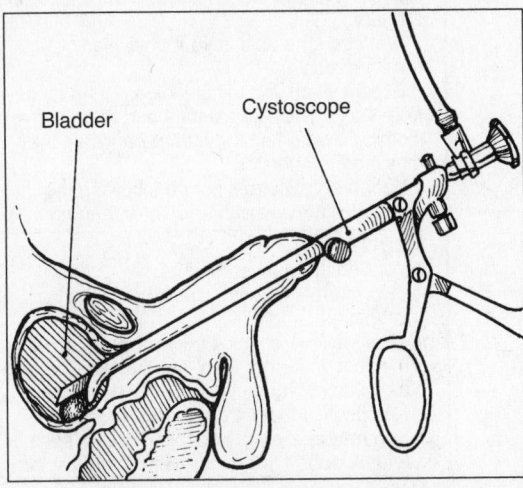

A lubricated cystoscope is inserted through the urethra into the bladder to allow removal of the stone. If needed, a catheter can be passed through the cystoscope.

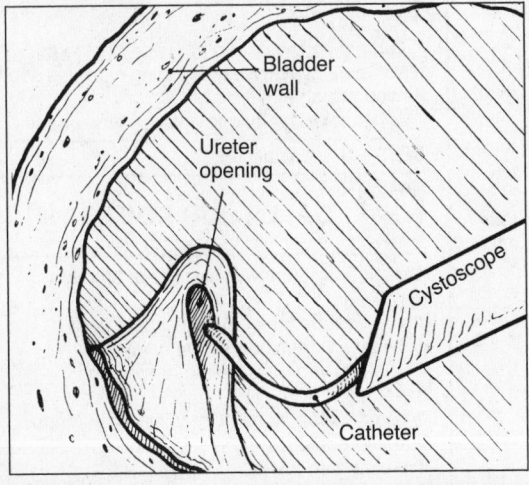

A catheter passed through the cystoscope toward the opening of the ureter. The catheter can be passed through the ureteral opening to remove other stones higher in the urinary tract.

SURGERIES

DILATATION AND CURETTAGE OF THE UTERUS (D & C)

 GENERAL INFORMATION

DEFINITION—Opening the cervix and scraping the lining (endometrium) and contents of the uterus. The D & C is often both a diagnostic and a therapeutic procedure.

BODY PARTS INVOLVED—Uterus; cervix; vagina (as route for surgery).

REASONS FOR SURGERY
• Diagnosis of abnormal bleeding or possible cancer inside the uterus.
• Incomplete spontaneous miscarriage.
• Treatment of minor diseases of the uterus.
• Prevent or stop hemorrhage or subsequent infection following miscarriage.
• Removal of membranes and placenta after childbirth in cases where they fail to deliver spontaneously (retained placenta).
• Elective abortion during early pregnancy.

SURGICAL RISK INCREASES WITH
• Obesity; smoking; alcoholism.
• Cervical infection or ongoing uterine infection.
• Recent or chronic illness; diabetes.
• Use of some prescription and nonprescription drugs. Inform your doctor of any drugs, medications, or vitamin and herb supplements you are using or have used in the last month.

 WHAT TO EXPECT

WHO OPERATES—Obstetrician-gynecologist, general surgeon or family doctor.

WHERE PERFORMED—Outpatient surgical facility or hospital.

DIAGNOSTIC TESTS
• Before surgery: Pap smear (see Glossary); pregnancy test; blood and hormonal studies.
• After surgery: Blood studies; Pap smear in 2 months.

ANESTHESIA—Local anesthesia by injection, or general anesthesia by injection and inhalation with an airway tube placed in the windpipe.

DESCRIPTION OF OPERATION
• The vagina is cleansed with an antiseptic solution.
• The cervix is carefully opened (dilated), either by inserting a series of tapered metal rods, each with a progressively larger diameter, into the cervical opening at the time of the procedure; or in advance by the use of laminaria (freeze-dried seaweed), which are placed in the cervix 8 to 12 hours prior to surgery. The laminaria will swell and gradually open the cervix to 1 to 2 centimeters.
• A curette is inserted into the uterus. The curette can be a suction device or a looped knife.
• The curette is used to scrape or suction the endometrium from the uterine wall.
• The instruments are removed.

POSSIBLE COMPLICATIONS
• Uterine infection (endometritis).
• Excessive bleeding.
• Inadvertent injury to the uterus, bladder or bowel.

AVERAGE HOSPITAL STAY—0 to 1 day.

PROBABLE OUTCOME—Tissue obtained successfully without complications in virtually all cases. Allow about 4 to 6 weeks for recovery from surgery.

 POSTOPERATIVE CARE

GENERAL MEASURES
• You may experience mild to moderate uterine cramping or backache for 2 to 3 days following surgery.
• Don't douche unless your physician recommends it.
• Expect slight vaginal bleeding during recovery from surgery. Use a sanitary pad to protect clothing. Avoid tampons temporarily, as they may lead to infection.
• Your first menstrual period following the procedure may be earlier or later than normal.

MEDICATION
• Your doctor may prescribe:
  - Hormones, if necessary to correct an imbalance.
  - Pain relievers. Don't take prescription pain medication longer than 4 to 7 days. Use only as much as you need.
  - Antibiotics to fight or prevent infection.
• You may use nonprescription drugs, such as acetaminophen, for minor pain. Avoid aspirin.

ACTIVITY
• Resume driving in 1 to 2 days.
• To help recovery and aid your well-being, resume daily activities, including work, as soon as you are able.
• Avoid sexual relations until spotting ceases.

DIET—No special diet.

 CALL YOUR DOCTOR IF

• Vaginal discharge increases or smells unpleasant.
• You experience pain that simple pain medication does not relieve quickly.
• Unusual vaginal swelling or bleeding develops.
• You develop signs of infection, including headache, muscle aches, dizziness or a general ill feeling and fever.
• New, unexplained symptoms develop.

DILATATION AND CURETTAGE
OF THE UTERUS (D & C)

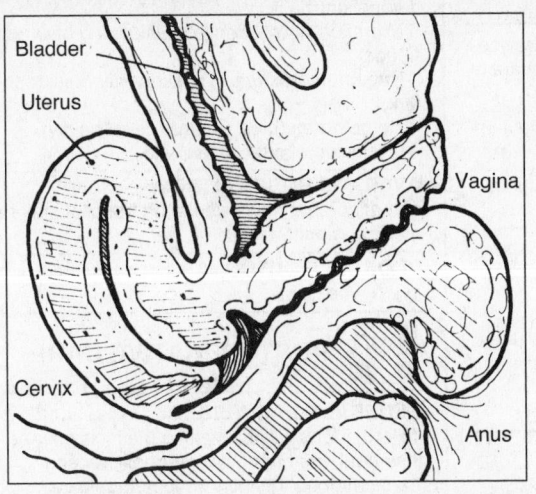

A side view of the female genital area.

Bladder

Uterus

Vagina

Cervix

Anus

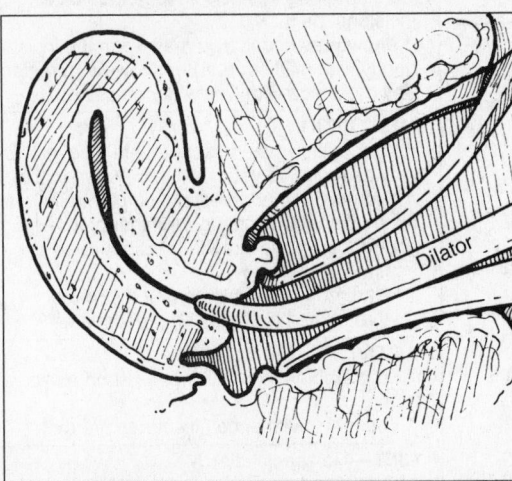

Forceps grasp the anterior portion of the cervix and a dilator is inserted into uterus.

Dilator

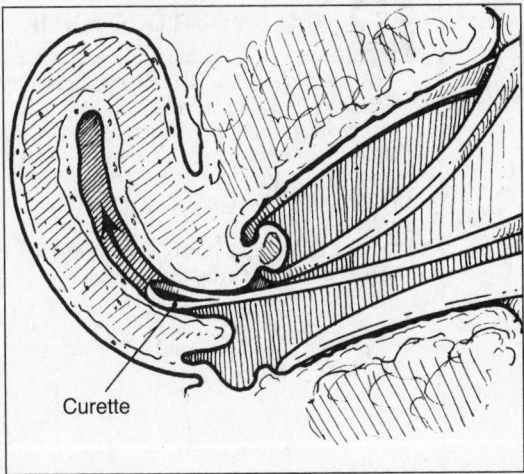

After the cervix has been dilated, a curette is passed into the cavity of the uterus. The curette is used to scrape or suction away the uterine lining for laboratory analysis or therapeutic reasons.

Curette

DEFIBRILLATOR IMPLANTATION

 GENERAL INFORMATION

DEFINITION—Permanent placement of device to automatically "shock" the heart in the event of a dangerous arrhythmia or cardiac arrest.

BODY PARTS INVOLVED—Heart, subclavian vein.

REASONS FOR SURGERY—To prevent fatal arrythmia or cardiac arrest.

SURGICAL RISK INCREASES WITH
* Age.
* Diabetes.
* Poor kidney function.
* High blood pressure.
* Poor nutrition.
* Chronic lung disease.
* Obesity.

 WHAT TO EXPECT

WHO OPERATES—Cardiologist, cardiothoracic surgeon.

WHERE PERFORMED—Hospital or outpatient facility.

DIAGNOSTIC TESTS
* Before surgery: Blood tests, chest x-ray, EKG (see Glossary).
* After surgery: EKG, chest x-ray.

ANESTHESIA—General anesthesia or local anaesthesia with sedation.

DESCRIPTION OF OPERATION
* The defibrillator is implanted in a manner similar to a pacemaker. The subclavian vein is accessed just under the clavicle. A wire is threaded into the vein and a catheter placed over the wire. The pacing wires are passed through the catheter and wedged into the ventricle of the heart. The wires are then connected to the defibrillator.
* A pocket is created between the skin and chest wall muscle (subcutaneous space) near the insertion site and the defibrillator is placed in the pocket.
* The pocket is closed with sutures and the defibrillator is tested to make sure it is functioning properly.

POSSIBLE COMPLICATIONS
* Bleeding around the insertion site or pocket.
* Infection.
* Migration (movement) or dislodging of wires (leads).
* Pneumothorax (air in chest cavity outside the lung).
* Hemothorax (bleeding into chest cavity).
* Occlusion of subclavian vein.

AVERAGE HOSPITAL STAY—Usually outpatient, but may need short hospital stay for medical monitoring.

PROBABLE OUTCOME—Expect full recovery in 2-3 weeks.

 POSTOPERATIVE CARE

GENERAL MEASURES
* Hard ridges will form along the incisions. As they heal, the ridges will gradually recede.
* Use heat on the incision to help relieve incisional pain.
* Shower as usual. You may wash the incisions gently with mild soap. After showering, replace any dressings with a new dry dressing.

MEDICATION
* Your doctor may prescribe pain relievers. Use only as much as you need to be comfortable.
* You may use nonprescription pain relievers such as acetaminophen for minor pain. Ask your doctor if it is okay to take ibuprofen or aspirin.
* Heart medications to control the rate or rhythm of the heart may be prescribed.

ACTIVITY
* Start ambulating (walking) as soon as you are home.
* You may swim once all sutures are out.

DIET—No special diet.

 CALL YOUR DOCTOR IF

* Pain, swelling, redness, drainage, or bleeding increases in the surgical area.
* You develop signs of infection, including headache, muscle aches, dizziness, fever, or a general ill feeling.
* You develop chest pain or shortness of breath.
* Arm becomes cold, numb, painful, or swollen.
* New unexplained symptoms develop

DEFIBRILLATOR IMPLANTATION

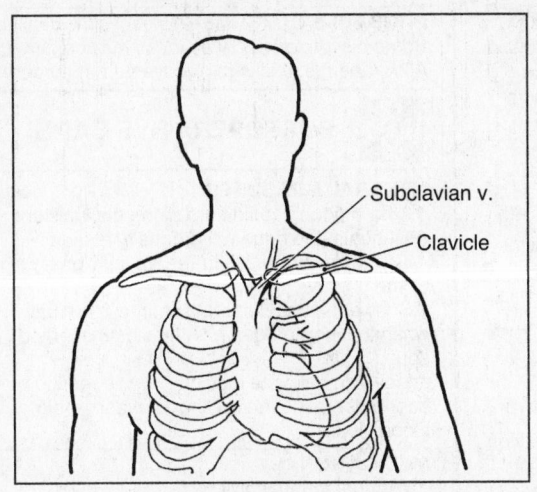

The subclavian vein can be accessed on either side right behind the clavicle.

Subclavian v.

Clavicle

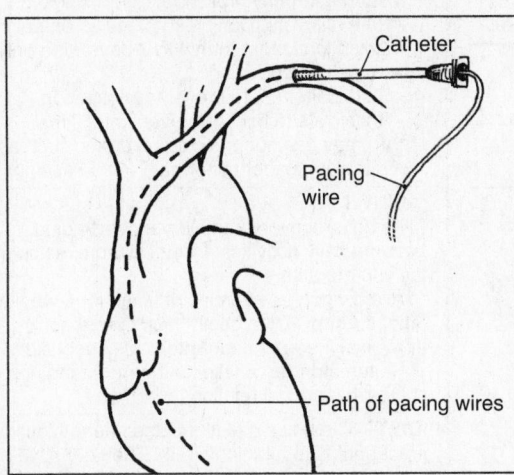

Once the vein is punctured, a catheter sheath is placed to allow insertion of the pacing wires into the heart muscle.

Catheter

Pacing wire

Path of pacing wires

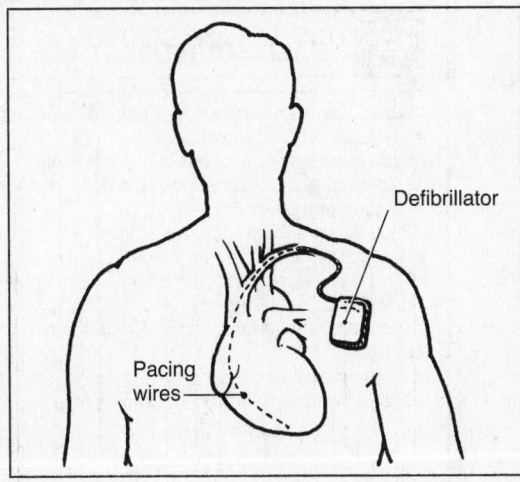

A subcutaneous pocket is created below the clavicle. The defibrillator is attached to the pacing wires and placed in the pocket.

Defibrillator

Pacing wires

DISK REMOVAL, RUPTURED
(Laminectomy)

 GENERAL INFORMATION

DEFINITION—Removal of part or all of an intervertebral disk that has protruded from its normal position.

BODY PARTS INVOLVED—Spine; intervertebral disk.

REASONS FOR SURGERY—Relief of painful symptoms caused by pressure on nerves or spinal cord.

SURGICAL RISK INCREASES WITH
• Adults over 60.
• Obesity; poor nutrition; smoking.
• Chronic illness, especially back pain or alcoholism.
• Diabetes.
• Use of some prescription and nonprescription drugs. Inform your doctor of any drugs, medications, or vitamin and herb supplements you are using or have used in the last month.

 WHAT TO EXPECT

WHO OPERATES—Neurosurgeon, orthopedist.

WHERE PERFORMED—Hospital.

DIAGNOSTIC TESTS
• Before surgery: Blood and urine studies; x-rays of back and lungs; CT scan and/or MRI; ECG (see Glossary for all).
• After surgery: Blood studies; back x-rays.

ANESTHESIA—General anesthesia by injection and inhalation with an airway tube placed in the windpipe.

DESCRIPTION OF OPERATION
• An incision is made over the protruded disk.
• The arches of the spine are cut away and removed to allow visualization of the disk.
• The protruding disk is scooped out.
• Sometimes, the vertebral bone around the affected area is joined together with normal bone taken from your hip area and inserted into the space from which the disk was removed. This procedure is called fusion.
• The skin is closed with sutures or clips, which usually can be removed about 1 week after surgery.

POSSIBLE COMPLICATIONS
• Excessive bleeding; blood clots.
• Surgical-wound infection.
• Injury to nerve roots, which can lead to paralysis.
• Incomplete disk removal.
• Unrelieved or worsened pain.
• Impaired bladder function (rare).

AVERAGE HOSPITAL STAY—2 to 6 days.

PROBABLE OUTCOME—Expect slow healing. Some discomfort and weakness may continue. Allow about 5 weeks for recovery from surgery.

 POSTOPERATIVE CARE

GENERAL MEASURES
• A hard ridge should form along the incision. As it heals, the ridge will gradually recede.
• Use warm compress to relieve incisional pain. Some patients prefer ice packs.
• Shower as usual after discharge. You may wash the incision gently with mild, unscented soap.
• Move and elevate legs often while resting in bed to decrease the likelihood of deep-vein blood clots.

MEDICATION
• Your doctor may prescribe:
  - Pain relievers. Don't take prescription pain medication longer than 4 to 7 days. Use only as much as you need.
  - Stool softeners to prevent constipation.
  - Antibiotics to fight or prevent infection.
• You may use nonprescription drugs, such as acetaminophen, for minor pain. Avoid aspirin.

ACTIVITY
• To help recovery and aid your well-being, resume daily activities, including work, as soon as you are able.
• Avoid vigorous exercise or lifting for 6 weeks after surgery. Then begin back exercises (physical therapy) under medical supervision.
• Resume driving 6 weeks after returning home.
• Resume sexual relations when able.

DIET—Clear liquid diet until the gastrointestinal tract begins to function again. Then eat a well-balanced diet to promote healing.

 CALL YOUR DOCTOR IF

• Pain, swelling, redness, drainage or bleeding increases in the surgical area.
• You develop signs of infection, including headache, muscle aches, dizziness or a general ill feeling and fever.
• You experience nausea, vomiting, constipation or abdominal swelling.
• You have weakness, numbness or pain in the back, buttocks or legs.
• You experience loss of bladder or bowel control.
• New, unexplained symptoms develop. Drugs used in treatment may produce side effects.

DISK REMOVAL, RUPTURED
(Laminectomy)

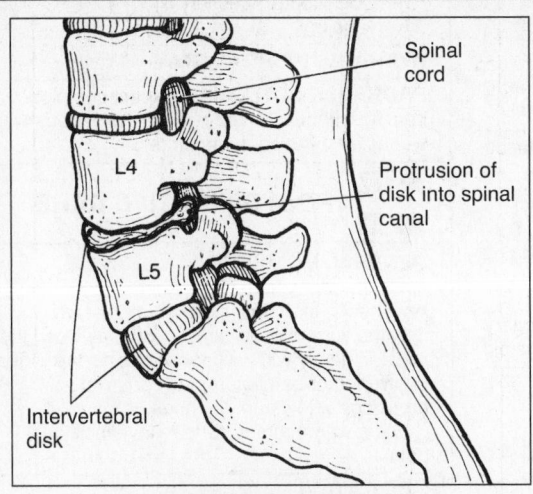

Spinal cord

Protrusion of disk into spinal canal

L4

L5

Intervertebral disk

An illustration of the bony spine, the spinal cord and the protruding intervertebral disk. This example shows the disk separating the 4th and 5th vertebral bodies.

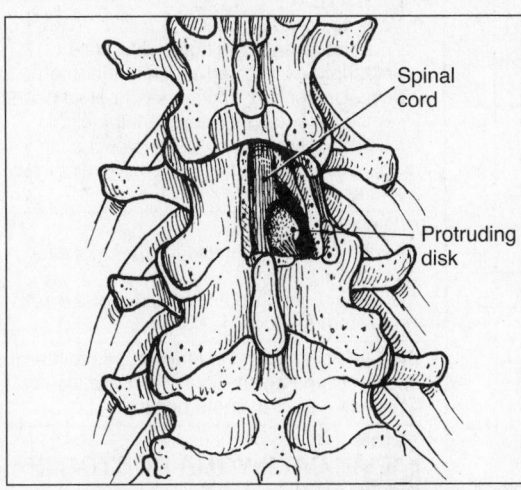

Spinal cord

Protruding disk

After the skin has been incised, the arches of the bone are located, cut away and partially or totally removed allowing the protruding disk to be scooped out.

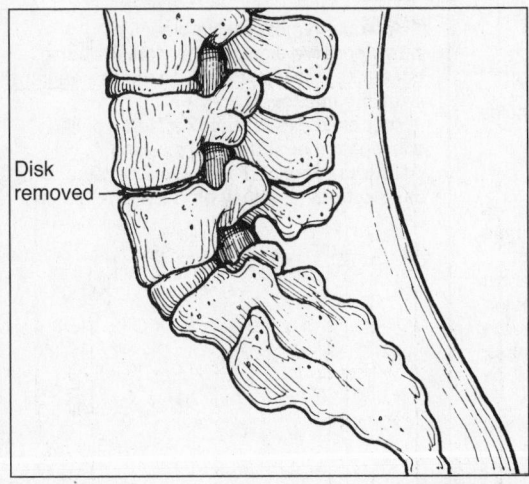

Disk removed

Appearance after the disk has been removed.

SURGERIES

DUCTUS ARTERIOSUS CLOSURE

GENERAL INFORMATION

DEFINITION—Closure of an abnormal opening in the ductus arteriosus, a blood vessel between the heart's aorta and the pulmonary artery that usually closes in the first few days of life.

BODY PARTS INVOLVED—Ductus arteriosus; pulmonary artery; aorta.

REASONS FOR SURGERY—For unknown reasons, closure does not always happen. The surgery is performed so that normal growth and development may occur. If the abnormal opening is large, surgery is performed during the first few days after birth. Otherwise, surgery may be delayed until the child is 1 to 2 years old.

SURGICAL RISK INCREASES WITH
* Preterm infants.
* Obesity.
* Recent or chronic illness.
* Diabetes.
* Use of some prescription and nonprescription drugs. Inform your doctor of any drugs, medications, or vitamin and herb supplements your child is using or has used in the last month.

WHAT TO EXPECT

WHO OPERATES
* Cardiovascular surgeon.
* Pediatric surgeon.

WHERE PERFORMED—Hospital.

DIAGNOSTIC TESTS
* Before surgery: Blood and urine studies; x-rays of chest; echocardiogram; cardiac catheterization (sometimes); ECG (see Glossary for all).
* During surgery: ECG monitor (see Glossary).
* After surgery: Blood studies.

ANESTHESIA—General anesthesia by injection and inhalation with an airway tube placed in the windpipe.

DESCRIPTION OF OPERATION
* An incision is made in the chest. The muscles are divided and the chest is spread open.
* The lung is deflated to expose the ductus arteriosus.
* The ductus arteriosus is tied tightly or clamped in two places, cut between the clamps and tied. The ends are sewn shut to prevent bleeding from the pulmonary artery or the aorta.
* Tubes are left in place to drain fluid. A catheter is left in place to remove air from the chest so that the lung can reinflate itself within 24 to 48 hours.
* The muscles are sewn together in layers with strong sutures.
* The skin is closed with sutures or clips, which usually can be removed about 1 week after surgery.

POSSIBLE COMPLICATIONS
* Excessive bleeding.
* Surgical-wound infection.
* Nerve injury.

AVERAGE HOSPITAL STAY—4 days.

PROBABLE OUTCOME—Expect complete healing without complications. Allow about 4 weeks for recovery from surgery.

POSTOPERATIVE CARE

GENERAL MEASURES
* A hard ridge should form along the incision. As it heals, the ridge will gradually recede.
* Bathe your child as usual. You may wash the incision gently with mild, unscented soap. After showering or bathing, replace any wet dressings with clean, dry ones.
* Use a warm compress to relieve incisional pain.

MEDICATION
* Your doctor may prescribe:
  - Pain relievers. Don't give your child prescription pain medication longer than 4 to 7 days. Use only as much as your child needs.
  - Antibiotics to fight or prevent infection.
* You may give your child nonprescription drugs, such as acetaminophen, for minor pain. Avoid aspirin.

ACTIVITY
* Avoid vigorous exercise for 6 weeks after surgery.
* Don't let your child ride in a car for 2 weeks after returning from the hospital.

DIET—Clear liquid diet until the gastrointestinal tract functions again. Then provide a well-balanced diet to promote healing.

CALL YOUR DOCTOR IF

* You observe excessive bleeding.
* You observe signs of infection, including headache, muscle aches, dizziness or a general ill feeling and fever.
* Your child experiences nausea, vomiting, constipation or abdominal swelling.
* New, unexplained symptoms develop. Drugs used in treatment may produce side effects.

DUCTUS ARTERIOSUS CLOSURE

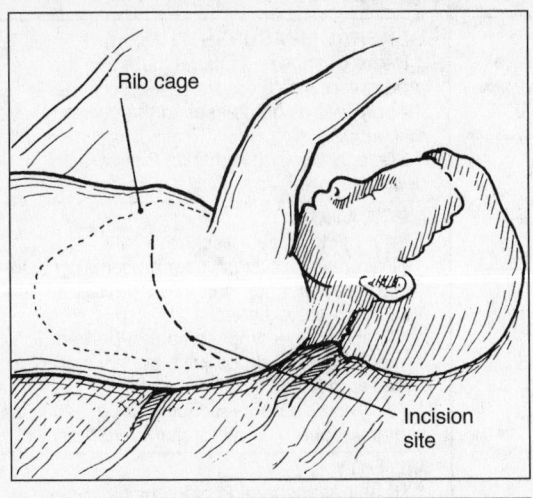

An illustration of the surgical site to expose the heart and great blood vessels. The patient is usually placed on the side with arm extended over the head.

Rib cage

Incision site

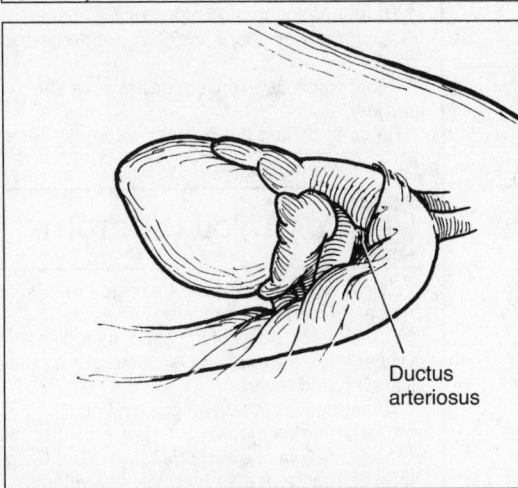

Shown is the ductus arteriosus, which is a blood vessel between the aorta and the pulmonary artery that usually closes at birth.

Ductus arteriosus

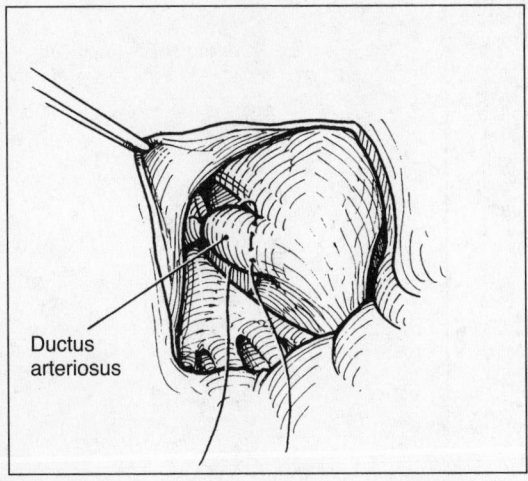

Ductus arteriosus is tied and ends sewn to prevent bleeding from the pulmonary artery or the aorta.

Ductus arteriosus

SURGERIES

ECTROPION REPAIR

GENERAL INFORMATION

DEFINITION—Repair of an ectropion (see Illness section) by removal of excess cartilage in the edge of the eyelid.

BODY PARTS INVOLVED—Lower eyelid.

REASONS FOR SURGERY
* Improved appearance.
* Relief of redness, irritation and discomfort.
* Reduced likelihood of infection in the membrane surrounding the eye.

SURGICAL RISK INCREASES WITH
* Smoking.
* Stress.
* Poor nutrition.
* Recent or chronic illness.
* Alcoholism.
* Diabetes.
* Use of some prescription and nonprescription drugs. Inform your doctor of any drugs, medications, or vitamin and herb supplements you are using or have used in the last month.

WHAT TO EXPECT

WHO OPERATES—Ophthalmologist.

WHERE PERFORMED—Hospital, ophthalmologist's office or outpatient surgical facility.

DIAGNOSTIC TESTS
* Before surgery: Blood and urine studies; eye examination.
* After surgery: Eye examination; laboratory examination of removed tissue.

ANESTHESIA—Local anesthesia by injection.

DESCRIPTION OF OPERATION
* An incision is made in the eyelid.
* The cartilage is cut close to the outer eyelid edge. A small wedge of cartilage is cut free and removed. The cartilage is sewn back together with fine sutures.
* Another wedge of cartilage is cut free and removed from the side of the eyelid close to the nose.
* The remaining cartilage is sewn together with fine sutures.
* The skin is closed with sutures, which usually can be removed about 10 days after surgery.

POSSIBLE COMPLICATIONS
* Surgical-wound infection.
* Recurrence.

AVERAGE HOSPITAL STAY—0 to 2 days.

PROBABLE OUTCOME—Expect complete healing without complications. Allow about 2 weeks for recovery from surgery.

POSTOPERATIVE CARE

GENERAL MEASURES
* Bathe or shower as usual, but keep the eye area dry for 4 to 5 days after surgery.
* Apply warm compresses to the eye to relieve discomfort.
* Sleep for several nights on 2 pillows to decrease swelling.

MEDICATION
* Your doctor may prescribe:
  - Pain relievers. Don't take prescription pain medication longer than 4 to 7 days. Use only as much as you need.
  - Antibiotic eye drops to fight or prevent infection. Keep drops cold, but not frozen, in the refrigerator.
* You may use nonprescription drugs, such as acetaminophen, for minor pain. Avoid aspirin.

ACTIVITY
* To help recovery and aid your well-being, resume daily activities, including work, as soon as you are able.
* Avoid vigorous exercise for 2 weeks after surgery.
* Resume driving 2 days after returning home.

DIET—No special diet.

CALL YOUR DOCTOR IF

* Pain, swelling, redness, drainage or bleeding increases in the surgical area.
* You develop signs of infection, including headache, muscle aches, dizziness or a general ill feeling and fever.
* You experience nausea or vomiting.
* Your vision changes.
* New, unexplained symptoms develop. Drugs used in treatment may produce side effects.

ECTROPION REPAIR

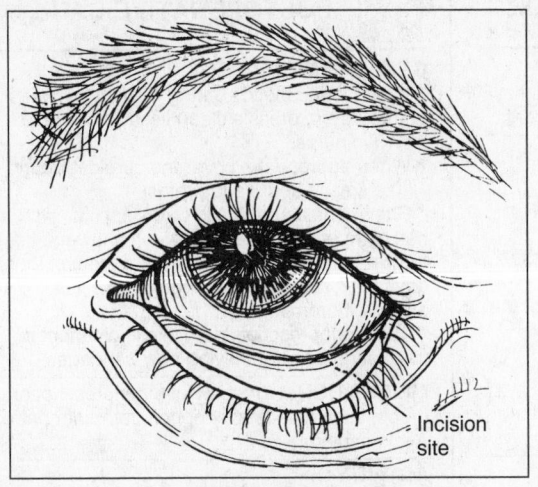

An illustration of the eye, eyelid and typical incision site for ectropion repair.

Incision site

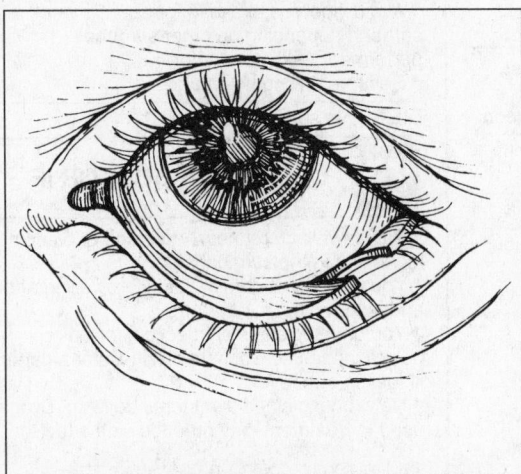

Cartilage is cut close to the outer eyelid edge. A small wedge of cartilage is cut free and removed.

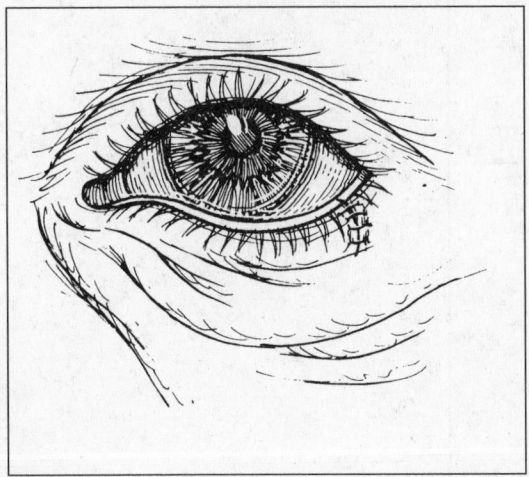

The cartilage is sewn back together and skin closed with small sutures, which are usually removed about 10 days after surgery.

ELECTROCAUTERIZATION
(Electrocoagulation; Electrosurgery; Fulguration)

 GENERAL INFORMATION

DEFINITION—Removal of abnormal or diseased tissue, or control of bleeding in small blood vessels, with controlled electric current.

BODY PARTS INVOLVED—Skin; blood vessels in surgical area.

REASONS FOR SURGERY
* Removal of lesions on the skin.
* Control of bleeding from small blood vessels during other surgeries.
* Stop bleeding from lesions in the lining of the stomach, small intestine or colon during endoscopy.
* Remove lesions in bladder.

SURGICAL RISK INCREASES WITH—None expected.

 WHAT TO EXPECT

WHO OPERATES—Family doctor, urologist, dermatologist, plastic and reconstructive surgeon, gastroenterologist or general surgeon.

WHERE PERFORMED—Hospital, outpatient surgical facility or doctor's office.

DIAGNOSTIC TESTS—Usually none.

ANESTHESIA—Local anesthesia by injection.

DESCRIPTION OF OPERATION—The procedure described here is used for dermatological lesions.
* Usually, a lesion is numbed with local anesthesia, and removed with a curette (see Glossary) or excised.
* Electrocauterization with an electric instrument destroys abnormal tissue that the curette does not remove.

POSSIBLE COMPLICATIONS
* Surgical-wound infection.
* Damage to underlying structure.
* Perforation (in bladder and bowel procedures).

AVERAGE HOSPITAL STAY—Usually none.

PROBABLE OUTCOME—Expect complete healing without complications. The scab will drop off spontaneously and the scar should be small. Allow 2 to 3 weeks for healing and recovery from surgery.

 POSTOPERATIVE CARE

GENERAL MEASURES
* If the wound bleeds during the first 24 hours after surgery, press a clean tissue or cloth to it for 10 minutes.
* When appropriate, cover the surgical wound with a small bandage to protect it.
* Shower as usual. Avoid baths until the wound has completely healed. Between showers, keep the wound dry with a bandage for the first 2 or 3 days after surgery. If a bandage gets wet, change it promptly.
* Apply nonprescription antibiotic ointment to the wound before applying new bandages.

MEDICATION—You may use nonprescription drugs, such as acetaminophen, for minor pain. Avoid aspirin.

ACTIVITY
* Avoid vigorous exercise for about 1 week after surgery, depending on other surgeries performed. Ask your doctor.
* Resume driving when able.

DIET—No special diet.

 CALL YOUR DOCTOR IF

* Pain, swelling, redness, drainage or bleeding increases in the surgical area.
* You develop abdominal pain or swelling after endoscopy.
* You develop signs of infection, including headache, muscle aches, dizziness or a general ill feeling and fever.
* New, unexplained symptoms develop. Drugs used in treatment may produce side effects.

ELECTROCAUTERIZATION
(Electrocoagulation; Electrosurgery; Fulguration)

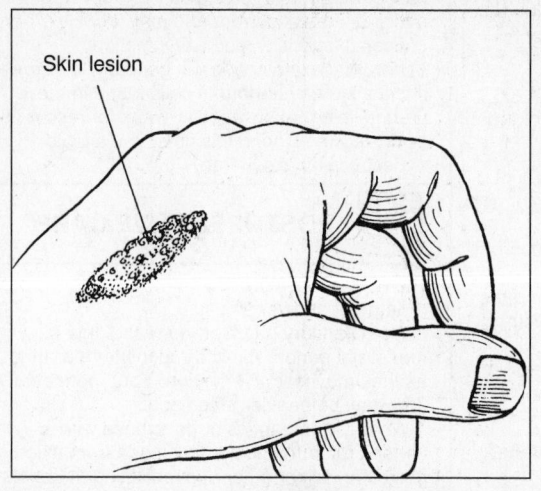

Skin lesion

After local anesthesia, the skin lesion is cleansed thoroughly.
- The location of the skin lesion in this illustration is on the hand and used as an example. The principles and techniques are similar for electrocauterization of skin lesions in other locations.

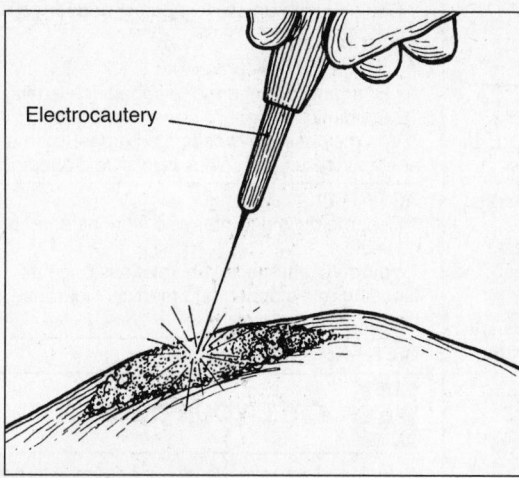

Electrocautery

The electrocautery destroys the cells of the skin lesion and prevents excessive bleeding.

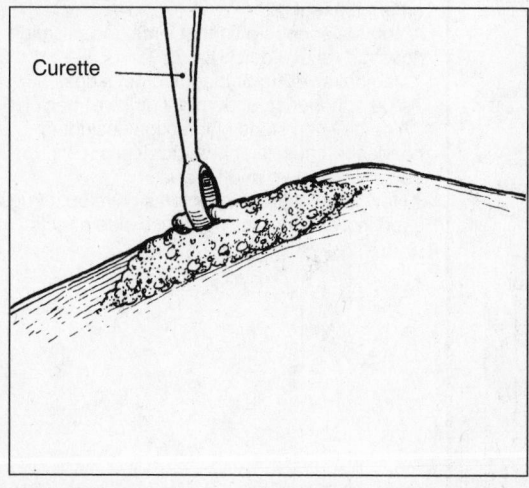

Curette

A curette removes the destroyed tissue. After tissue removal, the electrocautery is once again used to destroy cells at the base of the site where the lesion was removed.

SURGERIES

ENDOMETRIAL BIOPSY

GENERAL INFORMATION

DEFINITION—A diagnostic procedure that involves removal of tissue from the endometrium, the inner lining of the uterus.

BODY PARTS INVOLVED—Inner lining of the uterus; vagina (as route for surgery).

REASONS FOR SURGERY—Investigation of bleeding between menstrual periods or postmenopausal bleeding. Also used to investigate infertility. Laboratory examination of the removed tissue aids in diagnosis. If appropriate, the surgery is performed during the last few days of the patient's menstrual cycle. This is the best time to identify possible hormonal problems and, for patients undergoing fertility evaluation, to determine if ovulation is occurring.

SURGICAL RISK INCREASES WITH—None expected.

WHAT TO EXPECT

WHO OPERATES—Obstetrician-gynecologist, general surgeon or family doctor.

WHERE PERFORMED—Doctor's office; outpatient surgical facility; or hospital.

DIAGNOSTIC TESTS
* Before surgery: Pap smear; pregnancy test.
* After surgery: Laboratory examination of removed tissue.

ANESTHESIA—Usually none. Your doctor may prescribe a mild tranquilizer before surgery to calm you.

DESCRIPTION OF OPERATION
* A speculum is inserted into the vagina to hold it open and to bring the cervix into view. In some cases, it is necessary to use a tenaculum, a hooklike instrument that holds and helps stabilize the cervix.
* A small, straw-shaped instrument (or other biopsy instrument) is inserted through the cervix into the uterus. It is gently scraped against the inner lining of the uterus to gather tissue.
* An alternate method involves obtaining the tissue sample with a suction instrument; this procedure is sometimes referred to as vacuum aspiration.
* The instruments are removed. The surgery may cause slight pain, but it should be minor and temporary.

POSSIBLE COMPLICATIONS
* Excessive bleeding.
* Infection of the uterine lining (endometritis).
* Inadvertent injury to the uterus (rare).

AVERAGE HOSPITAL STAY—Usually none.

PROBABLE OUTCOME—Tissue obtained successfully without complications in virtually all cases. Laboratory testing can confirm whether ovulation has occurred, and may identify other causes of infertility, such as infection. Laboratory examination will generally determine if there are any abnormal cells found in the uterine lining. Allow about 1 week for recovery from surgery. During this time, you should expect vaginal discharge.

POSTOPERATIVE CARE

GENERAL MEASURES
* Bathe or shower as usual.
* Wear sanitary pads for the rest of this menstrual period. Avoid tampons temporarily, as they may lead to infection. Your menstrual flow may be heavier than usual.
* Wear cotton panties or pantyhose with a cotton crotch. Avoid panties made from nylon, polyester, silk or other nonventilating materials.
* Don't douche unless it is prescribed for you.

MEDICATION
* Your doctor may prescribe:
  - Hormones, if a hormone imbalance exists.
  - Antibiotics to fight or prevent infection.
* You may use nonprescription drugs, such as acetaminophen, for minor pain. Avoid aspirin.

ACTIVITY
* Resume daily activities and work as soon as possible.
* You may resume sexual relations once all bleeding has stopped and medical clearance is given.

DIET—No special diet.

CALL YOUR DOCTOR IF

* Vaginal discharge increases or begins to have an unpleasant odor.
* You experience pain that simple medication does not relieve quickly.
* Vaginal swelling or bleeding develops.
* You experience abdominal or lower back pain.
* You develop signs of infection, including headache, muscle aches, dizziness, or a general ill feeling and fever.
* New, unexplained symptoms develop. Drugs used in treatment may produce side effects.

ENDOMETRIAL BIOPSY

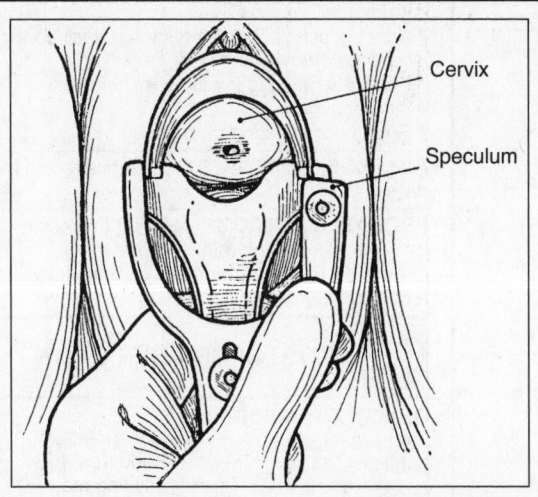

This view illustrates a female patient with extended legs in stirrups on an examining table to allow examination of the genital area.
- The speculum is inserted into the vagina to stretch it open and expose the cervix.

Cervix

Speculum

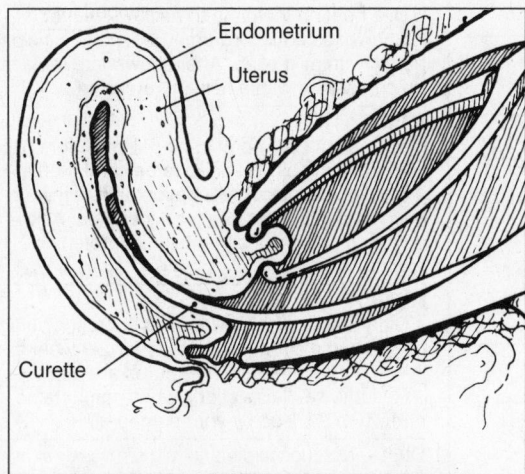

Endometrium

Uterus

Curette

Shown are the uterus, the endometrium (inner lining of the uterus), the operating curette and the forceps holding the upper lip of the cervix to allow introduction of the curette.

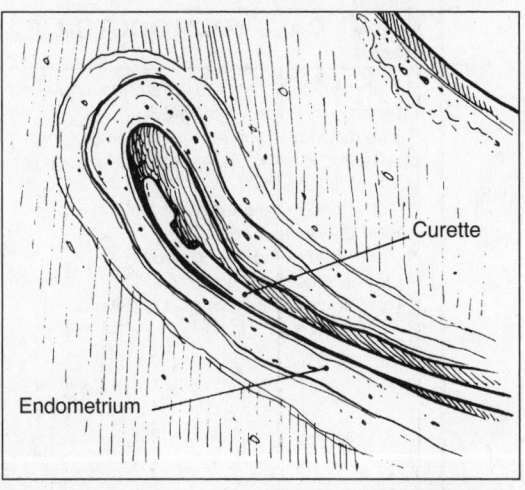

The curette removes a sample of the endometrium. The removed tissue is submitted to the laboratory for study.

Curette

Endometrium

SURGERIES

ENDOVASCULAR SURGERY

 ## GENERAL INFORMATION

DEFINITION—Repair of a narrowed (stenosed) or dilated (aneurysmal) artery using a special graft placed inside the artery. It is usually performed using a percutaneous (needle puncture) technique.

BODY PARTS INVOLVED—Various arteries in the body.

REASONS FOR SURGERY—To prevent rupture of an abdominal aortic aneurysm which usually results in massive hemorrhage and death, or to obtain better blood flow in a narrowed artery.

SURGICAL RISK INCREASES WITH
* Age.
* Diabetes.
* Poor kidney function.
* High blood pressure.
* Poor nutrition.
* Chronic lung disease.

 ## WHAT TO EXPECT

WHO OPERATES—General surgeon, vascular surgeon, cardiothoracic surgeon, interventional radiologist, or interventional cardiologist.

WHERE PERFORMED—Hospital.

DIAGNOSTIC TESTS
* Before surgery: Blood tests, chest x-ray, CT scan, and EKG (see Glossary).
* After surgery: Blood tests.

ANESTHESIA—General anesthesia, local anesthesia with sedation.

DESCRIPTION OF OPERATION
* The following is a description of an endo-vascular repair of an abdominal aortic aneurysm.
* The femoral artery is punctured in the groin and a large cannula (tube) is placed.
* The blood is thinned with anticoagulants.
* The endovascular graft is inserted through the cannula in the groin and positioned across the dilated aneurysmal portion of the abdominal aorta.
* A balloon inside the graft is inflated to seat the graft.
* The catheters and cannula are removed. The hole in the femoral artery may need to be repaired.

POSSIBLE COMPLICATIONS
* Bleeding from the groin site.
* Kidney failure.
* Poor circulation to the intestines which can lead to gangrene.
* Poor circulation to the lower extremities.
* Incisional hernia.
* Rupture or bleeding from the aorta.

AVERAGE HOSPITAL STAY—Usually 1 to 2 days.

PROBABLE OUTCOME—Expect full recovery in 2-3 weeks with no recurrence of the aneurysm. Stenotic (narrowed) lesions may reocclude in the future.

 ## POSTOPERATIVE CARE

GENERAL MEASURES
* A hard ridge may form in the groin over the puncture site. As it heals, the ridge will gradually recede.
* Use heat on the groin to help relieve pain.
* Shower as usual. You may wash the incisions gently with mild soap. After showering, replace any dressings with a new dry dressing.

MEDICATION
* Your doctor may prescribe pain relievers. Use only as much as you need to be comfortable.
* You may use nonprescription pain relievers such as acetaminophen for minor pain. Ask your doctor if it is okay to take ibuprofen or aspirin.

ACTIVITY
* Start ambulating (walking) as soon as you are home. Avoid strenuous activity for 2-3 weeks.
* You may swim once all sutures are out.
* Resume sexual relations when comfortable and when advised by your surgeon.

DIET—No special diet.

 ## CALL YOUR DOCTOR IF

* Pain, swelling, redness, drainage or bleeding increases in the surgical area.
* You develop signs of infection, including headache, muscle aches, dizziness fever, or a general ill feeling.
* You develop nausea and vomiting or abdominal pain.
* Prolonged constipation occurs.
* Legs are cold, numb, or painful.
* New unexplained symptoms develop.

ENDOVASCULAR SURGERY

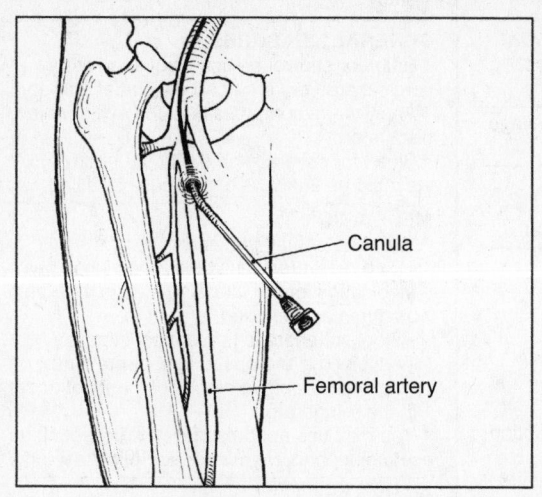

The femoral artery is accessed in the groin. A sheath or canula is placed to pass the graft.

Canula

Femoral artery

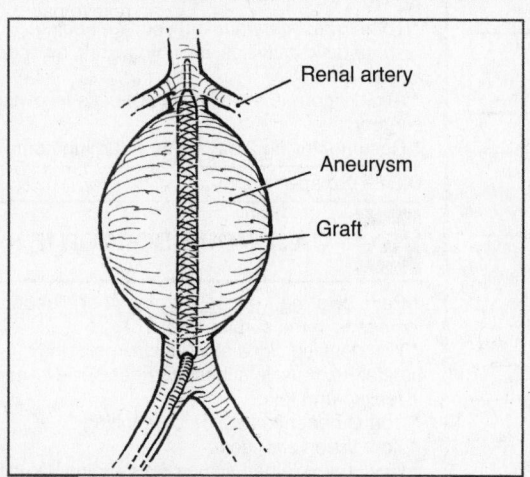

X-ray is used to position the graft in the exact location before the balloon is inflated.

Renal artery

Aneurysm

Graft

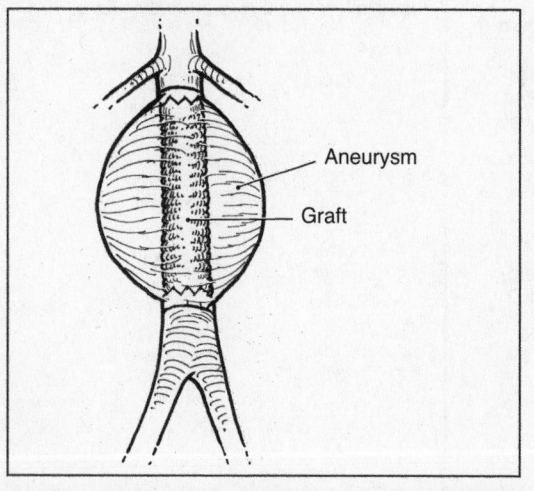

The graft is pressed into place inside the aorta when the balloon is inflated. The balloon is then deflated and removed allowing blood to flow through the graft.

Aneurysm

Graft

SURGERIES

ENTROPION REPAIR

GENERAL INFORMATION

DEFINITION—Shortening of excess tissue in the edge of the eyelid by removal of excess cartilage.

BODY PARTS INVOLVED—Skin and cartilage of the upper eyelid.

REASONS FOR SURGERY
* Improved appearance.
* Relief of redness, irritation and discomfort.

SURGICAL RISK INCREASES WITH
* Stress.
* Smoking.
* Poor nutrition.
* Recent or chronic illness.
* Alcoholism.
* Diabetes.
* Use of some prescription and nonprescription drugs. Inform your doctor of any drugs, medications, or vitamin and herb supplements you are using or have used in the last month.

WHAT TO EXPECT

WHO OPERATES—Ophthalmologist.

WHERE PERFORMED—Hospital, ophthalmologist's office or outpatient surgical facility.

DIAGNOSTIC TESTS
* Before surgery: Blood and urine studies; eye examination.
* After surgery: Laboratory examination of removed tissue.

ANESTHESIA—Local anesthesia by injection.

DESCRIPTION OF OPERATION
* An incision is made in the eyelid.
* The cartilage is partially cut about midway between the two sides of the eyelid.
* A small amount of the cartilage is cut free of connective tissue and removed.
* The remaining cartilage is closed with silk sutures. The skin is closed over the cartilage with fine sutures that usually can be removed about 10 days after surgery.

POSSIBLE COMPLICATIONS—Surgical-wound infection.

AVERAGE HOSPITAL STAY—1 to 2 days.

PROBABLE OUTCOME—Expect complete healing without complications. Allow about 2 weeks for recovery from surgery.

POSTOPERATIVE CARE

GENERAL MEASURES
* Bathe or shower as usual but keep the surgical area dry for 4 or 5 days after surgery.
* Apply warm compresses to the eye to relieve discomfort.
* Sleep for several nights with the head elevated on 2 pillows to decrease swelling.

MEDICATION
* Your doctor may prescribe:
  - Pain relievers. Don't take prescription pain medication longer than 4 to 7 days. Use only as much as you need.
  - Stool softeners to prevent constipation.
  - Antibiotic eye drops to fight or prevent infection. Keep eye drops cold, but not frozen, in the refrigerator.
* You may use nonprescription drugs, such as acetaminophen, for minor pain. Avoid aspirin.

ACTIVITY
* To help recovery and aid your well-being, resume daily activities, including work, as soon as you are able.
* Avoid vigorous exercise for 2 weeks following surgery.
* Resume driving 2 days after returning home.

DIET—No special diet.

CALL YOUR DOCTOR IF

* Pain, swelling, redness, drainage or bleeding increases in the surgical area.
* You develop signs of infection, including headache, muscle aches, dizziness or a general ill feeling and fever.
* You experience nausea or vomiting.
* Your vision changes.
* New, unexplained symptoms develop. Drugs used in treatment may produce side effects.

ENTROPION REPAIR

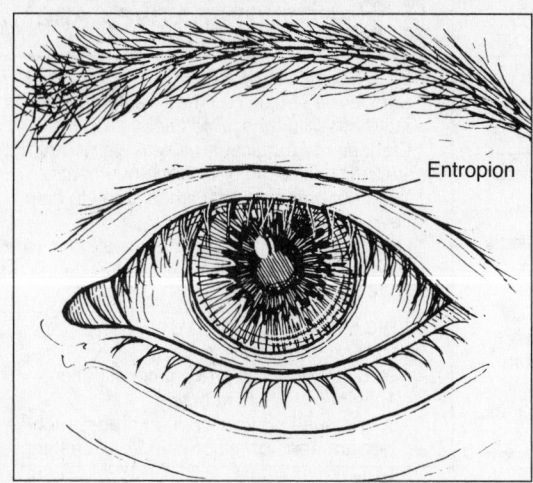

An illustration of excess tissue in the edge of the eyelid.

Entropion

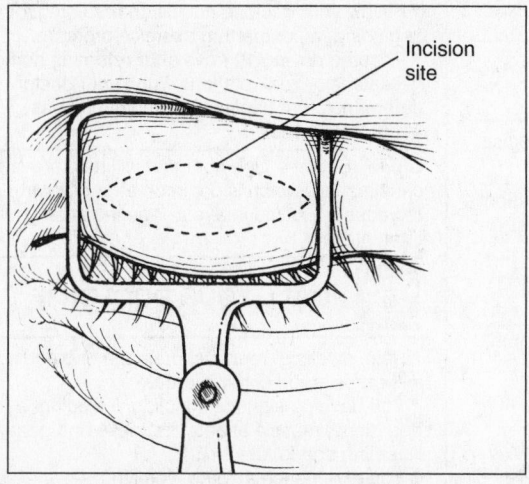

Incision site made in the skin overlying the eyelid.

Incision site

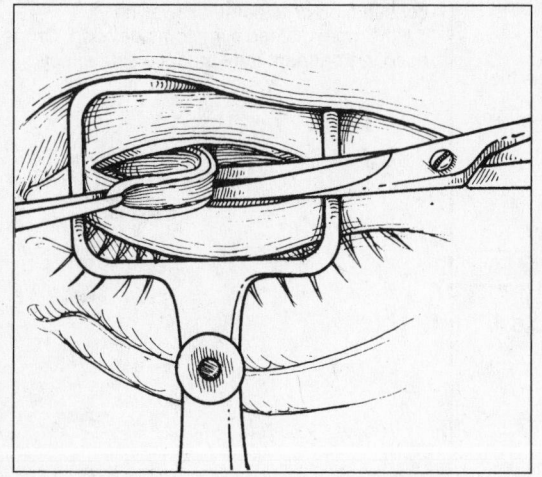

The cartilage in the upper eyelid is cut about midway between the two sides of the eyelid and removed.
 • Bleeding is controlled and skin is closed with small sutures, which can be removed in about 10 days following surgery.

SURGERIES

EPISIOTOMY
(Perineotomy)

GENERAL INFORMATION

DEFINITION—Surgical incision at the exterior of the vaginal opening to create enlargement.

BODY PARTS INVOLVED—Vagina; perineum.

REASONS FOR SURGERY—Usually performed during childbirth, just before the widest diameter of the baby's head passes through the outlet of the birth canal. This allows easier passage of the baby's head to reduce the potential of damage to the mother's vagina, bladder and rectum. Also helps expedite delivery in the case of forceps or vacuum use, or when there is maternal exhaustion or fetal distress, such as in a case of shoulder dystocia (when the shoulders of the baby get stuck after the head has already delivered).

SURGICAL RISK INCREASES WITH
- Obesity.
- Diabetes.

WHAT TO EXPECT

WHO OPERATES—Obstetrician-gynecologist, family doctor or midwife.

WHERE PERFORMED—Hospital or outpatient surgical facility.

DIAGNOSTIC TESTS
- Before surgery: Blood and urine studies.
- After surgery: Blood studies.

ANESTHESIA—Local anesthesia by injection.

DESCRIPTION OF OPERATION
- An incision is made in the perineum (the small area between the vaginal opening and the anus), just before the widest part of the baby's head is to be delivered. The size of the incision depends on how large an opening is required for the baby's head to pass through safely.
- The baby and placenta are delivered.
- The surgical area is repaired with sutures that will be absorbed by the body.

POSSIBLE COMPLICATIONS
- Excessive bleeding
- Surgical-wound infection (rare).
- Inadvertent injury to sphincter or rectum (rare).

AVERAGE HOSPITAL STAY—2 days.

PROBABLE OUTCOME—Expect complete healing without complications. Allow about 6 weeks for recovery from childbirth.

POSTOPERATIVE CARE

GENERAL MEASURES
- Shower as usual. You may wash the incision gently with mild, unscented soap.
- Cleanse the surgical area with warm (not hot) water after urination or bowel movements.
- Take hot baths several times a day to help relieve discomfort.
- Use ice packs made of gauze soaked in ice-cold witch hazel to relieve discomfort during the first 24 hours after delivery.

MEDICATION
- Your doctor may prescribe:
  - Stool softeners to prevent constipation.
  - Antibiotics to fight infection.
- You may use nonprescription drugs, such as acetaminophen, for minor pain. Avoid aspirin.

ACTIVITY
- Follow your doctor's advice on resuming, or beginning, a postpartum exercise program.
- Resume driving 10 days after returning home.
- Resume sexual relations when your doctor determines that healing is complete (usually about 3 to 6 weeks).

DIET—Eating a high-fiber diet will help prevent constipation, which is common after childbirth. Increase your fluid intake as you increase your fiber intake.

CALL YOUR DOCTOR IF

- Pain, swelling, redness, drainage or bleeding increases in the surgical area.
- You develop signs of infection, including headache, muscle aches, dizziness or a general ill feeling and fever.
- You experience nausea, vomiting, constipation or abdominal swelling.
- New, unexplained symptoms develop. Drugs used in treatment may produce side effects.

EPISIOTOMY
(Perineotomy)

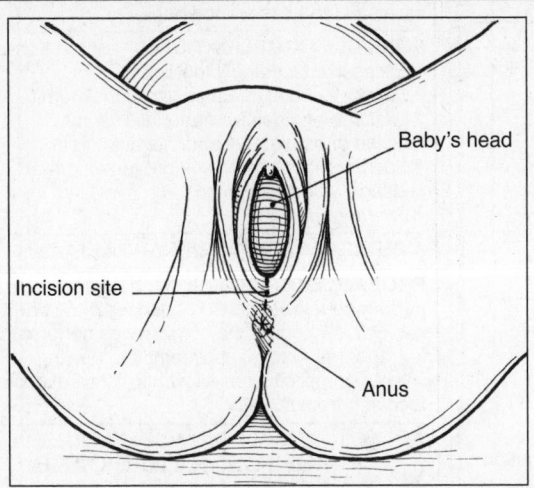

This view illustrates a female patient with extended legs in stirrups on an examining table to allow examination of the genital area.
  • The female genital area with a baby's head crowning at the entrance to the vagina and the incision site for the episiotomy.

Baby's head

Incision site

Anus

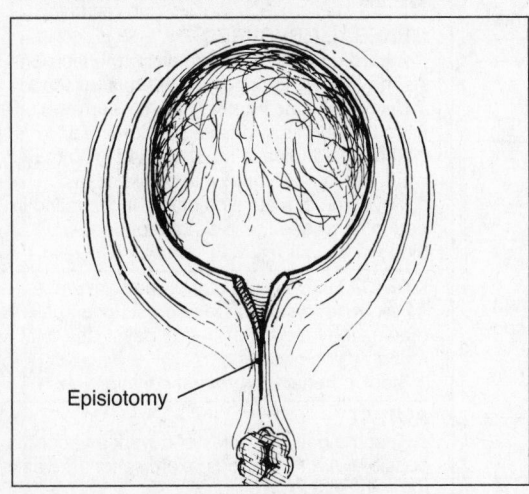

Incision is made in the perineum just before the widest part of the baby's head is delivered.

Episiotomy

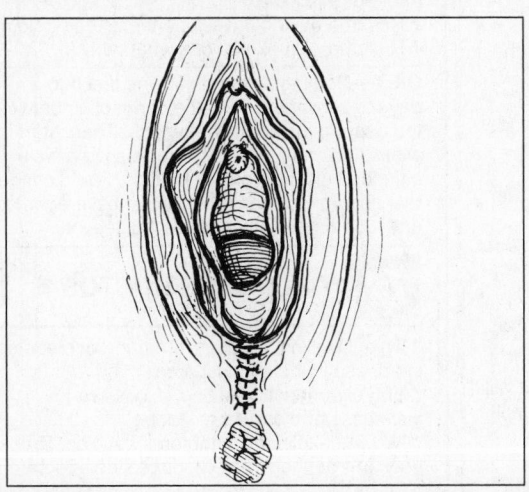

After the baby and placenta have been delivered, the episiotomy site is repaired with absorbable sutures.

SURGERIES

ESOPHAGECTOMY

GENERAL INFORMATION

DEFINITION—Removal of part of the esophagus, the tubular passage from the back of the throat to the stomach.

BODY PARTS INVOLVED—Esophagus; stomach; colon (sometimes).

REASONS FOR SURGERY
- Cancer of the esophagus.
- Burns and scarring of the esophagus.
- Opening a closure of the esophagus in a newborn (usually an inherited defect).

SURGICAL RISK INCREASES WITH
- Adults over 60; newborns and infants.
- Obesity; smoking; poor nutrition.
- Excess alcohol consumption.
- Chronic or recent illness, especially pneumonia or diabetes.
- Use of some prescription and nonprescription drugs. Inform your doctor of any drugs, medications, or vitamin and herb supplements you are using or have used in the last month.

WHAT TO EXPECT

WHO OPERATES—General surgeon or thoracic surgeon.

WHERE PERFORMED—Hospital.

DIAGNOSTIC TESTS
- Before surgery: Blood and urine studies; x-rays of chest and upper gastrointestinal tract; esophagogram; esophagoscopy; bronchoscopy (see Glossary for all).
- After surgery: Blood and urine studies; x-rays of chest and upper gastrointestinal tract.

ANESTHESIA—General anesthesia by injection and inhalation with an airway tube placed in the windpipe.

DESCRIPTION OF OPERATION
- Incisions are made in the abdomen and chest to expose the esophagus.
- The esophagus is isolated and examined.
- Abnormal tissues are removed. If the surgery is performed to treat cancer, nearby lymph glands are also removed.
- The bottom end of the remaining part of the esophagus is joined with the stomach; sometimes the colon is used to bridge the gap.
- The chest and abdomen are closed in layers. The skin is closed with sutures or clips, which can usually be removed about 1 week later.
- During the operation, a thin, plastic tube (called a jejunostomy tube) may be placed in your intestine and brought to the outside. It will be used to provide you with nourishment until you are able to take food by mouth.

- The operation can sometimes be done through an abdominal incision and a small incision at the base of the neck.

POSSIBLE COMPLICATIONS
- Excessive bleeding; blood clots.
- Surgical-wound infection; incisional hernia.
- Leakage of digestive material from new junction of esophagus and intestinal tract.
- Scarring at operation site prevents normal passage of food and fluids.
- Pneumonia.

AVERAGE HOSPITAL STAY—7 to 14 days.

PROBABLE OUTCOME—If the surgery was performed to treat cancer, chances of 5-year survival are poor. If the surgery was performed for other reasons, expect complete healing without complications. Allow 8 to 12 weeks for recovery from surgery.

POSTOPERATIVE CARE

GENERAL MEASURES
- A hard ridge should form along the incisions. As they heal, the ridges will gradually recede.
- Use an electric heating pad, a heat lamp or a warm compress to relieve incisional pain.
- Shower as usual after discharge. You may wash the incision gently with mild soap.
- Move and elevate legs often while resting in bed to decrease the likelihood of deep-vein blood clots.

MEDICATION—Your doctor may prescribe:
- Pain relievers. Don't take prescription pain medication longer than 4 to 7 days. Use only as much as you need.
- Stool softeners to prevent constipation.

ACTIVITY
- Resume daily activities and work as soon as possible. Avoid vigorous exercise for 12 weeks after surgery.
- Resume driving 3 weeks after returning home.
- Resume sexual relations when able.

DIET—Nothing by mouth for the first 6 to 7 days to allow healing of the connection between the esophagus and the stomach. Then, start with liquids and gradually progress to a well-balanced diet to promote healing. Avoid coffee, tea, cocoa, cola drinks, alcoholic beverages and any food or spice that cause indigestion.

CALL YOUR DOCTOR IF

- Pain, swelling, redness, drainage or bleeding increases in the surgical area.
- You experience vomiting, excessive weakness or black, tarry stools.
- New, unexplained symptoms develop. Drugs used in treatment may produce side effects.

ESOPHAGECTOMY

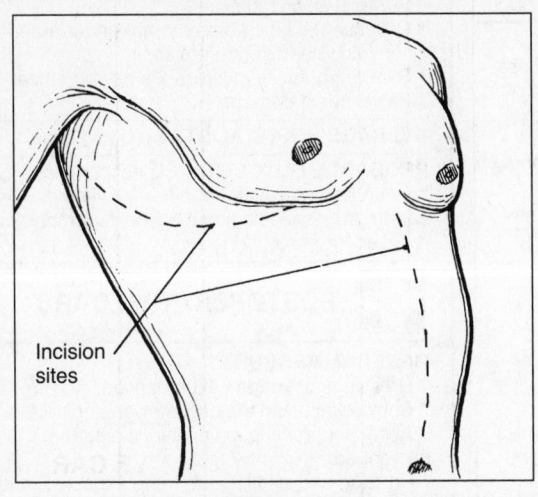

An illustration of the sites where incisions are made in order to expose the esophagus and the stomach.

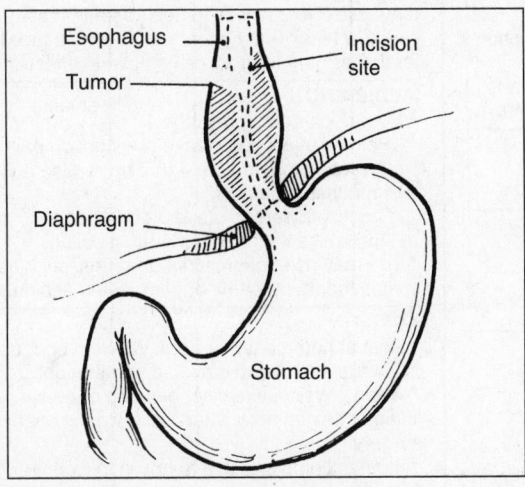

Esophagus

Tumor

Diaphragm

Incision site

Stomach

A portion of the esophagus is removed on both sides of the tumor or other defect.

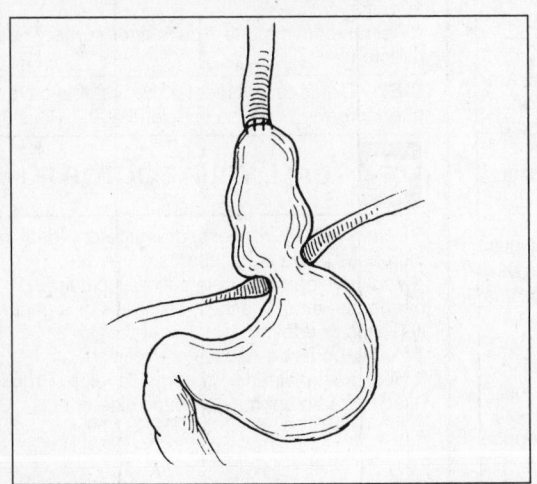

The bottom end of the remaining part of the esophagus is joined with the stomach; sometimes the colon is used to replace the missing portion of the esophagus.

SURGERIES

FACE LIFT & BLEPHAROPLASTY

GENERAL INFORMATION

DEFINITION
• Face lift (Rhytidectomy): Removal of excess skin, fat and tissue from the face in order to tighten sagging skin and eliminate wrinkles, jowls, or a double chin.
• Blepharoplasty: Removal of excess fat and skin from around the eyelids to reduce puffiness, bags under the eyes, and wrinkles.

BODY PARTS INVOLVED—Skin and underlying tissue of the face and eyelids.

REASONS FOR SURGERY
• Improved appearance of the face.
• Improved appearance and function of the eyelids.

SURGICAL RISK INCREASES WITH
• Obesity; smoking; poor nutrition.
• Recent or chronic illness.
• Diabetes.
• Alcoholism.
• Use of some prescription and nonprescription drugs. Inform your doctor of any drugs, medications, or vitamin and herb supplements you are using or have used in the last month.

WHAT TO EXPECT

WHO OPERATES—Plastic and reconstructive surgeon.

WHERE PERFORMED—Doctor's office, outpatient surgical facility or hospital.

DIAGNOSTIC TESTS
• Before surgery: Blood and urine studies.
• After surgery: Blood studies.

ANESTHESIA
• Local anesthesia by injection.
• General anesthesia by injection and inhalation with an airway tube placed in the windpipe.

DESCRIPTION OF OPERATION
• A number of different face lift procedures are available. Your doctor will explain the options.
• Usually a face lift involves incisions that are made where scarring will be less visible.
• Care is taken to clamp and tie tiny bleeding vessels during the procedure to prevent collection of scar tissue under the skin.
• Flaps of skin are cut away around the eyes and face. The skin is separated from underlying tissues. The muscles are tightened and excess fat and tissue are removed.
• The skin is closed with fine sutures, which usually can be removed about 1 week after surgery. Drains may be placed in the incision and left for a day.
• Compression dressingu are applied to reduce swelling and bleeding.

POSSIBLE COMPLICATIONS
• Excessive bleeding; blood clots.
• Surgical-wound infection.
• Collection of blood (hematoma) under areas where skin has been removed.
• Scarring or facial muscles are asymmetrical.
• Facial nerve damage.

AVERAGE HOSPITAL STAY—0 to 3 days.

PROBABLE OUTCOME—Expect complete healing and improved appearance without complications. Allow about 6 weeks or more for recovery from surgery.

POSTOPERATIVE CARE

GENERAL MEASURES
• Dressings or wraps will be applied.
• Shower as usual the day after or as directed.
• Apply nonprescription antibiotic ointment if prescribed.
• Bruising and swelling are to be expected, and may take 2 to 3 weeks to decrease. In most cases, it takes 3 to 6 months following a face lift for the surgery to produce its optimal effects.

MEDICATION
• Your doctor may prescribe:
  - Pain relievers. Don't take prescription pain medication longer than 4 to 7 days. Use only as much as you need.
  - Stool softeners to prevent constipation.
  - Antibiotics to fight or prevent infection.
• You may use nonprescription drugs, such as acetaminophen, for minor pain. Avoid aspirin.

ACTIVITY
• Rest at home after surgery. When in bed, use pillows to keep head elevated and straight.
• Avoid physical exercise, bending or heavy lifting or sexual activity for 1 to 2 weeks after surgery.
• Most patients are able to return to work in 7 to 10 days.
• Resume driving 3 to 7 days after surgery or as directed.

DIET—Liquid to soft diet for the first few days after surgery. Then, no special diet.

CALL YOUR DOCTOR IF

• Pain, swelling, redness, drainage or bleeding increases in the surgical area.
• You develop signs of infection, including headache, muscle aches, dizziness or a general ill feeling and fever.
• You experience nausea or vomiting.
• New, unexplained symptoms develop. Drugs used in treatment may produce side effects.

FACE LIFT & BLEPHAROPLASTY

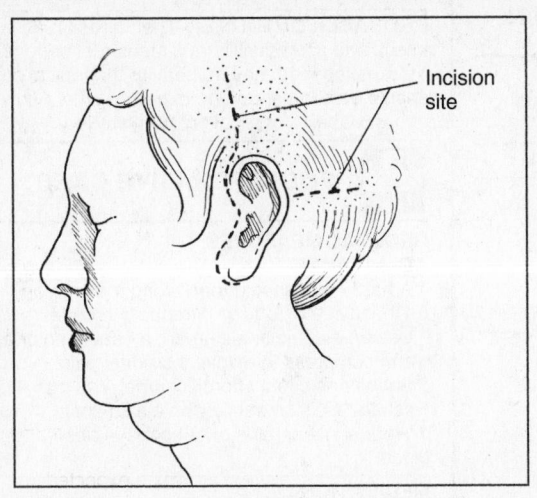

Incision site

Flaps of skin cut away around the eyes and face. Excess tissue is removed from underlying areas and excess skin is trimmed away.

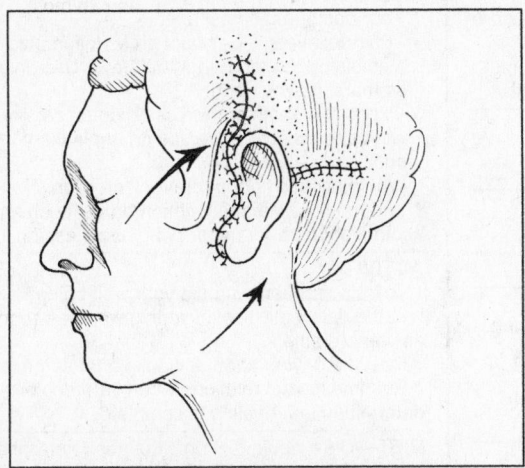

Skin is closed with fine sutures.

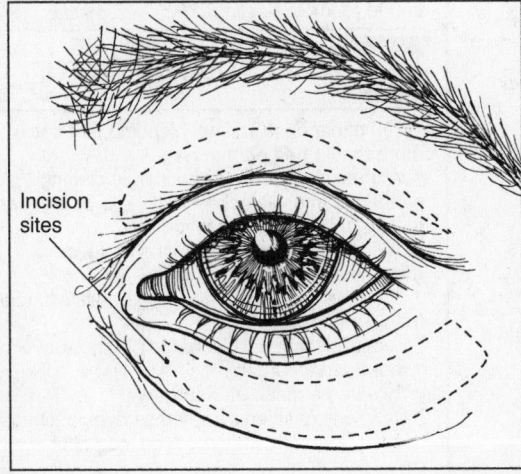

Incision sites

An illustration of excessive tissue surrounding the eye and the incision sites generally used.

FIBROID TUMOR REMOVAL
(Myomectomy)

 GENERAL INFORMATION

DEFINITION—Removal of fibroid tumors (leiomyoma, myoma) from the uterus through an incision in the lower abdomen.

BODY PARTS INVOLVED—Uterus.

REASONS FOR SURGERY
* Pelvic pain or back pain.
* Pressure on the bladder.
* Abnormal uterine bleeding; anemia.
* Difficulty in becoming pregnant.
* Discomfort with sexual intercourse.

SURGICAL RISK INCREASES WITH
* Obesity.
* Smoking.
* Poor nutrition, especially inadequate iron intake that has led to anemia.
* Recent or chronic illness.
* Diabetes.
* Use of some prescription and nonprescription drugs. Inform your doctor of any drugs, medications, or vitamin and herb supplements you are using or have used in the last month.

 WHAT TO EXPECT

WHO OPERATES—General surgeon or obstetrician-gynecologist.

WHERE PERFORMED—Hospital.

DIAGNOSTIC TESTS
* Before surgery: Blood studies; dilatation and curettage of the uterus (D & C); laparoscopy; x-rays of abdomen; barium-enema x-rays; intravenous pyelogram (see Glossary for all).
* After surgery: Blood studies.

ANESTHESIA—General anesthesia by injection and inhalation with an airway tube placed in the windpipe.

DESCRIPTION OF OPERATION
* One or more incisions are made in the lower abdomen.
* The muscles are separated and connective tissues are cut free to expose the uterus.
* Fibroid tumors are located; each tumor is removed separately, and each excision is repaired.
* The internal structures are closed in layers.
* The skin is closed with sutures or skin clips, which can be removed about 4 to 7 days later.

POSSIBLE COMPLICATIONS
* Excessive bleeding.
* Surgical-wound infection.
* Recurrence of the tumor.
* Perforation of the uterus or bowel during surgery.
* Bowel obstruction.

AVERAGE HOSPITAL STAY—2 to 3 days.

PROBABLE OUTCOME—The uterus is left intact, and you will still have menstrual periods. Your next period may be heavier than usual but should occur at about the expected time. Allow about 6 weeks for recovery from surgery.

 POSTOPERATIVE CARE

GENERAL MEASURES
* Don't smoke.
* A hard ridge should form along the incision. As it heals, the ridge will gradually recede.
* Use an electric heating pad, a heat lamp or a warm compress to relieve incisional pain.
* Shower as usual after discharge. You may wash the incision gently with a mild soap.
* Wear sanitary pads or tampons to absorb blood.

MEDICATION
* Your doctor may prescribe:
  - Pain relievers. Don't take prescription pain medication longer than 4 to 7 days. Use only as much as you need.
  - Vaginal creams or medicated douches, if vaginal discharge develops an unpleasant odor.
  - Antibiotics to fight or prevent infection.
* You may use nonprescription drugs, such as acetaminophen, for minor pain. Avoid aspirin.

ACTIVITY
* To help recovery and aid your well-being, resume daily activities, including work, as soon as you are able.
* Resume driving about 2 weeks after surgery.
* Resume sexual relations when your doctor determines that healing is complete.

DIET—Clear liquid diet until the gastrointestinal tract functions again. Then eat a well-balanced diet to promote healing.

 CALL YOUR DOCTOR IF

* You experience vaginal bleeding that soaks more than 1 pad per hour.
* You develop signs of infection, including headache, muscle aches, dizziness or a general feeling of ill health and fever.
* You have abdominal swelling or severe abdominal pain.
* The urge to urinate frequently persists longer than 1 month.
* Excessive vaginal discharge persists beyond 1 month after surgery.
* Symptoms recur after surgery.
* New, unexplained symptoms develop. Drugs used in treatment may produce side effects.

FIBROID TUMOR REMOVAL
(Myomectomy)

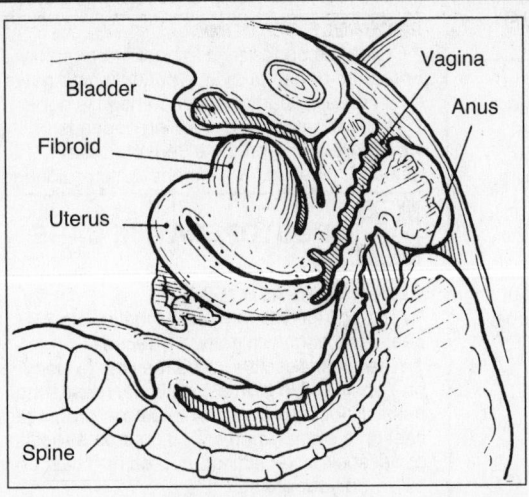

Bladder

Fibroid

Uterus

Vagina

Anus

Spine

An illustration of the female genital area seen through a cross section.
  • In this example, the fibroid tumor is on the front surface of the uterus.

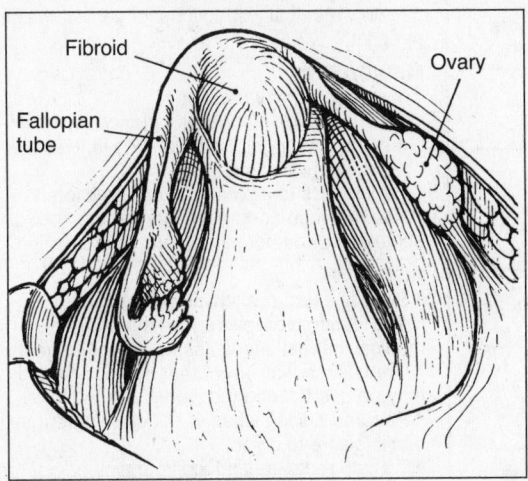

Fibroid

Fallopian tube

Ovary

After the skin has been incised and muscles retracted, the uterus and fibroid tumor are visible through the incision site.

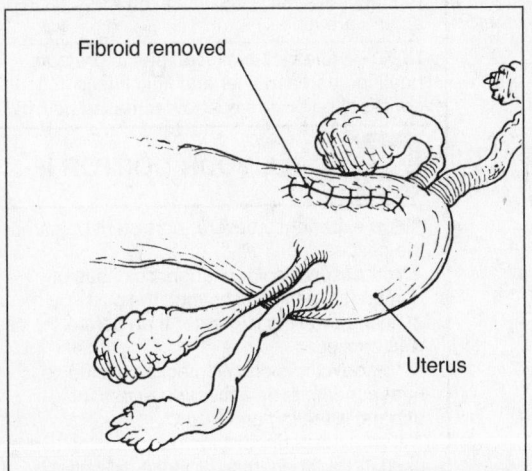

Fibroid removed

Uterus

The fibroid tumor is removed and the surgical site is repaired with absorbable sutures.

SURGERIES

FRACTURE REPAIR
(Fracture Reduction)

 GENERAL INFORMATION

DEFINITION—Realigning ends of a fractured (broken) bone. Open reduction is when an incision is made to fix the bone fragments. Closed reduction is when the bones are realigned by traction and fixed externally by a cast or splint.

BODY PARTS INVOLVED—Any bone in the body.

REASONS FOR SURGERY—Restoration of normal position and function of a broken bone.

SURGICAL RISK INCREASES WITH
- Adults over 60.
- Obesity; smoking; poor nutrition; alcoholism.
- Recent or chronic illness.
- Diabetes.
- Use of some prescription and nonprescription drugs. Inform your doctor of any drugs, medications, or vitamin and herb supplements you are using or have used in the last month.

 WHAT TO EXPECT

WHO OPERATES—Orthopedist, general surgeon or family doctor.

WHERE PERFORMED—Hospital, outpatient facility, doctor's office or emergency room.

DIAGNOSTIC TESTS
- Before surgery: Blood and urine studies; x-ray of affected area.
- During surgery: X-rays.
- After surgery: X-rays through cast or splint to determine if rejoined pieces remain in good position for healing.

ANESTHESIA
- Local anesthesia by injection.
- General anesthesia by injection and inhalation with an airway tube placed in the windpipe.

DESCRIPTION OF OPERATION
- In an open reduction, one or more incisions may be made in the skin over the fracture.
- The bone fragments are aligned as close as possible to their normal position.
- Sometimes, metal pins, screws or plates are used to re-join the areas of the fracture.
- Once the broken ends of bone are set, the affected part is kept rigid with a cast or splint.

POSSIBLE COMPLICATIONS
- Excessive bleeding.
- Improper alignment of joined bone ends.
- Failure of bones to heal (non-union).
- Pressure on nearby nerves; nerve damage.
- Infection.

AVERAGE HOSPITAL STAY—0 to 6 days.

PROBABLE OUTCOME
- Children's bones tend to heal more rapidly. Fractured bones of elderly patients may never heal properly, particularly if nutrition is poor.
- The time required for healing depends on the type of fracture and the extent of tissue damage. Healing time may be quite prolonged.

 POSTOPERATIVE CARE

GENERAL MEASURES
- A hard ridge will form along the incision. As it heals, the ridge will gradually recede.
- Whenever possible, raise the limb or body part enclosed in the cast. This decreases the possibility of swelling. For example, prop a leg cast on a pillow when in bed, and on a footstool or hassock when sitting; prop an arm cast on a pillow on your chest.
- Follow medical instructions for care of the cast or splint.

MEDICATION
- Your doctor may prescribe:
  - Pain relievers. Don't take prescription pain medication longer than 4 to 7 days. Use only as much as you need.
  - Antibiotics to fight or prevent infection.
- You may use nonprescription drugs, such as acetaminophen, for minor pain. Avoid aspirin.

ACTIVITY
- Special exercises, physical therapy or rehabilitation therapy may be needed. Follow all medical instructions to assure complete healing.
- Crutches, a walker or other mechanical aids may be used during recovery.
- Resume driving when your doctor determines that it is safe to do so.
- To help recovery and aid your well-being, resume daily activities, including work, as soon as you are able.

DIET—Eat a well-balanced diet to promote healing. Increase fiber and fluid intake if constipation occurs due to decreased activity.

 CALL YOUR DOCTOR IF

- You experience severe, persistent pain under the cast.
- You observe color change, coldness or numbness in tissues beyond the cast.
- Tissue swelling is greater than before the cast was applied.
- You develop signs of infection, including headache, muscle aches, dizziness, or a general ill feeling and fever.
- New, unexplained symptoms develop. Drugs used in treatment may produce side effects.

FRACTURE REPAIR
(Fracture Reduction)

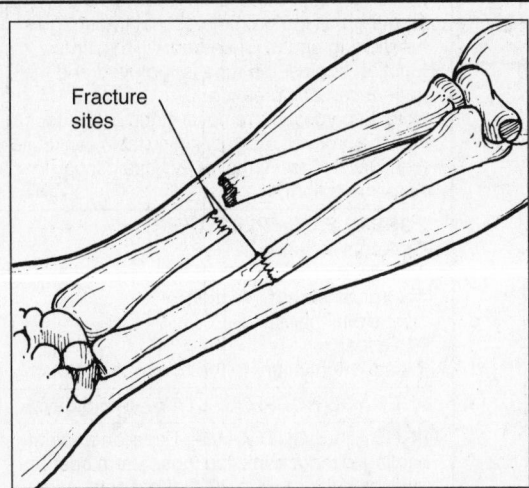

Fracture
sites

An illustration of fractures of the forearm bones.

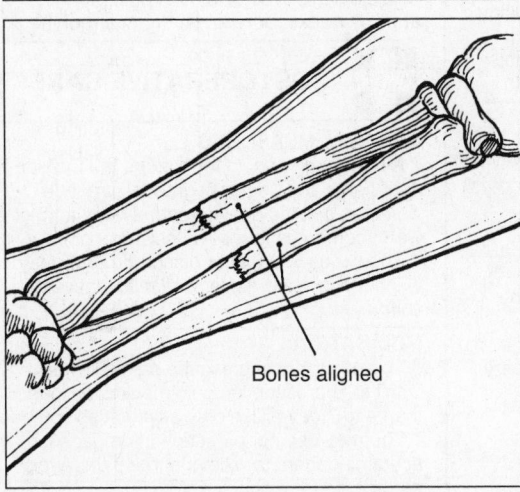

Bones aligned

When possible, the fractured bone ends are aligned by manipulation from the outside. If this cannot be done, the bone fragments can be aligned by surgical procedures to produce the same result.

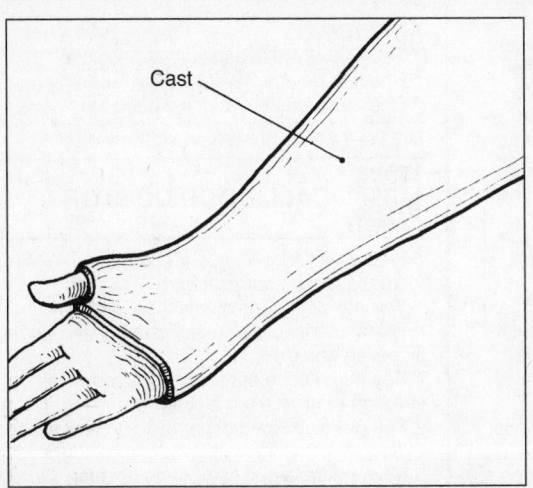

Cast

After the broken ends of bone are aligned, the affected part is held in place with a plaster cast or splint.

GALLBLADDER REMOVAL
(Cholecystectomy, Open)

 GENERAL INFORMATION

DEFINITION—Removal of the gallbladder though an incision in the abdomen.

BODY PARTS INVOLVED—Gallbladder; bile ducts.

REASONS FOR SURGERY
* Gallstones.
* Suspected gallbladder tumors.
* Chronic gallbladder infection.
* Sudden, severe infection of the gallbladder that does not respond rapidly to treatment.

SURGICAL RISK INCREASES WITH
* Obesity; smoking.
* Recent or chronic illness.
* Alcoholism; cirrhosis of the liver; diabetes; heart disease; or chronic obstructive pulmonary disease (COPD).
* Use of some prescription and nonprescription drugs. Inform your doctor of any drugs, medications, or vitamin and herb supplements you are using or have used in the last month.

 WHAT TO EXPECT

WHO OPERATES—General surgeon.

WHERE PERFORMED—Hospital.

DIAGNOSTIC TESTS
* Before surgery: Blood studies; x-rays of the gallbladder; ultrasound; ECG; radionuclide excretion scan (see Glossary for all).
* During surgery: Cholangiogram (see Glossary).
* After surgery: Blood studies.

ANESTHESIA—General anesthesia by injection and inhalation with an airway tube placed in the windpipe.

DESCRIPTION OF OPERATION
* An incision is made under the right rib cage or down the center of the abdomen. Abdominal muscles are separated to expose abdominal organs, which are inspected for undetected disease. Other surgeries may be performed at this time.
* The gallbladder is cut free and removed from under the liver.
* A cholangiogram is done to determine if gallstones are lodged in the bile ducts. If necessary, the gallstones are removed.
* The incision is closed with sutures, skin clips or staples, which usually can be removed about 1 week after surgery. Occasionally, a drainage tube is left in place to drain bile around the liver. If stones are removed from the bile duct, a second tube (T-tube) is placed to drain this duct and allow x-rays to be taken later of the bile duct.
* Sometimes, a tube running through the nose

to the stomach remains at least 1 to 2 days after surgery until the gastrointestinal tract begins functioning again. Once normal intestinal function begins, the tube is removed and the patient can begin eating.
Note: Laparoscopic removal of the gallbladder is now the preferable surgery in suitable candidates (see Gallbladder Removal By Laparoscopy in Surgery section).

POSSIBLE COMPLICATIONS
* Internal bleeding.
* Peritonitis.
* Surgical-wound infection.
* Incisional hernia.
* Bile leak.
* Inadvertent injury to the common bile duct.

AVERAGE HOSPITAL STAY—3 to 5 days.

PROBABLE OUTCOME—Expect complete healing without complications. The surgery relieves symptoms in 90% of patients. Allow about 6 weeks for recovery from surgery.

 POSTOPERATIVE CARE

GENERAL MEASURES
* A hard ridge should form along the incision. As it heals, the ridge will gradually recede.
* Use an electric heating pad, a heat lamp or a warm compress to relieve incisional pain.
* Shower as usual after discharge. You may wash the incision gently with mild, unscented soap.

MEDICATION
* Your doctor may prescribe pain relievers. Don't take prescription pain medication longer than 4 to 7 days. Use only as much as you need.
* You may use nonprescription drugs, such as acetaminophen, to relieve minor pain. Avoid aspirin.

ACTIVITY
* Take short walks as soon as possible.
* Resume driving 3 weeks after returning home.
* Resume sexual relations when able.

DIET—Your doctor will prescribe a diet.

 CALL YOUR DOCTOR IF

* Pain, swelling, redness, drainage or bleeding increases in the surgical area.
* You develop signs of infection, including headache, muscle aches, dizziness or a general ill feeling and fever.
* You experience constipation, abdominal swelling or unrelieved hiccups.
* You develop signs of jaundice (yellow skin or eyes).
* New, unexplained symptoms develop. Drugs used in treatment may produce side effects.

GALLBLADDER REMOVAL
(Cholecystectomy, Open)

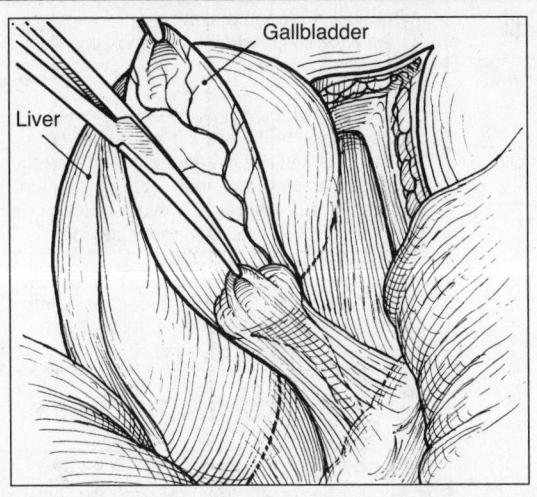

An illustration of the liver and gallbladder located just under the right rib cage. The liver must be retracted upward in order to expose the gallbladder.

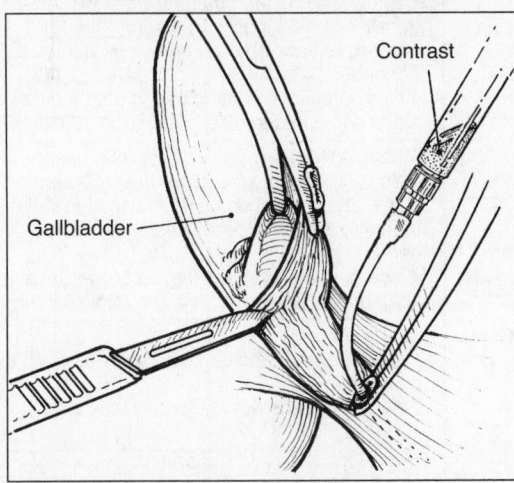

Gallbladder is cut free and removed. Catheter is inserted into bile duct to inject contrast dye for a cholangiography.

Occasionally, a drainage tube is left in place to drain bile around the liver.

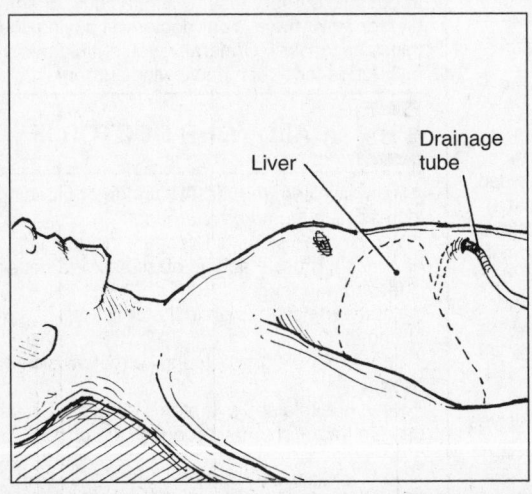

GALLBLADDER REMOVAL BY LAPAROSCOPY
(Laparoscopic Cholecystectomy)

 GENERAL INFORMATION

DEFINITION—Removal of the gallbladder with a laparoscope (a lighted scope attached to a video camera).

BODY PARTS INVOLVED—Gallbladder; bile ducts; liver.

REASONS FOR SURGERY
* Treatment of gallstones.
* Acute inflammation of the gallbladder.
* Benign and malignant tumors of the gallbladder.
* Chronic gallbladder infection.

SURGICAL RISK INCREASES WITH
* Obesity; smoking.
* Excess alcohol consumption.
* Recent or chronic illness.
* Cirrhosis of the liver.
* Diabetes.
* Use of some prescription and nonprescription drugs. Inform your doctor of any drugs, medications, or vitamin and herb supplements you are using or have used in the last month.

 WHAT TO EXPECT

WHO OPERATES—General surgeon.

WHERE PERFORMED—Hospital, outpatient surgical facility.

DIAGNOSTIC TESTS
* Before surgery: Blood studies, x-rays, ECG; ultrasound, radionuclide excretion scan (see Glossary for all).
* After surgery: Blood tests.

ANESTHESIA—General anesthesia by injection and inhalation with an airway tube placed in the windpipe.

DESCRIPTION OF OPERATION
* Four small incisions are made in the abdomen. A small needle is inserted into one incision to inflate the abdomen with air or carbon dioxide so the surgeon can see clearly.
* The laparoscope is inserted in one incision near the naval and the surgeon looks at a video monitor to see inside the abdomen. Surgical instruments are inserted into the other incisions.
* The gallbladder and the ducts running from it are located and separated. The gallbladder duct is clipped and the gallbladder is cut away and removed through one of the small incisions.
* The laparoscope and surgical instruments are removed and the carbon dioxide or air is allowed to escape from the abdomen.
* Small sutures under the skin and an adhesive bandage are used to close the wounds.

POSSIBLE COMPLICATIONS
* Surgical wound infection.
* Inadvertent injury to the common bile duct or to the small intestine.
* Bile leak.
* Excessive bleeding; blood clots.
* Unexpected findings such as adhesions, severe infection or inflammation may make it necessary to stop the laparoscopy procedure and use an open surgical procedure (see Gallbladder Removal in Surgery section).

AVERAGE HOSPITAL STAY—0 to 2 days.

PROBABLE OUTCOME—Expect complete healing without complications. Allow 1 to 2 weeks for recovery from surgery.

 POSTOPERATIVE CARE

GENERAL MEASURES
* Shower as usual. You may wash the incision gently with mild, unscented soap. After the shower, replace any wet dressings with clean, dry ones.
* Use an electric heating pad, a heat lamp or a warm compress to relieve any incisional pain.

MEDICATION
* Your doctor may prescribe pain relievers. Don't take prescription pain medication longer than 4 to 7 days. Use only as much as you need.
* You may use nonprescription drugs, such as acetaminophen, for minor pain. Avoid aspirin.

ACTIVITY
* Resume work and normal activity as soon as possible.
* Avoid vigorous activity for 6 weeks after surgery.

DIET—The use of a general anesthetic and abdominal surgery may require a liquid or soft diet for a few days. Your doctor will advise you if this is necessary. Generally, you should avoid fatty foods for a month following surgery.

 CALL YOUR DOCTOR IF

* Pain, swelling, redness, drainage or bleeding increases in the surgical areas.
* You develop signs of infection, including headache, muscle aches, dizziness or a general ill feeling and fever.
* You have severe pain in the chest or abdomen.
* You develop signs of jaundice (yellow skin or eyes).
* New, unexplained symptoms develop. Drugs used in treatment may produce side effects.

GALLBLADDER REMOVAL BY LAPAROSCOPY
(Laparoscopic Cholecystectomy)

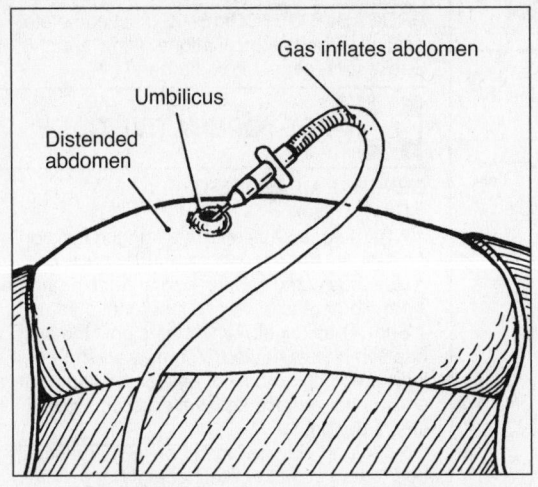

Distended abdomen

Umbilicus

Gas inflates abdomen

Carbon dioxide is used to inflate the abdomen to separate the organs.

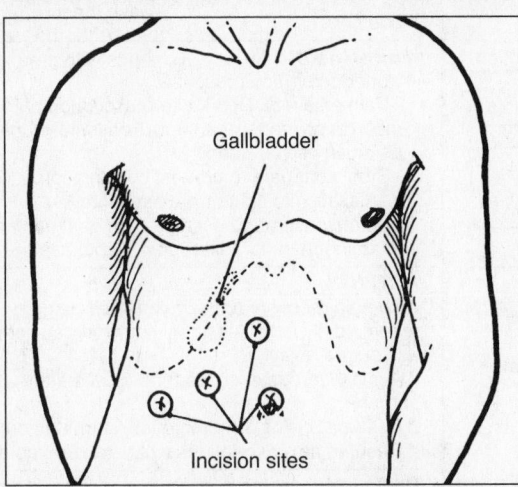

Gallbladder

Incision sites

Small incisions are made in the abdomen to allow insertion of the laparoscope and surgical instruments.

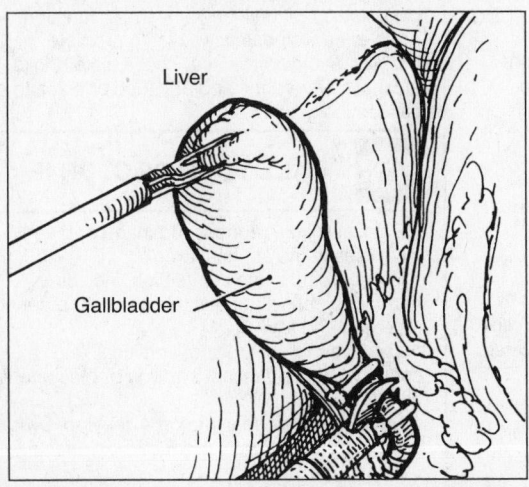

Liver

Gallbladder

The gallbladder is held in position while the cystic duct is separated and clipped. The gallbladder is cut away and removed.

SURGERIES

GASTROENTEROSTOMY FOR PYLORIC OBSTRUCTION

GENERAL INFORMATION

DEFINITION—Creation of an artificial passage between the stomach and the small intestine to bypass obstructions caused by ulcer scar tissue.

BODY PARTS INVOLVED—Stomach; duodenum; jejunum (usually).

REASONS FOR SURGERY—Restoration of normal function of the gastrointestinal tract.

SURGICAL RISK INCREASES WITH
* Adults over 60.
* Newborns and infants.
* Stress.
* Obesity.
* Smoking.
* Excess alcohol consumption.
* Poor nutrition.
* Recent or chronic illness.
* Diabetes.
* Use of some prescription and nonprescription drugs. Inform your doctor of any drugs, medications, or vitamin and herb supplements you are using or have used in the last month.

WHAT TO EXPECT

WHO OPERATES—General surgeon.

WHERE PERFORMED—Hospital.

DIAGNOSTIC TESTS
* Before surgery: Blood and urine studies; gastroscopy; x-rays of upper gastrointestinal tract; serum electrolytes (see Glossary).
* After surgery: Blood and urine studies.

ANESTHESIA—General anesthesia by injection and inhalation with an airway tube placed in the windpipe.

DESCRIPTION OF OPERATION
* An incision is made in the upper abdomen.
* The abdominal muscles are separated to expose the abdominal organs, which are inspected for any undetected disease. Other surgeries may be performed at this time.
* The stomach and jejunum are isolated. A small opening is made in each, and they are joined with sutures at the openings. Usually combined with vagotomy (see in Surgery section) to prevent further ulceration.
* The abdominal muscles are closed with sutures. The skin is closed with sutures or clips, which usually can be removed in about 1 week.

POSSIBLE COMPLICATIONS
* Excessive bleeding; surgical-wound infection.
* Spillage of stomach contents into abdomen.
* Slow digestion and emptying of the stomach.
* Incisional hernia.

AVERAGE HOSPITAL STAY—7 to 10 days.

PROBABLE OUTCOME—Expect complete healing without complications. Allow about 6 weeks for recovery from surgery.

POSTOPERATIVE CARE

GENERAL MEASURES
* Don't smoke.
* A hard ridge should form along the incision. As it heals, the ridge will gradually recede.
* Use an electric heating pad, a heat lamp or a warm compress to relieve incisional pain.
* Shower as usual. Avoid baths until the incision has completely healed. You may wash the incision gently with mild, unscented soap. After showering, replace any wet dressings with clean, dry ones.
* Move and elevate legs often while resting in bed to decrease the likelihood of deep-vein blood clots.

MEDICATION
* Your doctor may prescribe:
  - Pain relievers. Don't take prescription pain medication longer than 4 to 7 days. Use only as much as you need.
  - Stool softeners to prevent constipation.
  - Antibiotics to fight or prevent infection.
* You may use nonprescription drugs, such as acetaminophen, for minor pain. Avoid aspirin.

ACTIVITY
* To help recovery and aid your well-being, resume daily activities, including work, as soon as you are able.
* Avoid vigorous exercise for 6 weeks after surgery.
* Resume driving 1 month after returning home.
* Resume sexual relations when you feel able.

DIET—Nasogastric suction is used; followed by clear liquid diet until bowel starts to function. Then eat a well-balanced diet to promote healing. Avoid coffee, tea, cocoa, cola drinks, alcoholic beverages and any food or spice that causes indigestion.

CALL YOUR DOCTOR IF

* Pain, swelling, redness, drainage or bleeding increases in the surgical area.
* You develop signs of infection, including headache, muscle aches, dizziness or a general ill feeling and fever.
* You experience nausea, vomiting, constipation, abdominal swelling or black, tarry stools.
* New, unexplained symptoms develop. Drugs used in treatment may produce side effects.

GASTROENTEROSTOMY FOR PYLORIC OBSTRUCTION

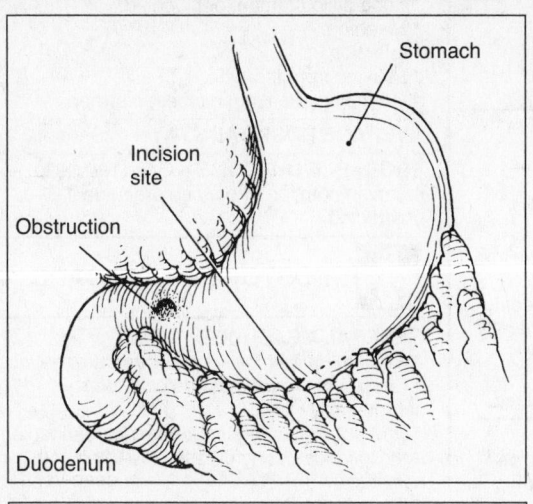

An illustration of a typical obstruction site in the lower end of the stomach, just before the duodenum (beginning of the first part of the intestine).

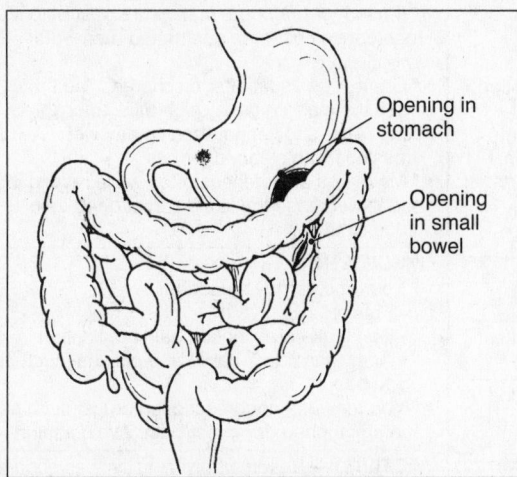

After the stomach and a small loop of small intestine are isolated, an opening is made in each.

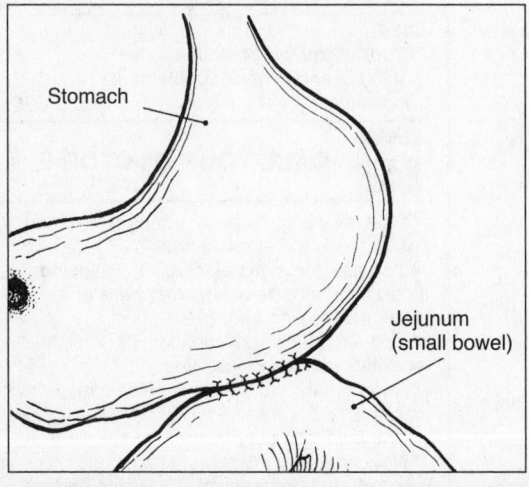

The cut end of the stomach is then joined with the surgically opened part of the jejunum, once again establishing a clear channel for the passage of food and fluids.

SURGERIES

GASTROSTOMY

GENERAL INFORMATION

DEFINITION—Making a surgical opening into the stomach for placement of a feeding or drainage tube.

BODY PARTS INVOLVED—Stomach; skin; structures of the abdominal wall.

REASONS FOR SURGERY
* Prevention of pneumonia in patients with swallowing disorders.
* Provide nutrition to those who cannot swallow.
* Blockage of esophagus.
* To provide access to the stomach for feeding or drainage of stomach contents. It is frequently used in patients who cannot or will not eat adequate amounts of food, or to drain the stomach when prolonged drainage is required.

SURGICAL RISK INCREASES WITH
* Obesity; poor nutrition.
* Recent or chronic illness, especially chronic lung disease.
* Diabetes.
* Excess alcohol consumption.
* Use of some prescription and nonprescription drugs. Inform your doctor of any drugs, medications, or vitamin and herb supplements you are using or have used in the last month.

WHAT TO EXPECT

WHO OPERATES—General surgeon or gastroenterologist.

WHERE PERFORMED—Hospital or outpatient surgical facility.

DIAGNOSTIC TESTS—Before surgery: Blood and urine studies; x-rays of gastrointestinal tract; endoscopy (see Glossary).

ANESTHESIA
* Local anesthesia by injection.
* General anesthesia by injection and inhalation with an airway tube placed in the windpipe.

DESCRIPTION OF OPERATION
* An incision is made in the abdominal wall.
* The stomach is isolated and an opening is made into it.
* The tube (usually polyvinylchloride or rubber) is secured by sutures around it to hold it in place.
* The other end of the tube is pulled to the outside through a separate puncture site.
* The abdominal incision is closed and the tube is stitched to the skin.
* The procedure may also be accomplished with gastroscopy (see Gastrostomy, Percutaneous Endoscopic in Surgery section).

POSSIBLE COMPLICATIONS
* Skin irritation around the gastrostomy tube.
* Tube dislodgement or clogging.
* Bleeding.
* Infection.
* Leaking from the tube.
* Cramping; bloating; nausea; diarrhea.

AVERAGE HOSPITAL STAY—0 to 1 day.

PROBABLE OUTCOME—Good results to maintain nutrition or provide drainage if obstructed.

POSTOPERATIVE CARE

GENERAL MEASURES
* Remain upright for 1/2 to 1 hour after eating.
* Keep skin around gastrostomy tube scrupulously clean.
* Prevent dislodging the tube by careful taping and vigilance during dressing, feeding and activities.
* If used for drainage, make sure gastrostomy tube doesn't become obstructed (use water irrigations).
* Shower as usual after discharge. You may wash the incision gently with mild, unscented soap. After showering, replace any wet dressings with clean, dry ones.
* Move and elevate legs often while resting in bed to decrease the likelihood of deep-vein blood clots.

MEDICATION
* Your doctor may prescribe:
  - Pain relievers.
  - Don't take prescription pain medication longer than 4 to 7 days. Use only as much as you need.
* You may use nonprescription drugs, such as acetaminophen, for minor pain. Avoid aspirin.

ACTIVITY—Resume normal activity as soon as possible to promote healing.

DIET
* Your doctor will prescribe a diet.
* Vitamin and mineral supplements (sometimes).

CALL YOUR DOCTOR IF

* Pain, swelling, redness, drainage or bleeding increases in the surgical area.
* You develop signs of infection, including headache, muscle aches, dizziness or a general ill feeling and fever.
* You experience constipation, abdominal swelling, nausea or vomiting.
* The skin around the the tube becomes raw or irritated.
* The tube falls out.
* New, unexplained symptoms develop. Drugs used in treatment may produce side effects.

GASTROSTOMY

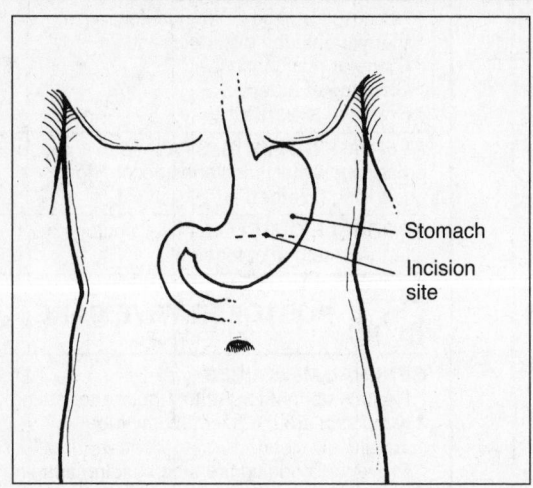

An illustration of the abdomen with proposed incision site for gastrostomy.

Stomach

Incision site

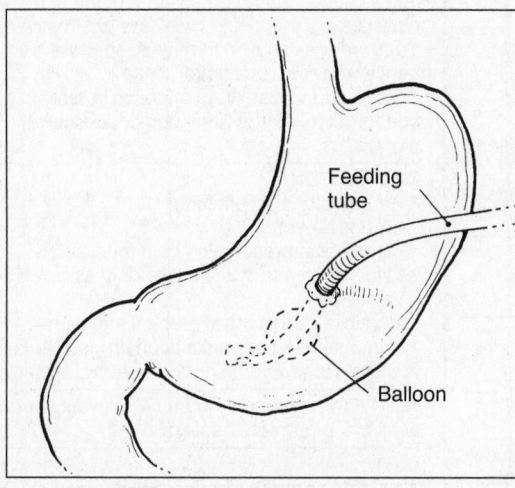

After the stomach has been located, a small opening is made into it and the stomach tube is pushed into the cavity of the stomach. The tube is secured by a balloon within the stomach.

Feeding tube

Balloon

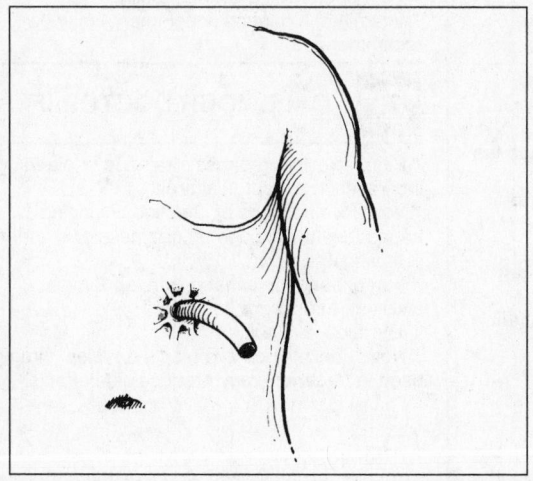

The other end of the tube is pulled to the outside through a separate small incision.

GASTROSTOMY, PERCUTANEOUS ENDOSCOPIC (P.E.G. Procedure)

 GENERAL INFORMATION

DEFINITION—Technique for placing a feeding tube without having to perform an open laparotomy (operation on the abdomen). This procedure is less costly and time consuming than a surgical gastrostomy (see in Surgery section).

BODY PARTS INVOLVED—Stomach; skin; structures of the abdominal wall.

REASONS FOR SURGERY
* To provide nutrition for those who cannot swallow.
* To provide nutrition to those who cannot or will not eat adequate amounts of food.
* Blockage of esophagus.
* Prevention of pneumonia in patients with swallowing disorders.

SURGICAL RISK INCREASES WITH
* Stress; obesity; poor nutrition.
* Recent or chronic illness, especially chronic lung disease.
* Diabetes.
* Excess alcohol consumption.
* Use of some prescription and nonprescription drugs. Inform your doctor of any drugs, medications, or vitamin and herb supplements you are using or have used in the last month.

 WHAT TO EXPECT

WHO OPERATES—General surgeon or gastroenterologist.

WHERE PERFORMED—Hospital or outpatient surgical facility.

DIAGNOSTIC TESTS—Before surgery: Blood and urine studies; x-rays of gastrointestinal tract.

ANESTHESIA—Local anesthesia (usually lidocaine injection).

DESCRIPTION OF OPERATION
* The endoscopist anesthetizes the throat with lidocaine or other local anesthesia.
* The endoscopist passes the endoscope to the appropriate point in the stomach.
* A small incision is made in the skin and an intravenous cannula is pushed through the skin into the stomach.
* A string is passed into the stomach through the cannula; the string is grasped inside the stomach and is brought back out through the mouth.
* The gastrostomy tube is tied to the string, then pulled back into the stomach and out through the abdominal wall.
* The gastrostomy tube is then fixed to the abdominal wall.

POSSIBLE COMPLICATIONS
* Abscess formation; wound infection.
* Inadvertent tube dislodgement.
* Catheter malfunction.
* Clogging of tube.
* Drainage around tube.

AVERAGE HOSPITAL STAY—0 to 1 day for procedure. Total time varies according to underlying disorder.

PROBABLE OUTCOME—Satisfactory alternate method of feeding.

 POSTOPERATIVE CARE

GENERAL MEASURES
* Remain upright for 1/2 to 1 hour after eating.
* Keep skin around gastrostomy tube scrupulously clean.
* Prevent dislodging the tube by careful taping and vigilance during dressing, feeding and activities.
* Shower as usual. You may wash the incision gently with mild, unscented soap.
* Move and elevate legs often while resting in to bed to decrease the likelihood of deep-vein blood clots.

MEDICATION
* Your doctor may prescribe:
  - Pain relievers.
  - Don't take prescription pain medication longer than 4 to 7 days. Use only as much as you need.
  - Antibiotics to fight or prevent infection.
* You may use nonprescription drugs, such as acetaminophen, for minor pain. Avoid aspirin.

ACTIVITY—Resume normal activity as soon as possible to promote healing.

DIET
* Your doctor will prescribe a diet.
* Vitamin and mineral supplements may be recommended.

 CALL YOUR DOCTOR IF

* Pain, swelling, redness, drainage or bleeding increases in the surgical area.
* You develop signs of infection, including headache, muscle aches, dizziness or a general ill feeling and fever.
* You experience constipation, abdominal swelling, nausea, or vomiting.
* The tube falls out.
* New, unexplained symptoms develop. Drugs used in treatment may produce side effects.

GASTROSTOMY, PERCUTANEOUS ENDOSCOPIC (P.E.G. Procedure)

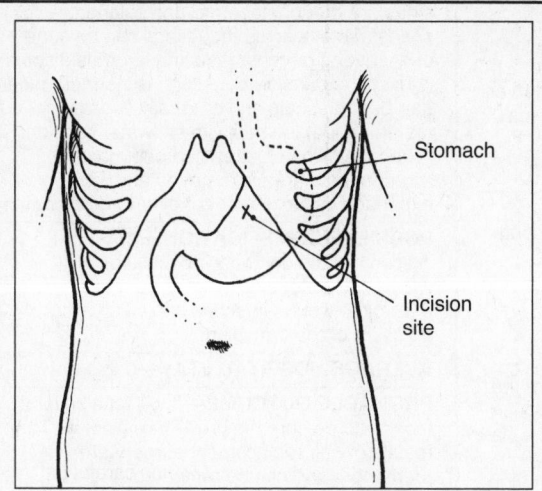

An illustration of the incision site in the abdomen over the position in the stomach chosen for the gastrostomy.

Stomach

Incision site

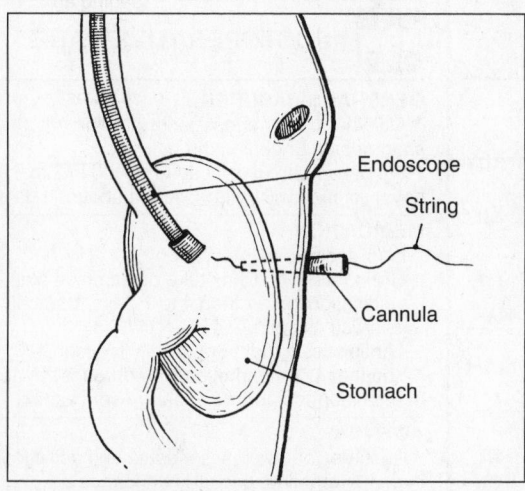

Shown are the endoscope at the upper end of the stomach and a tube inside the endoscope. The doctor makes a small incision into the skin and pushes an intravenous cannula through the skin into the stomach.

Endoscope

String

Cannula

Stomach

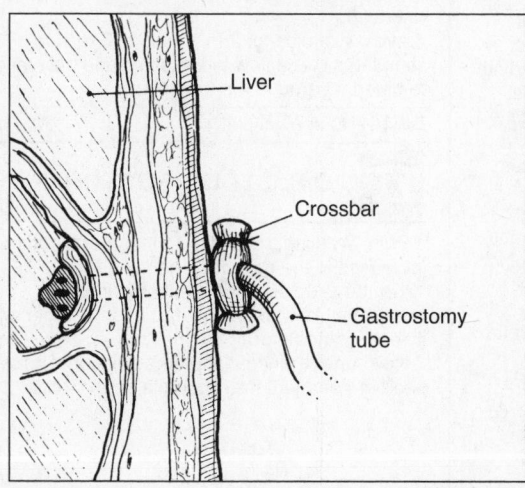

Final appearance with the feeding tube in place. The external end of the feeding tube is clamped to provide access for feeding in the future (not illustrated).

Liver

Crossbar

Gastrostomy tube

SURGERIES

HAIR TRANSPLANT

GENERAL INFORMATION

DEFINITION—Relocating hair-bearing skin, usually from the back of the head to the front. Multiple procedures are necessary with intervals in between, so that the total time involved may be 18 months or more.

BODY PARTS INVOLVED—Hair and scalp.

REASONS FOR SURGERY—To correct markedly receding hairlines or large bald spots caused by pattern baldness (see in Illness section), an inherited trait.

SURGICAL RISK INCREASES WITH
* Smoking.
* Recent or chronic illness; diabetes.
* Poor quality hair on the back and sides of the head.
* Hair transplants that are performed before hair loss has come to a standstill.
* Use of some prescription and nonprescription drugs. Inform your doctor of any drugs, medications, or vitamin and herb supplements you are using or have used in the last month.

WHAT TO EXPECT

WHO OPERATES—Plastic surgeon; other doctor with special training (sometimes).

WHERE PERFORMED—Doctor's office, outpatient surgical facility, special hair-transplant clinic or hospital (for more complex procedures).

DIAGNOSTIC TESTS
* Before surgery: Physical examination.
* After surgery: None required.

ANESTHESIA—Local anesthetic injected into both the donor and recipient sites. In complex procedures, more sedation may be necessary.

DESCRIPTION OF OPERATION—Several procedures are available. You and your doctor will decide the most appropriate one depending on the degree and location of your baldness:
* Punch grafts (plugs): A round graft is punched out of a donor site and fitted into a hole in the bald area. Each punch contains about 15 hairs plus skin and fatty tissue.
* Mini-plugs: About half the size of punch grafts and used to fill in spaces between larger grafts.
* Micro-plugs: Made by splitting one large plug into 4 to fill in spaces. Adds a more irregular natural look to hairline.
* Strip grafts: Similar to punch grafts except the graft is long and thin. May be used to finish hairline once plugs have filled in bald spot.
* Flaps: A flap of hair on the back or side is cut out and swiveled onto the bald spot. The cut edges of the donor site are brought together and stitched closed.

* Scalp reduction: An area of bald skin (2 inches by six inches) is cut out and the two sides are brought together and stitched. A series of these scalp reductions can be done over several months, reducing large bald spots.
* Tissue expansion: A balloon is inserted under hair-bearing scalp and gradually (weekly, for a 2 month period) inflated with saltwater solution. When the skin has stretched enough, the adjacent bald area is removed and the expanded tissue is brought over to cover it.

POSSIBLE COMPLICATIONS
* Scarring and decreased circulation.
* Excessive bleeding.
* Surgical-wound infection.
* Failure of the transplant.

AVERAGE HOSPITAL STAY—0 to 1 day.

PROBABLE OUTCOME—It will take several months to be sure the procedure worked. The results of hair replacement surgery are permanent and can be remarkable.

POSTOPERATIVE CARE

GENERAL MEASURES
* Ask your doctor about guidelines for shampooing or getting the hair wet.
* Bandages can usually be removed in 2 to 5 days; stitches will be removed in about 10 days.

MEDICATION
* Your doctor may prescribe:
  - Pain relievers. Don't take prescription pain medication longer than 4 to 7 days. Use only as much as you need.
  - Antibiotics to fight or prevent infection.
* You may use nonprescription drugs, such as acetaminophen, for minor pain. Avoid aspirin.

ACTIVITY
* Resume your normal schedule and activities, except swimming, once the bandages are removed.
* Avoid exercise for 2 to 3 weeks. Exercise stimulates blood flow to the scalp and may lead to bleeding around the transplants.

DIET—No special diet.

CALL YOUR DOCTOR IF

* Pain, swelling, redness, drainage or bleeding increases in the surgical area.
* You develop signs of infection, including headache, muscle aches, dizziness or a general ill feeling and fever.
* New, unexplained symptoms develop. Drugs used in treatment may produce side effects.

HAIR TRANSPLANT

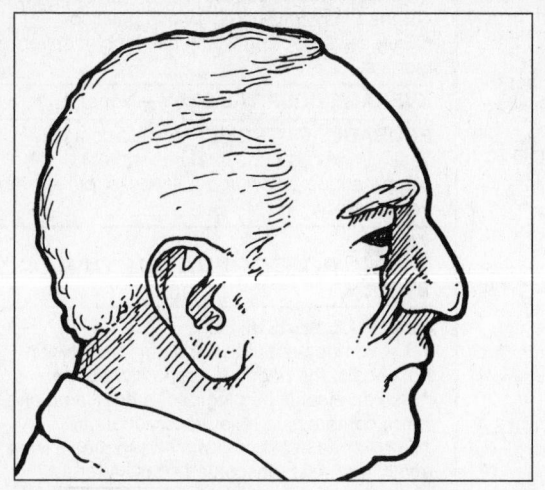

The surgical area before a plug transplant.

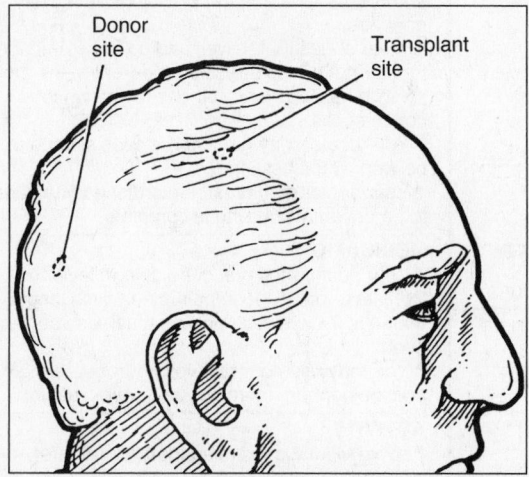

Donor site

Transplant site

A round plug is removed from a donor site and prepared for insertion into the transplant site.

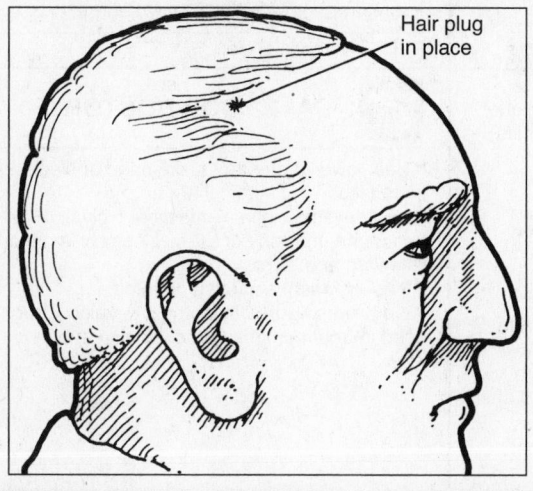

Hair plug in place

Hair plug is in place.

HAMMERTOE CORRECTION

GENERAL INFORMATION

DEFINITION—Removal of tendons and joining of middle joints in the toes to correct hammertoe, a deformity in which the toes bend downward. This causes the tops of the toes to become callused from rubbing against the inside of shoes. Hammertoe probably results from wearing shoes that do not fit properly, especially high-heeled shoes that place pressure on the front part of the foot and compress the smaller toes together tightly.

BODY PARTS INVOLVED—All toes except the big toes; tendons, blood vessels and nerves connected to these toes; overlying skin.

REASONS FOR SURGERY
* Relief of painful calluses.
* Prevention of permanent deformity.

SURGICAL RISK INCREASES WITH
* Obesity.
* Smoking.
* Excess alcohol consumption.
* Diabetes.
* Use of some prescription and nonprescription drugs. Inform your doctor of any drugs, medications, or vitamin and herb supplements you are using or have used in the last month.

WHAT TO EXPECT

WHO OPERATES—General surgeon (sometimes), podiatrist or orthopedic surgeon.

WHERE PERFORMED—Hospital or outpatient surgical facility.

DIAGNOSTIC TESTS
* Before surgery: Blood and urine studies; x-rays of feet.
* After surgery: Blood studies.

ANESTHESIA
* Local anesthesia by injection.
* Regional anesthesia by injection.

DESCRIPTION OF OPERATION
* After local anesthesia is injected, a tourniquet is applied above the ankle to keep the surgical area from bleeding.
* An incision is made through the skin.
* The tendons that attach to the toes are located, cut free of connective tissue to foot bones, and realigned so that they no longer bend downward.
* The middle joints of the affected toes are often fused together permanently with fine pins and wire sutures.
* The skin is closed with fine sutures, which usually can be removed about 7 to 10 days after surgery.
* A dressing is placed over the toes to help maintain their new position.

POSSIBLE COMPLICATIONS
* Excessive bleeding.
* Surgical-wound infection.
* Bones may return to previous position.
* Excessive swelling which can last for several months.

AVERAGE HOSPITAL STAY—None.

PROBABLE OUTCOME—Expect complete healing and relief of symptoms without complications. Allow about 4 weeks for recovery from surgery.

POSTOPERATIVE CARE

GENERAL MEASURES
* A hard ridge should form along the incision. As it heals, the ridge will gradually recede.
* Use an electric heating pad, a heat lamp or a warm compress to relieve incisional pain.
* Shower as usual. You may wash the incision gently with mild, unscented soap. After a shower, replace any wet dressings with clean, dry ones.
* Wear shoes that fit well and do not cramp the toes or put undue stress on the front of the foot.
* While healing, wear flat shoes and white cotton socks.
* Your doctor may prescribe a special shoe to be worn while healing.
* Your doctor may prescribe crutches or a cane to be used until healing is complete.

MEDICATION
* Your doctor may prescribe pain relievers. Don't take prescription pain medication longer than 4 to 7 days. Use only as much as you need.
* You may use nonprescription drugs, such as acetaminophen, for minor pain. Avoid aspirin.

ACTIVITY
* Avoid vigorous exercise for 6 weeks after surgery.
* Resume driving 1 week after returning home.

DIET—No special diet.

CALL YOUR DOCTOR IF

* Pain, swelling, redness, drainage or bleeding increases in the surgical area.
* You develop signs of infection, including headache, muscle aches, dizziness or a general ill feeling and fever.
* You experience nausea or vomiting.
* New, unexplained symptoms develop. Drugs used in treatment may produce side effects.

HAMMERTOE CORRECTION

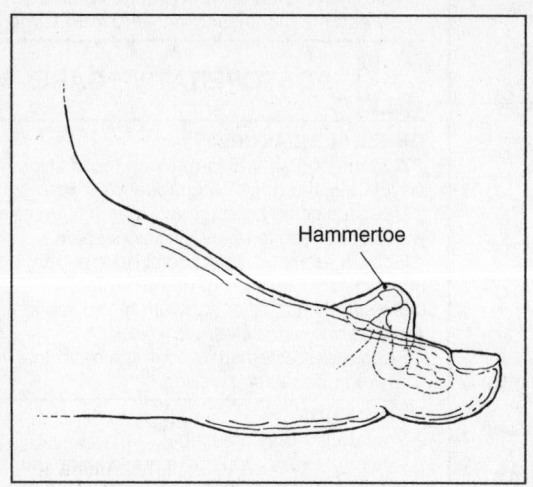

An illustration of a typical hammer toe (a deformity in which the toes bend downward).

Hammertoe

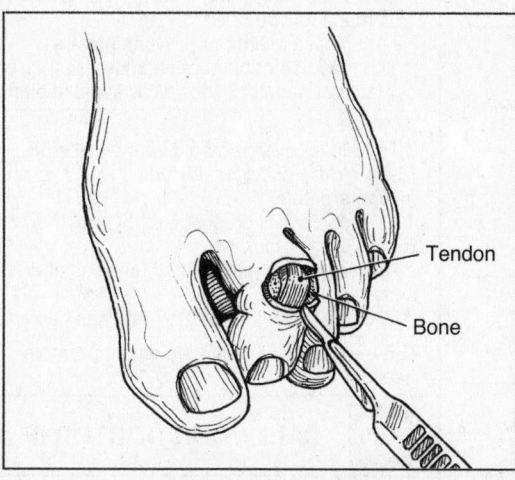

After local anesthesia is injected, tendons are located and divided so toes no longer bend downward.

Tendon

Bone

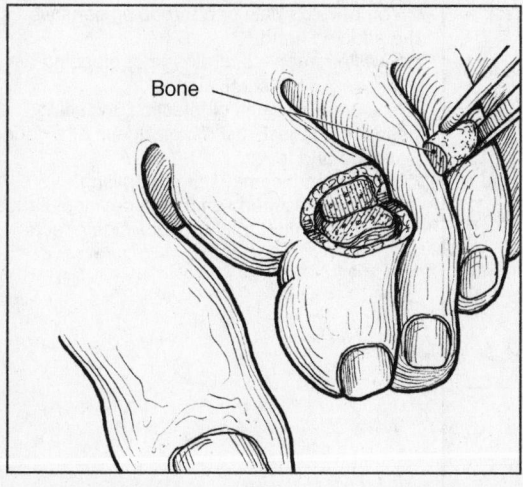

The portion of bone is removed and toes can return to normal shape.

Bone

HAND SURGERY

 GENERAL INFORMATION

DEFINITION—Any operation performed to restore or preserve the normal function of the hand.

BODY PARTS INVOLVED—Hand.

REASONS FOR SURGERY—Preservation or restoration of normal function of the hand that has been lost or impaired by disease, injury, or malformation.

SURGICAL RISK INCREASES WITH
* Obesity.
* Smoking.
* Poor nutrition.
* Excess alcohol consumption.
* Recent or chronic illness, especially diabetes, peripheral vascular disease and arthritis.
* Use of some prescription and nonprescription drugs. Inform your doctor of any drugs, medications, or vitamin and herb supplements you are using or have used in the last month.

 WHAT TO EXPECT

WHO OPERATES—General surgeon, hand surgeon, plastic surgeon, or orthopedic surgeon.

WHERE PERFORMED—Doctor's office, outpatient surgical facility, hospital or emergency room.

DIAGNOSTIC TESTS
* Before surgery: Blood and urine studies; x-rays of hands.
* After surgery: Blood studies.

ANESTHESIA
* Local anesthesia (sometimes) by injection.
* Regional anesthesia by injection.
* General anesthesia by injection and inhalation with an airway tube placed in the windpipe.

DESCRIPTION OF OPERATION
* The arm of the affected hand is elevated and wrapped with a blood-pressure cuff inflated to higher than normal blood pressure. This prevents the surgical area from bleeding.
* The procedures depend on the injury or disease in the hand.
* The wound is covered with gauze and padded dressings.

POSSIBLE COMPLICATIONS
* Excessive bleeding.
* Surgical-wound infection.
* Nerve damage.
* Scarring of tendons which limits motion.

AVERAGE HOSPITAL STAY—0 to 2 days.

PROBABLE OUTCOME—Expect complete healing of surgical wound. Success of surgery depends on the underlying problem or cause. Allow about 3 months for recovery from surgery.

 POSTOPERATIVE CARE

GENERAL MEASURES
* A hard ridge should form along the incision. As it heals, the ridge will gradually recede.
* Use an electric heating pad, a heat lamp or a warm compress to relieve incisional pain.
* Shower as usual, if you don't have a cast. You may wash the incision gently with mild, unscented soap. After showering, replace any wet dressings with clean, dry ones.
* Keep the affected arm above the heart to prevent or decrease swelling.

MEDICATION
* Your doctor may prescribe:
  - Pain relievers. Don't take prescription pain medication longer than 4 to 7 days. Use only as much as you need.
  - Antibiotics to fight or prevent infection.
* You may use nonprescription drugs, such as acetaminophen, for minor pain. Avoid aspirin.

ACTIVITY
* To help recovery and aid your well-being, resume daily activities, including work, as soon as you are able.
* Your doctor will prescribe a physical therapy rehabilitation program.
* Avoid vigorous exercise for 3 weeks after surgery.
* Resume driving when the hand has healed.

DIET—Eat a well-balanced diet to promote healing.

 CALL YOUR DOCTOR IF

* You develop pain or a throbbing sensation in the affected hand.
* Swelling, redness, drainage or bleeding increases in the surgical area.
* You develop signs of infection, including headache, muscle aches, dizziness or a general ill feeling and fever.
* You experience nausea or vomiting.
* New, unexplained symptoms develop. Drugs used in treatment may produce side effects.

HAND SURGERY

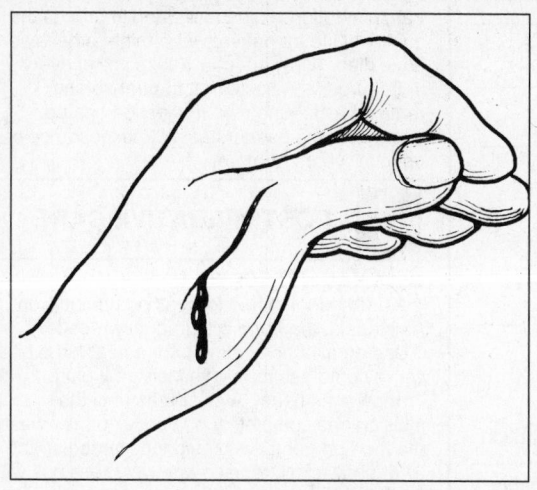

A typical hand injury with a deep laceration.
- Hand injuries may include severed nerves or blood vessels, severed or injured tendons or connective tissue, or amputated fingers.

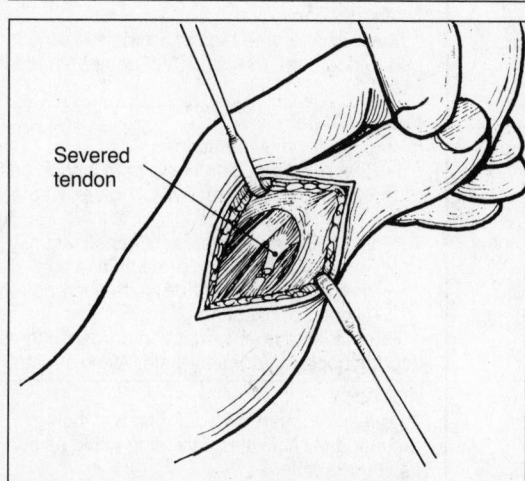

Severed tendon

The ragged injury is made into a clean surgical incision and muscles and connective tissue retracted for exposure. A severed tendon can be seen and repaired.

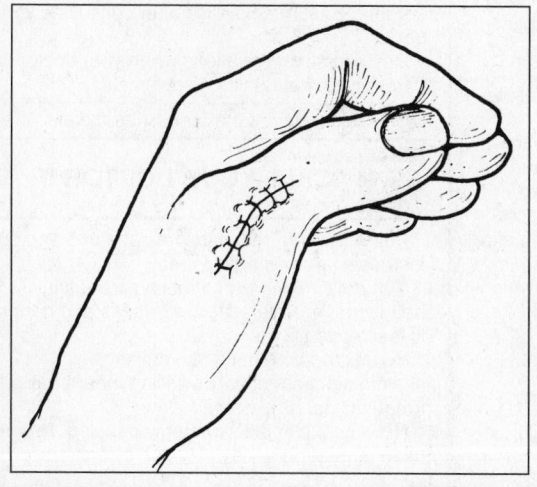

Skin is carefully closed after repair to the injured hand tissue. The hand and forearm are usually kept rigid with a plaster cast or splint.

SURGERIES

HEART TRANSPLANTATION

GENERAL INFORMATION

DEFINITION—Replacement of a diseased heart with a healthy heart.

BODY PARTS INVOLVED—Diseased or abnormal heart; healthy heart from donor.

REASONS FOR SURGERY
- Heart failure from coronary artery disease.
- Heart failure from cardiomyopathy.
- Valvular heart disease with congestive heart failure.
- Heart failure from severe congenital heart disease.

SURGICAL RISK INCREASES WITH
- Adults over 60; obesity; poor nutrition.
- Recent or chronic illness; diabetes.
- Alcoholism; smoking.
- Use of some prescription and nonprescription drugs. Inform your doctor of any drugs, medications, or vitamin and herb supplements you are using or have used in the last month.

WHAT TO EXPECT

WHO OPERATES—Cardiovascular surgeon.

WHERE PERFORMED—Hospital.

DIAGNOSTIC TESTS
- Before surgery: Blood and urine studies; chest x-ray; studies of the immune system; ECG; cardiac catheterization; ultrasound (see Glossary for all).
- During surgery: Cardiac monitoring.
- After surgery: Blood studies; ECG.

ANESTHESIA—General anesthesia by injection and inhalation with an airway tube placed in the windpipe.

DESCRIPTION OF OPERATION
- A healthy heart is obtained from a donor who has died from an accident or a disease other than heart disease, HIV, or hepatitis (see Glossary for both).
- An incision is made in the recipient's chest to expose the heart.
- A heart-lung machine sustains life while the diseased heart is cut free and removed, and until the donor heart has been transplanted.
- The donor heart is sewn into place. The aorta, pulmonary artery, superior vena cava and inferior vena cava are connected to the new heart.
- The skin is closed with sutures or clips, which are removed about 1 week after surgery.

POSSIBLE COMPLICATIONS
- Excessive bleeding; surgical-wound infection.
- Life-threatening general infections.
- Rejection of the transplanted heart.
- Cancer which develops as an adverse effect of immunosuppressant drugs.

AVERAGE HOSPITAL STAY—10 to 21 days.

PROBABLE OUTCOME—A successful transplantation prolongs life and improves the quality of life for patients who might otherwise have died. Allow about 6 weeks for recovery from surgery. Rejection of the transplant remains a life-long risk. If rejection can be controlled, the patient has a life expectancy of up to 10 years or more.

POSTOPERATIVE CARE

GENERAL MEASURES
- A hard ridge should form along the incision. As it heals, the ridge will gradually recede.
- Use an electric heating pad, a heat lamp or a warm compress to relieve incisional pain.
- Shower as usual. Avoid baths until the incision has completely healed. You may wash the incision gently with mild, unscented soap. After showering, replace any wet dressings with clean, dry ones.
- Move and elevate legs often while resting in bed to decrease the chance of deep-vein blood clots.

MEDICATION
- Your doctor may prescribe:
  - Pain relievers. Don't take prescription pain medication longer than 4 to 7 days. Use only as much as you need.
  - Stool softeners to prevent constipation.
  - Antibiotics to fight or prevent infection.
  - Immunosuppressant drugs to decrease the likelihood of rejection.
- You may use nonprescription drugs, such as acetaminophen, for minor pain. Avoid aspirin.

ACTIVITY
- To help recovery and aid your well-being, resume daily activities, including work, as soon as you are able.
- Avoid vigorous exercise for 6 weeks after surgery. Resume exercise after consulting your doctor.
- Resume sexual relations when your doctor determines that healing is complete.

DIET—Your doctor may prescribe a diet.

CALL YOUR DOCTOR IF

- Pain, swelling, redness, drainage or bleeding increases in the surgical area.
- You develop signs of infection, including headache, muscle aches, dizziness or a general ill feeling and fever.
- You experience nausea, vomiting, constipation, abdominal swelling, heartbeat irregularities, or extreme fatigue.
- New, unexplained symptoms develop. Drugs used in treatment may produce side effects.

HEART TRANSPLANTATION

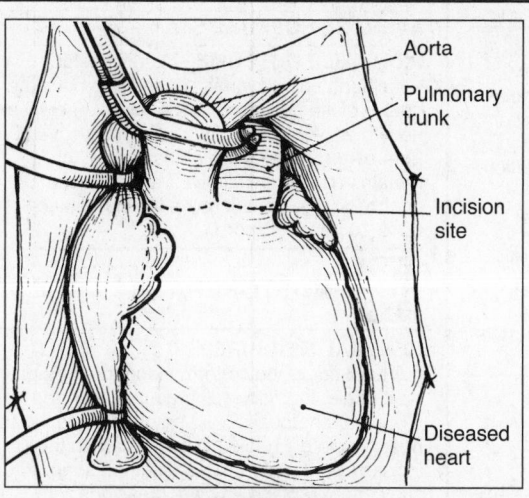

Aorta

Pulmonary trunk

Incision site

Diseased heart

An illustration of a diseased heart. The major blood vessels into and away from the heart are clamped and incision sites for the heart transplant indicated.

- A heart-lung machine sustains life while the diseased heart is cut free and removed, and until the donor heart has been transplanted.

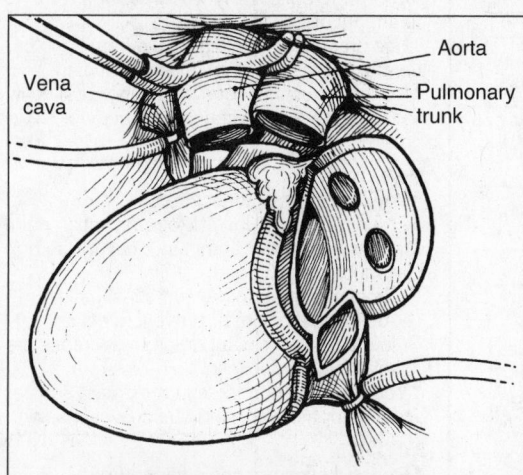

Vena cava

Aorta

Pulmonary trunk

After major vessels have been severed, the diseased heart is now ready to be removed from the chest and discarded.

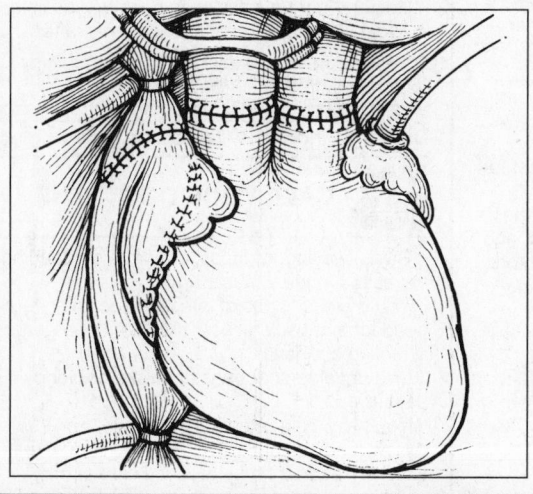

The donor heart is sewn in place. The aorta, pulmonary arteries, superior vena cava and inferior vena cava are connected to the new heart.

- The donor heart, which had been kept motionless by cooling, is now stimulated to resume beating with warming and a weak electrical current.

SURGERIES

HEART-LUNG TRANSPLANTATION

GENERAL INFORMATION

DEFINITION—Replacement of poorly functioning lungs and a damaged or healthy heart with donor organs. If the recipient's heart is normal, it may be extracted and donated to another patient in need of of a heart transplantation only (see Heart Transplantation in Surgery section).

BODY PARTS INVOLVED—Lungs, heart, trachea and blood vessels.

REASONS FOR SURGERY—Chronic lung disorders such as pulmonary hypertension, emphysema, cystic fibrosis and other lung conditions causing pulmonary fibrosis.

SURGICAL RISK INCREASES WITH
* Adults over 60; obesity; poor nutrition.
* Recent or chronic illness.
* Alcoholism; smoking.
* Diabetes.
* Use of some prescription and nonprescription drugs. Inform your doctor of any drugs, medications, or vitamin and herb supplements you are using or have used in the last month.

WHAT TO EXPECT

WHO OPERATES—Cardiovascular surgeon, thoracic surgeon.

WHERE PERFORMED—Hospital.

DIAGNOSTIC TESTS
* Before surgery: Blood and urine studies; studies of the immune system; ECG; cardiac catheterization; echocardiography, ultrasound; biopsy; pulmonary angiography; lung function studies (see Glossary for all).
* During surgery: Cardiac monitoring (see Glossary).
* After surgery: Repeat of some tests for monitoring of the new organs.

ANESTHESIA—General anesthesia by injection and inhalation, with an airway tube placed in the windpipe.

DESCRIPTION OF OPERATION
* An incision is made in the recipient's chest to expose the heart and lungs.
* A heart-lung machine sustains life while the diseased organs are cut free and removed, and until the donor organs have been transplanted.
* The donor organs are sewn into place. The new lungs are connected to the trachea.
* The skin is closed with sutures or clips, which usually can be removed about 1 week after surgery.

POSSIBLE COMPLICATIONS
* Excessive bleeding; blood clots.
* Surgical-wound infection.

* Life-threatening general infections.
* Rejection of transplanted organs.

AVERAGE HOSPITAL STAY—3 weeks.

PROBABLE OUTCOME—A successful transplantation prolongs life and improves the quality of life for patients who might otherwise have died. Allow about 6 weeks for recovery from surgery. Rejection of the transplant remains a risk indefinitely. If rejection can be controlled, the patient has a life expectancy of up to 10 years or more.

POSTOPERATIVE CARE

GENERAL MEASURES
* A hard ridge should form along the incision. As it heals, the ridge will gradually recede.
* Shower as usual. Avoid baths until the incision has completely healed. You may wash the incision gently with mild, unscented soap. After showering, replace any wet dressings with clean, dry ones.
* Use an electric heating pad, a heat lamp or a warm compress to relieve incisional pain.
* Move and elevate legs often while resting in bed to decrease the chance of deep-vein blood clots.

MEDICATION
* Your doctor may prescribe:
  - Pain relievers. Don't take prescription pain medication longer than 4 to 7 days. Use only as much as you need.
  - Stool softeners to prevent constipation.
  - Antibiotics to fight or prevent infection.
  - Immunosuppressant drugs to decrease the likelihood of rejection.
* You may use nonprescription drugs, such as acetaminophen, for minor pain. Avoid aspirin.

ACTIVITY
* Rehabilitation will begin after surgery.
* Resume normal activity as soon as possible.
* Avoid vigorous exercise for 6 weeks after surgery.
* Resume sexual relations when your doctor determines that healing is complete.

DIET—Your doctor will prescribe a diet.

CALL YOUR DOCTOR IF

* Pain, swelling, redness, drainage or bleeding increases in the surgical area.
* You develop signs of infection, including headache, muscle aches, dizziness or a general ill feeling and fever.
* You develop shortness of breath or bloody sputum.
* You have fluid retention.
* New, unexplained symptoms develop. Drugs used in treatment may produce side effects.

HEART-LUNG TRANSPLANTATION

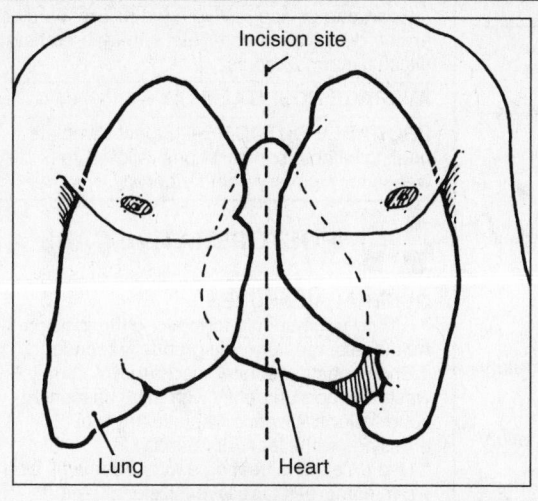

Illustration demonstrating surgical anatomy. Mid-line incision is made and recipient's heart and lungs are exposed.

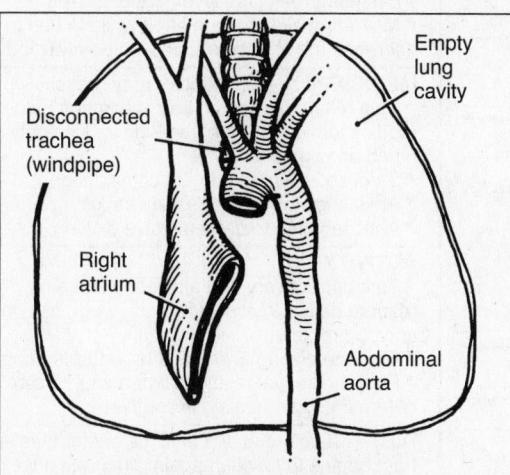

Recipient's heart and lungs are removed, leaving an empty cavity where new organs will be attached.

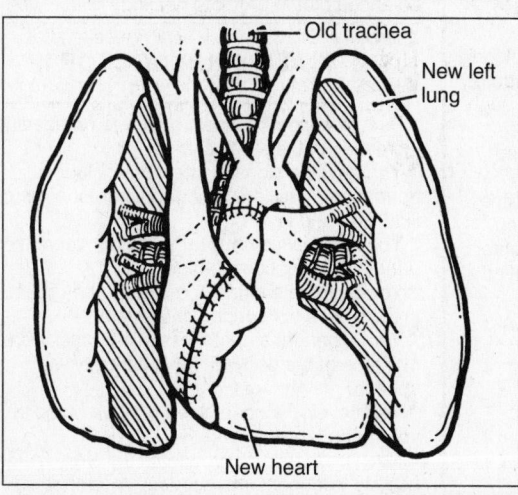

Donor's heart and lungs are sewn into position. The surgical site is examined for any leaks prior to closing of the chest.

HEART VALVE REPLACEMENT

GENERAL INFORMATION

DEFINITION—Replacement of one or more diseased heart valves with porcine (derived from swine) or artificial valves.

BODY PARTS INVOLVED—Valves that separate major sections of the heart.

REASONS FOR SURGERY—Prevention of complications resulting from valvular heart disease, especially congestive heart failure and bacterial endocarditis.

SURGICAL RISK INCREASES WITH
- Adults over 60.
- Obesity; smoking; poor nutrition.
- Recent illness such as acute upper respiratory infection.
- Alcoholism or chronic illness.
- Use of some prescription and nonprescription drugs. Inform your doctor of any drugs, medications, or vitamin and herb supplements you are using or have used in the last month.

WHAT TO EXPECT

WHO OPERATES—Cardiovascular surgeon.

WHERE PERFORMED—Hospital.

DIAGNOSTIC TESTS
- Before surgery: Blood and urine studies; x-rays of chest; ECG; cardiac catheterization (see Glossary for both).
- During surgery: ECG monitor.
- After surgery: Blood studies; ECG.

ANESTHESIA—General anesthesia by injection and inhalation with an airway tube placed in the windpipe.

DESCRIPTION OF OPERATION
- An incision is made in the chest, and the breastbone is divided. The chest is opened to expose the heart.
- A heart-lung machine circulates enough blood to sustain life throughout the surgical procedure.
- The diseased heart valves are located through delicate incisions made in the heart.
- Diseased valves are removed and replaced with artificial or porcine valves.
- The incisions in the heart are closed with fine sutures, and the chest cavity is reconstructed with wire sutures. The skin is closed with lighter sutures or clips, which usually can be removed about 1 week after surgery.
- Drains may be left in place for several days following the surgery.

POSSIBLE COMPLICATIONS
- Excessive bleeding; blood clots.
- Surgical-wound infection.
- Failure of the heart to resume normal heartbeat (rare).

- Clotting or infection of valve.
- Kidney damage or kidney failure.
- Heart attack; congestive heart failure; cardiac arrest; deep-vein blood clots; stroke; breathing difficulties; pneumonia.

AVERAGE HOSPITAL STAY—5 to 7 days.

PROBABLE OUTCOME—Expect complete healing without complications. Allow 4 to 6 weeks for recovery from surgery.

POSTOPERATIVE CARE

GENERAL MEASURES
- A hard ridge should form along the incision. As it heals, the ridge will gradually recede.
- Shower as usual after discharge. You may wash the incision gently with mild, unscented soap. After showering, replace any wet dressings with clean, dry ones.
- Use an electric heating pad, a heat lamp or a warm compress to relieve incisional pain.
- Move and elevate legs often while in bed to decrease the chance of deep-vein blood clots.

MEDICATION—Your doctor may prescribe:
- Pain relievers. Don't take prescription pain medication longer than 4 to 7 days. Use only as much as you need.
- Stool softeners to prevent constipation.
- Antibiotics to fight or prevent infection.
- Anticoagulant to prevent valve clotting.

ACTIVITY
- To help recovery and aid your well-being, resume daily activities, including work, as soon as you are able.
- Resume driving 5 weeks after returning home.
- Resume sexual relations when your doctor determines that healing is complete.

DIET—Clear liquid diet until the gastrointestinal tract begins to function again. Then eat a well-balanced diet to promote healing.

CALL YOUR DOCTOR IF

- Pain, swelling, redness, drainage or bleeding increases in the surgical area.
- You develop signs of infection, including headache, muscle aches, dizziness or a general ill feeling and fever.
- You experience nausea, vomiting, decreased urine output, or constipation.
- You develop shortness of breath, heartbeat irregularities, or sudden chest pain.
- You experience numbness or weakness on one side of the body, or have difficulty with speech.
- You develop a nose bleed or have blood in your urine.
- New, unexplained symptoms develop. Drugs used in treatment may produce side effects.

HEART VALVE REPLACEMENT

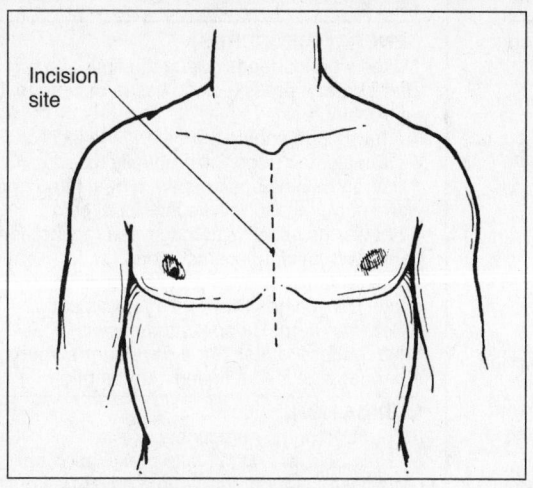

Incision site

An illustration of the incision site over the breast bone, which will be spread to allow exposure of the heart.
  • A heart-lung machine circulates enough blood to sustain life throughout the surgical procedure.

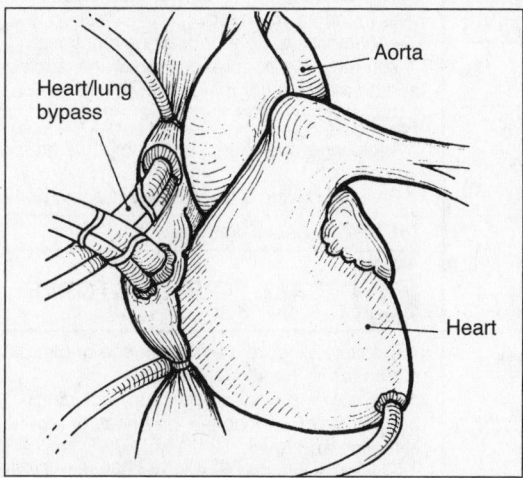

Aorta

Heart/lung bypass

Heart

The diseased heart valves are located through delicate incisions made in the heart.

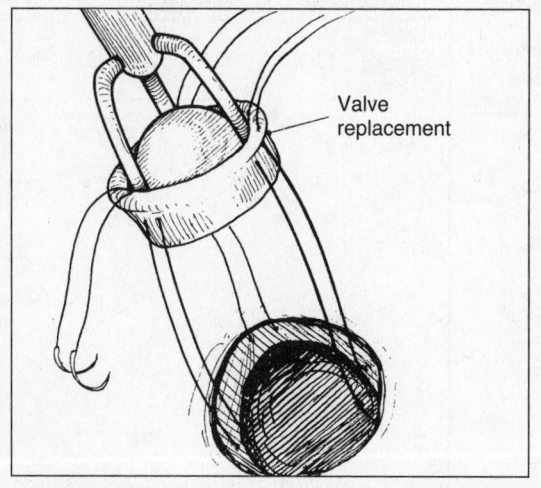

Valve replacement

Diseased valves are removed and replaced with artificial or porcine valves.
  • The incisions made in the heart are closed with fine sutures. The chest cavity is reconstructed with wire sutures in the chest muscle and breast bone.

SURGERIES

HEEL SPUR REMOVAL

GENERAL INFORMATION

DEFINITION—Removal of a heel spur, a sharp outgrowth on the bone of the heel.

BODY PARTS INVOLVED—Bottom of the heel bone.

REASONS FOR SURGERY—Relief of pain.

SURGICAL RISK INCREASES WITH
* Obesity.
* Smoking.
* Poor nutrition.
* Excess alcohol consumption.
* Recent or chronic illness.
* Diabetes.
* Use of some prescription and nonprescription drugs. Inform your doctor of any drugs, medications, or vitamin and herb supplements you are using or have used in the last month.

WHAT TO EXPECT

WHO OPERATES—General surgeon, orthopedist or podiatrist.

WHERE PERFORMED—Outpatient surgical facility or doctor's office.

DIAGNOSTIC TESTS
* Before surgery: Blood and urine studies; x-rays of both feet.
* After surgery: Blood studies; laboratory examination of removed tissue.

ANESTHESIA
* Local anesthesia by injection.
* Spinal anesthesia by injection (sometimes).

DESCRIPTION OF OPERATION
* Different surgical options are available for treatment. One option is described here. An incision is made over the spur.
* The spur is cut free and removed with special instruments.
* The skin is closed with sutures, which usually can be removed about 10 to 14 days after surgery.

POSSIBLE COMPLICATIONS
* Excessive bleeding.
* Surgical-wound infection.
* Numbness.
* Recurrence of the heel problem.
* Scar tissue from the incision becomes tender or painful.

AVERAGE HOSPITAL STAY—Usually none.

PROBABLE OUTCOME—Expect complete healing without complications. Allow about 6 months for complete recovery from surgery.

POSTOPERATIVE CARE

GENERAL MEASURES
* If the wound bleeds during the first 24 hours after surgery, press a clean tissue or cloth to it for 10 minutes.
* A hard ridge should form along the incision. As it heals, the ridge will gradually recede.
* Use an electric heating pad, a heat lamp or a warm compress to relieve incisional pain.
* Shower as usual. You may wash the incision gently with mild, unscented soap.
* Use crutches or a cane to walk until your doctor determines that healing is complete.
* Between baths, keep wound dry with a bandage for the first 2 or 3 days after surgery. If a bandage gets wet, change it promptly.

MEDICATION
* Your doctor may prescribe:
  - Pain relievers. Don't take prescription pain medication longer than 4 to 7 days. Use only as much as you need.
  - Antibiotics to fight or prevent infection.
* You may use nonprescription drugs, such as acetaminophen, for minor pain. Avoid aspirin.

ACTIVITY
* Avoid vigorous exercise for 3 months after surgery.
* Resume driving 1 week after returning home.

DIET—No special diet.

CALL YOUR DOCTOR IF

* Pain, swelling, redness, drainage or bleeding increases in the surgical area.
* You develop signs of infection, including headache, muscle aches, dizziness or a general ill feeling and fever.
* New, unexplained symptoms develop. Drugs used in treatment may produce side effects.

HEEL SPUR REMOVAL

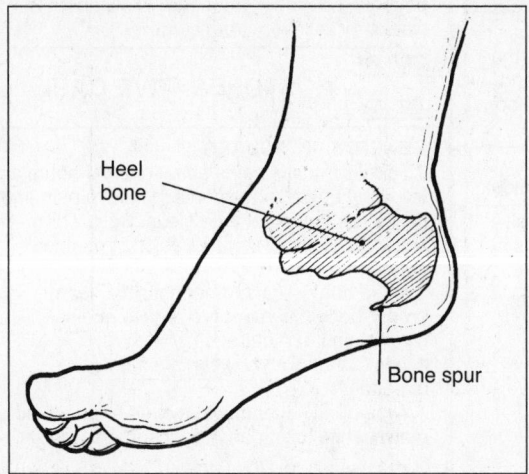

An illustration of a typical bone spur on the heel bone.

Heel bone

Bone spur

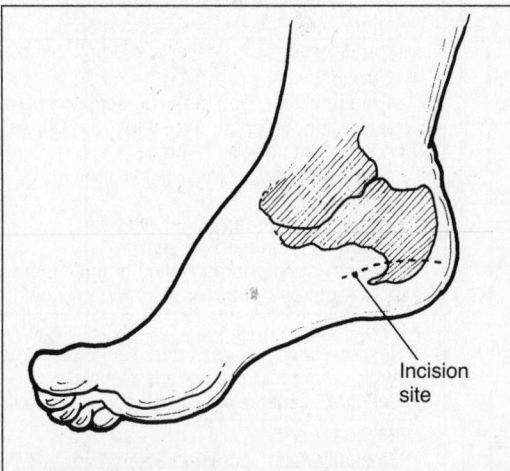

A typical incision site to enable removal of the bone spur, which is cut free and removed with special instruments.

Incision site

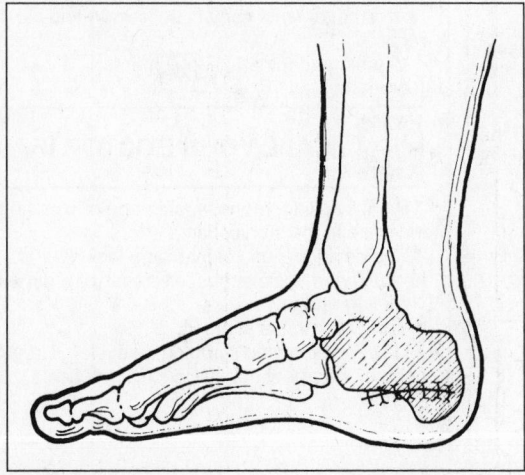

Skin is closed with sutures, which can usually be removed about 10 to 14 days after surgery.

HEMORRHOID BANDING

GENERAL INFORMATION

DEFINITION—Destruction of hemorrhoids (varicose veins that occur inside or outside the anus) by a technique that uses a rubber band over the stalk of the hemorrhoid to cut off blood flow.

BODY PARTS INVOLVED—Anus; rectum; dilated veins in anus and rectum (hemorrhoids).

REASONS FOR SURGERY—Pain, excessive bleeding, itching or prolapse of dilated veins in the rectum and anus.

SURGICAL RISK INCREASES WITH
• Obesity.
• Smoking.
• Poor nutrition.
• Adults over 60.
• Excess alcohol consumption.
• Recent or chronic illness.
• Diabetes.
• Inflammatory bowel disease.
• Use of some prescription and nonprescription drugs. Inform your doctor of any drugs, medications, or vitamin and herb supplements you are using or have used in the last month.

WHAT TO EXPECT

WHO OPERATES—Proctologist, colon-rectal surgeon or general surgeon.

WHERE PERFORMED—Doctor's office, hospital or outpatient surgical facility.

DIAGNOSTIC TESTS
• Before surgery: Blood and urine studies; anoscopy; sigmoidoscopy (see Glossary for both).
• After surgery: Blood studies.

ANESTHESIA
• Local anesthesia by injection.
• Spinal anesthesia by injection.
• General anesthesia by injection and inhalation with an airway tube placed in the windpipe.

DESCRIPTION OF OPERATION
• The doctor inserts several fingers to dilate the anal muscles. Sometimes anal muscles must be dilated vigorously to expose the hemorrhoids.
• The hemorrhoid is visualized and grasped with a special instrument.
• A small rubber band is slipped over the stalk of the hemorrhoid to bind it and cut off blood flow.

POSSIBLE COMPLICATIONS
• Excessive bleeding.
• Surgical-wound infection.
• Severe pain, especially with bowel movements.
• Urinary retention.

AVERAGE HOSPITAL STAY—0 to 1 day.

PROBABLE OUTCOME—Curable in most patients, no matter what age. Allow about 2 weeks for recovery from surgery.

POSTOPERATIVE CARE

GENERAL MEASURES
• Take warm sitz baths about every 4 hours and following bowel movements to relieve pain and help keep the rectal area clean. Sit in warm water for 10 to 20 minutes as often as it feels good.
• Avoid heavy lifting. If not possible, learn proper body mechanics to reduce strain contributing to recurrence.
• Don't strain with bowel movements or urination.
• Wipe gently after bowel movements with soft, moist, white toilet paper or absorbent, moist cotton.
• Expect drainage from the rectum for 2 to 3 weeks.

MEDICATION
• Your doctor may prescribe:
 - Pain relievers. Don't take prescription pain medication for longer than 4 to 7 days. Use only as much as you need.
 - Stool softeners or laxatives to prevent constipation.
 - Analgesic ointment to relieve pain.
 - Vitamins to encourage healing.
• You may use nonprescription drugs, such as acetaminophen, for minor pain. Avoid aspirin.

ACTIVITY
• Resume driving 1 week after returning home.
• Avoid sitting for long periods of time.
• Resume sexual relations as soon as you wish.

DIET
• No special diet. Increase dietary fiber and fluid intake to prevent constipation. Straining during bowel movements can cause hemorrhoids to recur.
• Vitamin and mineral supplements (sometimes).

CALL YOUR DOCTOR IF

• Pain, swelling, redness, drainage or bleeding increase in the surgical area.
• You develop signs of infection, including headache, muscle aches, dizziness or a general ill feeling and fever.
• You become constipated.
• New, unexplained symptoms develop. Drugs used in treatment may produce side effects.

HEMORRHOID BANDING

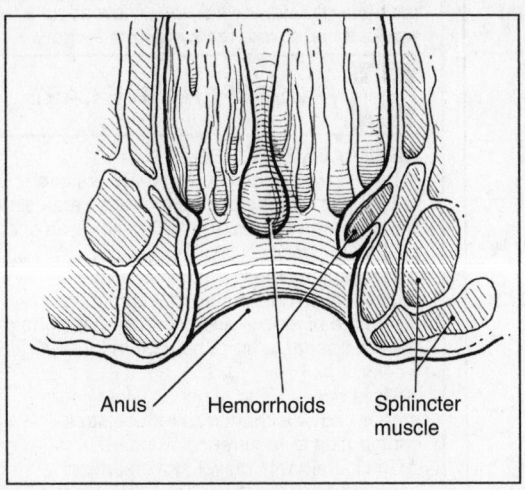

An illustration of a cross-sectional view of the region of the body containing the anus, the sphincter muscle of the anus and a view of an internal hemorrhoids just inside the anus.

Anus   Hemorrhoids   Sphincter muscle

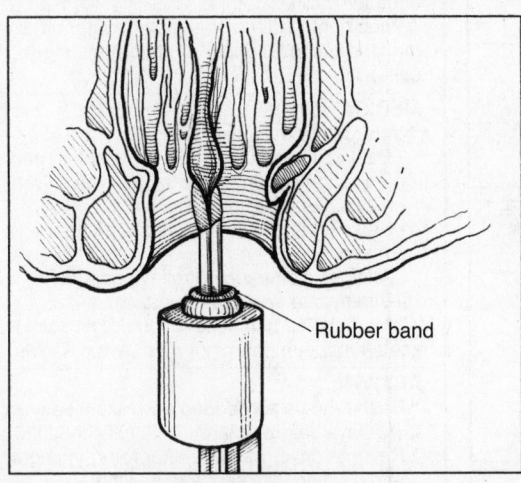

A hemorrhoid is found and grasped with a special instrument.

Rubber band

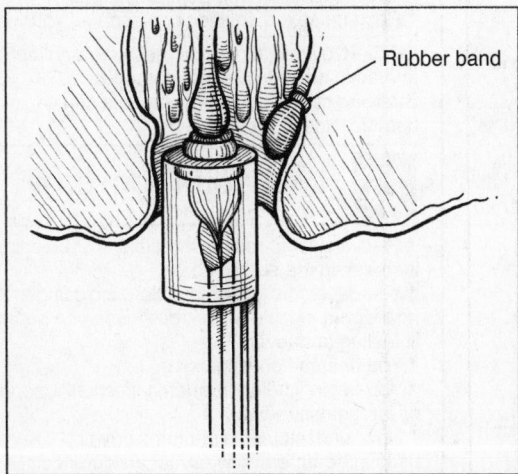

A small rubber band is slipped over the stalk of the hemorrhoid to bind it and cut off the blood flow.

Rubber band

SURGERIES

HEMORRHOID REMOVAL
(Hemorrhoidectomy)

 GENERAL INFORMATION

DEFINITION—Removal of hemorrhoids (varicose veins that occur inside or on the outside of the anus).

BODY PARTS INVOLVED—Dilated veins around the anus or just inside the rectum.

REASONS FOR SURGERY
- Relief of excessive itching, pain or bleeding.
- Relief of a painful thrombosed hemorrhoid (hemorrhoid containing a blood clot).

SURGICAL RISK INCREASES WITH
- Adults over 60.
- Obesity.
- Smoking.
- Poor nutrition.
- Excess alcohol consumption.
- Chronic illness.
- Inflammatory bowel disease.
- Bleeding problems.

 WHAT TO EXPECT

WHO OPERATES—Proctologist, colon-rectal surgeon or general surgeon.

WHERE PERFORMED—Outpatient surgical facility or hospital.

DIAGNOSTIC TESTS
- Before surgery: Blood and urine studies; anoscopy: sigmoidoscopy (see Glossary for both).
- After surgery: Blood studies.

ANESTHESIA
- Local anesthesia by injection.
- Spinal anesthesia by injection.
- General anesthesia by injection and inhalation with an airway tube placed in the windpipe.

DESCRIPTION OF OPERATION
- The dilated veins from around the anus and inside the rectum are cut free and removed, with care taken not to damage the sphincter muscle. Sometimes anal muscles must be dilated vigorously to expose the hemorrhoids.
- The surgical area may be sewn closed or left open, and medicated gauze is used to cover it.

POSSIBLE COMPLICATIONS
- Excessive bleeding.
- Surgical-wound infection.
- Urinary retention (common).
- Stricture of anus.
- Severe pain, especially with bowel movements.
- Constipation.

AVERAGE HOSPITAL STAY—2 to 3 days.

PROBABLE OUTCOME—Curable in most patients, no matter what age. Allow about 6 to 8 weeks for complete recovery from surgery.

 POSTOPERATIVE CARE

GENERAL MEASURES
- Take warm sitz baths every 4 hours or so relieve pain and help keep the rectal area clean. Sit in warm water for 10 to 20 minutes as often as it feels good.
- Use sanitary napkin/pad inside your underwear to help control fluid drainage, discharge of mucus and bleeding. It is normal to have a discharge from the rectum for several weeks.
- Avoid heavy lifting. If not possible, learn proper body mechanics to reduce strain contributing to recurrence.
- Don't strain with bowel movements or urination.
- Wipe gently after bowel movements with soft, moist, white toilet paper or absorbent, moist cotton.

MEDICATION
- Your doctor may prescribe:
  - Pain relievers. Don't take prescription pain medication for longer than 4 to 7 days. Use only as much as you need.
  - Stool softeners or laxatives to prevent constipation.
  - Analgesic ointment to relieve pain.
  - Vitamins to encourage healing.
- You may use nonprescription drugs, such as acetaminophen, for minor pain. Avoid aspirin.

ACTIVITY
- Rest at home as needed and take it easy for 7 to 10 days before you return to full schedule.
- Resume driving 1 week after returning home.
- Avoid sitting for long periods of time.
- Resume sexual relations as soon as you wish.

DIET—No special diet. Increase dietary fiber and fluid intake to prevent constipation. Straining during bowel movements can cause hemorrhoids to recur.

 CALL YOUR DOCTOR IF

- Pain, swelling, redness, drainage or bleeding increase in the surgical area.
- You develop signs of infection, including headache, muscle aches, dizziness or a general ill feeling and fever.
- You become constipated.
- You begin voiding frequently in small amounts or are unable to void.
- New, unexplained symptoms develop. Drugs used in treatment may produce side effects.

HEMORRHOID REMOVAL
(Hemorrhoidectomy)

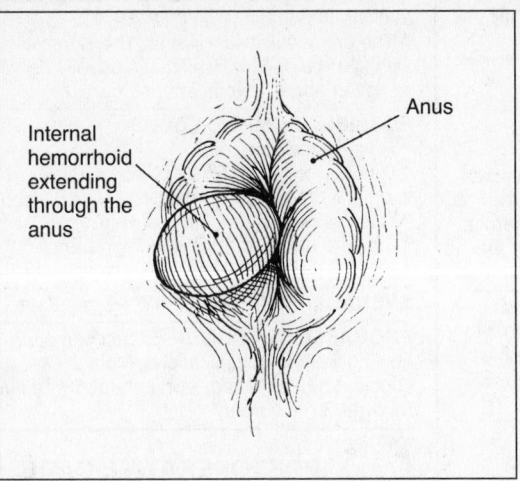

Internal
hemorrhoid
extending
through the
anus

Anus

An illustration of a typical internal hemorrhoid arising from inside the anus and extending through the anal opening.

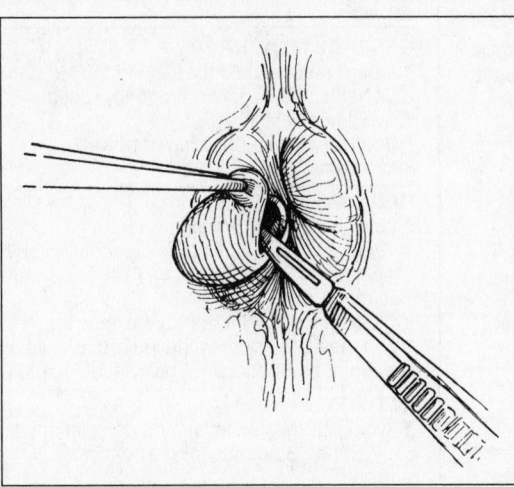

Dilated veins around the anus and inside the rectum are cut free and removed, with care taken not to damage the sphincter muscles.

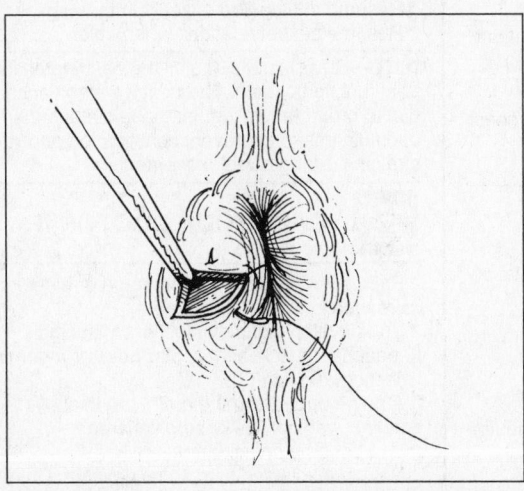

The surgical area is sewn closed or left open and medicated gauze is used to cover.

SURGERIES

HERNIA REPAIR, FEMORAL
(Femoral Herniorrhaphy)

GENERAL INFORMATION

DEFINITION—Closing or repairing a femoral hernia, an internal defect or weakness in the muscles of the abdominal wall. Sometimes, some fatty tissue or an intestine protrudes through the hernia defect, causing a noticeable bulge. If the intestine becomes trapped in the hernia defect, it is called an incarcerated hernia. If the intestine's blood supply is blocked by the hernia defect, it is called a strangulated hernia.

BODY PARTS INVOLVED—Groin (muscles and ligaments inside the lower abdomen next to the genitals); abdominal muscles; the opening allowing the femoral artery to pass from the abdomen to the leg.

REASONS FOR SURGERY
• Incarcerated hernia. This is an emergency!
• Strangulated hernia. This is an emergency!
• Uncomplicated hernia. Most surgeons recommend operating on a femoral hernia, even if no symptoms are present, in order to prevent the serious complications of incarceration or strangulation.

SURGICAL RISK INCREASES WITH
• Adults over 60; obesity; smoking.
• Excess alcohol consumption.
• Recent or chronic illness, especially chronic lung disease or diabetes.
• Use of some prescription and nonprescription drugs. Inform your doctor of any drugs, medications, or vitamin and herb supplements you are using or have used in the last month.

WHAT TO EXPECT

WHO OPERATES—General surgeon or urologist.

WHERE PERFORMED—Hospital or outpatient surgical facility.

DIAGNOSTIC TESTS
• Before surgery: Blood and urine studies; chest x-ray: ECG (see Glossary).
• After surgery: Blood studies.

ANESTHESIA
• Spinal anesthesia by injection.
• Local anesthesia by injection.
• General anesthesia by injection and inhalation with an airway tube placed in the windpipe.

DESCRIPTION OF OPERATION
• An incision is made in the groin area. The muscles and tissue are separated and the hernia sac is opened.
• The contents of the hernia sac are replaced in the abdominal cavity. The neck of the sac is sutured and a "plug" of plastic webbing is used to close the defect.
• The groin wall is sewn shut. The skin is closed with sutures or clips, which can usually be removed about 1 week after surgery.

POSSIBLE COMPLICATIONS
• Recurrence of hernia.
• Damage to the testicle's blood or nerve supply, if the patient is male.
• Compression of the femoral vein.
• Injury to nerve to groin and thigh area.
• Urinary retention.

AVERAGE HOSPITAL STAY—0 to 4 days.

PROBABLE OUTCOME—Expect complete healing without complications. Male virility should not be affected. Allow about 6 weeks for recovery from surgery.

POSTOPERATIVE CARE

GENERAL MEASURES
• A hard ridge should form along the incision. As it heals, the ridge will gradually recede.
• Avoid heavy lifting.
• Don't strain with urination or bowel movements.

MEDICATION
• Your doctor may prescribe:
  - Pain relievers. Don't take prescription pain medication longer than 4 to 7 days. Use only as much as you need.
  - Antibiotics to fight or prevent infection.
• You may use nonprescription drugs, such as acetaminophen, for minor pain. Avoid aspirin.

ACTIVITY
• Avoid vigorous exercise and don't lift anything heavier than 5 pounds for 6 weeks after surgery.
• Resume driving 3 to 4 weeks after surgery.
• Resume sexual relations when able.

DIET—Clear liquid diet until the gastrointestinal tract functions again. Then eat a well-balanced diet to promote healing. Increase dietary fiber and fluid intake to prevent constipation and straining during bowel movements.

CALL YOUR DOCTOR IF

• Pain, swelling, redness, drainage or bleeding increases in the surgical area.
• You develop signs of infection, including headache, muscle aches, dizziness or a general ill feeling and fever.
• A bulge appears in the groin, the thigh, scrotum, vaginal lips or surgical area.
• You become constipated.
• New, unexplained symptoms develop. Drugs used in treatment may produce side effects.

HERNIA REPAIR, FEMORAL
(Femoral Herniorrhaphy)

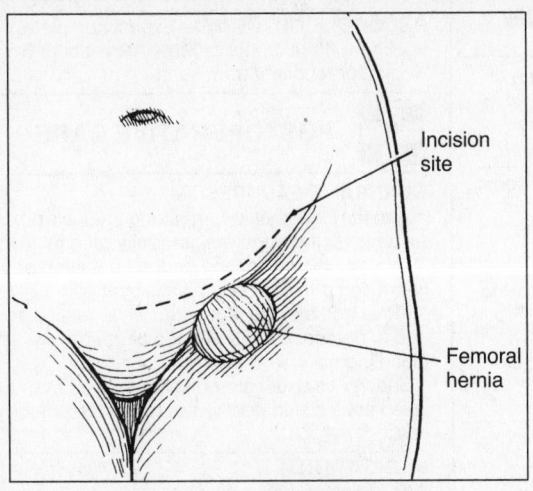

An illustration of a typical femoral hernia located in the groin.

Incision site

Femoral hernia

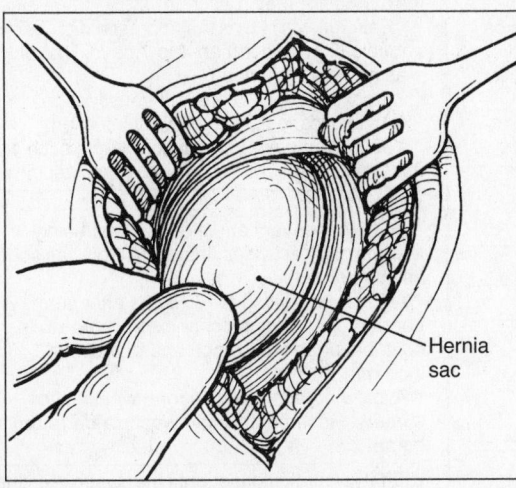

Skin has been incised and the muscles retracted disclosing the hernia sac.
- Contents of the hernia sac are replaced in the abdominal cavity.
- Muscles and fascia are used to cover the defect that allowed the hernia to protrude.
- Sometimes a plug of mesh or patch of mesh is used to bolster the defect.

Hernia sac

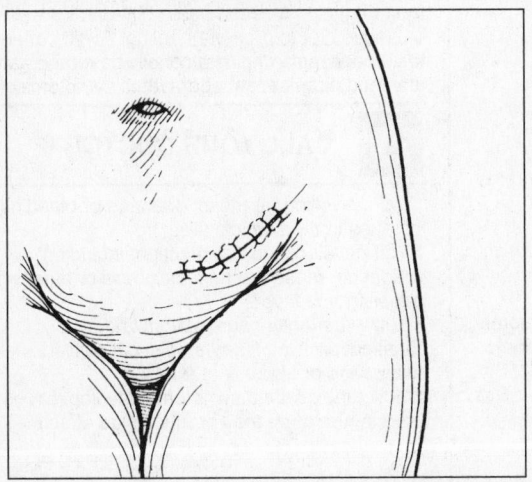

Muscle layers are sewn together followed by skin closure with sutures or clips, which can usually be removed about 1 week after surgery.

HERNIA REPAIR, HIATAL
(Hiatal Herniorrhaphy)

 GENERAL INFORMATION

DEFINITION—Closure of a hiatal hernia, an abnormal weakness or opening in the diaphragm, where the esophagus enters the abdomen.

BODY PARTS INVOLVED—Lower esophagus; diaphragm; upper part of stomach.

REASONS FOR SURGERY
• Relief of painful symptoms.
• Prevent the stomach from shifting upward into the chest cavity.
• Prevent the stomach from spilling digestive acid into the esophagus, causing infection, pain and scarring.

SURGICAL RISK INCREASES WITH
• Adults over 60; newborns and infants.
• Obesity or poor nutrition.
• Smoking, alcoholism.
• Recent or chronic illness, especially diabetes or chronic lung disease.
• Use of some prescription and nonprescription drugs. Inform your doctor of any drugs, medications, or vitamin and herb supplements you are using or have used in the last month.

 WHAT TO EXPECT

WHO OPERATES—General surgeon.

WHERE PERFORMED—Hospital.

DIAGNOSTIC TESTS
• Before surgery: Blood and urine studies; x-rays of chest and upper gastrointestinal tract; ECG; endoscopy (see Glossary for both).
• After surgery: Blood studies.

ANESTHESIA—General anesthesia by injection and inhalation with an airway tube placed in the windpipe.

DESCRIPTION OF OPERATION
• An incision is made in the abdomen or the chest.
• The hernia in the diaphragm is located and, in some cases, closed with sutures.
• The top of the stomach is wrapped around the lower part of the esophagus and sutured in place.
• The skin is closed with sutures or clips, which usually can be removed about 1 week after surgery.
• Laparoscopic repair is now available for some patients (see Laparoscopy in Surgery section).

POSSIBLE COMPLICATIONS
• Excessive bleeding or surgical-wound infection.
• Incisional hernia.
• Injury to esophagus or stomach.

AVERAGE HOSPITAL STAY—5 to 7 days.

PROBABLE OUTCOME—Expect complete healing without complications. Allow about 6 weeks for recovery from surgery.

 POSTOPERATIVE CARE

GENERAL MEASURES
• A hard ridge should form along the incision. As it heals, the ridge will gradually recede.
• Use an electric heating pad, a heat lamp or a warm compress to relieve incisional pain.
• Move and elevate legs often while resting in bed to decrease the likelihood of deep-vein blood clots.
• Shower as usual after discharge. You may wash the incision gently with mild, unscented soap.

MEDICATION
• Your doctor may prescribe:
 - Pain relievers. Don't take prescription pain medication longer than 4 to 7 days. Use only as much as you need.
 - Stool softeners to prevent constipation.
 - Antibiotics to fight or prevent infection.
• You may use nonprescription drugs, such as acetaminophen, for minor pain. Avoid aspirin.

ACTIVITY
• To help recovery and aid your well-being, resume daily activities, including work, as soon as you are able.
• Avoid heavy lifting for 6 weeks after surgery. Learn proper body mechanics to avoid strain contributing to recurrence and to prevent incisional hernia.
• Avoid vigorous exercise for 6 weeks after surgery. Resume driving 4 weeks after returning home.

DIET—Clear liquid diet until the gastrointestinal tract begins to function again. Then eat a well-balanced diet to promote healing. Avoid coffee, tea, cocoa, cola drinks, alcoholic beverages and any food or spice that aggravates symptoms.

 CALL YOUR DOCTOR IF

• Pain, swelling, redness, drainage or bleeding increase in the surgical area.
• You develop signs of infection, including headache, muscle aches, dizziness or a general ill feeling and fever.
• You experience nausea, vomiting, constipation, black tarry stools, difficulty in swallowing or abdominal swelling.
• New, unexplained symptoms develop. Drugs used in treatment may produce side effects.

HERNIA REPAIR, HIATAL
(Hiatal Herniorrhaphy)

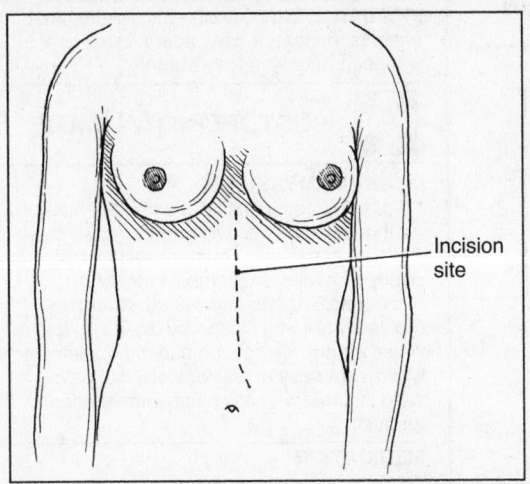

An illustration of a typical incision site to allow exposure of the lower end of the esophagus, the upper end of the stomach, and the diaphragm (a large muscle that separates the chest from the abdominal cavity).

Incision site

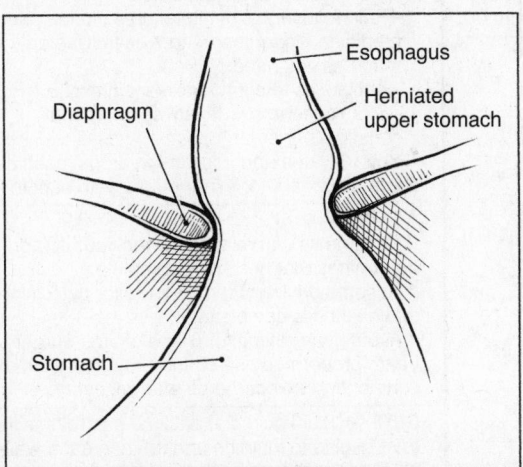

The herniated upper stomach through the widened opening in the diaphragm.

Esophagus

Herniated upper stomach

Diaphragm

Stomach

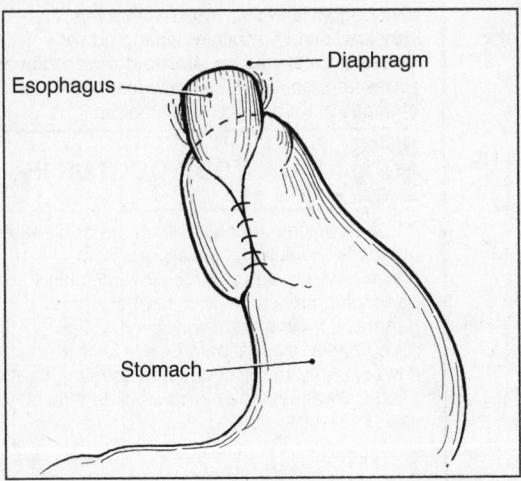

The top of the stomach is wrapped around the lower part of the esophagus and sutured in place.

Diaphragm

Esophagus

Stomach

SURGERIES

HERNIA REPAIR, INCISIONAL
(Incisional Herniorrhaphy)

GENERAL INFORMATION

DEFINITION—Repair of a defect in the abdominal wall created by a previous surgical incision.

BODY PARTS INVOLVED—Abdomen and intestines where previous surgery has been performed.

REASONS FOR SURGERY
* Possible strangulation of bowel.
* Painful lump in the abdomen.

SURGICAL RISK INCREASES WITH
* Obesity; poor nutrition.
* Excess alcohol consumption; smoking.
* Recent or chronic illness, especially chronic lung disease or diabetes.
* Use of some prescription and nonprescription drugs. Inform your doctor of any drugs, medications, or vitamin and herb supplements you are using or have used in the last month.

WHAT TO EXPECT

WHO OPERATES—General surgeon.

WHERE PERFORMED—Outpatient surgical facility or hospital.

DIAGNOSTIC TESTS
* Before surgery: Blood and urine studies; x-rays of the abdomen and chest; ECG (see Glossary).
* After surgery: Blood studies.

ANESTHESIA
* Local anesthesia by injection.
* Spinal anesthesia by injection.
* General anesthesia by injection and inhalation with an airway tube placed in the windpipe.

DESCRIPTION OF OPERATION
* An incision is made in the abdomen over the defect. The area is examined for protruding intestine.
* The intestine is replaced in the abdominal cavity. Usually, plastic mesh is used to strengthen the repair. The mesh can be used to cover the defect in the abdominal wall or the muscles can be closed and the mesh used to reinforce them.
* A drain is sometimes left in place for several days.
* The skin is closed with sutures or clips, which usually can be removed about 1 week after surgery.

POSSIBLE COMPLICATIONS
* Surgical-wound infection.
* Inadvertent injury to intestinal tract.
* Bowel obstruction.
* Recurrent hernia.

AVERAGE HOSPITAL STAY—0 to 4 days.

PROBABLE OUTCOME—Curable in most patients, no matter what age. Allow 2 to 4 weeks for recovery from surgery.

POSTOPERATIVE CARE

GENERAL MEASURES
* A hard ridge should form along the incision. As it heals, the ridge will gradually recede.
* Shower as usual. You may wash the incision gently with mild, unscented soap. After showering, change any wet dressings and replace them with clean, dry ones.
* Use an electric heating pad, a heat lamp or a warm compress to relieve incisional pain.
* Don't strain with bowel movements or urination.

MEDICATION
* Your doctor may prescribe:
  - Pain relievers. Don't take prescription pain medicine longer than 4 to 7 days. Use only as much as you need.
  - Antibiotics to fight or prevent infection.
  - Stool softeners or laxatives to prevent constipation.
* You may use nonprescription drugs, such as acetaminophen, for minor pain. Avoid aspirin.

ACTIVITY
* Resume sexual relations when your doctor determines that healing is complete.
* Resume driving when your doctor determines that healing is complete.
* Avoid heavy lifting for 6 weeks after surgery. Learn proper body mechanics to reduce strain contributing to recurrence after recovery.

DIET—Clear liquid diet until the gastrointestinal tract begins to function again. Then eat a well-balanced diet to promote healing. Increase dietary fiber and fluid intake to prevent constipation and straining during bowel movements. If you are overweight, consult your physician about a weight loss plan to reduce the chances of recurrence of the hernia.

CALL YOUR DOCTOR IF

* Pain, swelling, redness, drainage or bleeding occurs in the surgical area.
* You develop signs of infection, including headache, muscle aches, dizziness or a general ill feeling and fever.
* You become constipated.
* New, unexplained symptoms develop. Drugs used in treatment may produce side effects.

HERNIA REPAIR, INCISIONAL
(Incisional Herniorrhaphy)

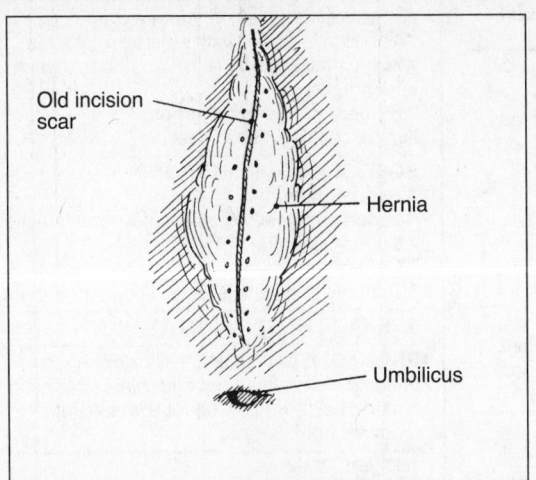

Old incision scar

Hernia

Umbilicus

An illustration of an incisional hernia in the abdominal wall protruding through an old incision scar.

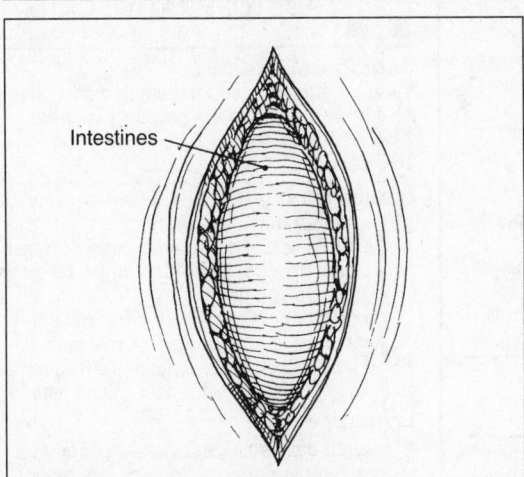

Intestines

Abdominal muscles retracted to reveal intestines pushing through the abdominal muscles.

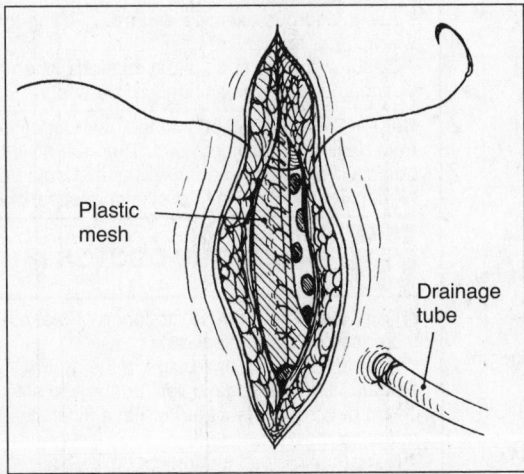

Plastic mesh

Drainage tube

The intestine is replaced in the abdominal cavity. Usually a plastic mesh is used to strengthen the repair.

HERNIA REPAIR, INGUINAL
(Inguinal Herniorrhaphy)

 GENERAL INFORMATION

DEFINITION—Closing or repairing a defect (opening) in the muscle layer of the abdominal wall in the inguinal (groin) area. A sac (of fatty tissue or an intestine) protrudes through the hernia defect, causing a noticeable bulge. If intestine or other abdominal contents are caught in the hernia and cannot be pushed back, it is called an incarcerated hernia. If the opening is so tight that it has cut off the blood supply to the incarcerated tissue, it is called a strangulated hernia.

BODY PARTS INVOLVED—Groin muscles and ligaments inside the lower abdomen next to the genitals; abdominal muscles.

REASONS FOR SURGERY
• Incarcerated hernia: This is an emergency!
• Strangulated hernia: This is an emergency!
• Uncomplicated hernia: Most doctors recommend operating on a hernia even if no hernia symptoms are present in order to prevent the serious complications of incarceration or strangulation.

SURGICAL RISK INCREASES WITH
• Adults over 60; newborns and infants.
• Excess alcohol consumption; smoking.
• Chronic lung disease, prostatism, constipation or family history of hernias.
• Use of some prescription and nonprescription drugs. Inform your doctor of any drugs, medications, or vitamin and herb supplements you are using or have used in the last month.

 WHAT TO EXPECT

WHO OPERATES—General surgeon or urologist.

WHERE PERFORMED—Hospital or outpatient surgical facility.

DIAGNOSTIC TESTS
• Before surgery: Blood and urine studies; x-rays of abdomen and chest; ECG (see Glossary).
• After surgery: Blood studies.

ANESTHESIA
• Spinal anesthesia by injection.
• Local anesthesia by injection.
• General anesthesia by injection and inhalation with an airway tube placed in the windpipe.

DESCRIPTION OF OPERATION
• There are options for performing this surgery. Described here is an open hernia repair:
• An incision is made in the abdomen. The abdominal muscles are separated.
• The hernia is located and any sac is reduced (pushed back into place) or removed.

• A plastic mesh is generally used to reinforce and cover the defect in the muscles.
• The skin is closed with sutures or staples, which usually can be removed about 1 week after surgery.
• Surgery may also be performed laparoscopically (see Glossary).

POSSIBLE COMPLICATIONS
• Recurrent hernia.
• Excessive bleeding; surgical-wound infection.
• Urinary retention.
• Constipation.
• Damage to testicle's blood supply or nerves.

AVERAGE HOSPITAL STAY—0 to 4 days.

PROBABLE OUTCOME—Curable in most patients, no matter what age. Male virility should not be affected. Allow about 6 weeks for recovery from surgery.

 POSTOPERATIVE CARE

GENERAL MEASURES
• A hard ridge should form along the incision. As it heals, the ridge will gradually recede.
• Don't strain with bowel movements or urination.

MEDICATION
• Your doctor may prescribe:
  - Pain relievers. Don't take prescription pain medication longer than 4 to 7 days. Use only as much as you need.
  - Stool softeners to prevent constipation.
  - Antibiotics to fight or prevent infection.
• You may use nonprescription drugs, such as acetaminophen, for minor pain. Avoid aspirin.

ACTIVITY
• Resume daily activities, including work, as soon as you are able (as long as it does not involve strenuous activity).
• Avoid vigorous exercise and heavy lifting for 6 weeks after surgery.
• Resume driving and sexual relations when your doctor determines healing is complete.

DIET—Clear liquid diet until the gastrointestinal tract begins to function again. Then eat a well-balanced diet to promote healing. It should be high in fiber and fluids to prevent constipation.

 CALL YOUR DOCTOR IF

• Pain, swelling, redness, drainage or bleeding increases in the surgical area.
• You develop pain or a bulge in the groin, scrotum, testicle, vaginal lips, or surgical area.
• You become constipated or have difficulty in urinating.
• New, unexplained symptoms develop.

HERNIA REPAIR, INGUINAL
(Inguinal Herniorrhaphy)

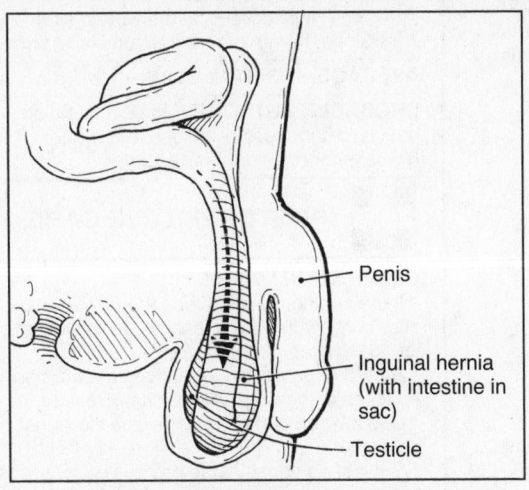

A side view of the male pelvic region.
• A typical inguinal hernia in which a loop of intestine has dropped down into the scrotum.

Penis

Inguinal hernia (with intestine in sac)

Testicle

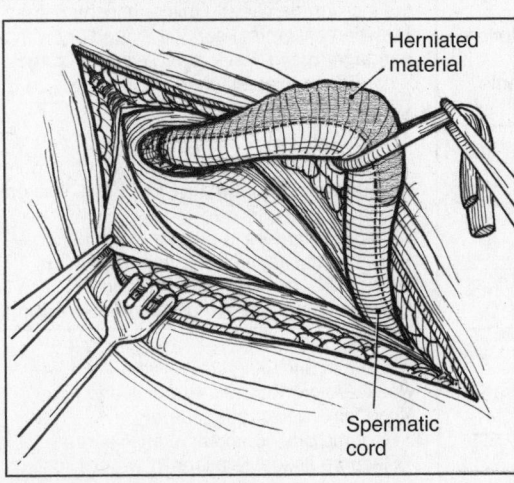

Herniated material

Spermatic cord

The hernia is located and the herniated material is pushed back into the abdomen. The sac is closed.

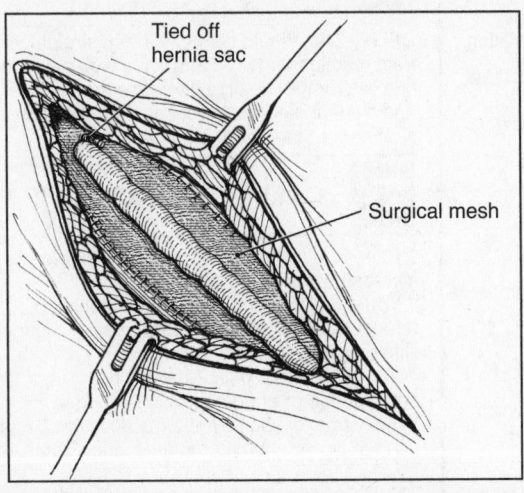

Tied off hernia sac

Surgical mesh

Mesh or other patch material is used to cover any defect and the outer muscles are closed over the top.

SURGERIES

HERNIA REPAIR, UMBILICAL

GENERAL INFORMATION

DEFINITION—Closure of an umbilical hernia, a weakening in the muscles around the umbilicus (navel) that allows abdominal contents to protrude prominently.

BODY PARTS INVOLVED—Abdominal muscular wall around the navel.

REASONS FOR SURGERY
* Improved appearance.
* Relief of pain.
* Prevention of incarceration or strangulation of the intestines (see Hernia Repair, Inguinal in Surgery section).

SURGICAL RISK INCREASES WITH
* Newborns and infants.
* Obesity; poor nutrition.
* Smoking; alcoholism.
* Recent or chronic illness, especially chronic lung disease.
* Diabetes.
* Use of some prescription and nonprescription drugs. Inform your doctor of any drugs, medications, or vitamin and herb supplements you are using or have used in the last month.

WHAT TO EXPECT

WHO OPERATES—General surgeon or pediatric surgeon.

WHERE PERFORMED—Hospital or outpatient surgical facility.

DIAGNOSTIC TESTS
* Before surgery: Blood and urine studies; abdominal and chest x-rays; ECG (see Glossary).
* After surgery: Blood studies.

ANESTHESIA
* Local anesthesia by injection.
* Spinal anesthesia by injection.
* General anesthesia by injection and inhalation with an airway tube placed in the windpipe.

DESCRIPTION OF OPERATION
* An incision is made slightly above or below the navel.
* Sometimes, an incision is made in the peritoneum to open the peritoneal cavity. The contents of the hernia sac are located and replaced in the abdominal cavity. The peritoneum is closed.
* The large abdominal muscle is pulled over the defect. The membrane covering the muscle is overlapped and tied to close the defect Plastic mesh (or other patch material) may be used to reinforce the muscles.
* The skin is closed with sutures or clips, which usually can be removed about 10 days after surgery. Drains may be placed temporarily around the incision to drain off excess fluid.

POSSIBLE COMPLICATIONS
* Excessive bleeding.
* Surgical-wound infection.
* Seroma (fluid collects at the wound site).
* Incisional hernia or recurrent umbilical hernia.

AVERAGE HOSPITAL STAY—0 to 1 day.

PROBABLE OUTCOME—Expect complete healing without complications. Allow about 3 to 6 weeks for recovery from surgery.

POSTOPERATIVE CARE

GENERAL MEASURES
* If the wound bleeds during the first 24 hours after surgery, press a clean tissue or cloth to it for 10 minutes.
* A hard ridge should form along the incision. As it heals, the ridge will gradually recede.
* Use a warm compress to relieve incisional pain.
* Shower as usual. Avoid baths. You may wash the incision gently with mild, unscented soap. Between showers, keep the wound dry with a bandage for the first 2 or 3 days after surgery. If a bandage gets wet, change it promptly.

MEDICATION
* Your doctor may prescribe:
  - Pain relievers. Don't use prescription pain medication longer than 4 to 7 days. Use only as much as you need.
  - Stool softeners to prevent constipation.
  - Antibiotics to fight or prevent infection.
* You may use nonprescription drugs, such as acetaminophen, for minor pain. Avoid aspirin.

ACTIVITY
* You can usually return to work in 2 to 4 weeks. Avoid vigorous exercise and heavy lifting for 6 weeks after surgery.
* Resume driving about 10 after surgery.
* Resume sexual relations in about 1 to 2 weeks, or as advised by your doctor.

DIET—Clear liquid diet until the gastrointestinal tract functions again. Then eat a well-balanced diet to promote healing. Increase dietary fiber and fluid intake to prevent constipation and straining during bowel movements.

CALL YOUR DOCTOR IF

* Pain, swelling, redness, drainage or bleeding increases in the surgical area.
* You develop signs of infection, including headache, muscle aches, dizziness or a general ill feeling and fever.
* You experience nausea, vomiting, constipation or abdominal swelling.
* New, unexplained symptoms develop. Drugs used in treatment may produce side effects.

HERNIA REPAIR, UMBILICAL

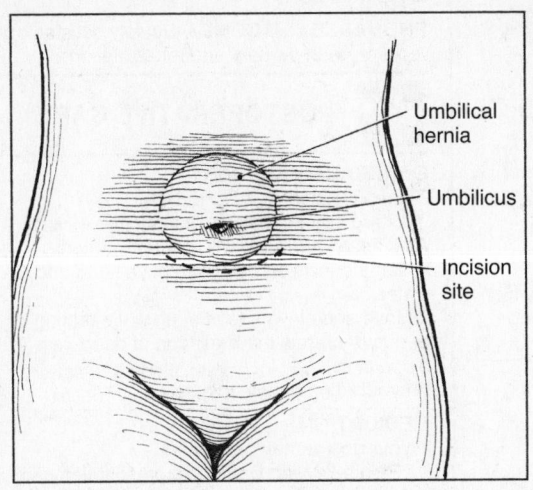

An illustration of a typical umbilical (navel) hernia and the incision site for the hernia repair.

- Umbilical hernia
- Umbilicus
- Incision site

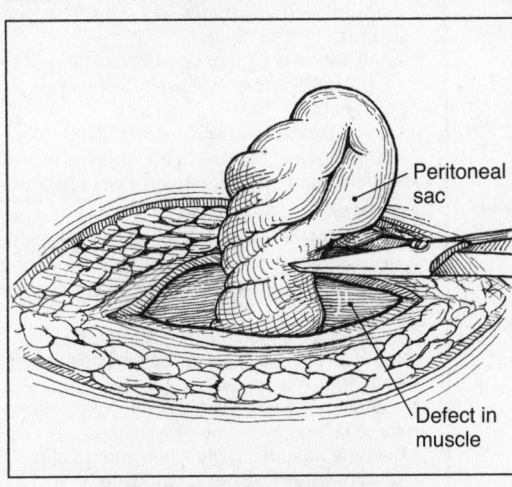

The incision is sometimes extended through the peritoneum to open the cavity.
- Contents of the hernia sac are located and replaced in the abdominal cavity.

- Peritoneal sac
- Defect in muscle

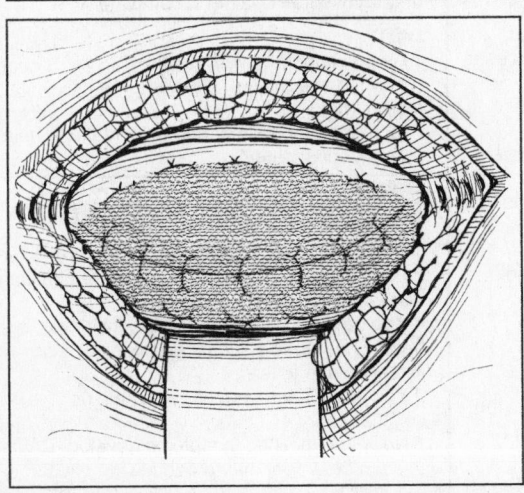

The peritoneum is closed. The large abdominal muscles will be pulled over the defect, when possible, and covered with mesh. Finally the skin is closed over the mesh.

HIP NAILING FOR HIP FRACTURE

GENERAL INFORMATION

DEFINITION—A surgical procedure to reattach the broken fragments of the fractured femur near the hip.

BODY PARTS INVOLVED—The head and neck of the femur and the acetabulum (the socket of the pelvis that receives the femur to form the hip joint).

REASONS FOR SURGERY
* To make early movement of the hip joint possible after fracture.
* To prevent prolonged bed confinement, which is usually dangerous in the elderly age group when hip fractures become more common.

SURGICAL RISK INCREASES WITH
* Adults over 60; obesity; poor nutrition.
* Smoking.
* Excess alcohol consumption.
* Recent or chronic illness.
* Diabetes.
* Use of some prescription and nonprescription drugs. Inform your doctor of any drugs, medications, or vitamin and herb supplements you are using or have used in the last month.

WHAT TO EXPECT

WHO OPERATES—Orthopedic surgeon; general surgeon (sometimes).

WHERE PERFORMED—Hospital.

DIAGNOSTIC TESTS—Before surgery: Blood and urine studies; x-rays of hip and lung.

ANESTHESIA—General anesthesia by injection and inhalation with an airway tube placed in the windpipe.

DESCRIPTION OF OPERATION
* After anesthesia, the area adjacent to the fractured hip is cleaned, shaven and draped.
* An incision is made at a point allowing access to the fractured parts.
* The broken fragments are realigned under direct vision and with x-ray.
* Plates are fitted to hold the nail to be inserted into the fractured fragments.
* The nail is hammered into the broken parts to hold them together and give strength to the injured area of the bone.
* The plate is attached to healthy bone to hold the nail in place.

POSSIBLE COMPLICATIONS
* Surgical-wound infection.
* Excessive bleeding.
* Blood clots breaking loose and traveling to the lungs (pulmonary embolism).
* Refracture at the hip.

AVERAGE HOSPITAL STAY—4 to 7 days, depending on the condition of the patient prior to hip fracture.

PROBABLE OUTCOME—Usually satisfactory recovery with surgery and rehabilitation.

POSTOPERATIVE CARE

GENERAL MEASURES
* Keep incision clean and dry.
* A hard ridge should form along the incision. As it heals, the ridge will gradually recede. Clean the incision daily with plain soap and water.
* Move and elevate legs often while resting in bed to decrease the likelihood of deep-vein blood clots.
* Avoid lifting heavy objects.

MEDICATION
* Your doctor may prescribe:
  - Pain relievers. Don't take prescription pain medication longer than 4 to 7 days. Use only as much as you need.
  - Antibiotics to fight or prevent infection.
  - Stool softeners or laxatives to prevent constipation.
  - Blood thinners to help prevent blood clots.
* You may use nonprescription drugs, such as acetaminophen, for minor pain. Avoid aspirin.

ACTIVITY
* A physical therapy program will be prescribed by your doctor. Usually you will start by using a walker, then crutches, followed by a cane if necessary.
* Avoid vigorous exercise for 12 weeks after surgery or until your doctor determines healing is complete.
* Your doctor will advise you when it is safe to resume driving.
* Resume sexual activity when your doctor determines that healing is complete.

DIET
* As prescribed by your doctor.
* Vitamin and mineral supplements (sometimes).
* Increase dietary fiber and fluid intake to help prevent constipation.

CALL YOUR DOCTOR IF

* Pain, swelling, redness, drainage or bleeding increases in the surgical area.
* You develop signs of infection, including headache, muscle aches, dizziness or a general ill feeling and fever.
* You experience nausea, vomiting, or constipation.
* New, unexplained symptoms develop. Drugs used in treatment may produce side effects.

HIP NAILING FOR HIP FRACTURE

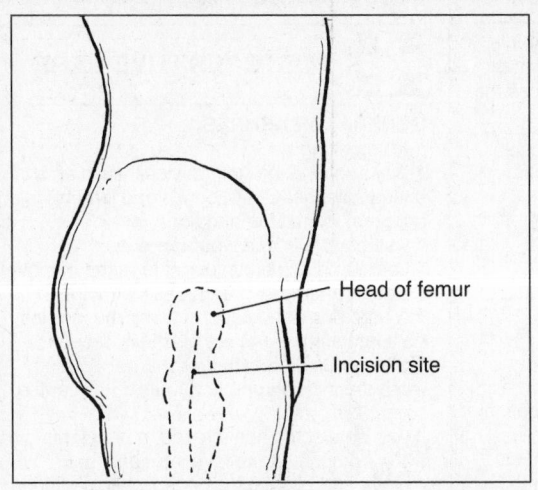

An illustration of an incision made over the affected hip showing the head of the femur that is fractured.

Head of femur

Incision site

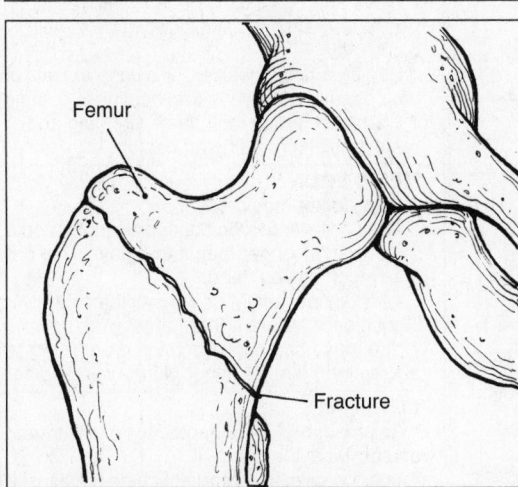

A closer view of the fractured femur.

Femur

Fracture

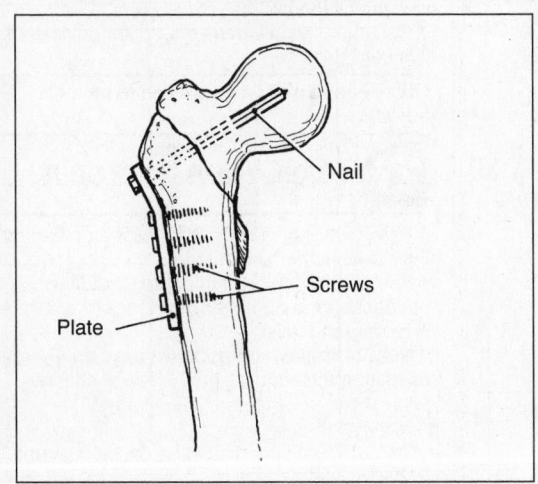

The bone fragments are realigned, and a plate, which is attached to healthy bone by a number of screws, is used to hold the nail in place. The nail is hammered into the broken parts of the femur, giving strength to the broken area of the bone.

Nail

Screws

Plate

HIP REPLACEMENT, TOTAL

GENERAL INFORMATION

DEFINITION—Surgical replacement of the hip joint. A metal ball replaces the worn head of the thigh bone and a cup (often plastic) replaces the worn socket.

BODY PARTS INVOLVED—Hip joint; muscles, ligaments, bones and bursa forming the hip joint.

REASONS FOR SURGERY—Diseased or injured hip with pain and stiffness causing an altered gait and impaired quality of life.

SURGICAL RISK INCREASES WITH
• Obesity; smoking.
• Excess alcohol consumption.
• Recent or chronic illness; diabetes.
• Use of some prescription and nonprescription drugs. Inform your doctor of any drugs, medications, or vitamin and herb supplements you are using or have used in the last month.

WHAT TO EXPECT

WHO OPERATES—Orthopedic surgeon.

WHERE PERFORMED—Hospital.

DIAGNOSTIC TESTS
• Before surgery: X-rays of joint; CT scan or MRI (see Glossary for both); joint aspiration (to check for active infection); blood and urine studies.
• During surgery: X-rays.
• After surgery: X-rays, blood tests, and examination of removed tissue.

ANESTHESIA
• General anesthesia by injection and inhalation with an airway tube placed in the windpipe.
• Spinal anesthesia by injection.

DESCRIPTION OF OPERATION
• An incision is made over the affected hip.
• The head and neck of the femur are removed.
• The femoral canal is reamed to accept the metal femoral component (head, neck and stem). The femoral component is cemented in place using a special form of bone cement.
• The acetabulum is shaped to accept a plastic cup. The cup is held in place with metal screws.
• The ball and socket are replaced into normal position.

POSSIBLE COMPLICATIONS
• Excessive bleeding; blood clots.
• Surgical-wound infection.
• Dislocation of hip.
• Pneumonia.
• Loosening of components.

AVERAGE HOSPITAL STAY—5 to 7 days.

PROBABLE OUTCOME—Expect complete healing without complications. Allow about 3 to 6 months for recovery from surgery.

POSTOPERATIVE CARE

GENERAL MEASURES
• No smoking.
• Buy and use self-help devices, such as a raised toilet seat, bath bench and long-handled grippers, to limit hip bending.
• Use handrails and wear low shoes.
• Learn and abide by your safe range of motion.
• Cough and deep breathe as instructed.
• A hard ridge should form along the incision. As it heals, the ridge will gradually recede.
• Shower as usual after discharge. You may wash the incision gently with mild, unscented soap.
• Use an electric heating pad, a heat lamp or a warm compress to relieve incisional pain.
• Move and elevate legs often while resting in bed to decrease the likelihood of deep-vein blood clots.
• Use crutches, a walker, or a cane to walk until your doctor determines that healing is complete.
• Physical therapy may hasten healing and restore strength. Ask your doctor.

MEDICATION
• Your doctor may prescribe:
  - Pain relievers. Don't take prescription pain medication longer than 4 to 7 days. Use only as much as you need.
  - Antibiotics to fight or prevent infection. Use antibiotics before future dental work.
• You may use nonprescription drugs, such as acetaminophen, for minor pain. Avoid aspirin.

ACTIVITY
• As prescribed and directed by your surgeon and physical therapist.
• Avoid very active sports such as tennis, skiing or contact sports.
• Resume driving when your doctor advises that it is safe to do so.

DIET—Eat a well-balanced diet to promote healing.

CALL YOUR DOCTOR IF

• Pain, swelling, redness, drainage or bleeding increases in the surgical area.
• You develop signs of infection, including headache, muscle aches, dizziness or a general ill feeling and fever.
• New, unexplained symptoms develop. Drugs used in treatment may produce side effects.

HIP REPLACEMENT, TOTAL

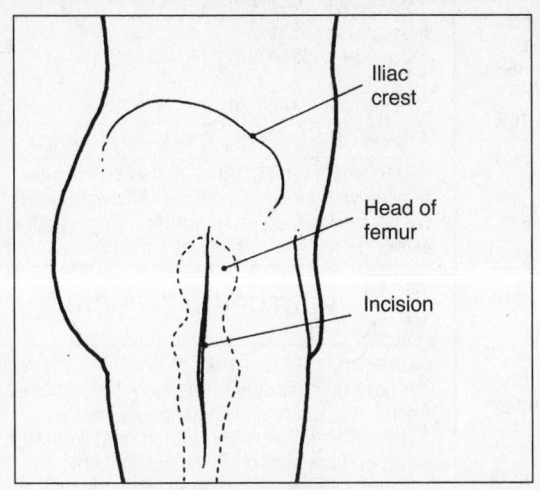

An illustration of an incision made over the affected hip showing the head of the femur that is diseased or injured.

Iliac crest

Head of femur

Incision

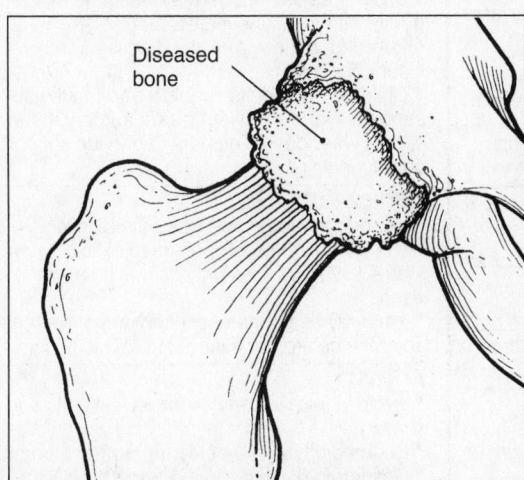

A closer view of a diseased hip joint. After the diseased bone has been removed, the artificial ball and socket are placed into normal position.

Diseased bone

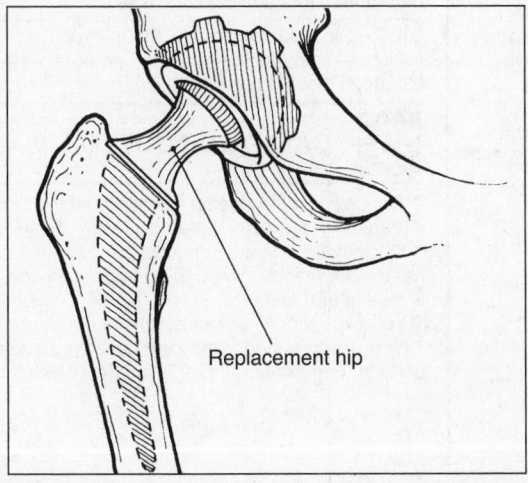

The appearance of the hip after the metal prosthesis has been inserted.

Replacement hip

HYDROCELECTOMY

GENERAL INFORMATION

DEFINITION—Removal of a hydrocele, fluid that has collected in a small sac usually on the testicle or in the membrane covering the testicle. Hydroceles frequently occur in infants, but may also occur in adults.

BODY PARTS INVOLVED—Scrotum; spermatic cord; membrane covering the testicle (tunica vaginalis); blood vessels and nerves connected to the scrotum.

REASONS FOR SURGERY
* In infants: completion of the repair of a congenital inguinal hernia, which frequently accompanies a congenital hydrocele.
* In adults: removal of an uncomfortable and unsightly scrotal cyst that may conceal a tumor in the testicle.

SURGICAL RISK INCREASES WITH
* Obesity; poor nutrition.
* Smoking; alcoholism.
* Chronic or recent illness.
* Diabetes.
* Use of some prescription and nonprescription drugs. Inform your doctor of any drugs, medications, or vitamin and herb supplements you are using or have used in the last month.

WHAT TO EXPECT

WHO OPERATES—General surgeon or urologist.

WHERE PERFORMED—Hospital or outpatient surgical facility.

DIAGNOSTIC TESTS
* Before surgery: Blood and urine studies; ultrasound (see Glossary).
* After surgery: Usually none.

ANESTHESIA
* General anesthesia by injection and inhalation with an airway tube placed in the windpipe in infants.
* Local anesthesia by injection.
* Spinal anesthesia by injection (sometimes).

DESCRIPTION OF OPERATION
* An incision is made in the scrotum over the testicle.
* The hydrocele is located and cut free from the scrotal contents.
* The hydrocele is incised, and the fluid inside it is drained. The skin edges of the hydrocele are tucked under and sewn together to prevent refilling.
* The scrotal contents are replaced. The skin is closed with fine suture material that will be absorbed by the body.

POSSIBLE COMPLICATIONS
* Excessive bleeding.
* Surgical-wound infection.
* Urinary retention.
* Damaged blood supply to the testicle.
* Twisting of the testicle.
* Recurrent hydrocele.

AVERAGE HOSPITAL STAY—0 to 1 day.

PROBABLE OUTCOME—Expect complete healing without complications. Allow about 2 weeks for recovery from surgery. Post-surgical swelling may last as long as 6 months.

POSTOPERATIVE CARE

GENERAL MEASURES
* A hard ridge should form along the incision. As it heals, the ridge will gradually recede.
* Use an electric heating pad, a heat lamp or a warm compress to relieve incisional pain.
* Shower as usual. You may wash the incision gently with mild, unscented soap. After showering, replace any wet dressings with clean, dry ones.
* Children and adults should wear an athletic supporter for 3 to 6 weeks after surgery. Infants should wear double diapers to provide support during healing.

MEDICATION
* Your doctor may prescribe pain relievers. Don't take prescription pain medication longer than 4 to 7 days. Use only as much as you need.
* You may use nonprescription drugs, such as acetaminophen, for minor pain. Avoid aspirin.

ACTIVITY
* Avoid vigorous exercise for 6 weeks after surgery.
* Resume driving 1 week after returning home.
* Resume sexual relations when your doctor determines that healing is complete.

DIET—Clear liquid diet until the gastrointestinal tract begins to function again. Then eat a well-balanced diet to promote healing.

CALL YOUR DOCTOR IF
* Pain, swelling, redness, drainage or bleeding increases in the surgical area.
* You develop signs of infection, including headache, muscle aches, dizziness or a general ill feeling and fever.
* You experience nausea or vomiting.
* New, unexplained symptoms develop. Drugs used in treatment may produce side effects.

HYDROCELECTOMY

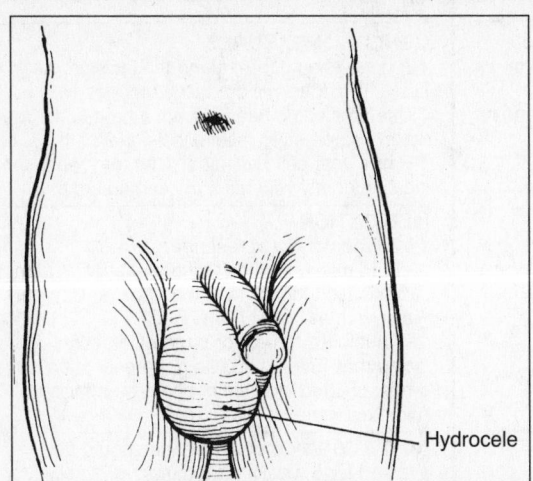

An illustration of a typical hydrocele distending one portion of the scrotum.

Hydrocele

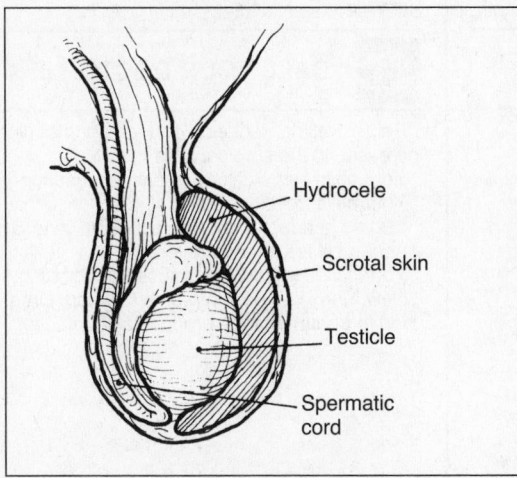

A hydrocele and surrounding tissues including the spermatic cord, testicle and scrotum.

Hydrocele

Scrotal skin

Testicle

Spermatic cord

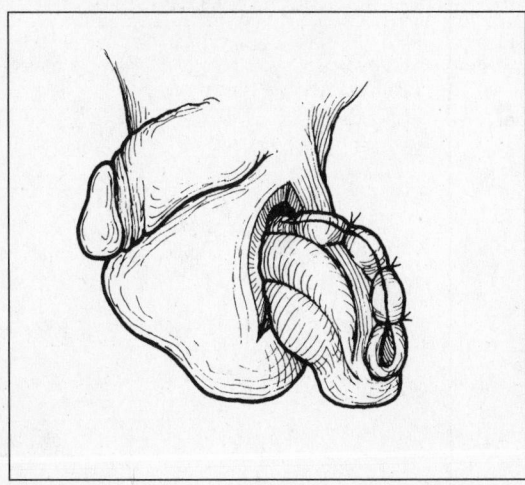

After the hydrocele has been incised and the fluid inside drained, the edges of the hydrocele are tucked under and sewn together to prevent refilling.
- The scrotal contents are then replaced and the skin closed with fine absorbable sutures that need not be removed.

SURGERIES

HYPOSPADIAS REPAIR & URETHROPLASTY

 ## GENERAL INFORMATION

DEFINITION—Creation of a new urethra to correct hypospadias, a congenital disorder in which the urethra opening is in an abnormal location on the penis. Surgery is usually done in infancy or early childhood.

BODY PARTS INVOLVED—Urethra.

REASONS FOR SURGERY
* Prevention of urinary-tract infections.
* Establishment of sexual function.
* Correction of abnormal urination patterns.

SURGICAL RISK INCREASES WITH
* Obesity.
* Poor nutrition.
* Recent or chronic illness.
* Diabetes.
* Use of some prescription and nonprescription drugs. Inform your doctor of any drugs, medications, or vitamin and herb supplements your child is using or has used in the last month.

 ## WHAT TO EXPECT

WHO OPERATES—Urologist.

WHERE PERFORMED—Hospital.

DIAGNOSTIC TESTS
* Before surgery: Blood and urine studies.
* After surgery: Blood studies; laboratory examination of removed tissue.

ANESTHESIA—General anesthesia by injection and inhalation, with an airway tube placed in the windpipe.

DESCRIPTION OF OPERATION
* An incision is made over the abnormal opening of the urethra.
* An instrument is passed through the urethra and extended along its full length. Abnormal scar tissue is cut free and removed. A new urethra is fashioned from existing tissue and sewn around a catheter, which will remain in place until healing is complete.
* After healing, the catheter is removed under anesthesia.
* The skin is closed with sutures that will be absorbed by the body.

POSSIBLE COMPLICATIONS
* Excessive bleeding.
* Surgical-wound infection.
* Scarring of urethra.

AVERAGE HOSPITAL STAY—2 to 7 days.

PROBABLE OUTCOME—Expect complete healing without complications. Allow about 3 months for recovery from surgery.

 ## POSTOPERATIVE CARE

GENERAL MEASURES
* A ridge should form along the incision. As it heals, the ridge will gradually recede.
* Use an electric heating pad, a heat lamp or a warm compress to relieve incisional pain.
* Bathe your child as usual. You may wash the incision gently with mild, unscented soap.

MEDICATION
* Your doctor may prescribe:
  - Pain relievers. Don't take prescription pain medication longer than 4 to 7 days. Use only as much as your child needs.
  - Antibiotics to fight or prevent infection.
* You may give your child nonprescription drugs, such as acetaminophen, for minor pain. Avoid aspirin.

ACTIVITY—Vigorous exercise should be avoided for 6 weeks after surgery.

DIET—No special diet.

 ## CALL YOUR DOCTOR IF

* Pain, swelling, redness, drainage or bleeding increases in the surgical area.
* Your child has difficulty or pain in urination.
* Your child develops signs of infection, including headache, muscle aches, dizziness or a general ill feeling and fever.
* Your child experiences nausea or vomiting.
* New, unexplained symptoms develop. Drugs used in treatment may produce side effects.

HYPOSPADIAS REPAIR & URETHROPLASTY

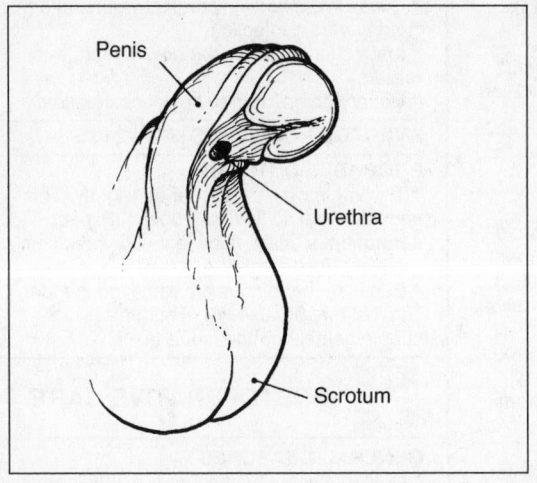

A typical hypospadias with opening of the urethra under the head of the penis.
- Openings of the urethra may occur in various other places on the penis other than its normal opening.

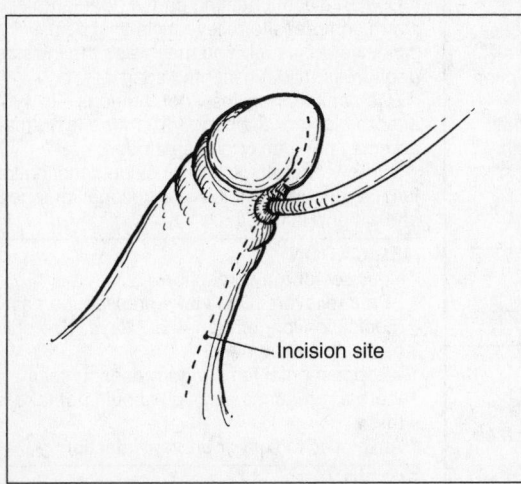

An instrument is placed through the urethra and is extended along its full length. Abnormal scar tissue is cut free and removed.
- A new urethra is fashioned from existing tissue and sewn around a catheter which will remain in place until healing is complete.

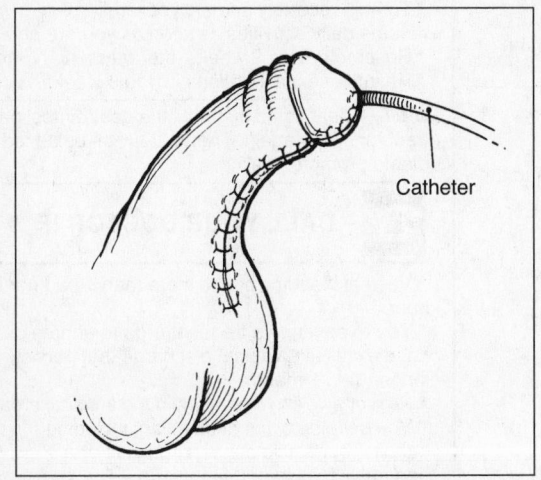

After healing, the catheter is removed under anesthesia.

HYSTERECTOMY (ABDOMINAL) WITH SALPINGO-OOPHORECTOMY

GENERAL INFORMATION

DEFINITION—Removal of the uterus, cervix, fallopian tubes and ovaries, through an incision in the abdomen.

BODY PARTS INVOLVED—Uterus; cervix; fallopian tubes; ovaries; vagina.

REASONS FOR SURGERY
* Uterus: Cancer or suspected cancer; fibroid tumors; chronic bleeding; prolapsed (dropped) uterus; endometriosis; chronic pelvic infection; severe menstrual pain; or voluntary sterilization.
* Fallopian tubes and ovaries: Cancer or suspected cancer of the ovaries; precancerous or twisted ovarian cysts; ovarian pregnancy; ovarian abscess; damage to the ovaries from severe endometriosis.

SURGICAL RISK INCREASES WITH
* Obesity; smoking.
* Iron-deficiency anemia; heart or lung disease; or diabetes.
* Use of some prescription and nonprescription drugs. Inform your doctor of any drugs, medications, or vitamin and herb supplements you are using or have used in the last month.

WHAT TO EXPECT

WHO OPERATES—General surgeon or obstetrician-gynecologist.

WHERE PERFORMED—Hospital.

DIAGNOSTIC TESTS
* Before surgery: Blood and urine studies; x-rays of abdomen and kidneys; dilatation and curettage of the uterus (D & C); ultrasound (see Glossary for both).
* After surgery: Blood studies.

ANESTHESIA—Spinal anesthesia or general anesthesia by injection and inhalation with an airway tube placed in the windpipe.

DESCRIPTION OF OPERATION
* An incision is made in the abdomen.
* The abdominal organs are examined.
* The uterus is freed from its attachments to the bladder and upper vagina. The uterus is removed along with the fallopian tubes and ovaries.
* The vagina is closed with sutures at its deeper end; the surgical wound is closed.
* The procedure may also be performed by laparoscopy (see in Surgery section).

POSSIBLE COMPLICATIONS
* Excessive bleeding; surgical-wound infection.
* Urinary tract infection.
* Inadvertent injury to the bowel, bladder or ureters.
* Urinary obstruction or bowel obstruction.

AVERAGE HOSPITAL STAY—2 to 5 days.

PROBABLE OUTCOME
* The vagina will be shortened slightly. This should cause no lasting problem. Expect permanent sterility. Allow about 6 weeks for recovery from surgery.
* Because the ovaries are removed, sudden surgical menopause will occur unless supplemental hormones are taken.

POSTOPERATIVE CARE

GENERAL MEASURES
* Use an electric heating pad, a heat lamp or a warm compress to relieve incisional pain.
* Shower as usual. You may wash the incision gently with mild, unscented soap.
* Use sanitary napkins—not tampons—to absorb blood or drainage (discharge is normal, and may have an unpleasant odor).
* Surgery aftereffects may include constipation, fatigue, urinary symptoms, emotional changes and weight gain.

MEDICATION
* Your doctor may prescribe:
  - Pain relievers. Don't take prescription pain medication longer than 4 to 7 days. Use only as much as you need.
  - Supplemental female hormones, unless there are reasons why you should not take them.
* Antibiotics to fight or prevent infection.

ACTIVITY
* To help recovery and aid your well-being, resume daily activities as soon as you are able.
* Resume driving 2 weeks after returning home.
* Resume sexual relations in 4 to 6 weeks.

DIET—Clear liquid diet until the gastrointestinal tract functions again. Then eat a well-balanced diet to promote healing.

CALL YOUR DOCTOR IF

* Vaginal bleeding soaks more than 1 pad per hour.
* You experience a frequent urge to urinate or have excessive vaginal discharge that persists longer than 1 month.
* Pain or swelling increases in the surgical area.
* You develop signs of infection, including headache, muscle aches, dizziness or a general ill feeling and fever.

HYSTERECTOMY (ABDOMINAL) WITH SALPINGO-OOPHORECTOMY

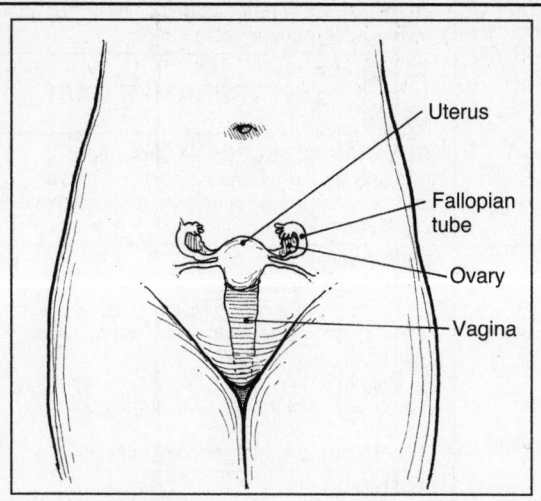

Shown are parts of the female reproductive tract including the uterus, fallopian tubes, ovaries and vagina.

Uterus

Fallopian tube

Ovary

Vagina

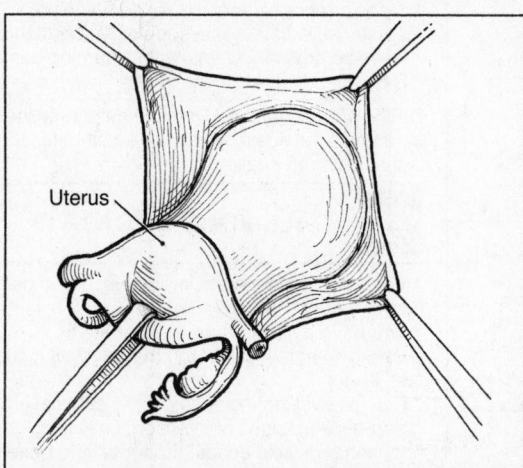

After an incision (either vertical or transverse) has been made in the lower abdomen and the muscles retracted, the uterus, cervix, fallopian tubes and ovaries are cut free and removed.

Uterus

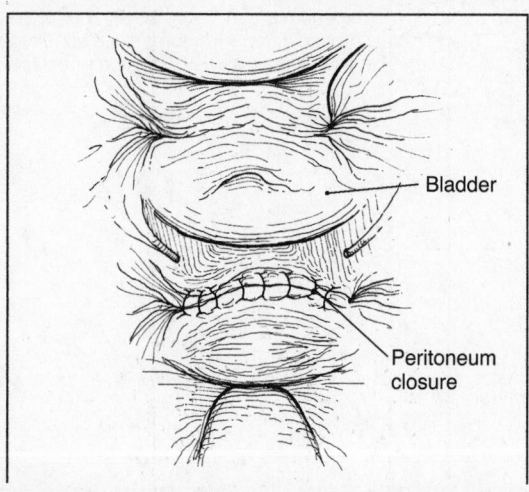

The peritoneum is closed with sutures.
 • The abdominal wall is closed in layers and the skin is closed with sutures that usually can be removed in 10 to 14 days (not illustrated).

Bladder

Peritoneum closure

SURGERIES

HYSTERECTOMY (VAGINAL)

GENERAL INFORMATION

DEFINITION—Removal of the uterus and cervix through an incision in the deepest recesses of the vagina. This surgery is frequently accompanied by reconstructive surgery (colporrhaphy), to repair weakened bladder.

BODY PARTS INVOLVED—Bladder muscles; rectal muscles; uterus; cervix; fallopian tubes; ovaries; vagina.

REASONS FOR SURGERY—Cancer or suspected cancer; fibroid tumors; chronic bleeding; prolapsed (dropped) uterus; endometriosis; chronic pelvic infection or severe menstrual pain.

SURGICAL RISK INCREASES WITH
* Obesity; smoking.
* Iron-deficiency anemia; heart or lung disease; or diabetes.
* Use of some prescription and nonprescription drugs. Inform your doctor of any drugs, medications, or vitamin and herb supplements you are using or have used in the last month.

WHAT TO EXPECT

WHO OPERATES—General surgeon or obstetrician-gynecologist.

WHERE PERFORMED—Hospital.

DIAGNOSTIC TESTS
* Before surgery: Blood and urine studies; x-rays of abdomen and kidneys; dilatation and curettage of the uterus (D & C); ultrasound (see Glossary for both).
* After surgery: Blood studies.

ANESTHESIA
* Spinal anesthesia by injection.
* General anesthesia by injection and inhalation with an airway tube placed in the windpipe.

DESCRIPTION OF OPERATION
* The deepest recesses of the vagina are opened. The cervix and uterus are cut free and removed. The rear part of the vagina is closed with sutures.
* A small foley catheter may be in the bladder for several days.
* The procedure may also be performed in conjunction with a laparoscopy (see in Surgery section) to remove the fallopian tubes or ovaries.

POSSIBLE COMPLICATIONS
* Excessive bleeding.
* Surgical-wound infection.
* Inadvertent injury to bladder, rectum or ureters.
* Urinary tract infection.

AVERAGE HOSPITAL STAY—1 to 3 days.

PROBABLE OUTCOME—The vagina will be shortened slightly. This should cause no lasting problem. Expect permanent sterility. Allow about 6 weeks for recovery from surgery.

POSTOPERATIVE CARE

GENERAL MEASURES—Use sanitary napkins—not tampons—to absorb blood or drainage (discharge is normal, and may have an unpleasant odor).

MEDICATION
* Your doctor may prescribe:
- Pain relievers. Don't take prescription pain medication longer than 4 to 7 days. Use only as much as you need.
- Supplemental female hormones, unless there are reasons why you should not take them.
* Antibiotics to fight or prevent infection.

ACTIVITY
* To help recovery and aid your well-being, resume daily activities as soon as you are able.
* Resume driving 2 weeks after returning home.
* Resume sexual relations in 4 to 6 weeks.

DIET—Clear liquid diet until the gastrointestinal tract functions again. Then eat a well-balanced diet to promote healing.

CALL YOUR DOCTOR IF

* Vaginal bleeding soaks more than 1 pad per hour.
* You have a frequent urge to urinate or excessive vaginal discharge that persists longer than 1 month.
* Pain or swelling increases in the surgical area.
* You develop signs of infection, including headache, muscle aches, dizziness or a general ill feeling and fever.
* You experience abdominal swelling or pain.
* New, unexplained symptoms develop. Drugs used in treatment may produce side effects.

HYSTERECTOMY (VAGINAL)

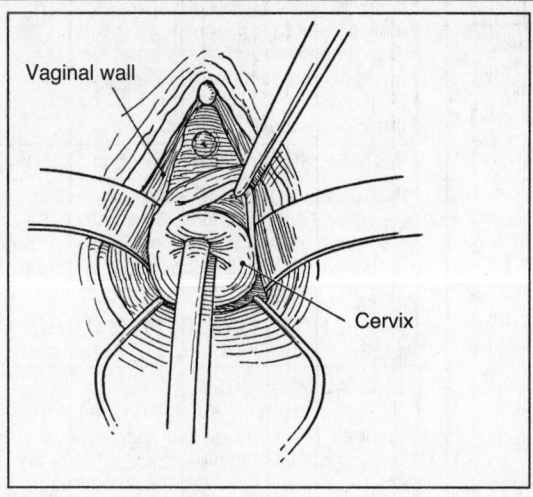

Vaginal wall

Cervix

This view illustrates a female patient with extended legs in stirrups on an examining table to allow examination of the genital area.
- An illustration of the vagina and cervix showing the first incision made to separate the cervix from the lowest layers of the bladder.

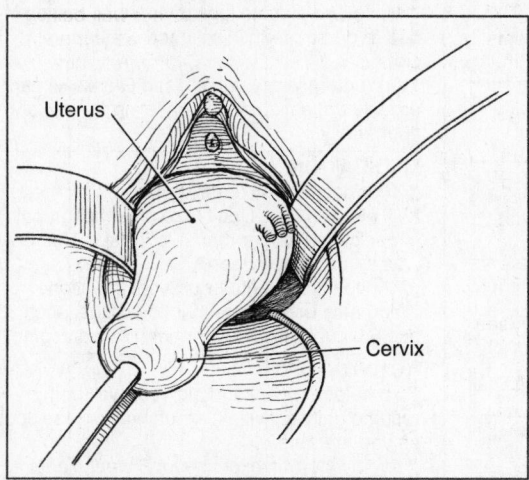

Uterus

Cervix

The deepest recesses of the vagina are opened. The cervix and uterus are cut free and removed. The bladder may also be repaired (not illustrated).

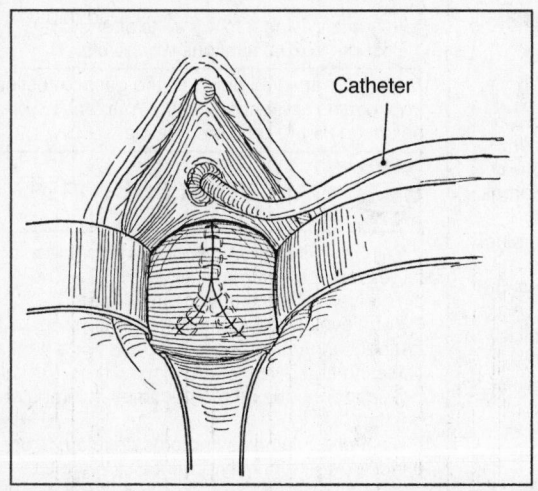

Catheter

A small catheter is left in the bladder to remain there several days until swelling subsides.

SURGERIES

ILEOSTOMY

GENERAL INFORMATION

DEFINITION—Creation of an opening in the ileum, the lower part of the small intestine. After surgery, all feces leave the body through this opening, which is called an "ostomy" or "stoma."

BODY PARTS INVOLVED—Ileum; cecum.

REASONS FOR SURGERY
* Ulcerative colitis.
* Multiple colon cancers.
* Colon surgery which weakens an area of the colon and necessitates a temporary bypass of the intestine until the colon has healed.

SURGICAL RISK INCREASES WITH
* Adults over 60; newborns and infants.
* Obesity; smoking; poor nutrition.
* Excess alcohol consumption.
* Recent or chronic illness, especially heart or lung disease or diabetes.
* Use of some prescription and nonprescription drugs. Inform your doctor of any drugs, medications, or vitamin and herb supplements you are using or have used in the last month.

WHAT TO EXPECT

WHO OPERATES—General surgeon; colon-rectal surgeon.

WHERE PERFORMED—Hospital.

DIAGNOSTIC TESTS
* Before surgery: Blood and urine studies; x-rays; ECG; sigmoidoscopy; colonoscopy (see Glossary for all).
* After surgery: Blood and urine studies.

ANESTHESIA—General anesthesia by injection and inhalation with an airway tube placed in the windpipe.

DESCRIPTION OF OPERATION
* An incision is made in the abdomen over the diseased intestinal tract.
* The muscles of the abdominal wall are separated to expose the abdominal organs, which are inspected for undetected disease. Other surgeries may be performed at this time.
* The ileum is clamped on both sides of the area to be opened and cut between the clamps. The part closer to the stomach is brought through another small incision in the abdominal wall to accept the stoma.
* The part of the intestinal tract below the ileum, usually around the diseased part of the intestine, is closed with sutures or is removed with the diseased colon. The abdominal contents are replaced. The muscles and skin are closed with sutures, which usually can be removed about 1 week after surgery.

POSSIBLE COMPLICATIONS
* Excessive bleeding.
* Surgical-wound infection; abscess.
* Incisional hernia.
* Skin irritation around the stoma.
* Intestinal obstruction.
* Scarring.
* Leakage of the ileal pouch.

AVERAGE HOSPITAL STAY—5 to 7 days.

PROBABLE OUTCOME—Expect complete cure without complications. Allow about 6 weeks for recovery. You will need to wear an external pouch to collect bowel movements.

POSTOPERATIVE CARE

GENERAL MEASURES
* A hard ridge should form along the incision. As it heals, the ridge will gradually recede.
* Shower as usual after discharge. You may wash the incision gently with mild soap.
* Move and elevate legs often while resting in bed to decrease the likelihood of deep-vein clots.
* An "enterostomy nurse" (see Glossary) can provide education and counseling for you and your family.

MEDICATION
* Your doctor may prescribe:
  - Pain relievers. Don't take prescription pain medication longer than 4 to 7 days. Use only as much as you need.
  - Antibiotics to fight or prevent infection.
* You may use nonprescription drugs, such as acetaminophen, for minor pain. Avoid aspirin.

ACTIVITY
* To help recovery and aid your well-being, resume daily activities, including work, as soon as you are able.
* Avoid vigorous exercise for 6 weeks after surgery.
* Resume driving 3 to 4 weeks after surgery.
* Resume sexual relations when able.

DIET—Clear liquid diet until the gastrointestinal tract begins to function again. Then eat a well-balanced diet to promote healing.

CALL YOUR DOCTOR IF

* Pain, swelling, redness, drainage or bleeding increases in the surgical area.
* You have abdominal swelling or pain.
* You develop signs of infection, including headache, muscle aches, dizziness or a general ill feeling and fever.
* Skin around the stoma becomes inflamed and painful.
* New, unexplained symptoms develop. Drugs used in treatment may produce side effects.

ILEOSTOMY

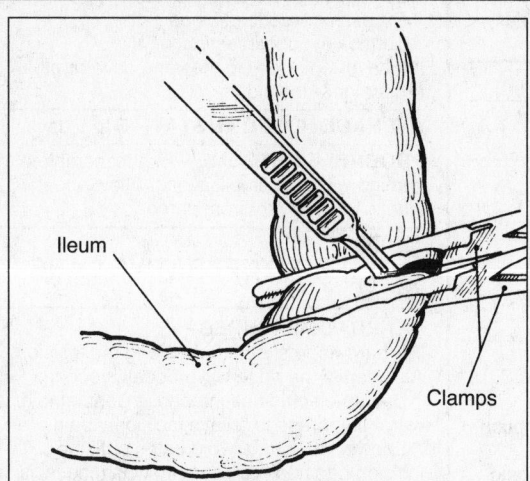

The muscles of the abdominal wall are separated to expose the abdominal organs, which are inspected for disease (not illustrated). The ileum is clamped on both sides of the area to be opened and cut between the clamps.

Ileum

Clamps

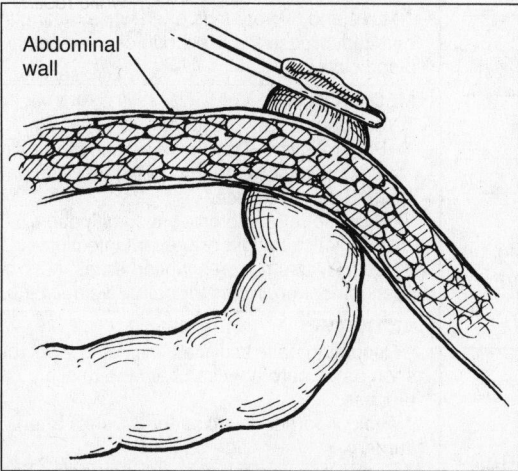

The part closer to the stomach is brought through another small incision in the abdominal wall to accept the stoma.
  • The part of the intestinal tract below the ileum, usually around the diseased part of the intestine, is removed with the diseased colon.

Abdominal wall

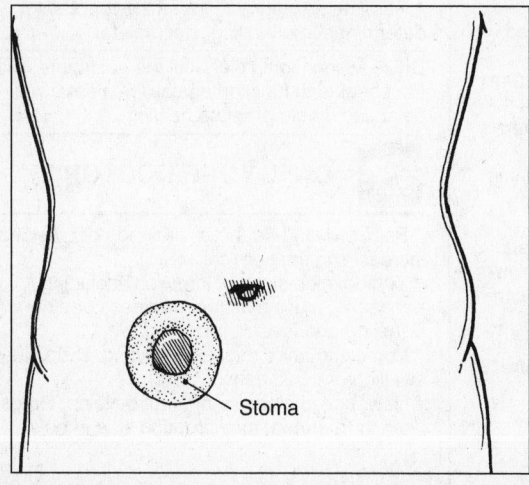

The stoma is shown in a frequently used location extending through the abdominal wall. After surgery, fecal contents will pass into an ileostomy bag.

Stoma

SURGERIES

KIDNEY REMOVAL
(Nephrectomy)

GENERAL INFORMATION

DEFINITION—Removal of a kidney.

BODY PARTS INVOLVED—Kidney; blood vessels connected to kidney; ureter.

REASONS FOR SURGERY
- Cancer or suspected cancer of the kidney.
- Severe kidney trauma.
- Dysfunctional kidney due to infection.

SURGICAL RISK INCREASES WITH
- Adults over 60; newborns and infants.
- Obesity; poor nutrition.
- Smoking; alcoholism.
- Recent or chronic illness.
- Diabetes.
- Use of some prescription and nonprescription drugs. Inform your doctor of any drugs, medications, or vitamin and herb supplements you are using or have used in the last month.

WHAT TO EXPECT

WHO OPERATES—General surgeon or urologist.

WHERE PERFORMED—Hospital.

DIAGNOSTIC TESTS
- Before surgery: Blood and urine studies; x-rays of kidneys, lower gastrointestinal tract and chest; ECG; ultrasound; cystoscopy; IVP; MRI; CT scan (see Glossary for all).
- After surgery: Blood studies.

ANESTHESIA—General anesthesia by injection and inhalation with an airway tube placed in the windpipe.

DESCRIPTION OF OPERATION
- An incision is made, usually in the left or right flank, but sometimes in the abdomen.
- The vein leading from the kidney is located, isolated and tied.
- The ureter is located, tied and cut away from the kidney.
- The artery that supplies blood to the kidney is tied and transected.
- The kidney is freed of adhesions or adjoining connective tissue and removed; surrounding lymph nodes may also be removed.
- All disconnected blood vessels are tied, and the muscles are closed with sutures. The skin is closed with sutures or clips, which usually can be removed in about 1 week after surgery.
- A urinary catheter (Foley) will be left in place for several days to make it easier to measure the amount of urine you are producing.
- Surgery may also be done by laparoscopy (see in Surgery section).

POSSIBLE COMPLICATIONS
- Excessive bleeding; blood clots.
- Surgical-wound infection.
- Inadvertent injury to the vena cava or other organs near the kidney.

AVERAGE HOSPITAL STAY—3 to 5 days.

PROBABLE OUTCOME—Expect complete healing without complications. Allow about 4 weeks for recovery from surgery.

POSTOPERATIVE CARE

GENERAL MEASURES
- A hard ridge should form along the incision. As it heals, the ridge will gradually recede.
- Use an electric heating pad, a heat lamp or a warm compress to relieve incisional pain.
- Shower as usual. Avoid baths until the incision has healed. You may wash the incision gently with mild, unscented soap.
- Move and elevate legs often while resting in bed to decrease the likelihood of deep-vein blood clots.

MEDICATION
- Your doctor may prescribe:
  - Pain relievers. Don't take prescription pain medication longer than 4 to 7 days. Use only as much as you need.
  - Stool softeners to prevent constipation.
  - Antibiotics to fight or prevent infection.
- You may use nonprescription drugs, such as acetaminophen, for minor pain. Avoid aspirin.

ACTIVITY
- Resuming daily activities, including work, as soon as you are able can help the healing process.
- Avoid vigorous exercise for 6 weeks after surgery.
- Resume driving 5 weeks after returning home.
- Resume sexual relations when your doctor determines that healing is complete.

DIET—Clear liquid diet until the gastrointestinal tract begins to function again. Then eat a well-balanced diet to promote healing.

CALL YOUR DOCTOR IF

- Pain, swelling, redness, drainage or bleeding increases in the surgical area.
- You develop signs of infection, including headache, muscle aches, dizziness or a general ill feeling and fever.
- You experience nausea, vomiting, abdominal swelling or constipation.
- New, unexplained symptoms develop. Drugs used in treatment may produce side effects.

KIDNEY REMOVAL
(Nephrectomy)

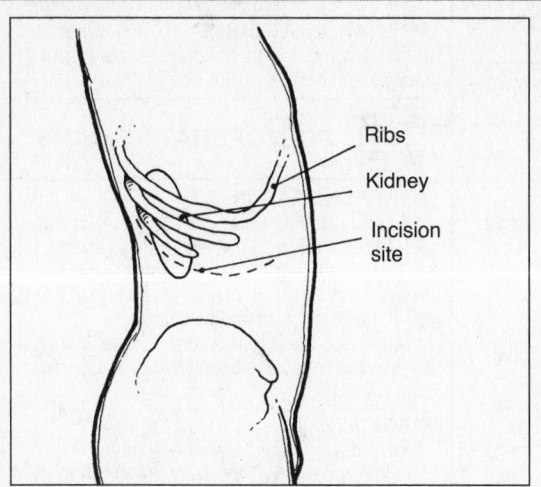

The usual incision for kidney removal in the flank below the last rib.

Ribs

Kidney

Incision site

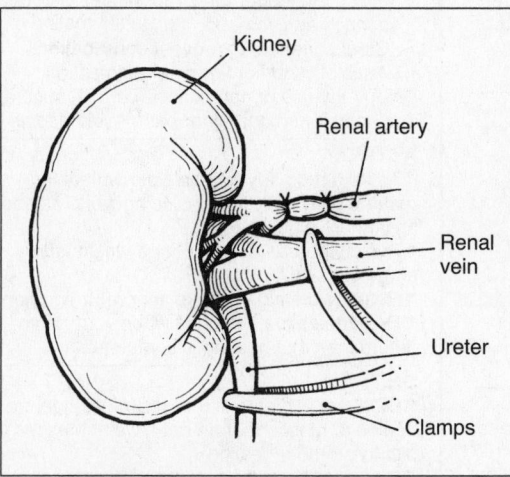

The vein leading from the kidney is located, isolated and tied.
- The ureter is located, tied and cut away from the kidney.
- The artery that supplies blood to the kidney is clamped in 2 places and cut between the clamps.
- The kidney is removed.

Kidney

Renal artery

Renal vein

Ureter

Clamps

SURGERIES

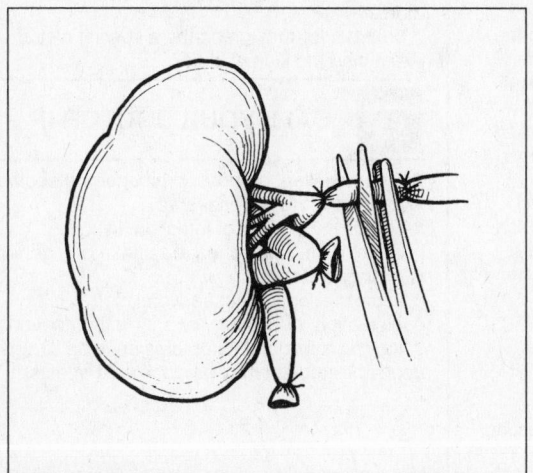

All disconnected blood vessels are tied. The abdominal muscles are closed (not illustrated).

KIDNEY STONE REMOVAL
(Ureterolithotomy)

GENERAL INFORMATION

DEFINITION—Removal of a kidney stone from one of the ureters.

BODY PARTS INVOLVED—Ureter; kidney.

REASONS FOR SURGERY—Restoration of normal urine flow in the ureter.

SURGICAL RISK INCREASES WITH
* Obesity; smoking; alcoholism.
* Poor nutrition.
* Recent or chronic illness.
* Diabetes.
* Use of some prescription and nonprescription drugs. Inform your doctor of any drugs, medications, or vitamin and herb supplements you are using or have used in the last month.

WHAT TO EXPECT

WHO OPERATES—Urologist or general surgeon.

WHERE PERFORMED—Hospital.

DIAGNOSTIC TESTS
* Before surgery: Blood and urine studies; x-rays of chest; ECG; intravenous pyelogram; ultrasound: CT scan (see Glossary for all).
* During surgery: Retrograde pyelogram (see Glossary).
* After surgery: Blood studies; urine tests.

ANESTHESIA—General anesthesia by injection and inhalation with an airway tube placed in the windpipe.

DESCRIPTION OF OPERATION
* An incision is made in the flank. The muscles are separated and the ureter is exposed.
* A small incision is made in the ureter. The kidney stone is pulled free and removed.
* After the ureter is closed, a tube is left in the wound for drainage, and a tube is inserted in the ureter to restore urine flow. This tube is removed after healing.
* Muscle layers are closed. The skin is closed with sutures or clips, which usually can be removed about 1 week after surgery.
* Some kidney stones may also be removed with lithotripsy (see in Surgery section), which involves the use of shockwaves to crush the stone so that it can be passed from the body with your urine.

POSSIBLE COMPLICATIONS
* Excessive bleeding.
* Surgical-wound infection.
* Urine leakage.
* Scarring at operative site causing obstruction or partial obstruction.

AVERAGE HOSPITAL STAY—4 to 5 days.

PROBABLE OUTCOME—Expect complete healing without complications. Allow about 2 weeks for recovery from surgery.

POSTOPERATIVE CARE

GENERAL MEASURES
* A hard ridge should form along the incision. As it heals, the ridge will gradually recede.
* Shower as usual. Avoid bathing until the incision has healed You may wash the incision gently with mild, unscented soap.
* Move and elevate legs often while resting in bed to decrease the likelihood of deep-vein blood clots.

MEDICATION
* Your doctor may prescribe:
  - Pain relievers. Don't take prescription pain medication longer than 4 to 7 days. Use only as much as you need.
  - Stool softeners to prevent constipation.
  - Antibiotics to fight or prevent infection.
* You may use nonprescription drugs, such as acetaminophen, for minor pain. Avoid aspirin.

ACTIVITY
* To help recovery and aid your well-being, resume daily activities, including work, as soon as you are able.
* Avoid vigorous exercise for 6 weeks after surgery.
* Resume driving 2 weeks after returning home.
* Resume sexual relations when your doctor determines that healing is complete.

DIET
* Clear liquid diet until the gastrointestinal tract begins to function. Then eat a well-balanced diet to promote healing.
* Increase daily water intake to 8 glasses or more.
* Your doctor may prescribe a special diet after examining the kidney stone.

CALL YOUR DOCTOR IF

* Pain, swelling, redness, drainage or bleeding increases in the surgical area.
* You develop signs of infection, including headache, muscle aches, dizziness or a general ill feeling and fever.
* You experience nausea, vomiting, constipation, or difficulty or pain with urination.
* New, unexplained symptoms develop. Drugs used in treatment may produce side effects.

KIDNEY STONE REMOVAL
(Ureterolithotomy)

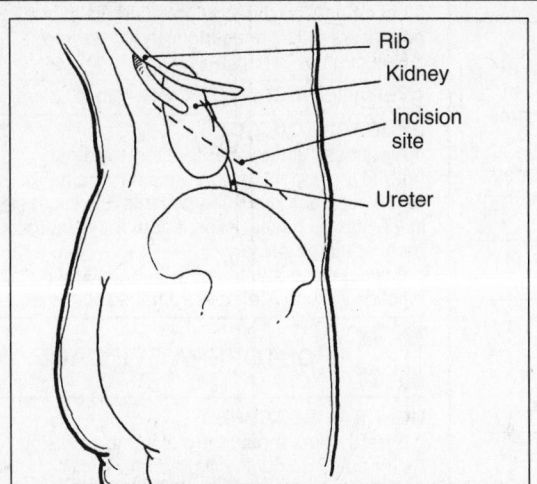

Incision site on the skin in the flank under the last rib.

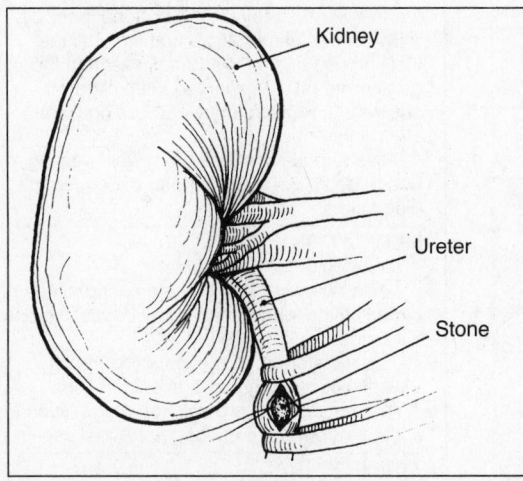

After a small incision has been made in the ureter, the kidney stone is pulled free and removed.

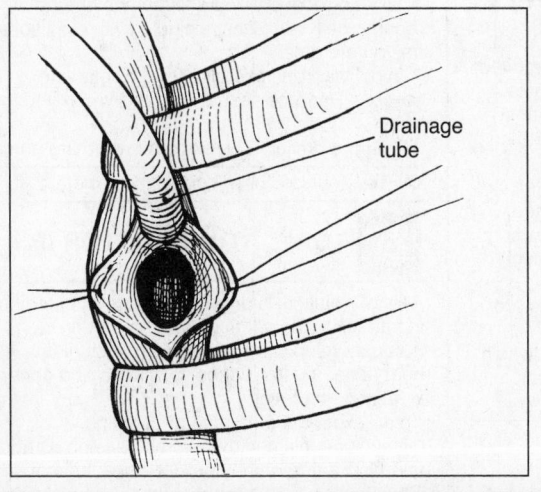

A tube is inserted for drainage. The tissues under the skin are closed with large absorbable sutures. The skin is closed with sutures or clips that usually can be removed about 1 week after surgery.

SURGERIES

KIDNEY TRANSPLANTATION

 GENERAL INFORMATION

DEFINITION—Replacement of a diseased kidney with a healthy kidney obtained from a healthy donor with compatible immunological characteristics. The donated kidney may come from a living relative or deceased donor.

BODY PARTS INVOLVED—Diseased kidney; healthy donor kidney; blood vessels to and from the kidney; ureters.

REASONS FOR SURGERY—Restoration of normal kidney function.

SURGICAL RISK INCREASES WITH
* Adults over 60.
* Obesity; poor nutrition.
* Recent or chronic illness; diabetes.
* Alcoholism; smoking.
* Use of some prescription and nonprescription drugs. Inform your doctor of any drugs, medications, or vitamin and herb supplements you are using or have used in the last month.

 WHAT TO EXPECT

WHO OPERATES—General surgeon or urologist with transplant experience and training.

WHERE PERFORMED—Hospital.

DIAGNOSTIC TESTS
* Before surgery: Blood and urine studies; x-rays of kidneys; ECG; CT scan; ultrasound.
* After surgery: Blood studies.

ANESTHESIA—General anesthesia by injection and inhalation with an airway tube placed in the windpipe.

DESCRIPTION OF OPERATION
* The diseased kidney from the recipient may be removed several weeks in advance. During this time, dialysis (see Glossary) provides artificial kidney function.
* Often, the recipients kidneys are not removed; they are left in place and the donor kidney is placed in the lower right part of the abdomen.
* A kidney is removed from the donor, then chilled and preserved for up to 12 hours.
* An incision is made in the abdomen of the recipient. The abdominal cavity is examined. The new kidney is placed and sewn in position.
* The blood vessels and ureters are connected to the new kidney.
* The peritoneum and abdominal muscles are closed.
* The skin is closed with sutures or clips, which usually can be removed about 1 week after surgery.

POSSIBLE COMPLICATIONS
* Excessive bleeding.
* Surgical-wound infection.

* Ureter leak; blockage of ureter.
* Occasionally, the new kidney does not function right away and continued dialysis is necessary until kidney function is restored.
* Rejection of transplant.

AVERAGE HOSPITAL STAY—7 to 10 days.

PROBABLE OUTCOME
* A successful transplant restores almost normal life expectancy in patients who might otherwise have died. Transplants are successful in 70-80% of cases. Allow about 4 weeks for recovery from surgery.
* A living donor continues with good kidney function and no ill effects from the procedure.

 POSTOPERATIVE CARE

GENERAL MEASURES
* A hard ridge should form along the incision. As it heals, the ridge will gradually recede.
* Use an electric heating pad, a heat lamp or a warm compress to relieve incisional pain.
* Shower as usual. Avoid bathing until the incision has healed. You may wash the incision gently with mild, unscented soap. After showering, replace any wet dressings with clean, dry ones.
* Move and elevate legs often while resting in bed to decrease the likelihood of deep-vein blood clots.

MEDICATION
* Your doctor may prescribe:
  - Pain relievers. Don't take prescription pain medication longer than 4 to 7 days. Use only as much as you need.
  - Stool softeners to prevent constipation.
  - Antibiotics to fight or prevent infection.
* You may use nonprescription drugs, such as acetaminophen, for minor pain. Avoid aspirin.

ACTIVITY
* To help recovery and aid your well-being, resume daily activities, including work, as soon as you are able.
* Avoid vigorous exercise for 6 weeks after surgery. Resume sexual relations when you feel able.
* Resume driving 2 weeks after returning home.

DIET—Your doctor will prescribe a diet.

 CALL YOUR DOCTOR IF

* Pain, swelling, redness, drainage or bleeding increases in the surgical area.
* You develop signs of infection, including headache, muscle aches, dizziness or a general ill feeling and fever.
* You experience nausea or vomiting.
* New, unexplained symptoms develop. Drugs used in treatment may produce side effects.

KIDNEY TRANSPLANTATION

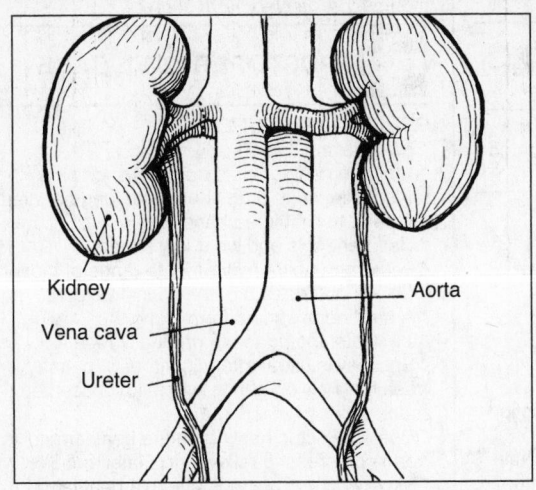

Shown are the kidneys and the adjoining body structures involved in the transplantation.

Kidney

Aorta

Vena cava

Ureter

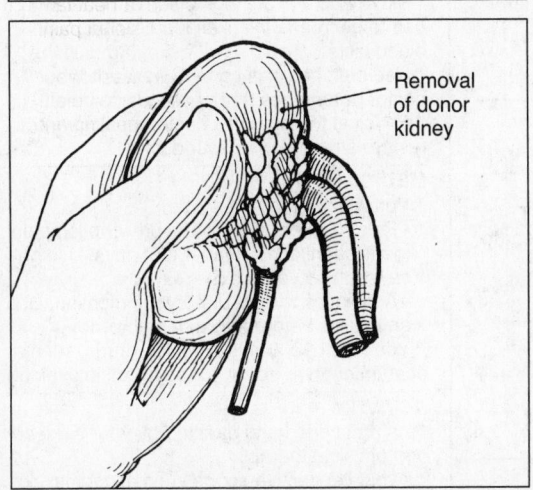

A kidney is removed from the donor, chilled and preserved for up to 12 hours.

Removal of donor kidney

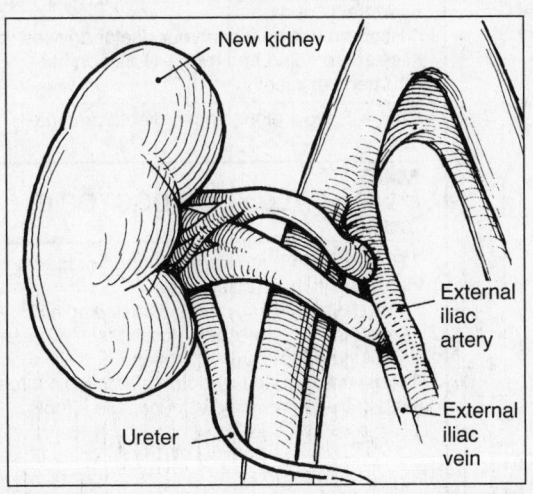

New kidney is placed and sewn into position. The blood vessels and ureters are connected to the new kidney.
- The abdominal muscles and skin are closed in layers (not illustrated).

New kidney

External iliac artery

External iliac vein

Ureter

KNEE REPLACEMENT, TOTAL

 GENERAL INFORMATION

DEFINITION—Surgical replacement of an injured or diseased knee to re-establish a pain-free, movable joint.

BODY PARTS INVOLVED—Knee joint; muscles, ligaments, bones, cartilage and bursa forming the knee joint.

REASONS FOR SURGERY—Diseased or injured knee causing chronic pain or disability impairing the quality of life.

SURGICAL RISK INCREASES WITH
* Obesity; smoking.
* Excess alcohol consumption.
* Recent or chronic illness.
* Diabetes.
* Use of some prescription and nonprescription drugs. Inform your doctor of any drugs, medications, or vitamin and herb supplements you are using or have used in the last month.

 WHAT TO EXPECT

WHO OPERATES—Orthopedic surgeon.

WHERE PERFORMED—Hospital.

DIAGNOSTIC TESTS
* Before surgery: X-rays of joint; MRI or CT scan (see Glossary for both); joint aspiration (to check for active infection); blood and urine studies.
* During surgery: X-rays.
* After surgery: X-rays, blood tests, and examination of tissue removed.

ANESTHESIA—General anesthesia by injection and inhalation with an airway tube placed in the windpipe.

DESCRIPTION OF OPERATION
* An incision is made into the affected knee.
* The arthritic or diseased surfaces of the femoral condyles and tibial plateau are removed.
* The above areas are replaced by durable prosthetic components that are fixed firmly in place with a special form of bone cement.
* The new knee joint may be hinged (for unstable knees) or unhinged.

POSSIBLE COMPLICATIONS
* Excessive bleeding; blood clots.
* Surgical-wound infection.
* Pneumonia.
* Limited range-of-motion of the knee.
* Loosening of joint components at a future time.

AVERAGE HOSPITAL STAY—3 to 5 days.

PROBABLE OUTCOME—Expect complete healing without complications. Allow about 6 months for recovery from surgery.

 POSTOPERATIVE CARE

GENERAL MEASURES
* No smoking.
* Buy and use self-help devices, such as a raised toilet seat, bath bench and long-handled grippers, to limit knee bending.
* Use handrails and wear low shoes.
* Learn and abide by your safe range of motion.
* Cough and deep breathe as instructed.
* A hard ridge should form along the incision. As it heals, the ridge will gradually recede.
* Shower as usual after discharge. You may wash the incision gently with mild, unscented soap.
* Use an electric heating pad, a heat lamp or a warm compress to relieve incisional pain.
* Move and elevate legs often while resting in bed to decrease the likelihood of deep-vein blood clots.
* Use crutches or a cane to walk until your doctor determines that healing is complete.
* Physical therapy may hasten healing and restore strength. Ask your doctor.

MEDICATION
* Your doctor may prescribe:
  - Pain relievers. Don't take prescription pain medication longer than 4 to 7 days. Use only as much as you need.
  - Antibiotics to fight or prevent infection. Use antibiotics before future dental work.
* You may use nonprescription drugs, such as acetaminophen, for minor pain. Avoid aspirin.

ACTIVITY
* As prescribed and directed by your surgeon and physical therapist.
* Avoid very active sports such as tennis, skiing or contact sports.
* Resume driving when your doctor advises that it is safe to do so and range-of-motion has returned sufficiently.

DIET—Eat a well-balanced diet to promote healing.

 CALL YOUR DOCTOR IF

* Pain, swelling, redness, drainage or bleeding increases in the surgical area.
* You develop signs of infection, including headache, muscle aches, dizziness or a general ill feeling and fever.
* New, unexplained symptoms develop. Drugs used in treatment may produce side effects.

KNEE REPLACEMENT, TOTAL

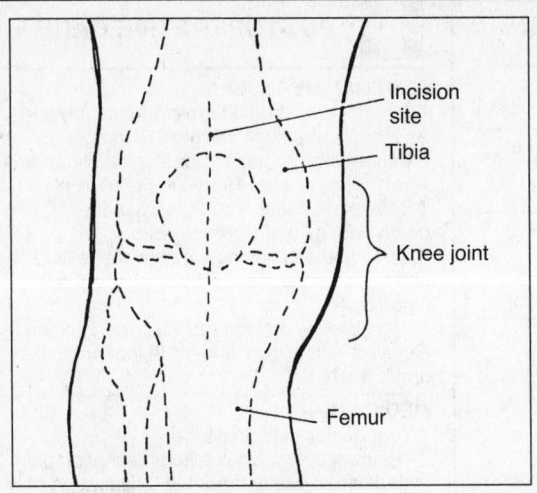

An illustration of the knee joint and a normal site for incision when a replacement procedure is planned.

- Incision site
- Tibia
- Knee joint
- Femur

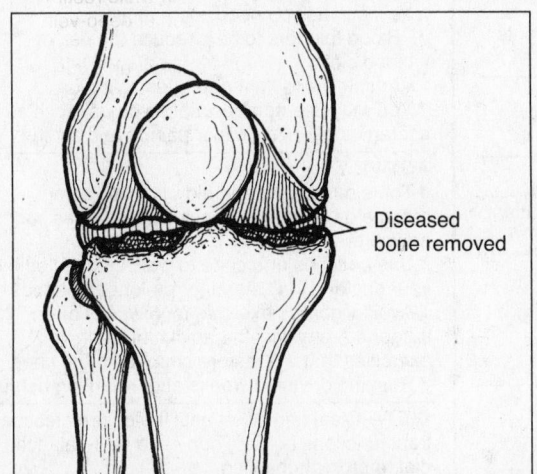

The diseased bone to be removed.

- Diseased bone removed

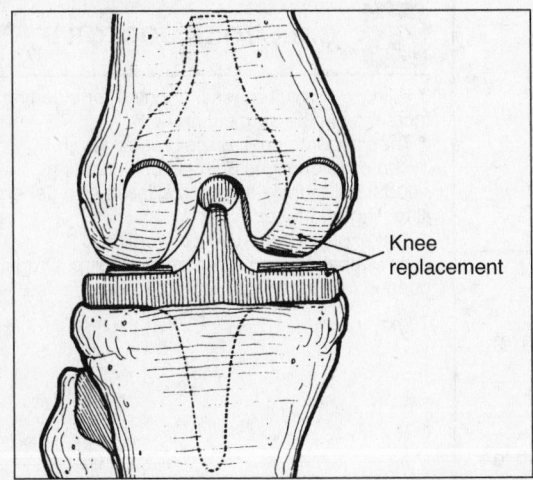

After the diseased surfaces of the femur and tibia have been removed, they are replaced by a durable prosthetic component fixed firmly in place with a special form of bone cement (sometimes).

- Knee replacement

SURGERIES

KNEECAP REMOVAL
(Patellectomy)

GENERAL INFORMATION

DEFINITION—Removal of the kneecap (patella).

BODY PARTS INVOLVED—Kneecap; knee joint; muscles and ligaments attached to kneecap.

REASONS FOR SURGERY
* Fracture of the kneecap.
* Recurrent dislocations of the kneecap.
* Painful degenerative arthritis in the kneecap.

SURGICAL RISK INCREASES WITH
* Obesity.
* Smoking.
* Poor nutrition.
* Recent or chronic illness.
* Diabetes.
* Use of some prescription and nonprescription drugs. Inform your doctor of any drugs, medications, or vitamin and herb supplements you are using or have used in the last month.

WHAT TO EXPECT

WHO OPERATES—Orthopedist.

WHERE PERFORMED—Hospital or outpatient surgical facility.

DIAGNOSTIC TESTS
* Before surgery: Blood and urine studies; x-rays of both knees.
* After surgery: Blood studies; x-rays of the affected knee.

ANESTHESIA
* Local anesthesia by injection.
* Spinal anesthesia by injection.
* General anesthesia by injection and inhalation with an airway tube placed in the windpipe.

DESCRIPTION OF OPERATION
* An incision is made around the kneecap.
* The muscles and tendons attached to the kneecap are cut, and the kneecap is removed.
* The muscles are sewn back together with strong suture material.
* The skin is closed with sutures or clips, which usually can be removed about 1 week after surgery.

POSSIBLE COMPLICATIONS
* Excessive bleeding.
* Surgical-wound infection.
* Blood clots which can break loose and travel to the lung.

AVERAGE HOSPITAL STAY—3 to 6 days.

PROBABLE OUTCOME—Expect complete healing without complications. Allow about 6 to 12 weeks for recovery from surgery.

POSTOPERATIVE CARE

GENERAL MEASURES
* A hard ridge should form along the incision. As it heals, the ridge will gradually recede.
* Use an electric heating pad, a heat lamp or a warm compress to relieve incisional pain.
* Shower as usual. You may wash the incision gently with mild, unscented soap.
* Move and elevate legs often while resting in bed to decrease the likelihood of deep-vein blood clots.
* While sleeping or sitting, keep the affected leg elevated with pillows under the foot or blocks under the bed.

MEDICATION
* Your doctor may prescribe:
  - Pain relievers. Don't take prescription pain medication longer than 4 to 7 days. Use only as much as you need.
  - Blood thinners to help reduce the risk of blood clots.
  - Antibiotics to fight or prevent infection.
* You may use nonprescription drugs, such as acetaminophen, for minor pain. Avoid aspirin.

ACTIVITY
* To help recovery and aid your well-being, resume daily activities, including work, as soon as you are able.
* Use crutches or a cane to walk as directed by your doctor. Don't stand for prolonged periods.
* Avoid vigorous exercise for 6 weeks after surgery. A physical therapist can teach you exercises that will restore strength to the knee.
* Resume driving 3 weeks after returning home.

DIET—Clear liquid diet until the gastrointestinal tract functions again. Then eat a well-balanced diet to promote healing.

CALL YOUR DOCTOR IF

* Pain, swelling, redness, drainage or bleeding increases in the surgical area.
* Toes become cold, discolored or numb.
* You develop signs of infection, including headache, muscle aches, dizziness or a general ill feeling and fever.
* You experience nausea or vomiting.
* New, unexplained symptoms develop. Drugs used in treatment may produce side effects.

KNEECAP REMOVAL
(Patellectomy)

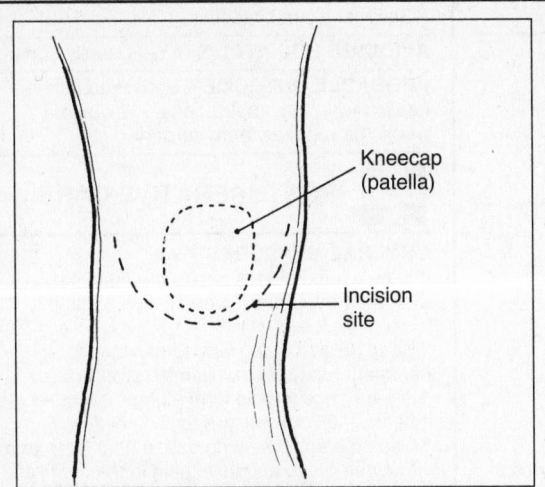

The kneecap and the proposed incision site for kneecap removal.

Kneecap
(patella)

Incision
site

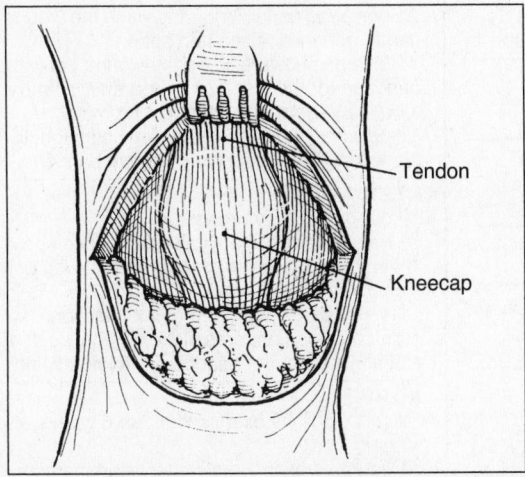

Muscles and tendons attached to the kneecap are cut and the kneecap is removed.

Tendon

Kneecap

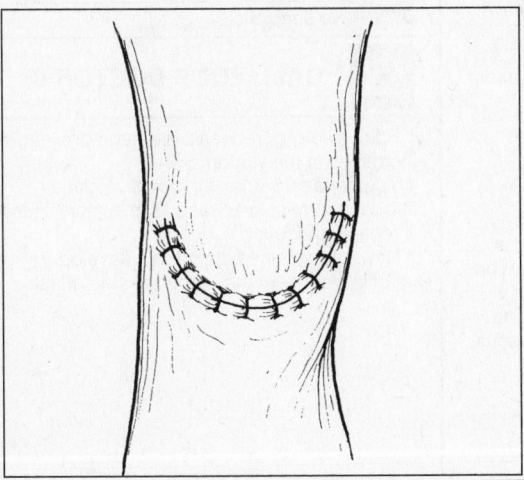

The muscles are sewn back together with strong suture material and the skin is closed with sutures or clips that usually can be removed about 1 week after surgery.

LACERATION REPAIR

GENERAL INFORMATION

DEFINITION—Repair of lacerations (open wounds in the skin extending to underlying tissue and sometimes muscle, blood vessels and nerves).

BODY PARTS INVOLVED—Skin; muscle; connective tissue.

REASONS FOR SURGERY
- Prevention of bleeding and infection.
- Examination to identify underlying injuries.
- Closure of the skin to hasten healing.

SURGICAL RISK INCREASES WITH
- Obesity.
- Smoking.
- Poor nutrition.
- Recent or chronic illness.
- Diabetes.
- Use of some prescription and nonprescription drugs. Inform your doctor of any drugs, medications, or vitamin and herb supplements you are using or have used in the last month.

WHAT TO EXPECT

WHO OPERATES—Family doctor, general surgeon, plastic and reconstructive surgeon, orthopedist or hand surgeon.

WHERE PERFORMED—Hospital, outpatient surgical facility or emergency room.

DIAGNOSTIC TESTS
- Before surgery: Blood and urine studies.
- After surgery: Blood studies.

ANESTHESIA
- Local anesthesia by injection.
- General anesthesia by a combination of injection and inhalation with an airway tube placed in the windpipe.

DESCRIPTION OF OPERATION
- The wound is cleansed and irrigated. The wound is inspected for possible tendon or nerve injury.
- The skin edges are examined. Shredded tissue and debris are removed. Sometimes, a ragged edge is trimmed for better cosmetic results.
- The underlying tissue is closed with sutures that will be absorbed by the body. The skin is closed with small sutures, which usually can be removed about 1 week after surgery.
- A bandage may be used to control bleeding.
- You may need an injection to prevent tetanus. Ask your doctor.

POSSIBLE COMPLICATIONS
- Excessive bleeding.
- Surgical-wound infection.

AVERAGE HOSPITAL STAY—Usually none.

PROBABLE OUTCOME—Expect complete healing without complications. Allow about 3 weeks for recovery from surgery.

POSTOPERATIVE CARE

GENERAL MEASURES
- If the wound bleeds during the first 24 hours after surgery, press a clean tissue or cloth to it for 10 minutes.
- Keep an arm or leg wound elevated for 24 hours after surgery to minimize swelling.
- A hard ridge should form along the wound. As it heals, the ridge will gradually recede.
- Use an electric heating pad, a heat lamp or a warm compress to relieve pain in the surgical area.
- Shower as usual. You may wash the wound gently with mild unscented soap.
- Between showers, keep the wound dry with a bandage for the first 2 or 3 days after surgery. If a bandage gets wet, change it promptly.
- Apply nonprescription antibiotic ointment to the wound before applying a clean bandage.

MEDICATION
- Your doctor may prescribe:
  - Pain relievers. Don't take prescription pain medication longer than 4 to 7 days. Use only as much as you need.
  - Antibiotics to fight or prevent infection.
- You may use nonprescription drugs, such as acetaminophen, for minor pain. Avoid aspirin.

ACTIVITY
- Avoid vigorous exercise for 3 to 6 weeks after surgery.
- Resume driving 2 days after returning home.

DIET—No special diet.

CALL YOUR DOCTOR IF

- Pain, swelling, redness, drainage or bleeding increases in the wound area.
- You develop signs of infection, including headache, muscle aches, dizziness or a general ill feeling and fever.
- New, unexplained symptoms develop. Drugs used in treatment may produce side effects.

LACERATION REPAIR

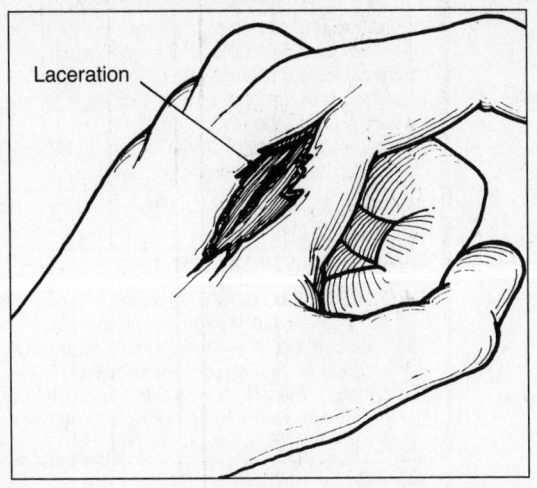

Laceration

A typical laceration on the side of the hand and finger.

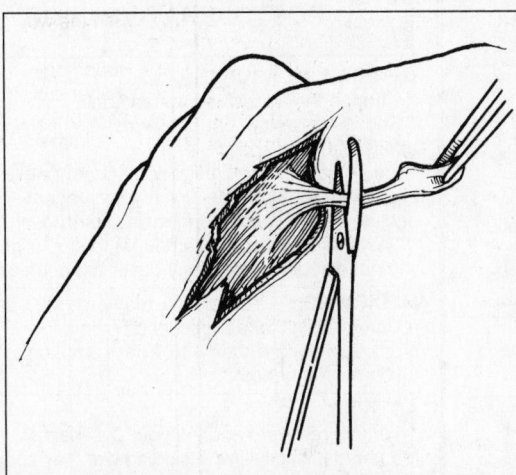

Shredded tissue and debris are removed. Sometimes a ragged edge of skin is trimmed for better cosmetic results.

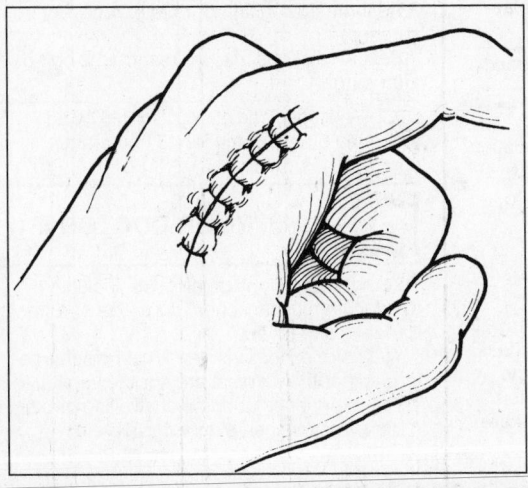

The underlying tissue is closed with sutures that will be absorbed by the body. Skin is closed with small sutures that usually can be removed about 1 week after surgery.

SURGERIES

LAPAROSCOPY

GENERAL INFORMATION

DEFINITION—Procedure that allows visual examination and some treatments of the pelvic and abdominal organs. The procedure is performed with a laparoscope, a fiber-optic instrument.

BODY PARTS INVOLVED—Abdomen and all its contents.

REASONS FOR SURGERY
- Evaluation and treatment of infertility in women.
- Evaluation of known or suspected endometriosis.
- Complications from pelvic disease.
- Masses or cysts in the pelvis.
- Undiagnosed pelvic or abdominal pain.
- Fibroid tumors of the uterus.
- Hysterectomy; voluntary sterilization.
- Diagnosis and treatment of an ectopic pregnancy (see Glossary).
- Diagnosis and treatment for a variety of abdominal disorders.

SURGICAL RISK INCREASES WITH
- Obesity; smoking; heart or lung disease.
- Advanced pregnancy.
- Previous abdominal surgery for intra-abdominal infections (such as ruptured appendicitis); previous bowel surgery.
- Use of some prescription and nonprescription drugs. Inform your doctor of any drugs, medications, or vitamin and herb supplements you are using or have used in the last month.

WHAT TO EXPECT

WHO OPERATES—General surgeon, obstetrician-gynecologist, gastroenterologist, or specially trained family doctors.

WHERE PERFORMED—Outpatient surgical facility or hospital.

DIAGNOSTIC TESTS—Before surgery: Blood studies.

ANESTHESIA
- General anesthesia by injection and inhalation with an airway tube placed in the windpipe.
- Local anesthesia (sometimes).

DESCRIPTION OF OPERATION
- A small incision is made in or below the patient's navel. A needle is inserted to inflate the abdomen with carbon dioxide.
- The operating table is tilted to allow the bowel and carbon dioxide to float up toward the chest. The laparoscope is then inserted through the incision and is used to examine the abdomen visually. Occasionally, other small incisions are made in order to insert other surgical instruments.

- The laparoscope is can also be used to used to perform surgeries, including gallbladder removal, appendectomy, tubal ligation, aspiration and excision of an ovarian cyst, and multiple other gynecological procedures.
- The laparoscope and any other instruments are removed, and the carbon dioxide is allowed to escape from the abdomen.
- Small sutures under the skin and an adhesive bandage are used to close the wound(s).

POSSIBLE COMPLICATIONS—Perforation of the bowel or liver (rare).

AVERAGE HOSPITAL STAY—0 to 2 days.

PROBABLE OUTCOME—Expect full recovery without complications. You may experience slight discomfort for 24 to 48 hours. You may have aches in your shoulders and chest from the carbon dioxide that was used to inflate your abdomen. No treatment is necessary. Allow 1 week for full recovery from surgery.

POSTOPERATIVE CARE

GENERAL MEASURES
- Change the adhesive bandage daily.
- Shower as usual. You may wash the incision gently with mild soap.
- If surgery was for sterilization and you were taking birth-control pills, finish your present package; then you no longer need birth-control.
- Use sanitary pad (not tampons) to stop slight vaginal bleeding which may occur after surgery.

MEDICATION—Your doctor may prescribe pain relievers. Don't take prescription pain medication longer than 4 to 7 days. Use only as much as you need.

ACTIVITY
- To help recovery and aid your well-being, resume daily activities, including work, as soon as you are able.
- Resume driving 24 hours after recovery from surgery.
- Sexual relations may be resumed 2 or 3 days after surgery.

DIET—No special diet. You should avoid carbonated beverages for 48 hours after surgery.

CALL YOUR DOCTOR IF

- You develop signs of infection, including headache, muscle aches, dizziness or a general ill feeling and fever.
- You have excessive bleeding or discharge from either the surgical area or the vagina.
- You experience abdominal swelling or pain.
- New, unexplained symptoms develop.

LAPAROSCOPY

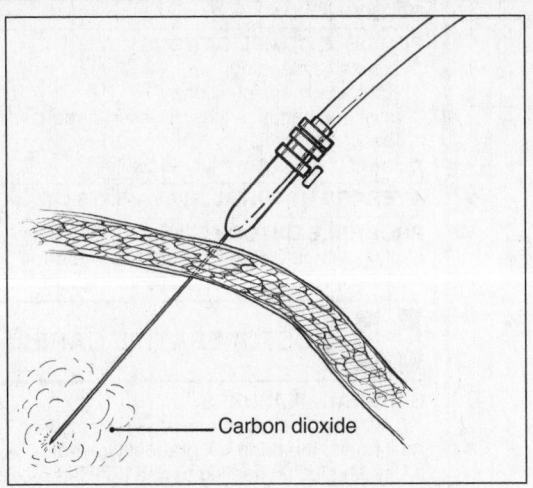

A hollow needle is inserted through the abdominal wall to inflate the abdomen with carbon dioxide.

Carbon dioxide

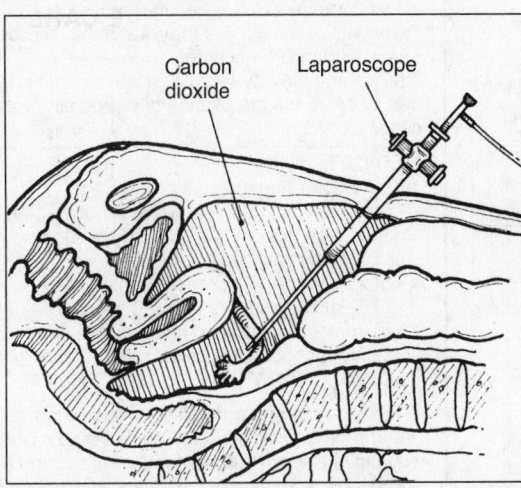

Carbon dioxide

Laparoscope

The laparoscope is inserted through a small incision to allow examination of the abdominal contents under direct vision.

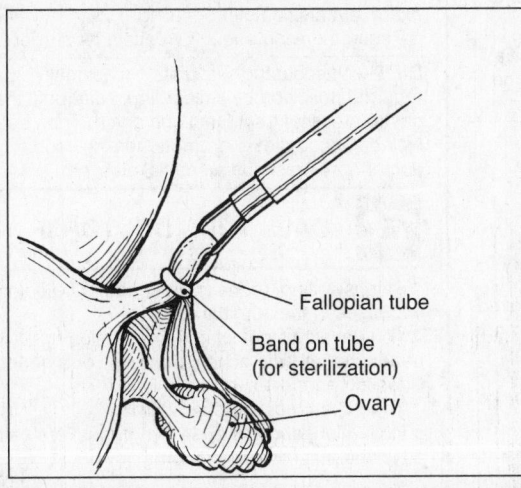

Fallopian tube

Band on tube (for sterilization)

Ovary

The laparoscope may be used to provide passage of other instruments for doctors to perform surgical procedures if necessary.
- After the laparoscope is removed, carbon dioxide is allowed to escape from the abdomen. The small amount remaining will be readily absorbed by the body.
- Sutures under the skin and adhesive bandages are used to close the wound (not illustrated).

SURGERIES

LAPAROTOMY

GENERAL INFORMATION

DEFINITION—Exploratory abdominal surgery to identify, diagnose, or treat a variety of conditions.

BODY PARTS INVOLVED—Skin; abdominal muscles; peritoneum; abdominal organs.

REASONS FOR SURGERY
* Diagnostic examination of the abdominal organs.
* Collection of tissue samples for diagnosis.
* Closure of hernias in the abdominal wall.
* Repair or removal of abnormal tissue.
* Removal of diseased organs.
* Correction of unsightly or disfiguring abnormalities.

SURGICAL RISK INCREASES WITH
* Stress; obesity; smoking.
* Excess alcohol consumption.
* Poor nutrition.
* Recent acute respiratory infection.
* Chronic illness.
* Diabetes.
* History of prior abdominal surgery, particularly if it occurred at the site of the current surgery.
* Use of some prescription and nonprescription drugs. Inform your doctor of any drugs, medications, or vitamin and herb supplements you are using or have used in the last month.

WHAT TO EXPECT

WHO OPERATES—General surgeon or obstetrician-gynecologist.

WHERE PERFORMED—Hospital.

DIAGNOSTIC TESTS
* Before surgery: Blood and urine studies; x-rays of kidneys and chest; ECG; ultrasound; MRI; CT scan; laparoscopy (see Glossary for all).
* After surgery: Blood studies.

ANESTHESIA—Spinal or general anesthesia by injection and inhalation with an airway tube placed in the windpipe.

DESCRIPTION OF OPERATION
* An incision is made in the abdomen. The abdominal muscles are separated, and the peritoneum (see Glossary) is opened.
* Blood vessels cut during the surgery are cauterized or clamped and tied. Wound edges are retracted with a special instrument.
* Fluid in the abdominal cavity is often removed for laboratory examination.
* The abdominal organs are examined. Other surgeries may be performed at this time.
* Samples of suspicious tissue are gathered or diseased areas are treated.
* The peritoneum is closed, and the muscles are reconstructed with heavy sutures.

* The skin is closed with sutures or clips, which usually can be removed about 3 to 7 days after surgery.

POSSIBLE COMPLICATIONS
* Excessive bleeding.
* Surgical-wound infection.
* Incisional hernia; excessive scar formation.
* Abscess formation.
* Bowel obstruction; injury to bowel.

AVERAGE HOSPITAL STAY—3 to 5 days.

PROBABLE OUTCOME—Expect complete healing without complications. Allow about 4 weeks for recovery from surgery.

POSTOPERATIVE CARE

GENERAL MEASURES
* A hard ridge should form along the incision. As it heals, the ridge will gradually recede.
* Use an electric heating pad, a heat lamp or a warm compress to relieve incisional pain.
* Shower as usual. You may wash the incision gently with mild, unscented soap.
* Move and elevate legs often while resting in bed to decrease the chance of deep-vein blood clots.

MEDICATION
* Your doctor may prescribe:
  - Pain relievers. Don't take prescription pain medication longer than 4 to 7 days. Use only as much as you need.
  - Stool softeners to prevent constipation.
  - Antibiotics to fight or prevent infection.
* You may use nonprescription drugs, such as acetaminophen, for minor pain. Avoid aspirin.

ACTIVITY
* To help recovery and aid your well-being, resume daily activities as soon as you are able.
* Avoid vigorous exercise for 6 weeks after surgery. Resume sexual relations when doctor's exam reveals complete healing.
* Resume driving about 3 weeks after surgery.

DIET—Nasogastric suction is occasionally required, followed by a clear liquid diet until the gastrointestinal tract functions again. Then eat a well-balanced diet to promote healing. Your doctor may prescribe a special diet.

CALL YOUR DOCTOR IF

* Pain, swelling, redness, drainage or bleeding increases in the surgical area.
* You develop signs of infection, including headache, muscle aches, dizziness or a general ill feeling and fever.
* You experience nausea, vomiting, constipation, abdominal swelling or severe pain.
* New, unexplained symptoms develop.

LAPAROTOMY

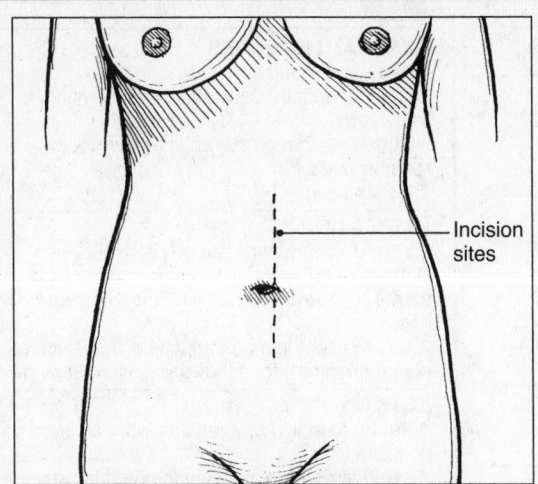

The incision site frequently used for a laparotomy (any opening made into the abdomen).

Incision sites

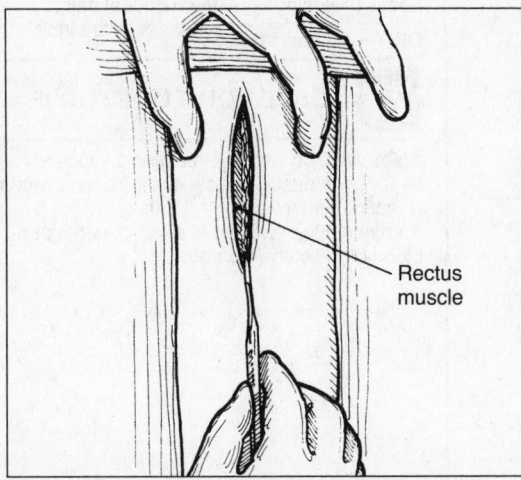

Wound edges are retracted with special instruments.
- Fluid in the abdominal cavity is often removed for laboratory examination.
- The abdominal organs are examined.
- Samples of suspicious tissue are gathered or diseased areas are treated (not illustrated).

Rectus muscle

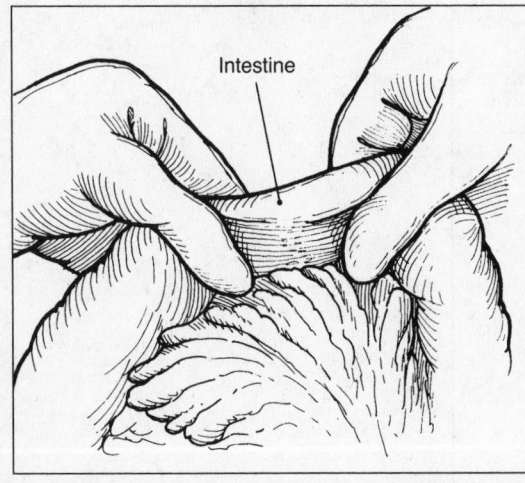

After inspection of all abdominal contents (the intestine is examined here between the surgeon's fingers), the abdominal contents are replaced into normal position. The muscles are closed, and the skin is closed with sutures that can be removed after 3 to 7 days.

Intestine

SURGERIES

LARYNGOSCOPY

GENERAL INFORMATION

DEFINITION—Procedure that allows visual examination and some treatment of the larynx (voice box).

BODY PARTS INVOLVED—Larynx, structure at the top of the windpipe that controls the voice.

REASONS FOR SURGERY
* To remove laryngeal polyps, singer's nodules and other benign growths.
* To remove enough tissue to biopsy.
* To assess vocal cord mobility.

SURGICAL RISK INCREASES WITH—None expected.

WHAT TO EXPECT

WHO OPERATES—Ear, nose and throat specialist (otolaryngologist).

WHERE PERFORMED—Hospital, outpatient surgical facility or doctor's office.

DIAGNOSTIC TESTS
* Before surgery: None.
* After surgery: Microscopic examination of removed tissue.

ANESTHESIA—Local anesthesia spray or general anesthesia.

DESCRIPTION OF OPERATION
* A fiberoptic laryngoscope is passed through the mouth and pharynx to extend to the larynx (voice-box).
* The larynx is examined visually by the operator.
* Specimens may be removed by snare to study for nodules, polyps or malignant changes.

POSSIBLE COMPLICATIONS
* Excessive bleeding.
* Swelling of tissues in the neck.
* Laryngospasm (closing of larynx).

AVERAGE HOSPITAL STAY—Usually no more than 1 day.

PROBABLE OUTCOME—Complete recovery if growth is benign. If growth is malignant, larynx removal may be necessary (see in Surgery section).

POSTOPERATIVE CARE

GENERAL MEASURES
* Keep your head elevated.
* Don't try to talk. Communicate by writing messages.
* Consult a speech therapist if your doctor recommends.
* No smoking.

MEDICATION
* Your doctor may prescribe pain relievers. Don't take prescription pain medication longer than 4 to 7 days. Use only as much as you need.
* You may use nonprescription drugs, such as acetaminophen, for minor pain. Avoid aspirin.

ACTIVITY
* Return to daily activities and work as soon as possible.
* Avoid strenuous exercise that would cause heavy breathing for several days.

DIET—No special diet.

CALL YOUR DOCTOR IF

* You develop signs of infection, including headache, muscle aches, dizziness or a general ill feeling and fever.
* You develop swelling in neck, coughing up of blood or difficulty in breathing.

LARYNGOSCOPY

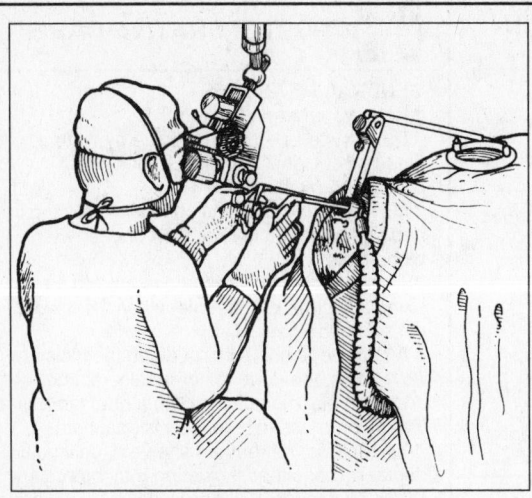

An illustration of a patient lying on his back. Instrumentation is in place and a rigid laryngoscope is passed through the mouth and pharynx to examine the larynx.

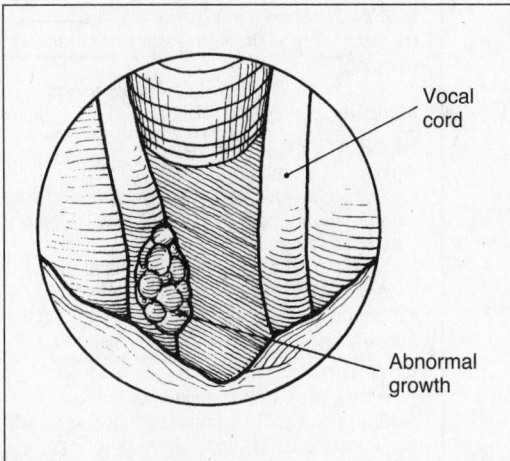

Vocal cord

Abnormal growth

An illustration of an abnormal growth on the patient's vocal cord.

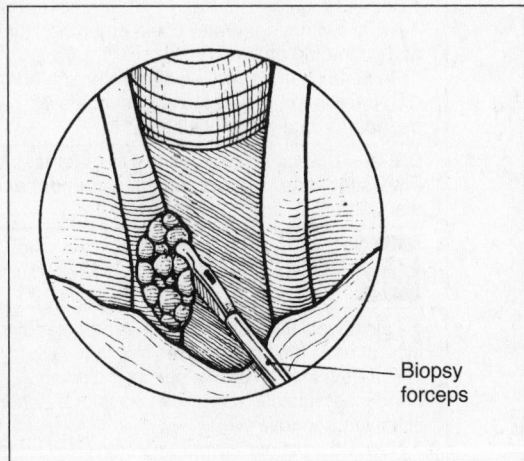

Biopsy forceps

Tissue specimens are removed with biopsy forceps to study for nodules, polyps or malignant changes.

LARYNX REMOVAL
(Laryngectomy)

 GENERAL INFORMATION

DEFINITION—Removal of the larynx.

BODY PARTS INVOLVED—Larynx (voice box); organ at the top of the windpipe that controls the voice.

REASONS FOR SURGERY—Cancer of the larynx.

SURGICAL RISK INCREASES WITH
* Adults over 60.
* Obesity; smoking; poor nutrition.
* Recent or chronic illness; alcoholism.
* Diabetes.
* Use of some prescription and nonprescription drugs. Inform your doctor of any drugs, medications, or vitamin and herb supplements you are using or have used in the last month.

 WHAT TO EXPECT

WHO OPERATES—Ear, nose and throat specialist (otolaryngologist).

WHERE PERFORMED—Hospital.

DIAGNOSTIC TESTS
* Before surgery: Blood and urine studies; laryngoscopy (see in Surgery section); CT scan; MRI; ECG (see Glossary for all).
* After surgery: Blood studies.

ANESTHESIA—General anesthesia by injection and inhalation with an airway tube placed in the windpipe.

DESCRIPTION OF OPERATION
* An incision is made in the neck. The muscles that attach the larynx to the windpipe are divided.
* The blood vessels and nerves that supply the larynx are located and cut.
* The larynx is cut free and removed with surrounding lymph node tissue (e.g., neck dissection) if indicated.
* A tracheostomy tube (see Glossary) is fitted and positioned.
* The muscles and skin edges are closed around the tube with sutures or clips, which usually can be removed about 1 week after surgery.

POSSIBLE COMPLICATIONS
* Excessive bleeding; surgical-wound infection.
* Inadvertent injury to the esophagus or trachea.
* Difficulty swallowing (usually temporary).

AVERAGE HOSPITAL STAY—5 to 7 days.

PROBABLE OUTCOME—Expect complete healing of the surgical wound. Allow about 4 weeks for recovery from surgery.

 POSTOPERATIVE CARE

GENERAL MEASURES
* Keep your head elevated.
* Don't try to talk. Communicate by writing messages. Consult a speech therapist if prescribed by doctor.
* Move and elevate legs often while resting in bed to decrease the likelihood of deep-vein blood clots.
* Treat crusting and secretions around the surgical wound with petroleum jelly, antibiotic ointment and gauze.
* A hard ridge should form along the incision. As it heals, the ridge will gradually recede.
* Use an electric heating pad, a heat lamp or a warm compress to relieve incisional pain.
* Take baths, rather than showers, until your doctor advises that showering may be resumed. When showering, it will be necessary to wear a bib-like cover over the opening to the tracheostomy to prevent water from entering the opening.
* Use a humidifier to add humidity to your home, especially your bedroom.

MEDICATION
* Your doctor may prescribe:
  - Pain relievers. Don't take prescription pain medication longer than 4 to 7 days. Use only as much as you need.
  - Stool softeners to prevent constipation.
  - Antibiotics to fight or prevent infection.
* You may use nonprescription drugs, such as acetaminophen, for minor pain. Avoid aspirin.

ACTIVITY
* To help recovery and aid your well-being, resume daily activities, including work, as soon as you are able.
* Avoid vigorous exercise for 6 weeks after surgery.
* Avoid swimming. Water could enter the stoma and you could drown.
* Resume driving 2 weeks after returning home.
* Rehabilitation may require learning new method for oral communication.

DIET—Tube or intravenous feedings for first 2 days after surgery. Then resume your normal diet gradually.

 CALL YOUR DOCTOR IF

* Pain, swelling, redness, drainage or bleeding increases in the surgical area.
* You develop signs of infection, including headache, muscle aches, dizziness or a general ill feeling and fever.
* New, unexplained symptoms develop. Drugs used in treatment may produce side effects.

LARYNX REMOVAL
(Laryngectomy)

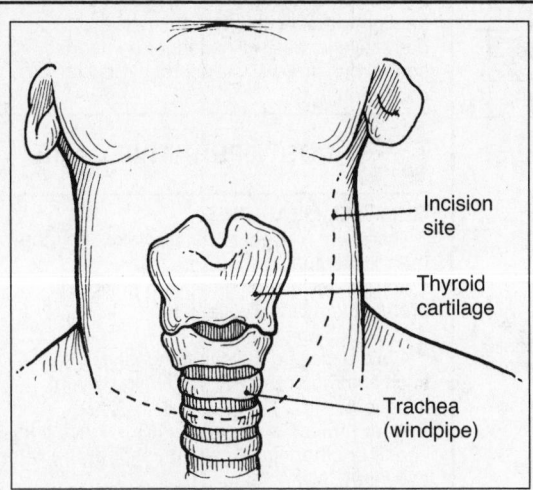

Structures in the neck. The larynx (voice box) is at the top of the windpipe.

Incision site

Thyroid cartilage

Trachea (windpipe)

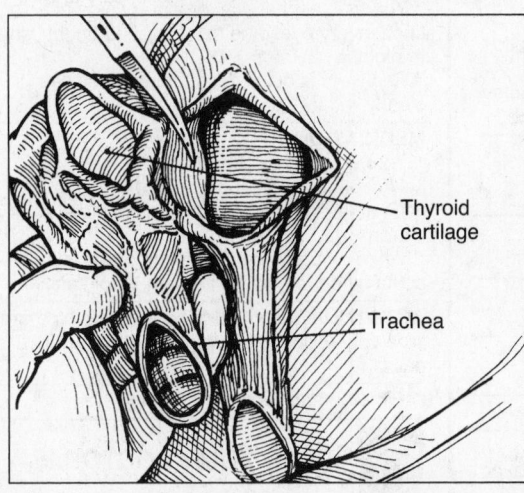

After an incision has been made in the neck, the muscles that attach the larynx to the windpipe are divided.
• The larynx has been cut free and removed

Thyroid cartilage

Trachea

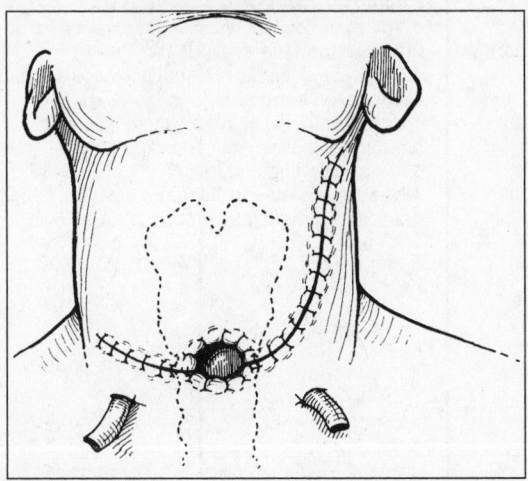

The trachea is sutured to the skin, allowing for a permanent tracheostomy. The muscle and skin edges are closed around the tube with sutures or clips that usually can be removed about 1 week after surgery.

SURGERIES

LASER IN-SITU KERATOMILEUSIS (LASIK)

GENERAL INFORMATION

DEFINITION—Removal of a thin layer of tissue from the center of the cornea in order to change the shape of the cornea and improve vision.

BODY PARTS INVOLVED—Cornea.

REASONS FOR SURGERY—To improve vision in patients with nearsightedness, farsightedness or astigmatism. The goal is to eliminate the need for corrective lenses (glasses or contacts).

SURGICAL RISK INCREASES WITH
* Vascular disease; autoimmune disease.
* Progressive myopia, hyperopia, or amblyopia (lazy eye).
* Women who are pregnant, nursing, or planning on becoming pregnant within 6 months.
* Active or recurrent eye disease, especially glaucoma.
* Diabetes.
* Use of some prescription and nonprescription drugs. Inform your doctor of any drugs, medications, or vitamin and herb supplements you are using or have used in the last month.

WHAT TO EXPECT

WHO OPERATES—Specially trained ophthalmologist.

WHERE PERFORMED—Doctor's office or outpatient surgical facility.

DIAGNOSTIC TESTS—Eye examination to determine degree of correction required.

ANESTHESIA—Topical anesthesia.

DESCRIPTION OF OPERATION
* The surgery involves folding back a thin layer of the outer corneal tissue.
* A thin layer of internal corneal tissue is then removed with the excimer laser. This causes the center of the cornea to flatten (for nearsightedness) or steepen (for farsightedness) or become more rounded (for astigmatism).
* Following removal of the tissue, the flap is replaced. It will usually adhere back in place without the need for sutures.

POSSIBLE COMPLICATIONS
* Infection.
* Difference in power between the two eyes.
* Double vision; hazy vision.
* Increased or decreased sensitivity to light.
* Loss of vision (rare).
* Over or under correction.

AVERAGE HOSPITAL STAY—None.

PROBABLE OUTCOME—Expect complete healing without complications. Usually, corrective lenses will no longer be needed, but sometimes they will still be required with less correction.

POSTOPERATIVE CARE

GENERAL MEASURES
* The entire procedure usually takes no more than 15 minutes.
* An eye patch should be worn at night to protect the eye while sleeping.
* Avoid rubbing the eye.
* Avoid exposing the eye to nonsterile water, such as bath or tap water, to help prevent infection.
* Wear protective eyewear while engaging in sports or other activities (e.g., shop work) where eye injury may occur.
* You may experience temporary side effects such as dry eyes and halos around bright lights at night.
* Recovery is quick. Most patients will see clearly within 1 or 2 days.

MEDICATION
* Your doctor may prescribe:
  - Antibiotics to fight or prevent infection.
  - Anti-inflammatory and moisturizing eye drops.
* You may use nonprescription drugs, such as acetaminophen, for minor pain. Avoid aspirin.

ACTIVITY—Resume driving only after you are sure your vision is adequate (usually within 2 days).

DIET—No special diet.

CALL YOUR DOCTOR IF

* You experience increased pain, redness, or drainage from the eye.
* You have decreased visual acuity or a loss of vision, even temporarily.
* You develop signs of infection, including headache, muscle aches, dizziness, or a general ill feeling and fever.
* New, unexplained symptoms develop. Drugs used in treatment may produce side effects.

LASER IN-SITU KERATOMILEUSIS (LASIK)

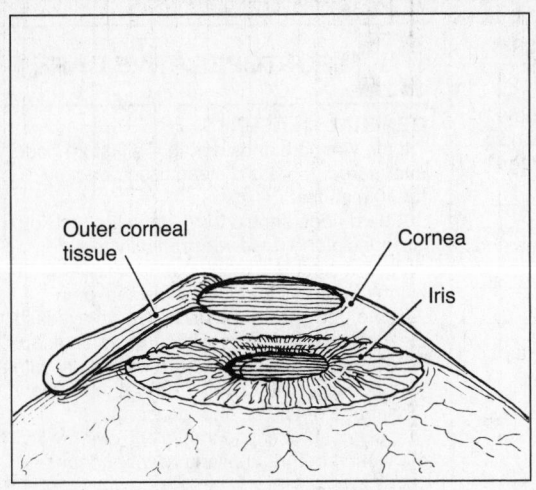

An illustration of the eye, showing a thin layer of outer corneal tissue which has been cut and folded back.

Outer corneal tissue

Cornea

Iris

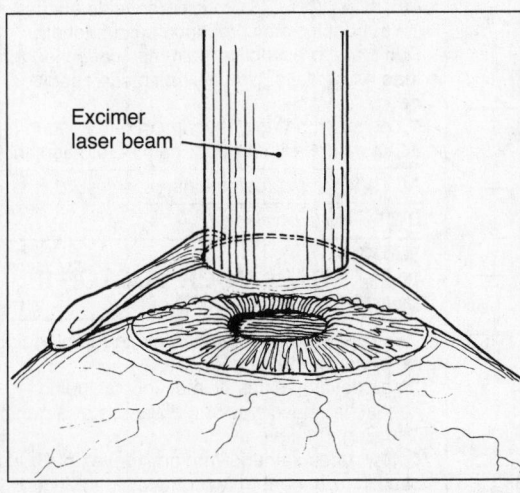

A thin layer of internal corneal tissue is then removed with an excimer laser.

• The laser beam can be used to change the shape of the cornea in a number of ways, depending on the type of refractive error which is affecting the patient's vision.

Excimer laser beam

SURGERIES

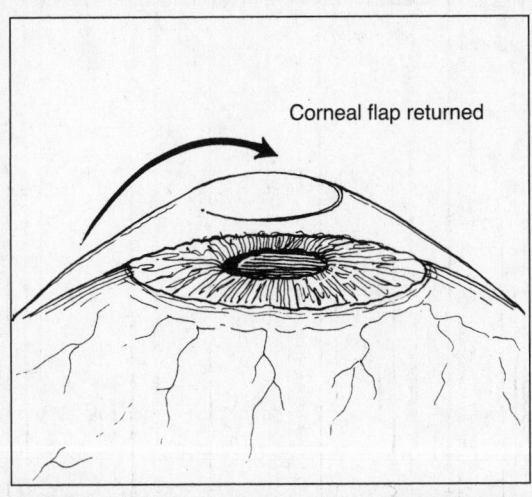

Following removal of the tissue, the flap is replaced. It will usually adhere back in place without the need for sutures.

Corneal flap returned

LIPOMA REMOVAL

GENERAL INFORMATION

DEFINITION—Removal of a lipoma (benign, fatty tumor). Lipomas vary in size. A lipoma can be pea-sized or larger than a grapefruit. Lipomas can be found anywhere on the body, but are most commonly found in the front and back of the chest and abdomen, or in the legs and arms.

BODY PARTS INVOLVED—Skin and underlying tissue, usually on the back, arms and legs.

REASONS FOR SURGERY
• Improved appearance.
• If lipoma is bothersome, e.g., at the belt-line.
• Diagnosis of lipoma is not certain.
• Prevention of cancer (rare).

SURGICAL RISK INCREASES WITH
• Recent or chronic illness.
• Diabetes.
• Use of some prescription and nonprescription drugs. Inform your doctor of any drugs, medications, or vitamin and herb supplements you are using or have used in the last month.

WHAT TO EXPECT

WHO OPERATES—Family doctor, general surgeon, dermatologist or plastic and reconstructive surgeon.

WHERE PERFORMED—Doctor's office or outpatient surgical facility.

DIAGNOSTIC TESTS
• Before surgery: Blood and urine studies; ultrasound; CT scan (see Glossary for both).
• After surgery: Laboratory examination of removed tissue.

ANESTHESIA
• Local anesthesia by injection.
• General anesthesia by injection and inhalation with an airway tube placed in the windpipe (for larger lipomas).

DESCRIPTION OF OPERATION
• An incision is made over the lipoma.
• The lipoma is cut free from surrounding connective tissue and removed.
• The skin is closed with sutures or clips, which usually can be removed about 1 week after surgery.
• Lipomas can also be removed by liposuction (see in Surgery section).

POSSIBLE COMPLICATIONS
• Excessive bleeding.
• Surgical-wound infection.
• Seroma (fluid collects under the skin).

AVERAGE HOSPITAL STAY—None.

PROBABLE OUTCOME—Expect complete healing without complications. Allow about 3 weeks for recovery from surgery.

POSTOPERATIVE CARE

GENERAL MEASURES
• If the wound bleeds during the first 24 hours after surgery, press a clean tissue or cloth to it for 10 minutes.
• A hard ridge should form along the incision. As it heals, the ridge will gradually recede.
• Use an electric heating pad, a heat lamp or a warm compress to relieve incisional pain.
• Bathe and shower as usual. You may wash the incision gently with mild, unscented soap.
• Between showers, keep the wound dry with a bandage for the first 2 or 3 days after surgery. If a bandage gets wet, change it promptly.
• Apply nonprescription antibiotic ointment to the wound before applying new bandages.

MEDICATION
• Your doctor may prescribe pain relievers. Don't take prescription pain medication longer than 4 to 7 days. Use only as much as you need.
• You may use nonprescription drugs, such as acetaminophen, for minor pain. Avoid aspirin.

ACTIVITY—No restrictions.

DIET—No special diet.

CALL YOUR DOCTOR IF

• Pain, swelling, redness, drainage or bleeding increases in the surgical area.
• You develop signs of infection, including headache, muscle aches, dizziness or a general ill feeling and fever.
• New, unexplained symptoms develop. Drugs used in treatment may produce side effects.

LIPOMA REMOVAL

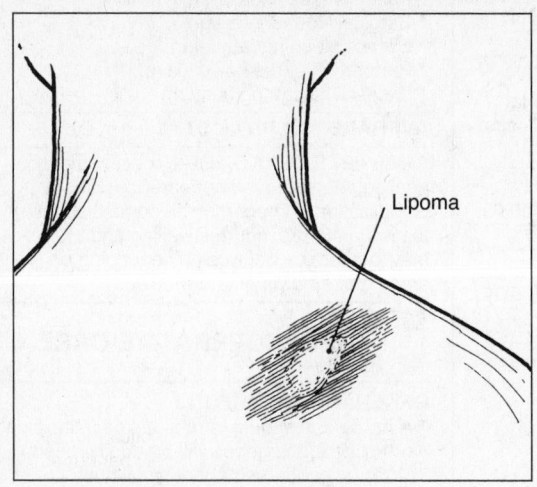

A typical lipoma situated just under the skin. Lipomas may be found in scattered locations over the entire body.

Lipoma

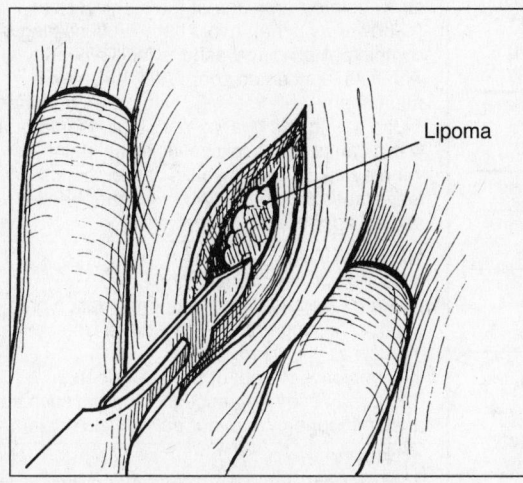

The lipoma is cut free from surrounding connective tissue and removed.

Lipoma

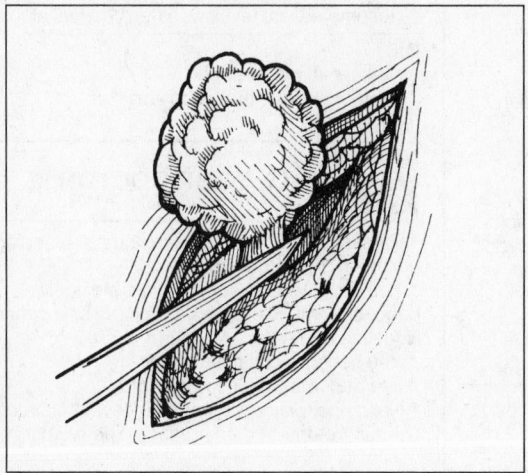

After the lipoma has been excised, the skin is closed with sutures or clips, which usually can be removed about 1 week after surgery (not illustrated).

LIPOSUCTION
(Suction Lipectomy)

GENERAL INFORMATION

DEFINITION—A surgical technique using suction equipment to permanently remove fat deposits, usually from the thighs, hips, buttocks, abdomen or chin.

BODY PARTS INVOLVED—Thighs and hips; buttocks; fat cells of the abdominal wall; chin or other small areas.

REASONS FOR SURGERY—Cosmetic improvement of fat deposits that are resistant to diet and/or exercise.

SURGICAL RISK INCREASES WITH
* Extreme obesity; smoking.
* Recent or chronic illness.
* Diabetes.
* Excess alcohol consumption.
* History of phlebitis.
* Use of some prescription and nonprescription drugs. Inform your doctor of any drugs, medications, or vitamin and herb supplements you are using or have used in the last month.

WHAT TO EXPECT

WHO OPERATES—Plastic surgeon.

WHERE PERFORMED—Outpatient surgical facility, hospital or doctor's office.

DIAGNOSTIC TESTS
* Before surgery: Blood and urine studies.
* After surgery: Blood and urine studies.

ANESTHESIA
* Local anesthesia and sedation for small areas.
* General anesthesia by injection and inhalation with an airway tube placed in the windpipe is usually used for larger areas of fat.

DESCRIPTION OF OPERATION
* The plastic surgeon marks areas to be operated on.
* Incisions (about 1/4 inch each) are made in suction areas.
* A suction tube, with one end attached to suction equipment, is repeatedly pushed through the incision into the excess fat and moved back and forth (20 to 30 times at each site) until the desired amount of fat is removed.
* Each incision is stapled or stitched closed, and a pressure dressing is placed over the wounds.
* Drains may be left in place under the skin for several days following surgery.

POSSIBLE COMPLICATIONS
* Nerve damage.
* Resuctioning in some areas may be necessary.

* Phlebitis (see Glossary).
* Surgical wound infection.
* Excess bleeding; anemia.
* Perforation of the bowel (rare).
* Excessive scarring (keloid).

AVERAGE HOSPITAL STAY—0 to 2 days.

PROBABLE OUTCOME—Expect complete healing and improved appearance without complications. There may be some discomfort following the procedure; swelling and bruising may last for several weeks, depending on the areas and amount of fat removed.

POSTOPERATIVE CARE

GENERAL MEASURES
* A hard ridge should form along each incision. As they heal, the ridges will gradually recede.
* Don't be concerned about small amounts of straw-colored drainage at the surgical sites.
* Shower as usual. Avoid baths until healing is complete. You may wash the incision gently with mild, unscented soap. After showering, replace any wet dressings with clean, dry ones.
* Use an electric heating pad, a heat lamp or a warm compress to relieve incisional pain.
* It may take several weeks or months for tenderness to subside. Allow time for healing and for appearance to improve.

MEDICATION
* Your doctor may prescribe:
  - Pain relievers. Don't take prescription pain medicine longer than 4 to 7 days. Use only as much as you need.
  - Antibiotics to fight or prevent infection.
* You may use nonprescription drugs, such as acetaminophen, for minor pain. Avoid aspirin.

ACTIVITY
* Resume driving 2 weeks after surgery.
* Resume sexual relations when you feel able to.

DIET
* No special diet required.
* Vitamin and mineral supplements (sometimes).

CALL YOUR DOCTOR IF

* Pain, swelling, redness, drainage or bleeding occurs in the surgical area.
* You develop signs of infection, including headache, muscle aches, dizziness or a general ill feeling and fever.
* You become constipated.
* Leg becomes swollen or painful.
* New, unexplained symptoms develop. Drugs used in treatment may produce side effects.

LIPOSUCTION
(Suction Lipectomy)

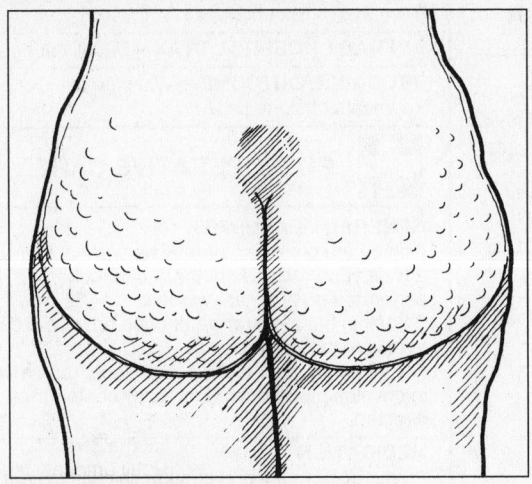

An illustration of fatty deposits under the skin in the buttocks area.

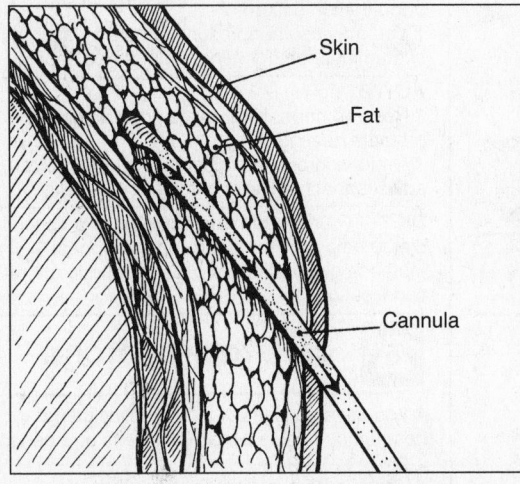

Skin

Fat

Cannula

Approximate 1 inch incisions are made in suction areas and a suction tube with one end attached to suction equipment is pushed through the incision into the excess fat and moved back and forth repeatedly.

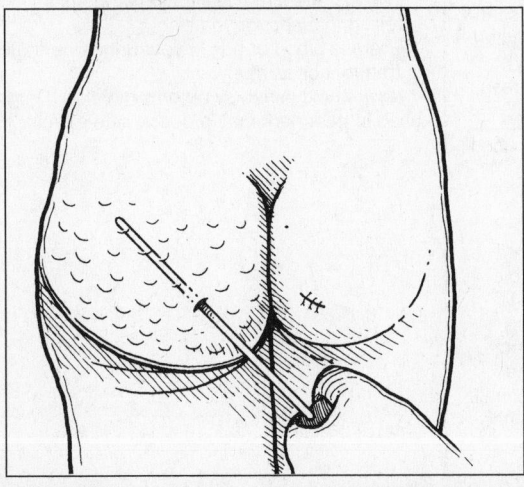

Liposuction complete on the patient's right side and progressing to the left side.

LITHOTRIPSY
(Shock Wave Treatment for Kidney Stones)

GENERAL INFORMATION

DEFINITION—A technique to crush kidney stones inside the body without a surgical incision. These stones are too large to pass by normal elimination. Seventy percent of patients pass stones spontaneously; 30% require urological treatment. This technique is one of the available treatments.

BODY PARTS INVOLVED—Kidney; ureter; bladder.

REASONS FOR SURGERY
* Kidney stones that are too large to pass by normal elimination. They are usually lodged in the kidney or upper third of the ureter.
* Relieve blocked urine flow.
* Decrease chance of infection.
* Relieve pain from kidney stone.
* Decrease chance of damage to kidney.

SURGICAL RISK INCREASES WITH
* Poor heart or respiratory function.
* Presence of a cardiac pacemaker.
* Pregnancy.
* Bleeding disorders.
* Use of some prescription and nonprescription drugs. Inform your doctor of any drugs, medications, or vitamin and herb supplements you are using or have used in the last month.

WHAT TO EXPECT

WHO OPERATES—Urologist.

WHERE PERFORMED—A special center for lithotripsy. Usually in an outpatient surgical facility of a regional referral center.

DIAGNOSTIC TESTS
* Before surgery: Cystoscopy (see in Surgery section), x-rays of kidneys; ultrasound; CT scan (see Glossary for both); blood and urine studies.
* During surgery: Ultrasound (see Glossary).
* After surgery: Blood and urine studies, x-rays, ultrasound (see Glossary).

ANESTHESIA—Usually none. Sedation is used in most cases.

DESCRIPTION OF OPERATION
* For one method, the patient rests in a tub of warm water after being sedated.
* Another method avoids the water by using a membrane coupling device applied directly to the skin overlying the kidney.
* The lithotripsy unit sends out high frequency sound waves directed toward the stone. The shock waves pulverize the stones and the small particles then pass spontaneously in your urine over 2-5 days.

POSSIBLE COMPLICATIONS—May require more than 1 treatment.

AVERAGE HOSPITAL STAY—Usually none.

PROBABLE OUTCOME—Mild pain as fragments of stone pass.

POSTOPERATIVE CARE

GENERAL MEASURES
* If you are pregnant, or may be pregnant, advise your doctor. Lithotripsy cannot be performed on pregnant women.
* Soak in tub of warm water once or twice a day to relieve mild back pain.
* Strain urine for 1 to 2 weeks. Place fragments in envelope to return to lithotripsy center or as directed.

MEDICATION
* Your doctor may prescribe antibiotics to fight or prevent infection.
* You may use nonprescription drugs, such as acetaminophen, for minor pain. Avoid aspirin.

ACTIVITY
* Resume normal activity as soon as possible to promote healing.
* Avoid vigorous exercise until your doctor advises that healing is complete.

DIET—Your doctor may recommend a special diet to help prevent recurrence of stones. Increase dietary fiber and fluid intake to prevent constipation.

CALL YOUR DOCTOR IF

* You develop signs of infection, including headache, muscle aches, dizziness or a general ill feeling and fever.
* You experience, constipation, abdominal swelling, nausea, or vomiting.
* There is blood or pus in your urine or urination is frequent or painful.
* New, unexplained symptoms develop. Drugs used in treatment may produce side effects.

LITHOTRIPSY
(Shock Wave Treatment for Kidney Stones)

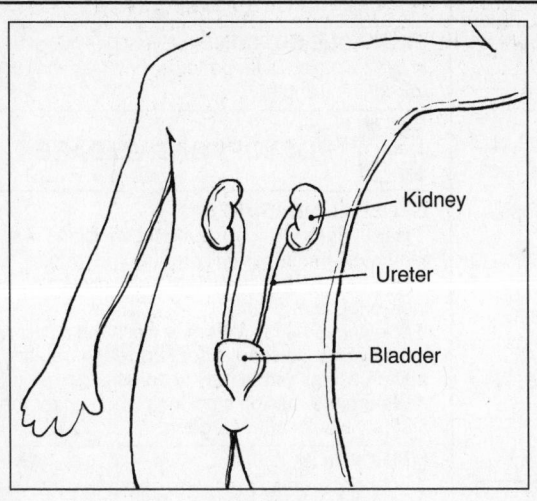

An illustration of the urinary tract.

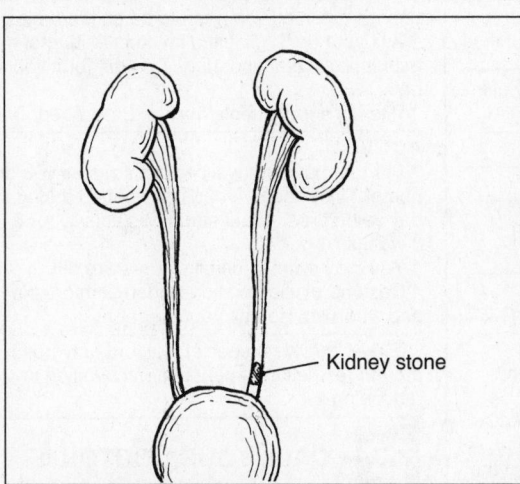

A stone is shown in the ureter leading from the left kidney.

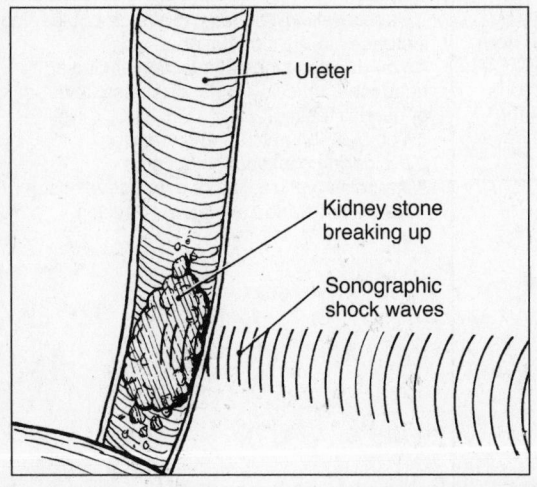

The lithotripsy unit turns out high frequency sound waves directed toward the stone. The shock waves pulverize the stone into small particles which then pass spontaneously in the patient's urine.

LIVER RESECTION

GENERAL INFORMATION

DEFINITION—Surgical removal of a portion of the liver.

BODY PARTS INVOLVED—Abdominal cavity, liver, gallbladder.

REASONS FOR SURGERY—Usually performed to remove an abnormal growth (tumor). May be necessary in trauma to stop excessive bleeding.

SURGICAL RISK INCREASES WITH
* Age.
* Diabetes.
* Poor kidney function.
* High blood pressure.
* Poor nutrition.
* Chronic lung disease.
* Obesity.
* Liver disease such as cirrhosis.

WHAT TO EXPECT

WHO OPERATES—General surgeon, vascular surgeon.

WHERE PERFORMED—Hospital.

DIAGNOSTIC TESTS
* Before surgery: Blood tests, chest x-ray, CT scan, EKG (see Glossary for these 2 terms).
* After surgery: Blood tests.

ANESTHESIA—General anesthesia.

DESCRIPTION OF OPERATION
* The abdomen is opened through a long vertical (up and down) or transverse incision.
* The portion of the liver to be removed is isolated and anatomical planes (sections of the liver) are identified to minimize bleeding.
* Blood vessels and bile ducts are ligated as the liver is separated.
* Up to three fourths of the liver can usually be removed safely with sufficient liver function from the remaining portion.
* Drains are usually left to minimize collections of bile and blood which typically ooze from the raw edge of the remaining liver for several days or weeks after surgery.

POSSIBLE COMPLICATIONS
* Bleeding from the remaining liver.
* Liver failure and or kidney failure.
* Poor circulation to the remaining liver.
* Prolonged bile leak.
* Incisional hernia.

AVERAGE HOSPITAL STAY—Usually 7-10 days with the first day or two in the intensive care unit.

PROBABLE OUTCOME—Expect full recovery in 8-12 weeks. Older patients may take longer to regain strength.

POSTOPERATIVE CARE

GENERAL MEASURES
* Hard ridges will form along the incisions. As they heal, the ridges will gradually recede.
* Use heat on the incision to help relieve incisional pain.
* Shower as usual. You may wash the incisions gently with mild soap. After showering, replace any dressings with a new dry dressing.
* Wear compression stockings when up for the first few weeks after surgery.

MEDICATION
* Your doctor may prescribe pain relievers. Use only as much as you need to be comfortable.
* Ask your doctor if it is okay to take ibuprofen, aspirin, or acetaminophen (Tylenol) for milder pain.
* Vitamin supplements may be prescribed.

ACTIVITY
* Start ambulating (walking) as soon as you are home. Take frequent naps as needed during the day when tired. Avoid strenuous activity for 6 to 8 weeks.
* You may swim once all sutures are out.
* Resume sexual relations when comfortable and when advised by your surgeon.

DIET—Usually no special diet, but may need protein restriction depending on condition of remaining liver.

CALL YOUR DOCTOR IF

* Pain, swelling, redness, drainage or bleeding increases in the surgical area.
* You develop signs of infection, including headache, muscle aches, dizziness, fever, or a general ill feeling.
* You develop nausea and vomiting.
* Prolonged constipation occurs.
* Jaundice (yellow skin or eyes) develops.
* New unexplained symptoms develop.

LIVER RESECTION

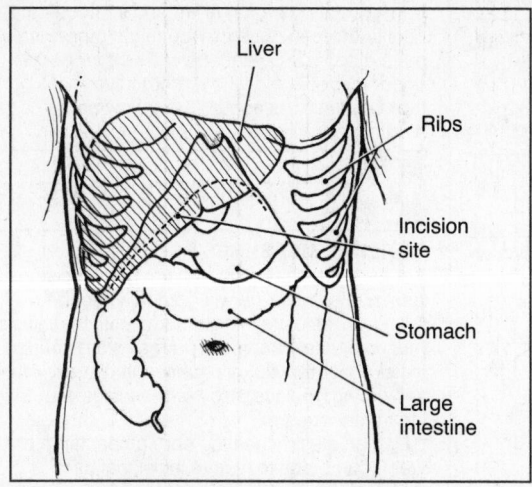

Liver

Ribs

Incision site

Stomach

Large intestine

An illustration of the anatomy of the liver and surrounding structures. An incision is usually made below the right rib margin.

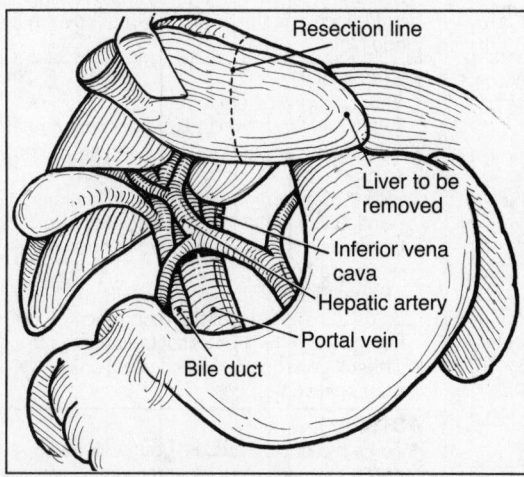

Resection line

Liver to be removed

Inferior vena cava

Hepatic artery

Portal vein

Bile duct

A line of resection is chosen to get adequate margins but maintain circulation in the remaining liver.

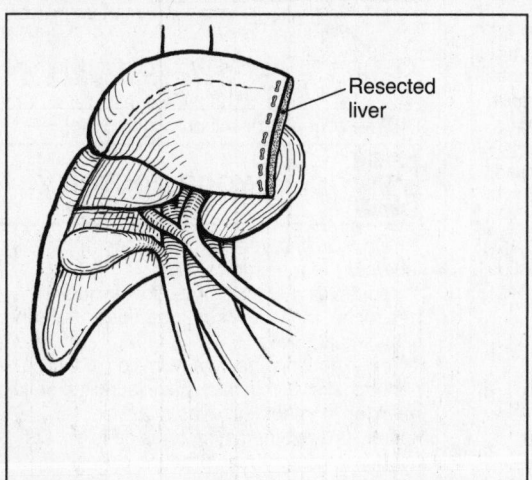

Resected liver

The resected liver margin is sutured to control bleeding.

SURGERIES

LIVER TRANSPLANTATION

GENERAL INFORMATION

DEFINITION—Replacement of a diseased liver with a healthy liver obtained from a donor with compatible immunological characteristics. In some cases, a segment of the liver of a living, related donor may be used.

BODY PARTS INVOLVED—Diseased or abnormal liver; healthy donor liver; blood vessels and bile ducts connected to liver.

REASONS FOR SURGERY—End-stage liver failure from liver cancer or other liver disease, such as chronic hepatitis or primary biliary cirrhosis (see Glossary for both).

SURGICAL RISK INCREASES WITH
* Adults over 60; infants.
* Obesity; smoking; poor nutrition.
* Excess alcohol consumption.
* Recent or chronic illness; diabetes.
* Kidney failure.
* Use of some prescription and nonprescription drugs. Inform your doctor of any drugs, medications, or vitamin and herb supplements you are using or have used in the last month.

WHAT TO EXPECT

WHO OPERATES—General surgeon with transplant experience and training.

WHERE PERFORMED—Hospital.

DIAGNOSTIC TESTS
* Before surgery: Immune-system and liver-matching procedures; studies of body systems.
* After surgery: Blood studies.

ANESTHESIA—General anesthesia by injection and inhalation with an airway tube placed in the windpipe.

DESCRIPTION OF OPERATION
* Liver is removed from donor, then chilled and preserved until surgery.
* An incision is made under the recipient's ribs. The abdominal muscles are separated or split, and the peritoneal cavity is opened.
* The liver and its bile ducts are isolated.
* The liver is cut free and removed. The donor liver is positioned and sewn in place. Blood vessels and bile ducts are connected.
* The peritoneum and abdominal muscles are closed. The skin is closed with sutures or clips, which usually can be removed about 1 week after surgery.

POSSIBLE COMPLICATIONS
* Excessive bleeding.
* Surgical-wound infection.
* Rejection of transplant.
* Bile-duct obstruction.
* Recurrence of hepatitis B or C in the new, previously healthy liver.

AVERAGE HOSPITAL STAY—3 weeks.

PROBABLE OUTCOME—A successful transplantation prolongs life and improves the quality of life in patients who might otherwise have died. The 5-year survival rate for people under 60 years old who undergo liver transplantation is about 75%. Allow about 6 months for recovery from surgery.

POSTOPERATIVE CARE

GENERAL MEASURES
* A hard ridge should form along the incision. As it heals, the ridge will gradually recede.
* Shower as usual. Avoid baths until the incision has completely healed. You may wash the incision gently with mild, unscented soap. After showering, replace any wet dressings with clean, dry ones.
* Use an electric heating pad, a heat lamp or a warm compress to relieve incisional pain.
* Move and elevate legs often while resting in bed to decrease the likelihood of deep-vein blood clots.

MEDICATION
* Your doctor may prescribe:
  - Pain relievers. Don't take prescription pain medication longer than 4 to 7 days. Use only as much as you need.
  - Stool softeners to prevent constipation.
  - Antibiotics to fight or prevent infection. Immunosuppressant drugs to decrease the likelihood of rejection.
  - Hepatitis B immunoglobulin (HBIg) or other drugs to help prevent the recurrence of hepatitis B after liver transplantation.
* Consult your doctor before using any nonprescription drugs.

ACTIVITY
* To help recovery and aid your well-being, resume daily activities as soon as you are able.
* Avoid vigorous exercise for 6 weeks after surgery.
* Resume driving when your doctor determines that healing is complete.

DIET—Your doctor will prescribe a diet.

CALL YOUR DOCTOR IF

* Pain, swelling, redness, drainage or bleeding increases in the surgical area.
* You develop signs of infection, including headache, muscle aches, dizziness or a general ill feeling and fever.
* You experience nausea, vomiting, constipation, abdominal swelling, back pain, jaundice; or fluid retention in abdomen, eyes or ankles.
* New, unexplained symptoms develop. Drugs used in treatment may produce side effects.

LIVER TRANSPLANTATION

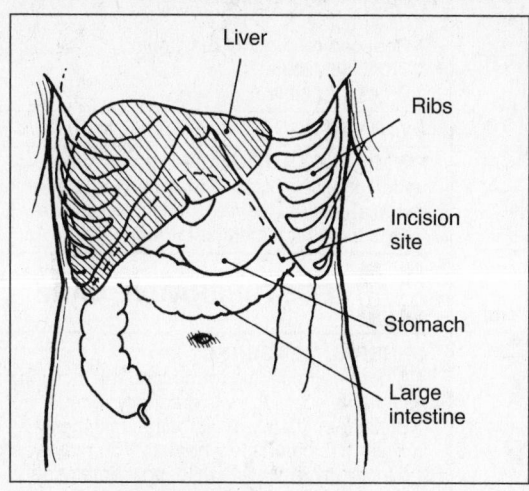

An illustration of the liver showing its anatomical relationship to other parts of the chest and abdomen.

Liver

Ribs

Incision site

Stomach

Large intestine

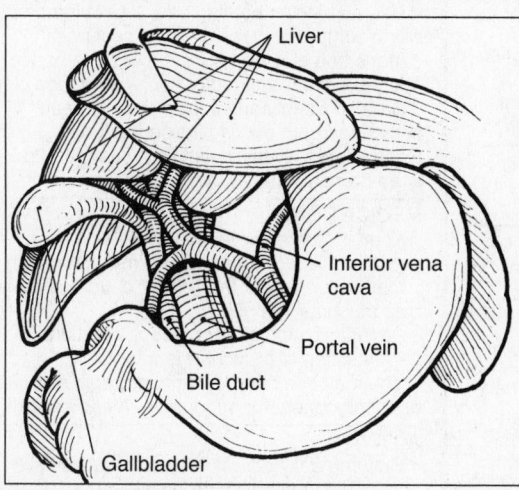

The liver and its bile ducts are isolated, cut free and removed.

Liver

Inferior vena cava

Portal vein

Bile duct

Gallbladder

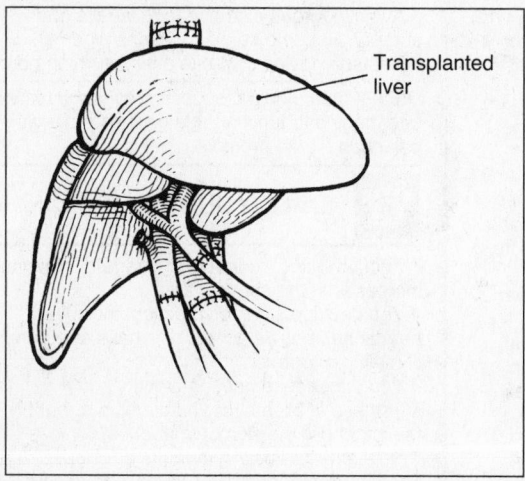

The donor liver is positioned and sewn into place. Blood vessels and bile ducts are connected.

Transplanted liver

SURGERIES

LUNG RESECTION
(Lobectomy; Pneumonectomy)

GENERAL INFORMATION

DEFINITION—Removal of tissue from the lungs. If part of a lung (usually called a lobe) is removed, the surgery is called lobectomy. If the entire lung is removed, the surgery is called pneumonectomy.

BODY PARTS INVOLVED—Lung; bronchial tubes; blood vessels in chest; ribs.

REASONS FOR SURGERY
• Cancer or suspected cancer of the lung.
• Diseased lobes of the lung caused by several chronic conditions, especially bronchiectasis.

SURGICAL RISK INCREASES WITH
• Adults over 60; obesity; poor nutrition.
• Excess alcohol consumption; smoking.
• Recent illness, especially upper-respiratory infection.
• Chronic illness, especially diabetes or lung disease.
• Use of some prescription and nonprescription drugs. Inform your doctor of any drugs, medications, or vitamin and herb supplements you are using or have used in the last month.

WHAT TO EXPECT

WHO OPERATES—Thoracic surgeon.

WHERE PERFORMED—Hospital.

DIAGNOSTIC TESTS
• Before surgery: Blood and urine studies; x-rays of chest and lungs; ECG; CT scan; bronchoscopy (see Glossary for all); pulmonary function studies.
• During surgery: ECG monitor.
• After surgery: Blood studies.

ANESTHESIA—General anesthesia by injection and inhalation with an airway tube placed in the windpipe.

DESCRIPTION OF OPERATION
• An incision is made in the chest. The ribs are spread apart for better exposure to the lungs.
• The blood supply to the diseased area is isolated and tied off.
• The diseased area is located and examined. The growth, the lobe in which it appears or the entire lung is cut free and removed along with lymph nodes in the area (if appropriate).
• A tube is inserted to drain fluid and air from the surgical area.
• The muscles are reconstructed with strong sutures. The skin is closed with sutures or clips, which usually can be removed about 1 week after surgery.

POSSIBLE COMPLICATIONS
• Excessive bleeding.

• Surgical-wound infection.
• Pneumonia.
• Reduced respiratory functioning.
• Bronchial fistula.
• Prolonged air leak.

AVERAGE HOSPITAL STAY—7 to 10 days.

PROBABLE OUTCOME—In some cases, underlying lung disease may be cured. In other cases, quality of life may be improved. Allow 6 weeks to several months for recovery.

POSTOPERATIVE CARE

GENERAL MEASURES
• A hard ridge should form along the incision. As it heals, the ridge will gradually recede.
• Shower as usual. Avoid baths until the incision has completely healed. You may wash the incision gently with mild, unscented soap.
• Use an electric heating pad, a heat lamp or a warm compress to relieve incisional pain.
• Move and elevate legs often while in bed to decrease the likelihood of deep-vein blood clots.
• Breathe deeply and cough often to keep secretions from pooling inside the lungs. Respiratory therapists can help you learn to keep bronchial tubes clear. Ask your doctor.

MEDICATION
• Your doctor may prescribe:
  - Pain relievers. Don't take prescription pain medication longer than 4 to 7 days. Use only as much as you need.
  - Antibiotics to fight or prevent infection.
  - A vaccine to prevent pneumonia.
• You may use nonprescription drugs, such as acetaminophen, for minor pain. Avoid aspirin.

ACTIVITY
• Resume daily activities as soon as you are able to aid the healing process.
• Avoid vigorous exercise for 6 weeks after surgery. Resume sexual relations when able.
• Resume driving 5 weeks after returning home.

DIET—Clear liquid diet until the gastrointestinal tract begins to function again. Then eat a well-balanced diet to promote healing.

CALL YOUR DOCTOR IF

• Pain, swelling, redness, drainage or bleeding increases in the surgical area.
• You develop signs of infection, including headache, muscle aches, dizziness or a general ill feeling and fever.
• You experience nausea, vomiting or shortness of breath, or you develop a "bubbly" feeling under the skin of your chest.
• New, unexplained symptoms develop. Drugs used in treatment may produce side effects.

LUNG RESECTION
(Lobectomy; Pneumonectomy)

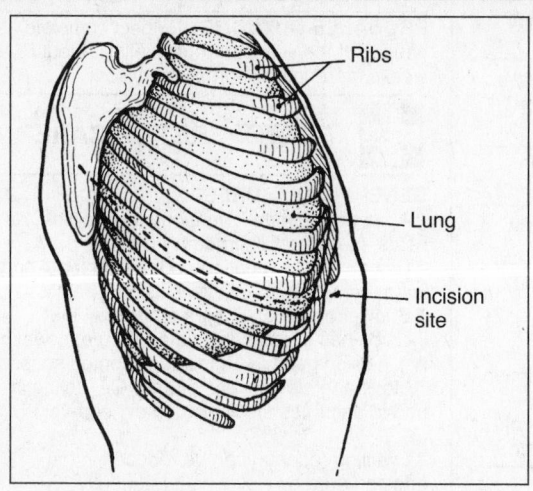

An illustration showing the usual incision site across the chest.

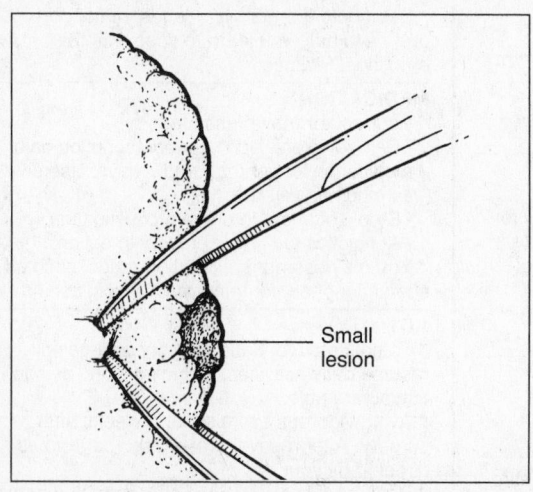

The diseased area on the lung is located and examined. The tumor, the lobe in which it appears, or the entire lung may be cut free and removed.

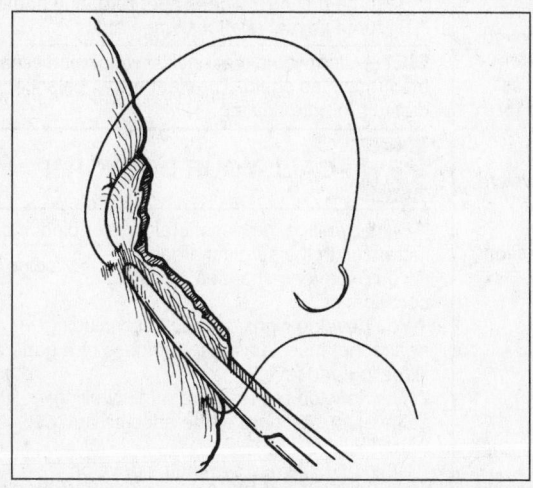

Muscles of the chest wall are reconstructed with strong sutures. A tube is usually left in place to drain fluid and air from the surgical area and to help the lung reinflate following surgery.

SURGERIES

MASTECTOMY, MODIFIED RADICAL
(Total Mastectomy)

GENERAL INFORMATION

DEFINITION—Complete removal of the breast, including the nipple, and removal of axillary nodes.

BODY PARTS INVOLVED—Breast; lymph glands.

REASONS FOR SURGERY—Cancer of the breast.

SURGICAL RISK INCREASES WITH
* Obesity or poor nutrition.
* Smoking; stress; adults over 60.
* Recent or chronic illness; diabetes.
* Use of some prescription and nonprescription drugs. Inform your doctor of any drugs, medications, or vitamin and herb supplements you are using or have used in the last month.

WHAT TO EXPECT

WHO OPERATES—General surgeon or oncological surgeon.

WHERE PERFORMED—Hospital.

DIAGNOSTIC TESTS
* Before surgery: Blood and urine studies; mammogram; needle biopsy (see Glossary for both).
* During surgery: Laboratory examination of removed tissue by frozen section.
* After surgery: Blood studies; laboratory examination of removed tissue.

ANESTHESIA—General anesthesia by injection and inhalation with an airway tube placed in the windpipe.

DESCRIPTION OF OPERATION
* An incision is made encompassing the entire breast.
* The underlying tissue is cut free and removed in one piece, along with the lymph glands from the armpit. Bleeding is controlled with sutures and electrocauterization. A tube is inserted for drainage, and will be left in place for 1 to 2 weeks.
* The skin is closed with sutures or clips, which usually can be removed about 1 week after surgery.
* See Breast Reconstruction in Surgery section.

POSSIBLE COMPLICATIONS
* Excessive bleeding.
* Surgical-wound infection.
* Depression.
* Accumulation of blood or serum under the skin in the surgical area.
* Limited shoulder motion; nerve damage.
* Lymphedema (see Glossary).
* Skin loss over mastectomy site.

AVERAGE HOSPITAL STAY—0 to 2 days.

PROBABLE OUTCOME—Expect complete healing of the surgical wound. Allow about 6 weeks for recovery from surgery.

POSTOPERATIVE CARE

GENERAL MEASURES
* A hard ridge may form along the incision. As it heals, the ridge will gradually recede.
* Use an electric heating pad, a heat lamp or a warm compress to relieve incisional pain.
* Shower as usual. Avoids baths until the incision has completely healed. You may wash the incision gently with mild, unscented soap.
* Move and elevate legs often while resting in bed to decrease the likelihood of deep-vein clots.
* Swelling (edema) can be reduced in the affected area by elevating it frequently.
* Seek help from family, friends, or support groups to help you learn to cope with the emotional feelings.

MEDICATION
* Your doctor may prescribe:
  - Pain relievers. Don't take prescription pain medication longer than 4 to 7 days. Use only as much as you need.
  - Stool softeners to prevent constipation.
  - Antibiotics to fight or prevent infection.
* You may use nonprescription drugs, such as acetaminophen, for minor pain. Avoid aspirin.

ACTIVITY
* To help recovery and aid your well-being, resume daily activities, including work, as soon as you are able.
* Avoid vigorous exercise for 6 weeks after surgery. After recovery, exercise your arm as directed by your doctor.
* Resume driving 2 weeks after returning home.
* Resume sexual relations when able.

DIET—Clear liquid diet until the gastrointestinal tract functions again. Then eat a well-balanced diet to promote healing.

CALL YOUR DOCTOR IF

* Pain, swelling, redness, drainage or bleeding increases in the surgical area.
* You experience nausea, vomiting or constipation.
* You develop signs of infection, including headache, muscle aches, dizziness or a general ill feeling and fever.
* You develop redness, warmth, swelling, stiffness or hardness in the affected arm or hand.
* New, unexplained symptoms develop.

MASTECTOMY, MODIFIED RADICAL
(Total Mastectomy)

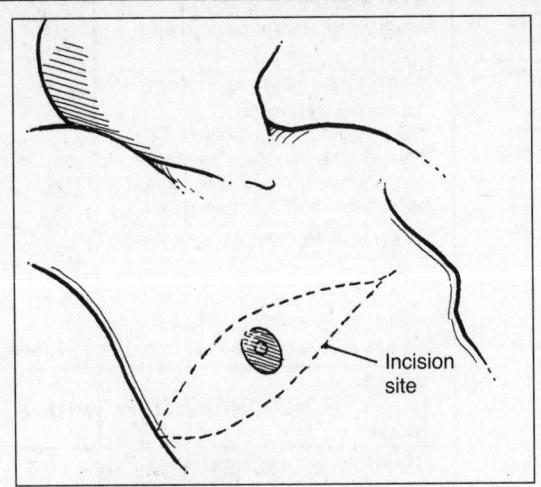

The usual site and elliptical form of the incision to remove the breast and underlying tissue.

Incision site

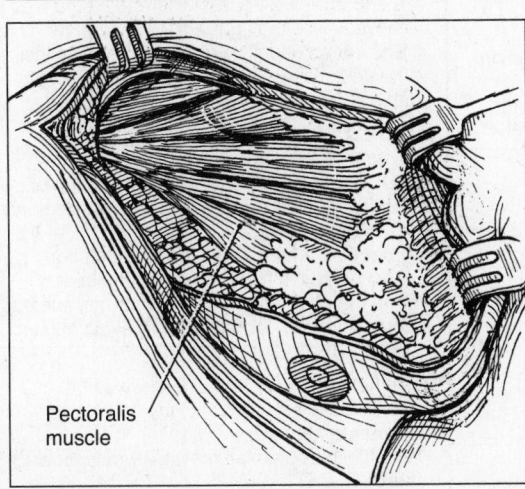

Underlying breast tissue is cut free and removed in one block with lymph glands from the armpit. The underlying muscle is left in place.

Pectoralis muscle

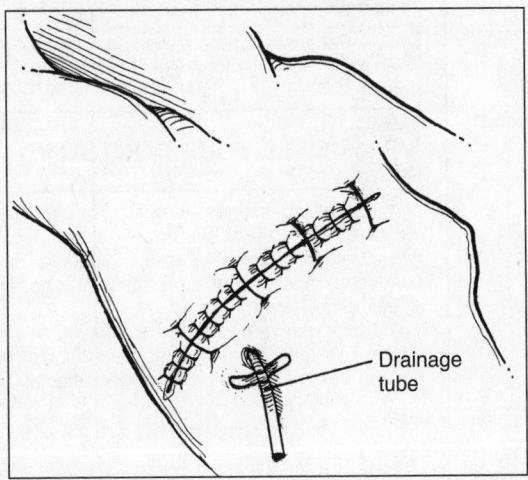

A tube is inserted for drainage. The tissues under the skin are closed with large, absorbable sutures. The skin is closed with sutures or clips that usually can be removed about 1 week after surgery.

Drainage tube

MASTECTOMY, PARTIAL (Lumpectomy)

GENERAL INFORMATION

DEFINITION—Removal of a lump from the female breast that is known or suspected to be cancerous. Lumpectomy is the least invasive procedure for breast cancer surgery, and is the most likely to leave the breast looking normal.

BODY PARTS INVOLVED—Breast.

REASONS FOR SURGERY—Cancer or suspected cancer of the breast. There is frequently more than one option for surgical treatment. Be sure you understand the rationale for any recommended procedure, the risks and benefits involved, as well as any possible alternative treatments.

SURGICAL RISK INCREASES WITH
* Obesity; smoking; stress.
* Poor nutrition.
* Recent or chronic illness.
* Diabetes.
* Use of some prescription and nonprescription drugs. Inform your doctor of any drugs, medications, or vitamin and herb supplements you are using or have used in the last month.

WHAT TO EXPECT

WHO OPERATES—General surgeon or oncological surgeon.

WHERE PERFORMED—Hospital.

DIAGNOSTIC TESTS
* Before surgery: Blood and urine studies; x-rays of chest; mammograms (see Glossary).
* During surgery: Laboratory examination of the removed lump by a pathologist.
* After surgery: Blood studies; laboratory examination of removed tissue; sometimes bone scans.

ANESTHESIA
* Local anesthesia by injection, accompanied by sedation.
* General anesthesia by injection and inhalation with an airway tube placed in the windpipe.

DESCRIPTION OF OPERATION
* An incision is made over the lump to be removed.
* The lump and a small surrounding area of normal tissue are cut free and removed. Bleeding is controlled with ties and electrocauterization.
* It is frequently necessary to perform axillary node dissection in conjunction with lumpectomy. If lymph node dissection is necessary, a separate incision in the axilla (under the armpit) is made to sample or significantly remove the axillary lymph nodes.

* The skin is closed with sutures or clips, which usually can be removed about 1 week after surgery.

POSSIBLE COMPLICATIONS
* Excessive bleeding.
* Surgical-wound infection.
* Need for additional surgery (sometimes).
* Lymphedema (see Glossary), if axillary lymph node dissection was performed.

AVERAGE HOSPITAL STAY—0 to 2 days.

PROBABLE OUTCOME—Expect complete healing of the surgical wound. Allow about 2 weeks for recovery from surgery. Radiation therapy is often required to complete treatment.

POSTOPERATIVE CARE

GENERAL MEASURES
* A firm area will appear where the lump was removed. This may remain for several months.
* Shower as usual. Avoid baths until the incision is healed. You may wash the incision gently with mild, unscented soap.

MEDICATION
* Your doctor may prescribe:
  - Pain relievers. Don't take prescription pain medication longer than 4 to 7 days. Use only as much as you need.
  - Stool softeners to prevent constipation.
  - Antibiotics to fight or prevent infection.
* You may use nonprescription drugs, such as acetaminophen, for minor pain. Avoid aspirin.

ACTIVITY
* To help recovery and aid your well-being, resume daily activities, including work, as soon as you are able.
* Avoid vigorous exercise for 2 weeks after surgery.
* Resume driving 1 day after returning home.

DIET—Eat lightly for the remainder of the day Then eat a well-balanced diet to promote healing.

CALL YOUR DOCTOR IF

* Pain, swelling, redness, drainage or bleeding increases in the surgical area.
* You develop signs of infection, including headache, muscle aches, dizziness or a general ill feeling and fever.
* You experience nausea or vomiting.
* New, unexplained symptoms develop. Drugs used in treatment may produce side effects.

MASTECTOMY, PARTIAL
(Lumpectomy)

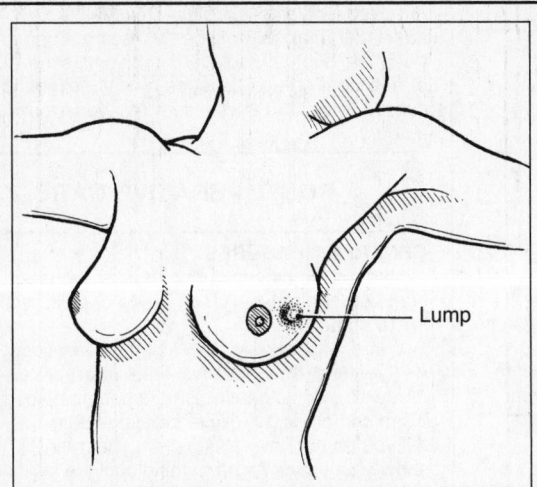

A breast lump in a typical location.

Lump

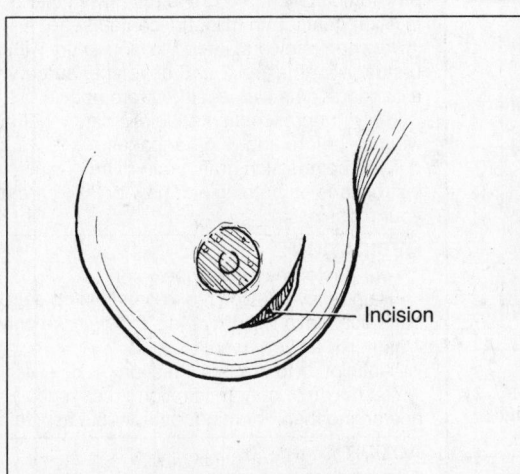

After the skin has been incised, the lump and a small surrounding area of normal tissue are cut free.

Incision

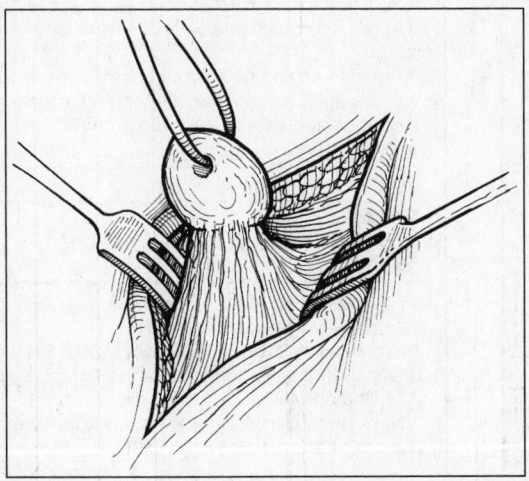

The lump is removed. Afterwards, the remaining breast is carefully palpated for any additional suspicious areas or suspicious lymph nodes.

SURGERIES

MELANOMA REMOVAL

GENERAL INFORMATION

DEFINITION—Removal of any lesion on the skin that might be malignant melanoma, the most dangerous form of skin cancer.

BODY PARTS INVOLVED—Skin.

REASONS FOR SURGERY—Treatment of malignant melanoma.

SURGICAL RISK INCREASES WITH
- Obesity; smoking; poor nutrition.
- Recent or chronic illness.
- Diabetes.
- Use of some prescription and nonprescription drugs. Inform your doctor of any drugs, medications, or vitamin and herb supplements you are using or have used in the last month.

WHAT TO EXPECT

WHO OPERATES—General surgeon, dermatologist or plastic and reconstructive surgeon.

WHERE PERFORMED—Hospital or outpatient surgical facility.

DIAGNOSTIC TESTS
- Before surgery: Blood and urine studies.
- During surgery: Microscopic examination of skin margins to determine how much skin to remove.
- After surgery: Laboratory examination of removed tissue. Possibly, CT scan; MRI; bone scans; PET scan (see Glossary for all).

ANESTHESIA
- Local anesthesia by injection.
- General anesthesia by injection and inhalation with an airway tube placed in the windpipe.

DESCRIPTION OF OPERATION
- Surgery is directed primarily toward cure and secondarily toward preservation of normal appearance.
- The tumor is removed along with a surrounding portion of normal, healthy skin to ensure complete removal of all cancer cells.
- Skin grafts (see in Surgery section) are frequently needed to close large skin defects.
- The skin is closed with fine suture material or clips, which usually can be removed about 10 days after surgery.

POSSIBLE COMPLICATIONS
- Surgical-wound infection.
- Excessive bleeding.
- Residual cancer due to not removing enough diseased skin.

AVERAGE HOSPITAL STAY—0 to 2 days.

PROBABLE OUTCOME—Expect complete healing of the surgical wounds. Examination of removed skin and tissue may reveal that additional treatment will be necessary. Further treatment such as radiation, additional surgery, or anticancer drugs depends on each patient's case. Allow about 2 weeks for recovery from surgery.

POSTOPERATIVE CARE

GENERAL MEASURES
- If the wound bleeds during the first 24 hours after surgery, press a clean tissue or cloth to it for 10 minutes.
- A hard ridge should form along the incisions. As they heal, the ridges will gradually recede.
- Use an electric heating pad, a heat lamp or a warm compress, to relieve incisional pain.
- If you do not have a skin graft, you may shower as usual. Avoid bathing until the incision has completely healed. You may wash the incision gently with mild, unscented soap.
- Between showers, keep the wound dry with a bandage for the first 2 or 3 days after surgery. If a bandage gets wet, change it promptly.
- Apply nonprescription antibiotic ointment to wounds before applying bandages.
- If you have a skin graft, you will be given instructions on bathing and how to take care of your dressings.

MEDICATION
- Your doctor may prescribe:
  - Pain relievers. Don't take prescription pain medication longer than 4 to 7 days. Use only as much as you need.
  - Antibiotics to prevent infection.
- You may use nonprescription drugs, such as acetaminophen, for minor pain. Avoid aspirin.

ACTIVITY
- To help recovery and aid your well-being, resume daily activities as soon as you are able.
- Avoid vigorous exercise for 2 weeks after surgery.
- Resume driving when your doctor determines you are able; this will vary depending on the size of the melanoma removed and the extent of the surgery.

DIET—No special diet.

CALL YOUR DOCTOR IF

- Pain, swelling, redness, drainage or bleeding increases in the surgical area.
- You develop signs of infection, including headache, muscle aches, dizziness or a general ill feeling and fever.
- New, unexplained symptoms develop. Drugs used in treatment may produce side effects.

MELANOMA REMOVAL

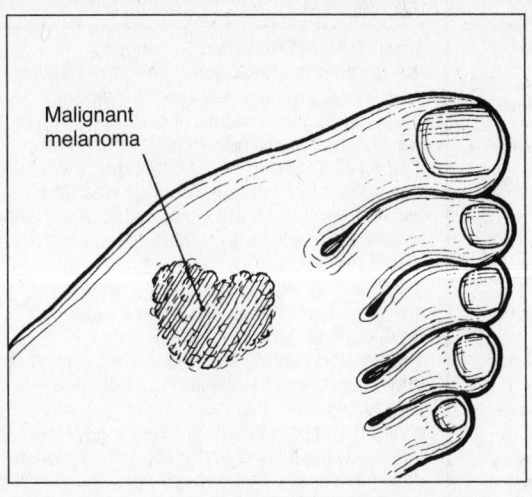

Malignant melanoma

A large lesion on the skin, in this case, on the top of the foot at the base of the toes.
- Melanomas may also appear on other skin locations.

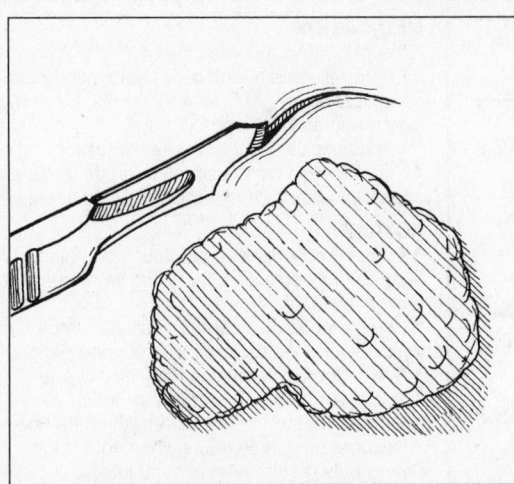

The tumor is removed along with the surrounding portion of normal, healthy skin (usually 2-3 centimeters) to ensure complete removal of all cancerous cells.

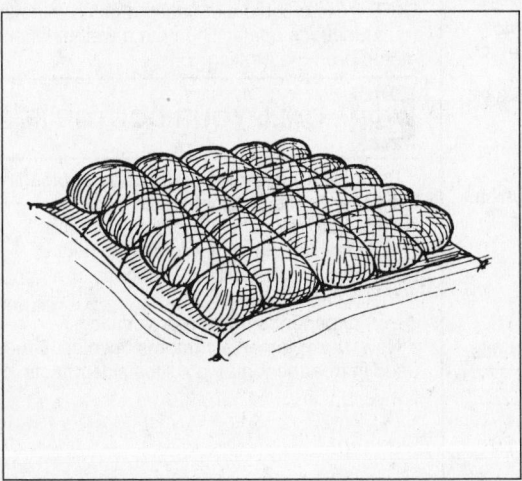

If possible, the skin is closed without grafting, but frequently a skin graft from another site must be used to completely close large lesion sites.
- Sutures used for closure or for skin grafting can usually be removed about 10 days after surgery.

MENISCECTOMY

GENERAL INFORMATION

DEFINITION—Removal of torn cartilage in the knee.

BODY PARTS INVOLVED—Knee and all its parts.

REASONS FOR SURGERY
* Prevention of permanent damage to the knee joint.
* Stop "locking" of knee joint.
* Relieve pain and swelling of knee.

SURGICAL RISK INCREASES WITH
* Obesity.
* Smoking.
* Recent or chronic illness.
* Diabetes.
* Use of some prescription and nonprescription drugs. Inform your doctor of any drugs, medications, or vitamin and herb supplements you are using or have used in the last month.

WHAT TO EXPECT

WHO OPERATES—Orthopedist.

WHERE PERFORMED—Hospital or outpatient surgical facility.

DIAGNOSTIC TESTS
* Before surgery: Blood and urine studies; x-rays of both knees; MRI; arthrogram (see Glossary for both).
* After surgery: X-rays of affected knee; blood studies.

ANESTHESIA
* Spinal anesthesia by injection.
* General anesthesia by injection and inhalation with an airway tube placed in the windpipe.

DESCRIPTION OF OPERATION
* The affected area can be approached by arthroscopy (see Glossary) or by incision into the knee joint. Either approach exposes the injured cartilage.
* If the torn cartilage can be repaired, it will be sutured. Or, if the torn cartilage cannot be repaired, the torn portion will be removed. Any injured ligaments are sewn together.
* The skin is closed with sutures or clips, which usually can be removed about 1 week after surgery.

POSSIBLE COMPLICATIONS
* Excessive bleeding; blood clots.
* Surgical-wound infection.
* Weakened knee joint and subsequent arthritis.

AVERAGE HOSPITAL STAY—0 to 2 days.

PROBABLE OUTCOME—Expect complete recovery without complications. Allow about 6 weeks for recovery from surgery.

POSTOPERATIVE CARE

GENERAL MEASURES
* A hard ridge should form along the incision. As it heals, the ridge will recede gradually.
* Use an electric heating pad, a heat lamp or a warm compress to relieve incisional pain.
* Shower as usual. Avoid baths until the incision has completely healed. You may wash the incision gently with mild, unscented soap. After showering, replace any wet dressings with clean, dry ones.
* Use an ice bag on the knee to reduce swelling. The ice bag should be used for 20 minutes, 4 to 5 times a day.
* Move and elevate legs often while resting in bed to decrease the likelihood of deep-vein blood clots.
* When sleeping or sitting, keep the affected leg elevated with pillows under the foot or blocks under the bed to help reduce pain and swelling.

MEDICATION
* Your doctor may prescribe:
  - Pain relievers. Don't take prescription pain medication longer than 4 to 7 days. Use only as much as you need.
  - Antibiotics to fight or prevent infection.
* You may use nonprescription drugs, such as acetaminophen, for minor pain. Avoid aspirin.

ACTIVITY
* To help recovery and aid your well-being, resume daily activities, including work, as soon as you are able.
* Use crutches or a cane to walk as directed by your doctor. Don't stand for prolonged periods.
* Avoid vigorous exercise for 4 weeks after surgery. A physical therapist can teach you exercises that will restore strength to the knee.
* Resume driving 3 weeks when your doctor determines that healing is complete.

DIET—Clear liquid diet until the gastrointestinal tract functions again. Then eat a well-balanced diet to promote healing.

CALL YOUR DOCTOR IF

* Pain, swelling, redness, drainage or bleeding increases in the surgical area.
* Toes become cold, discolored or numb.
* You develop signs of infection, including headache, muscle aches, dizziness or a general ill feeling and fever.
* You experience nausea or vomiting.
* New, unexplained symptoms develop. Drugs used in treatment may produce side effects.

MENISCECTOMY

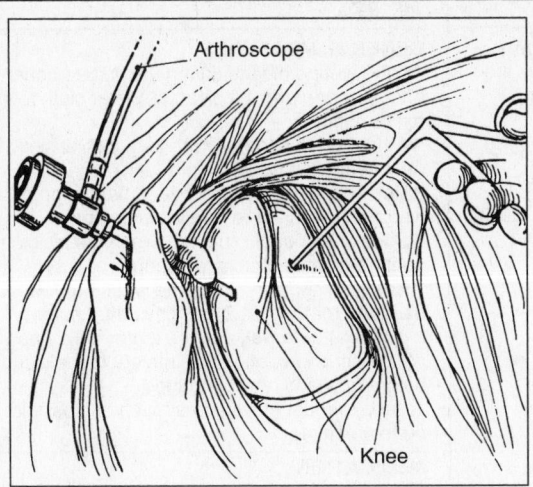

Arthroscope

Knee

An arthroscope inserted into a knee joint. The illustration shows surgical drapes around the joint.

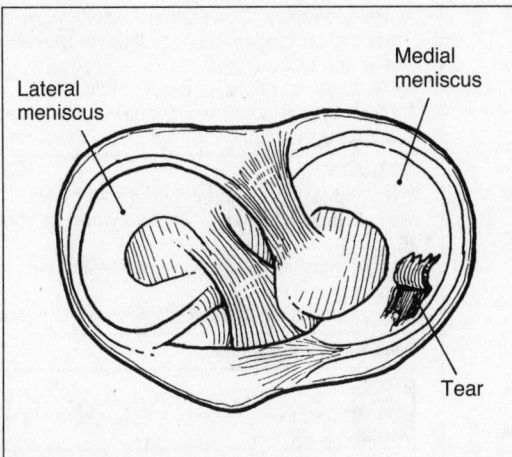

Medial meniscus

Lateral meniscus

Tear

The surgeon can visualize through the arthroscope any tear in either meniscus.

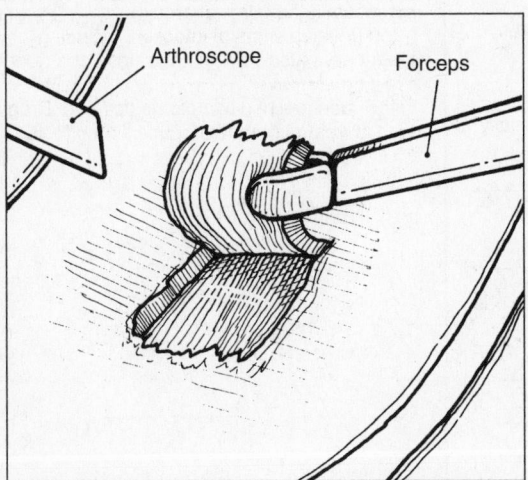

Arthroscope

Forceps

The torn meniscus is removed with forceps and extracted through the opening in the skin.
- Skin is closed with sutures or clips that usually can be removed about 1 week after surgery (not illustrated).

MORTON'S NEUROMA REMOVAL

 GENERAL INFORMATION

DEFINITION—Removal of Morton's neuroma, a small benign tumor in the nerve that serves the toes. Its cause is unknown and it produces severe pain.

BODY PARTS INVOLVED—A small tumor between the 2nd and 3rd toes or the 3rd and 4th toes. It may occur in either or both feet.

REASONS FOR SURGERY—Relief of pain caused by the neuroma.

SURGICAL RISK INCREASES WITH
* Obesity.
* Smoking.
* Poor nutrition.
* Recent or chronic illness.
* Diabetes.
* Use of some prescription and nonprescription drugs. Inform your doctor of any drugs, medications, or vitamin and herb supplements you are using or have used in the last month.

 WHAT TO EXPECT

WHO OPERATES—Orthopedist, podiatrist.

WHERE PERFORMED—Hospital, outpatient surgical facility, doctor's office or emergency room.

DIAGNOSTIC TESTS
* Before surgery: Blood and urine studies; x-rays of the foot.
* After surgery: Laboratory examination of removed tissue.

ANESTHESIA
* Local anesthesia by injection.
* General anesthesia by injection and inhalation with an airway tube placed in the throat.

DESCRIPTION OF OPERATION
* A tourniquet is wrapped around the leg to decrease bleeding in the surgical area.
* The neuroma is located, cut free from surrounding tissue and removed.
* The skin is closed with sutures, which usually can be removed about 10 to 14 days after surgery. The tourniquet is removed.

POSSIBLE COMPLICATIONS
* Excessive bleeding.
* Surgical-wound infection.
* Numbness in toes due to cut nerve (less bothersome for many patients than the previous pain caused by the neuroma).

AVERAGE HOSPITAL STAY—0 to 1 day.

PROBABLE OUTCOME—Expect complete healing without complications. Allow about 3 weeks for recovery from surgery.

 POSTOPERATIVE CARE

GENERAL MEASURES
* If the wound bleeds during the first 24 hours after surgery, press a clean tissue or cloth to it for 10 minutes.
* A hard ridge should form along the incision. As it heals, the ridge will gradually recede.
* Use an electric heating pad, a heat lamp or a warm compress to relieve incisional pain.
* Shower as usual. You may wash the incision gently with mild unscented soap.
* Between showers, keep the wound dry with a bandage for the first 2 or 3 days after surgery. If a bandage gets wet, change it promptly. Apply nonprescription antibiotic ointment to the wound before applying new bandages.
* Keep the foot elevated as much as possible during recovery.

MEDICATION
* Your doctor may prescribe:
  - Pain relievers. Don't take prescription pain medication longer than 4 to 7 days. Use only as much as you need.
  - Antibiotics to fight or prevent infection.
* You may use nonprescription drugs, such as acetaminophen, for minor pain. Avoid aspirin.

ACTIVITY
* To help recovery and aid your well-being, resume daily activities, including work, as soon as you are able.
* Avoid vigorous exercise for 6 weeks after surgery.
* Resume driving 1 week after returning home.

DIET—No special diet.

 CALL YOUR DOCTOR IF

* Pain, swelling, redness, drainage or bleeding increases in the surgical area.
* You develop signs of infection, including headache, muscle aches, dizziness or a general ill feeling and fever.
* New, unexplained symptoms develop. Drugs used in treatment may produce side effects.

MORTON'S NEUROMA REMOVAL

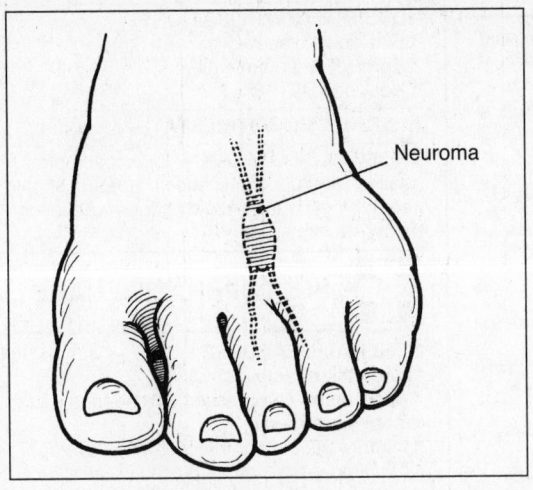

A typical location between the 3rd and 4th toes for a Morton's neuroma (a small benign tumor of nerve tissue).

Neuroma

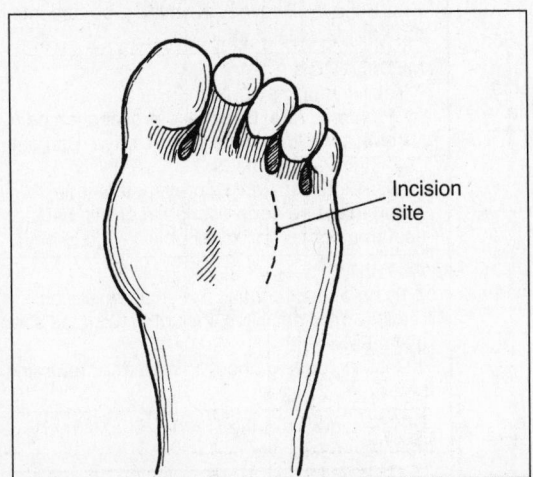

After a tourniquet has been wrapped around the leg to decrease bleeding in the surgical area, an incision is made through the skin.

Incision site

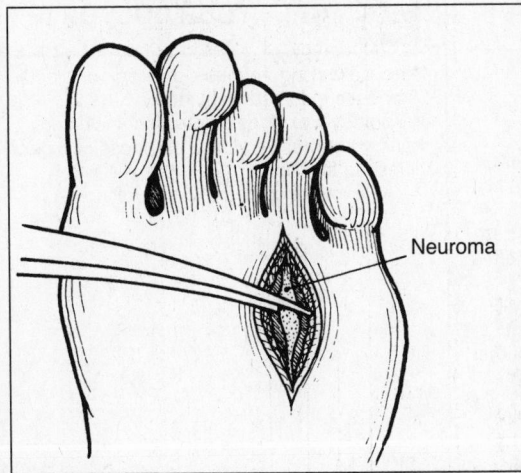

The neuroma is located, cut free from the surrounding tissue and removed.
- After removal, skin is closed with sutures that usually can be removed about 10 to 14 days after surgery (not illustrated).
- The tourniquet is removed to allow normal circulation to the leg and foot (not illustrated).

Neuroma

SURGERIES

MYRINGOTOMY

GENERAL INFORMATION

DEFINITION—Opening the eardrum (tympanic membrane) to remove fluid in the middle ear. This fluid consists of blood, pus, water and debris, and usually collects because of infection or allergy. Frequently, a small tube is inserted in the middle ear to maintain drainage.

BODY PARTS INVOLVED—Eardrum; middle ear; external ear canal (route for surgery).

REASONS FOR SURGERY
* Relief of pain caused by pressure.
* Prevent recurrent infections.
* Prevention of temporary or permanent hearing loss.

SURGICAL RISK INCREASES WITH
* Smoking.
* Recent illness, especially upper-respiratory infection.
* Chronic illness, especially diabetes.
* Previous perforation of the eardrum.
* Use of some prescription and nonprescription drugs. Inform your doctor of any drugs, medications, or vitamin and herb supplements you are using or have used in the last month.

WHAT TO EXPECT

WHO OPERATES—Ear, nose and throat specialist (otolaryngologist).

WHERE PERFORMED—Hospital or outpatient surgical facility.

DIAGNOSTIC TESTS
* Before surgery: Blood and urine studies; hearing tests; tympanogram (see Glossary).
* After surgery: Blood studies; hearing tests.

ANESTHESIA
* Local anesthesia by topical application.
* General anesthesia by injection and inhalation with an airway tube placed in the windpipe.

DESCRIPTION OF OPERATION
* An instrument called an ear speculum is placed in the external ear canal, and the operative microscope is positioned.
* An tiny incision is made around the eardrum, with care taken not to injure the small bones in the middle ear.
* The fluid is drained, and a tiny small tube (about the size of a grain of rice) is usually left in place to continue drainage.
* No sutures are placed in the eardrum. It will heal by itself, if infection is minimal or absent.
* The tube will prevent premature closure of the eardrum and allow the middle ear to heal. The tube will usually fall out by itself in 6 to 12 months. Occasionally, it will need to be surgically removed.

* The procedure is often repeated in the other ear.

POSSIBLE COMPLICATIONS
* Excessive bleeding.
* Surgical-wound infection.
* Hearing loss.

AVERAGE HOSPITAL STAY—0 to 1 day.

PROBABLE OUTCOME—Expect complete healing without complications. Hearing should improve noticeably. Allow about 4 weeks for recovery from surgery.

POSTOPERATIVE CARE

GENERAL MEASURES
* Keep the ear dry.
* Apply warm compresses or a heating pad to relieve discomfort.
* If future middle ear infections do develop, medicated drops can be placed in the ear canal where they will flow through the tube and into the ear to treat the infection.

MEDICATION
* Your doctor may prescribe:
  - Pain relievers. Don't take prescription pain medication longer than 4 to 7 days. Use only as much as you need.
  - Antibiotics to fight or prevent infection.
* You may use nonprescription drugs, such as acetaminophen, for minor pain. Avoid aspirin.

ACTIVITY
* To help recovery and aid your well-being, resume daily activities, including work, as soon as you are able.
* Resume driving about 1 week after returning home.

DIET—Liquid diet the first day after surgery, then no special diet.

CALL YOUR DOCTOR IF

* Pain, swelling, redness, drainage or bleeding increases in the surgical area.
* You develop signs of infection, including headache, muscle aches, dizziness or a general ill feeling and fever.
* You experience nausea or vomiting.

MYRINGOTOMY

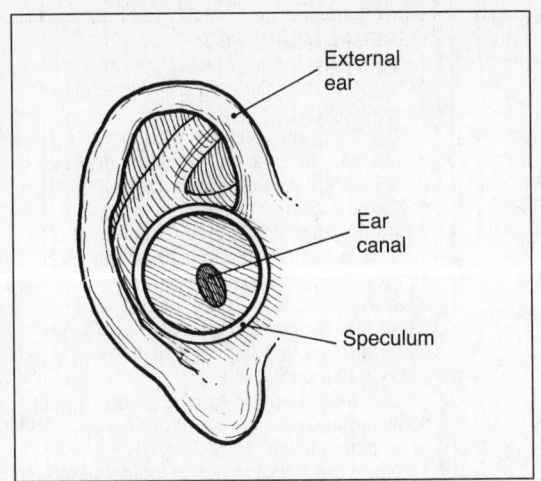

An illustration of parts of the ear, including cartilage and skin of the external ear. The ear canal, which goes from the outside inward to reach the eardrum, can be seen through a speculum inserted into the ear canal.

External ear

Ear canal

Speculum

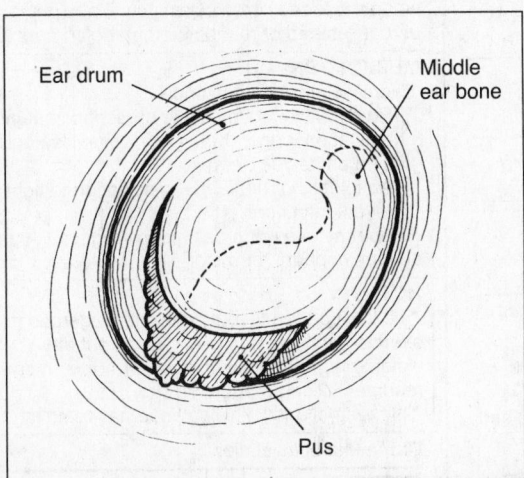

A tiny incision is made in a low section of the eardrum allowing fluid to drain.

Ear drum

Middle ear bone

Pus

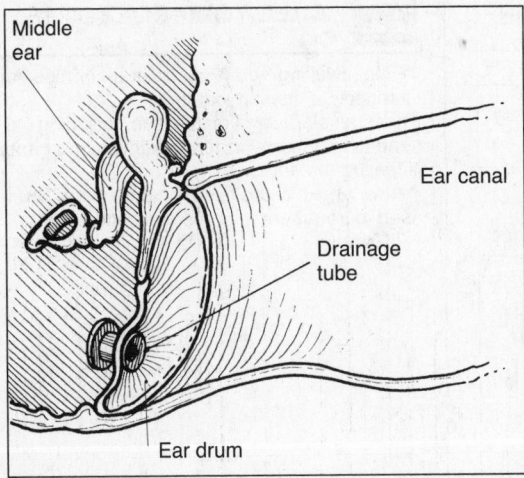

A drainage tube is usually left in place to continue drainage.
- No sutures are placed in the eardrum; it will heal by itself if infection is minimal or absent.
- The tubes will prevent premature closure of the eardrum and allow the middle ear to heal. Usually the tubes will come out by themselves 6 to 12 months following surgery.

Middle ear

Ear canal

Drainage tube

Ear drum

SURGERIES

NAIL REMOVAL

 GENERAL INFORMATION

DEFINITION—Removal of part or all of a toenail or fingernail.

BODY PARTS INVOLVED—Toenail, usually in the big toe; any fingernail.

REASONS FOR SURGERY
• Relief of painful symptoms of an ingrown toenail or fingernail, with or without an infection.
• Nails may be removed due to injury (with part of the nail torn away); splinters that cannot be removed without removing the nail; or warts under the nail.
• Nail infection (usually fungus).
• Correction of abnormal nail growth.

SURGICAL RISK INCREASES WITH
• Poor circulation in extremities.
• Diabetes.
• Use of some prescription and nonprescription drugs. Inform your doctor of any drugs, medications, or vitamin and herb supplements you are using or have used in the last month.

 WHAT TO EXPECT

WHO OPERATES—General surgeon, family doctor, dermatologist or podiatrist.

WHERE PERFORMED—Doctor's office or outpatient surgical facility.

DIAGNOSTIC TESTS—None required.

ANESTHESIA—Local anesthesia by injection.

DESCRIPTION OF OPERATION
• A section of skin is cut on the affected side of the toe.
• Part or all of the nail is pulled up along its bed and cut free of its underlying tissue.
• The nail bed along the affected side is scraped.
• A special nonstick bandage is applied tightly to prevent bleeding. Usually, no sutures are needed.

POSSIBLE COMPLICATIONS
• Excessive bleeding.
• Surgical-wound infection.

AVERAGE HOSPITAL STAY—None.

PROBABLE OUTCOME—Expect complete healing without complications. Allow about 3 weeks for recovery from surgery. The nail should eventually grow back.

 POSTOPERATIVE CARE

GENERAL MEASURES
• Keep the surgical area dry until after the dressing is changed for the first time at the doctor's office.
• After the dressing is changed for the first time, you may bathe or shower with the dressing on. After bathing, remove the wet dressing and replace it with a clean, dry one.
• After the dressing is changed the first time, soak the affected area in plain or salt water at 101 to 104F (38.3 to 40C) for 10 to 20 minutes several times a day to reduce pain and swelling.
• Elevate the affected area as much as possible for the first 24 to 48 hours following surgery, in order to help reduce pain.
• If a toenail is involved, avoid shoes that fit tightly, especially those with narrow toes. Wear white cotton socks.
• To prevent a recurrence of ingrown toenail, when the toenail grows back, cut it straight across instead of rounding off at the corners.

MEDICATION
• Your doctor may prescribe:
  - Pain relievers. Don't take prescription pain medication longer than 4 to 7 days. Use only as much as you need.
  - Antibiotics or antifungal medication to fight or prevent infection.
• You may use nonprescription drugs, such as acetaminophen, for minor pain. Avoid aspirin.

ACTIVITY
• Following toenail removal, avoid vigorous exercise until the nail heals. Don't put any weight on the affected foot for 24 hours, then resume walking gradually.
• No restrictions following fingernail removal.

DIET—No special diet.

 CALL YOUR DOCTOR IF

• Pain, swelling, redness, drainage or bleeding increases in the surgical area.
• You develop signs of infection, including headache, muscle aches, dizziness or a general ill feeling and fever.
• New, unexplained symptoms develop. Drugs used in treatment may produce side effects.

NAIL REMOVAL

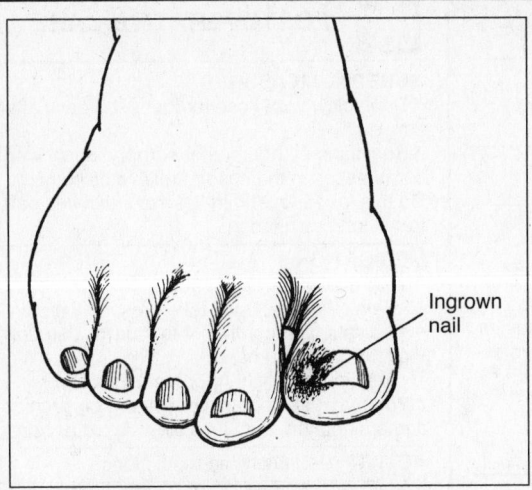

An ingrown toenail in the great toe.

Ingrown nail

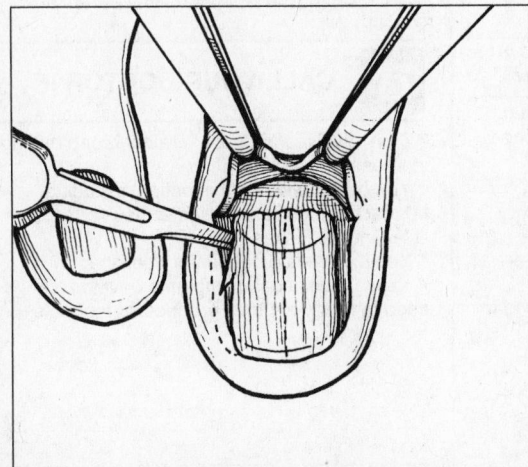

A section of the skin is cut on the affected side of the toe.
- Part or all of the nail is pulled up along its bed and cut free of its underlying tissue.

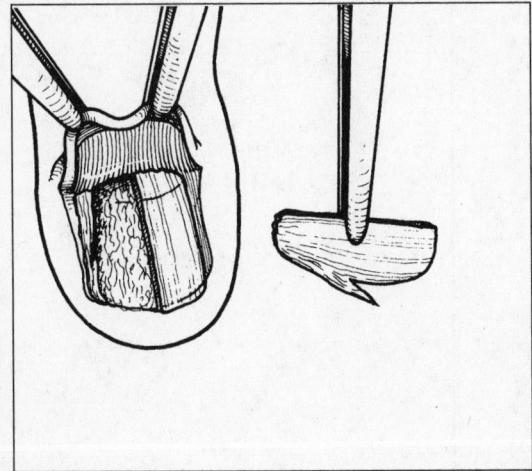

The toenail is removed and the nailbed along the affected side is scraped to prevent recurrence, if possible. The nailbed hardens slowly. A new nail usually grows to replace the removed one.

SURGERIES

NASAL POLYPS REMOVAL
(Nasal Polypectomy)

 GENERAL INFORMATION

DEFINITION—Removal of nasal polyps, accumulations of fluid under the membrane lining inside the nose.

BODY PARTS INVOLVED—Nose and its membrane lining.

REASONS FOR SURGERY—Restoration of normal breathing.

SURGICAL RISK INCREASES WITH—Use of some prescription and nonprescription drugs. Inform your doctor of any drugs, medications, or vitamin and herb supplements you are using or have used in the last month.

 WHAT TO EXPECT

WHO OPERATES—Ear, nose and throat specialist (otolaryngologist).

WHERE PERFORMED—Doctor's office, hospital or outpatient surgical facility.

DIAGNOSTIC TESTS—Often, none required. Sometimes, blood and urine studies are done before surgery.

ANESTHESIA
* Local anesthesia by topical application.
* Local anesthesia by injection.

DESCRIPTION OF OPERATION
* The nose is held open with a speculum.
* The polyps are located, clamped and removed with a wire loop.
* Bleeding is controlled with electrocautery.
* Petroleum jelly and gauze may be applied to the surgical area to prevent bleeding. Your doctor will remove this dressing, usually 3 to 4 days after surgery.

POSSIBLE COMPLICATIONS
* Excessive bleeding.
* Surgical-wound infection.

AVERAGE HOSPITAL STAY—0 to 1 day.

PROBABLE OUTCOME—Expect complete healing without complications. Allow about 2 weeks for recovery from surgery.

 POSTOPERATIVE CARE

GENERAL MEASURES
* Don't blow your nose for the first 3 days after surgery.
* Beginning 24 hours after surgery, apply warm compresses to the nose to relieve discomfort. Do this for 15 to 20 minutes several times daily, for as long as needed.

MEDICATION
* Your doctor may prescribe:
  - Pain relievers. Don't take prescription pain medication longer than 4 to 7 days. Use only as much as you need.
  - Antibiotics to fight or prevent infection.
* You may use nonprescription drugs, such as acetaminophen, to relieve pain. Avoid aspirin.

ACTIVITY—Usually, no restrictions.

DIET—Eat a well-balanced diet to promote healing.

 CALL YOUR DOCTOR IF

* Pain, swelling, redness, drainage or bleeding increase in the surgical area.
* You develop signs of infection, including headache, muscle aches, dizziness or a general ill feeling and fever.
* You experience nausea or vomiting.
* New, unexplained symptoms develop. Drugs used in treatment may produce side effects.

NASAL POLYPS REMOVAL
(Nasal Polypectomy)

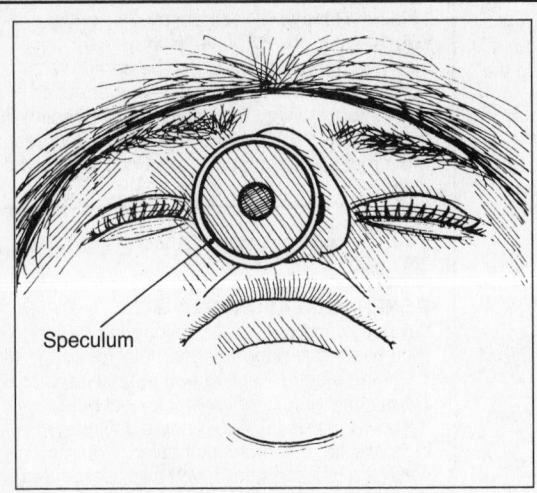

A speculum is used to visualize polyps inside the nose.

Speculum

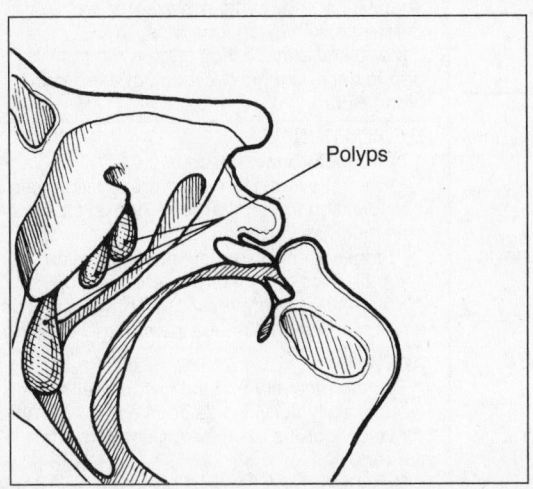

The polyps are visually located by the operator.

Polyps

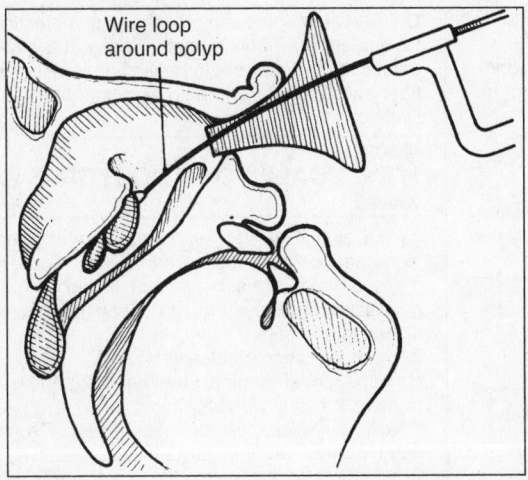

Wire loop around polyp

The polyps are clamped and removed with a wire snare.
- Following surgery, the nose is generally packed with petroleum jelly and gauze to prevent bleeding. This pack will be removed at a later time by your doctor.

NECK, RADICAL DISSECTION OF

 GENERAL INFORMATION

DEFINITION—Removal of the lymph nodes, a large muscle, and some of the nerves along the side of the neck.

BODY PARTS INVOLVED—Neck muscles; lymph glands; windpipe.

REASONS FOR SURGERY—Cancer in the oral cavity or neck, which will spread to other parts of the body if not removed.

SURGICAL RISK INCREASES WITH
• Adults over 60; obesity; smoking.
• Poor nutrition.
• Recent illness, especially respiratory illness.
• Alcoholism.
• Chronic illness, especially diabetes.
• Use of some prescription and nonprescription drugs. Inform your doctor of any drugs, medications, or vitamin and herb supplements you are using or have used in the last month.

 WHAT TO EXPECT

WHO OPERATES—Ear, nose and throat specialist (otolaryngologist) or general surgeon.

WHERE PERFORMED—Hospital.

DIAGNOSTIC TESTS
• Before surgery: Blood and urine studies; x-rays of chest; ECG; CT scan; needle biopsy; open biopsy (see Glossary for all).
• After surgery: Blood studies.

ANESTHESIA—General anesthesia by injection and inhalation with an airway tube placed in the windpipe.

DESCRIPTION OF OPERATION
• An incision shaped like an "H" is made in the neck. Skin flaps are separated from the underlying tissue.
• The lymph glands, muscles, jugular vein and connective tissue are cut free and removed.
• Sometimes, a tracheostomy (see in Surgery section) is performed. In other cases, part of the jaw and tongue are also removed.
• Tubes are left in the surgical area to drain secretions; the tubes are usually removed 3 to 5 days following surgery.
• The connective tissue is closed, and the skin is closed with sutures or clips, which usually can be removed about 1 week after surgery.

POSSIBLE COMPLICATIONS
• Excessive bleeding.
• Surgical-wound infection.
• Restricted breathing.
• Permanent weakness of lower lip.
• Inadvertent injury to the large blood vessels and nerves in the neck, tip of the lung, thoracic duct or laryngeal nerve.

AVERAGE HOSPITAL STAY—3 to 5 days.

PROBABLE OUTCOME—Expect complete healing. Removing tissue in the neck may cause some unavoidable disfigurement. However, some cancers can be cured completely with this surgery. Allow about 4 weeks for recovery from surgery. Depending on the muscles removed, you may have decreased movement in the shoulder area on the affected side.

 POSTOPERATIVE CARE

GENERAL MEASURES
• A hard ridge should form along the incision. As it heals, the ridge will gradually recede.
• Use an electric heating pad, a heat lamp or a warm compress to relieve incisional pain.
• Shower as usual. Avoid baths until the incisions have completely healed. You may wash the incision gently with mild, unscented soap. After showering, replace any wet dressings with clean, dry ones.
• Move and elevate legs often while resting in bed to decrease the likelihood of deep-vein blood clots.

MEDICATION
• Your doctor may prescribe:
  - Pain relievers. Don't take prescription pain medication longer than 4 to 7 days. Use only as much as you need.
  - Stool softeners to prevent constipation.
  - Antibiotics to fight or prevent infection.
• You may use nonprescription drugs, such as acetaminophen, to relieve pain. Avoid aspirin.

ACTIVITY
• To help recovery and aid in your well-being, resume daily activities as soon as you are able.
• Avoid vigorous exercise for 6 weeks after surgery.
• Resume driving 5 weeks after returning home.

DIET—Clear liquid diet until the gastrointestinal tract begins to function again. Then eat a well-balanced diet to promote healing. Increase your fiber and fluid intake to help decrease the likelihood of constipation.

 CALL YOUR DOCTOR IF

• Pain, swelling, redness, drainage or bleeding increases in the surgical area.
• You develop signs of infection, including headache, muscle aches, dizziness or a general ill feeling and fever.
• You experience nausea; vomiting; constipation; abdominal swelling; hoarseness; or have difficulty with breathing.
• New, unexplained symptoms develop. Drugs used in treatment may produce side effects.

NECK, RADICAL DISSECTION OF

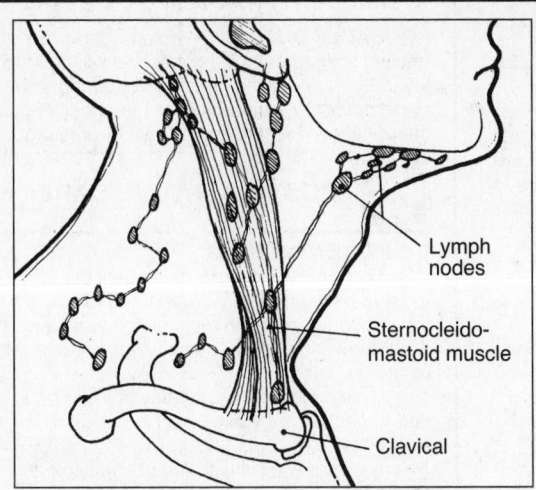

The lymph nodes, muscle and bone in the neck.

Lymph nodes

Sternocleido-mastoid muscle

Clavical

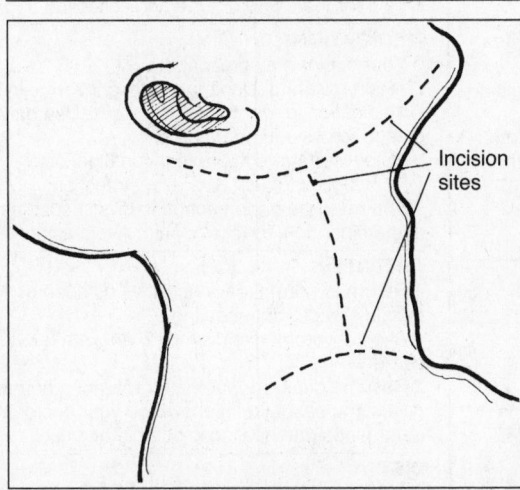

An illustration of the usual incision sites for radical neck dissection.

Incision sites

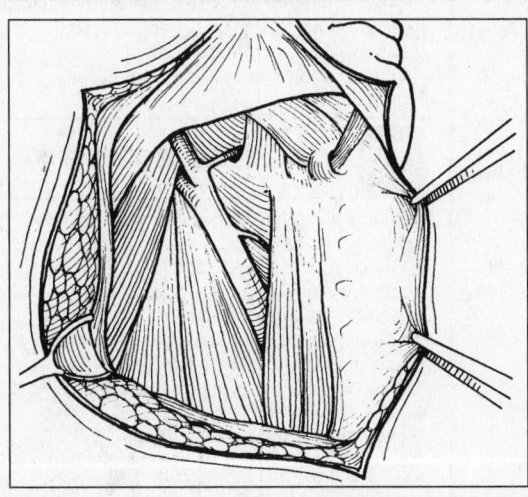

The lymph glands, muscles and connective tissue are cut free and removed.
- Only performed when laryngectomy is done.
- Tubes are left in the surgical area to drain secretions (not illustrated).
- The connective tissues are closed and the skin is closed with sutures or clips, which usually can be removed about 1 week after surgery (not illustrated).

NEPHROSTOMY, PERCUTANEOUS
(Nephrolithotomy, Percutaneous)

 GENERAL INFORMATION

DEFINITION—Creating a puncture wound through the skin and muscles of the back directly into the collecting system of the kidney (where urine is collected before traveling down the ureter to the bladder) and placing a tube for access or drainage.

BODY PARTS INVOLVED—Kidney; ureter.

REASONS FOR SURGERY
- To create an opening into the kidney to maintain temporary or permanent urinary drainage when there is a temporary blockage downstream toward the bladder.
- To provide access to remove or break up stones in the collecting system of the kidney.

SURGICAL RISK INCREASES WITH
- Adults over 60; newborns and infants.
- Obesity; smoking; poor nutrition.
- Recent or chronic illness, especially diabetes or alcoholism.
- Use of some prescription and nonprescription drugs. Inform your doctor of any drugs, medications, or vitamin and herb supplements you are using or have used in the last month.

 WHAT TO EXPECT

WHO OPERATES—General surgeon or urologist.

WHERE PERFORMED—Hospital.

DIAGNOSTIC TESTS
- Before surgery: Blood and urine studies; ultrasound; CT scan; IVP; cystoscopy (see Glossary for all).
- After surgery: Blood and urine studies.

ANESTHESIA—General anesthesia by injection and inhalation with an airway tube placed in the windpipe.

DESCRIPTION OF OPERATION
- An small incision is made, usually in the left or right flank, but sometimes in the abdomen.
- A special needle-like device is passed into the kidney.
- A catheter is passed through the puncture wound into the collecting system of the kidney.
- Stone removal may be accomplished with this procedure, or by pulverization by lithotripsy (see in Surgery section).
- Urine produced by this kidney reaches the outside through the catheter.

POSSIBLE COMPLICATIONS
- Excessive bleeding; blood clots.
- Surgical-wound infection.
- Inadvertent injury to the vena cava or other organs near the kidney.

AVERAGE HOSPITAL STAY—0 to 3 days.

PROBABLE OUTCOME—Expect complete healing without complications. You will need to wear a urine collection bag, either temporarily or permanently, depending on the underlying cause. Allow 4 weeks for recovery from surgery.

 POSTOPERATIVE CARE

GENERAL MEASURES
- Shower as usual. Avoid baths until the incision has completely healed You may wash the incision gently with mild, unscented soap. After showering, replace any wet dressings with clean, dry ones.
- Move and elevate legs often while resting in bed to decrease the likelihood of deep-vein blood clots.
- Your doctor will instruct you in emptying and caring for the catheter tube and collection bag.

MEDICATION
- Your doctor may prescribe:
  - Pain relievers. Don't take prescription pain medication longer than 4 to 7 days. Use only as much as you need.
  - Stool softeners to prevent constipation.
  - Antibiotics to fight or prevent infection.
- You may use nonprescription drugs, such as acetaminophen, to relieve pain. Avoid aspirin.

ACTIVITY
- Return to normal daily activities as soon as possible to promote healing.
- Avoid vigorous exercise for 2 weeks after surgery.
- Resume driving 1 week after returning home.
- Resume sexual relations when your doctor determines that healing is complete.

DIET
- Clear liquid diet until the gastrointestinal tract begins to function again. Then eat a well-balanced diet to promote healing.
- Vitamin and mineral supplements (sometimes).

 CALL YOUR DOCTOR IF

- Pain, swelling, redness, drainage or bleeding increases in the surgical area.
- You develop signs of infection, including headache, muscle aches, dizziness or a general ill feeling and fever.
- You experience constipation, abdominal swelling, nausea, or vomiting.
- The urine in the collection bag becomes red, cloudy, or foul-smelling.
- The catheter tube is dislodged.
- There is very little urine in the collection bag.
- New, unexplained symptoms develop.

NEPHROSTOMY, PERCUTANEOUS
(Nephrolithotomy, Percutaneous)

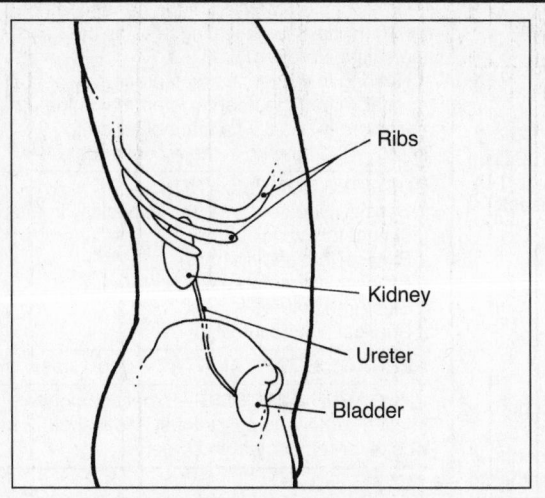

An illustration of a patient's right flank showing the kidney and surrounding structures.

Ribs

Kidney

Ureter

Bladder

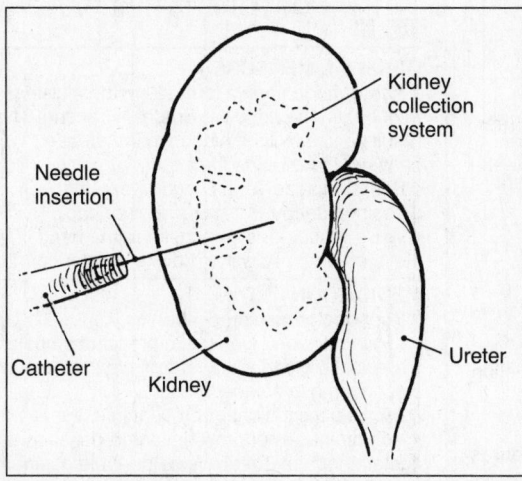

A special needle-like device is passed into the kidney. A catheter is passed through the puncture wound and into the collecting system of the kidney.

Kidney collection system

Needle insertion

Catheter

Kidney

Ureter

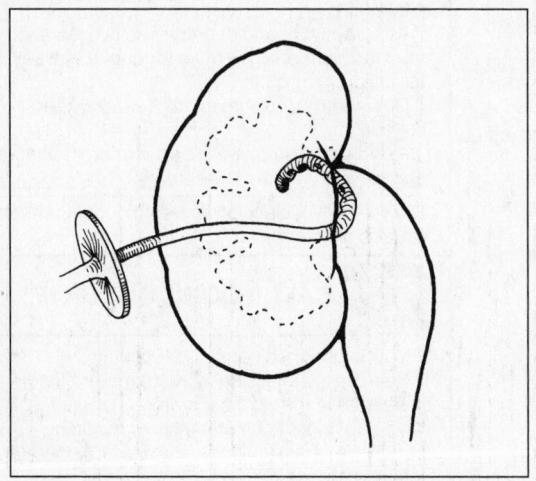

Urine produced by this kidney reaches the outside through the catheter.

SURGERIES

OTOPLASTY
(Ear Plastic Surgery)

GENERAL INFORMATION

DEFINITION—Cosmetic or reconstructive surgery on the outer ear.

BODY PARTS INVOLVED—Ears.

REASONS FOR SURGERY
- Improve appearance of the outer ear (usually to flatten protruding ears).
- To construct or repair a missing or badly damaged ear.

SURGICAL RISK INCREASES WITH
- Previous severe ear injury such as burn or extensive laceration.
- Diabetes.
- Use of some prescription and nonprescription drugs. Inform your doctor of any drugs, medications, or vitamin and herb supplements you are using or have used in the last month.

WHAT TO EXPECT

WHO OPERATES—Plastic surgeon, reconstructive surgeon, or otolaryngologist (ear, nose and throat specialist).

WHERE PERFORMED—Hospital; outpatient facility; well-equipped doctor's office.

DIAGNOSTIC TESTS
- Before surgery: Blood and urine studies.
- After surgery: Usually none necessary.

ANESTHESIA
- Local anesthesia by injection.
- General anesthesia by injection and inhalation with an airway tube placed in the windpipe.

DESCRIPTION OF OPERATION
To flatten protruding ears (several procedures are available, one is described here):
- A flap of skin is removed from the back of each ear.
- The underlying cartilage is remolded and the two edges of the wound stitched together. This brings the ear closer to the head.
- Bulky dressings are applied to the ear and left on for a few days. They are replaced by a headband that is worn for several weeks. Stitches are removed about a week after surgery.
For a missing or badly damaged ear:
- The procedure is extensive and complex and normally involves more than one operation with long intervals of healing in-between.
- A piece of rib cartilage is removed and sculptured to resemble a normal ear.
- The cartilage is transferred to a pocket of skin at the site where the ear will be located. Sometimes a skin graft is necessary.

- Dressings are applied to the ear and left on for 10-14 days until healing is completed and the stitches are removed.
- Hearing in the reconstructed ear may not be normal. When the hearing is normal in the other ear, there is usually no attempt made to improve the hearing in the reconstructed ear.

POSSIBLE COMPLICATIONS
- Sensitivity to cold weather, especially in the first year following surgery.
- Excessive bleeding (rare).
- Excessive scarring (keloid).
- Skin graft failure.
- Surgical wound infection (rare).

AVERAGE HOSPITAL STAY—0 to 1 day.

PROBABLE OUTCOME—Expect complete healing without complications. Allow about 2 weeks for recovery from surgery.

POSTOPERATIVE CARE

GENERAL MEASURES
- A hard ridge should form along the incision. As it heals, the ridge will gradually recede. The resulting scar will be hidden in the crease between the ear and the scalp.
- Bathe and shower as usual. Keep the dressings dry by wearing a shower cap.
- While resting or sleeping, keep the head elevated on 2 pillows to provide greater comfort.

MEDICATION
- Your doctor may prescribe:
  - Pain relievers. Don't take prescription pain medication longer than 4 to 7 days. Use only as much as you need.
  - Antibiotics to fight or prevent infection.
- You may use nonprescription drugs, such as acetaminophen, to relieve pain. Avoid aspirin.

ACTIVITY
- Resume work and everyday activity as soon as possible (usually 5 days for adults, 1 week for children).
- Resume mild exercise 2 to 3 weeks after surgery.
- Avoid vigorous exercise, swimming or contact sports for 6 weeks after surgery.

DIET—No special diet. Eat soft foods if chewing causes discomfort.

CALL YOUR DOCTOR IF

- You experience nausea or vomiting.
- Pain, swelling, redness, drainage or bleeding increases in the surgical area.
- You develop signs of infection, including headache, muscle aches, dizziness, general ill feeling or fever.
- New, unexplained symptoms develop.

OTOPLASTY
(Ear Plastic Surgery)

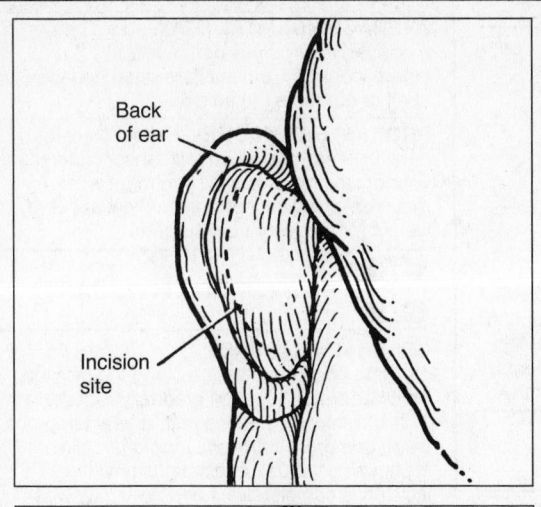

Back
of ear

Incision
site

Anatomy and incision site on the
back of the ear are identified and
marked prior to surgery.

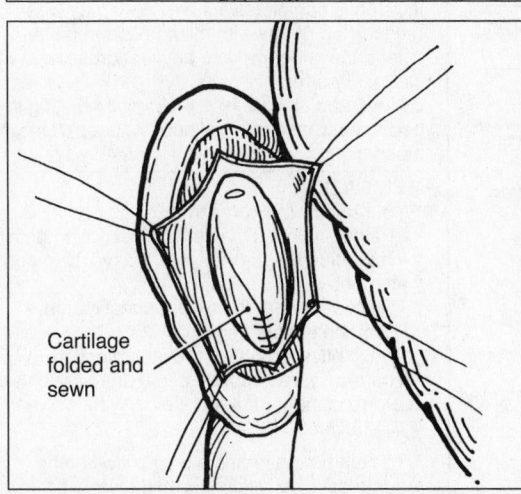

Cartilage
folded and
sewn

Skin is opened revealing underlying
cartilage, which is remolded to bring
ear closer to the head.

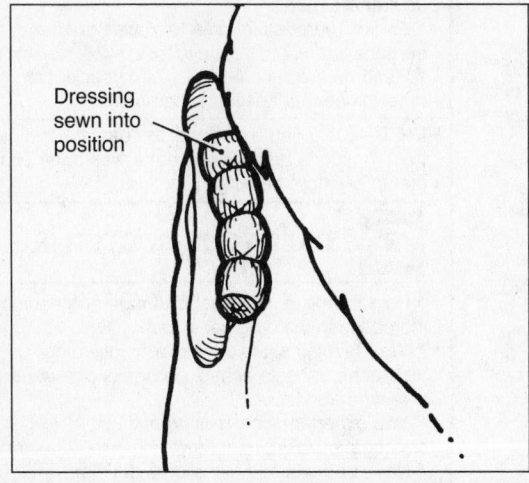

Dressing
sewn into
position

Skin is sewn closed and a dressing is
applied.

SURGERIES

OVARIAN CYST OR TUMOR REMOVAL

GENERAL INFORMATION

DEFINITION—Removal of cysts or tumors on an ovary.

BODY PARTS INVOLVED—Ovary, pelvis.

REASONS FOR SURGERY
* Cancer or suspected cancer in the ovaries.
* Rupture or twisting of an ovarian cyst.

SURGICAL RISK INCREASES WITH
* Adults over 60; stress; obesity.
* Poor nutrition; alcoholism; smoking.
* Recent or chronic illness, especially diabetes.
* Use of some prescription and nonprescription drugs. Inform your doctor of any drugs, medications, or vitamin and herb supplements you are using or have used in the last month.

WHAT TO EXPECT

WHO OPERATES—Obstetrician-gynecologist or general surgeon.

WHERE PERFORMED—Hospital.

DIAGNOSTIC TESTS
* Before surgery: Blood and urine studies; CT scan of pelvic organs; laparoscopy or culdoscopy; ultrasound; x-rays of chest, lower abdomen and lower intestinal tract; culdocentesis (see Glossary for all).
* During surgery: Laboratory examination of removed tissue by frozen section (see Glossary).
* After surgery: Blood studies.

ANESTHESIA—General anesthesia by injection and inhalation with an airway tube placed in the windpipe.

DESCRIPTION OF OPERATION
* An incision is made in the abdomen. The abdominal muscles are separated and the peritoneum is opened.
* Blood vessels supplying the ovaries are located, clamped and tied.
* The tumor or cyst in the ovary is located, cut free and removed or the cyst may be destroyed by electrocauterization (see Glossary).
* If examination reveals signs of cancer, the ovary is removed.
* The peritoneum is closed, and the abdominal muscles are sewn together with heavy sutures.
* The skin is closed with sutures or clips, which usually can be removed 10 days after surgery.
* This surgery, under many conditions, can be performed laparoscopically (see Glossary). Your doctor can determine which approach is best for your circumstances.

POSSIBLE COMPLICATIONS
* Excessive bleeding.
* Surgical-wound infection.
* Recurrent cancer.
* Excessive scarring (keloid).

AVERAGE HOSPITAL STAY—3 to 5 days. However, if surgery is performed laparoscopically, patients are often not admitted at all or go home the next day.

PROBABLE OUTCOME—Expect complete healing of surgical wound. If cancer is detected, your doctor will prescribe treatment with radiation or anticancer drugs. Allow about 4 weeks for recovery from surgery.

POSTOPERATIVE CARE

GENERAL MEASURES
* A hard ridge should form along the incision. As it heals, the ridge will gradually recede.
* Use an electric heating pad, a heat lamp or a warm compress to relieve incisional pain.
* Shower as usual. Avoid baths until the incision is completely healed. You may wash the incision gently with mild, unscented soap. After showering, replace any wet dressings with clean, dry ones.
* Move and elevate legs often while resting in bed to decrease the likelihood of deep-vein blood clots.

MEDICATION
* Your doctor may prescribe:
  - Pain relievers. Don't take prescription pain medication longer than 4 to 7 days. Use only as much as you need.
  - Stool softeners to prevent constipation. - Hormone supplements.
  - Antibiotics to fight or prevent infection.
* You may use nonprescription drugs, such as acetaminophen, for minor pain. Avoid aspirin.

ACTIVITY
* To help recovery and aid your well-being, resume daily activities, including work, as soon as you are able.
* Avoid vigorous exercise for 6 weeks after surgery.
* Resume sexual relations when your doctor determines that healing is complete.

DIET—Clear liquid diet until the gastrointestinal tract functions again. Then eat a well-balanced diet to promote healing.

CALL YOUR DOCTOR IF

* Pain, swelling, redness, drainage or bleeding increases in the surgical area.
* You develop signs of infection, including headache, muscle aches, dizziness or a general ill feeling and fever.
* You experience nausea, vomiting, constipation, abdominal swelling or hot flashes.
* New, unexplained symptoms develop.

OVARIAN CYST OR TUMOR REMOVAL

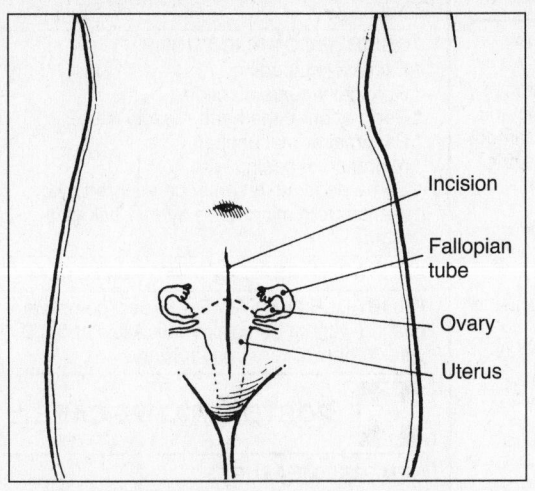

The organs of the female reproductive tract and the usual abdominal incision for this surgical procedure.

Incision

Fallopian tube

Ovary

Uterus

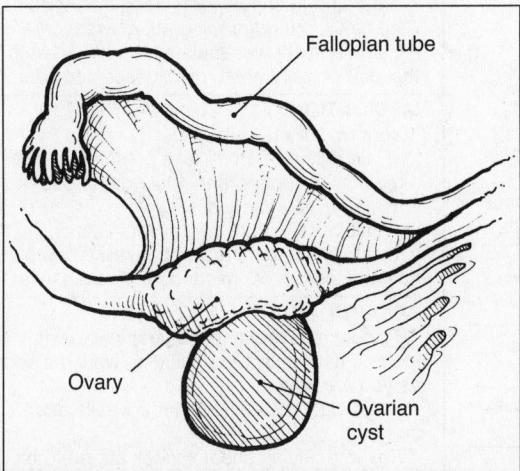

After the incision has been made through the skin and underlying tissue, the tumor or cyst in the ovary is located, cut free and removed.
  • If cancer is identified, a wider removal of tissue is indicated.

Fallopian tube

Ovary

Ovarian cyst

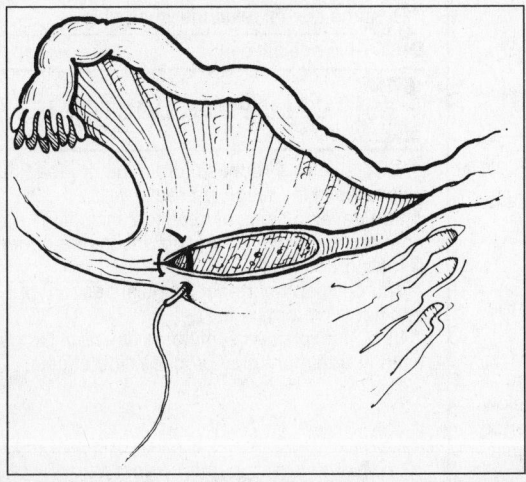

The bed of the ovarian cyst or tumor is sutured closed to prevent bleeding and adhesions.
  • The peritoneum is closed. The abdominal muscles are sewn together with heavy sutures and the skin is closed with sutures or clips, which usually can be removed about 10 days after surgery (not illustrated).

SURGERIES

PACEMAKER IMPLANTATION

GENERAL INFORMATION

DEFINITION—Placement of a temporary or permanent pacemaker into the chest wall. A pacemaker is an electronic device consisting of an electrode connected to the heart muscle and a regulatory device and power source implanted under the skin. It provides regular, mild electric shocks that stimulate the heart muscle and maintain normal heartbeat.

BODY PARTS INVOLVED—Veins in neck or under collarbone; tissue under the skin below the collarbone; heart.

REASONS FOR SURGERY
* Regulation of heartbeat that has slowed due to heart disease.
* Treatment of heart block.
* Following cardiac surgery to regulate heart rate.

SURGICAL RISK INCREASES WITH
* Adults over 60.
* Obesity.
* Smoking.
* Excess alcohol consumption.
* Recent or chronic illness.
* Diabetes.
* Use of some prescription and nonprescription drugs. Inform your doctor of any drugs, medications, or vitamin and herb supplements you are using or have used in the last month.

WHAT TO EXPECT

WHO OPERATES—Cardiovascular surgeon, cardiologist (sometimes).

WHERE PERFORMED—Outpatient surgical facility or hospital.

DIAGNOSTIC TESTS
* Before surgery: Blood and urine studies; x-rays of chest; ECG (see Glossary).
* During surgery: ECG; fluoroscopy (see Glossary for both).
* After surgery: ECG (see Glossary); x-rays of chest.

ANESTHESIA
* Local anesthesia by injection.
* General anesthesia by injection and inhalation with an airway tube placed in the windpipe.

DESCRIPTION OF OPERATION
* A needle is inserted in a vein under the collarbone. An electrode is passed through the vein into the heart. The implantation site is confirmed.
* The electrode is attached to the power and regulating units. A small incision is made below the collarbone, and the entire device is inserted into the incision and placed under the skin in a pouch created from tissue.

* The skin is closed with suture material, which usually can be removed about 1 week after surgery.

POSSIBLE COMPLICATIONS
* Excessive bleeding.
* Surgical-wound infection.
* Perforation of the heart muscle (rare).
* Pacemaker malfunction.
* Migration of pacing wire.
* Some pacemakers may be affected by radiation from microwave ovens. Ask your doctor.

AVERAGE HOSPITAL STAY—0 to 2 days.

PROBABLE OUTCOME—Expect complete healing without complications. Allow about 2 weeks for recovery from surgery.

POSTOPERATIVE CARE

GENERAL MEASURES
* A hard ridge should form along the incision. As it heals, the ridge will gradually recede.
* Bathe and shower as usual. You may wash the incision gently with mild, unscented soap.

MEDICATION
* Your doctor may prescribe:
  - Pain relievers. Don't take prescription pain medication longer than 4 to 7 days. Use only as much as you need.
  - Antibiotics to fight or prevent infection.
* You may use nonprescription drugs, such as acetaminophen, for minor pain. Avoid aspirin.

ACTIVITY
* To help recovery and aid your well-being, resume daily activities, including work, as soon as you are able.
* Avoid vigorous exercise for 2 weeks after surgery.
* Resume driving about 1 week after returning home.
* Resume sexual relations when able.

DIET—No special diet.

CALL YOUR DOCTOR IF

* Pain, swelling, redness, drainage or bleeding increases in the surgical area.
* You develop signs of infection, including headache, muscle aches, dizziness or a general ill feeling and fever.
* You develop heartbeat irregularities, or your original symptoms return.
* New, unexplained symptoms develop. Drugs used in treatment may produce side effects.

PACEMAKER IMPLANTATION

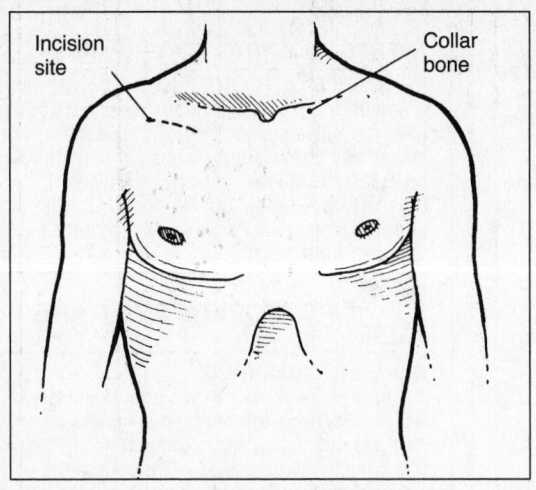

An illustration of the chest, collarbone and incision site generally used for pacemaker insertion.

Incision site

Collar bone

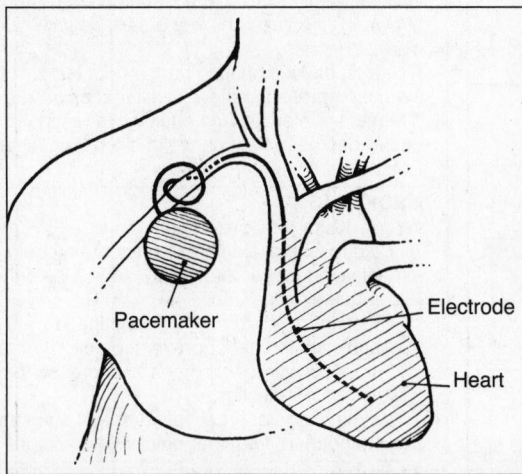

An electrode is passed through a vein near the incision site, which ends inside the heart cavity.
  • The electrode is attached to the power and regulating units. The entire device is inserted under the skin into a pouch created from tissue under the collarbone.

Pacemaker

Electrode

Heart

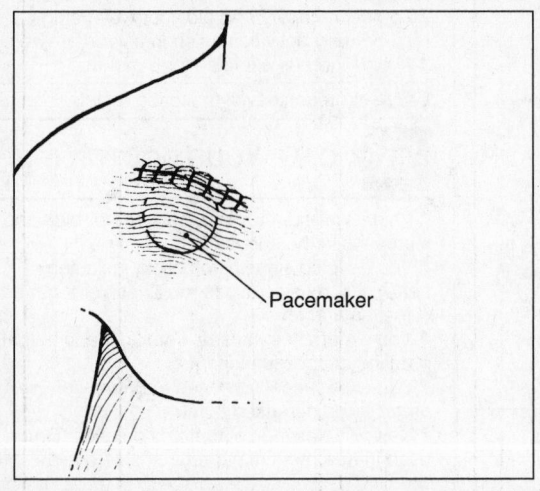

The pacemaker in place. The skin has been closed with sutures that usually can be removed about 1 week after surgery.

Pacemaker

PANCREAS TRANSPLANTATION

GENERAL INFORMATION

DEFINITION—Replacement of a diseased pancreas with a healthy pancreas obtained from a donor with compatible immunological characteristics. The duodenum is also replaced to allow drainage of pancreatic secretions into the gastrointestinal tract.

BODY PARTS INVOLVED—Diseased or abnormal pancreas and duodenum; healthy donor pancreas and duodenum.

REASONS FOR SURGERY—Prevention of complications of severe diabetes, such as kidney failure and damage to the retinas.

SURGICAL RISK INCREASES WITH
- Obesity; smoking; stress.
- Poor nutrition.
- Excess alcohol consumption.
- Recent or chronic illness; diabetes.
- Use of some prescription and nonprescription drugs. Inform your doctor of any drugs, medications, or vitamin and herb supplements you are using or have used in the last month.

WHAT TO EXPECT

WHO OPERATES—General surgeon.

WHERE PERFORMED—Hospital.

DIAGNOSTIC TESTS
- Before surgery: Evaluation of all body systems; immune-system and pancreas matching procedures.
- After surgery: Blood studies.

ANESTHESIA—General anesthesia by injection and inhalation with an airway tube placed in the windpipe.

DESCRIPTION OF OPERATION
- The pancreas is removed from the donor, chilled and preserved up to 12 hours until surgery.
- An incision is made under the ribs.
- The abdominal muscles are divided and the peritoneal cavity is entered.
- The pancreas and duodenum are cut free and removed.
- The donor pancreas and duodenum are positioned and connected to blood vessels.
- Sometimes, only the cells of the pancreas that produce insulin (islet cells) are transplanted. In some patients, this is all that is necessary to re-establish normal function.
- The peritoneum and muscles are closed. The skin is closed with sutures or clips, which usually can be removed in 1 week.

POSSIBLE COMPLICATIONS
- Excessive bleeding.
- Surgical-wound infection.
- Rejection of transplant.
- Development of a pancreatic fistula.
- Bowel leak.

AVERAGE HOSPITAL STAY—3 weeks.

PROBABLE OUTCOME—Islet-cell transplants are usually successful in giving young diabetics near-normal life expectancy. In adults, a successful transplant prolongs life and improves the quality of life for patients who might otherwise have died, but life expectancy is currently unknown. Allow about 6 months for recovery from surgery.

POSTOPERATIVE CARE

GENERAL MEASURES
- A hard ridge should form along the incision. As it heals, the ridge will gradually recede.
- Shower as usual. Avoid baths until the incision has completely healed. You may wash the incision gently with mild, unscented soap. After showering, replace any wet dressings with clean, dry ones.
- Use an electric heating pad, a heat lamp or a warm compress to relieve incisional pain.
- Move and elevate legs often while resting in bed to decrease the chance of deep-vein blood clots.

MEDICATION
- Your doctor may prescribe:
  - Pain relievers. Don't take prescription pain medication longer than 4 to 7 days. Use only as much as you need.
  - Stool softeners to prevent constipation.
  - Antibiotics to fight or prevent infection.
  - Immunosuppressant drugs to decrease the likelihood of rejection.
- You may use nonprescription drugs, such as acetaminophen, for minor pain. Avoid aspirin.

ACTIVITY
- To help recovery and aid your well-being, resume daily activities as soon as you are able.
- Avoid vigorous exercise for 6 months.

DIET—You doctor will prescribe a diet.

CALL YOUR DOCTOR IF

- Pain, swelling, redness, drainage or bleeding increases in the surgical area.
- You develop signs of infection, including headache, muscle aches, dizziness or a general ill feeling and fever.
- You experience nausea, vomiting, abdominal swelling or constipation.
- You experience increased frequency of urination or increased thirst.
- New, unexplained symptoms develop. Drugs used in treatment may produce side effects.

PANCREAS TRANSPLANTATION

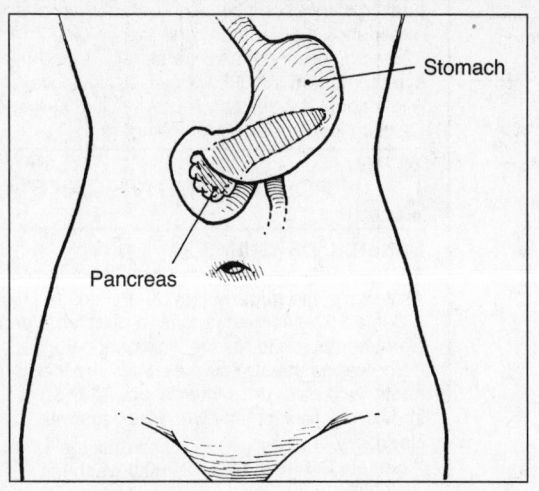

An illustration of the normal location and anatomy of the pancreas.

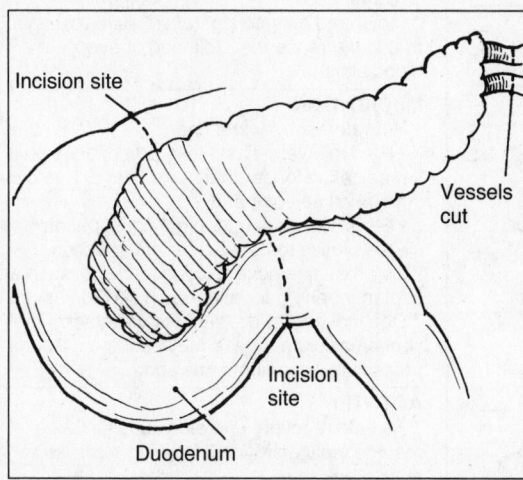

The diseased pancreas and the duodenum are cut free and removed.

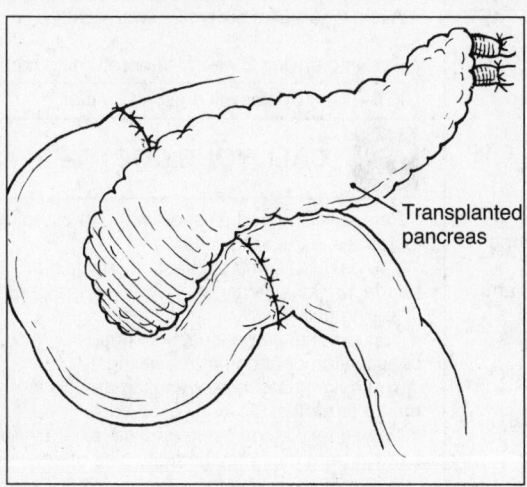

The donor pancreas and duodenum are positioned and connected to the blood vessels.
- Following transplant, muscles and skin are closed with sutures or clips that usually can be removed about 1 week after surgery (not illustrated).

PARATHYROIDECTOMY

GENERAL INFORMATION

DEFINITION—Removal of parathyroid tumors or the parathyroid glands.

BODY PARTS INVOLVED—The two pair (four in total) parathyroid glands (a part of the body's endocrine gland system).

REASONS FOR SURGERY
- Hyperparathyroidism (see Illness section).
- Parathyroid adenoma (a benign tumor).
- Parathyroid cancer (very rare).

SURGICAL RISK INCREASES WITH
- Obesity or smoking.
- Poor nutrition; alcoholism.
- Recent or chronic illness.
- Diabetes.
- Use of some prescription and nonprescription drugs. Inform your doctor of any drugs, medications, or vitamin and herb supplements you are using or have used in the last month.

WHAT TO EXPECT

WHO OPERATES—General surgeon.

WHERE PERFORMED—Hospital.

DIAGNOSTIC TESTS
- Before surgery: Blood and urine studies; x-rays of upper gastrointestinal tract; CT scan; ultrasound; fine needle biopsy; thyroid scan; (see Glossary for all).
- During surgery: Laboratory examination of removed tissue by frozen section (see Glossary).
- After surgery: Blood studies; laboratory examination of removed tissue.

ANESTHESIA—General anesthesia by injection and inhalation with an airway tube placed in the windpipe.

DESCRIPTION OF OPERATION
- An incision is made in the neck just under the Adam's apple. Layers of skin and muscle are lifted up. The parathyroid glands are located.
- If one gland is enlarged (adenoma), it is removed and the rest are left in place.
- If all the glands are equally enlarged, 3 or 3 1/2 of the glands are removed. This leaves enough parathyroid tissue to prevent hypoparathyroidism (low parathyroid hormone production).
- The muscle and skin layers are replaced and the surgical incision is closed.

POSSIBLE COMPLICATIONS
- Excessive bleeding; surgical-wound infection.
- Hypoparathyroidism.
- Inadvertent injury to thyroid gland or vocal-cord nerves.
- Recurrent hyperparathyroidism.
- Repeat surgery if not enough tissue removed.

AVERAGE HOSPITAL STAY—1 to 2 days.

PROBABLE OUTCOME—Expect complete healing without complications. You will probably experience a sore throat and raspy voice following surgery; these are usually temporary symptoms and should diminish as you recover. Allow about 4 weeks for recovery from surgery. Calcium levels may be low temporarily.

POSTOPERATIVE CARE

GENERAL MEASURES
- A hard ridge should form along the incision. As it heals, the ridge will gradually recede.
- Use an electric heating pad, a heat lamp or a warm compress to relieve incisional pain.
- Shower as usual. You may wash the incision gently with mild, unscented soap. After showering, replace any wet dressings with clean, dry ones.
- Elevate the head of your bed for the first 2 to 3 nights.
- Move and elevate legs often while resting in bed to decrease the likelihood of deep-vein blood clots.

MEDICATION
- Your doctor may prescribe:
  - Pain relievers. Don't take prescription pain medication longer than 4 to 7 days. Use only as much as you need.
  - Stool softeners to prevent constipation.
  - Antibiotics to fight or prevent infection.
- You may use nonprescription drugs, such as acetaminophen, for minor pain. Avoid aspirin.
- Don't take thiazide diuretics or antacids that contain calcium. These may cause a calcium, potassium or sodium imbalance.

ACTIVITY
- To help recovery and aid your well-being, resume daily activities, including work, as soon as you are able.
- Avoid vigorous activity for 6 weeks after surgery.
- Resume driving 2 weeks after returning home.

DIET—Your doctor will prescribe a diet.

CALL YOUR DOCTOR IF

- Pain, swelling, redness, drainage or bleeding increases in the surgical area.
- You develop signs of infection, including headache, muscle aches, dizziness or a general ill feeling and fever.
- You experience nausea, vomiting, constipation or abdominal swelling.
- You have numbness or tingling around the mouth or hands.
- New, unexplained symptoms develop. Drugs used in treatment may produce side effects.

PARATHYROIDECTOMY

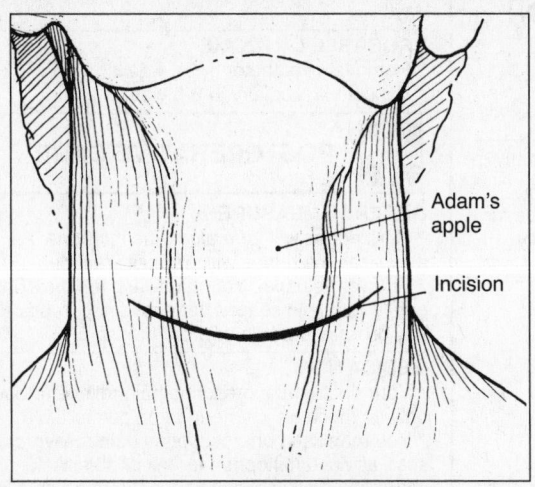

The incision site in the lower part of the neck below the protruding cartilage called the Adam's apple.

Adam's apple

Incision

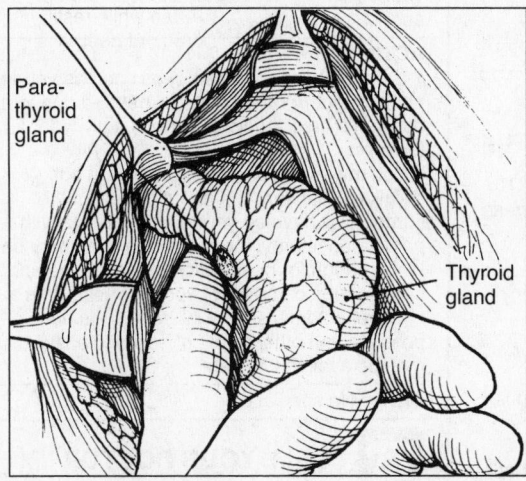

Para-thyroid gland

Thyroid gland

Parathyroid glands are located. Abnormal ones are removed. If the surgery is being performed because of overactivity of the parathyroid glands, rather than a tumor, all except one of the visualized parathyroid glands are cut free and removed.

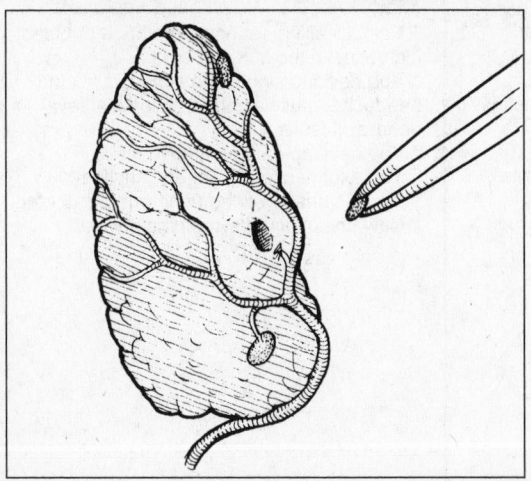

One parathyroid gland removed.
• After the surgery is finished, neck muscles are reapproximated, the tissue below the skin is closed with suture material and the skin is closed with clips.

SURGERIES

PENECTOMY
(Removal of Part or All of Penis)

 GENERAL INFORMATION

DEFINITION—Removal of part or all of the shaft and all of the head of the penis with creation of a new outlet for urine.

BODY PARTS INVOLVED—Penis, sometimes perineum.

REASONS FOR SURGERY—Usually done for malignant tumors of the penis. Occasionally done for trauma.

SURGICAL RISK INCREASES WITH
* Age.
* Diabetes.
* Poor kidney function.
* High blood pressure.
* Poor nutrition.
* Chronic lung disease.
* Obesity.

 WHAT TO EXPECT

WHO OPERATES—Urologist.

WHERE PERFORMED—Hospital.

DIAGNOSTIC TESTS
* Before surgery: Blood tests, chest x-ray, CT scan, cystoscopy, EKG (see Glossary for these 3 terms).
* After surgery: Blood tests.

ANESTHESIA—General anesthesia or spinal anesthesia.

DESCRIPTION OF OPERATION
* The shaft of the penis is encircled with a tourniquet to minimize bleeding. An incision is made through the skin and the urethra (tube that carries urine from the bladder to the outside) and corpora (blood filled cavities that facilitate erectile function) are identified. These are transected (cut) and vessels are ligated (sewn off).
* If enough shaft is remaining, the urethra is sutured to the skin edges. If insufficient shaft is left, the urethra is brought out through an opening in the perineum. Sphincter function (continence) is usually preserved but erectile function is usually lost.
* A foley catheter (see Glossary) is usually left in the bladder.

POSSIBLE COMPLICATIONS
* Bleeding from the surgery site.
* Urethral stricture (narrowing).
* Infection.

AVERAGE HOSPITAL STAY—Usually 3-5 days.

PROBABLE OUTCOME
* Removal of catheter in 7-14 days.
* Expect full recovery in 6-8 weeks.

 POSTOPERATIVE CARE

GENERAL MEASURES
* Hard ridges will form along the incisions. As they heal, the ridges will gradually recede.
* Shower as usual. You may wash the incisions gently with mild soap. After showering, replace any dressings with a new dry dressing.

MEDICATION
* Your doctor may prescribe pain relievers. Use only as much as you need to be comfortable.
* You may use nonprescription pain relievers such as acetaminophen for minor pain. Ask your doctor if it is okay to take ibuprofen or aspirin.

ACTIVITY
* Start ambulating (walking) as soon as you are home. Take frequent naps as needed during the day when tired. Avoid strenuous activity for 2 to 3 weeks.
* You may swim once all sutures are out.
* Talk to your surgeon about the effect the surgery will have on your sexual ability. With a partial penectomy, the remaining shaft may be long enough for penetration of the vagina and be able to become erect upon arousal. With a total penectomy, sexual intercourse is not possible, but other forms of sexual pleasure may be available to you.

DIET—No special diet.

 CALL YOUR DOCTOR IF

* Pain, swelling, redness, drainage or bleeding increases in the surgical area.
* You develop signs of infection, including headache, muscle aches, dizziness, fever, or a general ill feeling.
* You develop nausea and vomiting.
* You experience prolonged constipation, difficulty urinating or no urine out of catheter.
* New unexplained symptoms develop.

PENECTOMY
(Removal of Part or All of Penis)

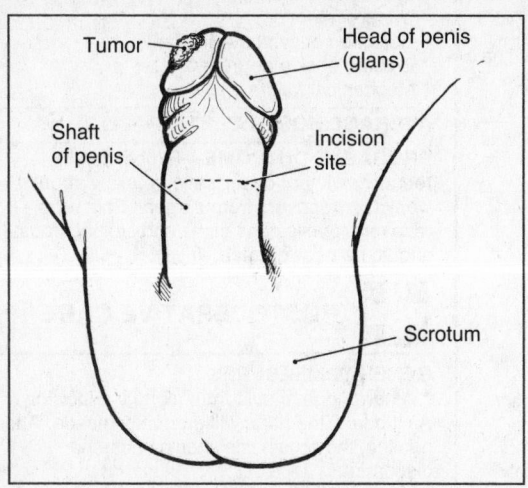

Tumor

Head of penis (glans)

Shaft of penis

Incision site

Scrotum

An illustration of the anatomy with a tumor on the glans.

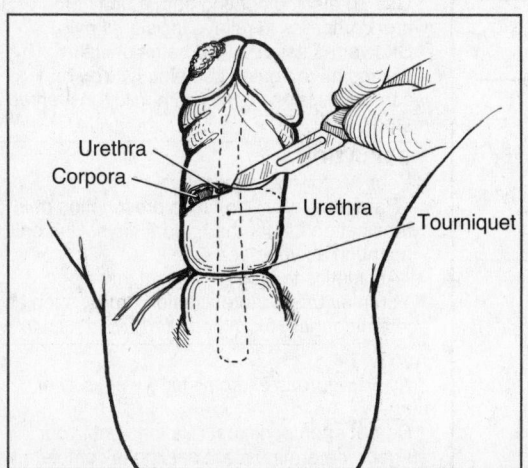

Urethra

Corpora

Urethra

Tourniquet

A tourniquet is applied to control bleeding and the incision is made through the shaft of the penis and urethra.

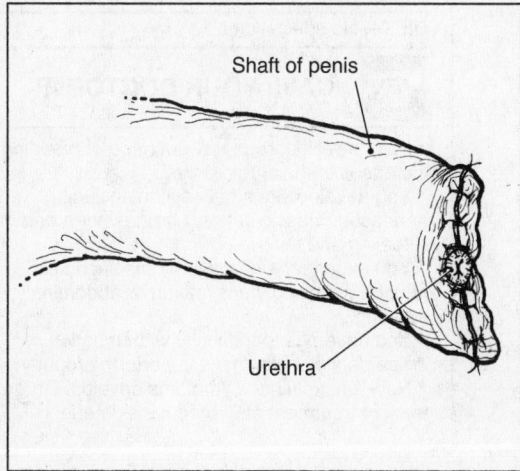

Shaft of penis

Urethra

The end of the shaft is closed and the urethra is sutured to the skin edges.

SURGERIES

PENILE IMPLANT

GENERAL INFORMATION

DEFINITION—Insertion of semiflexible plastic bars or an inflatable prosthesis in the penis. The former produces a permanent, partial erection. The latter can be inflated at will.

BODY PARTS INVOLVED—Penis.

REASONS FOR SURGERY—Impotence.

SURGICAL RISK INCREASES WITH
* Obesity.
* Smoking.
* Stress.
* Poor nutrition.
* Recent or chronic illness.
* Alcoholism.
* Diabetes.
* Use of some prescription and nonprescription drugs. Inform your doctor of any drugs, medications, or vitamin and herb supplements you are using or have used in the last month.

WHAT TO EXPECT

WHO OPERATES—Urologist.

WHERE PERFORMED—Hospital.

DIAGNOSTIC TESTS
* Before surgery: Blood and urine studies; chest x-ray; ultrasound (see Glossary).
* After surgery: Blood studies.

ANESTHESIA
* Spinal anesthesia by injection.
* General anesthesia by injection and inhalation with an airway tube placed in the windpipe.

DESCRIPTION OF OPERATION
Plastic Implant:
* An incision is made in the underside of the penis.
* The tissues on both sides of the urethra are expanded to allow placement of the implants.
* An implant is placed on each side of the urethra.
* The skin is closed with sutures that will be absorbed by the body.
Inflatable Prosthesis:
* Incisions are made in the underside of the penis, the side of the scrotum, and on the abdomen, several inches above the base of the penis.
* The penile tissue is stretched to allow placement of the prosthesis. The fluid reservoir for the prosthesis is implanted under the skin above the bladder at the base of the pelvis. The prosthesis can be inflated by applying pressure on the reservoir.
* The skin is closed with sutures that will be absorbed by the body.

POSSIBLE COMPLICATIONS
* Surgical-wound infection.
* Excessive bleeding.
* Urinary retention.
* Rejection of synthetic implants.
* Erosion of skin or urethra.
* Mechanical failure.

AVERAGE HOSPITAL STAY—1 to 2 days.

PROBABLE OUTCOME—Expect complete recovery without complications. Allow about 4 weeks for recovery from surgery. Following recovery, penile sensations and sexual arousal should be near normal.

POSTOPERATIVE CARE

GENERAL MEASURES
* A hard ridge should form along the incision. As it heals, the ridge will gradually recede. After healing, the prosthesis should cause no discomfort.
* Use an electric heating pad, a heat lamp or a warm compress to relieve incisional pain.
* Shower as usual. Avoid baths until the incisions have healed completely. You may wash the incisions gently with mild, unscented soap.

MEDICATION
* Your doctor may prescribe:
  - Pain relievers. Don't take prescription pain medication longer than 4 to 7 days. Use only as much as you need.
  - Antibiotics to fight or prevent infection.
* You may use nonprescription drugs, such as acetaminophen, for minor pain. Avoid aspirin.

ACTIVITY
* Avoid vigorous exercise for 6 weeks after surgery.
* Do not attempt sexual relations until your surgeon determines that healing is complete.
* Resume driving 1 week after returning home.

DIET—No special diet.

CALL YOUR DOCTOR IF

* Pain, swelling, redness, drainage or bleeding increases in the surgical area.
* You develop signs of infection, including headache, muscle aches, dizziness or a general ill feeling and fever.
* You experience new symptoms such as nausea, vomiting, constipation or abdominal swelling.
* You have pain or difficulty with urination.
* The penile implant fails to perform properly.
* New, unexplained symptoms develop. Drugs used in treatment may produce side effects.

PENILE IMPLANT

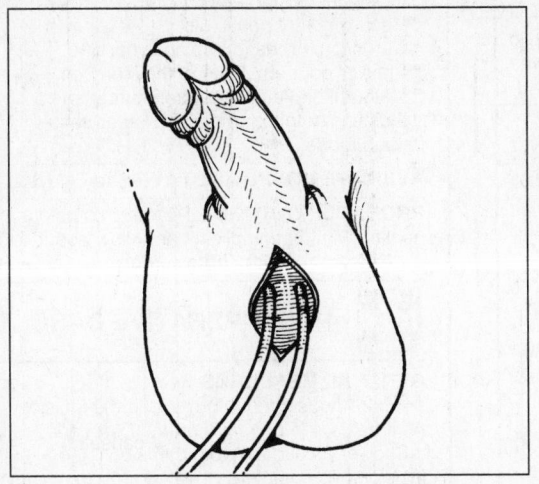

The incision for a penile implant, which may be either semi-rigid or an inflatable prosthesis. These drawings illustrate the inflatable form only. The equipment is different for a semi-rigid prosthesis but the principles and techniques for insertion are similar for both procedures.

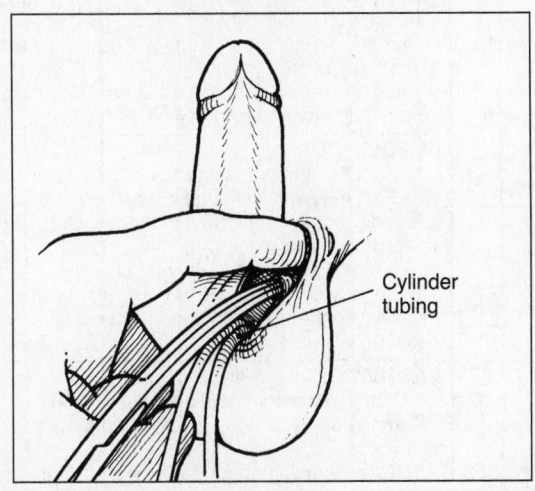

Cylinder tubing

After an incision has been made on the underside of the penis, the tissues on both sides of the urethra are expanded to allow placement of the implants.

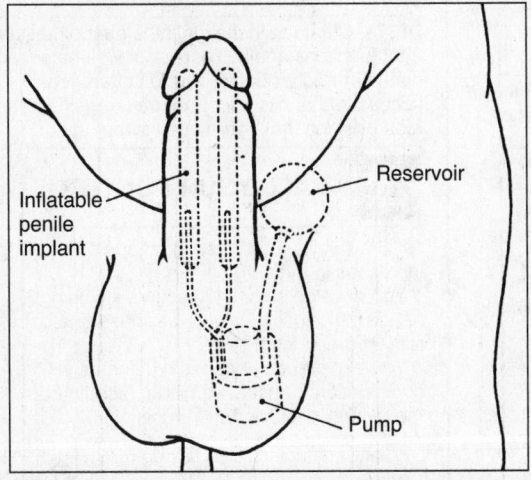

Inflatable penile implant

Reservoir

Pump

Implants in place, surgical incision closed with absorbable sutures.

PEPTIC ULCER SURGERY

GENERAL INFORMATION

DEFINITION—Surgery to decrease the acid production in the stomach in order to prevent ulcer formation.

BODY PARTS INVOLVED—Esophagus; stomach; duodenum; jejunum; vagus nerves.

REASONS FOR SURGERY—Treatment of complications of peptic ulcers:
* Bleeding.
* Intolerable pain.
* Blockage of stomach contents from emptying.
* Perforation. If an ulcer perforates, the contents of the gastrointestinal tract are dumped into the abdominal cavity, causing peritonitis. This is a medical emergency requiring immediate surgery.

SURGICAL RISK INCREASES WITH
* Adults over 60.
* Chronic illness, especially pancreatitis, hepatitis, alcoholism or diabetes.
* Poor nutrition, especially vitamin and mineral deficiencies.
* Use of any drugs that irritate the stomach.
* Use of some prescription and nonprescription drugs. Inform your doctor of any drugs, medications, or vitamin and herb supplements you are using or have used in the last month.

WHAT TO EXPECT

WHO OPERATES—General surgeon.

WHERE PERFORMED—Hospital.

DIAGNOSTIC TESTS
* Before surgery: Blood and urine studies; x-rays of abdomen; endoscopy (see Glossary).
* After surgery: Blood and urine studies; x-rays of abdomen.

ANESTHESIA—General anesthesia by injection and inhalation with an airway tube placed in the windpipe.

DESCRIPTION OF OPERATION—Any of the following procedures is used for this surgery:
* Vagotomy and pyloroplasty: The nerves that stimulate stomach-acid production are severed, and the outlet of the stomach that leads to the duodenum is enlarged.
* Gastric resection (antrectomy): The lower part of the stomach that produces acid is removed, and the remaining stomach is attached with sutures to the duodenum or the jejunum. This is usually combined with a vagotomy (cutting of the vagus nerve).
* Closure of perforated ulcer: The perforated ulcer is closed by various methods.
* Incisions that are made are closed with sutures or clips, which can usually be removed about 1 week after surgery.

POSSIBLE COMPLICATIONS
* Excessive bleeding; surgical-wound infection.
* Incisional hernia.
* Recurrence of peptic ulcer.
* Chronic diarrhea; dumping syndrome.
* Slow or poor emptying of the stomach.
* Malnutrition (lack of needed nutrients).
* Flushing, fainting or diarrhea after eating certain foods.

AVERAGE HOSPITAL STAY—3 to 7 days.

PROBABLE OUTCOME—Expect complete healing without complications. Allow about 4 to 6 weeks for recovery from surgery.

POSTOPERATIVE CARE

GENERAL MEASURES
* A hard ridge should form along the incision. As it heals, the ridge will gradually recede.
* Shower as usual. Avoid baths until the incision has completely healed. You may wash the incision gently with mild, unscented soap. After showering, replace any wet dressings with clean, dry ones.
* Use an electric heating pad, a heat lamp or a warm compress to relieve incisional pain.

MEDICATION
* Your doctor may prescribe:
  - Pain relievers. Don't take prescription pain medication longer than 4 to 7 days. Use only as much as you need.
  - Antibiotics to fight or prevent infection.
* You may use nonprescription drugs, such as acetaminophen, for minor pain. Do not take aspirin.

ACTIVITY
* To help recovery and aid your well-being, resume daily activities, including work, as soon as you are able.
* Resume driving about 2 weeks after returning home.

DIET—Clear liquid diet until the gastrointestinal tract functions again. Then eat a well-balanced diet to promote healing. Avoid coffee, tea, cocoa, cola drinks, alcoholic beverages and any food or spice that aggravates symptoms.

CALL YOUR DOCTOR IF

* Pain, swelling, redness, drainage or bleeding increases in the surgical area.
* You develop signs of infection, including headache, muscle aches, dizziness or a general ill feeling and fever.
* You experience abdominal pain or swelling; constipation; nausea; vomiting; bleeding from the rectum or black, tarry stools.
* New, unexplained symptoms develop. Drugs used in treatment may produce side effects.

PEPTIC ULCER SURGERY

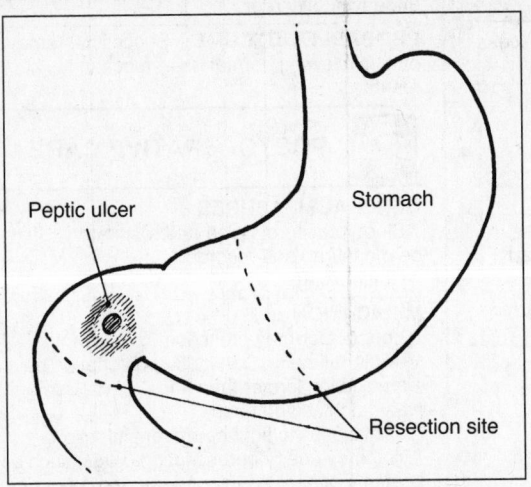

An illustration of the stomach with a peptic ulcer, the incision sites in the lower part of the stomach and the beginning portion of the duodenum.

Peptic ulcer

Stomach

Resection site

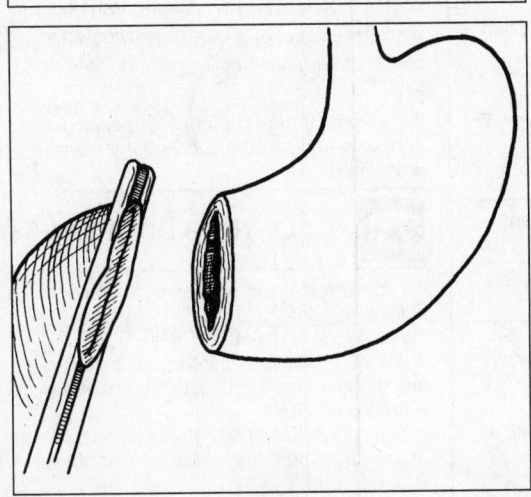

The part of the stomach that produces acid is removed along with the part of the stomach or duodenum that has a peptic ulcer or scarring from a healed or partially healed peptic ulcer.

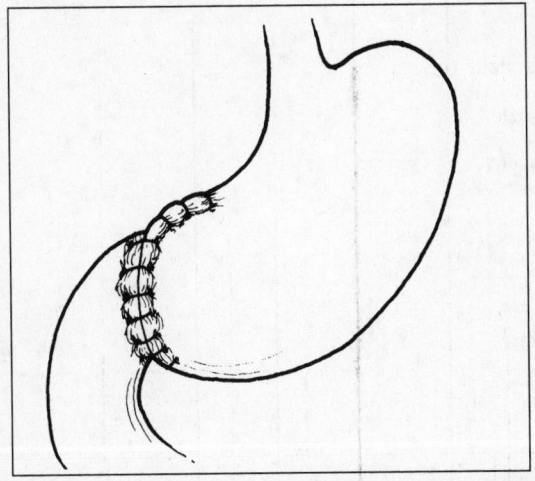

The remaining stomach is attached with sutures to the duodenum or sometimes to the jejunum located lower down in the small intestine.

PERICARDIOCENTESIS

GENERAL INFORMATION

DEFINITION—The needle aspiration of excess fluid from the pericardial sac.

BODY PARTS INVOLVED—Pericardium, a 2-layered membrane that surrounds the heart and the roots of the great blood vessels (aorta, pulmonary artery, pulmonary vein and vena cava).

REASONS FOR SURGERY—To remove abnormal fluid collections between the heart and the pericardium. The fluid may be there because the heart is inflamed, infected or injured (fluid may be blood).

SURGICAL RISK INCREASES WITH
* Obesity.
* Smoking.
* Excess alcohol consumption.
* Recent or chronic illness, especially chronic lung disease.
* Use of some prescription and nonprescription drugs. Inform your doctor of any drugs, medications, or vitamin and herb supplements you are using or have used in the last month.

WHAT TO EXPECT

WHO OPERATES—Cardiothoracic surgeon; cardiologist (sometimes).

WHERE PERFORMED—Hospital or outpatient surgical facility.

DIAGNOSTIC TESTS
* Before surgery: Chest x-rays; CT scan; ECG (see Glossary for both).
* During surgery: Chest x-rays.
* After surgery: Chest x-rays; fluid examination; ECG (see Glossary).

ANESTHESIA—Local anesthesia.

DESCRIPTION OF OPERATION
* Patient lies down on back with upper torso elevated about 60 degrees with arms supported by pillows.
* An I.V. is started and local anesthetic injected.
* The pericardiocentesis needle is inserted into chest wall between the left rib margin adjacent to the breastbone, usually into the space between the 5th and 6th ribs.
* The needle is advanced until fluid can be aspirated.

POSSIBLE COMPLICATIONS
* Heartbeat irregularities.
* Inadvertent organ or artery puncture (rare).
* Hemothorax (see Glossary).
* Pneumothorax (see Glossary).

AVERAGE HOSPITAL STAY—0 to 1 day for procedure. Total time varies according to underlying disorder.

PROBABLE OUTCOME—Successful removal of fluid allowing normal heart function to resume.

POSTOPERATIVE CARE

GENERAL MEASURES
* Blood pressure, pulse and respiratory rate will be measured and recorded.
* No smoking.

MEDICATION
* Your doctor may prescribe:
  - Pain relievers. Don't take prescription pain medication longer than 4 to 7 days. Use only as much as you need.
  - Antibiotics to fight or prevent infection.
* You may use nonprescription drugs, such as acetaminophen, for minor pain. Avoid aspirin.

ACTIVITY—Avoid vigorous exercise until your doctor determines healing is complete.

DIET
* Your doctor may prescribe a special diet.
* Vitamin and mineral supplements may be prescribed.

CALL YOUR DOCTOR IF

* You experience shortness of breath or chest pain, or you feel faint.
* You become anxious.
* You develop signs of infection, including headache, muscle aches, dizziness or a general ill feeling and fever.
* New, unexplained symptoms develop. Drugs used in treatment may produce side effects.

PERICARDIOCENTESIS

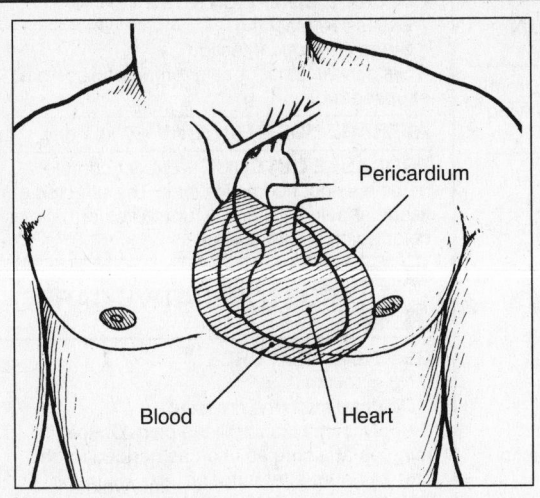

An illustration of the heart and surrounding structures.

Pericardium

Blood   Heart

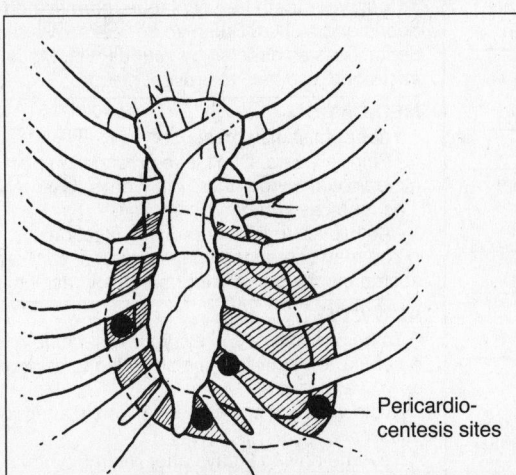

The muscles of the chest are pulled aside to illustrate possible sites for the pericardiocentesis needle to be placed into the pericardium.

Pericardio-centesis sites

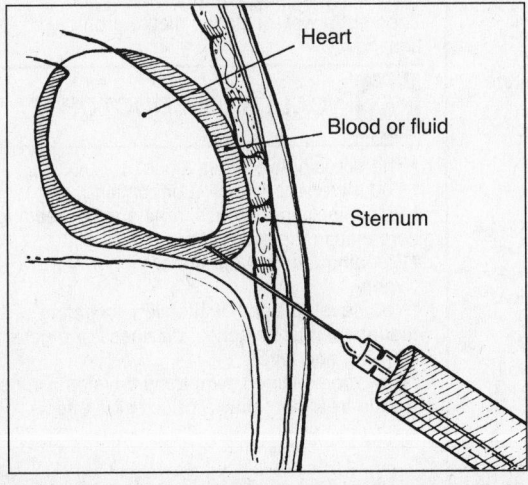

A needle attached to a syringe is advanced until the fluid can be aspirated. After fluid has been removed, the heart can function much more normally.

Heart

Blood or fluid

Sternum

PERIODONTAL SURGERY
(Pyorrhea Treatment)

 GENERAL INFORMATION

DEFINITION—Removal of infected tissue from the gums and reshaping of the bone underlying the gums.

BODY PARTS INVOLVED—Gums; surrounding bone.

REASONS FOR SURGERY—Prevention of the spread of gum infection.

SURGICAL RISK INCREASES WITH
* Adults over 60.
* Smoking.
* Excess alcohol consumption.
* Poor nutrition.
* Recent or chronic illness.
* Diabetes.
* Use of some prescription and nonprescription drugs. Inform your doctor of any drugs, medications, or vitamin and herb supplements you are using or have used in the last month.

 WHAT TO EXPECT

WHO OPERATES—Dentist or periodontist.

WHERE PERFORMED—Hospital, outpatient surgical facility or dentist's or periodontist's office.

DIAGNOSTIC TESTS
* Before surgery: Blood and urine studies; x-rays of the mouth.
* After surgery: Blood studies.

ANESTHESIA
* Local anesthesia by injection.
* General anesthesia (sometimes) by injection and inhalation with an airway tube placed in the windpipe.

DESCRIPTION OF OPERATION
* The diseased periodontal tissue is carefully cut free and removed.
* The gums are lifted or flapped away from the tooth and surrounding bone.
* The diseased root surfaces are cleaned or removed.
* The bone under the gum is reshaped, if necessary.
* A special type of fabric may be sewn around a tooth to cover a crater in the bone; the gum is then sewn over the fabric. After the bone and attachment to the root regenerate, the fabric is removed using a minor surgical procedure.
* Special dressings are applied that control bleeding and hasten healing. Your dentist will remove or replace dressings 5 to 10 days after surgery.

POSSIBLE COMPLICATIONS
* Excessive bleeding
* Surgical-wound infection.
* Sensitivity to hot or cold temperatures from exposed roots.

AVERAGE HOSPITAL STAY—0 to 1 day.

PROBABLE OUTCOME—Expect complete healing without complications. The affected gum tissue should heal and return to its normal pink color again in 2 to 3 weeks.

 POSTOPERATIVE CARE

GENERAL MEASURES
* No smoking.
* Do not disturb the dressing.
* Apply ice packs to relieve pain. Do this for 10 minutes at a time as often as needed for the first 24 hours after surgery.
* Keep your teeth free of plaque (germs, food debris and saliva). Brush your teeth and use dental floss as directed by your dentist. Mouth irrigations also help to prevent plaque.

MEDICATION
* Your dentist may prescribe:
  - Pain relievers. Don't take prescription pain medication longer than 4 to 7 days. Use only as much as you need.
  - Antibiotics to fight or prevent infection.
* You may use nonprescription drugs, such as acetaminophen, for minor pain. Avoid aspirin.

ACTIVITY
* To help recovery and aid your well-being, resume daily activities, including work, as soon as you are able.
* Avoid vigorous exercise for 3 weeks after surgery.
* Resume driving 2 days after returning home.

DIET—Clear liquid diet until healing occurs. Then eat a well-balanced diet to promote healing.

 CALL YOUR DOCTOR IF

* The dressing becomes loose.
* You experience nausea or vomiting.
* Pain, swelling, redness, drainage or bleeding increases in the surgical area.
* Bleeding recurs 48 hours or longer after surgery.
* You develop signs of infection, including headache, muscle aches, dizziness or a general ill feeling and fever.
* New, unexplained symptoms develop. Drugs used in treatment may produce side effects.

PERIODONTAL SURGERY
(Pyorrhea Treatment)

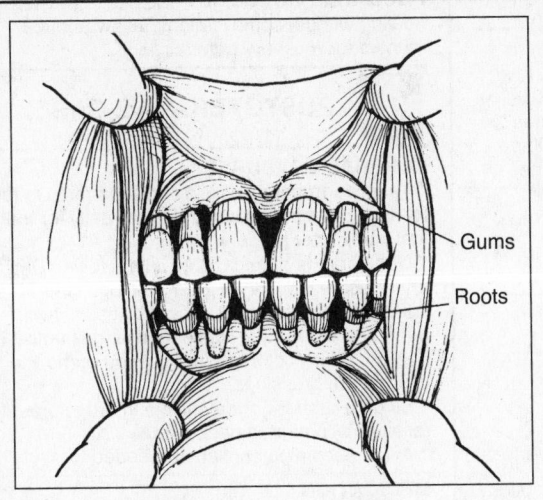

An illustration of the mouth, gums and roots of teeth.

Gums

Roots

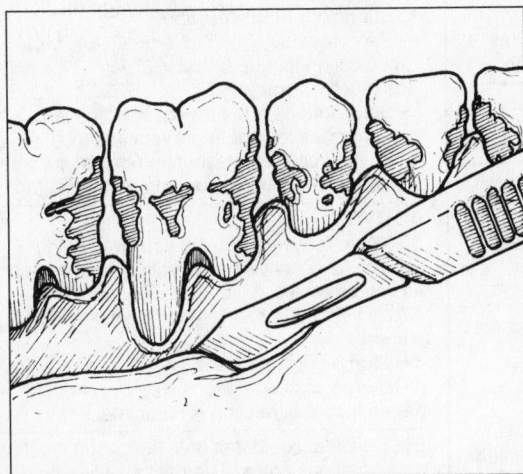

Periodontal tissue cut free and removed.

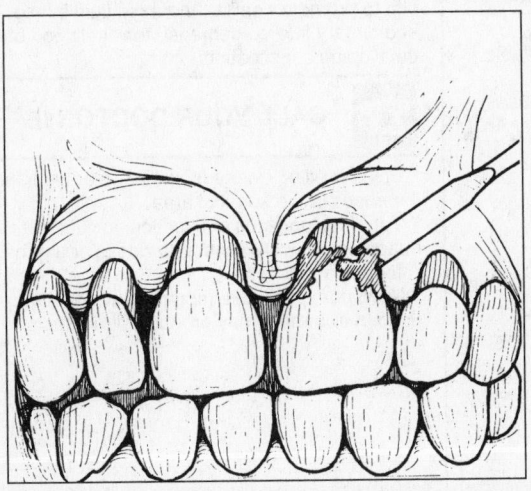

Special dressings are applied to control bleeding and hasten healing. These usually need to be removed or replaced 5 to 10 days after surgery.

PILONIDAL CYST REMOVAL

GENERAL INFORMATION

DEFINITION—Removal of a pilonidal cyst, a cyst that is located in area of the sacrum. In a pilonidal cyst, surface skin containing sweat glands, oil glands and hair follicles becomes trapped beneath the surface of the skin. The cyst often forms cavities, or openings to the outside, called sinuses. The cyst can also become infected, and an abscess can form.

BODY PARTS INVOLVED—Area over the tailbone.

REASONS FOR SURGERY—Relief of pain and prevention of the spread of infection.

SURGICAL RISK INCREASES WITH
* Obesity.
* Smoking.
* Recent or chronic illness.
* Diabetes.
* Use of some prescription and nonprescription drugs. Inform your doctor of any drugs, medications, or vitamin and herb supplements you are using or have used in the last month.

WHAT TO EXPECT

WHO OPERATES—General surgeon or proctologist.

WHERE PERFORMED—Hospital, outpatient surgical facility, doctor's office.

DIAGNOSTIC TESTS
* Before surgery: Blood and urine studies; chest x-ray; sigmoidoscopy (see Glossary).
* After surgery: Blood tests.

ANESTHESIA
* Local anesthesia by injection.
* General anesthesia by injection and inhalation with an airway tube placed in the windpipe.

DESCRIPTION OF OPERATION
* A variety of surgical treatments are available. One type is described here.
* The cyst and its cavities (also called sinuses) over the tailbone are identified with probes. An incision is made around the cyst.
* The cyst and all affected sinuses are removed.
* Bleeding is controlled with sutures or electrocauterization.
* The skin is usually left open to heal from the bottom out. This can take a period of 4 to 8 weeks.

POSSIBLE COMPLICATIONS
* Excessive bleeding.
* Surgical-wound infection.
* Slow healing.
* Recurrence of cyst.

AVERAGE HOSPITAL STAY—0 to 2 days.

PROBABLE OUTCOME—Expect complete healing without complications. Allow about 2 months for recovery from surgery.

POSTOPERATIVE CARE

GENERAL MEASURES
* Take warm baths to relieve discomfort. Do this for 15 to 20 minutes several times daily for the first week after surgery.
* Don't dry the surgical area with a towel. Drip dry or use a blow dryer after bathing.
* If the cyst is left open to heal by itself, it will drain and will require dressing changes until it is healed. Your doctor will instruct you on how to change the dressings.
* Sit on a rubber ring (available in drugstores) to relieve discomfort, if necessary.
* Avoid becoming constipated.

MEDICATION
* Your doctor may prescribe:
  - Pain relievers. Don't take prescription pain medication longer than 4 to 7 days. Use only as much as you need.
  - Stool softeners to prevent constipation.
  - Antibiotics to fight or prevent infection.
* You may use nonprescription drugs, such as acetaminophen, for minor pain. Avoid aspirin.

ACTIVITY
* To help recovery and aid your well-being, resume daily activities, including work, as soon as you are able.
* Avoid vigorous exercise for 6 weeks after surgery.
* Resume driving 1 week after returning home.
* Resume sexual relations when your doctor determines that healing is complete.

DIET—Clear liquid diet until the gastrointestinal tract functions again. Then eat a well-balanced diet to promote healing. Increase fluid intake and dietary fiber to decrease the likelihood of developing constipation.

CALL YOUR DOCTOR IF

* Pain, swelling, redness, drainage or bleeding increases in the surgical area.
* You develop signs of infection, including headache, muscle aches, dizziness or a general ill feeling and fever.
* New, unexplained symptoms develop. Drugs used in treatment may produce side effects.

PILONIDAL CYST REMOVAL

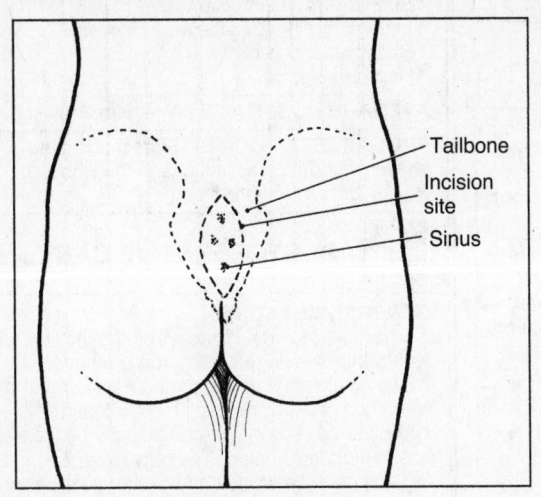

Tailbone

Incision site

Sinus

An illustration of several sinuses that tract from the deeper cysts to the skin surface.

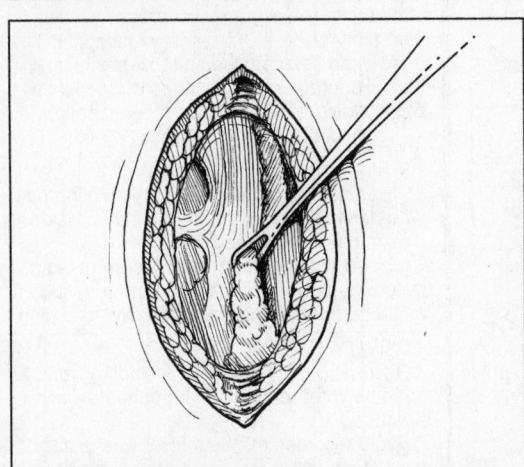

The cyst and all affected sinuses are identified and removed.

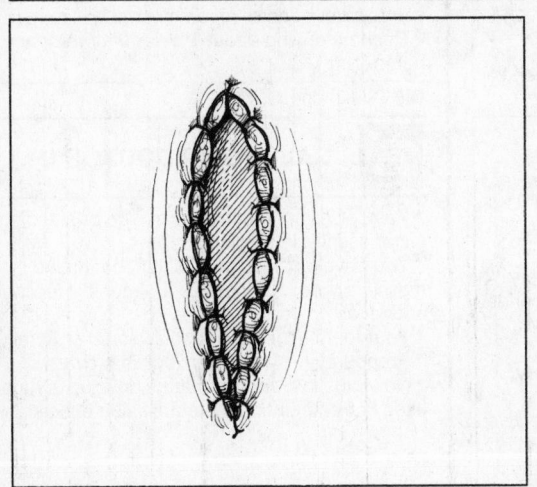

The skin is usually left open to heal slowly from the bottom. Some surgeons close the skin over the operative site at the time of surgery.

SURGERIES

POPLITEAL ARTERY EMBOLECTOMY

GENERAL INFORMATION

DEFINITION—Removal of a blood clot (embolus) that has blocked blood supply to the leg and foot.

BODY PARTS INVOLVED—Blood vessel in the leg that is called the femoral artery below the groin and the popliteal artery behind the knee; the heart is the usual source of the blood clot.

REASONS FOR SURGERY—Restoration of normal blood circulation in the legs. Re-establishing blood flow can restore muscular function, prevent gangrene and enable patients to return to normal or almost normal activities.

SURGICAL RISK INCREASES WITH
* Obesity; smoking.
* Rheumatic heart disease or coronary artery disease.
* Diabetes.
* Use of some prescription and nonprescription drugs. Inform your doctor of any drugs, medications, or vitamin and herb supplements you are using or have used in the last month.

WHAT TO EXPECT

WHO OPERATES—General surgeon or vascular surgeon.

WHERE PERFORMED—Outpatient surgical facility or hospital.

DIAGNOSTIC TESTS
* Before surgery: Blood and urine studies; chest x-ray; ECG; arteriogram (see Glossary for both).
* During surgery: Arteriogram (see Glossary) after blood clot is removed.
* After surgery: Blood studies; heart studies, such as sonogram (see Glossary).

ANESTHESIA
* Spinal anesthesia by injection.
* General anesthesia by injection and inhalation with an airway tube placed in the windpipe.

DESCRIPTION OF OPERATION
* An incision is usually made over the artery where the clot is lodged. Sometimes, however, the incision is made in the groin.
* The blood flow is controlled and the artery is opened above the blood clot.
* A special catheter is passed into the artery beyond the blood clot. The catheter is expanded with air beyond the clot and then withdrawn, forcing the clot out of the artery.
* An anticoagulant is injected into the artery, and normal blood circulation is restored.
* The artery is closed. Muscles and connective tissue are sewn together in layers. The skin is closed with sutures or clamps, which usually can be removed about 1 week after surgery.

POSSIBLE COMPLICATIONS
* Excessive bleeding.
* Surgical-wound infection.
* Inadvertent injury to the large nerves.
* Recurrent blood clot.
* Heart problems.

AVERAGE HOSPITAL STAY—0 to 3 days.

PROBABLE OUTCOME—Expect complete healing without complications. Allow about 3 weeks for recovery from surgery.

POSTOPERATIVE CARE

GENERAL MEASURES
* A hard ridge should form along the incision. As it heals, the ridge will gradually recede.
* Use an electric heating pad, a heat lamp or a warm compress to relieve incisional pain.
* Shower as usual. Avoid baths until the incision has completely healed. You may wash the incision gently with mild, unscented soap. After showering, replace any wet dressings with clean, dry ones.
* Move and elevate legs often while resting in bed to decrease the likelihood of deep-vein blood clots.

MEDICATION
* Your doctor may prescribe:
  - Pain relievers. Don't take prescription pain medication longer than 4 to 7 days. Use only as much as you need.
  - Blood thinners to prevent recurrent clots.
* You may use nonprescription drugs, such as acetaminophen, for minor pain. Avoid aspirin.

ACTIVITY
* Resuming daily activities, including work, as soon as you are able can help the healing process.
* Avoid vigorous exercise for 3 weeks after surgery, but start a walking exercise program as soon as your doctor recommends.
* Resume driving about 1 week after returning home.

DIET—No special diet.

CALL YOUR DOCTOR IF

* Pain, swelling, redness, drainage or bleeding increases in the surgical area.
* You develop signs of infection: headache, muscle aches, dizziness or a general ill feeling and fever.
* Your foot becomes cold, discolored or numb.
* Preoperative symptoms don't improve.
* New, unexplained symptoms develop. Drugs used in treatment may produce side effects.

POPLITEAL ARTERY EMBOLECTOMY

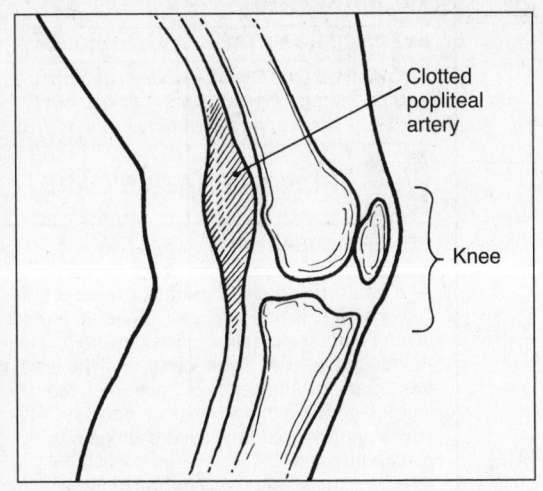

An illustration of a clot in the popliteal artery extending behind the knee.

Clotted popliteal artery

Knee

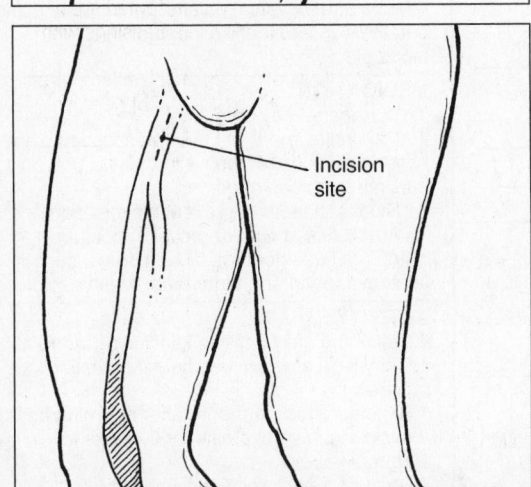

An incision for a special catheter is made inside the upper thigh at the inguinal level.

Incision site

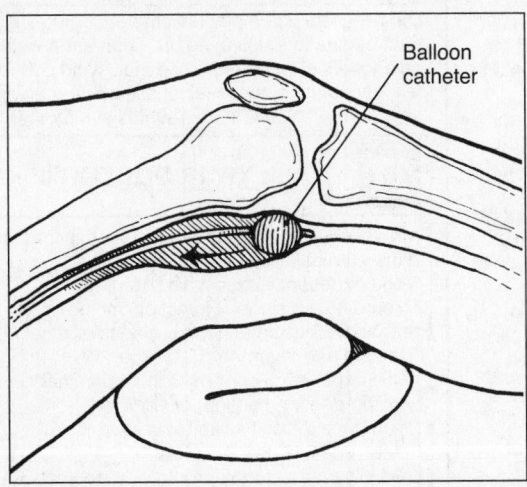

The catheter is passed into the artery beyond the blood clot. It is expanded with air and then withdrawn, forcing the clots out of the artery.

- After the clot has been removed, muscles and connective tissues are sewn together in layers. The skin is closed with sutures or clamps.

Balloon catheter

SURGERIES

PROSTATE GLAND REMOVAL, SUPRAPUBIC

GENERAL INFORMATION

DEFINITION—Removal of an abnormal or enlarged prostate gland through an opening in the lower abdomen.

BODY PARTS INVOLVED—Prostate gland; bladder; rectum; urethra.

REASONS FOR SURGERY
• Restoration of normal passage of urine.
• Cancer of the prostate.

SURGICAL RISK INCREASES WITH
• Adults over 60.
• Stress; smoking; obesity.
• Poor nutrition.
• Recent illness, especially upper-respiratory infection.
• Alcoholism or chronic illness.
• Diabetes.
• Use of some prescription and nonprescription drugs. Inform your doctor of any drugs, medications, or vitamin and herb supplements you are using or have used in the last month.

WHAT TO EXPECT

WHO OPERATES—Urologist.

WHERE PERFORMED—Hospital.

DIAGNOSTIC TESTS
• Before surgery: Blood and urine studies; chest x-ray; kidney function studies; intravenous pyelogram; ultrasound; cystoscopy; ECG (see Glossary for all); prostate biopsy.
• After surgery: Blood studies.

ANESTHESIA
• Spinal anesthesia by injection.
• General anesthesia by injection and inhalation with an airway tube placed in the windpipe.

DESCRIPTION OF OPERATION
• An incision is made in the lower abdomen.
• The bladder and urethra are opened, and the enlarged parts of the prostate gland cut free and removed.
• Two catheters are placed in the bladder, and a tube to drain secretions is placed next to the bladder. The urethra and bladder are closed with sutures. One of the catheters will pass through the penis, and the other will be brought out through the incision along with the drain.
• The catheters and drains will usually remain in place for several days.
• The muscles are repositioned and sewn in place. The skin is closed with sutures or clips, which usually can be removed about 1 week after surgery.

POSSIBLE COMPLICATIONS
• Excessive bleeding.
• Surgical-wound infection.

• Inability to control urinary stream.
• Impotence.
• Sterility (sometimes).

AVERAGE HOSPITAL STAY—3 to 5 days.

PROBABLE OUTCOME—Expect complete healing without complications. Allow about 6 weeks for recovery from surgery.

POSTOPERATIVE CARE

GENERAL MEASURES
• A hard ridge should form along the incision. As it heals the ridge will gradually recede.
• Use an electric heating pad, a heat lamp or a warm compress to relieve incisional pain.
• Shower as usual. Avoid baths until the incision has completely healed. You may wash the incision gently with mild, unscented soap. After showering, replace any wet dressings with clean, dry ones.
• Move and elevate legs often while resting in bed to decrease the likelihood of deep-vein blood clots.

MEDICATION
• Your doctor may prescribe:
  - Pain relievers. Don't take prescription pain medication longer than 4 to 7 days. Use only as much as you need.
  - Stool softeners to prevent constipation.
  - Antibiotics to fight or prevent infection.
• You may use nonprescription drugs, such as acetaminophen, for minor pain. Avoid aspirin.

ACTIVITY
• Resuming daily activities, including work, as soon as you are able can help the healing process.
• Resume driving 1 month after returning home.
• Avoid vigorous exercise for 6 weeks following surgery.
• Resume sexual relations when able.

DIET—Clear liquid diet until the gastrointestinal tract begins to function again. Then eat a well-balanced diet to promote healing. Avoid coffee, tea, cocoa, cola drinks, alcoholic beverages and any food or spice that aggravates symptoms.

CALL YOUR DOCTOR IF

• Pain, swelling, redness or drainage increases in the surgical area.
• You experience excessive bleeding.
• You develop signs of infection, including headache, muscle aches, dizziness or a general ill feeling and fever.
• You experience constipation, abdominal swelling or pain, nausea, or vomiting.
• You have difficulty with urination.
• New, unexplained symptoms develop. Drugs used in treatment may produce side effects.

PROSTATE GLAND REMOVAL, SUPRAPUBIC

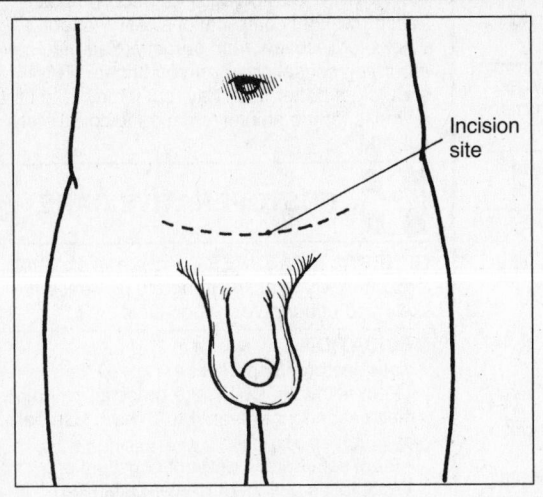

An illustration of the usual incision site for prostatectomy.

Incision site

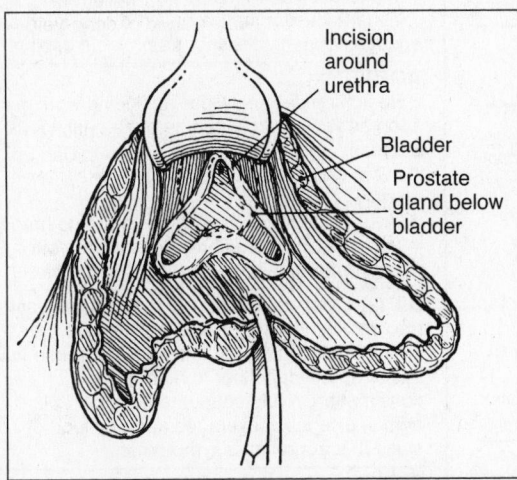

Incision around urethra

Bladder

Prostate gland below bladder

The bladder and urethra are opened and the enlarged parts of the prostate gland cut free and removed.

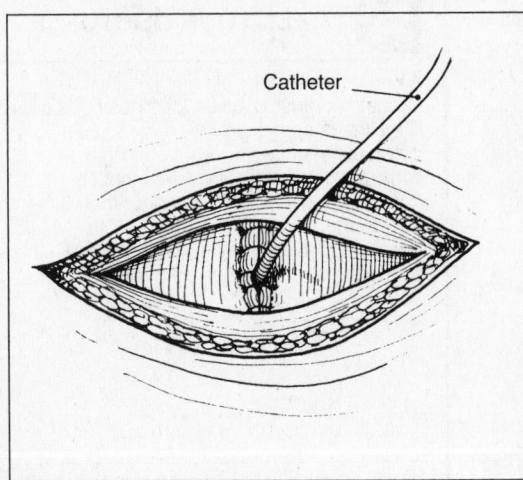

Catheter

Two catheters are placed in the bladder and a tube to drain secretions is placed next to the bladder. The urethra and bladder are closed with sutures.
  • One of the catheters will pass through the penis and the other will be brought out through the incision along with the drain (not illustrated).

PROSTATE GLAND REMOVAL, TRANSURETHRAL

GENERAL INFORMATION

DEFINITION—Removal of part of an enlarged prostate gland with a cystoscope, an instrument that is passed up through the urethra.

BODY PARTS INVOLVED—Penis; prostate gland; urethra; bladder.

REASONS FOR SURGERY—Restoration of normal passage of urine.

SURGICAL RISK INCREASES WITH
• Obesity; smoking.
• Poor nutrition.
• Recent or chronic illness.
• Alcoholism.
• Diabetes.
• Use of some prescription and nonprescription drugs. Inform your doctor of any drugs, medications, or vitamin and herb supplements you are using or have used in the last month.

WHAT TO EXPECT

WHO OPERATES—Urologist.

WHERE PERFORMED—Hospital.

DIAGNOSTIC TESTS
• Before surgery: Blood and urine studies; x-rays of kidneys and chest; kidney-function studies; ECG; intravenous pyelogram (IVP); ultrasound (see Glossary for all).
• After surgery: Blood studies.

ANESTHESIA
• Spinal anesthesia by injection.
• General anesthesia by injection and inhalation with an airway tube placed in the windpipe.

DESCRIPTION OF OPERATION
• A cystoscope (a thin, scope with lenses and a light at its tip) is passed up through the urethra to the prostate gland.
• The prostate gland is examined for tumors and signs of infection.
• An electrosurgical loop is inserted through the cystoscope tip and cuts away the diseased parts of the prostate gland.
• The cystoscope is removed. A catheter may be placed in the bladder for a day or two.

POSSIBLE COMPLICATIONS
• Excessive bleeding.
• Inability to control urinary stream (incontinence).
• Urinary retention.
• Impotence (sometimes).
• Sterility.
• Epididymitis.

AVERAGE HOSPITAL STAY—2 to 3 days.

PROBABLE OUTCOME—Expect complete healing without complications. Allow about 3 weeks for recovery from surgery. You may have a burning sensation when you urinate. This should get better each day, but it may take up to 6 weeks for the painful urination to completely subside.

POSTOPERATIVE CARE

GENERAL MEASURES—Move and elevate legs often while resting in bed to decrease the likelihood of deep-vein blood clots.

MEDICATION
• Your doctor may prescribe:
- Pain relievers. Don't take prescription pain medication longer than 4 to 7 days. Use only as much as you need.
- Stool softeners to prevent constipation.
- Antibiotics to fight or prevent infection.
• You may use nonprescription drugs, such as acetaminophen, for minor pain. Avoid aspirin.

ACTIVITY
• Resuming daily activities, including work, as soon as you are able can help the healing process.
• Avoid vigorous exercise for 2 weeks after surgery.
• Resume driving 1 week after returning home.
• Try to resume sexual relations when your doctor determines that healing is complete.

DIET—Clear liquid diet until the gastrointestinal tract begins to function again. Then eat a well-balanced diet to promote healing. Increase fluid intake and dietary fiber to help prevent constipation. Avoid coffee, tea, cocoa, cola drinks, alcoholic beverages and any food or spice that aggravates symptoms.

CALL YOUR DOCTOR IF

• You develop signs of infection, including headache, muscle aches, dizziness or a general ill feeling and fever.
• You experience nausea, vomiting, constipation, or difficulty with urination.
• You remain impotent for longer than 3 months after surgery.
• New, unexplained symptoms develop. Drugs used in treatment may produce side effects.

PROSTATE GLAND REMOVAL, TRANSURETHRAL

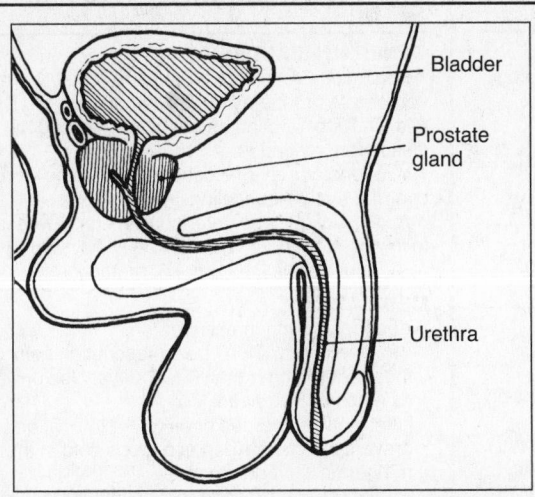

Bladder

Prostate gland

Urethra

A side view of the bladder, urethra and prostate gland in the male.

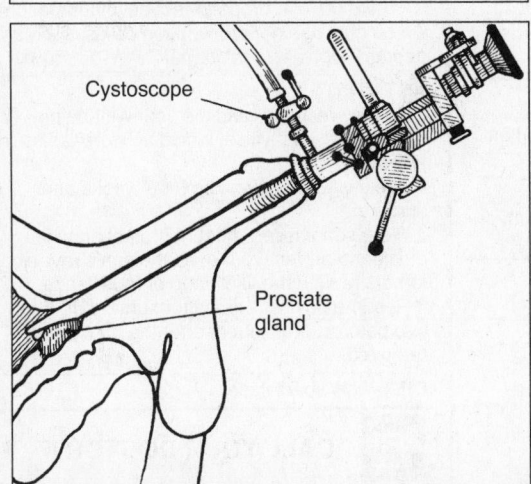

Cystoscope

Prostate gland

The cystoscope is passed through the urethra to the segment where the prostate gland is located.
  • A miniature telescope and light inside the cystoscope make the prostate gland visible through the cystoscope.

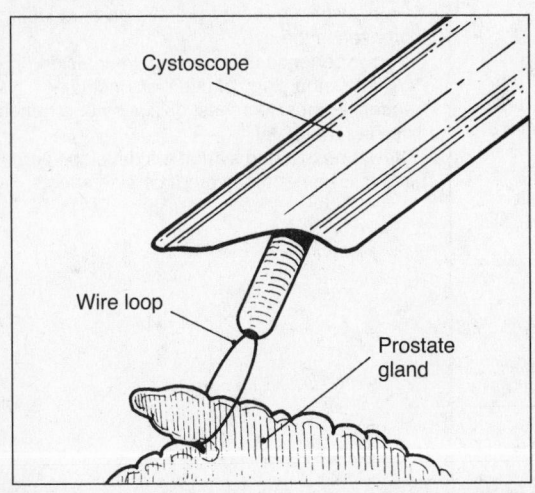

Cystoscope

Wire loop

Prostate gland

A wire snare is passed through the cystoscope tip to remove part of the diseased or enlarged prostate gland.

PTERYGIUM EXCISION

 ## GENERAL INFORMATION

DEFINITION—Removal of a pterygium, an abnormal tissue that grows from the inner edge of the sclera (white outer coat enclosing the eyeball) and extends over a portion of the cornea.

BODY PARTS INVOLVED—Eye; cornea; conjunctiva (the membrane covering the eye).

REASONS FOR SURGERY
* Restoration or protection of normal vision.
* Improved appearance.

SURGICAL RISK INCREASES WITH
* Recent or chronic illness.
* Diabetes.
* Use of some prescription and nonprescription drugs. Inform your doctor of any drugs, medications, or vitamin and herb supplements you are using or have used in the last month.

 ## WHAT TO EXPECT

WHO OPERATES—Ophthalmologist.

WHERE PERFORMED—Hospital or outpatient surgical facility.

DIAGNOSTIC TESTS
* Before surgery: Complete eye examination.
* After surgery: Complete eye examination.

ANESTHESIA
* Local anesthesia by topical application, usually accompanied by sedation.
* Local anesthesia by injection, usually accompanied by sedation.

DESCRIPTION OF OPERATION
* An incision is made in the conjunctiva around the pterygium.
* The pterygium is cut and brought upward, clear of the cornea.
* The lower edge of the pterygium is cut free and the entire pterygium is removed.
* A autograft is fashioned from an area of the conjunctiva underneath the eyelid and is placed to cover the area from where the pterygium was removed.
* Fine sutures are used to attach the graft and to close the membrane from where the graft was taken; the sutures will dissolve and will be absorbed by the body.

POSSIBLE COMPLICATIONS
* Surgical-wound infection.
* Recurrence of the pterygium.
* Scarring.

AVERAGE HOSPITAL STAY—Usually none.

PROBABLE OUTCOME—Expect complete healing without complications. Allow about 3 weeks for recovery from surgery.

 ## POSTOPERATIVE CARE

GENERAL MEASURES
* Beginning 24 hours after surgery, apply warm compresses to the eye to relieve discomfort. Do this for 10 to 15 minutes each hour as long as discomfort continues.
* Your doctor may prescribe a patch to be worn over the eye while healing.
* Avoid sunlight whenever possible for 6 weeks following surgery. If you must be in the sun, wear dark sunglasses with UV protection.

MEDICATION
* Your doctor may prescribe:
  - Pain relievers. Don't take prescription pain medication longer than 4 to 7 days. Use only as much as you need.
  - Antibiotic eye drops or ointment to fight or prevent infection. Keep eye drops cold in the refrigerator, but not frozen.
  - Steroidal eye drops to reduce inflammation.
* You may use nonprescription drugs, such as acetaminophen for minor pain. Avoid aspirin.

ACTIVITY
* To help recovery and aid your well-being, resume daily activities, including work, as soon as you are able.
* Avoid vigorous exercise for 3 weeks after surgery.
* Wear sunglasses with UV protection when outside to protect your eyes the sun's rays and to help reduce the likelihood of recurrence.
* Resume driving 1 day after surgery or, if an eye patch is prescribed, after the patch is removed.

DIET—No special diet.

 ## CALL YOUR DOCTOR IF

* Pain, swelling, redness, drainage or bleeding increases in the eye.
* You experience difficulty with your vision.
* You develop signs of infection, including headache, muscle aches, dizziness or a general ill feeling and fever.
* New, unexplained symptoms develop. Drugs used in treatment may produce side effects.

PTERYGIUM EXCISION

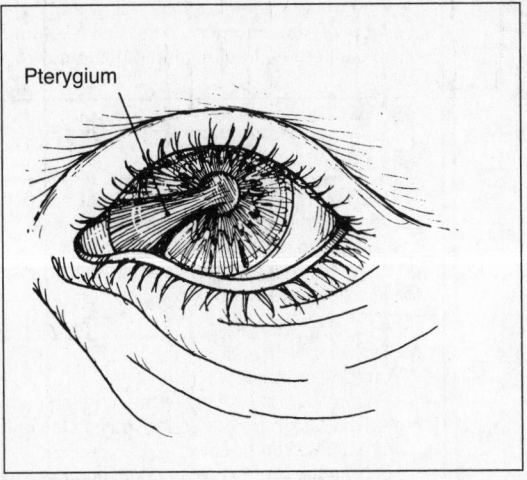

Pterygium

An illustration of a typical pterygium extending from the edge of the eye inward to attach to the cornea.

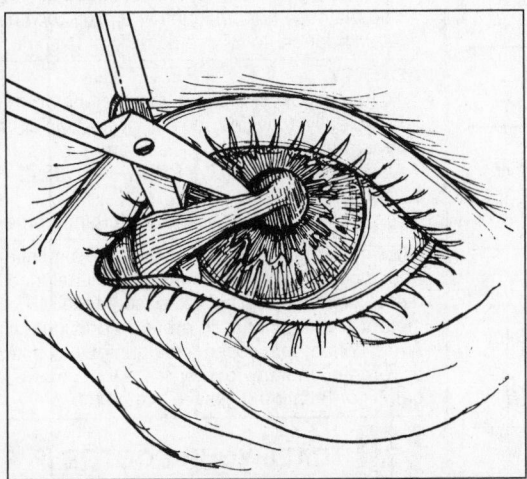

An incision is made in the conjunctiva around the pterygium.
- The pterygium is cut and brought upward clear of the cornea.

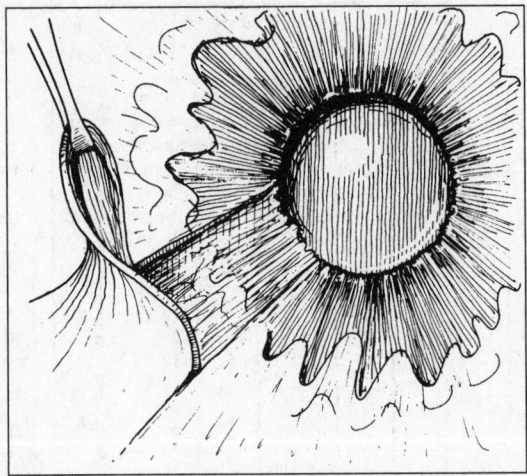

The lower edge of the pterygium is cut free and the entire growth is removed.
- Open areas in the membrane covering the eye are closed with fine sutures that will dissove and be absorbed by the body.

RECTAL OR COLON POLYP REMOVAL
(Polypectomy)

 GENERAL INFORMATION

DEFINITION—Removal of a polyp from the membrane lining inside the rectum or colon.

BODY PARTS INVOLVED—Membrane lining of the rectum and colon.

REASONS FOR SURGERY
- Removal of a possible source of cancer.
- Removal of tissue to see if cancer is present.
- To remove the source of rectal bleeding.

SURGICAL RISK INCREASES WITH
- Obesity.
- Smoking.
- Poor nutrition.
- Recent or chronic illness.
- Diabetes.
- Use of some prescription and nonprescription drugs. Inform your doctor of any drugs, medications, or vitamin and herb supplements you are using or have used in the last month.

 WHAT TO EXPECT

WHO OPERATES—General surgeon; colon-rectal surgeon; gastroenterologist; family doctor.

WHERE PERFORMED—Hospital; outpatient surgical facility; doctor's office.

DIAGNOSTIC TESTS
- Before surgery: Blood and urine studies; x-rays of lower gastrointestinal tract; sigmoidoscopy; colonoscopy (see Glossary for both).
- After surgery: Blood studies; laboratory examination of removed tissue.

ANESTHESIA—Intravenous sedative and narcotic pain killer.

DESCRIPTION OF OPERATION
- The colon is cleansed the night before by drinking various solutions.
- A colonoscope or sigmoidoscope (see Glossary for both) is inserted through the rectum into the sigmoid colon. You may feel mild cramping.
- The polyp is located and removed with a wire snare.
- Bleeding is controlled with electric current or pressure applied with gauze soaked in epinephrine (see Glossary).

POSSIBLE COMPLICATIONS
- Excessive bleeding.
- Inadvertent perforation of the colon resulting in infection.

AVERAGE HOSPITAL STAY—Usually none.

PROBABLE OUTCOME—Expect complete healing without complications. Allow 2 to 3 days for recovery from surgery. If the polyp is found to be cancerous, treatment and outcome will vary.

 POSTOPERATIVE CARE

GENERAL MEASURES—Your first bowel movement may be red or maroon and may contain blood clots. If bowel movements continue to have this appearance, or if you have liquid blood in your stool, contact your doctor right away.

MEDICATION
- Your doctor may prescribe:
  - Pain relievers. Don't take prescription pain medication longer than 4 to 7 days. Use only as much as you need.
  - Stool softeners to prevent constipation.
- You may use nonprescription drugs, such as acetaminophen, to relieve pain. Avoid aspirin.

ACTIVITY
- To help recovery and aid your well-being, resume daily activities, including work, as soon as you are able.
- Avoid vigorous exercise for 4 weeks after surgery.
- Resume driving 3 days after returning home.

DIET—Clear liquid diet until the gastrointestinal tract functions again. Then eat a well-balanced diet to promote healing. Increase intake of dietary fiber and fluids to prevent constipation. Avoid coffee, tea, cocoa, cola drinks, alcoholic beverages and any food or spice that causes painful or irritating digestive symptoms.

 CALL YOUR DOCTOR IF

- You develop signs of infection, including headache, muscle aches, dizziness or a general ill feeling and fever.
- You experience nausea, vomiting, constipation, abdominal swelling or pain.
- You experience weakness, dizziness or a rapid pulse upon standing (symptoms of internal bleeding).
- New, unexplained symptoms develop. Drugs used in treatment may produce side effects.

RECTAL OR COLON POLYP REMOVAL
(Polypectomy)

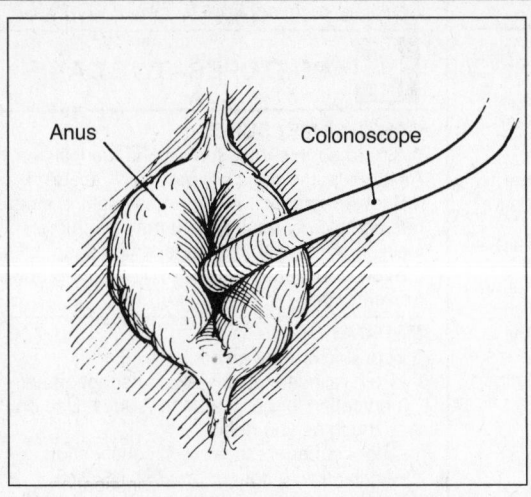

An illustration of a flexible colonoscope inserted into the anus.

Anus

Colonoscope

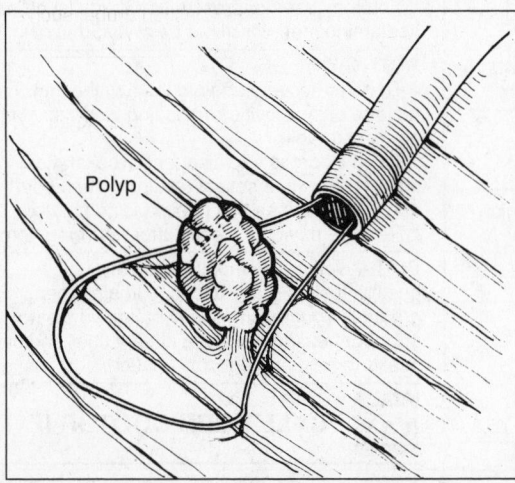

The colonoscope or sigmoidoscope is advanced to reach the sigmoid colon where polyps (when present) are usually located.
  • The polyp is removed with a wire snare.

Polyp

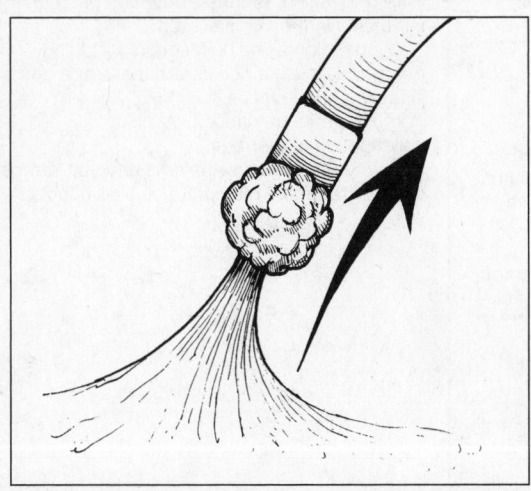

After the polyp has been removed, bleeding of the remaining stump is controlled with electric current.

SURGERIES

RECTOVAGINAL FISTULA REPAIR

GENERAL INFORMATION

DEFINITION—Repair of a fistula (an abnormal tract) between the rectum and vagina that usually results from diverticulitis, cervical cancer, inflammatory bowel disease, radiation therapy or surgical procedures.

BODY PARTS INVOLVED—Vagina; rectum; connective tissue; blood vessels and nerves in the perineum.

REASONS FOR SURGERY
• Prevention of fecal matter from contaminating the vagina or urinary tract.
• Discomfort and embarrassment caused by feces and gas passing through the vagina.

SURGICAL RISK INCREASES WITH
• Obesity; smoking.
• Poor nutrition; alcoholism.
• Recent or chronic illness.
• Diabetes.
• Use of some prescription and nonprescription drugs. Inform your doctor of any drugs, medications, or vitamin and herb supplements you are using or have used in the last month.

WHAT TO EXPECT

WHO OPERATES—Obstetrician-gynecologist, proctologist, colon-rectal surgeon or general surgeon.

WHERE PERFORMED—Hospital.

DIAGNOSTIC TESTS
• Before surgery: Blood and urine studies; x-rays of lower gastrointestinal tract and kidneys.
• After surgery: Blood studies.

ANESTHESIA—General anesthesia by injection and inhalation with an airway tube placed in the windpipe.

DESCRIPTION OF OPERATION
• The abdomen is explored and the involved area of the colon is isolated. The colon is separated from the vaginal opening.
• The segment of colon involved is resected (removed) and the colon is sewn back together.
• Sometimes, a temporary colostomy (see in Surgery section) is necessary for proper healing. This is closed at a later time.
• The skin and muscles are closed with sutures. The skin sutures are removed in about a week.

POSSIBLE COMPLICATIONS
• Excessive bleeding.
• Surgical-wound infection.
• Failure to heal completely.

AVERAGE HOSPITAL STAY—5 to 7 days.

PROBABLE OUTCOME—Expect complete healing without complications. Allow about 6 weeks for recovery from surgery.

POSTOPERATIVE CARE

GENERAL MEASURES
• A hard ridge should form along the incision. As it heals, the ridge will gradually recede.
• Shower as usual. Avoid baths until the incision has completely healed. You may wash the incision gently with mild, unscented soap.
• Avoid constipation and straining during bowel movements.

MEDICATION
• Your doctor may prescribe:
  - Pain relievers. Don't take prescription pain medication longer than 4 to 7 days. Use only as much as you need.
  - Stool softeners to prevent constipation.
  - Antibiotics to fight or prevent infection.
• You may use nonprescription drugs, such as acetaminophen, for minor pain. Avoid aspirin.

ACTIVITY
• To help recovery and aid your well-being, resume daily activities, including work, as soon as you are able.
• Avoid vigorous exercise for 6 weeks after surgery. Resume sexual relations when your doctor determines that healing is complete.
• Resume driving 3 weeks after returning home.

DIET—Nothing by mouth until the gastrointestinal tract functions again. Then, gradually progress to a well-balanced diet to promote healing. Increase dietary fiber and fluid intake to help prevent constipation.

CALL YOUR DOCTOR IF

• Pain, swelling, redness, drainage or bleeding increases in the surgical area.
• You develop signs of infection, including headache, muscle aches, dizziness or a general ill feeling and fever.
• You experience nausea, vomiting, constipation or diarrhea.
• New, unexplained symptoms develop. Drugs used in treatment may produce side effects.

RECTOVAGINAL FISTULA REPAIR

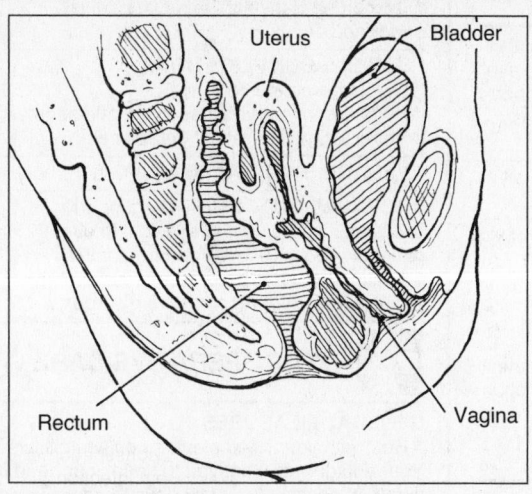

An illustration of the side view of the normal female urogenital tract.

Uterus

Bladder

Rectum

Vagina

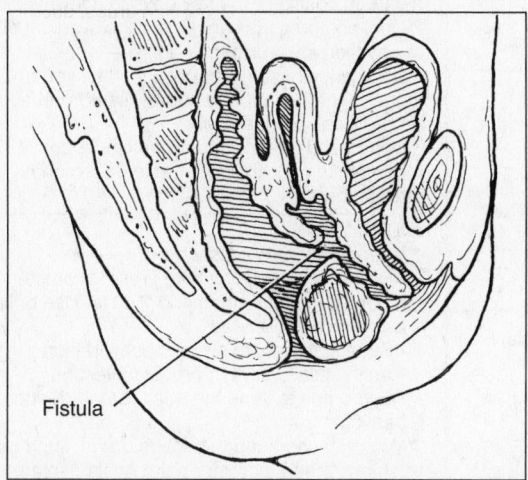

A view of a fistula (an abnormal tract) which has formed between the rectum and the vagina.

Fistula

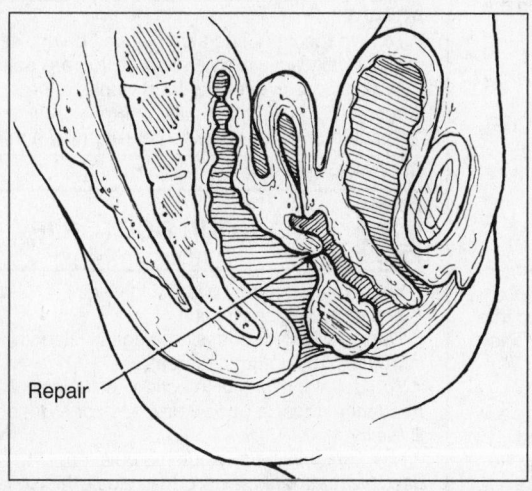

The involved area of the colon is isolated and separated from the vagina. The segment of the colon involved is removed and the colon is then sewn back together.

Repair

SURGERIES

RETINAL DETACHMENT REPAIR

GENERAL INFORMATION

DEFINITION—Reattachment of a retina that has become separated from the rest of the eye. The retina is the light-sensitive area at the back of the eye. See Retinal Detachment in Illness section.

BODY PARTS INVOLVED—The eye and all its parts.

REASONS FOR SURGERY—Prevention of vision loss.

SURGICAL RISK INCREASES WITH
* Obesity; smoking; alcoholism.
* Poor nutrition.
* Recent or chronic illness, especially diabetes.
* Use of some prescription and nonprescription drugs. Inform your doctor of any drugs, medications, or vitamin and herb supplements you are using or have used in the last month.

WHAT TO EXPECT

WHO OPERATES—Ophthalmologist.

WHERE PERFORMED—Hospital or outpatient surgical facility.

DIAGNOSTIC TESTS
* Before surgery: Complete eye examination.
* After surgery: Complete eye examination.

ANESTHESIA
* Local anesthesia by injection or topical application.
* General anesthesia by injection and inhalation with an airway tube placed in the windpipe.

DESCRIPTION OF OPERATION—Your doctor will choose one or more of the following procedures, depending on how severe the detachment is.
* Laser photocoagulation: Tears or holes in the retina are repaired with laser beams that coagulate the eye tissue and cause it to readjust to its normal position.
* Cryopexy: The membrane lining the eye is cut. A cryosurgical probe is placed around the detached retina. The probe applies extreme cold, causing eye tissue to coagulate and to adhere to its normal position.
* Diathermy: Heat from an electric current is applied to seal a tear in the retina.
* Pneumatic retinopexy: If the tear or tears which caused the retina to detach are in the upper part of the eye, a gas can be injected into the eye to push the retina back into place. The tears can then be repaired with laser photocoagulation or cryopexy.
* Scleral buckling: If a large area of the retina is detached, it is often necessary to drain fluid from under the retina and then place a silicone

band or sponge on the outside of the eye to push it against the retina.
* If a cornea transplant is required, it is performed.

POSSIBLE COMPLICATIONS
* Surgical-wound infection.
* Partial or total vision loss in the affected eye from recurrence of retinal detachment.

AVERAGE HOSPITAL STAY—Usually none.

PROBABLE OUTCOME—Surgery is successful in preserving eyesight in over 90% of patients. About 10% will require another operation, which is usually successful. Allow about 2 weeks for recovery from surgery.

POSTOPERATIVE CARE

GENERAL MEASURES
* Rest with your head elevated on two pillows. Your doctor may want you to keep your head in a certain position for a few days to a few weeks.
* Cool compresses can reduce the swelling of the eyelids and surrounding tissue.
* Use dark glasses in bright light until you no longer need to keep the pupils dilated with eye drops. Don't rub the eyes.
* Don't bend over or strain with lifting, bowel movements or urination for at least 6 months after surgery.

MEDICATION
* Your doctor may prescribe:
  - Pain relievers. Don't take prescription pain medication longer than 4 to 7 days. Use only as much as you need.
  - Stool softeners to prevent constipation.
  - Antibiotics to fight or prevent infection.
  - Eye drops to keep the pupil dilated during healing.
* You may use nonprescription drugs, such as acetaminophen for minor pain. Avoid aspirin.

ACTIVITY
* To help recovery and aid your well-being, resume daily activities as soon as you are able.
* Avoid vigorous exercise for 6 weeks after surgery.
* Resume driving 4 weeks after returning home.

DIET—No special diet.

CALL YOUR DOCTOR IF

* You experience any change in vision.
* You develop constipation.
* Pain, swelling, redness, drainage or bleeding increases in the surgical area.
* You develop signs of infection, including headache, muscle aches, dizziness or a general ill feeling and fever.
* New, unexplained symptoms develop. Drugs used in treatment may produce side effects.

RETINAL DETACHMENT REPAIR

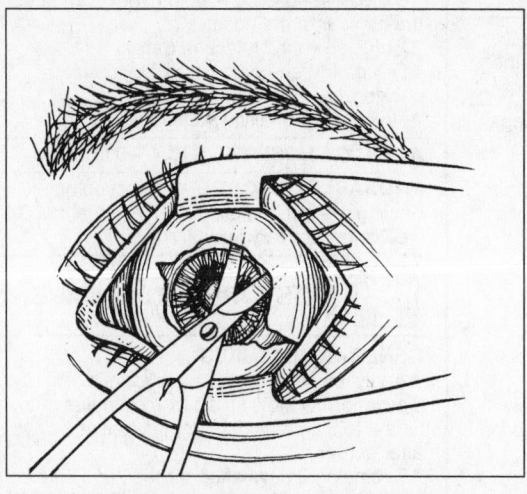

An illustration of the relationship of parts of the eye.
- Scissors cutting the sclera (the membrane lining the eye).

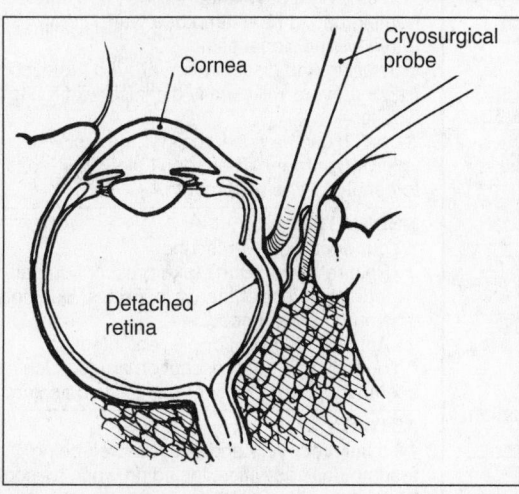

Cyrosurgical probe is placed around the detached retina. The probe applies extreme cold causing eye tissue to coagulate and adhere to its normal position.

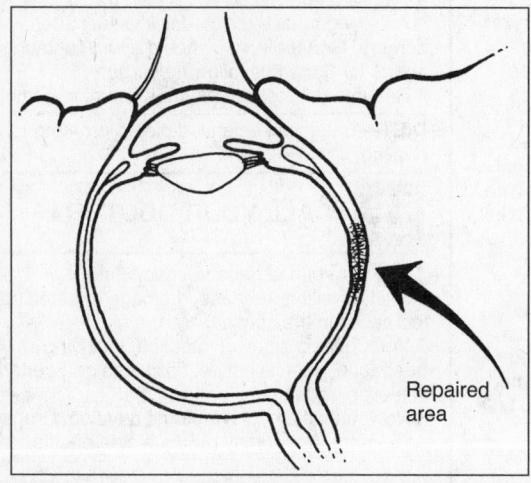

The retina returned to normal position after the detached retina has been secured in its proper position.

SURGERIES

RHINOPLASTY & SEPTOPLASTY

GENERAL INFORMATION

DEFINITION—Reconstruction of the nose (rhinoplasty) and removal of deformities of the septum (septoplasty).

BODY PARTS INVOLVED—Nose, including nasal cartilage and bone and mucous membrane of the septum.

REASONS FOR SURGERY
• Opening of blocked nasal passages.
• Improved appearance.

SURGICAL RISK INCREASES WITH
• Obesity; smoking.
• Poor nutrition.
• Excess alcohol consumption.
• Recent or chronic illness.
• Diabetes.
• Use of some prescription and nonprescription drugs. Inform your doctor of any drugs, medications, or vitamin and herb supplements you are using or have used in the last month.

WHAT TO EXPECT

WHO OPERATES—Plastic and reconstructive surgeon or an ear, nose and throat specialist.

WHERE PERFORMED—Hospital or outpatient surgical facility.

DIAGNOSTIC TESTS
• Before surgery: Blood and urine studies; x-rays of facial bones.
• After surgery: Blood studies.

ANESTHESIA
• Local anesthesia by injection.
• General anesthesia by injection and inhalation with an airway tube placed in the windpipe.

DESCRIPTION OF OPERATION
• The nostril is held open with a speculum.
• An incision is made in the nose. To minimize visual scarring, the incision is usually made from within the nostrils; external cuts may be made if the shape of the nostrils is being changed.
• The bone or cartilage is fractured, trimmed and molded into the desired shape. If the goal is to increase the length of the nose, or to elevate the bridge, cartilage or bone from elsewhere in the body may be used as an implant. A synthetic material may also be used for the implant.
• The mucous membrane is closed with fine sutures, which usually can be removed about 10 days after surgery. Bandages are applied.
• For some procedures, petroleum-jelly-coated packing gauze or plastic splints are used to hold the septum in place during healing (up to 2 weeks).

POSSIBLE COMPLICATIONS
• Excessive bleeding.
• Excessive scarring (keloid) which can affect the contour of the nose.
• Surgical-wound infection (rare).
• Discomfort and pain caused by gauze packing.
• Recurrence of airway obstruction.

AVERAGE HOSPITAL STAY—0 to 1 day.

PROBABLE OUTCOME—Expect complete healing without complications. Allow about 3 weeks for recovery from surgery.

POSTOPERATIVE CARE

GENERAL MEASURES
• Apply ice packs to the nose to relieve discomfort. Do this for 10 to 20 minutes at a time 4 to 8 times a day during the first 2 days after surgery.
• Beginning 2 days after surgery, use an electric heating pad, a heat lamp or a warm compress to relieve incisional pain.
• Swelling and discoloration around the eyes (racoon eyes) will usually diminish within 2 to 3 weeks.
• Don't blow the nose at all for the first week following surgery. Then, don't blow your nose forcefully for the next month.

MEDICATION
• Your doctor may prescribe:
  - Pain relievers. Don't take prescription pain medication longer than 4 to 7 days. Use only as much as you need.
  - Antibiotics to fight or prevent infection.
• You may use nonprescription drugs, such as acetaminophen, for minor pain. Avoid aspirin.

ACTIVITY
• To help recovery and aid your well-being, resume daily activities, including work, as soon as you are able.
• Avoid vigorous exercise for 3 weeks after surgery. Generally, you should avoid contact sports for 6 months following surgery.
• Resume driving 1 week after returning home.

DIET—Eat a well-balanced diet to promote healing.

CALL YOUR DOCTOR IF

• You experience nausea or vomiting.
• Pain, swelling, redness, drainage or bleeding increases in the surgical area.
• You develop signs of infection, including headache, muscle aches, dizziness or a general ill feeling and fever.
• New, unexplained symptoms develop. Drugs used in treatment may produce side effects.

RHINOPLASTY & SEPTOPLASTY

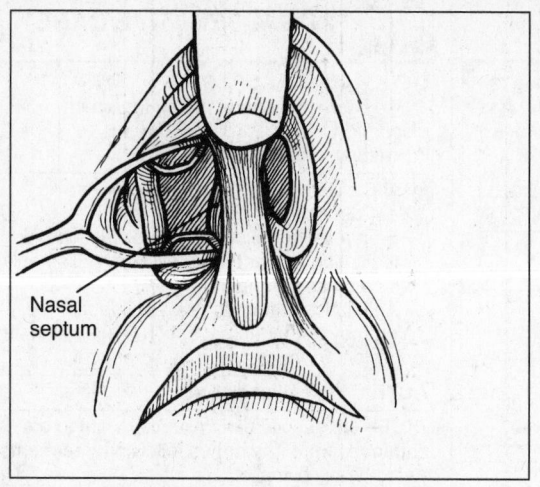

Nasal
septum

An illustration of the mouth and nose
with a speculum opening one side of
the nose.

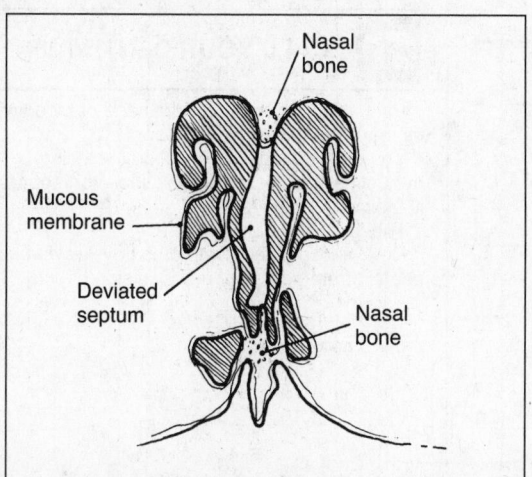

Nasal
bone

Mucous
membrane

Deviated
septum

Nasal
bone

An incision is made inside the nose.
The bone or cartilage is fractured,
trimmed and molded into the desired
shape.

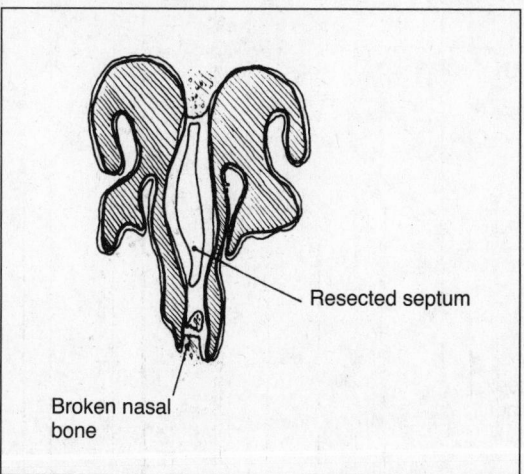

Resected septum

Broken nasal
bone

Resected septum closed with fine
sutures that usually can be removed
about 10 days after surgery.

ROOT CANAL TREATMENT
(Endodontic Therapy)

GENERAL INFORMATION

DEFINITION—A dental procedure designed to save a tooth in which the living tissue (pulp) has died or is chronically diseased. The procedure cleans out dead or dying nerve tissue, as well as any infection, from the inside of a tooth.

BODY PARTS INVOLVED—Teeth and pulp.

REASONS FOR SURGERY—To avoid extraction of the affected tooth.

SURGICAL RISK INCREASES WITH
* Diabetes.
* Use of some prescription and nonprescription drugs. Inform your doctor of any drugs, medications, or vitamin and herb supplements you are using or have used in the last month.

WHAT TO EXPECT

WHO OPERATES—Endodotist (tooth pulp specialist); general dentist.

WHERE PERFORMED—Dentist's office.

DIAGNOSTIC TESTS
* Before surgery: X-rays.
* During surgery: X-rays.
* After surgery: X-rays.

ANESTHESIA—Local anesthetic.

DESCRIPTION OF OPERATION
* Root canal therapy is usually done in 1 to 2 appointments.
* A hole is drilled into the pulp so that any infected matter can be removed.
* The root canals are enlarged and shaped with long, fine-tipped instruments.
* Medicated cotton and a temporary filling are placed in the cavity.
* After a week, or at the next appointment, the filling is removed and the cavity is filled with special material, gutta percha, and the root is sealed.

POSSIBLE COMPLICATIONS
* Pain and swelling.
* Surgical-wound infection.
* Persistent or recurring abscess.

AVERAGE HOSPITAL STAY—Usually none.

PROBABLE OUTCOME—Expect complete healing without complications. Allow about 2 weeks for recovery from surgery. Complete healing may take several months, but there should be no symptoms or discomfort. The tooth should function as long as a normal tooth would. Teeth that undergo root canal treatment usually require a crown.

POSTOPERATIVE CARE

GENERAL MEASURES
* Use warm, salt-water rinses for mouth discomfort.
* Brush and floss teeth as usual.

MEDICATION
* Your dentist may prescribe:
  - Pain relievers. Don't take prescription pain medication longer than 2 or 3 days. Use only as much as you need.
  - Antibiotics to fight or prevent infection.
* You may use nonprescription drugs, such as ibuprofen, for minor pain. Avoid aspirin.

ACTIVITY—No restrictions.

DIET—No special diet. You may want to eat soft foods for a day or two following treatments. Avoid heavy biting.

CALL YOUR DENTIST IF

* Pain, swelling, redness, drainage or bleeding increases in the surgical area.
* You develop signs of infection, including headache, muscle aches, dizziness or a general ill feeling and fever.
* The tooth feels loose.
* New, unexplained symptoms develop. Drugs used in treatment may produce side effects.

ROOT CANAL TREATMENT
(Endodontic Therapy)

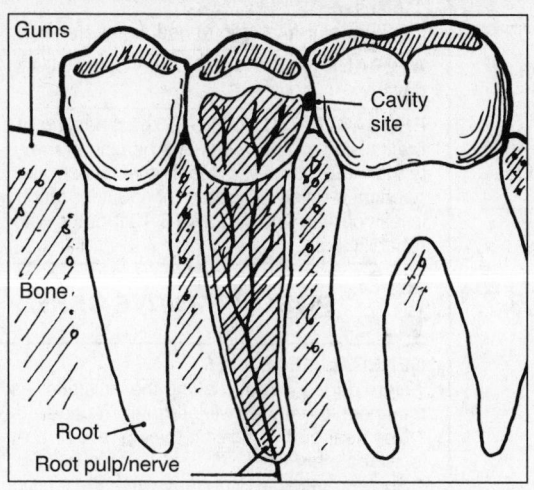

Cavity site is identified.

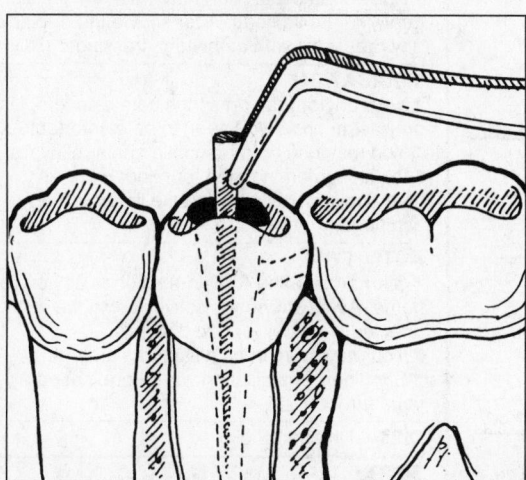

Cavity is drilled and root canal is enlarged.

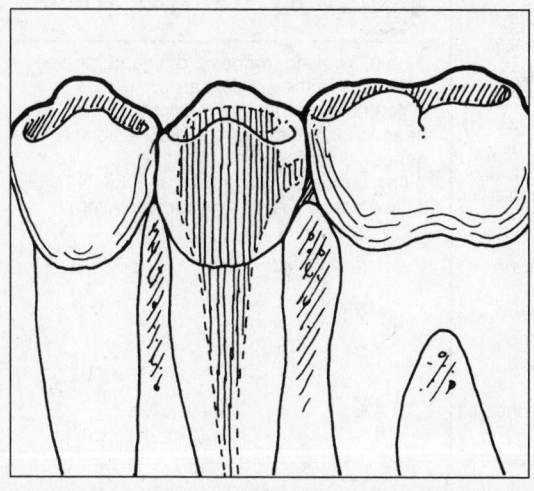

Canal is filled with special material to seal it off.

ROTATOR CUFF REPAIR

GENERAL INFORMATION

DEFINITION—Repair of the tendinous insertions of several shoulder muscles after they are torn by acute trauma or repeated injury. The rotator cuff is a group of muscles and tendons that form a cuff over the shoulder. They hold the arm in its "ball and socket" joint and help the shoulder to rotate.

BODY PARTS INVOLVED—Scapula (wing bone) and several of its muscles, humerus (upper arm bone).

REASONS FOR SURGERY—To alleviate or diminish pain in the shoulder and increase strength in movements requiring shoulder motion. Repair also decreases chances of shoulder dislocation.

SURGICAL RISK INCREASES WITH
* Age.
* Diabetes.
* Poor kidney function.
* High blood pressure.
* Poor nutrition.
* Chronic lung disease.
* Obesity.

WHAT TO EXPECT

WHO OPERATES—Orthopedic surgeon.

WHERE PERFORMED—Hospital.

DIAGNOSTIC TESTS
* Before surgery: Blood tests, MRI, possible arthrogram (see Glossary).
* After surgery: Possible arthrogram.

ANESTHESIA—General anesthesia.

DESCRIPTION OF OPERATION
* There are three approaches to a repair. The recommended approach will depend on the extent of the injury and the experience of the operating surgeon.
* One approach is to repair the torn cuff using an arthroscope. In this surgery small puncture sites are utilized to mobilize the torn tendons and re-anchor them to the top of the humerus.
* A second approach is to assess the tear using an arthroscope and then repair the torn tendon through a mini incision.
* A third approach is the traditional open surgery through an incision extending over the shoulder joint. Again the torn tendons are mobilized and, if possible, fixed to the upper humerus using sutures or staples. Sometimes the end of the scapula (acromion) is trimmed and scar tissue is removed.
* Sometimes the tendons cannot be reattached because they have retracted too much.
* The shoulder is usually immobilized with a sling after surgery.

POSSIBLE COMPLICATIONS
* Bleeding in the joint or from the surgical site.
* Infection.
* Failure of the tendon to heal to the bone

AVERAGE HOSPITAL STAY—Usually 0-3 days.

PROBABLE OUTCOME—Expect healing of the incision in 2-3 weeks and healing of the tendon in 8-10 weeks. Most patients experience good pain relief. Full return of shoulder function is less certain and can take 8-12 months with rehabilitation.

POSTOPERATIVE CARE

GENERAL MEASURES
* Hard ridges will form along the incisions. As they heal, the ridges will gradually recede.
* Use heat on the incision to help relieve incisional pain.
* Shower as usual. You may wash the incisions gently with mild soap. After showering, replace any dressings with a new dry dressing.

MEDICATION
* Your doctor may prescribe pain relievers. Use only as much as you need to be comfortable.
* You may use nonprescription pain relievers such as acetaminophen for minor pain. Ask your doctor if it is okay to take ibuprofen or aspirin.

ACTIVITY
* Start ambulating (walking) as soon as you are home. Avoid strenuous activity using the affected shoulder for 6 to 8 weeks.
* You may swim once all sutures are out.
* Shoulder rehabilitation will be prescribed by your surgeon.

DIET—No special diet.

CALL YOUR DOCTOR IF

* Pain, swelling, redness, drainage, or bleeding increases in the surgical area.
* You develop signs of infection, including headache, muscle aches, dizziness, fever, or a general ill feeling.
* Arm becomes cold, numb, painful, or swollen.
* New unexplained symptoms develop.

ROTATOR CUFF REPAIR

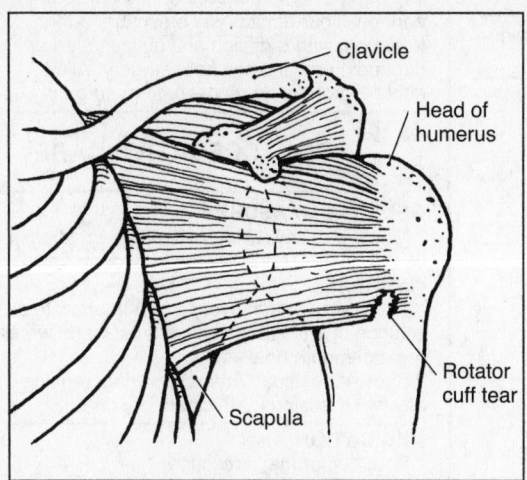

An illustration of the shoulder anatomy with a small rotator cuff tear.

Clavicle

Head of humerus

Rotator cuff tear

Scapula

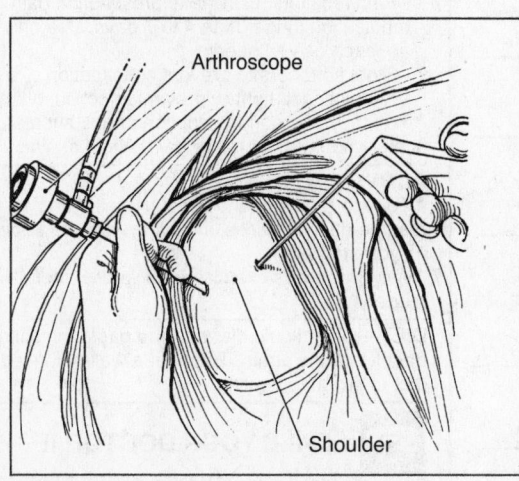

The surgery can be performed open or using arthroscopy. The illustration shows an arthroscope and an instrument inserted through small puncture wounds to repair the torn cuff.

Arthroscope

Shoulder

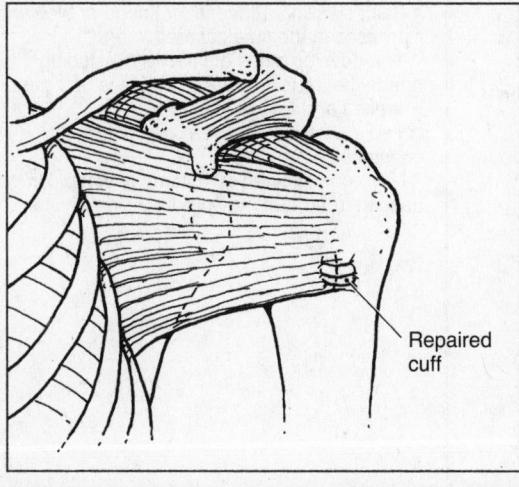

The cuff is fixed back to the humerus with staples or sutures.

Repaired cuff

SALIVARY GLAND TUMOR REMOVAL

GENERAL INFORMATION

DEFINITION—Removal of a cancerous tumor of the salivary glands.

BODY PARTS INVOLVED—Salivary glands under the tongue (sublingual) or under the jawbone (submaxillary or parotid).

REASONS FOR SURGERY—Cancer or suspected cancer of the sublingual, parotid or submaxillary salivary glands.

SURGICAL RISK INCREASES WITH
• Adults over 60.
• Obesity.
• Smoking.
• Excess alcohol consumption.
• Poor nutrition.
• Recent or chronic illness.
• Diabetes.
• Use of some prescription and nonprescription drugs. Inform your doctor of any drugs, medications, or vitamin and herb supplements you are using or have used in the last month.

WHAT TO EXPECT

WHO OPERATES—Ear, nose and throat specialist (otolaryngologist) or general surgeon.

WHERE PERFORMED—Hospital.

DIAGNOSTIC TESTS
• Before surgery: Blood and urine studies; x-rays of the head, neck, upper gastrointestinal tract and chest.
• After surgery: Blood studies.

ANESTHESIA—General anesthesia by injection and inhalation with an airway tube placed in the windpipe.

DESCRIPTION OF OPERATION
• Incisions are made in the skin over the tumor.
• The tumor is isolated, cut free and removed.
• The tissue is examined to determine if the tumor is benign or cancerous.
• If the tumor is benign, the skin over the tumor is closed with fine silk sutures.
• A plastic drain tube may be placed in the incision and left for several days.
• If the tumor is cancerous, a radical neck dissection (see in Surgery section) is usually performed.

POSSIBLE COMPLICATIONS
• Excessive bleeding.
• Surgical-wound infection.
• Facial nerve injury.
• Fistula (see Glossary) from salivary gland.

AVERAGE HOSPITAL STAY—1 to 2 days.

PROBABLE OUTCOME—Expect complete healing without complications. You may experience some permanent numbness of the earlobe. Your doctor may prescribe further treatment with radiation and anticancer drugs depending on findings from surgery. Allow about 3 months for recovery from surgery.

POSTOPERATIVE CARE

GENERAL MEASURES
• Move and elevate legs often while resting in bed to decrease the likelihood of deep-vein blood clots.
• Rinse your mouth every 2 to 3 hours with a solution of 1 teaspoon salt in 8 oz. warm water. A clean mouth heals faster.
• Shower as usual. After showering, replace any wet dressings with clean, dry ones.

MEDICATION
• Your doctor may prescribe:
  - Pain relievers. Don't take prescription pain medication longer than 4 to 7 days. Use only as much as you need.
  - Stool softeners to prevent constipation.
  - Antibiotics to fight or prevent infection.
• You may use nonprescription drugs, such as acetaminophen, for minor pain. Avoid aspirin.

ACTIVITY
• To help recovery and aid your well-being, resume daily activities, including work, as soon as you are able.
• Avoid vigorous exercise for 3 weeks after surgery.

DIET—Clear liquid diet until the gastrointestinal tract functions again. Then eat a well-balanced diet to promote healing.

CALL YOUR DOCTOR IF

• Pain, swelling, redness, drainage or bleeding increases in the surgical area.
• You develop signs of infection, including headache, muscle aches, dizziness or a general ill feeling and fever.
• You experience nausea, vomiting or constipation.
• New, unexplained symptoms develop. Drugs used in treatment may produce side effects.

SALIVARY GLAND TUMOR REMOVAL

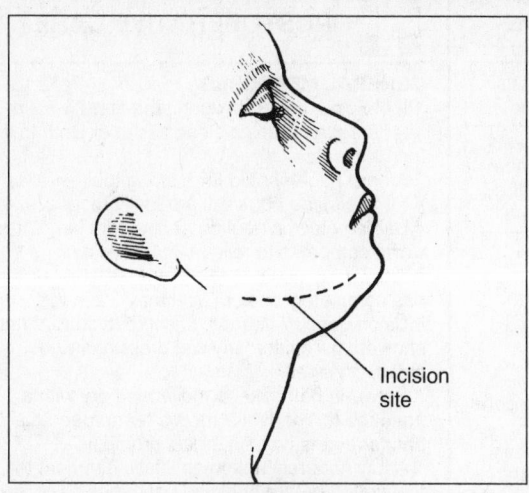

An illustration of the submaxillary area with the dotted line indicating the incision site for submaxillary gland removal.

Incision site

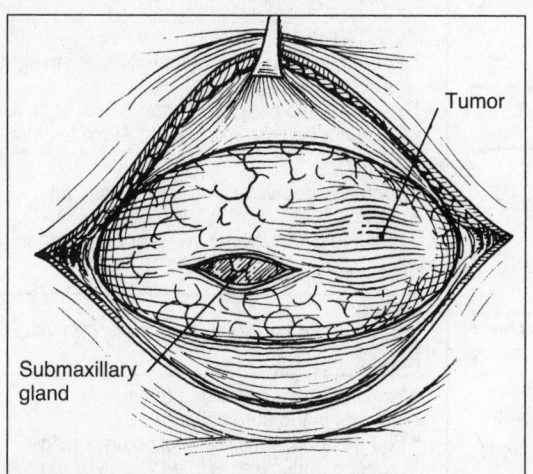

Incisions are made through the skin and tissues under the skin to expose the tumor.

Tumor

Submaxillary gland

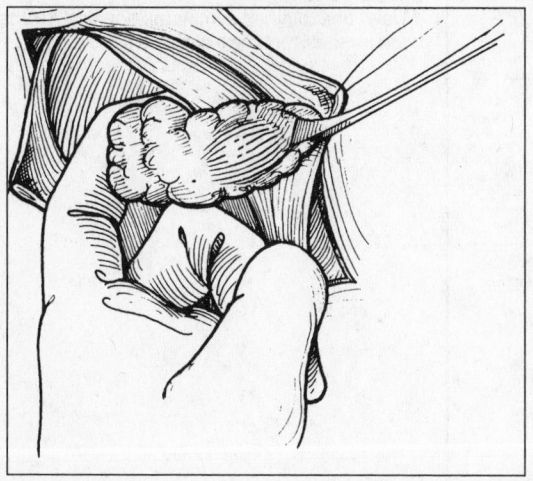

The tumor is isolated, cut free and scooped out with a finger or surgical instrument.

SURGERIES

SEBACEOUS CYST REMOVAL
(Epidermoid Cyst Removal)

 GENERAL INFORMATION

DEFINITION—Removal of benign sebaceous cysts, sometimes called epidermoid cysts.

BODY PARTS INVOLVED—Sebaceous cysts, usually occurring on the skin of the trunk, face, scalp and neck. They often appear behind the ear.

REASONS FOR SURGERY
• Prevention of infections.
• Improved appearance.

SURGICAL RISK INCREASES WITH
• Any bleeding disorder.
• Diabetes.
• Use of some prescription and nonprescription drugs. Inform your doctor of any drugs, medications, or vitamin and herb supplements you are using or have used in the last month.

 WHAT TO EXPECT

WHO OPERATES—Family doctor, general surgeon or dermatologist.

WHERE PERFORMED—Doctor's office or outpatient surgical facility.

DIAGNOSTIC TESTS
• Before surgery: Usually none.
• After surgery: Laboratory examination of removed tissue.

ANESTHESIA—Local anesthesia by injection.

DESCRIPTION OF OPERATION
• An incision is made over the cyst, with care taken not to rupture its confining wall. Leakage from the cyst can cause inflammation and delayed healing.
• The cyst and its contents are removed intact.
• The skin is closed with sutures or clips, which usually can be removed about 1 week after surgery.

POSSIBLE COMPLICATIONS
• Excessive bleeding.
• Surgical-wound infection.
• Recurrence of the cyst, if the cyst wall is not completely removed.

AVERAGE HOSPITAL STAY—Usually none.

PROBABLE OUTCOME—Expect complete healing without complications. Allow about 2 to 3 weeks for healing to be fairly complete.

 POSTOPERATIVE CARE

GENERAL MEASURES
• If the wound bleeds during the first 24 hours after surgery, press a clean tissue or cloth to it for 10 minutes.
• A hard ridge should form along the incision. As it heals, the ridge will gradually recede.
• Use an electric heating pad, a heat lamp or a warm compress to relieve incisional pain.
• Shower as usual. Avoid baths until the incision has completely healed. You may wash the incision gently with mild, unscented soap. After showering, replace any wet dressings with clean, dry ones.
• Between baths, keep the wound dry with a bandage for the first 2 days after surgery. If a bandage gets wet, change it promptly.
• Apply nonprescription antibiotic ointment to the wound before applying bandages.

MEDICATION
• Your doctor may prescribe antibiotics to fight or prevent infection.
• You may use nonprescription drugs, such as acetaminophen, for minor pain. Avoid aspirin.

ACTIVITY
• Avoid vigorous exercise for 2 weeks after surgery.
• Resume driving when you feel well enough to.

DIET—No special diet.

 CALL YOUR DOCTOR IF

• Pain, swelling, redness, drainage or bleeding increases in the surgical area.
• You develop signs of infection, including headache, muscle aches, dizziness or a general ill feeling and fever.
• New, unexplained symptoms develop. Drugs used in treatment may produce side effects.

SEBACEOUS CYST REMOVAL
(Epidermoid Cyst Removal)

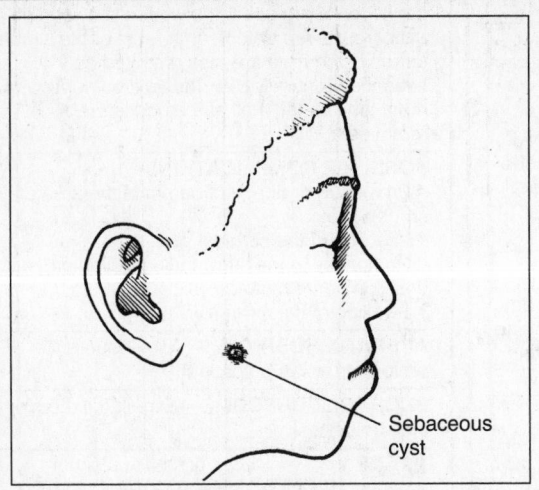

An illustration of a typical sebaceous cyst. In this case, on the side of the face.

Sebaceous cyst

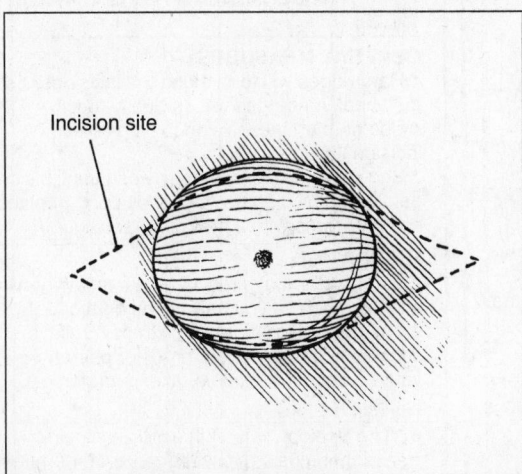

An incision is made over the cyst with care taken not to rupture its capsule (soft tissue lining the surface of the cyst).

Incision site

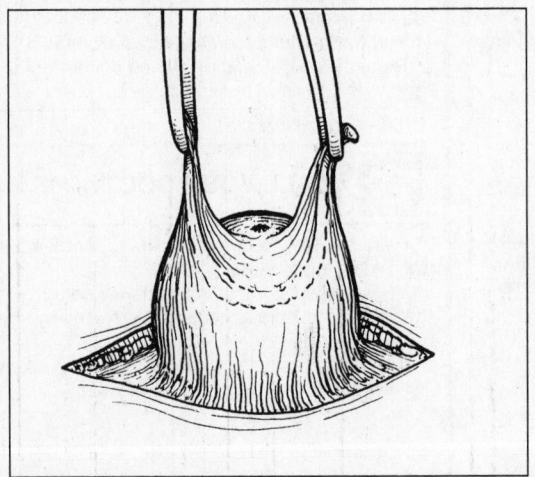

The cyst and its contents are removed intact.

SENTINEL NODE BIOPSY

GENERAL INFORMATION

DEFINITION—Removal of one or more lymph nodes usually in the axilla (armpit) to assess the possible spread of cancer. This is most frequently done with breast cancer but is also done with melanoma and several other solid cancers. The sentinel node is the lymph node where the cancer cells are most likely to go.

BODY PARTS INVOLVED—Axillary lymph nodes. Occasionally groin, chest, or intraabdominal lymph nodes.

REASONS FOR SURGERY—To identify any spread of cancer cells which assists in staging (describing the extent of cancer) and treating the disease.

SURGICAL RISK INCREASES WITH
* Age.
* Diabetes.
* Obesity.

WHAT TO EXPECT

WHO OPERATES—General surgeon.

WHERE PERFORMED—Hospital or outpatient surgical center.

DIAGNOSTIC TESTS
* Before surgery: Only those needed to workup primary cancer. EKG (see Glossary) in elderly patients or previous history of heart disease.
* After surgery: Laboratory examination of the removed node(s).

ANESTHESIA—General anesthesia.

DESCRIPTION OF OPERATION
* The sentinel node can be identified by a radioactive marker or with a blue dye. Frequently both methods are employed to increase the accuracy.
* Prior to surgery a radioactive substance is injected around the tumor or the area where the tumor was removed. In the breast it is sometimes injected around the nipple. A scan may be done to track the progress of the radioactive material.
* After general anaesthesia, a blue dye is injected and and incision is made in the nodal area of concern. A probe is used to track and locate a node which has collected the greatest amount of radioactive substance and the blue dye is tracked in addition, usually to the same one or few nodes.

* The identified node(s) are removed and sent for immediate review by the pathologist. If no cancer cells are seen, the wound is closed. If cancer cells are detected, the rest of the lymph nodes in the area are also removed and examined routinely over the next day or two. A drain may be left if all of the nodes are removed.

POSSIBLE COMPLICATIONS
* Prolonged drainage of serum in the area of surgery.
* Infection of the surgical site.
* Numbness in the surrounding region or possible nerve damage.
* Swelling of the extremity.

AVERAGE HOSPITAL STAY—Usually performed as an outpatient.

PROBABLE OUTCOME—Expect full recovery in 3-4 weeks.

POSTOPERATIVE CARE

GENERAL MEASURES
* Hard ridges will form along the incisions. As they heal, the ridges will gradually recede.
* Use heat on the incision to help relieve incisional pain.
* Shower as usual. You may wash the incisions gently with mild soap. After showering, replace any dressings with a new dry dressing.

MEDICATION
* Your doctor may prescribe pain relievers. Use only as much as you need to be comfortable.
* You may use nonprescription pain relievers such as acetaminophen for minor pain. Ask your doctor if it is okay to take ibuprofen or aspirin.

ACTIVITY
* Start ambulating (walking) as soon as you are home. Take frequent naps as needed during the day when tired.
* You may swim once all sutures are out.
* Resume sexual relations when comfortable and when advised by your surgeon.

DIET—No special diet.

CALL YOUR DOCTOR IF

* Pain, swelling, redness, drainage, or bleeding increases in the surgical area.
* You develop signs of infection, including headache, muscle aches, dizziness, fever, or a general ill feeling.
* Arm becomes cold, numb, painful, or swollen.
* New unexplained symptoms develop.

SENTINEL NODE BIOPSY

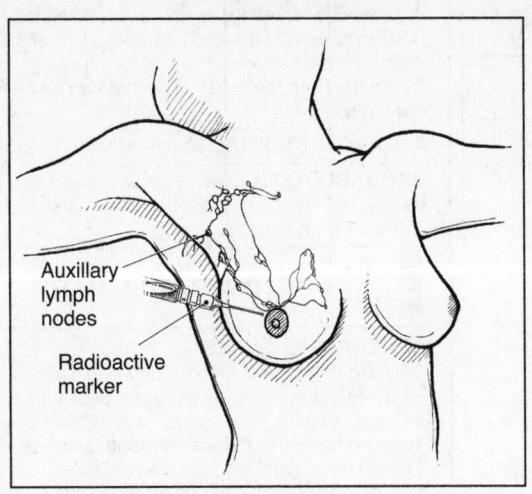

Blue dye and/or a radioactive marker are injected near the tumor or around the areola.

Auxillary lymph nodes

Radioactive marker

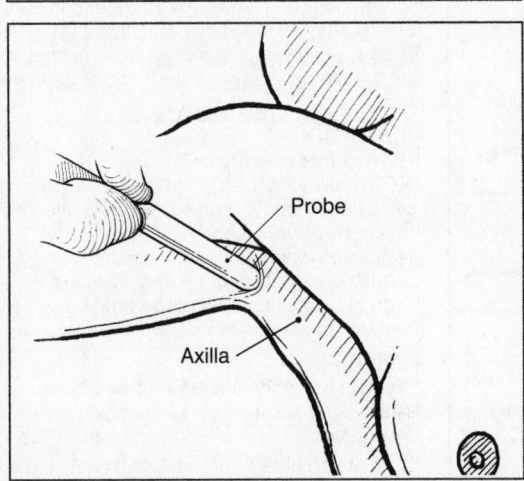

A probe similar to a gieger counter is used to locate lymph nodes that take up the radioactive marker.

Probe

Axilla

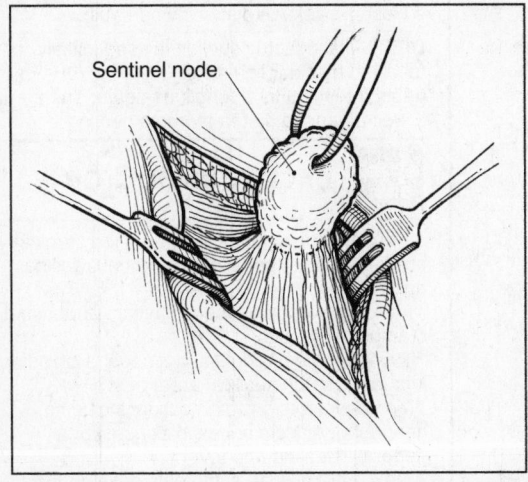

The lymph node(s) containing radioactive marker and/or blue dye is carefully dissected free from the surrounding tissue and examined for cancer cells.

Sentinel node

SIGMOID COLON REMOVAL
(Sigmoid Colectomy)

 GENERAL INFORMATION

DEFINITION—Removal of part or all of the sigmoid colon.

BODY PARTS INVOLVED—Sigmoid colon, the part of the large intestine (colon) that extends from the descending colon to the rectum.

REASONS FOR SURGERY
- Diverticulitis with bleeding or infection.
- Cancer or precancerous polyps.
- Volvulus (see Glossary).
- Colon stricture.
- Rectovaginal fistula.
- Prolapse of rectum.

SURGICAL RISK INCREASES WITH
- Adults over 60 years; newborns and infants.
- Obesity or smoking.
- Poor nutrition.
- Excess alcohol consumption.
- Chronic illness; recent illness such as acute, recurrent diverticulitis.
- Diabetes.
- Use of some prescription and nonprescription drugs. Inform your doctor of any drugs, medications, or vitamin and herb supplements you are using or have used in the last month.

 WHAT TO EXPECT

WHO OPERATES—General surgeon.

WHERE PERFORMED—Hospital.

DIAGNOSTIC TESTS
- Before surgery: Blood and urine studies; x-rays of upper and lower gastrointestinal tract; ECG; endoscopy; proctoscopy; colonoscopy (see Glossary for all).
- After surgery: Blood studies.

ANESTHESIA—General anesthesia by injection and inhalation with an airway tube placed in the windpipe.

DESCRIPTION OF OPERATION
- An incision is made in the abdomen, and the abdominal muscles are opened.
- The sigmoid colon is isolated and clamps are placed at each end.
- All of the diseased sigmoid colon is cut free and removed. The two healthy ends are brought back together and joined.
- The abdominal contents are replaced into the abdomen, and the muscles are closed. The skin is closed with sutures or skin clips, which usually can be removed about 1 week after surgery.
- If surgery is performed to treat infection or tumor, a temporary colostomy (see Surgery section) may be necessary.

POSSIBLE COMPLICATIONS
- Excessive bleeding; deep-vein blood clots.
- Surgical-wound infection; abscess formation.
- Bowel obstruction.
- Leaking from the repair area that can result in peritonitis.

AVERAGE HOSPITAL STAY—7 to 10 days.

PROBABLE OUTCOME—Expect complete healing without complications. Allow 6 weeks for recovery from surgery.

 POSTOPERATIVE CARE

GENERAL MEASURES
- A hard ridge should form along the incision. As it heals, the ridge will gradually recede.
- Use an electric heating pad, a heat lamp or a warm compress to relieve incisional pain.
- Shower as usual. Avoid baths until the incision has completely healed. After showering, replace any wet dressings with clean, dry ones.
- Move and elevate legs often while resting in bed to help decrease the likelihood of deep-vein clots.

MEDICATION
- Your doctor may prescribe:
  - Pain relievers. Don't take prescription pain medication longer than 4 to 7 days. Use only as much as you need.
  - Stool softeners to prevent constipation.
  - Antibiotics to fight or prevent infection.
- You may use nonprescription drugs, such as acetaminophen, for minor pain. Avoid aspirin.

ACTIVITY
- To help recovery and aid your well-being, resume daily activities as soon as you are able.
- Avoid heavy lifting or vigorous exercise for 6 weeks after surgery.
- Resume driving 3 weeks after returning home.
- Resume sexual relations when able.

DIET—Nasogastric suction is used initially, followed by clear liquid diet until the gastrointestinal tract functions again. Then, eat a well-balanced diet to promote healing.

 CALL YOUR DOCTOR IF

- You develop signs of leaking in the surgical area: fever, fast pulse or abdominal swelling and pain.
- You experience nausea, vomiting, abdominal cramps or bloating.
- Pain, swelling, redness, drainage or bleeding increases in the surgical area.
- You develop signs of infection, including headache, muscle aches, dizziness, or a general ill feeling and fever.
- New, unexplained symptoms develop.

SIGMOID COLON REMOVAL
(Sigmoid Colectomy)

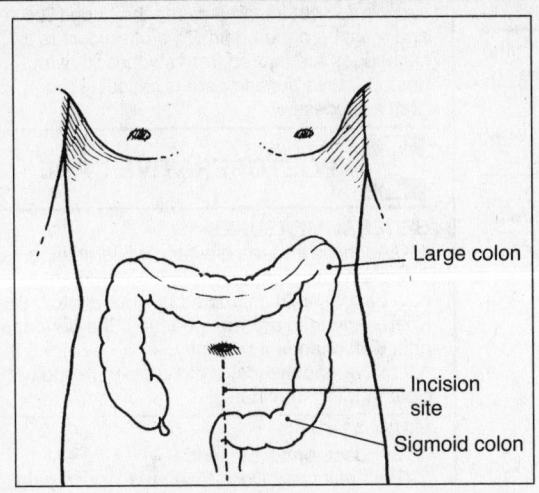

An illustration of the large intestine, sigmoid colon and the usual incision site for this surgical procedure.

Large colon

Incision site

Sigmoid colon

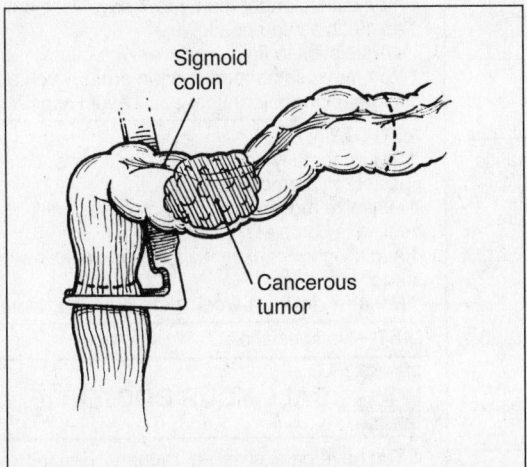

The sigmoid colon is isolated and clamps are placed at each end.
- All of the diseased sigmoid colon is cut free and removed.

Sigmoid colon

Cancerous tumor

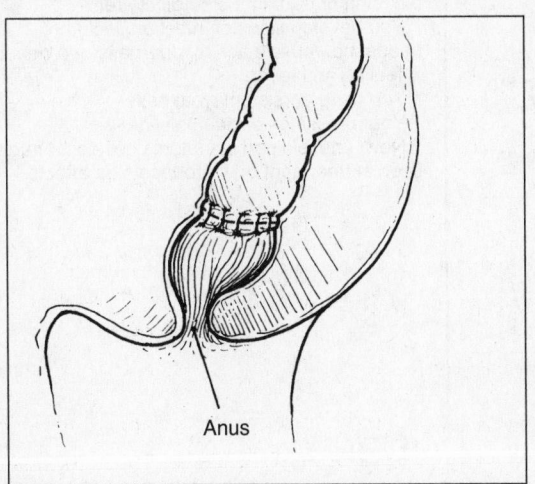

The two healthy ends of the colon are repositioned and joined whenever possible.

Anus

SURGERIES

SKIN GRAFT

GENERAL INFORMATION

DEFINITION—Taking skin from one area of the body and attaching it to another area where no skin exists.

BODY PARTS INVOLVED—Skin (donor sites and recipient sites).

REASONS FOR SURGERY—Extensive wounds, burns or certain surgeries may require skin grafts for healing to occur.

SURGICAL RISK INCREASES WITH
• Adults over 60.
• Newborns and infants.
• Obesity; smoking.
• Poor nutrition.
• Anemia.
• Recent or chronic illness.
• Diabetes.
• Use of some prescription and nonprescription drugs. Inform your doctor of any drugs, medications, or vitamin and herb supplements you are using or have used in the last month.

WHAT TO EXPECT

WHO OPERATES—General surgeon or plastic and reconstructive surgeon.

WHERE PERFORMED—Hospital, outpatient surgical facility or emergency room (rarely).

DIAGNOSTIC TESTS
• Before surgery: Blood and urine studies.
• After surgery: Blood studies.

ANESTHESIA
• Local anesthesia by injection.
• General anesthesia by injection and inhalation with an airway tube placed in the windpipe.

DESCRIPTION OF OPERATION
• Skin is removed from a donor site. The donor site is covered with gauze.
• Debris is cleared from the recipient site.
• The skin from the donor site is placed on the recipient site and fastened at each corner with sutures. Bandages are applied. New blood vessels begin growing from the recipient area into the transplanted skin within 36 hours.

POSSIBLE COMPLICATIONS
• Excessive bleeding.
• Surgical-wound infection.
• Collection of serum under recipient site that prevents growth of new blood vessels.
• Loss of grafted skin.

AVERAGE HOSPITAL STAY—2 to 12 days, depending on extent of surgery.

PROBABLE OUTCOME—Allow about 6 weeks for recovery from surgery. Most skin grafts are successful, but in some cases they don't "take" and must be done again. This often occurs if skin edges are injured from stitches. Skillful postoperative nursing care is critical to the graft's success.

POSTOPERATIVE CARE

GENERAL MEASURES
• Keep the graft area elevated while healing.
• Apply nonprescription antibiotic ointment to new bandages, if instructed by your doctor. Keep bandages dry while bathing. If a bandage gets wet, change it promptly.
• If the wound bleeds, press a clean tissue or cloth to it for 10 minutes.

MEDICATION
• Your doctor may prescribe:
  - Pain relievers. Don't take prescription pain medication longer than 4 to 7 days. Use only as much as you need.
  - Antibiotics to fight or prevent infection.
• You may use nonprescription drugs, such as acetaminophen, for minor pain. Avoid aspirin.

ACTIVITY
• Return to daily activities and work as soon as possible to promote healing.
• Minimize movement of the graft site until healing is complete.
• Avoid vigorous exercise for 6 weeks following surgery.
• Resume driving 1 week after returning home.

DIET—No special diet.

CALL YOUR DOCTOR IF

• You have pain, swelling, redness, drainage, bleeding or odor in the surgical area.
• You develop signs of infection, including headache, muscle aches, dizziness or a general ill feeling and fever.
• You have persistent weakness.
• Your dressings accidentally get wet.
• New, unexplained symptoms develop. Drugs used in treatment may produce side effects.

SKIN GRAFT

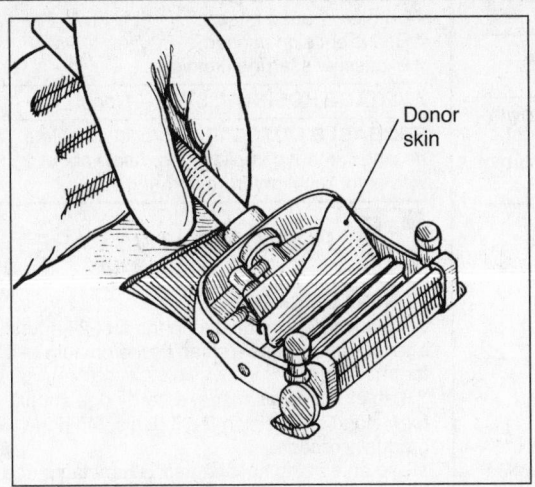

Donor skin

A thin layer of skin to be used for grafting is removed with a dermatome (skin cutting instrument).

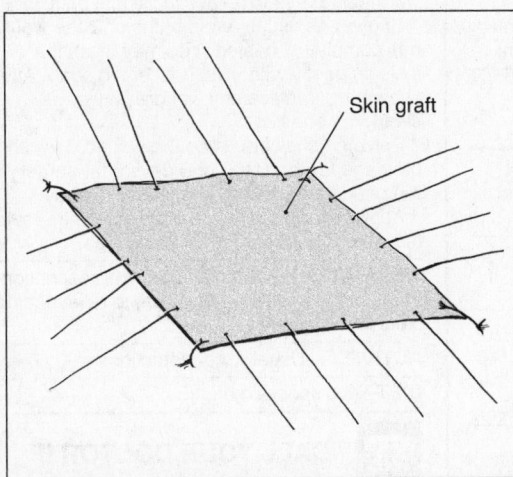

Skin graft

After skin has been removed from donor site, it is placed over the recipient site and fastened to normal skin around the periphery.

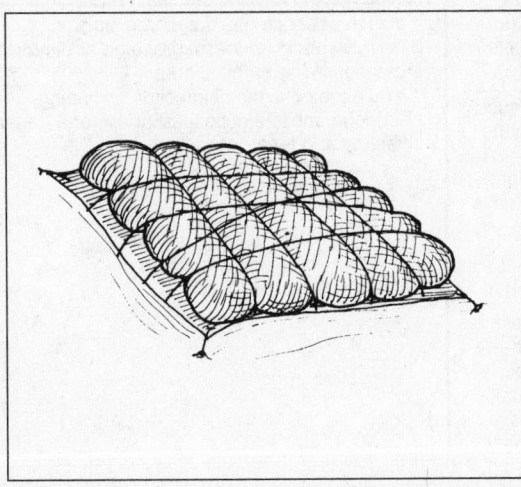

Pressure bandages are applied over the skin graft. The new blood vessels begin growing from the recipient area into the transplanted skin within 36 hours.

SKIN LESION REMOVAL

GENERAL INFORMATION

DEFINITION—Removal or ablation of any benign or cancerous lesion on the skin.

BODY PARTS INVOLVED—Abnormal growth on the skin. The most common are warts, moles, skin cancers, molluscum contagiosum or actinic keratosis.

REASONS FOR SURGERY
* Diagnosis of the abnormal growth.
* Removal of any abnormality suspected to be cancerous.
* Concern about appearance.
* Irritation of the lesion due to clothing.

SURGICAL RISK INCREASES WITH
* Adults over 60.
* Obesity; poor nutrition; anemia.
* Recent or chronic illness; diabetes.
* Use of some prescription and nonprescription drugs. Inform your doctor of any drugs, medications, or vitamin and herb supplements you are using or have used in the last month.

WHAT TO EXPECT

WHO OPERATES—Family doctor, dermatologist, general surgeon or plastic and reconstructive surgeon.

WHERE PERFORMED—Hospital, emergency room, doctor's office or outpatient surgical facility.

DIAGNOSTIC TESTS
* Before surgery: Blood and urine studies.
* After surgery: Laboratory examination of removed tissue.

ANESTHESIA
* Local anesthesia by injection.
* General anesthesia by injection and inhalation with an airway tube placed in the windpipe (for large excisions, skin grafts, or for procedures on young children).

DESCRIPTION OF OPERATION—Techniques to remove or ablate abnormal growths from the skin include:
* Scraping the abnormality away (curettement).
* Cutting with scissors, especially if the lesion is on a stalk.
* Freezing warts and benign superficial keratoses (cryotherapy).
* Using heat (electrosurgery).
* Incising the skin with a cold scalpel, removing the lesion and sewing the skin edges together.
* The technique chosen depends on the nature of the lesion and the condition of the patient. If sutures or clips are used to close the wound, they can usually be removed about 1 week after surgery.
* Skin grafting is sometimes required.

POSSIBLE COMPLICATIONS
* Excessive bleeding.
* Surgical-wound infection.
* Recurrent skin cancer.
* Excessive scarring (keloid).

AVERAGE HOSPITAL STAY—None.

PROBABLE OUTCOME—Expect complete healing without complications. Allow about 2 weeks for recovery from surgery.

POSTOPERATIVE CARE

GENERAL MEASURES
* If the wound bleeds during the first 24 hours after surgery, press a clean tissue or cloth to it for 10 minutes.
* If an incision was made, a hard ridge should form along the incision. As it heals, the ridge will gradually recede.
* Use an electric heating pad, a heat lamp or a warm compress to relieve incisional pain.
* Shower as usual. Avoid baths until the wound has completely healed. You may wash the incision gently with mild, unscented soap. After showering, replace any wet dressings with clean, dry ones.
* Between showers, keep the wound dry with a bandage for the first 2 or 3 days after surgery. If the bandage gets wet, change it promptly.
* Apply a nonprescription antibiotic ointment to the wound before applying bandages.

MEDICATION—You may use nonprescription drugs, such as acetaminophen, to relieve minor pain. Avoid aspirin.

ACTIVITY—Usually, no restrictions.

DIET—No special diet.

CALL YOUR DOCTOR IF

* You experience nausea or vomiting.
* Pain, swelling, redness, drainage or bleeding increases in the surgical area.
* You develop signs of infection, including headache, muscle aches, dizziness or a general ill feeling and fever.

SKIN LESION REMOVAL

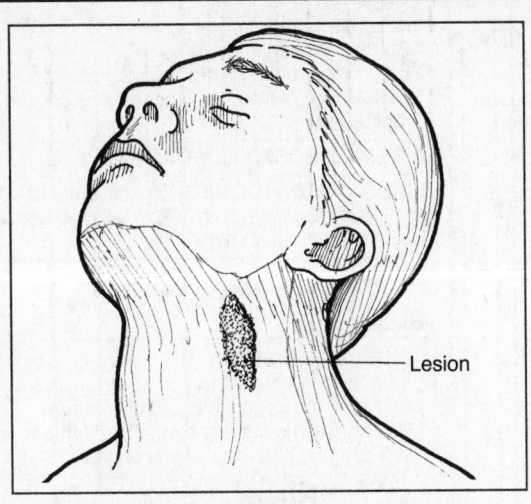

An illustration of a skin lesion on the neck to be removed surgically.

Lesion

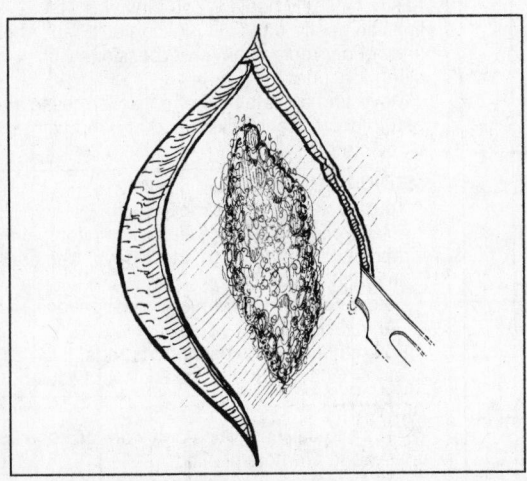

An incision is made around the lesion in an ellipse for easier closure.

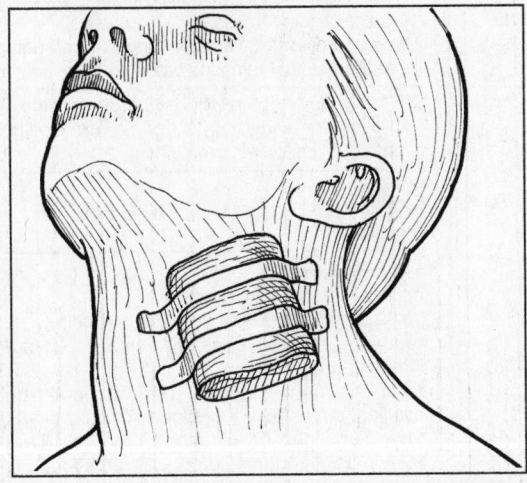

The skin is closed and a bandage has been applied.

SURGERIES

SMALL-BOWEL RESECTION

GENERAL INFORMATION

DEFINITION—Removal of diseased, injured, or abnormal section of the small bowel (small intestine).

BODY PARTS INVOLVED—Small intestine, including the mesentery (blood supply) around it.

REASONS FOR SURGERY
- Tumor, gangrene, narrowing or obstruction in the small intestine.
- Trauma, such as from a wound.

SURGICAL RISK INCREASES WITH
- Adults over 60.
- Obesity.
- Smoking.
- Poor nutrition.
- Previous abdominal surgery.
- Recent or chronic illness.
- Diabetes.
- Use of some prescription and nonprescription drugs. Inform your doctor of any drugs, medications, or vitamin and herb supplements you are using or have used in the last month.

WHAT TO EXPECT

WHO OPERATES—General surgeon.

WHERE PERFORMED—Hospital.

DIAGNOSTIC TESTS
- Before surgery: Blood and urine studies; x-rays of chest and gastrointestinal tract; CT; MRI; colonoscopy (see Glossary for all).
- After surgery: Blood studies.

ANESTHESIA
- Spinal anesthesia by injection.
- General anesthesia by injection and inhalation with an airway tube placed in the windpipe.

DESCRIPTION OF OPERATION
- Operative procedures will vary depending on the cause.
- An incision is made in the abdomen.
- The muscles are separated or cut, and the abdominal cavity is entered.
- The intestine is examined for disease.
- The small intestine is clamped above and below the diseased section. The diseased section between the clamps is cut free and removed.
- The two open ends of the remaining small bowel are fastened together with sutures or staples. Occasionally, a temporary ileostomy (see Surgery section) is necessary.
- The peritoneum and muscles are closed with sutures. The skin is closed with sutures or clips, which usually can be removed about 1 week after surgery.

POSSIBLE COMPLICATIONS
- Excessive bleeding.
- Deep-vein blood clots.
- Abscess formation.
- Surgical-wound infection.
- Leak where bowel is put back together.
- Recurrence of intestinal obstructions caused by adhesions.

AVERAGE HOSPITAL STAY—7 to 10 days.

PROBABLE OUTCOME—Expect complete healing of surgical wound. Allow about 6 weeks for recovery from surgery.

POSTOPERATIVE CARE

GENERAL MEASURES
- A hard ridge should form along the incision. As it heals, the ridge will gradually recede.
- Use an electric heating pad, a heat lamp or a warm compress to relieve incisional pain.
- Shower as usual. Avoid baths until the incision has completely healed. You may wash the incision gently with mild, unscented soap. After showering, replace any wet dressings with clean, dry ones.
- Move and elevate legs often while resting in bed to decrease the likelihood of deep-vein blood clots.

MEDICATION
- Your doctor may prescribe:
  - Pain relievers. Don't take prescription pain medication longer than 4 to 7 days. Use only as much as you need.
  - Stool softeners to prevent constipation.
  - Antibiotics to fight or prevent infection.
- You may use nonprescription drugs, such as acetaminophen, for minor pain. Avoid aspirin.

ACTIVITY
- Return to daily activities and work as soon as possible to promote healing.
- Avoid vigorous exercise for 6 weeks after surgery.
- Resume driving 3 weeks after returning home.
- Resume sexual relations when you feel able to.

DIET—Intravenous feeding with nasogastric suctioning for several days, then return slowly to a diet your doctor will prescribe.

CALL YOUR DOCTOR IF

- Pain, swelling, redness, drainage or bleeding increases in the surgical area.
- You develop signs of infection, including headache, muscle aches, dizziness or a general ill feeling and fever.
- You experience nausea, vomiting, abdominal swelling, constipation, or bloody or tarry stools.
- New, unexplained symptoms develop. Drugs used in treatment may produce side effects.

SMALL-BOWEL RESECTION

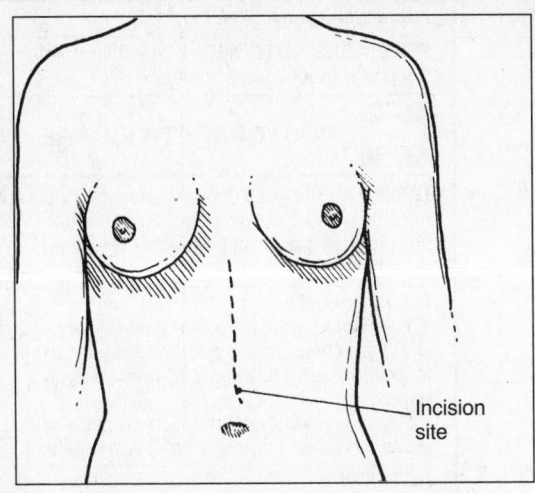

An illustration of a typical incision site for small bowel removal.

Incision site

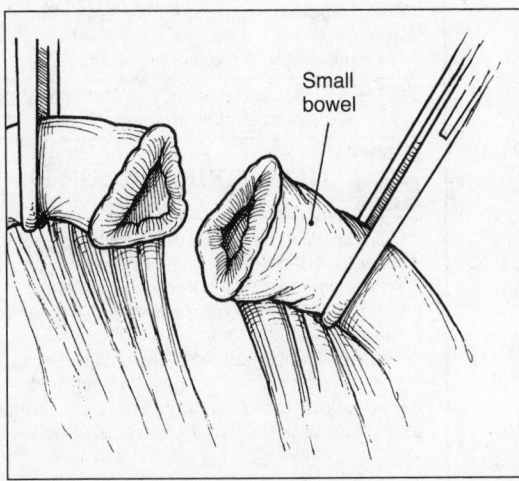

Small bowel

After the abdominal muscles are separated, the abdominal cavity is entered and the intestinal tract is examined for disease.
 • The small intestine is clamped above and below the diseased section. The diseased section between the clamps is cut free and removed.

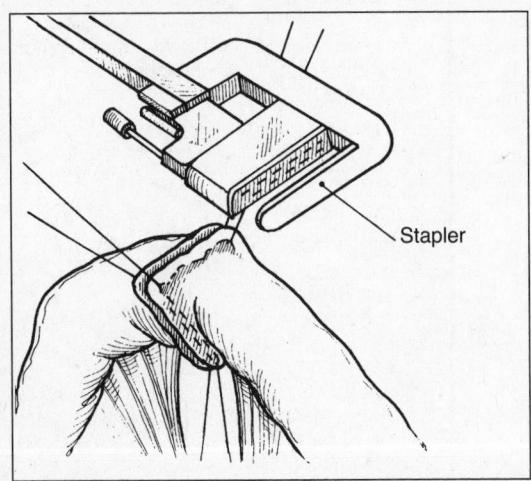

Stapler

The 2 open ends of the remaining small bowel are fastened together with sutures or staples.

SPINAL TAP
(Lumbar Puncture)

 GENERAL INFORMATION

DEFINITION—Removal of spinal fluid from the spinal canal, either for laboratory analysis or prior to surgery with spinal anesthesia.

BODY PARTS INVOLVED—Skin; muscles; covering of spinal cord (meninges); vertebral column.

REASONS FOR PROCEDURE
• Diagnosis of disorders of the central nervous system that may involve the brain, spinal cord, or their coverings.
• Injection of spinal anesthesia.
• Myelogram (see Glossary).

SURGICAL RISK INCREASES WITH
• Recent or chronic illness.
• Alcoholism.
• Increased intracranial pressure due to any cause.
• Central nervous system infection.
• Severe arthritis in spine.
• Diabetes.
• Use of some prescription and nonprescription drugs. Inform your doctor of any drugs, medications, or vitamin and herb supplements you are using or have used in the last month.

 WHAT TO EXPECT

WHO OPERATES—General surgeon, family doctor, neurologist, neurosurgeon, anesthesiologist or internist.

WHERE PERFORMED—Hospital, outpatient surgical facility or emergency room.

DIAGNOSTIC TESTS
• Before surgery: Blood and urine studies.
• During surgery: Pressure of spinal fluid measured with a manometer (see Glossary).
• After surgery: Laboratory examination of removed fluid.

ANESTHESIA—Local anesthesia by injection.

DESCRIPTION OF OPERATION
• The patient is positioned on his side with the knees drawn as close to the chest as possible.
• A hollow needle is inserted in the back between the 2nd and 3rd lumbar vertebrae.
• The spinal canal is penetrated with the needle. Fluid pressure is measured and then fluid is removed.
• The surgical wound will heal by itself.

POSSIBLE COMPLICATIONS
• Surgical wound infection.
• Headaches (common during the first 24 hours after the procedure).
• Meningitis (rare).

AVERAGE HOSPITAL STAY—Usually 6 to 24 hours in the surgical facility.

PROBABLE OUTCOME—Expect complete healing without complications.

 POSTOPERATIVE CARE

GENERAL MEASURES—Moving the head and neck as little as possible for 12 hours after surgery helps prevent headache. Resume activity slowly.

MEDICATION
• Your doctor may prescribe pain relievers. Don't take prescription pain medication longer than 4 to 7 days. Use only as much as you need.
• You may use nonprescription drugs, such as acetaminophen, for minor pain. Avoid aspirin.

ACTIVITY
• Avoid vigorous exercise for 2 weeks after surgery.
• Resume driving 3 days after returning home.

DIET—No special diet. Increase fluid intake to help prevent post-spinal-tap headaches.

 CALL YOUR DOCTOR IF

• Pain, swelling, redness, drainage or bleeding increases in the needle insertion area.
• You develop signs of infection, including headache, muscle aches, dizziness or a general ill feeling and fever.
• You experience nausea or vomiting.
• You develop pain or stiffness in your neck.
• New, unexplained symptoms develop. Drugs used in treatment may produce side effects.

SPINAL TAP
(Lumbar Puncture)

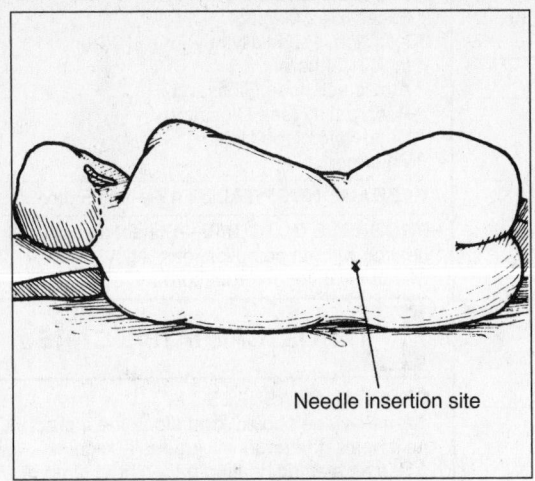

An illustration of a typical needle insertion site and the mid-spine.

Needle insertion site

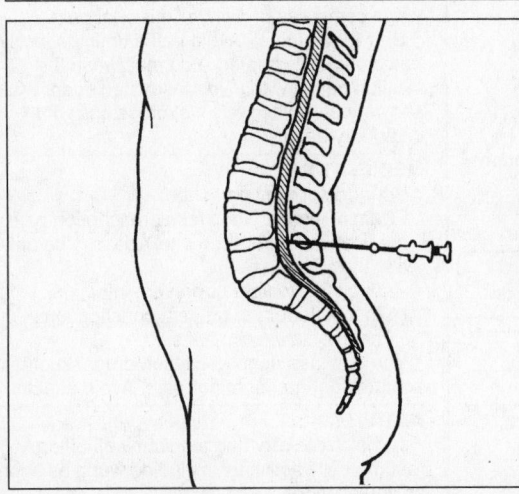

The needle is inserted between sinus processes of the bone into the cavity of the spinal canal, which surrounds the spine and is filled with fluid.

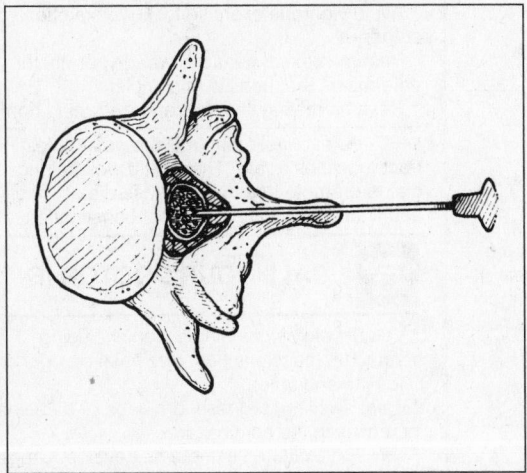

The spinal canal is penetrated with the needle. The fluid pressure is measured, then fluid is removed for laboratory examination.

SURGERIES

SPLEEN REMOVAL
(Splenectomy)

 GENERAL INFORMATION

DEFINITION—Removal of the spleen.

BODY PARTS INVOLVED—The spleen, a large organ on the left side of the upper abdominal cavity next to the stomach.

REASONS FOR SURGERY
- Injury to the spleen causing rupture and bleeding.
- Various blood diseases, including spherocytosis, thrombocytopenia or lymphatic leukemia (see Glossary for all).
- Splenic-vein thrombosis caused by esophageal varices (see Glossary).
- Benign or cancerous tumors.

SURGICAL RISK INCREASES WITH
- Adults over 60.
- Newborns and infants.
- Obesity.
- Smoking.
- Excess alcohol consumption.
- Poor nutrition.
- Recent or chronic illness.
- Diabetes.
- Use of some prescription and nonprescription drugs. Inform your doctor of any drugs, medications, or vitamin and herb supplements you are using or have used in the last month.

 WHAT TO EXPECT

WHO OPERATES—General surgeon.

WHERE PERFORMED—Hospital.

DIAGNOSTIC TESTS
- Before surgery: Blood and urine studies; x-rays of abdomen; CT scan (see Glossary).
- After surgery: Blood studies.

ANESTHESIA—General anesthesia by injection and inhalation with an airway tube placed in the windpipe.

DESCRIPTION OF OPERATION
- An incision is made in the abdomen.
- The spleen is located and isolated.
- Blood vessels to the spleen are cut and tied off.
- The spleen is rotated and removed from its bed where it is attached to the coverings of the stomach, kidney and diaphragm (see Glossary).
- If the spleen has been ruptured, the abdomen is explored to identify any other injured organs or blood vessels. Other surgeries may be performed at this time.
- The muscles are closed in layers. The skin is closed with sutures or skin clips, which usually can be removed in about 1 week.

POSSIBLE COMPLICATIONS
- Excessive bleeding.
- Infection, especially in young children.
- Incisional hernia.
- Atelectasis (see Glossary).
- Pancreatitis (see Glossary).
- Deep-vein blood clots.
- Pneumonia.

AVERAGE HOSPITAL STAY—3 to 5 days.

PROBABLE OUTCOME—Expect complete healing without complications. Allow about 4 weeks for recovery from surgery.

 POSTOPERATIVE CARE

GENERAL MEASURES
- A hard ridge should form along the incision. As it heals, the ridge will gradually recede.
- Use an electric heating pad, a heat lamp or a warm compress to relieve incisional pain.
- Shower as usual. Avoid baths until the incision has completely healed. You may wash the incision gently with mild, unscented soap. After showering, replace any wet dressings with clean, dry ones.

MEDICATION
- Your doctor may prescribe:
  - Pain relievers. Don't take prescription pain medication longer than 4 to 7 days. Use only as much as you need.
  - Antibiotics to fight or prevent infection.
  - Stool softeners to prevent constipation.
  - Pneumonia vaccinations.
- You may use nonprescription drugs, such as acetaminophen, for minor pain. Avoid aspirin.

ACTIVITY
- To help recovery and aid your well-being, resume daily activities, including work, as soon as you are able.
- Avoid vigorous exercise for 6 weeks after surgery.
- Resume sexual relations when your doctor determines that healing is complete.
- Resume driving 4 weeks after returning home.

DIET—Clear liquid diet until the gastrointestinal tract functions again. Then eat a well-balanced diet to promote healing. Increase dietary fiber and fluid intake to help prevent constipation.

 CALL YOUR DOCTOR IF

- You develop signs of infection, including headache, muscle aches, dizziness or a general ill feeling and fever.
- Pain, swelling, redness, drainage or bleeding increases in the surgical area.
- New, unexplained symptoms develop. Drugs used in treatment may produce side effects.

SPLEEN REMOVAL
(Splenectomy)

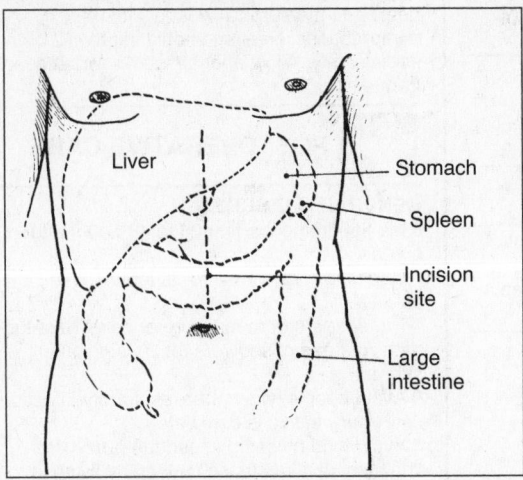

Liver
Stomach
Spleen
Incision site
Large intestine

An illustration of the spleen, other internal organs and the usual incision site for a spleen removal. An alternate incision is under the left rib cage.

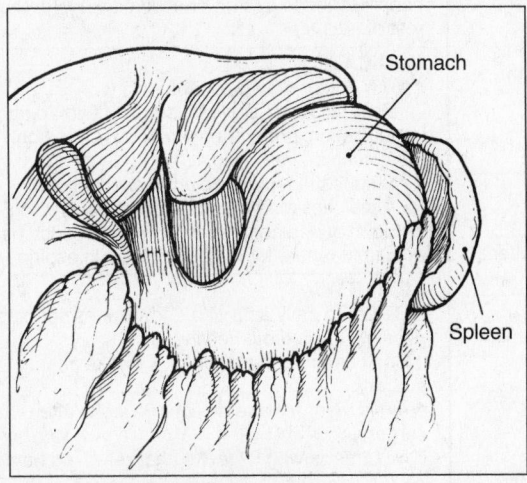

Stomach
Spleen

The spleen is rotated and removed from its bed where it's attached to the coverings of the stomach, kidney and diaphragm.

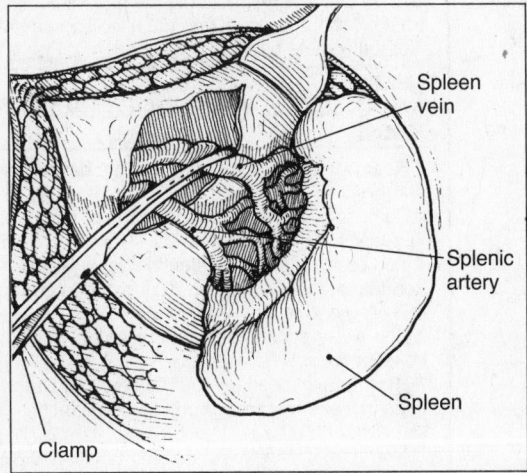

Spleen vein
Splenic artery
Spleen
Clamp

Blood vessels that supply the spleen are clamped and tied and the spleen is removed.

STAPES REMOVAL
(Stapedectomy)

GENERAL INFORMATION

DEFINITION—Removal of the stapes, one of the bones in the middle ear that transmit sound waves to the inner ear. The stapes is also called the stirrup.

BODY PARTS INVOLVED—External ear canal; eardrum; middle ear; stapes.

REASONS FOR SURGERY—Improvement of hearing ability or prevention of continued hearing loss, usually due to otosclerosis (see in Illness section).

SURGICAL RISK INCREASES WITH
- Obesity.
- Smoking.
- Poor nutrition.
- Recent or chronic illness.
- Diabetes.
- Use of some prescription and nonprescription drugs. Inform your doctor of any drugs, medications, or vitamin and herb supplements you are using or have used in the last month.

WHAT TO EXPECT

WHO OPERATES—Ear, nose and throat specialist (otolaryngologist).

WHERE PERFORMED—Hospital or outpatient surgical facility.

DIAGNOSTIC TESTS
- Before surgery: Blood and urine studies; hearing tests.
- After surgery: Hearing tests.

ANESTHESIA—General anesthesia by injection and inhalation with an airway tube placed in the windpipe.

DESCRIPTION OF OPERATION
- If both ears are affected, surgery is usually done on separate occasions.
- The operating microscope is positioned, and an incision is made in the middle ear.
- The small bones in the ear are identified, and the stapes is isolated and removed.
- Sometimes, a prosthesis made of stainless steel wire and cellulose sponge is inserted to replace the stapes.
- Blood and fluid are suctioned gently from the ear.
- The wound is closed with fine sutures, which can usually be removed about 1 week after surgery.

POSSIBLE COMPLICATIONS
- Excessive bleeding.
- Surgical-wound infection.

AVERAGE HOSPITAL STAY—3 to 5 days.

PROBABLE OUTCOME—Expect complete healing of the surgical wound without complications. Hearing should improve immediately. Allow about 3 weeks for recovery from surgery.

POSTOPERATIVE CARE

GENERAL MEASURES
- Lie flat during the first 24 to 48 hours after surgery.
- Don't blow your nose for at least 1 week after surgery.
- Protect ears from moisture or cold. Take tub baths instead of showers for 2 weeks after surgery.
- Avoid people with upper-respiratory infections until your healing is complete.
- Avoid loud noises and sudden pressure changes, such as those caused by flying in nonpressurized aircraft or scuba diving, for the rest of your life.

MEDICATION
- Your doctor may prescribe:
  - Pain relievers. Don't take prescription pain medication longer than 4 to 7 days. Use only as much as you need.
  - Stool softeners to prevent constipation.
  - Antibiotics to fight or prevent infection.
- You may use nonprescription drugs, such as acetaminophen, for minor pain. Avoid aspirin.

ACTIVITY
- Return to daily activities and work as soon as possible to promote healing.
- Don't strain, bend or lift for 3 weeks after surgery.
- Avoid vigorous exercise for 6 weeks after surgery.
- Resume driving 3 weeks after returning home.

DIET—Clear liquid diet until the gastrointestinal tract functions again. Then eat a well-balanced diet to promote healing.

CALL YOUR DOCTOR IF

- Hearing does not improve within 2 days after surgery.
- Pain, swelling, redness, drainage or bleeding increases in the surgical area.
- You develop signs of infection, including headache, muscle aches, dizziness or a general ill feeling and fever.
- You experience nausea, vomiting or constipation.
- New, unexplained symptoms develop. Drugs used in treatment may produce side effects.

STAPES REMOVAL
(Stapedectomy)

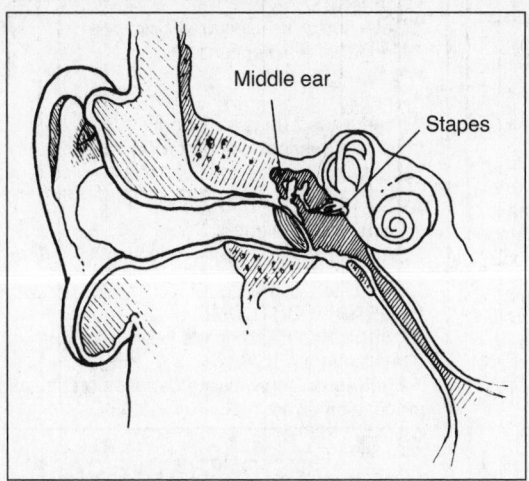

Middle ear

Stapes

An illustration of the outer ear, middle ear and the stapes (one of the bones in the middle ear that transmits sound waves to the inner ear). The stapes is also called the stirrup.

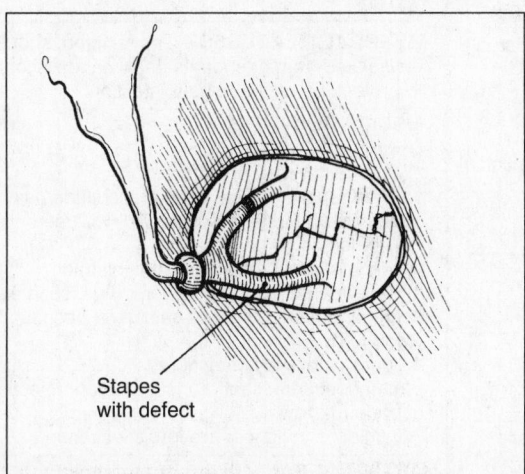

Stapes with defect

Appearance of the middle ear structure as seen through an operating microscope. Small bones in the ear are identified and the stapes is isolated and removed.

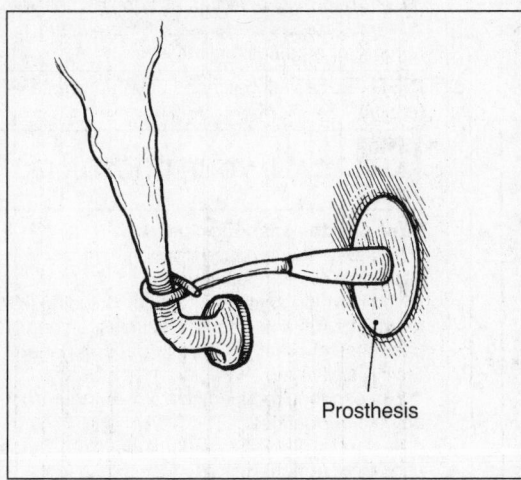

Prosthesis

Sometimes a prosthesis made of stainless steel wire and cellulose sponge is inserted to replace the defective stapes.

SURGERIES

STEM CELL TRANSPLANT

GENERAL INFORMATION

DEFINITION—Transplantation of stem cells (see Glossary) from a donor for introduction into the bloodstream of a recipient. The donor may be a different person than the recipient (allogenic transplant), or may be the same person as the recipient (autologous transplant). The topic of stem cell transplantation is a very complicated one and the information contained herein provides only an overview of the subject. Consult your doctor for additional information.

BODY PARTS INVOLVED—The subclavian vein or internal jugular vein of the donor and the recipient.

REASONS FOR SURGERY—Replenishment of stem cells which have become weakened or been destroyed by one of the following:
* Acute leukemia or aplastic anemia.
* Multiple myeloma.
* High-dose chemotherapy treatment of some types of cancer.

SURGICAL RISK INCREASES FOR BOTH DONOR AND RECIPIENT WITH
* Obesity; smoking; poor nutrition.
* Recent or chronic illness; diabetes.
* Use of some prescription and nonprescription drugs. Inform your doctor of any drugs, medications, or vitamin and herb supplements you are using or have used in the last month.

WHAT TO EXPECT

WHO OPERATES—Specially trained oncologist or hematologist. Catheter in vein placed by surgeon or anesthesiologist.

WHERE PERFORMED—Hospital or outpatient surgical facility.

DIAGNOSTIC TESTS
* Before surgery: Blood studies of both donor and recipient.
* After surgery: Blood studies in recipient to determine success of transplant.

ANESTHESIA—Local anesthetic for catheter placement.

DESCRIPTION OF OPERATION
* Before surgery, the donor is examined for communicable diseases.
* Stem cells are usually removed through venous access lines which are placed in surgery under local anesthesia and heavy sedation.
* The stem cells are filtered and then injected into the recipient's vein.

POSSIBLE COMPLICATIONS
Donor: None expected.
Recipient:
* Rejection of transplanted stem cells.
* Uncontrolled infections.
* Bleeding problems.
* Anemia.
* If the transplant is autologous (from oneself), there is a possibility of receiving cancer cells back in the new marrow, especially in leukemia.

AVERAGE HOSPITAL STAY
* **Donor:** Outpatient.
* **Recipient:** Varies from outpatient to several months.

PROBABLE OUTCOME
* **Donor:** Expect complete healing without complications.
* **Recipient:** Survival rate depends on disease process involved.

POSTOPERATIVE CARE

GENERAL MEASURES—The recipient should be isolated from attendants, family and visitors to protect the recipient from infection.

MEDICATION—
Donor:
* Your doctor may prescribe:
  - Pain relievers. Don't take prescription pain medication longer than 4 to 7 days. Use only as much as you need.
  - Antibiotics to fight or prevent infection.
* You may use nonprescription drugs, such as acetaminophen, for minor pain. Avoid aspirin.
Recipient:
* Your doctor may prescribe:
  - Immunosuppressant drugs to prevent rejection of bone marrow.
  - Antibiotics to fight or prevent infection.

ACTIVITY—For both donor and recipient:
* Return to daily activities as soon as possible.
* Avoid vigorous exercise for 6 weeks after surgery or as medically advised.

DIET—Eat a well-balanced diet to promote healing.

CALL YOUR DOCTOR IF

For both donor and recipient:
* You experience nausea or vomiting; or develop a rash or flushing.
* You develop signs of infection, including headache, muscle aches, dizziness, a cough, shortness of breath, a sore throat or a general ill feeling and fever.
* You experience bleeding from your gums or any of your orifices.
* New, unexplained symptoms develop. Drugs used in treatment may produce side effects.

STEM CELL TRANSPLANT

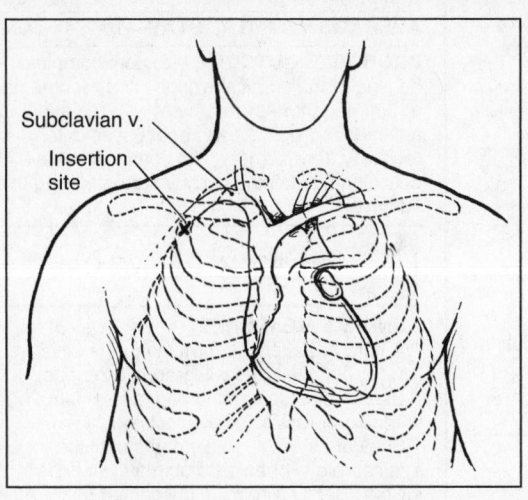

Illustration showing anatomy of region catheter is usually placed.

Subclavian v.

Insertion site

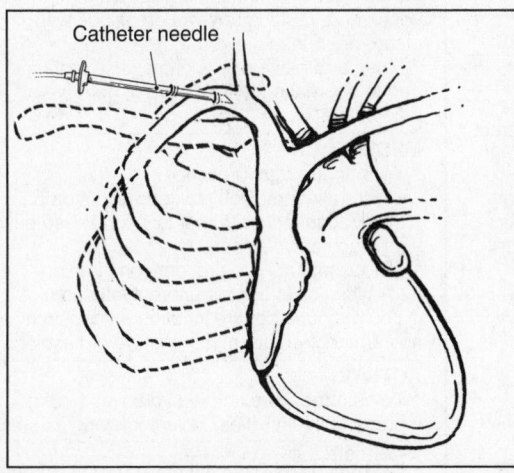

Catheter needle

The subclavian vein is punctured with a needle and a soft plastic catheter is threaded into the vein.

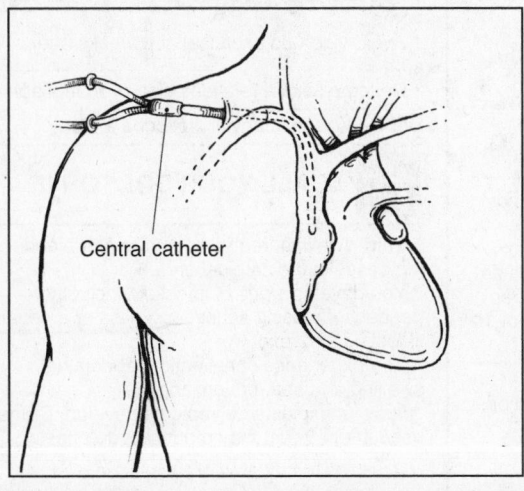

The catheter is used to withdraw blood for stem cells and replace unused portions of the blood.

Central catheter

STOMACH CANCER SURGERY

GENERAL INFORMATION

DEFINITION—Removal of cancerous tissue (gastric carcinoma) in the stomach.

BODY PARTS INVOLVED—Stomach; small intestine; esophagus (sometimes).

REASONS FOR SURGERY—Cancer of the stomach.

SURGICAL RISK INCREASES WITH
- Adults over 60.
- Obesity; poor nutrition; smoking.
- Alcoholism.
- Recent or chronic illness; diabetes.
- Use of some prescription and nonprescription drugs. Inform your doctor of any drugs, medications, or vitamin and herb supplements you are using or have used in the last month.

WHAT TO EXPECT

WHO OPERATES—General surgeon.

WHERE PERFORMED—Hospital.

DIAGNOSTIC TESTS
- Before surgery: X-rays of gastrointestinal tract and chest; blood and urine studies; ECG; endoscopy; CT scan; (see Glossary for all).
- During surgery: Laboratory examination of removed tissue by frozen section (see Glossary).
- After surgery: Blood studies; laboratory examination of removed tissue.

ANESTHESIA—General anesthesia by injection and inhalation with an airway tube placed in the windpipe.

DESCRIPTION OF OPERATION
- An incision is made below the ribs.
- Abdominal muscles are cut or retracted, the peritoneum is opened and the stomach is isolated.
- Usually, the entire stomach is removed. The esophagus is attached to a pouch made of small intestine, to create a new "stomach." The nearby lymph nodes and omentum (see Glossary) are removed; sometimes the spleen is also removed.
- If any stomach is left the remaining stump of stomach is joined to a loop of small intestine (usually the jejunum) for normal digestive flow.
- The peritoneum is closed and the muscles are sewn together. The skin is closed with sutures or clips, which usually can be removed about 10 days after surgery.

POSSIBLE COMPLICATIONS
- Excessive bleeding; surgical-wound infection.
- Incisional hernia.
- Chronic diarrhea; dumping syndrome.
- Malnutrition.

- Poor emptying of stomach.
- Ulcer disease.

AVERAGE HOSPITAL STAY—10 to 14 days.

PROBABLE OUTCOME—Expect complete healing of the surgical wound. Your doctor may recommend further treatment with radiation and anticancer drugs. Allow about 6 weeks for recovery from surgery. It is common to have difficulty maintaining body weight following this surgery.

POSTOPERATIVE CARE

GENERAL MEASURES
- A hard ridge should form along the incision. As it heals, the ridge will gradually recede.
- Use an electric heating pad, a heat lamp or a warm compress to relieve incisional pain.
- Shower as usual. Avoid baths until the incision has completely healed. You may wash the incision gently with mild, unscented soap. After showering, replace any wet dressings with clean, dry ones.
- Move and elevate legs often while resting in bed to decrease the likelihood of deep-vein blood clots.

MEDICATION
- Your doctor may prescribe:
  - Pain relievers. Don't take prescription pain medication longer than 4 to 7 days. Use only as much as you need.
  - Stool softeners to prevent constipation.
  - Antibiotics to fight or prevent infection.
- You may use nonprescription drugs, such as acetaminophen, for minor pain. Avoid aspirin.

ACTIVITY
- To help recovery and aid your well-being, resume daily activities, including work, as soon as you are able.
- Resume driving 3 to 4 weeks after returning home.
- Avoid vigorous exercise for 6 weeks after surgery.
- Resume sexual relations when you feel able.

DIET—Your doctor will prescribe a diet.

CALL YOUR DOCTOR IF

- Pain, swelling, redness, drainage or bleeding increases in the surgical area.
- You develop signs of infection, including headache, muscle aches, dizziness or a general ill feeling and fever.
- You experience constipation, abdominal swelling, nausea, or vomiting.
- New, unexplained symptoms develop. Drugs used in treatment may produce side effects.

STOMACH CANCER SURGERY

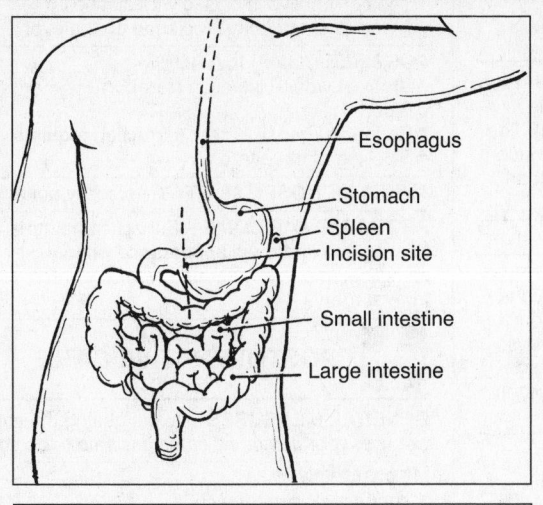

An illustration of the digestive system which shows the esophagus, stomach, spleen, large and small intestines, and a typical incision site for stomach cancer surgery.

Esophagus

Stomach

Spleen

Incision site

Small intestine

Large intestine

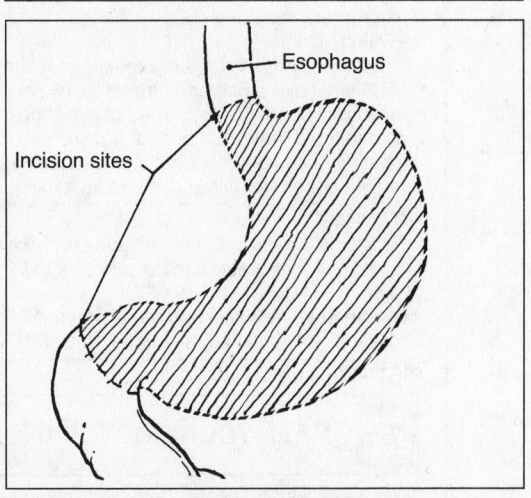

Esophagus

Incision sites

The abdominal muscles are cut and retracted; the peritoneum is opened and the stomach is isolated (not shown).
  • Incisions are made in the lower part of the esophagus and the top of the small intestine, and the entire stomach is removed.

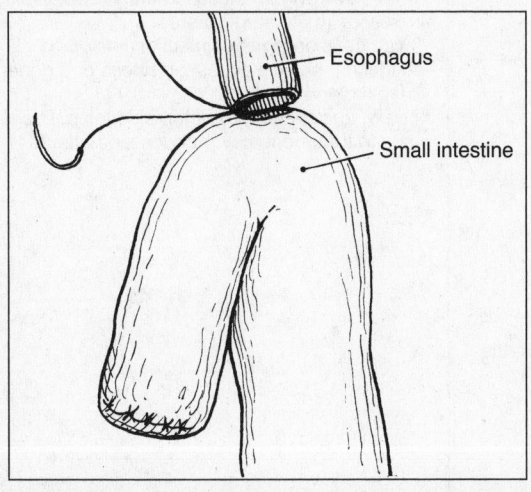

Esophagus

Small intestine

The esophagus is attached to a pouch made of small intestine, to create a new "stomach".
  • Not shown: The peritoneum is closed and the muscles are sewn together. The skin is closed with sutures or clips which usually can be removed about 10 days after surgery.

SURGERIES

STRABISMUS SURGERY
(Squint Repair)

GENERAL INFORMATION

DEFINITION—Surgery to strengthen or weaken the muscles that regulate movement of the eyeball (see Strabismus in Illness section). The surgery will vary with the extent of the deviation of the movement, and may require more than one operation.

BODY PARTS INVOLVED—Eyes.

REASONS FOR SURGERY—Realign the eyes to restore single binocular vision and a balance in the appearance of the eyes. The procedure is usually performed in children while the eye is still developing to save vision in the affected eye. In adults, the surgery is for reconstruction reasons only.

SURGICAL RISK INCREASES WITH
* Poor nutrition.
* Recent or chronic illness.
* Diabetes.
* Use of some prescription and nonprescription drugs. Inform your doctor of any drugs, medications, or vitamin and herb supplements you are using or have used in the last month.

WHAT TO EXPECT

WHO OPERATES—Ophthalmologist.

WHERE PERFORMED—Hospital, outpatient surgical facility.

DIAGNOSTIC TESTS
* Before surgery: Special eye examinations to determine the amount of deviation. Tests performed will depend on the age of the patient; usually an older child or an adult can cooperate with instructions for visual testing, while an infant cannot.
* After surgery: Eye examinations may be repeated as necessary.

ANESTHESIA—General anesthesia by injection and inhalation with an airway tube placed in the windpipe.

DESCRIPTION OF OPERATION
* The head is wrapped in sterile towels, leaving the eyes exposed.
* The eye muscle is exposed by cutting through the conjunctiva and fascia and a special instrument (called a squint hook) holds the whole width of the muscle.
* If the muscle is to be lengthened, it is cut close to its root and reattached with absorbable stitches to the surface layers of the eye at a distance determined by the initial tests.
* If the muscle is to be shortened, it is cut close to its root and a section is removed. The two ends are then stitched together.

* The conjunctiva is closed with stitches.
* A pad or shade may be placed on the eye.

POSSIBLE COMPLICATIONS
* Surgical-wound infection (rare).
* Bleeding.
* Repeat surgery if further correction required.
* Swelling of the eyelid.

AVERAGE HOSPITAL STAY—Usually none.

PROBABLE OUTCOME—Expect complete healing and improved appearance without complications. Allow about 2 weeks for recovery from surgery.

POSTOPERATIVE CARE

GENERAL MEASURES—Avoid getting the eye wet until your doctor indicates it is safe to do so.

MEDICATION
* Your doctor may prescribe:
  - Pain relievers.
  - Antibiotic drops to fight or prevent infection.
  - Steroidal eye drops or ointment to relieve inflammation. Keep both types of eye drops cold in the refrigerator, but not frozen.
* You may use nonprescription drugs, such as acetaminophen, for minor pain. Avoid aspirin.

ACTIVITY
* Rest until the effects of the anesthesia wear off. The eye may water and be sensitive to light at first.
* Most normal activities can be resumed in about a week. Avoid swimming for 10 days.

DIET—No special diet.

CALL YOUR DOCTOR IF

* Pain, swelling, redness, drainage or bleeding increases in the surgical area.
* You develop signs of infection, including headache, muscle aches, dizziness or a general ill feeling and fever.
* New, unexplained symptoms develop. Drugs used in treatment may produce side effects.

STRABISMUS SURGERY
(Squint Repair)

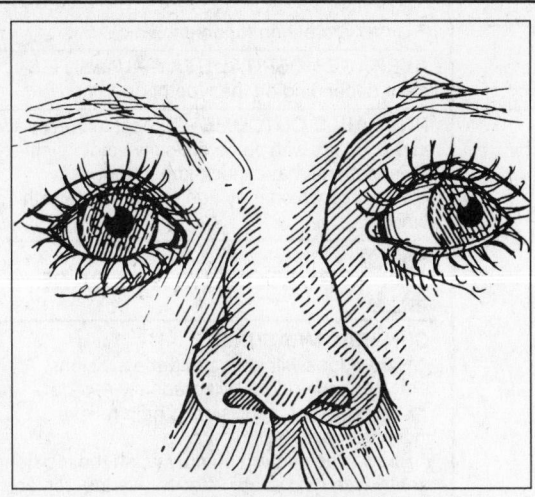

An infant's left eye demonstrates an external deviation.

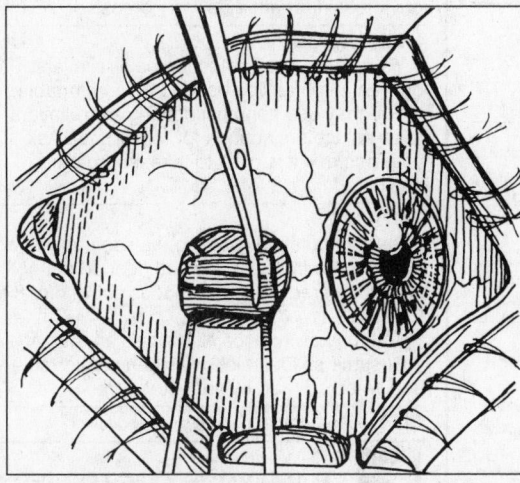

The eye muscle is surgically exposed and cut.

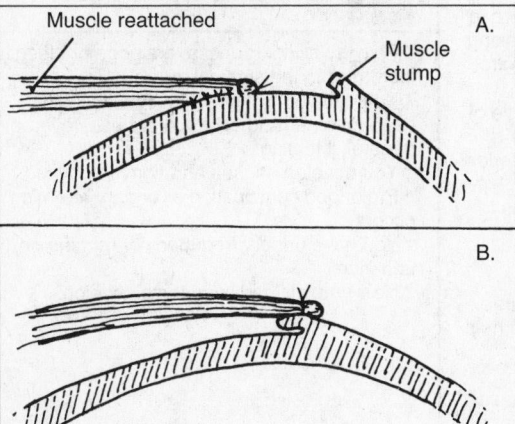

Muscle reattached

Muscle stump

A.

B.

A. Muscle shortening.

B. Muscle lengthening.

STRESS INCONTINENCE OPERATIONS

 GENERAL INFORMATION

DEFINITION—Operations to relieve uncontrolled leakage of urine from the bladder

BODY PARTS INVOLVED—Abdominal cavity, bladder, urethra, and vagina.

REASONS FOR SURGERY—To improve quality of life in women who leak urine either spontaneously or with stress such as lifting or coughing and to prevent excoriation (red, sore skin) and breakdown of the skin of the perineum.

SURGICAL RISK INCREASES WITH
* Age.
* Diabetes.
* Poor kidney function.
* High blood pressure.
* Poor nutrition.
* Chronic lung disease.
* Obesity.

 WHAT TO EXPECT

WHO OPERATES—Urologist or gynecologist.

WHERE PERFORMED—Hospital.

DIAGNOSTIC TESTS
* Before surgery: Blood tests and cystogram (see Glossary).
* After surgery: Blood tests (sometimes).

ANESTHESIA—General anesthesia or spinal anaesthesia.

DESCRIPTION OF OPERATION
* There are multiple operations that have been designed to control incontinence. Most are variations of ways to alter the angle that the urethra exits the bladder. Advancing age and vaginal deliveries cause relaxation of the perineal muscles (those between the urethral opening and the rectum), causing the urethra to exit the bladder at a more obtuse angle, making it difficult for the sphincter to completely control the flow urine.
* The simplest operation to change the angle of the urethra is called an anterior repair. This is done through the vagina, tightening the anterior wall by pulling the sidewalls in for support.
* More complex operations involve incisions in the lower abdomen to create a sling with sutures to pull the urethra forward. These involve more extensive surgery and recovery but tend to also be more successful and durable than the simple operations. Your doctor will help you decide which operation is best for your individual situation.
* A catheter is left in the bladder for 1-2 weeks after the operation.

POSSIBLE COMPLICATIONS
* Bleeding.
* Infection.
* Urinary retention (unable to void).

AVERAGE HOSPITAL STAY—Usually 2-5 days depending on the type of operation.

PROBABLE OUTCOME—Expect full recovery in 6-8 weeks with some difficulty voiding initially. Most patients have much improvement in continence which may again deteriorate with time.

 POSTOPERATIVE CARE

GENERAL MEASURES
* Hard ridges will form along the incisions. As they heal, the ridges will gradually recede.
* Use heat on the incision to help relieve incisional pain.
* Shower as usual. You may wash the incisions gently with mild soap. After showering, replace any dressings with a new dry dressing.

MEDICATION
* Your doctor may prescribe pain relievers. Use only as much as you need to be comfortable.
* You may use nonprescription pain relievers such as acetaminophen for minor pain. Ask your doctor if it is okay to take ibuprofen or aspirin.

ACTIVITY
* Start ambulating (walking) as soon as you are home. Take frequent naps as needed during the day when tired. Avoid strenuous activity for 6 to 8 weeks.
* You may swim once all sutures are out.
* Resume sexual relations when comfortable and when advised by your surgeon.

DIET—No special diet.

 CALL YOUR DOCTOR IF

* Pain, swelling, redness, drainage or bleeding increases in the surgical area.
* You develop signs of infection, including headache, muscle aches, dizziness, fever, or a general ill feeling.
* You develop nausea and vomiting.
* Prolonged constipation or urinary retention occurs.
* You have urinary frequency or burning on urination.
* New unexplained symptoms develop.

STRESS INCONTINENCE OPERATIONS

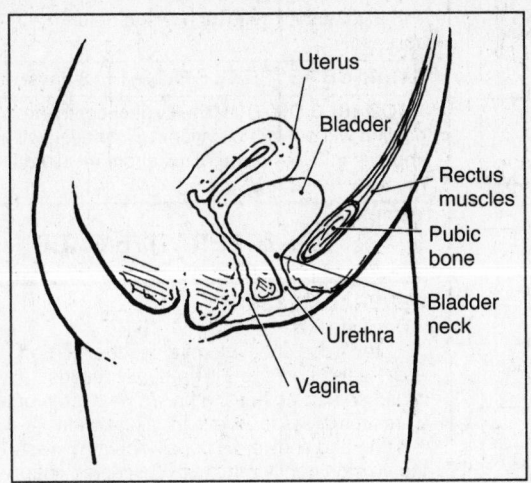

A cross sectional view of the bladder and surrounding structures.

Uterus

Bladder

Rectus muscles

Pubic bone

Bladder neck

Urethra

Vagina

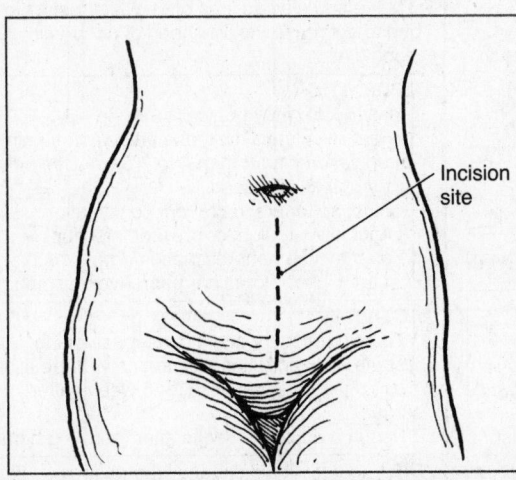

An incision is made through the skin and muscles of the lower abdomen either vertical (as shown) or transverse.

Incision site

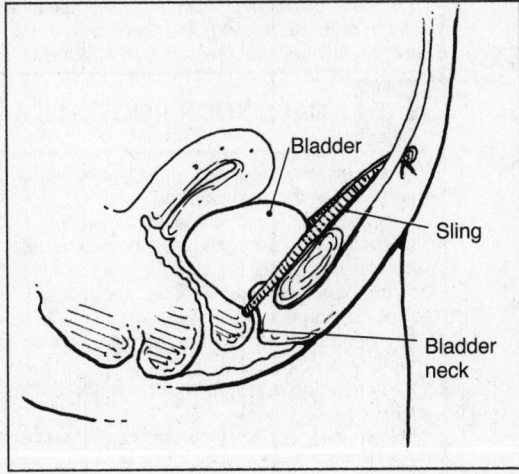

A sling is constructed to change the angle of the urethra as it exits the bladder (bladder neck).

Bladder

Sling

Bladder neck

SYMPATHECTOMY, CERVICODORSAL

GENERAL INFORMATION

DEFINITION—Interruption of the sympathetic nerve chain at the base of the neck near the spine.

BODY PARTS INVOLVED—Cervicodorsal sympathetic nerves (part of the autonomic nervous system) that control contraction and expansion of small arteries in the arms; lungs; upper ribs.

REASONS FOR SURGERY
* Relieve post-traumatic pain complex.
* Restoration of normal blood supply to the arms. Removing part of the sympathetic nervous system stops spasms in the blood vessels that can cause or aggravate decreased circulation.

SURGICAL RISK INCREASES WITH
* Obesity; smoking; alcoholism.
* Recent or chronic illness.
* Atherosclerosis.
* Diabetes.
* Use of some prescription and nonprescription drugs. Inform your doctor of any drugs, medications, or vitamin and herb supplements you are using or have used in the last month.

WHAT TO EXPECT

WHO OPERATES—General surgeon, neurosurgeon or vascular surgeon.

WHERE PERFORMED—Hospital.

DIAGNOSTIC TESTS
* Before surgery: Blood and urine studies; x-rays of chest; ECG (see Glossary); diagnostic sympathetic nerve block.
* After surgery: Blood studies; x-rays of chest.

ANESTHESIA—General anesthesia by injection and inhalation with an airway tube placed in the windpipe.

DESCRIPTION OF OPERATION
* An incision is made in the armpit.
* The muscles are divided, and part of the 3rd rib is removed.
* One lung is allowed to collapse temporarily to allow easier entry into the chest cavity.
* The cervical and dorsal sympathetic nerve chains are identified and divided.
* The lung is re-expanded. The muscles and skin edges are closed with sutures or clips, which usually can be removed about 1 week after surgery.
* This procedure can now be done via a thoracoscope (an optical instrument with a lighted tip).

POSSIBLE COMPLICATIONS
* Excessive bleeding.
* Surgical-wound infection.
* Inadvertent injury to lung tissue or lung collapse.

AVERAGE HOSPITAL STAY—1 to 3 days.

PROBABLE OUTCOME—Expect complete healing without complications. Circulation will improve in 3 to 4 days. Allow about 4 weeks for recovery from surgery.

POSTOPERATIVE CARE

GENERAL MEASURES
* Don't smoke.
* A hard ridge should form along the incision. As it heals, the ridge will gradually recede.
* Use an electric heating pad, a heat lamp or a warm compress to relieve incisional pain.
* Bathe and shower as usual. You may wash the incision gently with mild, unscented soap.
* Move and elevate legs often while resting in bed to decrease the likelihood of deep-vein blood clots.

MEDICATION
* Your doctor may prescribe:
  - Pain relievers. Don't take prescription pain medication longer than 4 to 7 days. Use only as much as you need.
  - Stool softeners to prevent constipation.
  - Antibiotics to fight or prevent infection.
* You may use nonprescription drugs, such as acetaminophen, for minor pain. Avoid aspirin.

ACTIVITY
* To help recovery and aid your well-being, resume daily activities as soon as you are able.
* Avoid vigorous exercise for 6 weeks after surgery.
* Resume driving 2 weeks after returning home.

DIET—Clear liquid diet until the gastrointestinal tract functions again. Then eat a well-balanced diet to promote healing. After recovery, eat a low-fat, low-salt diet (see diets in Appendix).

CALL YOUR DOCTOR IF

* Pain, swelling, redness, drainage or bleeding increases in the surgical area.
* You develop signs of infection, including headache, muscle aches, dizziness or a general ill feeling and fever.
* You experience constipation, abdominal swelling, nausea, or vomiting.
* You experience coldness, discoloration or numbness in the hand.
* You develop a cough, shortness of breath or chest pain.
* New, unexplained symptoms develop. Drugs used in treatment may produce side effects.

SYMPATHECTOMY, CERVICODORSAL

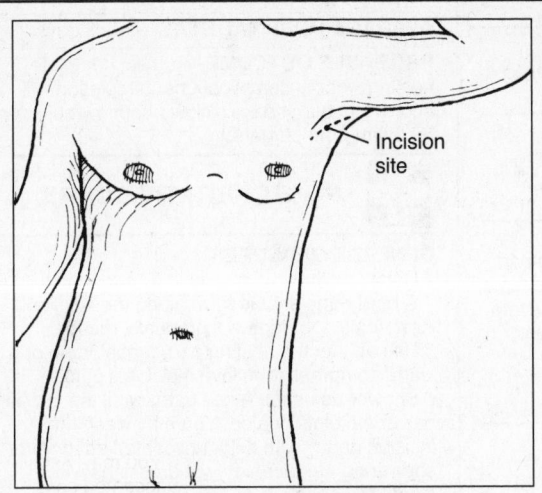

An illustration of the usual incision site for a cervicodorsal sympathectomy.

Incision site

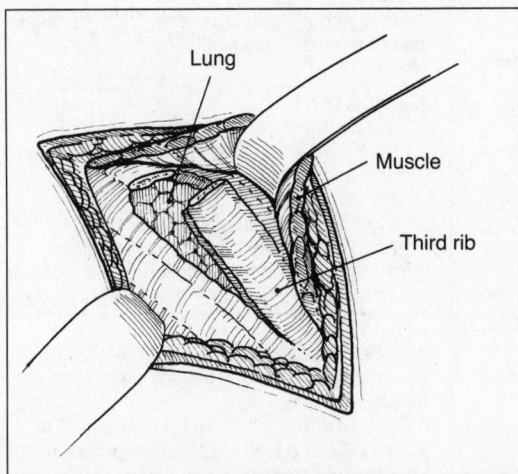

Lung

Muscle

Third rib

Muscles attached to ribs are divided and part of the 3rd rib is removed. One portion of the lung is allowed to temporarily collapse to allow easier entry into the chest cavity.

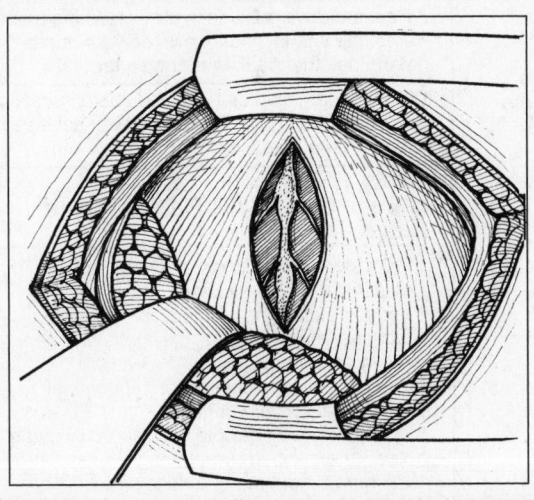

The cervical and dorsal sympathetic nerve chains are identified and divided.
• Following the operation, the ribs are reconstructed and held in place with heavy sutures. The lung is re-expanded and the muscles and skin edges are closed with sutures or clips (not illustrated).

SURGERIES

SYMPATHECTOMY, LUMBAR

GENERAL INFORMATION

DEFINITION—Removing a section of the sympathetic nerves located near the spinal cord in the lower back.

BODY PARTS INVOLVED—The lumbar sympathetic nerves (part of the autonomic nervous system) that control contraction and expansion of small arteries in the legs.

REASONS FOR SURGERY
• Improve blood flow to the legs. Removing part of the sympathetic nervous system stops spasms in the blood vessels that can cause or aggravate decreased blood flow and cause severe pain.
• Relieve symptoms of reflex sympathetic dystrophy.
• Nonhealing ulcers in legs or feet.

SURGICAL RISK INCREASES WITH
• Obesity; smoking.
• Recent or chronic illness.
• Atherosclerosis.
• Diabetes.
• Use of some prescription and nonprescription drugs. Inform your doctor of any drugs, medications, or vitamin and herb supplements you are using or have used in the last month.

WHAT TO EXPECT

WHO OPERATES—General surgeon, neurosurgeon or vascular surgeon.

WHERE PERFORMED—Hospital.

DIAGNOSTIC TESTS
• Before surgery: Blood and urine studies; lumbar sympathetic nerve block.
• After surgery: Blood studies.

ANESTHESIA—General anesthesia by injection and inhalation with an airway tube placed in the windpipe.

DESCRIPTION OF OPERATION
• A short, horizontal incision is made on the abdomen slightly above and to the side of the navel. The muscles are separated.
• The lumbar sympathetic chain of nerves is located, cut free, and a short segment is removed.
• The muscles are sewn together with large sutures.
• The skin is closed with sutures or clips, which usually can be removed about 1 week after surgery.

POSSIBLE COMPLICATIONS
• Excessive bleeding.
• Surgical-wound infection.
• Incisional hernia (rare).
• Inadvertent injury to the ureter (rare).
• May result in impotence.

• Incomplete resection of nerves due to accessory fibers.

AVERAGE HOSPITAL STAY—3 to 5 days.

PROBABLE OUTCOME—Expect complete healing without complications. Circulation will improve in 3 to 4 days. Allow about 4 weeks for recovery from surgery.

POSTOPERATIVE CARE

GENERAL MEASURES
• Don't smoke.
• A hard ridge should form along the incision. As it heals, the ridge will gradually recede.
• Use an electric heating pad, a heat lamp or a warm compress to relieve incisional pain.
• Shower as usual. Avoid baths until the incision has completely healed. You may wash the incision gently with mild, unscented soap. After showering, replace any wet dressings with clean, dry ones.
• Move and elevate legs often while resting in bed to decrease the likelihood of deep-vein blood clots.

MEDICATION
• Your doctor may prescribe:
  - Pain relievers. Don't take prescription pain medication longer than 4 to 7 days. Use only as much as you need.
  - Stool softeners to prevent constipation.
  - Antibiotics to fight or prevent infection.
• You may use nonprescription drugs, such as acetaminophen, for minor pain. Avoid aspirin.

ACTIVITY
• To help recovery and aid your well-being, resume daily activities, including work, as soon as you are able.
• Avoid vigorous exercise for 6 weeks after surgery. Start a walking exercise program when your doctor prescribes it.
• Resume driving 2 weeks after returning home.
• Resume sexual relations when your doctor determines that healing is complete.

DIET—Clear liquid diet until the gastrointestinal tract functions again. Then eat a well-balanced diet to promote healing.

CALL YOUR DOCTOR IF

• Pain, swelling, redness, drainage or bleeding increases in the surgical area.
• You develop signs of infection, including headache, muscle aches, dizziness or a general ill feeling and fever.
• You experience constipation, abdominal swelling, nausea or vomiting.
• Your foot becomes cold, discolored or numb.
• New, unexplained symptoms develop. Drugs used in treatment may produce side effects.

SYMPATHECTOMY, LUMBAR

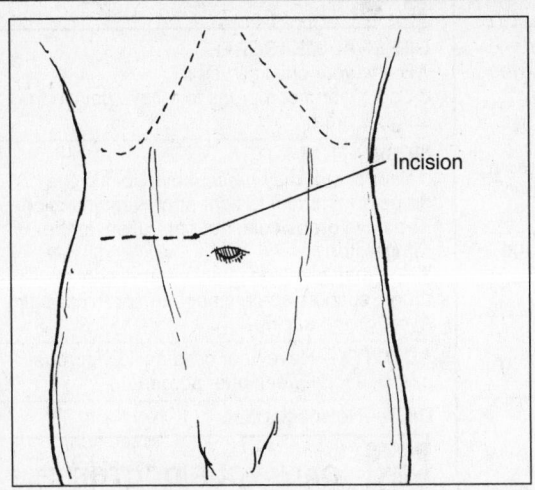

An illustration of a typical incision site to allow access to the sympathetic chain.

Incision

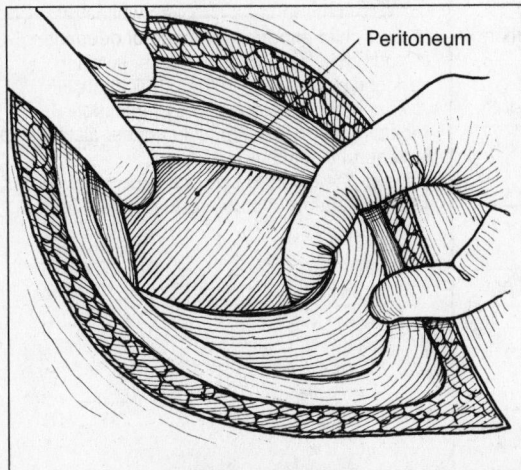

Muscles overlying the spine are separated.

Peritoneum

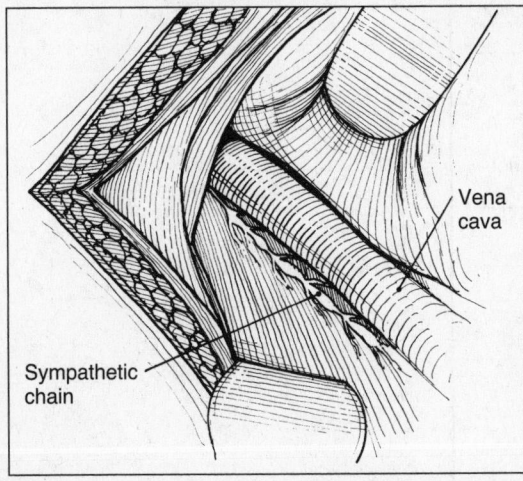

The lumbar sympathetic chain of nerves is located, cut free and removed.

Vena cava

Sympathetic chain

TEAR DUCT, OPENING OF

GENERAL INFORMATION

DEFINITION—Opening of tear ducts (also called lacrimal ducts) in the corners of the eyes closer to the nose. They may be blocked by infection or foreign material, or may be incompletely open in newborns. This is a common problem, affecting 6% of newborns. In 90% of these cases, however, the ducts open spontaneously by 1 year of age.

BODY PARTS INVOLVED—Tear glands and tear ducts, usually in newborns, infants or young children.

REASONS FOR SURGERY—Infection or complete blockage that does not respond to simple treatment.

SURGICAL RISK INCREASES WITH
• Obesity.
• Poor nutrition.
• Recent or chronic illness.
• Diabetes.
• Use of some prescription and nonprescription drugs. Inform your doctor of any drugs, medications, or vitamin and herb supplements your child is using or has used in the last month.

WHAT TO EXPECT

WHO OPERATES—Ophthalmologist or pediatric surgeon.

WHERE PERFORMED—Hospital or outpatient surgical facility.

DIAGNOSTIC TESTS
• Before surgery: Blood and urine studies.
• After surgery: Blood studies.

ANESTHESIA
• Local anesthesia by injection or topical application (sometimes).
• General anesthesia by injection and inhalation with an airway tube placed in the windpipe.

DESCRIPTION OF OPERATION
• The tear duct is expanded, probed and irrigated until fluid flows freely through it. The procedure is repeated on the other tear duct.
• Sutures are not needed. Bleeding should not be a problem.

POSSIBLE COMPLICATIONS—Surgical-wound infection.

AVERAGE HOSPITAL STAY—0 to 1 day.

PROBABLE OUTCOME—Expect complete healing without complications. Allow about 10 days for recovery from surgery.

POSTOPERATIVE CARE

GENERAL MEASURES
• Bathe your child as usual.
• Use a warm compress to relieve pain in the surgical area.

MEDICATION
• Your doctor may prescribe antibiotic eye drops or ointment to fight or prevent infection. Keep eye drops cold, but not frozen, in the refrigerator.
• You may give your child nonprescription drugs, such as acetaminophen, for minor pain. Avoid giving aspirin.

ACTIVITY—Have your child avoid vigorous exercise for 1 week after surgery.

DIET—No special diet.

CALL YOUR DOCTOR IF

• Your child experiences nausea or vomiting.
• Your child has increased pain, swelling, redness or drainage in the surgical area.
• Your child develops signs of infection, including headache, muscle aches, dizziness or a general ill feeling and fever.
• New, unexplained symptoms develop. Drugs used in treatment may produce side effects.

TEAR DUCT, OPENING OF

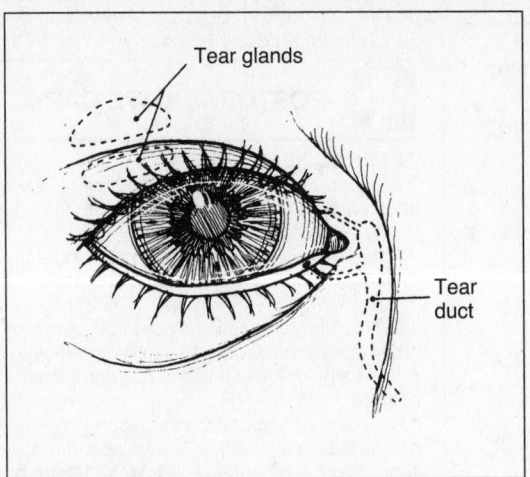

An illustration of tear glands, tear duct and other parts of the eye.

Tear glands

Tear duct

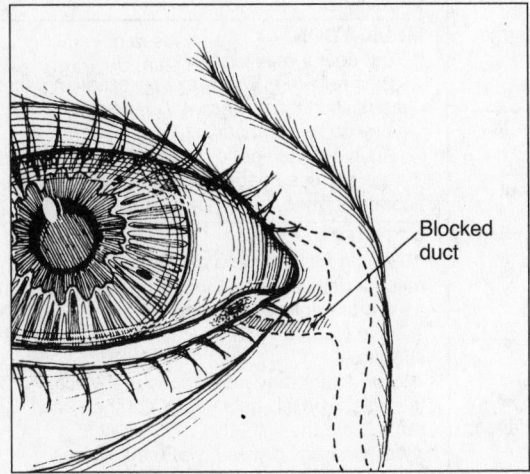

The blocked tear duct is identified.

Blocked duct

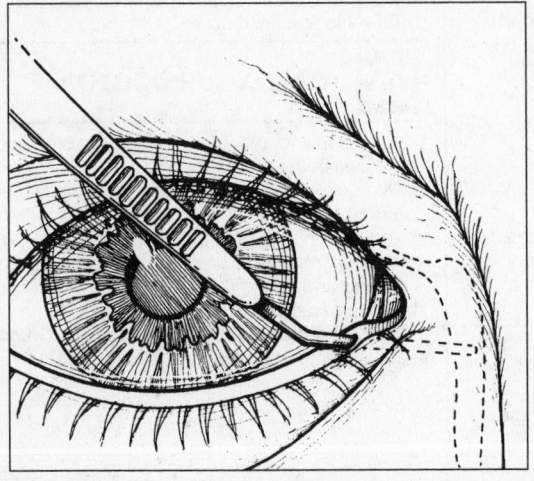

The blocked duct is expanded, probed and irrigated until fluid freely flows through it.

SURGERIES

TENDON REPAIR

GENERAL INFORMATION

DEFINITION—Reattaching tendons (see Glossary) to their connective tissue, or sewing sections of cut or torn tendons together.

BODY PARTS INVOLVED—Injured tendons, most frequently in the hand, foot, ankle, wrist, shoulder, hip, knee and elbow.

REASONS FOR SURGERY—Restoration of normal function of joints or tissue surrounding tendons.

SURGICAL RISK INCREASES WITH
- Adults over 60.
- Obesity; smoking; alcoholism.
- Poor nutrition.
- Recent or chronic illness.
- Diabetes.
- Use of some prescription and nonprescription drugs. Inform your doctor of any drugs, medications, or vitamin and herb supplements you are using or have used in the last month.

WHAT TO EXPECT

WHO OPERATES—Orthopedic surgeon, hand surgeon or general surgeon.

WHERE PERFORMED—Hospital, outpatient surgical facility or emergency room.

DIAGNOSTIC TESTS
- Before surgery: Blood and urine studies; x-rays of the injured part.
- After surgery: Blood studies.

ANESTHESIA
- Local anesthesia by injection.
- Spinal anesthesia by injection.
- General anesthesia by injection and inhalation with an airway tube placed in the windpipe.

DESCRIPTION OF OPERATION
- An incision is made over the injured tendon.
- The severed ends of the tendon are located and sewn together. If the tendon has been destroyed, a tendon graft may be required to bridge the gap.
- If necessary, tendons are reattached to surrounding connective tissue.
- The surgical area is examined for injuries to nerves and blood vessels.
- The skin is closed with sutures, which usually can be removed about 10 days after surgery.
- Usually, the injured part is kept rigid with a splint or plaster cast.

POSSIBLE COMPLICATIONS
- Excessive bleeding.
- Surgical-wound infection.
- Partial loss of function in joint served by the injured tendon(s).
- Repeat rupture of tendon.

AVERAGE HOSPITAL STAY—0 to 1 day.

PROBABLE OUTCOME—Expect complete healing without complications. Allow about 3 to 6 months for recovery from surgery.

POSTOPERATIVE CARE

GENERAL MEASURES
- If the wound bleeds during the first 24 hours after surgery, press a clean tissue or cloth to it for 10 minutes.
- A hard ridge should form along the incision. As it heals, the ridge will gradually recede.
- Use an electric heating pad, a heat lamp or a warm compress to relieve incisional pain.
- Shower as usual after the splint is removed. Avoid baths until the incision has completely healed.
- Between showers, keep the wound dry with a bandage for the first 2 or 3 days after the splint is removed. If a bandage gets wet, change it promptly.

MEDICATION
- Your doctor may prescribe:
  - Pain relievers. Don't take prescription pain medication longer than 4 to 7 days. Use only as much as you need.
  - Antibiotics to fight or prevent infection.
- You may use nonprescription drugs, such as acetaminophen, for minor pain. Avoid aspirin.

ACTIVITY
- To help recovery and aid your well-being, resume daily activities, including work, as soon as you are able.
- Avoid vigorous exercise for 6 weeks after surgery.
- Your doctor may refer you to a physical therapist who will help you strengthen and rehabilitate the limb.
- Ask your doctor when you may resume driving; will vary depending upon area repaired.

DIET—No special diet.

CALL YOUR DOCTOR IF

- Pain, swelling, redness, drainage or bleeding increases in the surgical area.
- Skin below the cast becomes cold, discolored or numb.
- You develop signs of infection, including headache, muscle aches, dizziness or a general ill feeling and fever.
- You experience nausea or vomiting.
- New, unexplained symptoms develop. Drugs used in treatment may produce side effects.

TENDON REPAIR

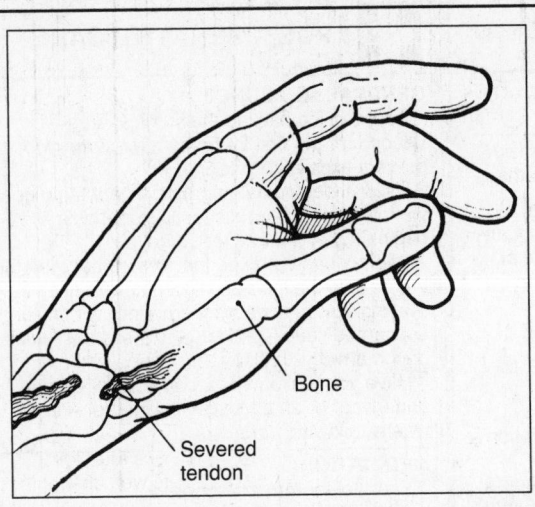

An illustration of a typical severed tendon in the wrist.

Bone

Severed tendon

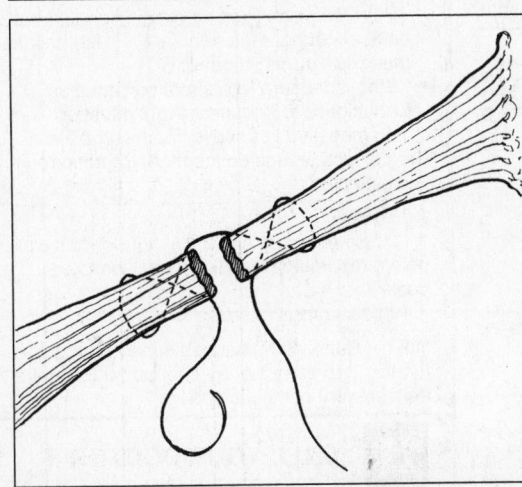

Severed ends of a tendon are located and sewn together.

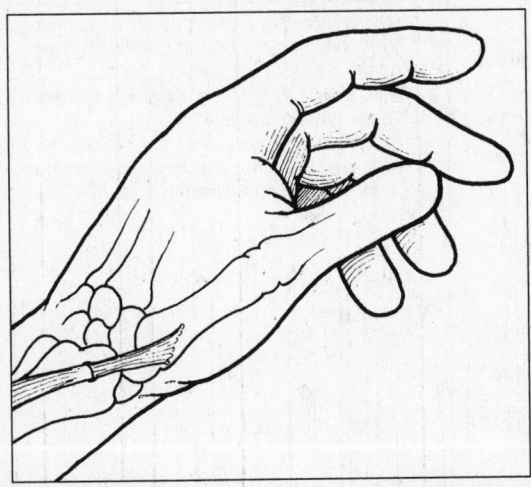

If necessary, tendons are reattached to surrounding connective tissue.

TESTICLE FIXATION
(Orchiopexy)

 GENERAL INFORMATION

DEFINITION—Fastening an undescended or twisted testicle in its normal position.

BODY PARTS INVOLVED—Scrotum; testicle; vas deferens; blood vessels and nerves in the scrotum.

REASONS FOR SURGERY—Placement of an undescended testicle in its normal position, or correction of a twisted testicle. Usually done before a boy is age 5.

SURGICAL RISK INCREASES WITH
• Congenital disorders.
• Chronic illness.
• Diabetes.
• Use of some prescription and nonprescription drugs. Inform your doctor of any drugs, medications, or vitamin and herb supplements your child is using or has used in the last month.

 WHAT TO EXPECT

WHO OPERATES—Urologist or general surgeon.

WHERE PERFORMED—Hospital.

DIAGNOSTIC TESTS
• Before surgery: Blood and urine studies; ultrasound (see Glossary).
• After surgery: Blood studies.

ANESTHESIA
• Spinal anesthesia by injection.
• Local anesthesia by injection.

DESCRIPTION OF OPERATION
• An incision is made in the scrotum or groin area.
• The blood supply and nerves leading to the testicle are located and carefully preserved.
• If the testicle has not descended from the abdomen, the surgeon reaches into the inguinal canal with special instruments and gently pulls it down.
• The testicle and its blood supply and nerves are pulled to the bottom of the scrotum and sewn in place.
• The skin is closed with sutures that will be absorbed by the body.

POSSIBLE COMPLICATIONS
• Excessive bleeding.
• Surgical-wound infection.
• Damage to blood supply to the testicle; death of the testicle.

AVERAGE HOSPITAL STAY—0 to 2 days.

PROBABLE OUTCOME—Expect complete healing without complications. Allow about 3 weeks for recovery from surgery.

 POSTOPERATIVE CARE

GENERAL MEASURES
• Apply an ice pack to the surgical area as needed for the first 24 hours after surgery to prevent excessive swelling.
• Use an electric heating pad, a heat lamp or a warm compress to relieve incisional pain beginning 24 hours after surgery.
• Use sponge baths or showers, rather than tub baths, until the incision has completely healed. The incision may be washed gently with mild, unscented soap. Replace any dressings which become wet with clean, dry ones.
• Have your child wear 2 pairs of jockey type underwear or an athletic supporter for 4 to 6 weeks following surgery.

MEDICATION
• Your doctor may prescribe:
  - Pain relievers. Pain medication should not be used longer than 4 to 7 days. Use only as much as your child need.
  - Stool softeners to prevent constipation.
  - Antibiotics to fight or prevent infection.
• You may give your child nonprescription drugs, such as acetaminophen, for minor pain. Avoid aspirin.

ACTIVITY
• To help recovery and aid in your child's well-being, resume daily activities as soon as possible.
• Avoid vigorous exercise for 6 weeks.

DIET—Eat a well-balanced diet to promote healing. Increase dietary fiber and fluid intake to help prevent constipation.

 CALL YOUR DOCTOR IF

• Your child experiences nausea or vomiting.
• Your child has discomfort or difficulty in urination.
• Pain, swelling, redness, drainage or bleeding increases in the surgical area.
• Your child develops signs of infection, including headache, muscle aches, dizziness or a general ill feeling and fever.

TESTICLE FIXATION
(Orchiopexy)

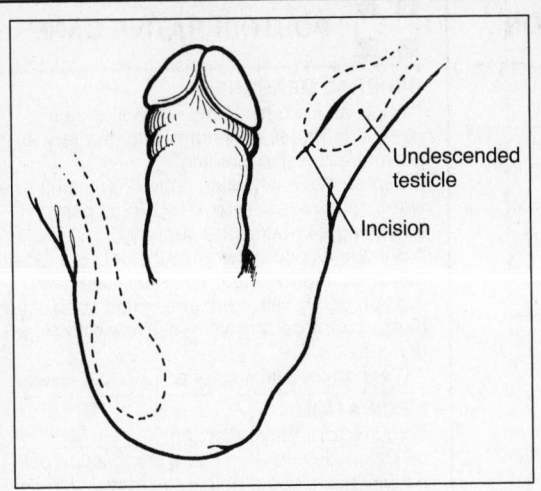

An illustration of an undescended testicle on the patient's left side and a typical incision site into the scrotum.

Undescended testicle

Incision

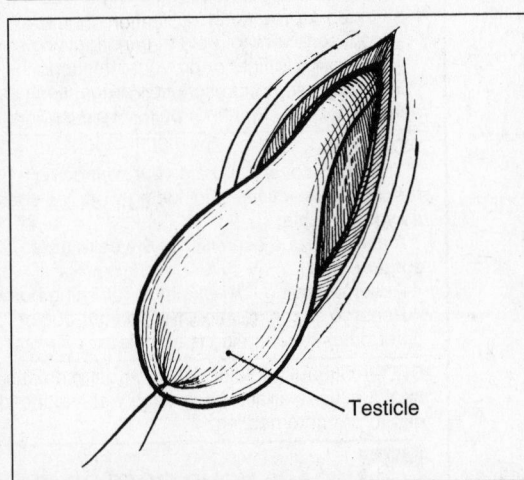

The blood supply and nerves leading to the testicle are carefully preserved.
 • The surgeon reaches into the inguinal canal with special instruments and gently pulls the testicle down into the scrotum.

Testicle

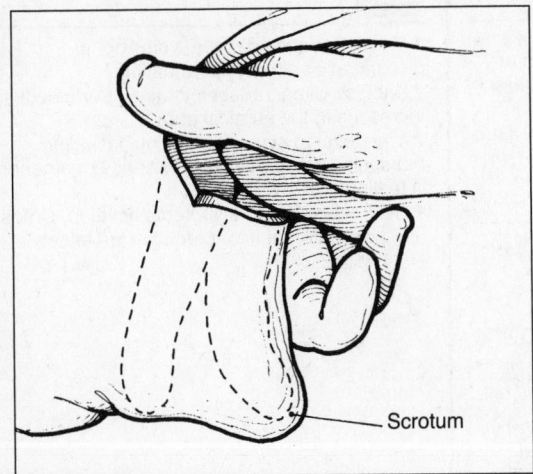

The testicle, its blood supply and nerves are pulled to the bottom of the scrotum and sewn into place.

Scrotum

SURGERIES

TESTICLE REMOVAL (Orchiectomy)

GENERAL INFORMATION

DEFINITION—Removal of one of the testicles (orchiectomy).

BODY PARTS INVOLVED—Scrotum; testicle; vas deferens; blood vessels and nerves in the scrotum.

REASONS FOR SURGERY
- Cancer or gangrene of the testicle.
- Prostate cancer.
- Undescended testicle.

SURGICAL RISK INCREASES WITH
- Adults over 60.
- Smoking.
- Recent or chronic illness.
- Diabetes.
- Use of some prescription and nonprescription drugs. Inform your doctor of any drugs, medications, or vitamin and herb supplements you are using or have used in the last month.

WHAT TO EXPECT

WHO OPERATES—Urologist or general surgeon.

WHERE PERFORMED—Hospital.

DIAGNOSTIC TESTS
- Before surgery: Blood and urine studies; x-rays; CT scan; ultrasound; ECG (see Glossary for all).
- After surgery: Blood studies; laboratory studies of the removed testicle.

ANESTHESIA
- Local anesthesia by injection.
- Spinal anesthesia by injection.
- General anesthesia by injection and inhalation with an airway tube placed in the windpipe.

DESCRIPTION OF OPERATION
- An incision is made in the inguinal region or scrotum. The blood supply and nerves leading to the testicle are located and cut free.
- The testicle is cut free from surrounding tissue and removed.
- The skin is closed with sutures that will be absorbed by the body.

POSSIBLE COMPLICATIONS
- Excessive bleeding.
- Surgical-wound infection.
- Urinary retention.

AVERAGE HOSPITAL STAY—0 to 2 days.

PROBABLE OUTCOME—Expect complete healing without complications. Allow about 3 weeks for recovery from surgery. Removal of one testicle should not interfere with normal sexual function or the ability to have children.

POSTOPERATIVE CARE

GENERAL MEASURES
- Apply an ice pack to the surgical area as needed for the first 24 hours after surgery to prevent excessive swelling.
- Use an electric heating pad, a heat lamp or a warm compress to relieve incisional pain beginning 24 hours after surgery.
- Shower as usual. Avoid baths until the incision has completely healed. You may wash the incision gently with mild, unscented soap. After bathing, replace any wet dressings with clean, dry ones.
- Wear an athletic supporter for 4 to 6 weeks.

MEDICATION
- Your doctor may prescribe:
  - Pain relievers. Don't take prescription pain medication longer than 4 to 7 days. Use only as much as you need.
  - Stool softeners to prevent constipation.
  - Antibiotics to fight or prevent infection.
- You may use nonprescription drugs, such as acetaminophen, for minor pain. Avoid aspirin.

ACTIVITY
- To help recovery and aid your well-being, resume daily activities, including work, as soon as you are able.
- Avoid vigorous exercise for 6 weeks after surgery.
- Resume driving 2 weeks after returning home.
- Resume sexual relations when your doctor determines that healing is complete.

DIET—Clear liquid diet until the gastrointestinal tract functions again. Then eat a well-balanced diet to promote healing.

CALL YOUR DOCTOR IF

- You experience nausea, vomiting, or discomfort or difficulty in urination.
- Pain, swelling, redness, drainage or bleeding increases in the surgical area.
- You develop signs of infection, including headache, muscle aches, dizziness or a general ill feeling and fever.
- New, unexplained symptoms develop. Drugs used in treatment may produce side effects.

TESTICLE REMOVAL
(Orchiectomy)

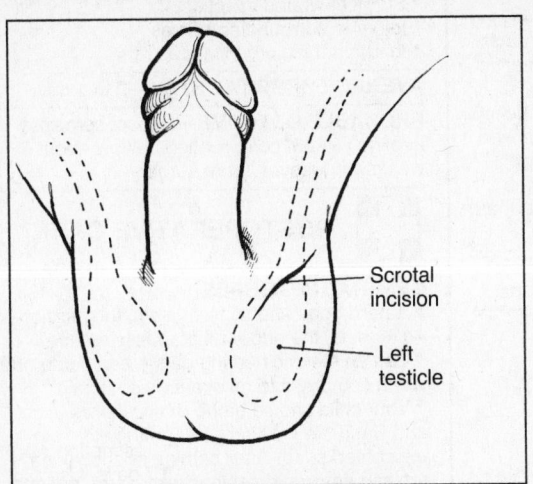

An illustration of the penis, scrotum, testicle and incision site for removal of a testicle.
- Sometimes the incision for this operation is made higher up in the groin.
- Usually the incision is made in the scrotum.

Scrotal incision

Left testicle

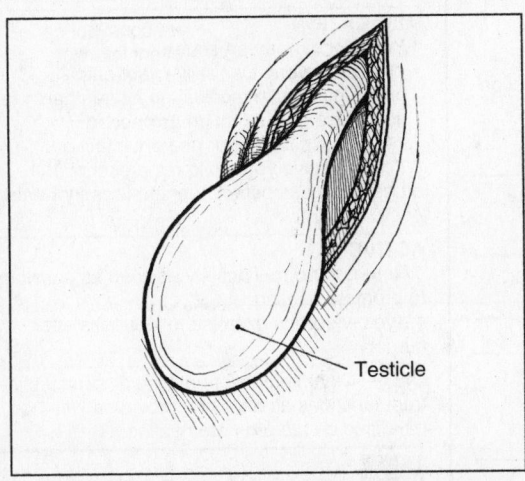

The blood supply, vas deferens (carries sperm for testicle) and nerves leading to the testicle are located and cut free. The testicle is then cut free from surrounding tissue.

Testicle

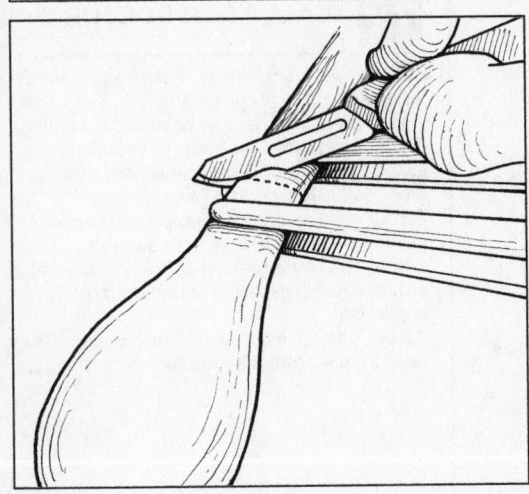

The excised testicle is removed.
- The skin is closed with sutures that will be absorbed by the body.

SURGERIES

THYROGLOSSAL DUCT & CYST REMOVAL

GENERAL INFORMATION

DEFINITION—Removal of a thyroglossal duct that has a cyst. The cyst results from remnants of the thyroid gland that do not descend normally during early fetal development. The cyst usually appears during childhood, attached to the hyoid bone by the duct. The duct then passes upward to its origin at the base of the tongue. Surgery is usually performed when the patient is between 6 and 10 years old.

BODY PARTS INVOLVED—Thyroglossal cyst; remnants of the thyroglossal duct; hyoid bone.

REASONS FOR SURGERY
• Prevention of infections.
• Relief of pressure on the airway that causes difficulty in breathing or swallowing.

SURGICAL RISK INCREASES WITH
• Obesity.
• Poor nutrition.
• Recent or chronic illness.
• Other congenital disorders.
• Diabetes.
• Use of some prescription and nonprescription drugs. Inform your doctor of any drugs, medications, or vitamin and herb supplements you are using or have used in the last month.

WHAT TO EXPECT

WHO OPERATES—General surgeon or ear, nose and throat specialist (otolaryngologist).

WHERE PERFORMED—Hospital.

DIAGNOSTIC TESTS
• Before surgery: Blood and urine studies; ultrasound; CT scan (see Glossary).
• After surgery: Blood studies.

ANESTHESIA—General anesthesia by injection and inhalation with an airway tube placed in the windpipe.

DESCRIPTION OF OPERATION
• An incision is made in the neck over the thyroglossal cyst.
• The cyst is cut free of muscle and connective tissue. The part of the hyoid bone to which the cyst is attached is cut, and the cyst and bone are removed.
• The thyroglossal duct is located, tied, cut and removed.
• The neck muscles are closed with fine sutures.
• The skin is closed with either sutures or clips, which usually can be be removed about 4 to 7 days after surgery.

POSSIBLE COMPLICATIONS
• Excessive bleeding.
• Surgical-wound infection.
• Injury to surrounding nerves.
• Inadvertent injury to larynx (rare).

AVERAGE HOSPITAL STAY—0 to 1 day.

PROBABLE OUTCOME—Expect complete healing without complications. Allow about 6 weeks for recovery from surgery.

POSTOPERATIVE CARE

GENERAL MEASURES
• A hard ridge should form along the incision. As it heals, the ridge will gradually recede.
• Use an electric heating pad, a heat lamp or a warm compress to relieve incisional pain.
• Your child should bathe or shower as usual, and wash the incision gently with mild, unscented soap. After bathing or showering, replace any wet dressings with clean, dry ones.

MEDICATION
• Your doctor may prescribe:
  - Pain relievers. Don't give your child prescription pain medication longer than 4 to 7 days. Use only as much as needed.
  - Antibiotics to fight or prevent infection.
• You may give your child nonprescription drugs, such as acetaminophen, for minor pain. Avoid aspirin.

ACTIVITY
• Return to normal activity as soon as possible to promote healing.
• Avoid vigorous exercise for 3 weeks after surgery.

DIET—Clear liquid diet until the gastrointestinal tract functions again. Then provide a well-balanced diet to promote healing.

CALL YOUR DOCTOR IF

• Pain, swelling, redness, drainage or bleeding increases in the surgical area.
• Your child experiences nausea or vomiting.
• Your child develops signs of infection, including headache, muscle aches, dizziness or a general ill feeling and fever.
• Your child develops hoarseness that doesn't go away within 2 weeks after surgery.
• Your child experiences difficulty in breathing or has a harsh vibrating sound during respiration.
• New, unexplained symptoms develop. Drugs used in treatment may produce side effects.

THYROGLOSSAL DUCT & CYST REMOVAL

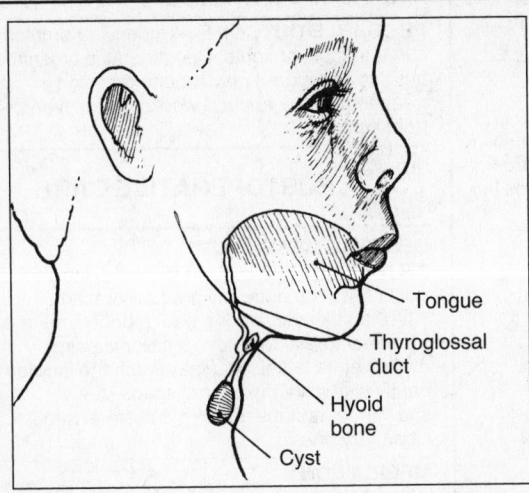

An illustration of the tongue, thyroglossal duct, hyoid bone and a cyst in the thyroglossal duct.

Tongue

Thyroglossal duct

Hyoid bone

Cyst

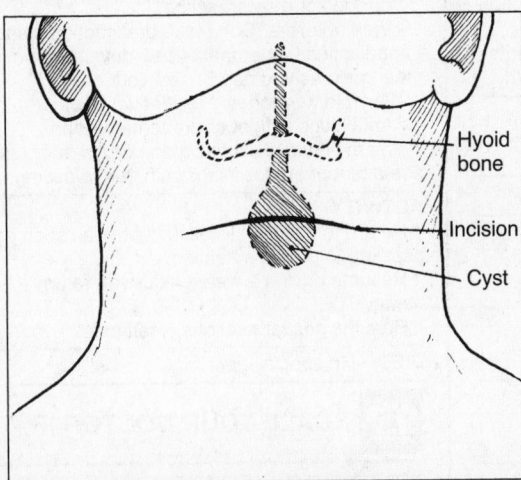

The skin is incised directly over the cyst.

Hyoid bone

Incision

Cyst

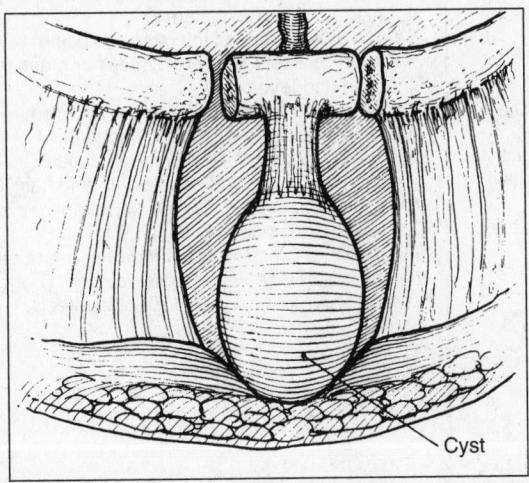

The cyst is cut free of muscle, connective tissue and part of the hyoid bone to which the cyst is attached. The cyst and bone are removed.
- Muscles and connective tissue are returned to their normal positions (not illustrated).

Cyst

THYROID GLAND REMOVAL
(Thyroidectomy)

 GENERAL INFORMATION

DEFINITION—Removal of part or all of the thyroid gland.

BODY PARTS INVOLVED—Thyroid gland, the organ in the neck below the Adam's apple that controls the body's metabolism; lymph nodes in the neck.

REASONS FOR SURGERY
* Hyperthyroidism.
* Benign or cancerous tumors of the thyroid.
* Goiter (see Glossary).

SURGICAL RISK INCREASES WITH
* Adults over 60.
* Obesity; poor nutrition.
* Smoking.
* Untreated hyperthyroidism (see Glossary).
* Diabetes.
* Use of some prescription and nonprescription drugs. Inform your doctor of any drugs, medications, or vitamin and herb supplements you are using or have used in the last month.

 WHAT TO EXPECT

WHO OPERATES—General surgeon.

WHERE PERFORMED—Hospital.

DIAGNOSTIC TESTS
* Before surgery: Blood studies; ultrasound; CT scan; needle biopsy; radioactive-iodine uptake and scan (see Glossary for all).
* After surgery: Blood studies.

ANESTHESIA—General anesthesia by injection and inhalation with an airway tube placed in the windpipe.

DESCRIPTION OF OPERATION
* An incision is made in the neck following natural skin lines.
* Neck muscles are cut or retracted.
* Blood supply to the thyroid gland is clamped.
* The thyroid gland is cut free and removed, and a drain is left in place. In certain cases, some normal thyroid gland tissue is left intact.
* If cancer is present, some lymph nodes may be removed around the thyroid.
* The muscles are closed and the skin is closed with sutures or clips, which can usually be removed in 2 to 10 days after surgery.

POSSIBLE COMPLICATIONS
* Hoarseness or loss of voice, if vocal-cord nerves are damaged during surgery.
* Hypothyroidism (see Glossary).
* Hypoparathyroidism (see Glossary).
* Excessive bleeding.
* Surgical-wound infection.

AVERAGE HOSPITAL STAY—0 to 3 days.

PROBABLE OUTCOME—Underlying problem cured in most patients. Cancer that is present but has not spread may require radiation treatment. Allow about 6 weeks for recovery from surgery.

 POSTOPERATIVE CARE

GENERAL MEASURES
* A hard ridge should form along the incision. As it heals, the ridge will gradually recede.
* Use an electric heating pad, a heat lamp or a warm compress to relieve incisional pain.
* Shower as usual. You may wash the incision gently with mild, unscented soap. After showering, replace any wet dressings with clean, dry ones.

MEDICATION
* Your doctor may prescribe:
  - Pain relievers. Don't take prescription pain medication longer than 4 to 7 days. Use only as much as you need.
  - Thyroid hormones.
  - Antibiotics to fight or prevent infection.
* You may use nonprescription drugs, such as acetaminophen, for minor pain. Avoid aspirin.

ACTIVITY
* Return to daily activities and work as soon as possible to promote healing.
* Resume driving 2 weeks after you return home.
* Resume sexual relations when able.

DIET—No special diet.

 CALL YOUR DOCTOR IF

* Pain, swelling, redness, drainage or bleeding increases in the surgical area.
* You develop signs of infection, including headache, muscle aches, dizziness or a general ill feeling and fever.
* You develop symptoms of hypothyroidism, including excessive weakness, fatigue, intolerance to cold, menstrual irregularities, constipation, or dry and coarse skin and hair.
* You develop symptoms of hypoparathyroidism (see Glossary), including dry hair, brittle fingernails; dry, scaly skin or irregular heartbeat.
* New, unexplained symptoms develop. Drugs used in treatment may produce side effects.

THYROID GLAND REMOVAL
(Thyroidectomy)

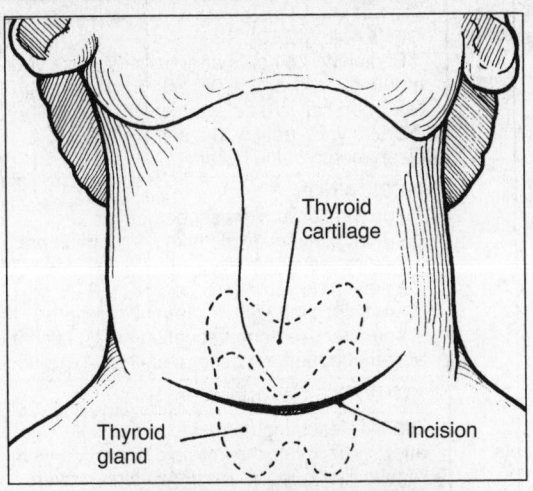

An illustration of structures in the neck and the typical incision site for thyroid gland removal.

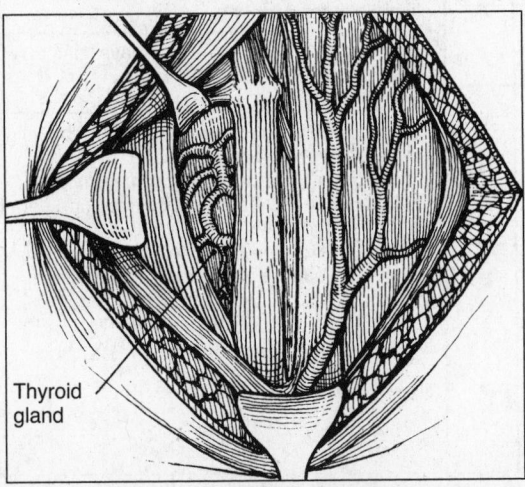

Muscles and connective tissue are retracted revealing the thyroid gland.

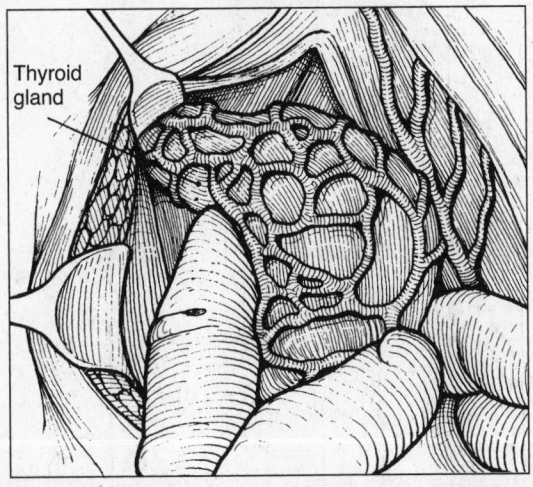

The blood supply to the thyroid gland is clamped and all or part of the gland is cut free and removed.
- The remaining tissue is replaced in its normal position. The skin is closed with sutures or clips (not illustrated).

TONGUE, CHEEK OR GUM BIOPSY

 GENERAL INFORMATION

DEFINITION—Removal of tissue from the oral cavity.

BODY PARTS INVOLVED—Tongue; cheek; gums; roof of mouth; salivary glands under the tongue.

REASONS FOR SURGERY—Usually performed to determine if any unusual lesion in the mouth is cancerous. Laboratory examination of the removed tissue aids in diagnosis.

SURGICAL RISK INCREASES WITH
- Adults over 60.
- Smoking.
- Excess alcohol consumption.
- Diabetes.
- Use of some prescription and nonprescription drugs. Inform your doctor of any drugs, medications, or vitamin and herb supplements you are using or have used in the last month.

 WHAT TO EXPECT

WHO OPERATES—Dentist, oral surgeon, general surgeon or ear, nose and throat specialist.

WHERE PERFORMED—Hospital, outpatient surgical facility or doctor's, dentist's or oral surgeon's office.

DIAGNOSTIC TESTS
- Before surgery: Blood and urine studies; CT scan; MRI (see Glossary for both).
- After surgery: Laboratory examination of removed tissue.

ANESTHESIA
- Local anesthesia by injection.
- General anesthesia (sometimes) by injection and inhalation with an airway tube placed in the windpipe.

DESCRIPTION OF OPERATION
- The area where the tissue is to be gathered is numbed with a local anesthetic.
- Abnormal tissue and a small amount of healthy surrounding tissue is removed.
- Small stitches may be needed to close the incision. These usually can be removed in 3 to 5 days after surgery.

POSSIBLE COMPLICATIONS
- Excessive bleeding.
- Surgical-wound infection.

AVERAGE HOSPITAL STAY—None.

PROBABLE OUTCOME—Tissue obtained successfully without complications in virtually all cases. Allow about 2 weeks for recovery from surgery.

 POSTOPERATIVE CARE

GENERAL MEASURES
- Beginning 24 hours after surgery, rinse your mouth every 1 or 2 hours with a solution of 1/2 teaspoon salt in 8 oz. warm water.
- Brush your teeth with a soft toothbrush. A clean mouth heals faster.

MEDICATION
- Your doctor may prescribe:
  - Pain relievers. Don't take prescription pain medication longer than 4 to 7 days. Use only as much as you need.
  - Antibiotics to fight or prevent infection.
- You may use nonprescription drugs, such as acetaminophen, for minor pain. Avoid aspirin.

ACTIVITY—No restrictions.

DIET—Resuming normal food and fluid intake after surgery will ensure rapid healing. If your regular diet is too difficult, try a high-protein liquid diet for 2 or 3 days.

 CALL YOUR DOCTOR IF

- Pain, swelling, redness, drainage or bleeding increases in the surgical area.
- You develop signs of infection, including headache, muscle aches, dizziness or a general ill feeling and fever.
- New, unexplained symptoms develop. Drugs used in treatment may produce side effects.

TONGUE, CHEEK OR GUM BIOPSY

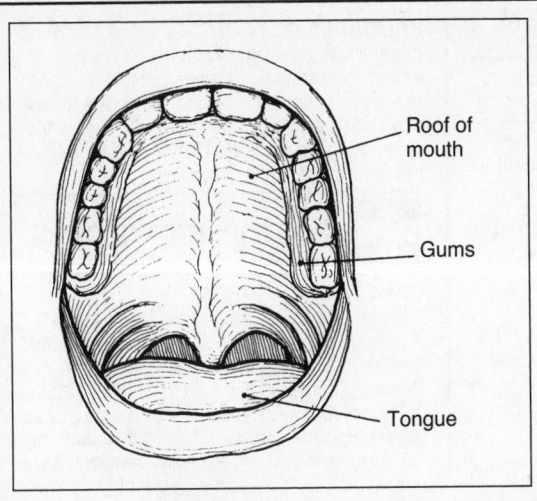

An illustration of the roof of the mouth, gums, teeth and tongue.

Roof of mouth

Gums

Tongue

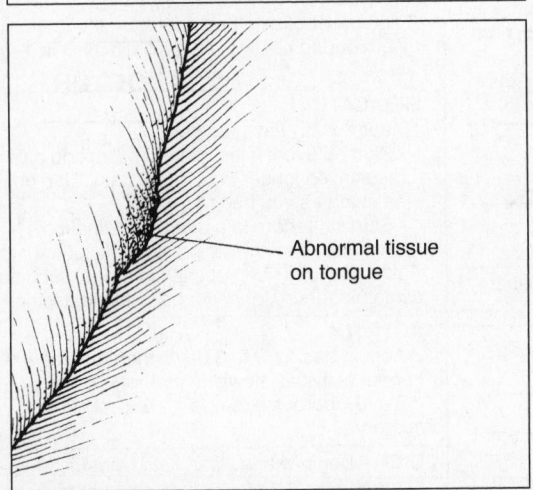

The abnormal tissue on the edge of the tongue illustrated here.

Abnormal tissue on tongue

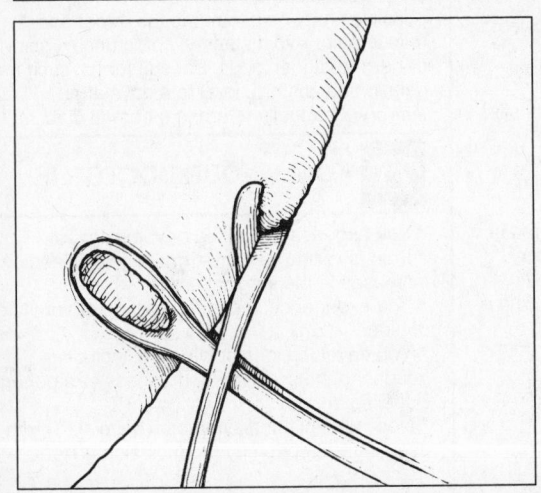

After injecting a local anesthetic, the abnormal tissue and a small amount of healthy surrounding tissue is removed.

• Small stitches may be needed to close the incision. If so, they usually can be removed in 3 to 5 days after surgery (not illustrated).

SURGERIES

TONSIL & ADENOID REMOVAL
(Tonsillectomy & Adenoidectomy)

 GENERAL INFORMATION

DEFINITION—Removal of the tonsils and adenoids.

BODY PARTS INVOLVED—Tonsils; adenoids; opening from the nose into the throat; back of the throat.

REASONS FOR SURGERY
In tonsils:
• More than 5 attacks of tonsillitis in 1 year.
• Peritonsillar abscess (see Glossary).
In adenoids:
• Obstruction of air through the nose.
• Infections in the middle ear.

SURGICAL RISK INCREASES WITH
• Obesity; smoking.
• Poor nutrition.
• Recent or chronic illness.
• Diabetes.
• Use of some prescription and nonprescription drugs. Inform your doctor of any drugs, medications, or vitamin and herb supplements you are using or have used in the last month.

 WHAT TO EXPECT

WHO OPERATES—Ear, nose and throat specialist or general surgeon.

WHERE PERFORMED—Hospital or outpatient surgical facility.

DIAGNOSTIC TESTS
• Before surgery: Blood and urine studies.
• After surgery: Laboratory examination of removed tissue; blood studies.

ANESTHESIA—General anesthesia by injection and inhalation with an airway tube placed in the windpipe.

DESCRIPTION OF OPERATION
• Several techniques are available; one is described here.
• The mouth is held open to expose the tonsils.
• The tonsils are grasped with clamps and pulled toward the middle of the mouth. The tonsils are cut free of surrounding membrane and removed.
• Bleeding is controlled by pressure, sutures or clamps and ties or with use of electrocautery (see Glossary).
• The adenoids are located and removed with a special instrument.

POSSIBLE COMPLICATIONS
• Excessive bleeding, sometimes requiring another operation.
• Adenoid-tissue regrowth.
• Nausea and dehydration.

AVERAGE HOSPITAL STAY—0 to 2 days.

PROBABLE OUTCOME—Expect complete healing without complications. You will experience moderate nasal congestion and drainage, a sore throat and earaches for a few days after surgery. Allow about 3 weeks for recovery from surgery. During this time, avoid becoming hot, tired or excited.

 POSTOPERATIVE CARE

GENERAL MEASURES
• Bathe or shower as usual.
• Use ice packs or popsicles to relieve pain.
• Minimize talking in the first 2 to 3 days following surgery.
• Try not to cough, clear the throat, cry or sing for 1 week after surgery.
• The pain in your throat may worsen before it improves.
• You may notice a bad odor from the nose or mouth during healing. This will diminish in 1 to 2 weeks.

MEDICATION
• Your doctor may prescribe:
  - Pain relievers. Don't take prescription pain medication longer than 4 to 7 days. Use only as much as you need.
  - Stool softeners to prevent constipation.
  - Antibiotics to fight or prevent infection.
• You may use nonprescription drugs, such as acetaminophen, for minor pain. Avoid aspirin.

ACTIVITY
• Rest in bed for 2 to 3 days, then resume normal activities slowly to promote healing.
• Avoid vigorous exercise for 6 weeks after surgery.

DIET—Begin with a clear, liquid diet following surgery. Sucking on ice chips or eating popsicles may help to numb the throat and relieve pain. Avoid steamy, hot, crunchy, spicy, or hard-to-digest foods. Eat soft foods, such as gelatin and custard, for 3 to 4 days after surgery. Gradually return to a normal diet.

 CALL YOUR DOCTOR IF

• You experience nausea or vomiting.
• Pain, swelling, redness, drainage or bleeding increases in the surgical area.
• You experience coughing, spitting or vomiting of blood.
• You develop signs of infection, including headache, muscle aches, dizziness or a general ill feeling and fever.
• New, unexplained symptoms develop. Drugs used in treatment may produce side effects.

TONSIL & ADENOID REMOVAL
(Tonsillectomy & Adenoidectomy)

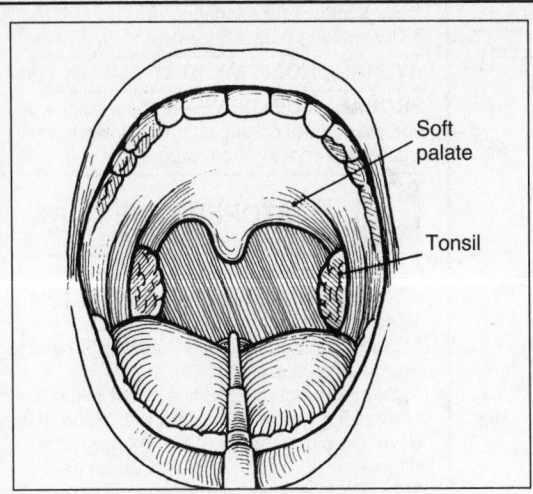

An illustration of the roof of the mouth, tongue (pushed downward by a retractor), the soft and hard palate, and tonsils.

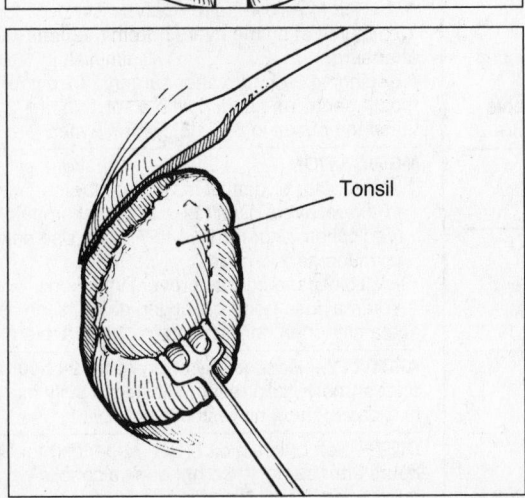

The tonsils are grasped with clamps and pulled toward the middle of the mouth. The tonsils are cut free of surrounding membrane and tension is applied to the base of the tonsil.

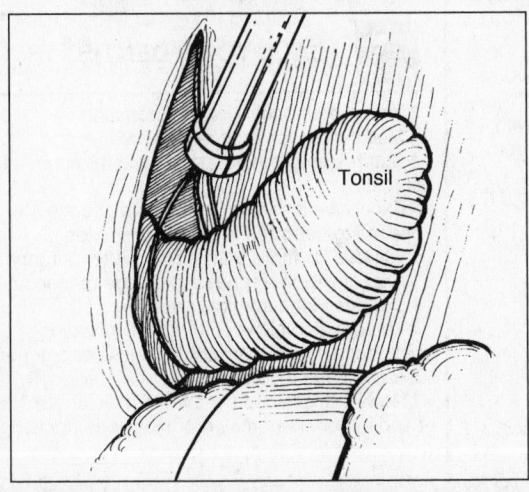

The base of the tonsil is generally reached with a wire snare that cuts through the tonsil allowing easy removal.

- Bleeding is controlled by pressure sutures, electrocautery or clamps and ties.
- Frequently, the adenoids will be removed at the same time (which are not shown in this illustration). Adenoids are tissues similar anatomically to tonsillar tissue and are located in the back of the throat up behind the hard palate toward the rear opening into the nose.

SURGERIES

TOOTH EXTRACTION

 GENERAL INFORMATION

DEFINITION—Removal (extraction) of a tooth.

BODY PARTS INVOLVED—Teeth; gums; bones in jaw.

REASONS FOR SURGERY
Routine removals:
* Loss of supporting tissue, bone or gums.
* Infection of the nerve in the tooth.
* Fractured teeth that cannot be restored.

Impacted-tooth removals:
* Infection and pain around the lower wisdom teeth.
* Pain upon closing the jaws.
* Destruction or erosion of nearby teeth and bone due to growth of surrounding tissue.
* Lack of space for normal tooth growth.

SURGICAL RISK INCREASES WITH
* Smoking.
* Poor nutrition.
* Diabetes.
* Use of some prescription and nonprescription drugs. Inform your doctor of any drugs, medications, or vitamin and herb supplements you are using or have used in the last month.

 WHAT TO EXPECT

WHO OPERATES—Dentist or oral surgeon.

WHERE PERFORMED—Hospital, outpatient surgical facility or dentist's or oral surgeon's office.

DIAGNOSTIC TESTS
* Before surgery: Blood and urine studies; x-rays of mouth.

ANESTHESIA
* Local anesthesia by injection.
* General anesthesia by injection and inhalation with an airway tube placed in the windpipe.

DESCRIPTION OF OPERATION
* For impacted teeth, the gum is incised over the tooth to be removed.
* For all extractions, the tooth is grasped with special instruments, rotated and elevated from the surrounding gum and bone.
* A gauze sponge is packed into the space left by the extracted tooth.
* Sometimes, sutures are used to close the gum edges. They usually come out by themselves, but may need removal in 3 or 4 days after surgery.

POSSIBLE COMPLICATIONS
* Excessive bleeding.
* Surgical-wound infection.
* Dry sockets (see Glossary).

AVERAGE HOSPITAL STAY—Usually none.

PROBABLE OUTCOME—Expect complete healing without complications. Allow about 3 weeks for recovery from surgery.

 POSTOPERATIVE CARE

GENERAL MEASURES
* Do not smoke or use drinking straws for the next 24 hours.
* Keep your mouth closed firmly on the gauze sponge. Don't spit.
* Change the gauze sponge about every 30 minutes if it becomes soaked with blood. If not, leave it in place for about 3 to 4 hours after surgery.
* Use ice to relieve pain. Apply an ice pack for 10 minutes at a time every hour for 12 hours after surgery.
* Beginning 24 hours after surgery, rinse your mouth gently as needed with a solution of 1/2 teaspoon of salt in 8 oz. lukewarm water.

MEDICATION
* Your doctor or dentist may prescribe:
  - Pain relievers. Don't take prescription pain medication longer than 4 to 7 days. Use only as much as you need.
  - Antibiotics to fight or prevent infection.
* You may use nonprescription drugs, such as acetaminophen, for minor pain. Avoid aspirin.

ACTIVITY—Rest quietly at home for 24 hours after surgery, then resume limited activity for 1 or 2 days. Then, no restrictions.

DIET—Soft or liquid diet (See Appendix) for 24 hours after surgery. Do not drink alcoholic beverages during this time.

 CALL YOUR DENTIST IF

* You experience nausea or vomiting.
* Medication does not relieve pain.
* Sutures drop out during the first 48 hours after surgery.
* Excessive bleeding (one gauze sponge becoming deep red in 10 to 15 minutes) continues for more than 4 hours after surgery.
* Pain, swelling, redness, drainage or bleeding increases in the surgical area.
* You develop signs of infection, including headache, muscle aches, dizziness or a general ill feeling and fever.
* New, unexplained symptoms develop. Drugs used in treatment may produce side effects.

TOOTH EXTRACTION

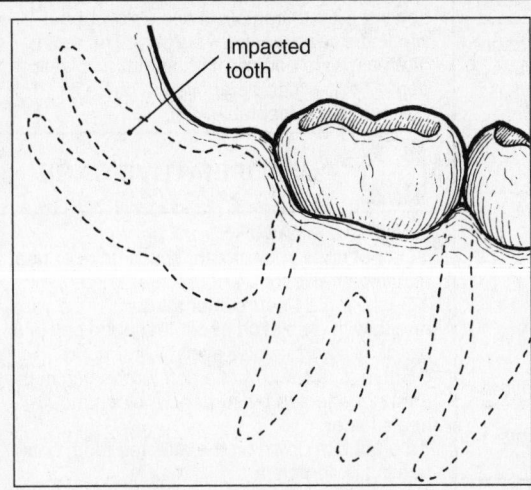

Impacted tooth

A bony impacted tooth.

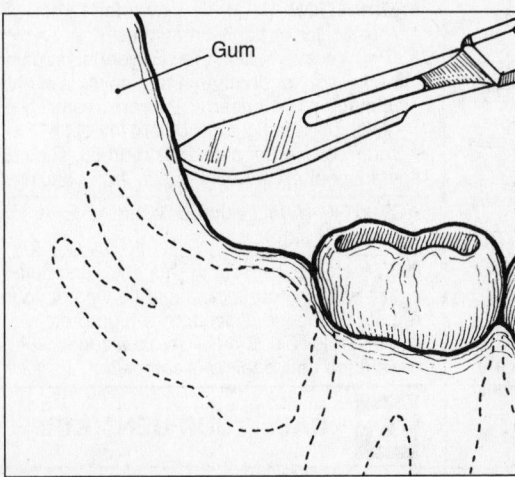

Gum

The gum is incised over the tooth to be removed.

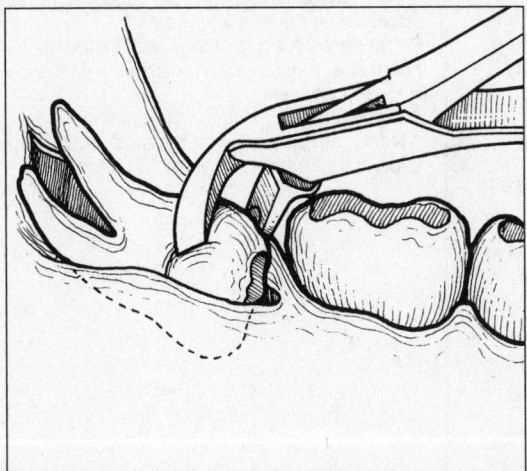

Tooth to be extracted is grasped with special instruments, rotated and elevated from the gum and bone. If sutures are used to close the surgical site, they may need removal 3 to 4 days after surgery.

SURGERIES

TOOTH REPLANTATION

GENERAL INFORMATION

DEFINITION—Replanting a tooth that has been knocked out of its normal position. Best results are obtained when the tooth is replanted within 2 hours after injury.

BODY PARTS INVOLVED—Mouth; teeth; gums.

REASONS FOR SURGERY—Prevention of permanent loss of a tooth.

SURGICAL RISK INCREASES WITH
• Smoking; poor nutrition.
• Recent or chronic illness.
• Poor dental hygiene or gum disease.
• Diabetes.
• Use of some prescription and nonprescription drugs. Inform your doctor of any drugs, medications, or vitamin and herb supplements you are using or have used in the last month.

WHAT TO EXPECT

WHO OPERATES—Oral surgeon or dentist.

WHERE PERFORMED—Hospital, oral surgeon's or dentist's office, outpatient surgical facility, doctor's office or emergency room.

DIAGNOSTIC TESTS—Before surgery: Usually none, because of the need for immediate surgery.

ANESTHESIA—Local anesthesia by injection.

DESCRIPTION OF OPERATION
• If you or your child has a tooth knocked out, try to find the tooth, wash it and replace it in the socket as quickly as possible. Go to your dentist as soon as possible.
• If you cannot replace the tooth in its socket, wash it and keep it wet. Go to your dentist immediately.
• Usually the root canal nerve of the tooth is removed and filled with plastic material before the tooth is reinserted. Some dentists simply place the tooth back into the socket immediately.
• The replanted tooth is anchored to neighboring teeth with wire or plastic.

POSSIBLE COMPLICATIONS
• Excessive bleeding.
• Surgical-wound infection.
• Rejection of tooth (rare if surgery is performed within 2 hours after injury).

AVERAGE HOSPITAL STAY—0 to 1 day.

PROBABLE OUTCOME—Expect complete healing without complications. Allow about 4 weeks for recovery from surgery. The tooth often appears normal. If it darkens, a plastic dental veneer can be applied to make it cosmetically acceptable.

POSTOPERATIVE CARE

GENERAL MEASURES
• Do not rinse your mouth, spit, smoke or use drinking straws for 24 hours after surgery.
• Beginning 24 hours after surgery, rinse your mouth with a solution of 1/2 teaspoon salt in 8 oz. of lukewarm water every 1 or 2 hours.
• Brush your teeth with a soft toothbrush in the area not affected by surgery. A clean mouth heals faster.
• Do not bite down on the affected tooth until healing is complete.

MEDICATION
• Your doctor or dentist may prescribe:
  - Pain relievers. Don't take prescription pain medication longer than 4 to 7 days. Use only as much as you need.
  - Antibiotics to fight or prevent infection.
• You may use nonprescription drugs, such as acetaminophen, for minor pain. Avoid aspirin.

ACTIVITY—Avoid vigorous exercise for 6 weeks after surgery.

DIET—Resuming your normal food and fluid intake will promote more rapid healing. If your regular diet is too difficult, try a high-protein liquid diet for 2 or 3 days. Avoid alcoholic beverages until healing is complete.

CALL YOUR DENTIST IF

• Pain, swelling, redness, drainage or bleeding increases in the surgical area.
• You develop signs of infection, including headache, muscle aches, dizziness or a general ill feeling and fever.
• You experience nausea or vomiting.
• New, unexplained symptoms develop. Drugs used in treatment may produce side effects.

TOOTH REPLANTATION

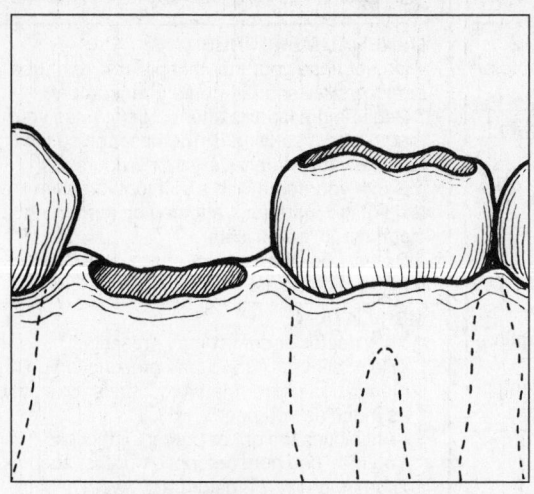

An illustration of teeth, gums and a socket left by a missing tooth.

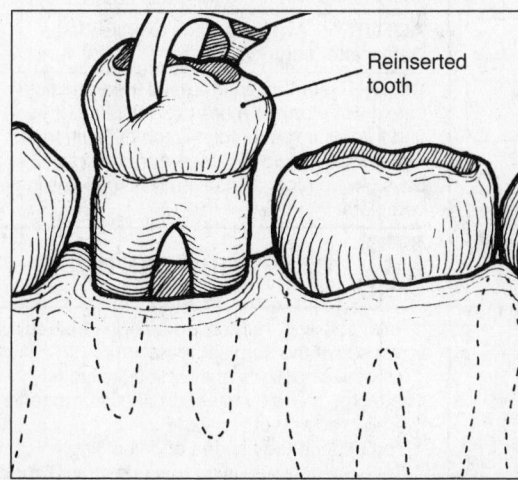

Reinserted tooth

The root canal nerve of the tooth is removed and filled with plastic material before the tooth is reinserted.

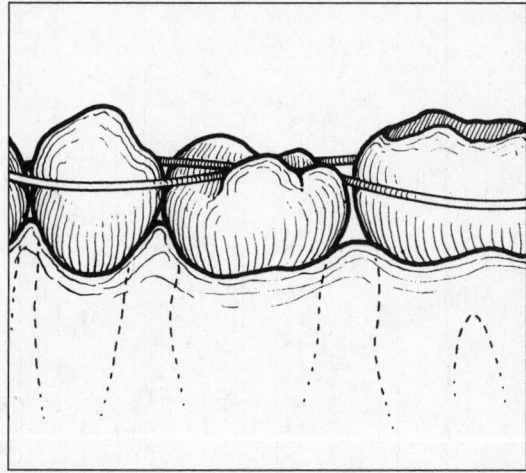

The replanted tooth is anchored to neighboring teeth with wire or plastic.

TOOTH TRANSPLANTATION

 GENERAL INFORMATION

DEFINITION—Replacement of an injured or diseased first or second molar with a third molar (wisdom tooth).

BODY PARTS INVOLVED—Mouth; teeth; gums.

REASONS FOR SURGERY—Restoration of normal tooth function.

SURGICAL RISK INCREASES WITH
• Recent or chronic illness.
• Smoking.
• Diabetes.
• Use of some prescription and nonprescription drugs. Inform your doctor of any drugs, medications, or vitamin and herb supplements you are using or have used in the last month.

 WHAT TO EXPECT

WHO OPERATES—Dentist or oral surgeon.

WHERE PERFORMED—Dentist's or oral surgeon's office, outpatient surgical facility or hospital.

DIAGNOSTIC TESTS
• Before surgery: Blood and urine studies.
• After surgery: Blood studies.

ANESTHESIA
• Local anesthesia by injection.
• General anesthesia (sometimes) by injection and inhalation, with an airway tube placed in the windpipe.

DESCRIPTION OF OPERATION
• A wisdom tooth is pulled.
• Sometimes, the root of the pulled tooth may be shortened for better fit.
• The socket where the tooth will be transplanted is enlarged.
• The wisdom tooth is inserted in the socket and secured to neighboring teeth. This provides support during healing.

POSSIBLE COMPLICATIONS
• Excessive bleeding.
• Surgical-wound infection.
• Rejection of transplanted tooth (rare).

AVERAGE HOSPITAL STAY—0 to 1 day.

PROBABLE OUTCOME—Expect complete healing without complications. Allow about 1 month for recovery from surgery.

 POSTOPERATIVE CARE

GENERAL MEASURES
• Do not rinse your mouth, spit, smoke or use drinking straws for 24 hours after surgery.
• Beginning 24 hours after surgery, rinse your mouth with a solution of 1/2 teaspoon salt in 8 oz. lukewarm water every 1 or 2 hours.
• Brush your teeth with a soft toothbrush in the area of the mouth not affected by surgery. A clean mouth heals faster.
• Do not bite down on the affected tooth until healing is complete.

MEDICATION
• Your doctor or dentist may prescribe:
  - Pain relievers. Don't take prescription pain medication longer than 4 to 7 days. Use only as much as you need.
  - Antibiotics to fight or prevent infection.
• You may use nonprescription drugs, such as acetaminophen, for minor pain. Avoid aspirin.

ACTIVITY—Avoid vigorous exercise for 3 weeks after surgery.

DIET—Resuming your normal food and fluid intake will promote more rapid healing. If you find that your regular diet is too difficult, try a high-protein liquid diet (see Appendix) for 2 or 3 days. Avoid alcoholic beverages until healing is complete.

 CALL YOUR DENTIST IF

• Pain, swelling, redness, drainage or bleeding increases in the surgical area.
• You develop signs of infection, including headache, muscle aches, dizziness or a general ill feeling and fever.
• You experience nausea and vomiting.
• New, unexplained symptoms develop. Drugs used in treatment may produce side effects.

TOOTH TRANSPLANTATION

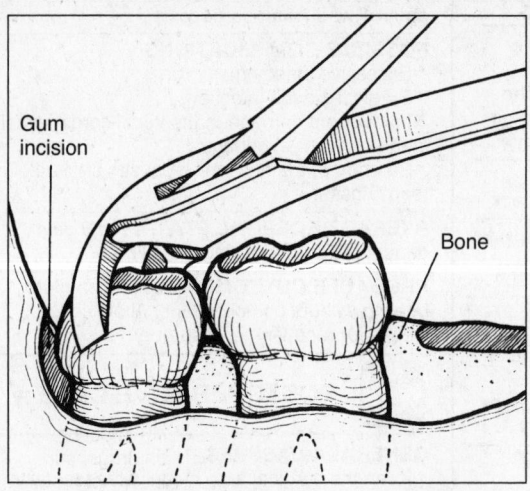

Gum incision

Bone

Shown here are the gums, bones and lower teeth, with forceps grasping the tooth to be transplanted.

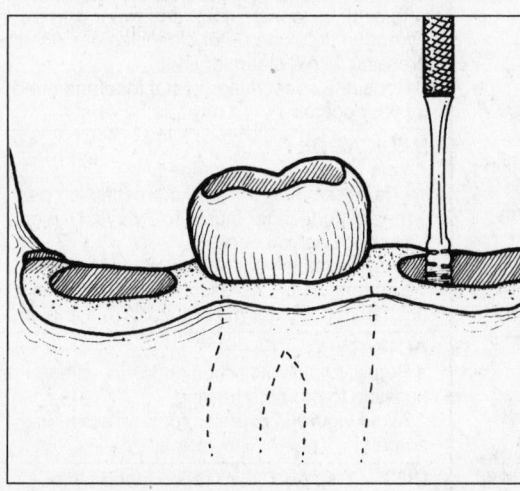

The socket where the tooth will be transplanted is enlarged.

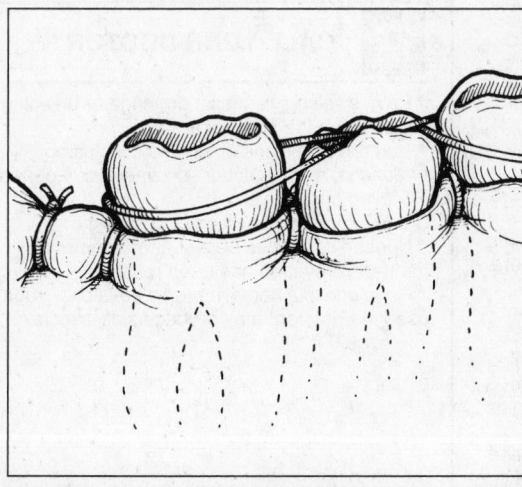

In this example, the wisdom tooth, having been removed, is inserted in the socket and secured to neighboring teeth to provide support during healing.

SURGERIES

TRACHEOSTOMY

GENERAL INFORMATION

DEFINITION—Creation of an opening in the windpipe (trachea) that will function as an airway either temporarily or permanently. The opening bypasses obstructions that prevent air from being inhaled or exhaled.

BODY PARTS INVOLVED—Windpipe; muscles, blood vessels and nerves in the neck.

REASONS FOR SURGERY
- Restoration of normal breathing.
- Control of secretions from the nose and throat, particularly in patients who are unconscious.
- Creation of an open airway in patients who require prolonged breathing assistance.
- Creation of an airway in patients whose larynx is removed.

SURGICAL RISK INCREASES WITH
- Newborns and infants.
- Adults over 75.
- Obesity; smoking; poor nutrition.
- Recent illness, especially upper-respiratory infection.
- Alcoholism or chronic illness.
- Diabetes.
- Use of some prescription and nonprescription drugs. Inform your doctor of any drugs, medications, or vitamin and herb supplements you are using or have used in the last month.

WHAT TO EXPECT

WHO OPERATES—Ear, nose and throat specialist or general surgeon.

WHERE PERFORMED—Hospital, outpatient surgical facility or emergency room.

DIAGNOSTIC TESTS—Blood and urine studies and x-rays of chest before and after surgery if necessary.

ANESTHESIA
- Local anesthesia (in emergencies) by injection.
- General anesthesia (when time allows) by injection and inhalation with an airway tube placed in the windpipe.

DESCRIPTION OF OPERATION
- An incision is made in the neck. The muscles and connective tissue around the windpipe are divided.
- A section at the front of the windpipe is cut free and removed or a flap is created.
- A tracheostomy tube is fitted into the opening in the windpipe to function as an airway. The patient will breathe through this tube as long as it is in place. Supplemental oxygen and mechanical assisted breathing can be supplied if necessary.

- The skin is closed around the tube with sutures or clips, which usually can be removed about 1 week after surgery.

POSSIBLE COMPLICATIONS
- Excessive bleeding.
- Surgical-wound infection.
- Inadvertent damage to the vocal cords, vocal-cord nerves or esophagus.
- Scarring of trachea which causes stricture (see Glossary).

AVERAGE HOSPITAL STAY—1 to 3 days, depending on underlying condition.

PROBABLE OUTCOME—Expect complete healing without complications. Allow about 2 weeks for recovery from surgery.

POSTOPERATIVE CARE

GENERAL MEASURES
- Keep the surgical area clean. Cleanse daily with mild, unscented soap and water or with hydrogen peroxide. After cleansing, replace the dressing with a clean, dry one.
- Consult a speech therapist if recommended by your doctor.

MEDICATION
- Your doctor may prescribe:
  - Pain relievers. Don't take prescription pain medication longer than 4 to 7 days. Use only as much as you need.
  - Antibiotics to fight or prevent infection.
- You may use nonprescription drugs, such as acetaminophen, for minor pain. Avoid aspirin.

ACTIVITY
- Return to daily activities and work as soon as possible to promote healing.
- Avoid vigorous exercise for 6 weeks after surgery.

DIET—Your doctor will recommend a diet.

CALL YOUR DOCTOR IF

- Pain, swelling, redness, drainage or bleeding increases in the surgical area.
- You develop signs of infection, including headache, muscle aches, dizziness or a general ill feeling and fever.
- You experience nausea or vomiting.
- Speech difficulties persist after a temporary tracheostomy tube has been removed.
- New, unexplained symptoms develop. Drugs used in treatment may produce side effects.

TRACHEOSTOMY

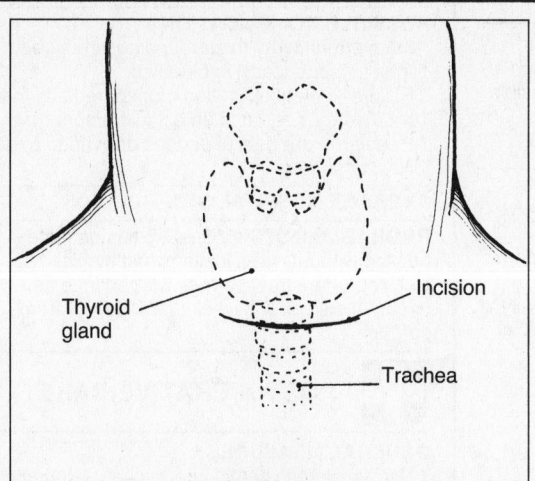

An illustration of structures in the neck and the usual incision site through the skin.

Thyroid gland

Incision

Trachea

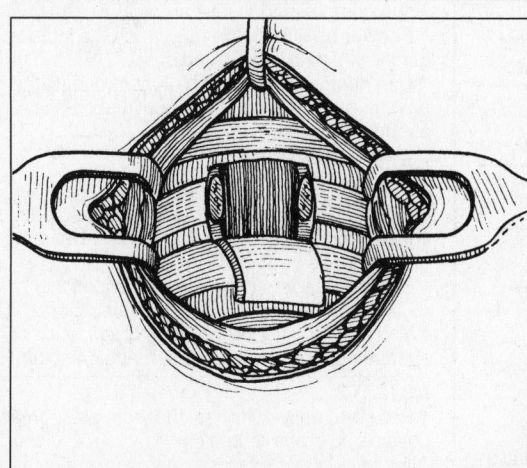

A section at the front of the windpipe is incised and widened.

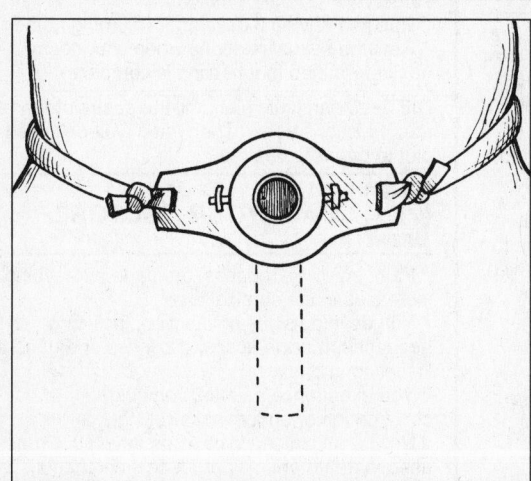

A tracheostomy tube is fitted into the opening in the windpipe to function as an airway. As long as the tracheostomy tube is in place and open, the patient will breathe through it instead of through the mouth or nose.

TUBAL LIGATION

GENERAL INFORMATION

DEFINITION—A method of sterilization that involves blocking the Fallopian tubes in such a way that the ovum (egg) becomes inaccessible for fertilization.

BODY PARTS INVOLVED—Fallopian tubes.

REASONS FOR SURGERY—Prevention of unwanted pregnancy. It is important to receive professional counseling before deciding to undergo this surgery. Sterilization is considered a permanent form of birth control. In some cases, it can be surgically reversed, generally at a considerable cost and with increased risk for subsequent pregnancies (e.g., ectopic pregnancy).

SURGICAL RISK INCREASES WITH
- Obesity; smoking; poor nutrition.
- Recent or chronic illness; diabetes.
- Use of some prescription and nonprescription drugs. Inform your doctor of any drugs, medications, or vitamin and herb supplements you are using or have used in the last month.

WHAT TO EXPECT

WHO OPERATES—Obstetrician-gynecologist or general surgeon.

WHERE PERFORMED—Hospital or outpatient surgical facility.

DIAGNOSTIC TESTS
- Before surgery: Blood and urine studies.
- After surgery: Blood studies.

ANESTHESIA
- Local anesthesia by injection.
- Spinal anesthesia by injection.
- General anesthesia by injection and inhalation with an airway tube placed in the windpipe.

DESCRIPTION OF OPERATION
- One of several techniques is used to expose the Fallopian tubes for surgery. The most common is laparoscopy, which involves two small incisions, and the use of a scope instrument with a fiberoptic light. Other methods used are: minilaparotomy, which involves a vaginal approach and an incision just at or above the pubic hairline; laparotomy, which requires a standard surgical incision through the abdomen; and posterior colpotomy (rare) which utilizes an approach through the rear of the vagina.
- Once the Fallopian tubes are exposed, a small section of each tube is cut free and removed. The severed ends are tied (ligated) or blocked completely by coagulation using an electric current. In some cases, the tubes are clamped using a clip or band.

- The skin is closed with sutures or clips, which can usually be removed 1 week after surgery.

POSSIBLE COMPLICATIONS
- Inadvertent injury to surrounding structures.
- Infection or excessive bleeding.
- Failure of the sterilization procedure (less than 1%). This may result in an ectopic pregnancy.
- Heavier, more painful periods or ovarian cysts following surgery.

AVERAGE HOSPITAL STAY—0 to 1 day.

PROBABLE OUTCOME—Expect complete healing without complications and sterility for life. Your menstrual periods will continue as usual. Allow about 2 weeks for recovery from surgery.

POSTOPERATIVE CARE

GENERAL MEASURES
- Use an electric heating pad, a heat lamp or a warm compress to relieve surgical-wound pain.
- Shower as usual. You may wash the incision gently with mild, unscented soap.
- Use another method of birth control until the next menstrual period in case ovulation has already occurred.

MEDICATION
- Your doctor may prescribe:
  - Pain relievers. Don't take prescription pain medication longer than 4 to 7 days. Use only as much as you need.
  - Stool softeners to prevent constipation.
  - Antibiotics to fight or prevent infection.
- You may use nonprescription drugs, such as acetaminophen, for minor pain. Avoid aspirin.

ACTIVITY
- Return to daily activities and work as soon as possible to promote healing.
- Avoid vigorous exercise for 2 weeks after surgery.
- Resume driving 3 days after returning home.
- Resume sexual relations when your doctor has determined that healing is complete.

DIET—Clear liquid diet until the gastrointestinal tract functions again. Then eat a well-balanced diet to promote healing.

CALL YOUR DOCTOR IF

- Pain, swelling, redness, drainage or bleeding increases in the surgical area.
- You develop signs of infection, including headache, muscle aches, dizziness or a general ill feeling and fever.
- You experience nausea, vomiting, constipation or abdominal swelling.
- New, unexplained symptoms develop. Drugs used in treatment may produce side effects.

TUBAL LIGATION

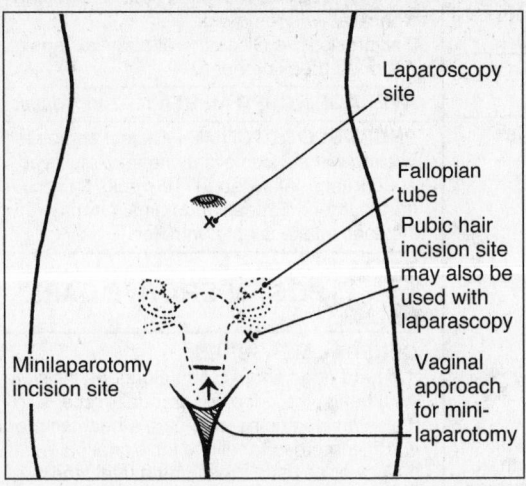

An illustration of structures of the female abdomen and pelvis showing 3 possible sites for a tubal ligation. One is a laparoscopy site, the other a vaginal approach, the third an incision at about the top of the pubic hairline.

Laparoscopy site

Fallopian tube

Pubic hair incision site may also be used with laparascopy

Vaginal approach for mini-laparotomy

Minilaparotomy incision site

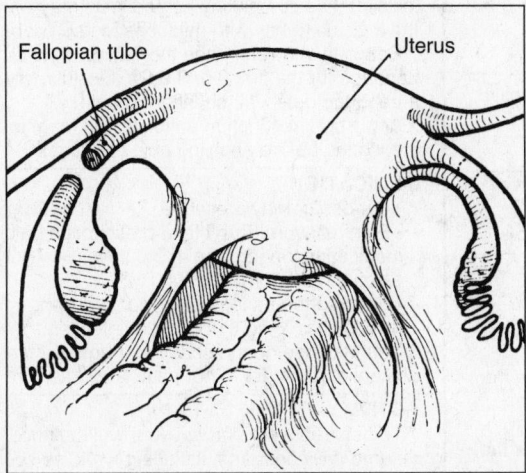

Once the fallopian tubes are exposed, a small section of each tube is cut free and removed.

Fallopian tube

Uterus

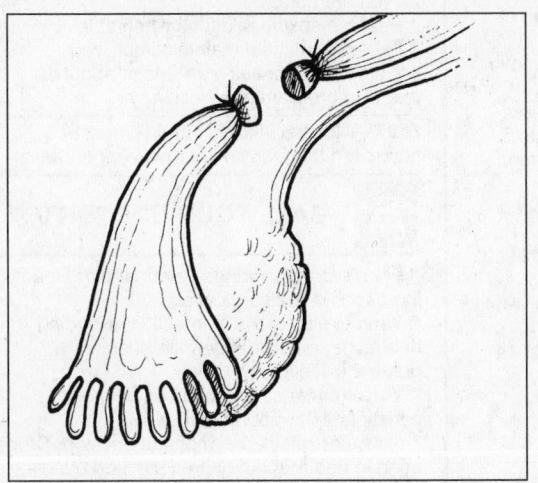

The severed ends are tied.

SURGERIES

TUMMY TUCK
(Abdominoplasty)

 GENERAL INFORMATION

DEFINITION—Removal of excess skin and fat from the abdomen.

BODY PARTS INVOLVED—Fat between skin and muscles in abdomen; skin.

REASONS FOR SURGERY
- Improved appearance.
- Reduce incidence of fungal infections in overlapping tissue.

SURGICAL RISK INCREASES WITH
- Smoking; alcoholism; poor nutrition.
- Previous abdominal surgery.
- Recent or chronic illness, especially diabetes.
- Use of some prescription and nonprescription drugs. Inform your doctor of any drugs, medications, or vitamin and herb supplements you are using or have used in the last month.

 WHAT TO EXPECT

WHO OPERATES—Plastic and reconstructive surgeon.

WHERE PERFORMED—Hospital.

DIAGNOSTIC TESTS
- Before surgery: Blood and urine studies.
- After surgery: Blood studies.

ANESTHESIA—General anesthesia by injection and inhalation with an airway tube placed in the windpipe.

DESCRIPTION OF OPERATION
- A large, elliptical incision, usually running from hip to hip, is made in the abdomen. Another incision is usually made around the navel so that it can be moved to a new position after the excess skin has been removed.
- Excessive skin and the underlying apron of excess fat are cut free and removed. Liposuction may also be performed to remove some of the excess fat.
- The navel is reattached in its new location.
- Drains are left under the operative site to prevent accumulation of blood and fluid from tissue drainage.
- Both edges of the skin are gently stretched and carefully sewn together with sutures. Bandages and a firm, elastic dressing similar to a girdle may be placed over the abdomen and buttocks to help hold the stitches together while healing takes place.
- Sutures can usually be removed in 10 to 14 days.

POSSIBLE COMPLICATIONS
- Wide or excessive scars (keloid).
- Excessive bleeding.
- Surgical-wound infection.
- Blood or serum collection beneath the flap where fat was removed.
- Necrosis (see Glossary) of surgical flaps.
- Wound breaking open.

AVERAGE HOSPITAL STAY—2 to 5 days.

PROBABLE OUTCOME—Expect complete healing without complications and improved appearance. Allow about 10 weeks for recovery from surgery. Excess abdominal fat may return if caloric intake is not controlled.

 POSTOPERATIVE CARE

GENERAL MEASURES
- A hard ridge should form along the incision. As it heals, the ridge will gradually recede.
- Use an electric heating pad, a heat lamp or a warm compress to relieve incisional pain.
- Shower as usual. Avoid baths until the incision has completely healed. You may wash the incision gently with mild, unscented soap.
- Between showers, keep the wound dry with a bandage for the first 2 or 3 days after surgery. If a bandage gets wet, change it promptly.
- Apply nonprescription antibiotic ointment to the wound before applying new bandages.

MEDICATION
- Your doctor may prescribe:
  - Pain relievers. Don't take prescription pain medication longer than 4 to 7 days. Use only as much as you need.
  - Stool softeners to prevent constipation.
  - Antibiotics to fight or prevent infection.
- You may use nonprescription drugs, such as acetaminophen, for minor pain. Avoid aspirin.

ACTIVITY
- To help recovery and aid your well-being, resume daily activities, including work, as soon as you are able.
- Resume sexual relations when able.
- Exercise will help maintain improved appearance. Consult your doctor about an exercise program after recovery.

DIET—No special diet, but diet must be controlled to maintain improved appearance.

 CALL YOUR DOCTOR IF

- Pain, swelling, redness, drainage or bleeding increases in the surgical area.
- You develop signs of infection, including headache, muscle aches, dizziness or a general ill feeling and fever.
- You experience nausea, vomiting, constipation or abdominal swelling.
- New, unexplained symptoms develop. Drugs used in treatment may produce side effects.

TUMMY TUCK
(Abdominoplasty)

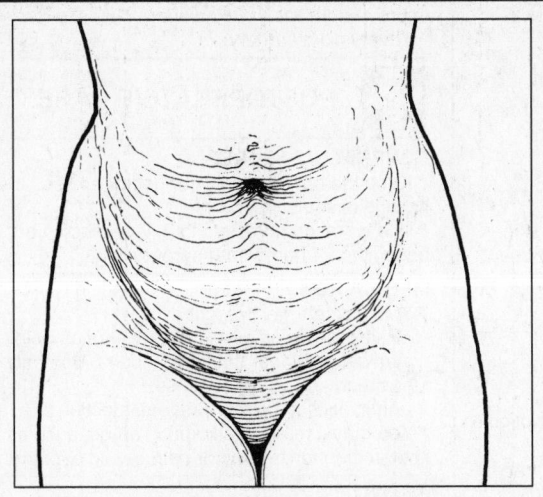

An illustration of typical distribution of excess skin and fat in the lower abdomen.

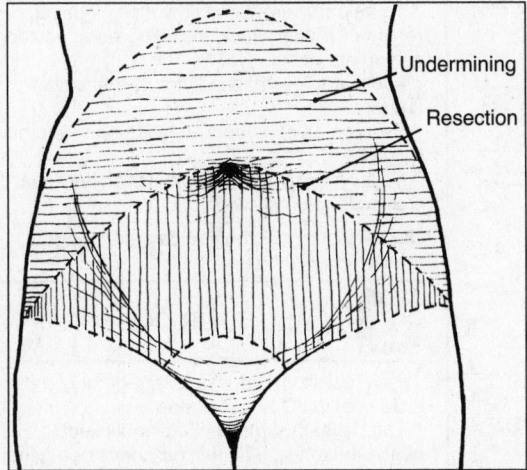

Undermining

Resection

A large elliptical incision is made in the lower abdomen.
- Excessive skin and the underlying apron of excess fat are cut and removed.

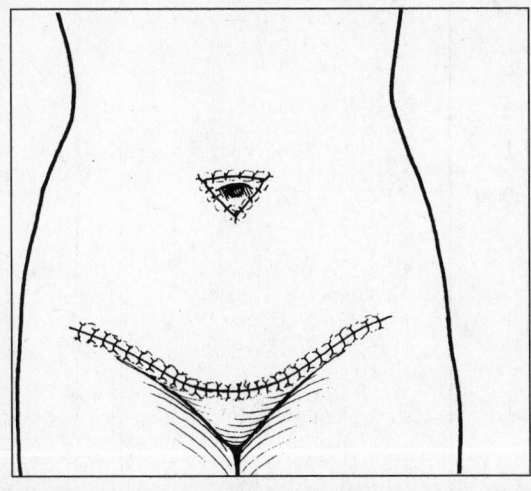

Drains are usually left under the operative site to prevent accumulation of blood and fluid from tissue drainage.
- Both edges of the skin are gently stretched and carefully sewn together with sutures, which can usually be removed in 10 to 14 days.

TYMPANOPLASTY

GENERAL INFORMATION

DEFINITION—Repair, removal or bypass of an obstruction or defect in the middle ear that prevents sound waves from reaching the inner ear. This is called conductive hearing loss, which can be total or partial. Usually, it is caused by chronic infection in the middle ear.

BODY PARTS INVOLVED—Eardrum (tympanic membrane); middle ear cavity; skin separating middle ear from inner ear; inner ear.

REASONS FOR SURGERY—Restoration of, or improvement in, hearing ability.

SURGICAL RISK INCREASES WITH
• Recent or chronic illness.
• Diabetes.
• Use of some prescription and nonprescription drugs. Inform your doctor of any drugs, medications, or vitamin and herb supplements you are using or have used in the last month.

WHAT TO EXPECT

WHO OPERATES—Ear, nose and throat specialist (otolaryngologist).

WHERE PERFORMED—Hospital.

DIAGNOSTIC TESTS
• Before surgery: Blood and urine studies; hearing tests.
• After surgery: Hearing tests.

ANESTHESIA—General anesthesia by injection and inhalation with an airway tube placed in the windpipe.

DESCRIPTION OF OPERATION
• An instrument called an ear speculum is placed in the external ear canal, and the operating microscope is positioned.
• The middle ear is entered through an incision in the eardrum.
• Depending on the type of defect, one of the following procedures is performed:
Repair of a defect in the eardrum.
Closure of the defect in the eardrum with a graft.
Fenestration, which is the creation of a new opening into a part of the inner ear. This method is used to treat otosclerosis (see Illness section).

POSSIBLE COMPLICATIONS
• Excessive bleeding.
• Surgical-wound infection.
• Recurrence of hole in the eardrum.

AVERAGE HOSPITAL STAY—0 to 2 days.

PROBABLE OUTCOME—Expect complete healing without complications. Hearing should improve noticeably. Allow about 4 weeks for recovery from surgery.

POSTOPERATIVE CARE

GENERAL MEASURES
• Keep the ear dry until your doctor advises that healing is complete.
• Use warm compresses to relieve discomfort beginning 24 hours after surgery.

MEDICATION
• Your doctor may prescribe:
- Pain relievers. Don't take prescription pain medication longer than 4 to 7 days. Use only as much as you need.
- Antibiotics to fight or prevent infection.
• You may use nonprescription drugs, such as acetaminophen, for minor pain. Avoid aspirin.

ACTIVITY
• To help recovery and aid your well-being, resume daily activities, including work, as soon as you are able.
• Avoid vigorous exercise for 4 weeks after surgery.
• Resume driving about 2 weeks after returning home.
• No swimming until your doctor advises that it is all right to do so.

DIET—Liquid diet the first day after surgery, then no special diet.

CALL YOUR DOCTOR IF

• Pain, swelling, redness, drainage or bleeding increases in the surgical area.
• You develop signs of infection, including headache, muscle aches, dizziness or a general ill feeling and fever.

TYMPANOPLASTY

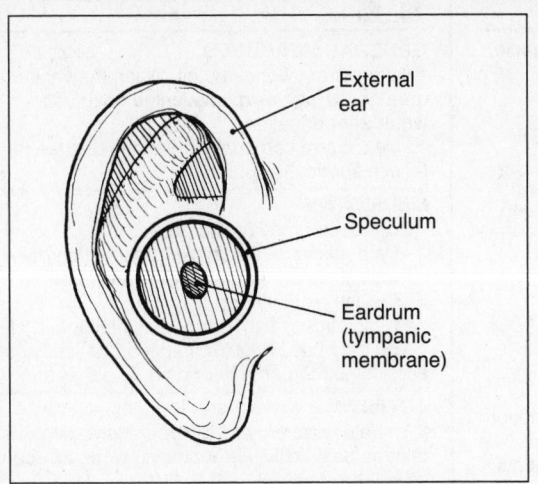

An illustration of the external ear with a speculum in place showing the appearance of the eardrum through the ear speculum.

External ear

Speculum

Eardrum (tympanic membrane)

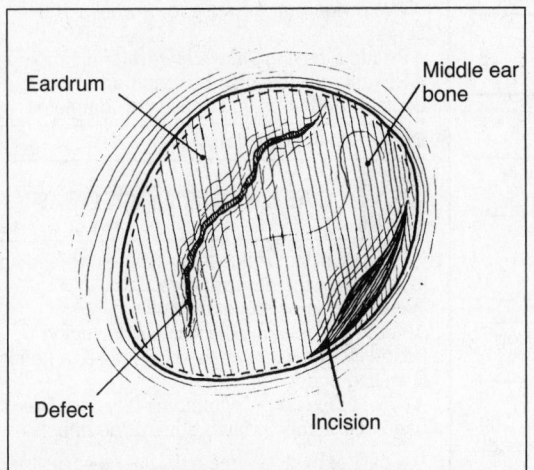

The middle ear is entered through an incision in the eardrum.

Eardrum

Middle ear bone

Defect

Incision

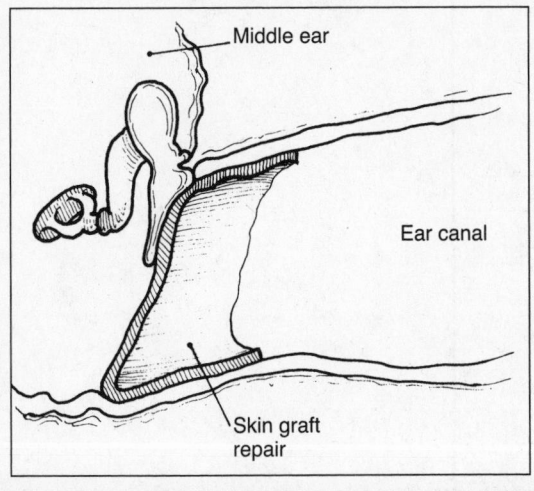

A graft repair of the defect once again seals off the middle and inner ear from air and debris in the ear canal.

Middle ear

Ear canal

Skin graft repair

SURGERIES

URETHRAL CARUNCLE REMOVAL

GENERAL INFORMATION

DEFINITION—Removal of a urethral caruncle, a small benign tumor that develops at the opening of the female urethra.

BODY PARTS INVOLVED—Urethra; vagina (route for surgery).

REASONS FOR SURGERY—Treatment of excessive bleeding or discomfort.

SURGICAL RISK INCREASES WITH
* Adults over 60.
* Obesity; smoking.
* Poor nutrition.
* Recent or chronic illness.
* Alcoholism.
* Diabetes.
* Use of some prescription and nonprescription drugs. Inform your doctor of any drugs, medications, or vitamin and herb supplements you are using or have used in the last month.

WHAT TO EXPECT

WHO OPERATES—Urologist or obstetrician-gynecologist.

WHERE PERFORMED—Hospital, outpatient surgical facility or doctor's office.

DIAGNOSTIC TESTS
* Before surgery: Pap smear (see Glossary); pelvic examination; blood and urine studies.
* After surgery: Pelvic examination.

ANESTHESIA—Local anesthesia by injection and topical application.

DESCRIPTION OF OPERATION
* The vagina is held open with a speculum. The caruncle is located, cleansed and anesthetized with local anesthesia.
* The caruncle is then removed with electrocauterization or a scalpel.
* Bleeding is controlled with pressure or electrocauterization.

POSSIBLE COMPLICATIONS
* Excessive bleeding.
* Surgical-wound infection.

AVERAGE HOSPITAL STAY—Usually none.

PROBABLE OUTCOME—Expect complete healing without complications. Allow about 2 weeks for recovery from surgery.

POSTOPERATIVE CARE

GENERAL MEASURES
* Bathe or shower as usual. Wash the vaginal area gently with mild, unscented soap and water after urination.
* Use a warm compress in the genital area to relieve surgical-wound pain.

MEDICATION
* Your doctor may prescribe:
  - Pain relievers. Don't take prescription pain medication longer than 4 to 7 days. Use only as much as you need.
  - Antibiotics to fight or prevent infection.
* You may use nonprescription drugs, such as acetaminophen, for minor pain. Avoid aspirin.

ACTIVITY
* To help recovery and aid your well-being, resume daily activities, including work, as soon as you are able.
* Avoid vigorous exercise for 2 weeks after surgery.
* Resume driving 3 days after returning home.
* Sexual relations may be resumed when your doctor determines that healing is complete.

DIET—No special diet.

CALL YOUR DOCTOR IF

* Pain, swelling, redness, drainage or bleeding increases in the surgical area.
* Urination is painful or difficult.
* You develop signs of infection, including headache, muscle aches, dizziness or a general ill feeling and fever.
* New, unexplained symptoms develop. Drugs used in treatment may produce side effects.

URETHRAL CARUNCLE REMOVAL

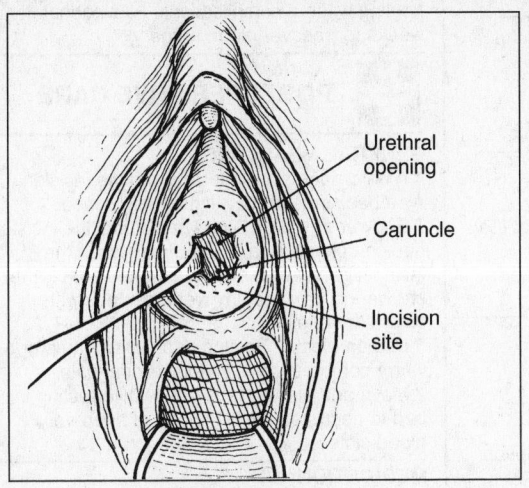

View of the vagina, held open with a speculum, showing the caruncle to be removed and the usual incision site.

Urethral opening

Caruncle

Incision site

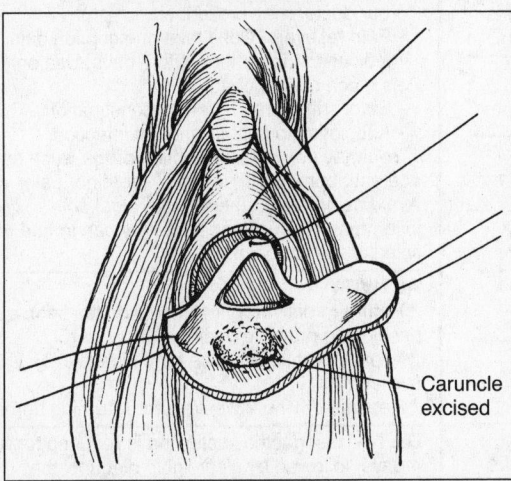

Caruncle is removed with electrocauterization or by cutting with a scalpel.

Caruncle excised

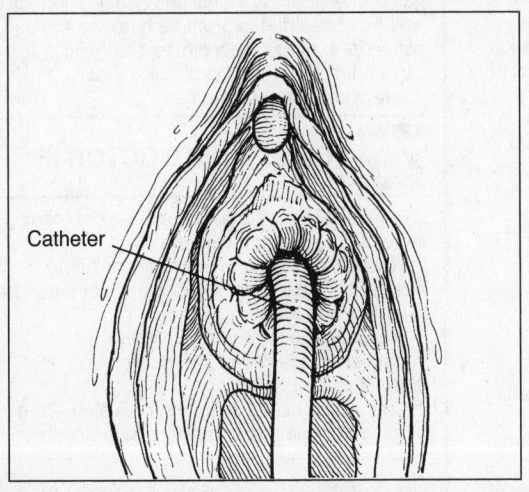

After repair, a catheter may be left inside the bladder until healing begins.

Catheter

VAGOTOMY

GENERAL INFORMATION

DEFINITION—Disconnecting branches of the vagus nerve to slow acid production in the stomach. Usually, this surgery is performed before other surgeries such as gastroenterostomy (see in Surgery section).

BODY PARTS INVOLVED—Stomach; branches of the vagus nerve.

REASONS FOR SURGERY—Treatment of the complications of peptic ulcers such as: obstruction of digestive flow; ulcer perforation; bleeding of an ulcer; or intolerable pain.

SURGICAL RISK INCREASES WITH
* Obesity or smoking.
* Poor nutrition.
* Recent or chronic illness.
* Diabetes.
* Use of some prescription and nonprescription drugs. Inform your doctor of any drugs, medications, or vitamin and herb supplements you are using or have used in the last month.

WHAT TO EXPECT

WHO OPERATES—General surgeon.

WHERE PERFORMED—Hospital.

DIAGNOSTIC TESTS
* Before surgery: Blood and urine studies; x-rays of gastrointestinal tract; gastroscopy; gastroduodenoscopy; ECG (see Glossary).
* After surgery: Blood studies; tissue studies.

ANESTHESIA—General anesthesia by injection and inhalation with an airway tube placed in the windpipe.

DESCRIPTION OF OPERATION
* An incision is made in the abdomen, and the abdominal muscles are separated.
* The vagus nerve is identified, and the branches that control stomach-acid production are isolated, divided and clipped. Segments of the vagus nerve are removed for laboratory study.
* The abdominal muscles are sewn together in layers. The skin is closed with sutures or clips, which usually can be removed about 7 to 10 days after surgery.

POSSIBLE COMPLICATIONS
* Excessive bleeding.
* Surgical-wound infection.
* Incisional hernia.
* Dumping syndrome.
* Diarrhea.
* A sensation of flushing or fainting after eating some foods.
* Recurrent ulcer due to incomplete vagotomy.

AVERAGE HOSPITAL STAY—3 to 5 days.

PROBABLE OUTCOME—Expect complete healing without complications. Allow about 6 weeks for recovery from surgery.

POSTOPERATIVE CARE

GENERAL MEASURES
* A hard ridge should form along the incision. As it heals, the ridge will gradually recede.
* Shower as usual. Avoid baths until the incision has completely healed. You may wash the incision gently with mild, unscented soap. After showering, replace any wet dressings with clean, dry ones.
* Use an electric heating pad, a heat lamp or a warm compress to relieve incisional pain.
* Move and elevate legs often while resting in bed to decrease the likelihood of deep-vein blood clots.

MEDICATION
* Your doctor may prescribe:
  - Pain relievers. Don't take prescription pain medication longer than 4 to 7 days. Use only as much as you need.
  - Stool softeners to prevent constipation.
  - Antibiotics to fight or prevent infection.
* You may use nonprescription drugs, such as acetaminophen and antacids, for minor pain. Avoid aspirin and other nonsteroidal anti-inflammatory drugs because they can irritate the lining of the stomach.

ACTIVITY
* Return to daily activities and work as soon as possible to promote healing.
* Avoid vigorous exercise for 6 weeks after surgery.
* Resume driving 2 weeks after returning home.

DIET—Nasogastric suctioning is required for 3-4 days, followed by clear liquid diet until the gastrointestinal tract functions again. Then eat a well-balanced diet to promote healing. Avoid coffee, tea, cocoa, cola drinks, alcoholic beverages and any food or spice that aggravates ulcer symptoms.

CALL YOUR DOCTOR IF

* Pain, swelling, redness, drainage or bleeding increases in the surgical area.
* You develop signs of infection, including headache, muscle aches, dizziness or a general ill feeling and fever.
* You experience nausea, vomiting, constipation, diarrhea, black tarry stools or abdominal swelling.
* New, unexplained symptoms develop. Drugs used in treatment may produce side effects.

VAGOTOMY

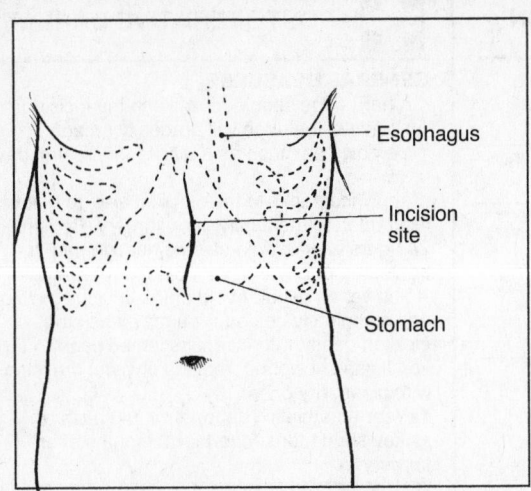

An illustration of the esophagus, stomach, rib cage and a typical incision site.

Esophagus

Incision site

Stomach

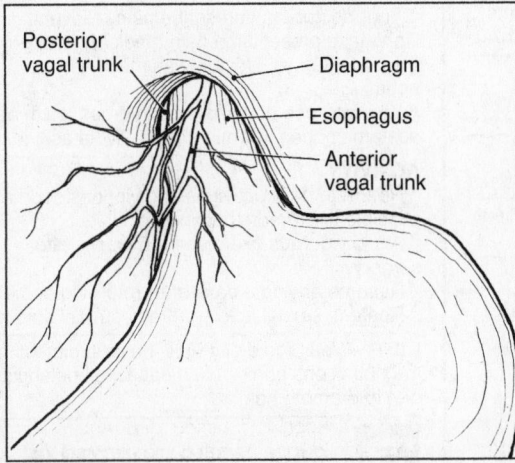

The vagas nerve is identified.

Posterior vagal trunk

Diaphragm

Esophagus

Anterior vagal trunk

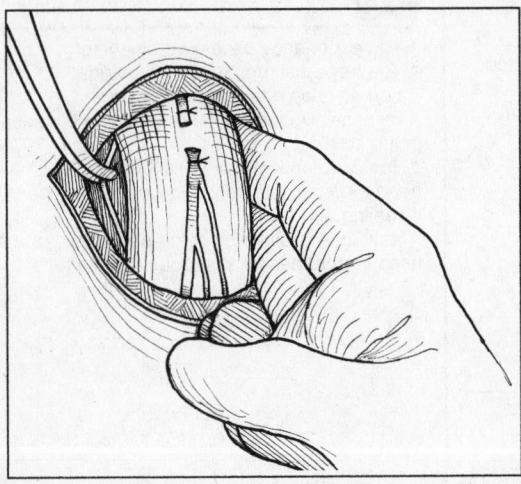

The abdominal muscles that were opened to gain access to the vagas nerve are repaired in layers.
- The branches that control stomach acid production are isolated, divided and clipped.
- The overlying muscles and skin are repaired with sutures or clips (not illustrated).

SURGERIES

VARICOCELE REMOVAL
(Varicocelectomy)

GENERAL INFORMATION

DEFINITION—Removal of a varicocele, a swelling in the scrotum caused by veins that have become distended and twisted.

BODY PARTS INVOLVED—Scrotum and its contents (usually the left testis); varicocele.

REASONS FOR SURGERY
* Relief of discomfort in the scrotum.
* Reduced congestion of the venous system around the testicles.
* Improved quality and quantity of sperm production (sometimes).

SURGICAL RISK INCREASES WITH
* Recent or chronic illness.
* Obesity.
* Diabetes.
* Use of some prescription and nonprescription drugs. Inform your doctor of any drugs, medications, or vitamin and herb supplements you are using or have used in the last month.

WHAT TO EXPECT

WHO OPERATES—General surgeon or urologist.

WHERE PERFORMED—Hospital or outpatient surgical facility.

DIAGNOSTIC TESTS
* Before surgery: Blood and urine studies; ultrasound (see Glossary).
* After surgery: Blood studies.

ANESTHESIA
* Local anesthesia by injection.
* Spinal anesthesia by injection.

DESCRIPTION OF OPERATION
* An incision is made in the scrotum.
* The spermatic cord is identified.
* Abnormal veins are cut and tied. The twisted, dilated vein or veins that form the varicocele are cut free and removed. The artery and normal-appearing veins are protected.
* The skin is closed with sutures that will be absorbed by the body.
* A snug bandage is placed over the incision.

POSSIBLE COMPLICATIONS
* Excessive bleeding.
* Surgical-wound infection.
* Difficulty with urination.
* Inadvertent injury to the spermatic cord.

AVERAGE HOSPITAL STAY—0 to 1 day.

PROBABLE OUTCOME—Expect complete healing without complications. Allow about 1 week for recovery from surgery.

POSTOPERATIVE CARE

GENERAL MEASURES
* A hard ridge should form along the incision. As it heals, the ridge will gradually recede.
* Lie down as much as possible for the first day or two.
* Apply ice packs to the surgical area to relieve discomfort immediately after surgery. Beginning 24 hours later use an electric heating pad, a heat lamp or a warm compress to relieve pain.
* Shower as usual. Avoid baths until the incision has completely healed. You may wash the incision gently with mild, unscented soap. After you finish showering, replace any wet dressings with clean, dry ones.
* Wear an athletic supporter or two pairs of jockey shorts for support for 2 months after surgery.

MEDICATION
* Your doctor may prescribe pain relievers. Don't take prescription pain medication longer than 4 to 7 days. Use only as much as you need.
* You may use nonprescription drugs, such as acetaminophen, for minor pain. Avoid aspirin.

ACTIVITY
* Return to daily activities and work as soon as possible to promote healing.
* Avoid vigorous exercise for 6 weeks after surgery.
* Resume driving 3 days after returning home.
* Resume sexual activity when you feel able to.

DIET—Clear liquid diet until the gastrointestinal tract functions again. Then eat a well-balanced diet to promote healing.

CALL YOUR DOCTOR IF

* You experience excessive bleeding.
* You have discomfort with urination.
* You develop nausea or vomiting.
* Pain, swelling, redness or drainage increases in the surgical area.
* You develop signs of infection, including headache, muscle aches, dizziness or a general ill feeling and fever.
* New, unexplained symptoms develop. Drugs used in treatment may produce side effects.

VARICOCELE REMOVAL
(Varicocelectomy)

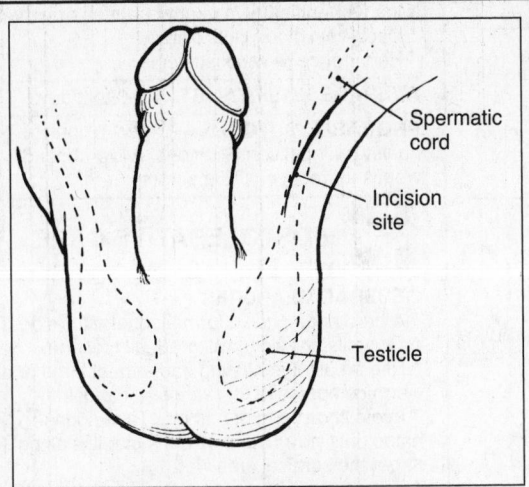

An illustration of the penis, scrotum, spermatic cord, testicle and a typical incision site.

Spermatic cord

Incision site

Testicle

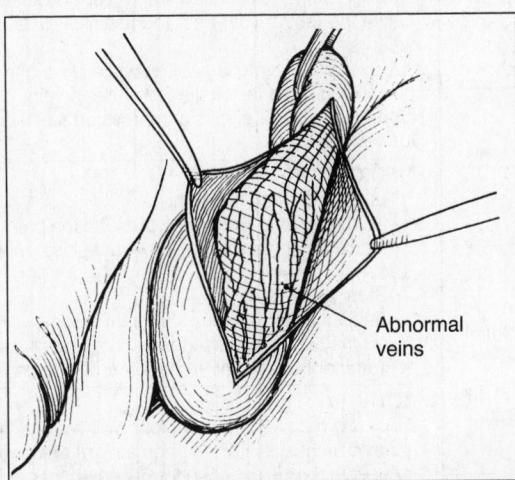

The open cord revealing the abnormal veins.

Abnormal veins

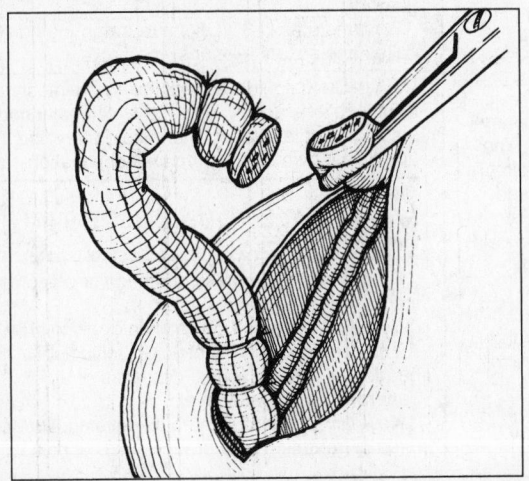

Abnormal veins are cut and tied. The twisted, dilated vein or veins that form the varicocele are cut free and removed.
  • The skin is closed with sutures that will be absorbed by the body (not illustrated).

SURGERIES

VARICOSE VEIN REMOVAL

GENERAL INFORMATION

DEFINITION—Removal of varicose veins, which are veins in the leg that have become abnormally swollen or dilated.

BODY PARTS INVOLVED—Diseased veins in the legs, usually in the greater and lesser saphenous veins.

REASONS FOR SURGERY
* Improvement of appearance.
* Relief of pain or pressure symptoms.
* Treatment of recurrent superficial phlebitis (see Glossary).
* Help heal venous statis ulcers (see Glossary).

SURGICAL RISK INCREASES WITH
* Obesity; smoking; poor nutrition.
* Excess alcohol consumption.
* Adults over 60.
* History of phlebitis (blood clots); diabetes.
* Use of some prescription and nonprescription drugs. Inform your doctor of any drugs, medications, or vitamin and herb supplements you are using or have used in the last month.

WHAT TO EXPECT

WHO OPERATES—Vascular or general surgeon; plastic surgeon.

WHERE PERFORMED—Outpatient surgical facility or hospital.

DIAGNOSTIC TESTS
* Before surgery: Blood and urine studies; chest x-ray; ultrasound; ECG; doppler venous studies (see Glossary for all).
* After surgery: Blood studies.

ANESTHESIA
* Local anesthesia by injection.
* Spinal anesthesia by injection.
* General anesthesia by injection and inhalation with an airway tube placed in the windpipe.

DESCRIPTION OF OPERATION
* An incision is made over the top of the saphenous-femoral vein system (see Glossary).
* The large, diseased veins are identified. The upper and lower ends of each diseased vein are cut and tied. A thin wire instrument is passed through the vein, beginning at the ankle and extending upward through the inside of the vein; the wire is used to strip (remove) the entire vein.
* After the main veins have been removed, smaller veins are identified; incisions are made and the smaller veins are tied individually and removed.
* The skin is closed with sutures, which usually can be removed about 1 week after surgery.
* The legs are wrapped snugly in elastic bandages.

POSSIBLE COMPLICATIONS
* Excessive bleeding; surgical-wound infection.
* Inadvertent injury to nearby arteries or nerves.
* Deep-vein blood clots (rare).
* Recurrence of varicose veins.

AVERAGE HOSPITAL STAY—0 to 2 days.

PROBABLE OUTCOME—Expect complete healing without complications. Allow about 6 weeks for recovery from surgery.

POSTOPERATIVE CARE

GENERAL MEASURES
* A hard ridge should form along the incision. As it heals, the ridge will gradually recede.
* Use an electric heating pad, a heat lamp or a warm compress to relieve incisional pain.
* Avoid showering or bathing. Take sponge baths until your doctor advises that it is all right to get the surgical area wet.
* Keep your legs elevated whenever possible. Raise the foot of your bed and use foot rests when sitting.
* Move and elevate legs often while resting in bed to decrease the likelihood of deep-vein blood clots. Wear elastic compression stockings for 4-6 weeks.

MEDICATION
* Your doctor may prescribe:
  - Pain relievers. Don't take prescription pain medication longer than 4 to 7 days. Use only as much as you need.
  - Stool softener laxatives.
  - Antibiotics to fight or prevent infection.
* You may use nonprescription drugs, such as acetaminophen, for minor pain. Avoid aspirin.

ACTIVITY
* To help recovery and aid your well-being, resume daily activities as soon as you are able.
* Avoid vigorous exercise for 6 weeks after surgery.
* Resume driving 3 weeks after returning home.
* Resume sexual relations when able.

DIET—Clear liquid diet until the gastrointestinal tract functions again. Then eat a well-balanced diet to promote healing. Increase dietary fiber and fluid intake to help prevent constipation.

CALL YOUR DOCTOR IF

* Pain, swelling, redness, drainage or bleeding increases in the surgical area.
* Your foot becomes cold, numb or discolored.
* You develop signs of infection, including headache, muscle aches, dizziness or a general ill feeling and fever.
* New, unexplained symptoms develop. Drugs used in treatment may produce side effects.

VARICOSE VEIN REMOVAL

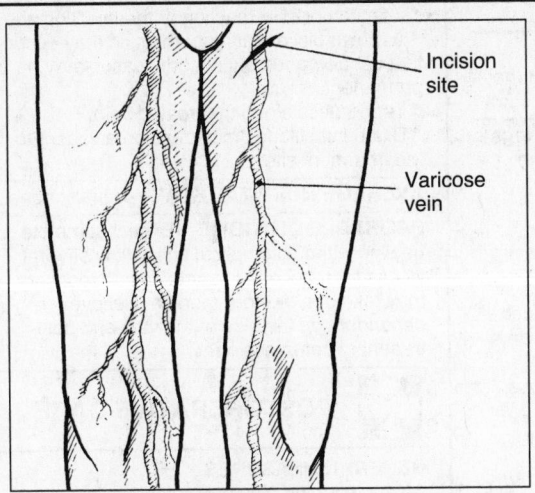

Incision site

Varicose vein

An illustration of diseased veins in the legs, usually the greater and lesser saphenous veins.

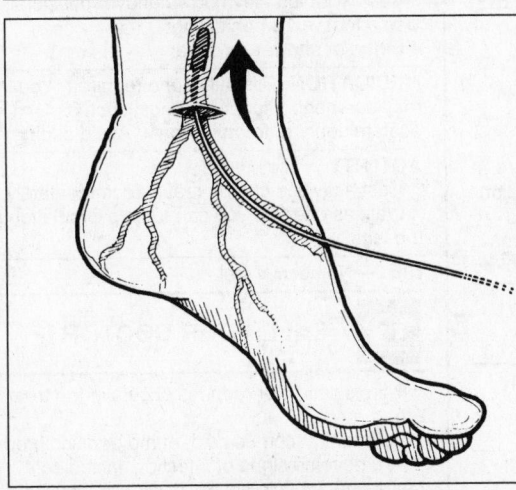

The large diseased veins are identified.
- The upper and lower ends of each diseased vein are cut and tied and a thin wire instrument is passed through the inside of the vein; the wire is used to strip (remove) the entire vein (see lower illustration).

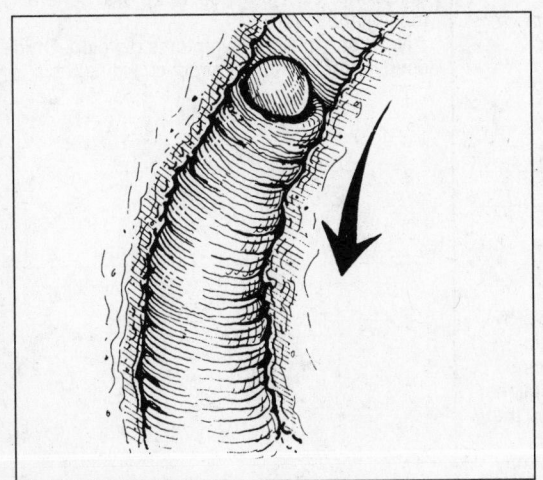

- After the main veins have been removed, smaller veins are identified, incisions are made into the skin and smaller veins are tied individually and removed.
- After surgery, the legs are wrapped snugly in elastic bandages.

VARICOSE VEIN SCLEROTHERAPY

 ## GENERAL INFORMATION

DEFINITION—Use of a special injected chemical solution to collapse veins so that they no longer carry blood.

BODY PARTS INVOLVED—Veins in the legs, usually on the backs of the calves or on the insides of the leg. Spider veins (superficial, small veins in skin) usually form a linear, discrete or grouped pattern.

REASONS FOR SURGERY
• To relieve symptoms of varicose veins (swelling, distortion or twisting of a vein) such as pain, aching, fatigue or swelling of feet and ankles.
• As a follow-up treatment following varicose vein removal (see in Surgery section).
• As an early treatment to prevent the development of larger varicose veins.
• To improve cosmetic appearance of the legs.

SURGICAL RISK INCREASES WITH
• Obesity; smoking.
• Excess alcohol consumption.
• Adults over 60.
• History of thrombophlebitis, deep-vein thrombosis or pulmonary embolism.
• Diabetes.
• Use of some prescription and nonprescription drugs. Inform your doctor of any drugs, medications, or vitamin and herb supplements you are using or have used in the last month.

 ## WHAT TO EXPECT

WHO OPERATES—General surgeon, family doctor, dermatologist, vascular surgeon or plastic surgeon.

WHERE PERFORMED—Outpatient surgical facility, doctor's office.

DIAGNOSTIC TESTS
• Before surgery: Normally a physical examination is sufficient, but your doctor may perform a tourniquet test to evaluate the problem or special x-rays (venography).
• After surgery: None expected.

ANESTHESIA—None required.

DESCRIPTION OF OPERATION
• A special solution (called a sclerosant) is injected into the vein or veins. This causes inflammation in the lining of the vein, and eventual fibrosis (scar tissue formation), which leads to the vein's obliteration. The blood is forced to reroute itself through healthier veins. Complete treatment may take several injections.
• After injection, firm pressure is applied so that the walls of the vein are pressed together.
• In some cases, a compression bandage may be required.

POSSIBLE COMPLICATIONS
• Varicose veins may recur.
• Infection or skin reaction at the injection site.
• A brown discoloration of the skin may occur that usually fades but in some cases may be permanent.
• Tenderness along the treated vein.
• Dilated capillaries may develop adjacent to the treatment site.

AVERAGE HOSPITAL STAY—Usually none.

PROBABLE OUTCOME—Expect complete healing without complications. Allow several weeks for recovery; in some cases, recovery may take one or more months. Recovery is dependent on the size of the vein and post-treatment compression.

 ## POSTOPERATIVE CARE

GENERAL MEASURES
• Keep your leg elevated whenever possible. Use a foot rest when sitting.
• Bathe or shower as usual.

MEDICATION—Usually none required. You may use nonprescription drugs, such as acetaminophen, for minor pain. Avoid aspirin.

ACTIVITY
• Most activities can be resumed immediately.
• Walk as often as you can to help circulation in the legs.

DIET—No special diet.

 ## CALL YOUR DOCTOR IF

• Pain, swelling or redness occurs in the treated area.
• Your foot becomes cold, numb or discolored.
• You develop signs of infection, including headache, muscle aches, dizziness, general ill feeling and fever.
• New, unexplained symptoms develop. Drugs used in treatment may produce side effects.

VARICOSE VEIN SCLEROTHERAPY

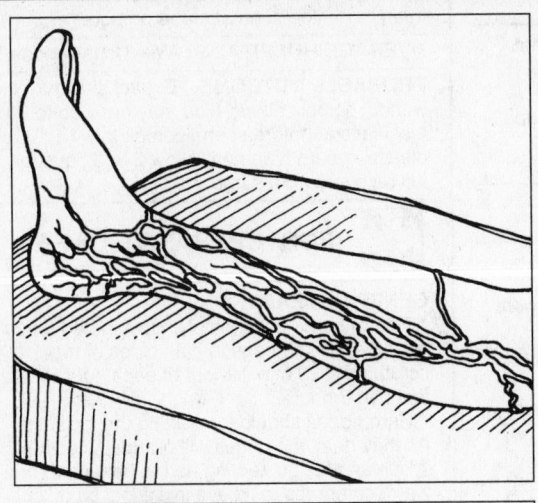

Leg is prepared and positioned for treatment.

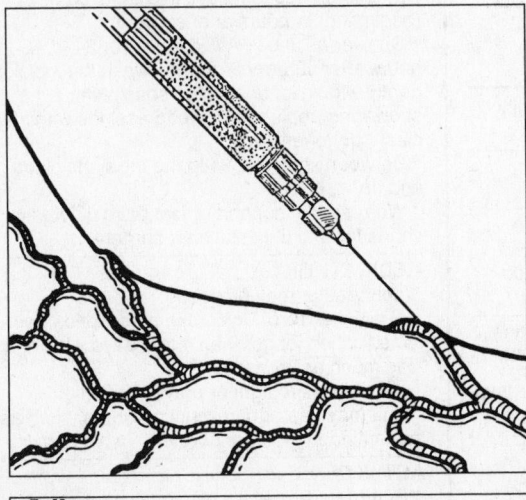

A special solution is injected into a vein.

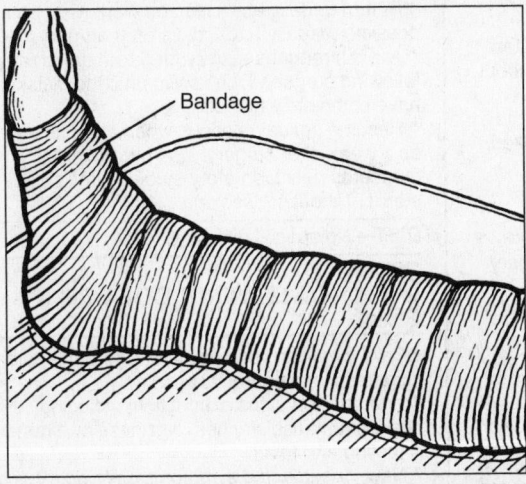

Bandage

In severe cases, a compression bandage may be required.

SURGERIES

VASECTOMY

GENERAL INFORMATION

DEFINITION—A method of sterilization that involves cutting and tying the vas deferens (sperm channels inside the scrotum). The surgery stops the flow of sperm and provides a safe, effective form of birth control without affecting sexual desire or ability.

BODY PARTS INVOLVED—Scrotum; vas deferens.

REASONS FOR SURGERY
• Voluntary sterilization.
• Recurrent epididymitis (see Glossary) when caused by chronic prostate infection.

SURGICAL RISK INCREASES WITH
• Recent or chronic illness; diabetes.
• Use of some prescription and nonprescription drugs. Inform your doctor of any drugs, medications, or vitamin and herb supplements you are using or have used in the last month.

WHAT TO EXPECT

WHO OPERATES—General surgeon, family doctor, or urologist.

WHERE PERFORMED—Doctor's office, outpatient surgical facility or hospital.

DIAGNOSTIC TESTS
• Before surgery: None required.
• After surgery: Sperm studies, at least twice during 10 weeks after surgery.

ANESTHESIA—Local anesthesia by injection.

DESCRIPTION OF OPERATION
• The scrotum is shaved at home before surgery.
• Incisions are made on both sides of the scrotum. The vas deferens is identified, tied in two places and cut between the ties.
• The divided vas deferens is returned to the scrotum.
• The edges of incised skin are reconstructed with fine sutures, which usually fall out in about 7 days.
• Another method for vasectomy is called the no-scalpel technique. It requires 2 specialized instruments and avoids the usual surgical incisions. It requires no sutures to close the surgical site, and may result in fewer complications. Some men may not be appropriate candidates for this type of surgery because of differences in scrotal anatomy.

POSSIBLE COMPLICATIONS
• Collection of blood in scrotum.
• Excessive bleeding; surgical-wound infection.
• Epididymitis (see Glossary).
• Sperm granuloma (benign lump in the surgical area).
• Small possibility of re-establishing fertility.

• Pregnancy may still occur in about 1% of cases (often as a result of unprotected intercourse too soon after the procedure).

AVERAGE HOSPITAL STAY—Usually none.

PROBABLE OUTCOME—Expect sterility without complications. You may have up to 30 ejaculations before sperm completely disappears from semen. Allow 2 to 3 days for full recovery from surgery.

POSTOPERATIVE CARE

GENERAL MEASURES
• Return home immediately. Rest in bed for 24 hours. Apply ice bags to both sides of the scrotum for 20 minutes out of each hour for the first 6 to 8 hours.
• Hard ridges should form along the incisions. As they heal, the ridges will gradually recede.
• Use an electric heating pad, a heat lamp or a warm compress to relieve incisional pain (beginning 24 hours after surgery).
• Shower as usual. Avoid baths for 24 to 48 hours after surgery. You may wash the incisions gently with mild, unscented soap. After showering, replace any wet dressings with clean, dry ones.
• Between showers, keep the incisions clean and dry.
• Wear scrotal support or two pairs of jockey shorts for 4 to 6 weeks after surgery.

MEDICATION
• Your doctor may prescribe:
  - Pain relievers. Don't take prescription pain medication longer than 4 to 7 days. Use only as much as you need.
  - Antibiotics to fight or prevent infection.
• You may use nonprescription drugs, such as acetaminophen, for minor pain. Avoid aspirin.

ACTIVITY
• Return to daily activities and work as soon as possible (usually 2 to 3 days after surgery).
• Avoid strenuous activity for 5 to 7 days following surgery. Don't swim until the incisions have completely healed.
• Resume sexual relations when able, as soon as 1 week after surgery. Use birth-control measures until laboratory studies confirm sterility (about 12 weeks).

DIET—No special diet.

CALL YOUR DOCTOR IF

• Pain, swelling, redness, drainage or bleeding increases in the surgical area.
• You develop signs of infection, including headache, muscle aches, dizziness or a general ill feeling and fever.
• New, unexplained symptoms develop.

VASECTOMY

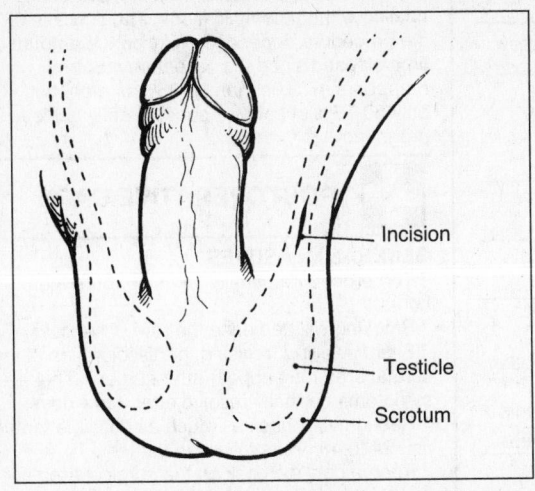

The penis, scrotum and testicles showing a typical incision site for a vasectomy.

Incision

Testicle

Scrotum

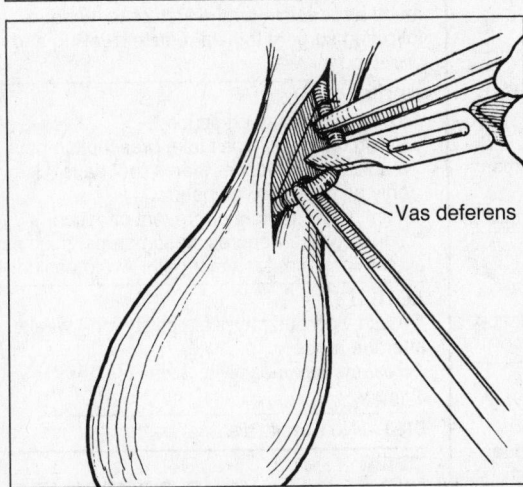

The vas deferens is identified, tied in 2 places and cut between the ties.

Vas deferens

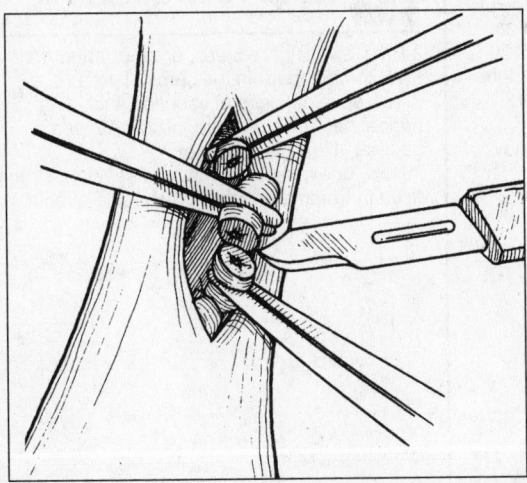

The divided vas deferens is returned to the scrotum and the edges of incised skin are reconstructed with fine sutures that usually fall out in about 7 days (not illustrated).

SURGERIES

VASECTOMY REVERSAL

GENERAL INFORMATION

DEFINITION—A procedure to restore the flow of sperm through the vas deferens (the tubes that carry the sperm from the testicle to the urethra). There are two types of vasectomy reversal: a vasovasostomy and a vasoepididymostomy.

BODY PARTS INVOLVED—Scrotum; vas deferens.

REASONS FOR SURGERY—Restores male reproduction ability (fertility).

SURGICAL RISK INCREASES WITH
• Diabetes.
• Use of some prescription and nonprescription drugs. Inform your doctor of any drugs, medications, or vitamin and herb supplements you are using or have used in the last month.

WHAT TO EXPECT

WHO OPERATES—Urologist.

WHERE PERFORMED—Doctor's office, outpatient surgical facility, or a hospital.

DIAGNOSTIC TESTS—Usually none. For men over 40, an ECG (see Glossary) may be performed.

ANESTHESIA
• Local anesthesia by injection.
• Regional anesthesia by injection.
• General anesthesia by injection and inhalation with an airway tube placed in the windpipe.

DESCRIPTION OF OPERATION
• The area around the scrotum is anesthetized.
• The previously cut ends of the vas deferens are located and trimmed back to normal tissue.
• The ends are then sewn back together with very fine sutures.
• When too much scarring or inflammation has occurred in the epididymis, sperm can be blocked from getting to the vas deferens. If this blockage has occurred, connecting the two ends of the vas deferens will not prove successful, and bypassing the blockage via a vasoepididymostomy must be performed.
• A vasoepididymostomy is performed by connecting the vas deferens directly to the epididymis.

POSSIBLE COMPLICATIONS
• Infection.
• Scrotal hematoma (black and blue bruised scrotum).
• Scarring where the ends are connected, causing continued blockage.
• Epididymitis (see Glossary).
• Urinary retention.

AVERAGE HOSPITAL STAY—0 to 1 day.

PROBABLE OUTCOME—Expect complete healing without complications. The success of the procedure depends largely on the amount of time elapsed since the vasectomy. Sperm reappears in more than 80-95% of men, but only 50-75% of couples subsequently achieve pregnancy.

POSTOPERATIVE CARE

GENERAL MEASURES
• The procedure usually takes no more than 5 hours.
• Smoking will decrease the rate of success.
• Slight swelling, bruising, or discoloration of the scrotal area may appear after surgery. These symptoms normally resolve after a few days.
• Rest on your back as much as possible for the first 24 to 48 hours following surgery.
• Keep a cold ice pack on the surgical area as much as possible for the first 24 to 48 hours following surgery to help reduce swelling and bruising.

MEDICATION
• Your doctor may prescribe:
  - Pain relievers. Don't take prescription pain medication for longer than 4 to 7 days. Use only as much as you need.
  - Antibiotics to fight or prevent infection.
• You may use nonprescription drugs, such as acetaminophen, for minor pain. Avoid aspirin.

ACTIVITY
• Avoid vigorous physical activity for 4 weeks after the surgery.
• Resume sexual activity 3 weeks after the surgery.

DIET—No special diet.

CALL YOUR DOCTOR IF

• Pain, swelling, redness, or other abnormal symptoms appear in the surgical area.
• You develop signs of infection, including headache, muscle aches, dizziness, or a general ill feeling and fever.
• New, unexplained symptoms develop. Drugs used in treatment may produce side effects.

VASECTOMY REVERSAL

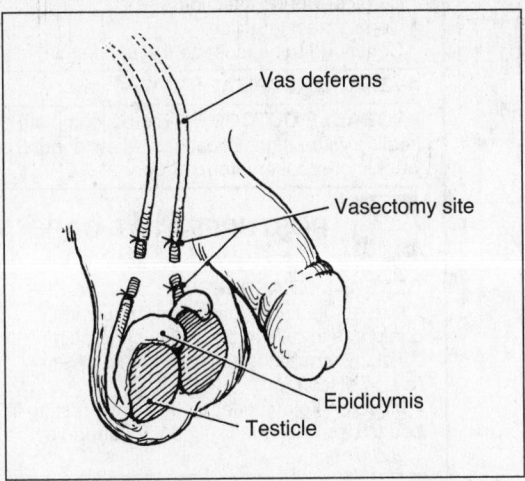

Vas deferens

Vasectomy site

Epididymis

Testicle

An illustration showing the site of a previous vasectomy. The vas deferens has previously been cut and tied to prevent the flow of sperm from the testicles to the urethra.

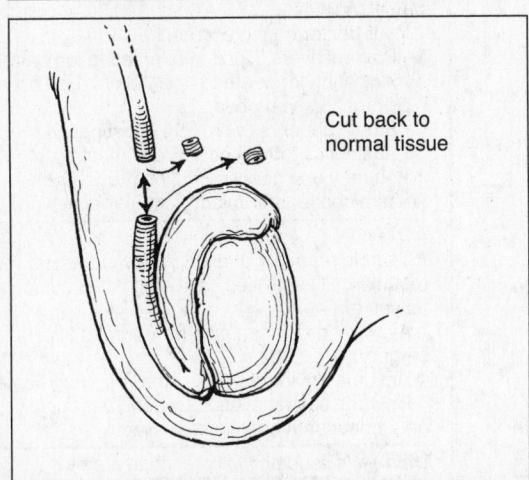

Cut back to normal tissue

The previously cut ends of the vas deferens have been located and trimmed back to reveal normal tissue.

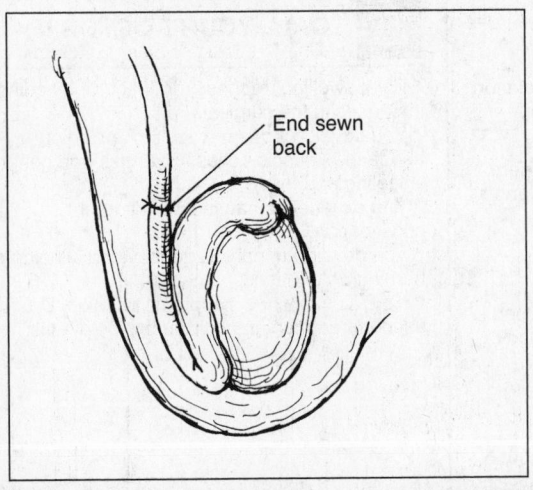

End sewn back

The ends are sewn back together with very fine sutures.

SURGERIES

VESICOVAGINAL FISTULA REPAIR

 GENERAL INFORMATION

DEFINITION—Repair of a vesicovaginal fistula, an abnormal tract between the bladder and the vagina that usually results from tearing in childbirth, as a complication of cervical uterine surgery (e.g., vaginal hysterectomy), or as a complication of cervical cancer (particularly when radiation therapy is used).

BODY PARTS INVOLVED—Vagina and bladder.

REASONS FOR SURGERY
* Control of urine flow from the bladder.
* Prevention of vaginal and urinary tract infections.

SURGICAL RISK INCREASES WITH
* Adults over 60.
* Obesity or smoking.
* Poor nutrition.
* Recent or chronic illness.
* Alcoholism.
* Previous pelvic surgery.
* Diabetes.
* Use of some prescription and nonprescription drugs. Inform your doctor of any drugs, medications, or vitamin and herb supplements you are using or have used in the last month.

 WHAT TO EXPECT

WHO OPERATES—Obstetrician-gynecologist, urologist or general surgeon.

WHERE PERFORMED—Hospital.

DIAGNOSTIC TESTS
* Before surgery: Blood and urine studies; pelvic exam; cystoscopy (see Glossary) with biopsy (sometimes).
* After surgery: Blood studies; laboratory examination of removed tissue.

ANESTHESIA
* Spinal anesthesia by injection.
* General anesthesia by injection and inhalation with an airway tube placed in the windpipe.

DESCRIPTION OF OPERATION
* A speculum is used to hold the vagina open.
* Scar tissue around the fistula is cut free and removed; this tissue is often sent to the laboratory for examination.
* Healthy tissue is interposed between the 2 layers of the fistula.
* The bladder wall and vaginal wall are closed with sutures that will be absorbed by the body.
* The bladder is filled with sterile water to search for leaks. If leaks exist, further repairs are made. If no leaks are found, a catheter is placed in the bladder.
* The catheter usually can be removed about 5 to 7 days after surgery.

POSSIBLE COMPLICATIONS
* Excessive bleeding.
* Surgical-wound infection.
* Urinary tract infection.
* Continued urine leakage through fistula.

AVERAGE HOSPITAL STAY—6 days.

PROBABLE OUTCOME—Expect complete healing without complications. Allow about 6 weeks for recovery from surgery.

 POSTOPERATIVE CARE

GENERAL MEASURES
* Use an electric heating pad, or a warm compress to relieve surgical-wound pain.
* Take warm baths several times a day to relieve discomfort.
* Move and elevate legs often while resting in bed to decrease the likelihood of deep-vein blood clots.

MEDICATION
* Your doctor may prescribe:
  - Pain relievers. Don't take prescription pain medication longer than 4 to 7 days. Use only as much as you need.
  - Stool softeners to prevent constipation.
  - Antibiotics to fight or prevent infection.
* You may use nonprescription drugs, such as acetaminophen, for minor pain. Avoid aspirin.

ACTIVITY
* To help recovery and aid your well-being, resume daily activities, including work, as soon as you are able.
* Avoid vigorous exercise for 6 weeks after surgery.
* Resume driving 3 weeks after returning home.
* Resume sexual relations when your doctor determines that healing is complete.

DIET—Your doctor will prescribe a diet.

 CALL YOUR DOCTOR IF

* Pain, swelling, redness, drainage or bleeding increases in the surgical area.
* You develop signs of infection, including headache, muscle aches, dizziness or a general ill feeling and fever.
* You experience nausea, vomiting or constipation.
* You develop urinary frequency and stinging or burning on urination.
* New, unexplained symptoms develop. Drugs used in treatment may produce side effects.

VESICOVAGINAL FISTULA REPAIR

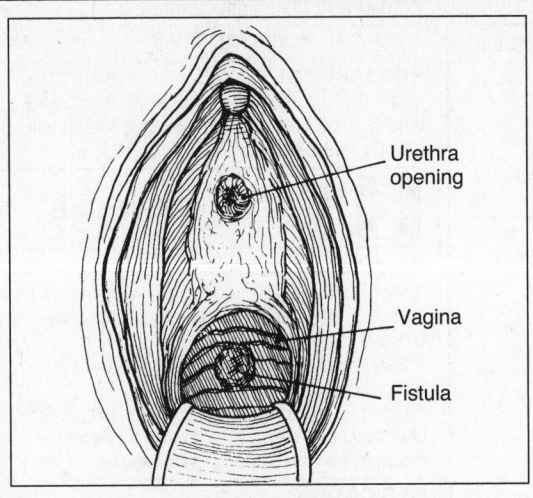

The vagina with a retractor in place to expose the fistula, an abnormal tract between the bladder and the vagina that usually results from tearing in childbirth, as a complication of cervical uterine surgery (e.g., vaginal hysterectomy), or as a complication of cervical cancer (particularly when radiation therapy is used).

Urethra opening

Vagina

Fistula

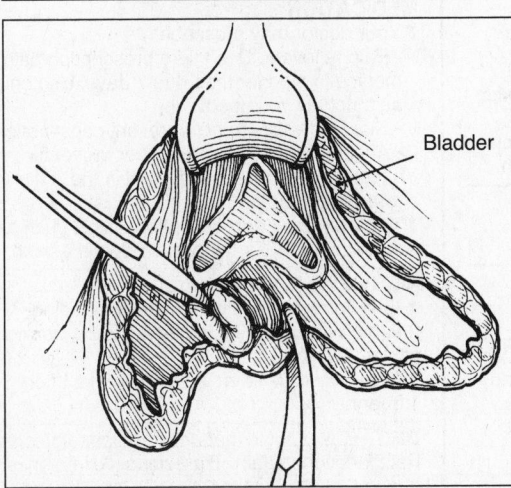

Scar tissue around the fistula is cut free and removed. Healthy tissue is interposed between the 2 layers of the fistula.
• The bladder wall and vaginal wall are both closed with absorbable sutures.

Bladder

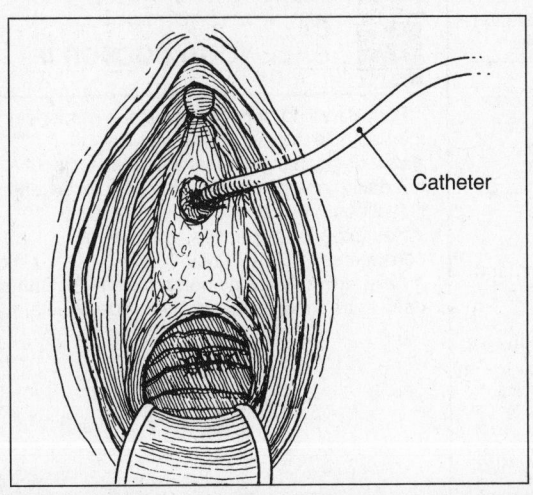

The bladder is filled with sterile water to search for leaks. If leaks exist, further repairs are made. If no leaks are found, a catheter is placed in the bladder and the opening closed with sutures.

Catheter

VITRECTOMY

GENERAL INFORMATION

DEFINITION—Removal of fluid from the eyeball that has clouded and blocked light from reaching the retina, causing loss of vision. A chemical solution is injected to replace the removed fluid.

BODY PARTS INVOLVED—Eye and all its parts.

REASONS FOR SURGERY—Restoration of normal vision or prevention of continued vision loss resulting from disease that blocks light from reaching the retina. These include: bleeding, injury or infection inside the eyeball; diabetes; sickle-cell disease; complications of cataract surgery; or glaucoma.

SURGICAL RISK INCREASES WITH
- Adults over 60.
- Obesity or smoking.
- Poor nutrition.
- Recent or chronic illness.
- Alcoholism.
- Diabetes.
- Use of some prescription and nonprescription drugs. Inform your doctor of any drugs, medications, or vitamin and herb supplements you are using or have used in the last month.

WHAT TO EXPECT

WHO OPERATES—Ophthalmologist.

WHERE PERFORMED—Hospital.

DIAGNOSTIC TESTS
- Before surgery: Eye examination; blood and urine studies.
- After surgery: Eye examination.

ANESTHESIA
- Local anesthesia by injection.
- General anesthesia by injection and inhalation with an airway tube placed in the windpipe.

DESCRIPTION OF OPERATION
- A small instrument is inserted behind the cornea. The instrument is used to cut free and remove the clouded vitreous fluid and scar tissue.
- This surgery often causes a retinal detachment. Usually this is corrected by injecting gas into the vitreous cavity.
- A chemical solution that promotes healing and stimulates normal vitreous fluid production is injected.
- If sutures are needed to close the surgical wound, they will be absorbed by the body.

POSSIBLE COMPLICATIONS
- Surgical-wound infection in the eye.
- Recurrent retinal detachment.

AVERAGE HOSPITAL STAY—Usually none.

PROBABLE OUTCOME—Expect complete healing without complications. Allow about 6 weeks for recovery from surgery. Vision will greatly improve by then.

POSTOPERATIVE CARE

GENERAL MEASURES
- Move and elevate legs often while resting in bed to decrease the likelihood of deep-vein blood clots.
- Use warm compresses over the eyes to relieve discomfort.
- Don't lift heavy objects, bend over or strain with bowel movements until your doctor determines that healing is complete.

MEDICATION
- Your doctor may prescribe:
  - Pain relievers. Don't take prescription pain medication longer than 4 to 7 days. Use only as much as you need.
  - Stool softeners to help prevent constipation.
  - Antibiotic eye drops to fight or prevent infection. Keep eye drops cold in the refrigerator; do not freeze.
- You may use nonprescription drugs, such as acetaminophen, for minor pain. Avoid aspirin.

ACTIVITY
- To help recovery and aid your well-being, resume daily activities, including work, as soon as you are able.
- Avoid vigorous exercise for 6 weeks after surgery.

DIET—Clear liquid diet until the gastrointestinal tract functions again. Then eat a well-balanced diet to promote healing.

CALL YOUR DOCTOR IF

- Pain, swelling, redness, drainage or bleeding increases in the surgical area.
- You develop signs of infection, including headache, muscle aches, dizziness or a general ill feeling and fever.
- You experience nausea, vomiting or constipation.
- New, unexplained symptoms develop. Drugs used in treatment may produce side effects.

VITRECTOMY

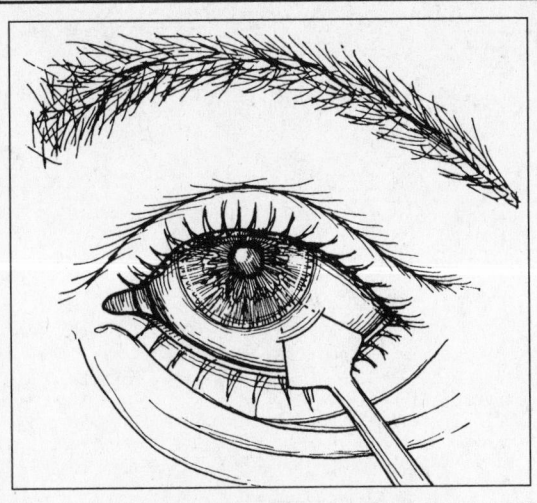

An illustration of the various structures of the eye.

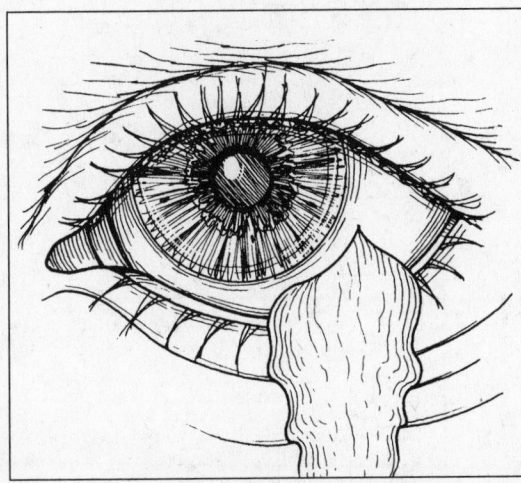

A small instrument is inserted behind the cornea to cut free and remove the clouded vitreous fluid and scar tissue.
- Occasionally gas is injected into the vitreous cavity to help prevent the complication of retinal detachment.

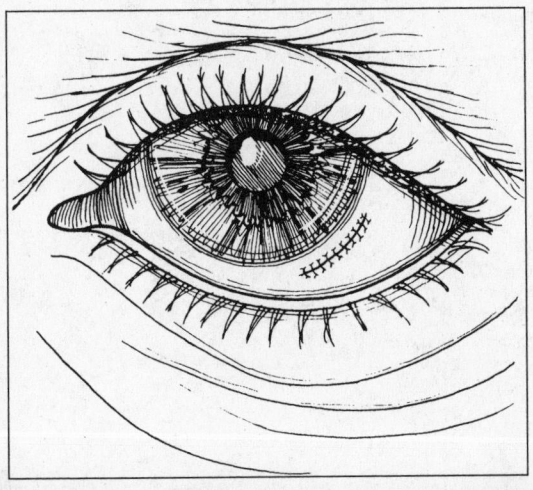

Sutures to close the incision can be removed in 4 to 6 days.

Appendix

DIETS

Adult Diet, Standard
Allergy/Food Sensitivity Diet
Bland Diet
High-Fiber Diet
Lactose Intolerance Diet
Liquid Diet, Clear
Liquid Diet, Full
Low-Fat/Low-Cholesterol Diet
Low-Salt Diet
Weight Loss Diet
Weight Loss Suggestions

GENERAL TOPICS

Breast Self-Examination
Condom Usage
Exercise and Physical Fitness
  Benefits
Immunizations, Childhood
R.I.C.E. Therapy
Safe Use of Medicine
Sexually Transmitted Diseases
Skin Self-Examination
Stress, How to Cope
Testicular Self-Examination

ADULT DIET, STANDARD

The United States Department of Agriculture provides these Dietary Guidelines for the general public to eat more healthfully. (Individuals with a chronic health condition, those who want to lose weight or athletes with special needs should consult a health care provider and/or dietician to determine what type of diet plan is appropriate for them.)

The website, www.mypyramid.gov, will help you choose the foods and amounts that are right for you (one specific diet doesn't fit all individuals) and your activity levels (30 minutes of daily exercise is recommended).

For good health, an individual should:
• Consume a sufficient amount of fruits and vegetables while staying within energy needs.

2 cups of fruit and 2 1/2 cups of vegetables per day are recommended for a typical 2,000-calorie a day intake, with higher or lower amounts depending on the calorie level.

Choose a variety of fruits and vegetables each day. Select from all five vegetable subgroups (dark green, orange, legumes, starchy vegetables, and other vegetables) several times a week.
• Consume 6 ounces of grains a day. In general, at least half the grains should come from whole grains (3 or more ounce-equivalents), and the rest of the grains coming from enriched or whole-grain products.
• Consume 3 cups per day of fat-free or low-fat milk or equivalent milk products (cheese. yogurt).

Food groups to choose from:
• **Grains:** Bread, pasta, oatmeal, breakfast cereals, tortillas, and grits are examples of grain products. Grains are divided into 2 subgroups: Whole grains contain the entire grain kernel—the bran, germ, and endosperm; refined grains have been milled, a process that removes the bran and germ.
• **Milk, Yogurt, Cheese:** All fluid milk products and many foods made from milk are considered part of this food group. Foods made from milk that retain their calcium content are part of the group, while foods made from milk that have little to no calcium, such as cream cheese, cream, and butter, are not. Most milk group choices should be fat-free or low-fat.
• **Vegetables:** Any vegetable or 100% vegetable juice counts as a member of the vegetable group. Vegetables may be raw or cooked; fresh, frozen, canned, or dried/dehydrated; and may be whole, cut-up, or mashed.
• **Fruits:** Fruit or 100% fruit juice counts as part of the fruit group. Fruits may be fresh, canned, frozen, or dried, and may be whole, cut-up, or pureed.
• **Meat, Poultry, Fish, Dry Beans, Peas, Eggs, Nuts:** Most meat and poultry choices should be lean or low-fat. Fish, nuts, and seeds contain healthy oils, so choose these foods frequently instead of meat or poultry. Dry beans and peas are part of this group as well as the vegetable group.
• **Fats and Oils:** Solid fats include butter, stick margarine, shortening, and lard. Oils are fats that are liquid at room temperature, like the vegetable oils used in cooking.
• **Sugar and Salt:** Choose and prepare foods with little added sugars and salt (sodium). Read food labels and avoid products high in sugar and sodium. Limit salt intake to less than 2,300 mg (one teaspoon) daily.

Menu ideas (for someone on a 2,000 calories-per-day diet)

BREAKFAST: 1 1/2 cups oat bran flakes with 4 ounces fat-free milk; a medium-sized banana; drink may be coffee or tea (without any added sugar or cream).
LUNCH: 1 small whole wheat bagel topped with 2 ounces lean turkey breast lunch meat, 2 romaine lettuce leaves, 1 tomato slice and reduced-fat dressing; 10 baby carrots
DINNER: 3 ounces broiled lean beef steak with herbal seasoning; 1 large sweet potato with 2 teaspoons low fat margarine; 1/2 cup cooked broccoli; beverage is 8 ounce glass of fat-free milk
3 SNACKS: 1/2 cup natural applesauce; 1/3 cup almonds
        1 cup nonfat pudding
        1 cup low-fat frozen yogurt; 1 medium-sized peach

BREAKFAST: 1 cup of oatmeal; 1 cup of low-fat yogurt; 1/2 cup of berries; drink may be coffee or tea (without any added sugar or cream).
LUNCH: Fill 2 whole wheat tortillas with 1 ounce cooked chicken breast, 1/4 cup refried beans, 1/4 cup onion and tomato, 2 tablespoons light, shredded cheese, and 1/4 cup romaine lettuce
DINNER: 1 1/2 cups cooked whole wheat pasta; 1/2 cup low fat pasta sauce, 1/2 cup cooked mushrooms, 1/4 cup cooked onions and 2 ounces cooked extra lean ground turkey breast; beverage is 8 ounce glass of fat-free milk.
3 SNACKS: A medium-sized banana
        1/4 cup unsalted peanuts, a medium-sized apple
        6 ounces fat-free yogurt; 1 cup grapes

ALLERGY/FOOD SENSITIVITY DIET
(continued on next page)

The diet is individually tailored to omit those foods that cause an immediate or delayed allergic reaction.

The diet may be recommended once a recognized relationship has been established between a particular food or foods and a symptomatic reaction. Common signs and symptoms of food allergies include skin reactions (itching, erythema, hives, eczema, edema) or reactions of the gastrointestinal tract (vomiting, diarrhea, abdominal pain). Systemic anaphylactic reactions could include sneezing, wheezing, conjunctivitis, palpitations, cardiac arrhythmia, shock, or collapse. Reactions can be immediate, or take up to 72 hours to appear.

This information describes some of the more common food allergies (wheat, eggs, milk, corn). Other common food allergens include: Seafood, nuts, legumes, chocolate, cola, citrus fruit, beef, white potatoes, pork, chicken, oatmeal, rye, mustard, garlic, tomatoes, and cucumbers. The wheat-, egg-, corn-, and milk-free diets commonly use an "elimination" approach to assess potential food allergens and intolerances. Elimination diets must be planned carefully and monitored regularly.

WHEAT SENSITIVITY
Avoid foods containing wheat and wheat products. These include:
- **Milk/Dairy:** Flavored milk drinks: malted milk, chocolate milk, Ovaltine.
- **Meat/Meat Substitutes:** Meat loaf, croquettes; meats, fish, and poultry breaded or prepared with wheat flour; hot dogs, sausage, luncheon meats; canned meat dishes with sauce; casseroles made with wheat-based ingredients.
- **Breads & Grains:** All dry or cooked wheat cereals, wheat germ, wheat bran; graham flour; all commercial breads, crackers, muffins, and biscuits (unless 100% rye), soy, corn, or specifically labeled "wheat free"; French toast, waffles, pancakes; flour tortillas; pasta, except those specifically labeled "wheat free."
- **Fruits & Vegetables:** Breaded, fried vegetables; scalloped tomatoes.
- **Desserts/Sweets:** All commercial cookies, cakes, pies, doughnuts, pastries; commercial pie fillings, custards, puddings thickened with wheat flour; commercial ice cream, ice cream cones; prepared cake and cookie mixes.
- **Beverages:** Coffee substitutes, Postum; flavored instant coffee mixes; instant coffee (unless 100% coffee); beer, gin, whiskey.
- **Miscellaneous:** Pretzels, seasoned potato and corn chips; cream soups; cream-cheese dips, salad dressings (thickened with wheat); commercially prepared baked beans; soy sauce; commercially prepared gravies and sauces (usually thickened with wheat flour).

EGG SENSITIVITY
Avoid all products containing eggs. These include:
- **Milk/Dairy:** Eggnog, Ovaltine, malted milk.
- **Meat/Meat Substitutes:** Meatloaf, meat balls, croquettes; breaded or batter-dipped meat, fish, poultry; egg substitutes containing eggs or egg whites; soufflé, quiche.
- **Breads & Grains:** Breads and rolls with glazed crust; muffins, sweet rolls, doughnuts; French toast, pancakes, waffles; some commercial cake, cookie, muffin mixes; egg noodles.
- **Fruits & Vegetables:** Batter dipped fruits or vegetables; fruit fritters.
- **Desserts/Sweets:** Cream pies; meringues, custards; french ice cream; commercially prepared cookies and cakes; candies made with almond paste, cream, chocolate, fondant, marshmallow; macaroons.
- **Beverages:** Some root beer; malted drinks.
- Miscellaneous: Salad dressings and mayonnaise unless egg-free; egg-based sauces such as hollandaise; broth, consommé, bouillon, egg-drop soup, noodle soup, stocks clarified with egg; Simplesse.

MILK SENSITIVITY
Avoid all products containing milk. These include:
- **Milk/Dairy:** Cow's milk in all forms: fresh, dry, evaporated, condensed, buttermilk; chocolate milk, cocoa, milkshakes, malted milk, eggnog; Ovaltine; flavored instant coffee mixes; yogurt; whey.
- **Meat/Meat Substitutes:** Meatloaf, cold cuts, hot dogs; creamed meats, fish, poultry; scrambled eggs, quiche, souffles; all cheeses.
- **Breads & Grains:** Commercial breads or rolls made with milk; muffins, pancakes, French toast, waffles; prepared mixes made with milk or milk products; macaroni and cheese; pasta in cream sauce.
- **Fruits & Vegetables:** Mashed, scalloped, au gratin potatoes; vegetables with cheese or cream sauce.
- **Desserts/Sweets:** Custards, puddings; cream pies; ice cream, sherbet, frozen yogurt; candies made with chocolate, caramel, or milk ingredients; cakes and cookies made with milk or milk ingredients; whipped cream.
- **Beverages:** All milk-based beverages as noted above.
- **Miscellaneous:** Butter, margarine; sour cream; milk gravy, cream sauces, cheese sauce; salad dressings made with milk or milk-based ingredients; egg substitutes made with milk-based ingredients; Simplesse.

ALLERGY/FOOD SENSITIVITY DIET
(continued from previous page)

CORN SENSITIVITY

Avoid food containing corn, corn syrup, and cornstarch. This includes:

• **Milk/Dairy:** Chocolate milk, milkshakes, milk substitutes, cheese spreads, soy milk.

• **Meat/Meat Substitutes:** Bacon, ham, cold cuts, sausage, enchiladas, tacos, tostados, tamales, commercial entrees except those specifically labeled corn-free, commercial peanut butter.

• **Breads & Grains:** Corn bread, muffins, or rolls; English muffins, corn chips, corn tortillas, graham crackers, hominy, grits, packaged mixes of all types, corn fritters, pizza crust sprinkled with cornmeal, Cheerios, Corn Chex, Toasties, presweetened ready-to-eat cereals.

• **Fruits & Vegetables:** Sweetened fruit juice and juice products; fruits canned in heavy syrup, fruit desserts thickened with cornstarch, Harvard beets, corn, mixed vegetables, succotash, potatoes fried in corn oil, polenta.

• **Desserts/Sweets:** Cakes, candied fruits, cream pie, ice cream, pastries, sherbet.

• **Beverages:** Carbonated beverages containing corn syrup, presweetened ice tea, sweetened fruit punch, ale, beer, whiskey, gin.

• **Miscellaneous:** All commercial soups, homemade soup thickened with cornstarch, cane sugar, corn syrup, imitation maple syrup, Karo syrup, confectioners sugar, jam, jelly, and preserves, corn oil, corn oil margarine, baking powder, corn starch, chewing gum, distilled vinegar, MSG (monosodium glutamate), popcorn, yeast.

WHEAT, EGG, MILK, CORN-FREE DIET — SAMPLE MENU

	Suggested Meal Plan	Suggested Foods and Beverages
BREAKFAST		
	Citrus fruit or juice	orange juice (1/2 cup)
	Cereal	oatmeal (1 cup)
	Meat/meat substitute	peanut butter (no added corn syrup) (1 Tbsp)
	Bread - margarine	rice cakes (2)
	Beverage	coffee
LUNCH (can be noon or evening meal)		
	Meat/meat substitute	lean beef patty (no fillers) (3 oz)
	Potato/substitute	baked potato (1)
	Bread	Rye-Krisp crackers (4)
	Vegetable and/or salad	tossed salad (1 cup)/vinegar/olive oil (2 Tbsp)
	Dessert	apple (1)
	Beverage	iced tea
DINNER (can be evening or noon meal)		
	Soup or juice	turkey rice soup (1 cup)
	Meat/meat substitute	baked chicken (3 oz)
	Potato/substitute	rice (1/2 cup)
	Vegetable and/or salad	green beans (1/2 cup)
	Bread - margarine	slice 100% rye bread
	Dessert	gelatin dessert (1/2 cup)
	Beverage	coffee
SNACK		
	Fruit or juice	orange (1)
	Bread	rice cakes

If planned carefully, allergy diets are generally adequate in all nutrients. The exception would be the milk-free diet, which is inadequate in calcium and possibly vitamin D, and will likely require supplementation. The elimination diets can be deficient in calories, carbohydrates, vitamins and minerals; therefore, long-term use is not advised and monitoring of nutritional sufficiency is essential.

NOTE: These diets should be utilized under the prescription and careful guidance of a health care provider and/or dietitian.

Adapted from the Southwest Diet Manual 1999

BLAND DIET
(continued on next page)

This diet is designed to provide adequate nutrition during treatment of inflammatory or ulcerative conditions of the esophagus, stomach, and intestines. It is intended to decrease irritation of the mucosa, aid in physical comfort, and provide increased dietary variety as individual tolerance improves.

The basic food groups are used for planning nutritionally adequate meals. The diet may vary due to individual food intolerances and the patient's lifestyle. Active mucosal irritants are avoided. These include caffeine, coffee, decaffeinated coffee, tea, cocoa, carbonated beverages containing caffeine, alcohol, chocolate, pepper, chili powder, and any other foods that cause individual discomfort. Some patients find acid fruits and fruit juices too irritating for regular use. Most foods stimulate gastric secretions and are therefore not useful as buffers to gastric acid. Three to five small moderate meals per day are recommended, if tolerable. Avoid bedtime snacks, which can stimulate acid production during the night.

There is no scientific evidence that foods other than those listed above will contribute to the formation or continuation of ulcerative disease.

The bland diet will meet the requirements for all essential nutrients. Food intolerances or habits that limit variety and quantity of food selection may cause some nutrient deficiencies. Patients on this diet will need to be individually assessed to determine if nutritional supplementation is necessary. Chronic or severe blood loss may lead to iron deficiency.

FOOD LISTS

Food Group	Foods Allowed	Foods to Avoid
Milk & Dairy	Milk (whole, low fat or fat-free), dry or instant milk, evaporated milk, buttermilk or yogurt.	Chocolate milk or cocoa.
Meats & Meat Substitutes	Lean and tender meats with visible fat r emoved; beef, veal, lamb, fresh pork (cooked medium to well done). Poultry; fresh, frozen or canned fish or shellfish; organ meats— liver and sweetbreads; eggs, cottage cheese, cheese.	Fried or smoked meats, processed ham, sausage,spiced or highly seasoned meats fried eggs.
Breads & Grains	Enriched breads, cooked or ready-to-eat cereals, tortillas, rolls, English muffins, melba toast, rusks, zwieback, saltines, crackers, pasta, rice.	Fried tortillas, fry bread.
Fruits & Vegetables	All fruit, juices and vegetables as tolerated; baked (without skin), boiled, mashed, diced or creamed potatoes, yams.fried or hash brown potatoes.	Citrus fruits, gas forming vegetables,
Desserts & Sweets	Custard, vanilla or fruit-flavored puddings, tapioca pudding, sherbet, ice cream, frozen yogurt, or ice milk (except chocolate and peppermint), fruit ices, flavored and plain gelatin, Junket, plain or iced cakes, sponge cake, angel food or pound cake, cookies without chocolate or peppermint, sugar, jam, jelly, honey, syrup.	Any foods containing chocolate, cocoa, or seasonings not allowed.

BLAND DIET
(continued from previous page)

FOOD LISTS

Food Group	Foods Allowed	Foods to Avoid
Beverages	Decaffeinated tea, cereal beverages such as Postum and Pero, juices as allowed, caffeine-free carbonated beverages.	Coffee, tea or other drinks that contain caffeine; decaffeinated coffee; chocolate drinks; alcoholic beverages.
Miscellaneous	Salt, lemon and lime juice, vanilla and other extracts and flavorings, sage, cinnamon, thyme, mace, all-spice, paprika, vinegar, prepared mustard.	Pepper, chili powder, cocoa or chocolate.

SAMPLE MENU

	Suggested Meal Plan	Suggested Foods and Beverages
BREAKFAST		
	Fruit juice	apricot nectar (1/2 cup)
	Cereal with milk	oatmeal (1/2 cup)
	Meat/meat substitute	soft cooked egg (1)
	Bread/margarine	slice of toast, margarine (1 tsp)
	Beverage	low-fat milk (1 cup), decaffeinated tea
DINNER (noon or evening meal)		
	Meat/meat substitute	meat loaf (3 oz), no gravy
	Vegetable	green beans (1/2 cup)
		cooked carrots (1/2 cup)
	Potato/potato substitute	whipped potatoes (1/2 cup)
	Dessert	lemon sponge pudding (1/2 cup)
	Bread/margarine	dinner roll (1), margarine (1 tsp)
	Beverage	low-fat (1%) milk (1 cup)
SUPPER (noon or evening meal)		
	Soup or juice	vegetable bean soup (1 cup)
	Meat/meat substitute	baked chicken (3 oz)
	Potato/potato substitute	noodles (1/2 cup)
	Vegetable	green peas (1/2 cup)
	Dessert	applesauce (1/2 cup)
	Bread/margarine	slice of bread, margarine (1 tsp)
	Beverage	low-fat (1%) milk, decaffeinated tea

GLUTEN-RESTRICTED DIET
(continued on next page)

This diet is designed to eliminate the protein gluten found in barley, buckwheat, bulgur, millet, oats, quinoa, rye, spelt, triticale, wheat germ, wheat, or their derivatives for individuals with gluten-sensitive enteropathy or celiac sprue and dermatitis herpetiformis. The gliadin component of gluten is believed to be the trigger for intolerance.

All protein sources are acceptable except those containing gluten. Products made from the flours or starches of arrowroot, corn, potato, rice, and soybean replace products made from wheat, rye, oats, and barley and those cereals and grains listed above.

Tips on Reading Labels:

The following terms listed on product labels may mean there is gluten in the product: Flour or Cereal Products; Hydrolyzed Vegetable Protein (HVP) or Texturized Vegetable Protein (TVP); Malt or Malt Flavoring; Modified Starch or Modified Food Starch; Soy Sauce or Soy Sauce Solids (may contain wheat); Starch; Vegetable Protein; Vegetable Gum.

Those from wheat, rye, oat, or barley sources must be excluded from the diet. Only those from arrowroot, corn, potato, soy, or tapioca are permitted. Specific ingredient information may be obtained from manufacturers or the Celiac Sprue Association, P.O. Box 31700, Omaha. NE 68131; (877) 272-4272; website: www.csaceliacs.org or other celiac websites. Gluten-free products are available from some stores. Ask your pharmacist about medications; some drugs contain gluten. This diet should be adequate in all nutrients. An added effort will need to be made to ensure adequate fiber.

FOOD LISTS

Food Group	Foods Allowed	Foods to Avoid
Breads/Grains	Cornflakes; cornmeal; hominy; rice; puffed rice; grits; Cream of Rice; or Rice Krispies. Food items made from from rice, corn, or soybean flours, or gluten-free wheat starch, arrowroot, or tapioca. Homemade broth, vegetable, or cream soups made with allowed ingredients.	All products made from barley; buckwheat; bulgur; millet; oats; quinoa; rye; spelt; triticale wheat germ or wheat; cereals containing malt flavorings; prepared cake, cookie, bread, biscuit, muffin, pancake, or waffle mixes.
Fruits/ Vegetables	All except items listed to avoid.	Any thickened or prepared (e.g., some pie fillings). Any creamed or breaded vegetables.
Milk/Dairy	All except items listed to avoid.	Commercial chocolate milk with cereal addition; malted milk; instant milk drinks; cocoa mix; nondairy cream substitutes; processed cheese, cheese foods, and spreads containing a gluten source; cheese containing oat gum.
Desserts/ Sweets	Ices; homemade ice-cream; custard; junket; rice pudding; tapioca; gelatin; cakes, cookies, and pastries prepared with gluten-free wheat starch; syrup; jelly; jam; hard candies; molasses; plain chocolate candies; marshmallows.	All others unless labeled gluten-free. Read labels.

GLUTEN-RESTRICTED DIET
(continued from previous page)

FOOD LISTS (continued)

Food Group	Foods Allowed	Foods to Avoid
Meat/Meat Substitutes	All unprocessed meats, eggs, dried beans, and legumes, nuts, peanut butter, soybeans.	Any prepared with stabilizers or fillers, poultry, and fish, such as frankfurters, luncheon meats, sandwich spreads, sausages and canned meats; breaded fish, poultry or meats; poultry or meat prepared with hydrolyzed or texturized vegetable protein (HVP,TVP).
Beverages	Carbonated beverages, fruit juices, tea, coffee, decaffeinated coffee to which no wheat flour was added, sports beverages.	Postum, Ovaltine, ale, beer, root beer.
Miscellaneous	Herbs; spices; pickles; vinegar; popcorn; potato chips; homemade broth; vegetable or cream soup made with allowed ingredients; jelly; jam; honey, corn syrup; butter or margarine.	Commercial salad dressings except pure mayonnaise; chip dips; some catsup; chili sauce; soy sauce; steak sauce; mustard; horseradish; sauces and gravies with gluten sources; some dry seasoning mixes; pickles; distilled white vinegar; stabilizers; some chewing gum; malt or malt flavoring unless derived from corn; baking powder.

SAMPLE MENU

	Suggested Meal Plan	Suggested Foods and Beverages
BREAKFAST		
	Fruit juice	apricot nectar (1/2 cup)
	Cereal	cream of rice (1 cup)
	Meat/meat substitute	poached egg (1)
	Bread - margarine	rice cake (1)/margarine (1 tsp)
	Milk/beverage	1% milk (1 cup); coffee or tea
DINNER (noon or evening meal)		
	Meat/meat substitute	beef patty (no fillers) (3 oz)
	Potato/potato substitute	mashed potato (1/2 cup)
	Vegetable and/or salad	frozen peas (1/2 cup), lettuce/tomato salad (1 cup) salad dressing (1 Tbsp)
	Bread - margarine	slice gluten-free bread/margarine (1 tsp)
	Dessert	fresh apple (1)
	Beverage	coffee or tea
SUPPER (noon or evening meal)		
	Soup or juice	tomato juice (1/2 cup)
	Meat/meat substitute	baked chicken (3 oz)
	Potato/potato substitute/	rice (1/2 cup)
	Vegetable and/or salad	spinach (1/2 cup)
	Bread - margarine	corn tortilla (1)
	Dessert	rice pudding (1/2 cup)
	Milk/beverage	1% milk (1 cup), coffee or tea

HIGH-FIBER DIET
(continued on next page)

This diet is designed to emphasize foods rich in dietary fiber as a part of preventive and/or therapeutic nutrition. High-fiber diets may be used in the treatment of irritable bowel syndrome, uncomplicated diverticulosis, and constipation.

The high fiber diet has an emphasis on fiber-rich foods such as fruits, legumes, vegetables, whole-grain breads, and high fiber cereals. The Daily Reference Value for fiber is 25 gm (based on 2000 calorie-per-day diet). The American Diabetes Association has reported that up to 40 gm fiber daily or 25 gm per 1000 Kcal may be beneficial (National Cancer Institute recommends 25 to 30 gm a day). A maximum of 50 gm of fiber per day is suggested.

Dietary fiber is the component found in many foods that cannot be digested by the enzymes in the intestinal tract. Adequate fluid intake is important when following a high-fiber diet due to the water binding capacity of fiber. Fiber should be increased in the diet slowly to avoid unpleasant side effects (gas, abdominal bloating, cramps). Unprocessed wheat bran can increase fiber intake. Its intake should be increased slowly. It can be added to milk, cereal, yogurt, and other recipes and mixes. Dietary fiber can be divided into two separate categories: water-insoluble fiber and water-soluble fiber.

• Water-insoluble fiber:
Water-insoluble components, such as cellulose, hemicellulose, and lignin, remain essentially unchanged during digestion. Foods containing water-insoluble fiber include the following: fruits, vegetables, cereals, and whole grain products. Research suggests that insoluble fiber may be beneficial in the prevention and/or treatment of constipation and diverticular disease and may decrease the risk of colon cancer.

• Water-soluble fiber:
Water-soluble fiber, such as gum, pectin, and mucilages, does dissolve in water and is found in oats, beans, barley, and some fruits and vegetables. Some studies show that this type of fiber may improve blood glucose and cholesterol levels and appetite regulation.

It is believed that with a varied, well-balanced diet, mineral or nutrient imbalances are unlikely to happen in those consuming a high-fiber diet.

DIETARY FIBER CONTENT OF FOODS IN COMMONLY SERVED PORTIONS

FOOD GROUP

	Breads (1 slice)	Cereals (1 oz.)	Pasta (1 cup)	Rice (1/2 cup)	Legumes (1/2 cup)
Less 1 gm	bagel, white French	Rice-Krispies, Special K, cornflakes		white	
1-1.9 gm	whole-wheat flour tortilla	oatmeal, Nutri-Grain, Cheerios	macaroni, spaghetti	brown	
2-2.9 gm	bran muffin	Wheaties, Shredded-Wheat, Total			
3-3.9 gm	corn tortilla	Cream of Wheat, Honey-Bran	whole-wheat spaghetti		lentils
4-4.9 gm		Bran Chex, 40% Bran-Flakes, Raisin Bran			lima beans, dried peas
5-5.9 gm		Corn Bran			
More 6 gm		All-Bran, Bran Buds, 100% Bran			kidney beans, baked beans, navy beans

HIGH-FIBER DIET
(continued from previous page)

DIETARY FIBER CONTENT OF FOODS IN COMMONLY SERVED PORTIONS

FOOD GROUP

	Vegetables (1/2 cup)	Fruits 1 (medium unless stated)
Less 1 gm	cucumber, lettuce (1 cup) green pepper, mushrooms, onions	grapes (20), watermelon (1 cup) plums
1-1.9 gm	asparagus, green beans, cabbage, potato (no skin), celery, cauliflower, sweet potato	apricots (3), grapefruit (1/2), peach with skin, pineapple (1/2 cup)
2-2.9 gm	broccoli, spinach, Brussels sprouts, carrots, corn, potato (with skin)	apple without skin, banana, orange
3-3.9 gm	peas	apple with skin, pear with skin, raspberries (1/2 cup)
4-4.9 gm		
5-5.9 gm		
More 6 gm		

SAMPLE MENU

	Suggested Meal Plan	Suggested Foods and Beverages
BREAKFAST	Fruit juice	prune juice (1/2 cup)
	Cereal	All Bran cereal (1/2 cup)
	Meat/Meat substitute	poached egg (1)
	Bread and spread	slice whole grain toast & tsp margarine
	Beverage	1% milk (1/2 cup) & coffee or tea
LUNCH (can be noon or evening meal)	Meat/Meat substitute	meat loaf (3 oz)
	Potato/Potato substitute	baked potato (1)
	Vegetable and/or salad	lima beans (1/2 cup), tossed salad (1 cup), dressing (1 Tbsp)
	Bread and spread	slice rye bread & margarine (1 tsp)
	Dessert/coffee or tea	fig cookies (4), coffee or tea
DINNER (can be evening or noon meal)	Soup or juice	lentil soup (1/2 cup)
	Meat/Meat substitute	baked chicken (3 oz)
	Vegetable and/or salad	banana squash (1/2 cup), tossed salad (1 cup), dressing (1 Tbsp)
	Bread and spread	slice rye bread & margarine (1 tsp)
	Dessert	baked apple with cinnamon
	Beverage	1% milk (1 cup), coffee or tea

Adapted from the Southwest Diet Manual 1999

LACTOSE INTOLERANCE DIET
(continued on next page)

This diet is designed to minimize gastrointestinal (GI) disturbances such as abdominal cramps, bloating, flatulence, increased GI motility, and diarrhea associated with ingestion of the carbohydrate lactose.

This diet is individualized to provide the appropriate amount of lactose that a lactose-intolerant individual may tolerate. Milk and milk products including whey and milk solids are limited.

Current research indicates that most lactose-intolerant individuals can consume 15–30 grams of lactose per day (about 2 cups milk) without experiencing severe symptoms. Tolerance level is highly individualized. There are a number o

FOOD LISTS

Food Group	Foods Allowed	Foods to Avoid
Milk/dairy	Milk substitutes and non-dairy products. Milk treated with lactose reducing enzymes; soy milk; as tolerated: buttermilk, acidophilus milk, yogurt.	Milk or milk products in excess of allowed amounts. Avoid or decrease intake if intolerance develops.
Meats/meat substitute	Any meat, fish and poultry except those listed to avoid, peanut butter, kosher hot dogs, dried beans, eggs. Cheeses as tolerated: blue, brick, Swiss, Camembert, cheddar, Colby, mozzarella, muenster, provolone.	All other cheese and cheese products. Creamed meats, luncheon meats, hot dogs, other processed meats with added lactose, breaded meats or fish or poultry, any menu item that contain foods to avoid.
Breads/grains	Breads, cereals, crackers, quick breads (such as muffins, biscuits, etc.) in moderation if made with milk, rice, pasta, no-lactose cereals.	Excessive use of commercial products with added milk or lactose. milk or cream-based soups or pasta; cooked or dry cereal with milk, French toast, macaroni and cheese.
Fruits/vegetables	Any fresh, canned or frozen (prepared without milk, lactose or cheese).	Fruit juice products containing lactose and dietetic fruits with added lactose, vegetables in cream or cheese sauce, potatoes made with milk or cheese.
Desserts/Sweets	Sugar, honey, jelly, jams, plain sugar candies (such as gumdrops, jelly beans, marshmallows), Angel food cake, fruit ices, gelatin, commercial mixes or baked products containing milk in moderation, nondairy frozen desserts.	Cream candies, tablet candies containing lactose, cream pies, products with cream fillings, cream cheese or sour cream, commercial puddings, artificial sweeteners containing lactose, toffee, caramels.
Beverages	Coffee, tea, carbonated beverages, cereal beverages, sports beverages, alcoholic beverages (if allowed by your doctor). Isomil, Pregestimil, Prosobee.	Cocoa, ovaltine, cocoa malt, cocoa mixes, beverages containing cream, flavored instant coffee mixes.

LACTOSE INTOLERANCE DIET
(continued from previous page)

FOOD LISTS (continued)

Food Group	Foods Allowed	Foods to Avoid
Miscellaneous	Condiments, pure flavorings, popcorn, nuts, salt, vinegar, spice blends with lactose lactalbumin, citric acid, MSG, margarine, butter, bacon, lard, mayonnaise, vegetable oils, vegetable shortenings, most oil based commercial salad, dressings, nondairy whipped cream, broth-type soups.	Cream sauces, milk gravies, gum, ascorbic acid tablets, spices, lactate, lactic acid, added, whey, salad dressing with added milk or cheese not allowed, sour cream (alone, or in spreads and dips, cream cheese and cheese spreads, whipped cream, milk or cream soups.

SAMPLE MENU

	Suggested Meal Plan	Suggested Foods and Beverages
BREAKFAST		
	Fruit juice	orange juice w/calcium (1 cup)
	Cereal	shredded wheat (1/2 cup)
	Meat/Meat substitute	soft cooked egg (1)
	Bread and spread	slice wheat toast with margarine
	Milk	lactose-free, low fat milk (1 cup)
	Beverage	coffee or tea
LUNCH (can be noon or evening meal)		
	Meat/Meat Substitute	baked chicken (3 oz)
	Potato/Potato Substitute	brown rice (1/2 cup)
	Vegetable	spinach (1/2 cup),
	Salad	lettuce & tomato salad (1 cup).salad dressing (1 Tbsp)
	Bread and spread	slice wheat bread with margarine (1 tsp)
	Dessert	angel food cake (1 slice) with strawberries (1/2 cup)
	Beverage	coffee or tea
DINNER (can be evening or noon meal)		
	Soup or juice	apple juice (1/2 cup)
	Meat/Meat substitute	lean roast beef (3 oz)
	Vegetable	cooked carrots (1/2 cup)
	Salad	three bean salad (1/2 cup)
	Bread and spread	dinner roll (1). margarine/honey (1 tsp each)
	Dessert	fruit sorbet (1/2 cup)
	Beverage	coffee or tea

Adapted from the Southwest Diet Manual 1999

LIQUID DIET, CLEAR

   This diet is often used to minimize digestion within the gastrointestinal tract. Fluid and energy are provided in a form that minimizes digestion.
The diet consists of clear liquids or foods that are fluid at body temperature. This diet is also residue-free which minimizes fecal output.
   Due to the extremely restrictive nature of this diet, use should be limited to three days or less. For prolonged use, an appropriate low-residue supplement is recommended for nutritional support. Large intakes of beverages high in simple sugars, electrolytes, or amino acids may produce nausea, diarrhea, or dehydration. Liquids such as apple or grape juice, broth, and some fruit punches may need to be diluted before use with vulnerable patients.

FOOD LISTS

Food Groups	Foods Allowed	Foods to Omit
Milk/Dairy	None	All
Meat/Meat Substitute	None	All
Breads/Grains	None	All
Fruits/Vegetables All others	grape or cranberry or strained juices such as orange, lemonade or grapefruit, pulp-free fruit ices.	Clear fruit juices, such as: apple,
Desserts/Sweets	Clear, flavored gelatin, Popsicles, clear fruit ices, sugar, honey, sugar substitute, hard candy.	All others
Beverages	Clear coffee or tea, carbonated beverages, sports drinks.	All others including milk, nectars, cream, juices with pulp.
Miscellaneous	High-protein broth or gelatin, iodized salt, clear broth or bouillon.	All others

SAMPLE MENU

BREAKFAST	Grape juice Clear broth Flavored gelatin Black coffee
LUNCH (can be noon or evening meal)	Apple juice Clear beef broth Flavored gelatin Clear tea
DINNER (can be evening or noon meal)	Cranberry juice Clear chicken broth Flavored gelatin Clear tea

Adapted from the Southwest Diet Manual 1999

APPENDIX

LIQUID DIET, FULL

This diet is intended for the patient who cannot chew or swallow solid foods or as a transition from the clear liquid to a soft or general diet. It contains foods which are liquid or will become liquid at body temperature and are free from irritants. If the milk based foods in this diet are poorly tolerated in patients, the use of low-lactose foods or a lactase product may prove beneficial.

FOOD LISTS

Food Groups	Foods Allowed	Foods to Avoid
Milk & Dairy	All milk and milk drinks such as milk shakes and eggnogs made from commercial mix; yogurt that is plain or flavored (no seeds or fruit). All beverages including high-protein, high-calorie oral supplements.	Cheese, cottage cheese.
Meat/Meat Substitutes	Eggnogs, custards.	All others.
Breads / Grains	Thin, cooked cereal such as farina, grits, oatmeal.	All others.
Fruits / Vegetables	Vitamin C sources (daily): Strained citrus and tomato juices. Vitamin A sources (alternate days): Strained carrot juice.	All others.
Desserts and Sweets	Custards, puddings, plain gelatin, plain ice cream, ice milk, sherbet, sugar, hard candy, honey, Popsicles, syrup, frozen yogurt.	All others.
Miscellaneous	Butter, margarine, cream, nondairy creamer.	All others.

SAMPLE MENU

Suggested Meal Plan	Suggested Foods and Beverages
BREAKFAST	
Fruit juice	orange juice, strained
Cereal	Farina
Meat/Meat substitute	custard
Milk/Dairy	2% Milk
Beverage	coffee
LUNCH (can be noon or evening meal)	
Soup	strained cream soup
Juice	tomato juice
Salad	lime gelatin
Dessert	ice cream
Beverage	ginger ale
SNACK Milk/Dairy	1 milk shake
DINNER (can be evening or noon meal)	
Soup	strained cream soup
Juice	peach nectar
Dessert	Popsicle
Beverage	chocolate milk
SNACK Juice	cranberry juice
Milk/Dairy	vanilla pudding, 2% milk

Adapted from the Southwest Diet Manual 1999

LOW-FAT/LOW-CHOLESTEROL DIET (continued on next page)

The low-fat/low-cholesterol diets are designed to improve serum lipid profiles for the treatment and prevention of coronary heart disease (CHD). Foods high in total fat, saturated fat, and cholesterol are controlled. Total cholesterol intake is restricted. Limited amounts of monounsaturated and polyunsaturated fats are used as replacements for saturated fats. Calories need to be adjusted to achieve or maintain desired body weight. Lean meat, fish, skinless poultry, and non- or low-fat dairy products are included as well as plant sources of protein, such as legumes, dried beans, and dried peas. High-fat meats and poultry, organ meats, egg yolks, and cheese are limited. Foods high in complex carbohydrates and fiber such as fruits, vegetables, whole-grain products, and legumes are emphasized.

The National Cholesterol Education Program (NCEP) guidelines indicate that a serum total cholesterol should be measured in all adults over the age of 20 at least once every 5 years. Total cholesterol levels below 200 mg/dL are classified as "desirable blood cholesterol," those 200-239 mg/dL as "borderline high cholesterol" and those 240 mg/dL and over as "high blood cholesterol." Serum (blood-level) high density lipoprotein cholesterol (HDL-C) of at least 35 mg/dL is desirable. Elevated total serum cholesterol should be confirmed by repeat testing per your health care provider's recommendation. The goals of therapy are to reduce serum cholesterol to less than 200 mg/dL and Low Density Lipoprotein (LDL) to less than 130 mg/dL for people with other heart disease risk factors and to 160 mg/dL for clients with no other risk factors.

Step I Diet Therapy of Blood Cholesterol

Nutrient	Recommended Intake
Total Fat	Less than 30% of Total Calories
Saturated Fat	8 to 10% of Total Calories
Polyunsaturated Fat	Up to 10 % of Total Calories
Monounsaturated Fat	10 to 15 % of Total Calories
Carbohydrates	At least 55% of Total Calories
Protein	Approximately 15% of Total Calories
Cholesterol	Less than 300 mg
Total Calories	To achieve and maintain desirable weight

Note: Step II Diet therapy reduces saturated fat to less than 7% of calories and cholesterol to less than 200 mg.

After starting the diet plan, patients should be checked at 4 to 6 weeks and then 3 months for cholesterol levels and diet adherence. It usually takes 6 months for results. Drug therapy may be recommended if cholesterol levels are still high.

Cholesterol is found only in animal products.

Saturated fats are often solid at room temperature and are usually found in animal products such as meats, poultry, butter, cheese, and ice cream. Plant sources of saturated fats include palm oil, palm kernel oil, and coconut oil. Monounsaturated fats are found in products, such as olive oil, peanuts, flaxseed oil, and canola (rapeseed) oil. Polyunsaturated fats are usually liquid at room temperature and are found in safflower, sunflower, corn, soybean and cottonseed oils, seeds, and certain nuts.

Along with cholesterol testing, all adults should be evaluated for other CHD risk factors such as hypertension, smoking, diabetes, and obesity.

FOOD LISTS—STEP I DIET

Milk/Dairy

• Allowed: Skim (nonfat) or 1% fat milk (liquid, powdered, or evaporated), nonfat or low-fat yogurt, nonfat or low-fat cottage cheese, nonfat or low-fat cheese, nonfat sour cream; and nonfat cream cheese.

• Avoid: Whole milk (over 3% fat) (liquid, evaporated, or condensed); 2% milk, cream; half-and-half; imitation milk products; most nondairy creamers; whipped toppings; whole milk yogurt; regular cottage cheese (4% fat); natural cheeses made from whole milk (cheddar, Swiss, blue, Camembert, etc.); low-fat or regular cream cheese; low-fat or regular sour cream; low-fat sour cream. NOTE: If 2% milk is used, decrease added fat by 1 teaspoon for each cup of milk.

Meat/Meat Substitute

• Allowed: Cooked dried beans; split peas; lentils; pinto beans; poultry without the skin; fish; tuna packed in water; lean beef (extra lean ground beef, eye of round, sirloin, round tip, round, top round, tenderloin, top loin); lean pork (tenderloin, leg, shoulder); lamb (arm, leg, loin, rib); luncheon meats (1 gram of fat or less per ounce); egg whites (2 egg whites will equal 1 whole egg); low-cholesterol egg substitutes.

LOW-FAT/LOW-CHOLESTEROL DIET
(continued from previous page)

• Avoid: Fried meats or meat substitutes; fatty cuts of beef, pork or lamb; goose; duck; liver; kidney; brains; or other organ meats; sausages; bacon; regular luncheon meats; peanut butter (except as allowed under Miscellaneous); or egg yolks beyond allotment.

Breads & Grains
• Allowed: Whole-grain breads (oatmeal, whole wheat, rye, bran, multigrain, etc.); English muffins; bagels; pita bread; rice; pasta; homemade baked goods low in fat; low-fat crackers (rice cakes, popcorn cakes, Rye Krisp, Melba toast, pretzels, breadsticks); or hot or cold cereals (with 1 to 2 grams of fat or less per serving).
• Avoid: High-fat baked goods (pies, cakes, doughnuts, croissants, pastries, muffins, biscuits); fry bread; high-fat crackers; egg noodles; granola type cereals; cereals with more than 2 grams of fat per serving; pasta and rice prepared with cream; butter; and cheese sauces.

Vegetables
• Allowed: Any fresh, frozen, canned. or dried.
• Avoid: Vegetables prepared in butter, cream, and other sauces; fried vegetables.

Fruits
• Allowed: Any fresh, frozen, canned, or dried.
• Avoid: Coconuts, avocados, and olives except as allowed under Miscellaneous.

Desserts & Sweets (Limit to control calories)
• Allowed: Sugar; jelly; jam; honey; molasses; low-fat or fat-free frozen desserts (such as sherbet, sorbet, ices, nonfat frozen yogurt, and Popsicles); angel food cake; low-fat or fat-free cakes and cookies (such as vanilla wafers, graham crackers, ginger snaps [and others with less than 2 grams of fat per serving]); baking cocoa; low-fat or fat-free candy (such as jelly beans or hard candy); low-fat or fat-free puddings; gelatin desserts.
• Avoid: Ice cream; high-fat cakes, pies, and cookies (most commercially made); chocolate; puddings made with whole milk; and nut candies.

Beverages
• Allowed: Juices, tea, coffee, decaffeinated coffee, carbonated drinks, and most alcoholic drinks.
• Avoid: Milkshakes; ice cream floats; eggnog; alcoholic drinks containing milk, cream, or coconut.

Miscellaneous
• Allowed: Limit fat based on total number of calories consumed.
   Limit: (1 tsp per serving) Unsaturated vegetable oils (corn, olive, canola, flaxseed, safflower, sesame, soybean, or sunflower); margarine or shortening made from unsaturated vegetable oils; mayonnaise and salad dressings made from unsaturated oils (1 Tbsp); diet margarine (2 tsp); olives (10 small or 5 large); avocado (1/8 medium or 2 Tbsp); seeds and nuts (1 Tbsp seeds, 6 almonds, 20 small peanuts); peanut butter (2 tsp).
   No Limit: Vegetable oil sprays; fat-free mayonnaise and salad dressings, fat-free sour cream; herbs, spices, pepper, and salt substitute (with health care provider's approval); mustard; catsup; vinegar; lemon and lime juice; fat-free sauces; cream sauces made with allowed ingredients.
• Avoid: Butter; coconut oil; palm oil; palm kernel oil; lard; bacon fat; salad dressings made with egg yolk; fried snack foods (potato chips, cheese curls, tortilla chips); regular cream sauces.

Step 1 Diet	Suggested Meal Plan	Suggested Foods and Beverages
BREAKFAST	Citrus fruit or juice	grapefruit half
	Cereal	bran flakes (1/2 cup)
	Meat/meat substitute	low cholesterol egg substitute (1/4 cup)
	Bread/margarine	2 slices whole wheat toast, jelly (1 tsp)
	Milk/beverage	1% milk (1 cup), coffee
LUNCH (can be noon or evening meal)		
	Meat/meat substitute	3 oz baked chicken breast
	Potato/potato substitute	sweet potato (1/2 cup)
	Vegetable and/or salad	fat-free green beans (1/2 cup)
		garden salad (1 cup). low-fat dressing (2 Tbsp)
	Bread and spread	whole wheat rolls (2). honey (2 tsp)
	Dessert	strawberries (1 cup)
	Beverage	iced tea
DINNER (can be evening or noon meal)		
	Soup or juice	vegetable juice (1/2 cup)
	Meat/meat substitute	fat-free meatballs (3 oz), tomato sauce (1/2 cup)
	Potato/substitute	spaghetti (1/2 cup)
	Vegetable and/or salad	broccoli (1/2 cup), spinach salad (1 cup), low-fat dressing (2 Tbsp)
	Bread and spread	slice Italian bread margarine (1 tsp)
	Dessert	fruit sorbet (1/2 cup)
	Milk/beverage	1% milk (1 cup), coffee or tea

LOW-SALT DIET
(continued on next page)

Salt is sodium chloride. Over 90% of sodium in an average diet is in the form of salt. Many persons will benefit from reductions in salt intake, including hypertensive (high blood pressure) individuals, blacks, and middle- and older-aged adults. Reducing salt intake can also help prevent hypertension in otherwise health individuals.

The Dietary Guidelines for Americans recommends the salt intake for most individuals as no more than 2,300 milligrams (mg) a day. This is about one teaspoon. The aim of a low-salt diet is to consume no more than 1,500 mg (about 2/3 of a teaspoon) of sodium per day. An increased dietary intake of potassium is also recommended (4,700 mg a day). Dietary potassium can lower blood pressure and blunt the effects of salt on blood pressure in some individuals. These diet changes can be made gradually rather than trying to change all at once.

On average, the natural salt content of food accounts for only about 10% of total intake, while discretionary salt use (i.e., salt added at the table or while cooking) provides another 5-10% of total intake. Approximately 75% is derived from salt added by manufacturers. In addition, foods served by food establishments may be high in sodium.

It is important to read the food label and determine the sodium content of food, which can vary by several hundreds of milligrams in similar foods. Food labels list sodium rather than salt content. When reading a Nutrition Facts Panel on a food product, look for the sodium content. Foods that are low in sodium (less than 140 mg) are low in salt.

Salt substitutes should be approved by your health care provider. Salt-free herbs and spices may be used freely.

FOOD LISTS

Milk and Dairy Products
• Allowed: Any milk—white, low-fat, skim, chocolate and cocoa; yogurt; natural cheese (limit 1 oz per day), low sodium cheese, cottage cheese, substitute for 8 oz of milk: 4 oz evaporated milk, 4 oz condensed milk, or 1/3 cup dry milk powder.
• Avoid: Buttermilk, malted milk, instant cocoa or milk mixes, processed cheese.

Meats and Meat Substitutes
• Allowed: Fresh or fresh frozen: beef, lamb, pork, veal, and game; chicken, turkey, Cornish hen or other poultry; any fresh-water or fresh-frozen unbreaded fish and shellfish; low-sodium canned tuna or salmon; unsalted or low sodium peanut butter; eggs, dried beans and peas, unsalted nuts.
• Avoid: Any meat, fish or poultry that is smoked, cured, salted, or canned, such as bacon, dried beef, corned beef, cold cuts, ham, turkey ham, hot dogs, sausages, sardines, anchovies, pickled items (herring, meats, or eggs), koshered meats and poultry, imitation crab, frozen/boxed entrees with more than 500 mg sodium per serving, salted nuts or peanut butter.

Breads and Grains
• Allowed: Enriched white, wheat, rye, and pumpernickel bread; hard rolls, bagels, English muffins, cooked cereal without salt; dry cereals low in sodium; unsalted crackers and breadsticks; corn or flour tortillas; biscuits, muffins, cornbread, pancakes, and waffles all made with low-sodium baking powder; low-sodium or homemade bread crumbs; rice, noodles, barley, spaghetti, macaroni, and other pastas; homemade bread stuffing.
• Avoid: Breads and rolls with salted tops; quick breads; hot or dry cereals with added salt; crackers with salted tops; pancakes, waffles, muffins, biscuits, and cornbread with salt, baking powder, self-rising flour or instant mixes; regular bread crumbs or cracker crumbs; commercial stuffing.

Vegetables
• Allowed: Fresh, frozen, and low-sodium or unsalted canned vegetables; regular canned, drained vegetables (limit to 1/2 cup serving per day); unsalted tomato sauce, low-sodium or unsalted vegetable juice; salt-free potato chips.
• Avoid: Regular canned vegetables (over 1/2 cup per day); vegetable juices; sauerkraut; pickled vegetables and others prepared in brine; instant potato products with added salt or sodium.

Fruits (3-4 or more servings a day)
• Allowed: All fruits and juices
• Avoid: None except salted prunes (saladitos).

Desserts/Sweets
• Allowed: Any sweets like sugar, honey, jam, jelly, syrup, marmalade, hard candy; limit regular baked products (cake, pie, cookies) to 1 serving a day.
• Avoid: More than 1 serving a day of regular baked products.

LOW-SALT DIET
(continued from previous page)

Beverages
• Allowed: Coffee, tea, soft drinks with less than 35 mg sodium per serving; alcoholic beverages (if your health care provider approves).
• Avoid: Commercially softened water as beverage or in food preparation.

Miscellaneous
• Allowed: Salt-free butter or margarine; vegetable oils, shortening, and mayonnaise; salt-free salad dressings; salt substitute (with health care provider's approval); pepper, herbs, and spices; flavorings; vinegar and lemon or lime juice; salt-free seasonings; low-sodium condiments: catsup, chili sauce, mustard, and pickles; fresh-ground horseradish; homemade or salt-free soups; low-sodium baking powder; unsalted snacks: nuts, seeds, pretzels, chips, and popcorn.
• Avoid: Light-salt; garlic salt, celery salt, onion salt, and seasoned salt; sea salt, rock salt, and kosher salt; seasonings containing salt and sodium compounds; monosodium glutamate (MSG, Accent); regular catsup, chili sauce, mustard, pickles, relishes, olives, and horseradish; Kitchen Bouquet; gravy and sauce mixes; barbecue sauce, soy and teriyaki sauce; Worcestershire and steak sauce; salted snack foods: nuts, seeds, pretzels, chips, and popcorn; commercially prepared convenience foods; regular canned or dried soups.

SAMPLE MENU
(approximately 1,500 mg salt; 4,700 mg potassium)

	Suggested Meal Plan	Suggested Foods and Beverages
BREAKFAST		
	Fruit or fruit juice	orange juice (6 oz)
		cantaloup (1/2 cup)
	Cereal	shredded wheat cereal (1 cup)
	Bread and spread	slice white toast, unsalted margarine (1 tsp)
	Beverage	1% milk (1 cup), coffee or tea (no sugar or cream)
LUNCH (can be noon or evening meal)		
	Meat/meat substitute	turkey (2 oz in a sandwich)
		swiss cheese (1 oz)
	Vegetable or salad	tomato slice (1) and lettuce leaves (2)
		baby carrots (8)
	Bread and spread	2 slices whole-wheat bread, mayonnaise (1 Tbsp)
	Dessert	fig bar cookies (2)
	Beverage	coffee or tea (no sugar or cream)
DINNER (can be evening or noon meal)		
	Meat/meat substitute	baked salmon (3 oz)
	Potato/potato substitute	long grain brown rice (1/2 cup)
	Vegetable and/or salad	tossed salad (1 1/2 cups), oil and vinegar dressing (2 Tbsp)
		asparagus spears (6)
	Bread and spread	whole wheat dinner roll (1 medium), unsalted margarine (1 tsp)
	Dessert	slice angel food cake, strawberries (1/2 cup), whipped cream (2 Tbsp)
	Beverage	coffee or tea (no sugar or cream)
SNACK	Fruit	banana (1 medium)
	Meat/meat substitute	unsalted dry roasted almonds (1/4 cup)

WEIGHT LOSS DIET
(continued on next page)

This is a simple "exchange list" diet for individuals who want to lose weight. The goal of diet therapy is to reduce caloric intake to a level that can be safely and comfortably tolerated. Usually diets that provide 1,200 to 1,500 calories a day are acceptable for most people. However, you and your health care provider should determine the appropriate amount of calories required for your weight, height, activity level and general health. The example shown is for a 1,400 calories per day menu. It may be modified by adding more food portions.

Plan your breakfast, lunch, and dinner meals by selecting items from the appropriate food list. This sample diet allows you one fruit portion, one starch, and one milk for breakfast. You may choose cereal with banana and milk. Coffee or tea is a "free" item. Amounts of each portion are indicated in each food list. Portions can be interchanged among breakfast, lunch, and dinner as long as the total for the day doesn't exceed those indicated. For example, you can eat all your fruits for breakfast if desired, but don't exceed four portions for the day.

SUGGESTED MEAL PLANS FOR 1400 CALORIES PER DAY DIET
DAILY PORTIONS FROM FOOD LISTS

(See lists below and following page)

BREAKFAST	LUNCH	DINNER	SNACK
1 Fruit	2 Meats	2 Meats	1 Starch
1 Starch/Bread	1 Vegetable	1 Fat	1 Fruit
1 Milk	1 Fat	2 Starch/Bread	1 Milk
	2 Starch/Bread	1 Vegetable	
	1 Fruit	1 Fruit	
	(raw vegetable as desired)	(raw vegetable as desired)	

FOOD LISTS (continued on next page)

FRUIT LIST (60 calories, 15 grams carbohydrates)
(A portion is 1 small piece or 1/2 cup unless listed)

Apples (juice or sauce)	Fruit cocktail	Plums (2)
Apricots (4)	Grapefruit or juice	Prunes (3)
Apricots, dried (7 halves)	Grapes (15)	Prune juice (1/4 cup)
Banana (1/2)	Grape juice	Raspberries (1 cup)
Blackberries (3/4 cup)	Lemon	Raisins (2 Tbsp)
Blueberries (3/4 cup)	Orange/orange juice	Rhubarb
Cantaloupe (1/3)	Peach	Strawberries (10)
Cherries	Pear	Tangerine
Dates (2)	Pineapple	Watermelon (1 cup)

VEGETABLE LIST (25 calories, 5 grams carbohydrates, 2 grams protein)
(A portion is 1 cup raw or 1/2 cup cooked)

Artichoke	Celery	Peppers
Asparagus	Cucumber	Peas
Beans (green, wax or sprouts)	Eggplant	Pumpkin
Beets	Endive	Radish
Broccoli	Mixed Vegetables	Rutabaga
Brussels Sprouts	Mushrooms	Spinach
Cabbage or Sauerkraut	Okra	Squash
Cauliflower	Onions	Tomato
Carrot	Parsnips	Turnips

Note: Some vegetables are shown in the Starch List.

WEIGHT LOSS DIET
(continued from previous page)

FOOD LISTS (continued on next page)

STARCH LIST (80 calories, 15 grams carbohydrates, 2-3 grams protein, 1-2 grams fat)
(A portion is 1/4 cup or as listed)

Angel Food Cake (1 oz)	Cornbread (1 in. cube)	Popcorn, fat free (3 cups)
Bagel (small or 1 oz)	Cornstarch (2 Tbsp)	Potato, white (1/2 cup)
Beans, canned (1/3 cup)	English Muffin (1/2)	Potato, sweet (1/3 cup)
Biscuit (1)	Gelatin (1/2 cup)	Pretzels (5 small)
Bread (1 slice)	Graham Crackers (2)	Rice (1/3 cup)
Bun (1/2)	Lentils, canned (1/3 cup)	Ricecakes (2)
Cereal (3/4 cup, dry;	Matzo crackers (3/4 oz)	Saltines (6)
1/2 cup, hot)	Pancakes (1)	Taco Shell (1)
Corn (1/2 cup)	Pasta (1/2 cup)	Tortilla (one 6-inch)
Cookies (fat-free,1 or 2 small)	Pita bread (1/2)	

MEAT OR MEAT SUBSTITUTE LIST (55-70 calories, 7 grams protein, 3-5 grams fat)
(A portion is 1 ounce or 1/4 cup or as listed)

Beef (lean cuts)	Eggs (3 per week)	Pork (chops, ham, roast)
Cheese (skim milk types)	Fish (all types)	Shellfish
Cold cuts or frankfurters	Lamb (leg, roasted)	Soybeans, cooked (1/3 cup)
(95% fat-free)	Peanut Butter (1 Tbsp)	Veal
Cottage Cheese (1/3 cup)	Poultry (no skin)	

FAT LIST (45 calories, 5 grams fat)
(Use nonfat or low-fat products when they are available.)

Bacon, crisp (1 slice)	Gravy (2 Tbsp)	Oils (1 teaspoon)
Cheese, cream (1 Tbsp)	Margarine* (1 teaspoon)	Olives (5 small)
Coconut (1 Tbsp)	Mayonnaise* (1 teaspoon)	Salad Dressings* (1 Tbsp)
Cream, light (2 Tbsp)	Nuts (6 to 10)	Seeds (1 Tbsp)

* Portion amounts may be increased if using nonfat products (e.g., mayonnaise, 2 Tbsp)

MILK LIST (80 calories, 12 grams carbohydrates, 8 grams protein)

Fat-free milk (1 cup)   Yogurt (1 cup plain, nonfat, unsweetened except with sugar substitute)

FREE ITEMS (you may have these as desired)

Beverages: Coffee, tea, sugar-free beverages
Pickles, except sweet pickles
Bouillon and consommés
All spices, herbs, flavorings and artificial sweeteners
Catsup, mustard, soy sauce, vinegars
Worcestershire sauce

Sugar-free gelatin
Salad greens
Nonstick pan spray
Sugar substitutes
Lemon or lime juice

ADDITIONAL INFORMATION

• Purchase fruits fresh, fresh-frozen or canned unsweetened, or in natural juices. All juices should be unsweetened.
• Vegetable and fruit portions are for the edible amounts of the item.
• Allowed amounts of meats are after cooking; amounts shown are for edible parts only (excluding bones). Be sure to trim all extra fat away from meat prior to cooking. Remove skin from all poultry. Roasting or broiling of meats is preferred.
• If salt intake is limited, avoid foods high in sodium (pickles) and don't use salt at the table.
• Even though the diet should meet your nutritional needs, a vitamin and mineral supplement may be recommended by your doctor.
• Everyone on a diet will experience an occasional setback. This doesn't mean failure. Long-term success is still possible.
• Combine your diet with behavior modification to help you maintain the weight loss.

WEIGHT LOSS SUGGESTIONS

Weight control diets are designed to provide a specific calorie level calculated to meet an individual's requirement to attain optimal body weight. Weight loss of 1-2 pounds per week is generally optimal. An exercise program is also highly recommended. Try to get 30 to 60 minutes of exercise each day.

The U.S. Department of Agriculture's Food Guide Pyramid diet plan can be used as a guide to healthy eating and is likely to produce desired weight loss. Weight loss diets of greater than 1200 calories per day are generally adequate in all nutrients except iron, as long as the diet is planned to include a variety of foods from all food groups.

FOOD GUIDE PYRAMID — DAILY SERVINGS
* Fats, Oils, & Sweets (Use Sparingly): These foods provide calories and little else nutritionally. Most people should use these foods sparingly.
* Milk, Yogurt, Cheese (2-3 Servings) & Meat, Poultry, Fish, Dry Beans, Eggs, Nuts (2-3 Servings): Most of these foods come from animals. These foods are important for protein, calcium, iron and zinc.
* Vegetables (3-5 Servings) & Fruits (2-4 Servings): All of these foods are from plants. Most people need to eat more of these foods for the vitamins, minerals and fiber they supply.
* Bread, Cereal, Rice and Pasta (6-11 Servings): All of these foods are from grains. Individuals need the most of these foods each day.

BEHAVIORAL STRATEGIES IN MANAGEMENT OF WEIGHT CONTROL
Individuals seeking to make a lifetime commitment to improve their eating and exercise habits can succeed at long-term weight loss. Most of the successful long-term weight-loss programs include several components; behavior modification; exercise; nutrition; social support; and cognitive changes, including goal setting, assertiveness training, and coping with mistakes and motivation. Emphasis should be placed on slow, progressive weight loss.

The following is a list of behavior modification techniques which can be used to promote healthy eating, lifestyle and in turn, weight loss.

BEHAVIOR MODIFICATION TECHNIQUES
* Evaluate what behaviors, activities or feelings trigger eating.
* Don't use food as a reward for desired behavior.
* Drink plenty of noncaloric fluids, including water daily.
* Change usual eating places, avoid eating while involved in other activities.
* Make an effort to eat breakfast and small, frequent meals.
* Eat fresh fruits and raw vegetables at least 4 times daily.
* Exercise along with television exercise programs or during commercials when watching television.
* Eat slowly, putting your utensil down between bites.
* Weight should be checked on a weekly basis only.
* Clean high-calorie, low-nutrient foods out of cupboards.
* Keep busy so the focus is not food.
* Shop from a healthy food list and not when hungry.
* Leave the table soon after eating and don't feel a need to finish everything.
* Trim fat off meat and skin off poultry.
* Place a photo of a thinner you on the mirror.
* Plan ahead, especially when attending social events.
* Keep records of intake and/or weight loss progress.
* When weight drops, give away clothes that no longer fit.
* Break the habit of nibbling while cooking or cleaning up from meals.
* Try low-fat and low-calorie food items (the taste keeps improving).

BREAST SELF-EXAMINATION

FINDING BREAST CANCER EARLY

• There have been many advances made in diagnosing and treating breast cancer. More and more women are surviving the disease. In many cases, breast cancers found early and treated promptly have a better chance for a cure.

• Tools to detect breast cancer include exams by a medical professional, mammography, ultrasound, and breast self-examination (BSE). BSE has come under some debate about how effective it is. Studies have shown that there is no difference in the number of lives saved among women who did perform a BSE and those who did not. In addition, they have found that BSE may increase unneeded biopsies and anxiety.

• The American Cancer Society continues to recommend that BSE be performed monthly beginning at age 20. BSE will help a woman under age 40 learn what her breasts feel like under normal conditions. If a lump or other change is discovered, she can see her health care provider about it. There is some added benefit to women over age 40 in doing a BSE. Exams by a medical professional and mammography should have the most emphasis in early detection of breast cancer.

• Several products have been approved by the Food & Drug Administration (FDA) to help women perform monthly breast self-examinations. They may help make the exams easier for some women. Ask your health care provider about their use.

WHEN TO EXAMINE YOUR BREASTS

• Follow the same procedure once a month a few days to about a week after your period ends, when your breasts are usually not tender or swollen. Breast tissue in adult women changes throughout the month as it responds to hormone levels occurring during the menstrual cycle. Some women have normally lumpy breasts, but they can still learn the pattern of the lumps and should be able to detect new or unusual lumps.

• After menopause, check your breasts on the same day of each month. After a hysterectomy, ask your health care provider about the best time of the month.

BREAST EXAM WHILE LYING DOWN ON YOUR BACK

• To examine your right breast, put a pillow or folded towel under your right shoulder. Place your right hand under your head—this distributes breast tissue more evenly on the chest.

• Use the finger pads of the three middle fingers of your left hand. Press gently and firmly. A ridge of firm tissue in the lower curve of each breast is normal. Then move around the breast in 1) a circular pattern, 2) up and down line, or 3) in a wedge pattern. Always use the same pattern each month. Now repeat the procedure on your left breast with a pillow under your left shoulder and the left hand under your head. Notice how your breast structure feels.

• Check the area under each arm (with your elbow slightly bent). The lymph glands are in this area. They may become swollen if you are sick. If you feel a small lump that moves freely, check it daily for a few days. If it doesn't go away, call your health care provider.

• Any discharge from the nipple, clear or bloody, should be reported to your health care provider.

BREAST EXAM IN THE SHOWER

Examine your breasts during a shower (hands glide easier over wet skin). With the fingers flat, move the hand gently over every part of each breast. Use your right hand to examine the left breast, left hand for the right breast. Check for any lump, hard knot, or thickening.

BREAST EXAM IN FRONT OF A MIRROR

Inspect your breasts with arms at your sides. Next, raise your arms high overhead. Look for any changes in each breast (swelling, dimpling, or changes in the nipple).

SIGNS OF POSSIBLE PROBLEMS IN YOUR BREASTS

• Lumps, hard knots, or thickening in the breast.
• Unusual swelling, warmth, redness, or darkening that does not go away.
• Change in the size or shape of your breast.
• Dimpling or puckering of the skin.
• Itchy, scaly, sore, or rash on the nipple.
• Pulling in of the nipple or other parts of the breast.
• Nipple discharge that starts suddenly.
• Pain in one spot that does not vary or change with your monthly cycle.

WHAT TO DO

• It is important to see your health care provider as soon as possible if you find any suspicious changes in your breasts. Don't be frightened. Most breast lumps or changes are not cancer.

• Remember that a monthly breast exam is not a substitute for the other two critical parts of the guidelines for early breast cancer detection. The American Cancer Society recommends an annual mammogram after age 40, and an exam by a medical professional every three years for women ages 20–39, and annually for women over age 40. Ask your health care provider about when you should schedule a mammogram and a breast exam.

• To learn more: American Cancer Society, 1599 Clifton Rd., Atlanta, GA 30329, (800) ACS-2345; website: www.cancer.org or National Cancer Institute, (800) 4-CANCER; website: www.nci.nih.gov.

CONDOM USAGE
(continued on next page)

 GENERAL INFORMATION

WHO SHOULD USE A CONDOM?
• Condoms are used for both birth control and reducing the risk of disease. Some people think that other forms of birth control will also protect them against disease. This is not true. Even if you use another form of birth control, you need a condom to help reduce the risk of getting STDs (sexually transmitted diseases) including the human immunodeficiency virus (HIV) infection.
• Condoms do not make sex 100% safe, but, if properly used, they can reduce the chance of contracting STDs. This can mean protection not only for you and your partner, but also for any children you may have in the future.

CHOOSING A CONDOM
Read the label and look for the following:
• The condoms should be made of latex (rubber) or made of polyurethane.
• It should say that the condoms are to prevent disease, and if used properly, latex condoms help reduce risk of HIV transmission and many other STDs. If the package doesn't say anything about preventing disease, the condoms may not provide the protection you need. Novelty condoms, for example, will not be labeled for either disease- or pregnancy-prevention. Condoms that don't cover the entire penis are not labeled for disease prevention and should not be used for this purpose. For proper protection, a condom must unroll to cover the entire penis.
• Check the expiration date (EXP followed by date). The condom should not be purchased or used after that date.
• Condoms are available in many stores and from vending machines. If buying condoms from vending machines, check for proper labeling. Do not buy condoms from a vending machine located where it may be subject to extreme temperatures or direct sunlight.
• Condoms should be stored in a cool, dry place out of direct sunlight. Closets or drawers usually make good storage places. Condoms should not be kept in a pocket, wallet, or purse for more than a few hours at a time because they may be exposed to extreme temperatures.

HOW TO USE A CONDOM
• When opening a condom, handle the package gently. Don't use teeth, sharp fingernails, scissors, or other sharp instruments. These may damage the condom. Make sure you can see what you're doing!
• After you open the package, inspect the condom. If the material sticks to itself or is gummy, the condom is no good. Check the condom top for other obvious damage such as brittleness, tears, and holes. Do not unroll the condom to check it; this could damage it.
• Use a new condom at the beginning of every sexual act (vaginal or anal intercourse and oral sex).
• Put the condom on as soon as the penis is erect and before any contact is made between the penis and any part of the partner's body. Don't delay condom use. Studies have shown that while pre-ejaculatory fluid is not semen, it does contain HIV.
• If the condom does not have a reservoir tip, pinch the tip enough to leave a half-inch space for semen to collect. Make sure to squeeze out any air in the tip to help keep the condom from breaking.
• While holding the condom by the rim (and pinching the half-inch tip, if needed), place the condom on top of the penis. Then, continuing to hold it by the rim, unroll it all the way to the base of the penis. If you are using water-based lubricant, you can put more on the outside of the condom.
• If you feel the condom break, stop right away, withdraw, and put on a new condom.
• After ejaculation and before the penis gets soft, grip the rim of the condom and carefully withdraw.
• To remove the condom, gently pull it off the penis, being careful the semen doesn't spill out.
• Wrap the used condom in a tissue and throw it in the trash. Because condoms may cause problems in sewers, don't flush them down the toilet. Then wash your hands with soap and warm water.

PRECAUTION
Condoms provide good protection for vaginal and oral sex (where the penis is in contact with the mouth). The protection they give for anal sex is questionable. The Surgeon General of the Public Health Service has said, "Condoms provide some protection, but anal intercourse is simply too dangerous a practice." Condoms may be more likely to break during anal intercourse than during other types of sex. This is due to the greater amount of friction and other stresses involved. Even if the condom doesn't break, anal intercourse is very risky because it can cause rectal tissue to tear and bleed. This allows disease germs to pass more easily from one partner to another.

APPENDIX

CONDOM USAGE
(continued from previous page)

SPERMICIDES

Spermicides (gels, creams, foams, or films), which kill sperm, are used for birth control, either alone or with barrier contraceptives such as the diaphragm or cervical cap. A spermicide called nonoxynol 9 has been widely used with condoms to supposedly help reduce the risk of STD transmission. Studies now show that nonoxynol 9 does not reduce the risk of transmission of the human immunodeficiency virus (HIV) or other STDs during intercourse. Some condoms come with nonoxynol-9 already added but they are not recommended for prevention of STDs. The best STD and HIV barrier is a latex condom without nonoxynol-9. Nevertheless, a condom that is lubricated with nonoxynol-9 is safer than unprotected sex with no condom at all. Condom packages are required to be labeled with the expiration date of the spermicide, and they should not be used after that date. In females, frequent use of spermicides containing nonoxynol 9 can cause vaginal irritation and lesions (sores), which may actually increase the possibility of transmitting an STD from an infected partner.

LUBRICANTS

Lubricants may help prevent condoms from breaking during use. They may prevent irritation that might increase the chance of infection. Some condoms come lubricated with dry silicone, jelly, or cream, or you can add water-based lubricants specifically made for this purpose (for example, K-Y Lubricating Jelly). If you use a separate lubricant, never use a product that contains oils, fats, or greases such as a petroleum-based jelly (for example, Vaseline), baby oil or lotion, hand or body lotion, cooking shortening, or oily cosmetics such as cold creams. These can seriously weaken latex, causing a condom to tear easily. If you use a spermicide, you do not necessarily need to use a lubricant because some spermicide acts as a lubricant.

TO LEARN MORE

Centers for Disease Control and Prevention STD Hotline (800) 227-8922; website: www.cdc.gov/std.

EXERCISE AND PHYSICAL FITNESS BENEFITS

 GENERAL INFORMATION

DESCRIPTION
Exercise is a part of a healthy lifestyle at any age. It helps you feel and look better, aids in weight loss, and can lower the risk for many common diseases. Exercise can be fun—even though it may not seem fun at first. Talk to your health care provider about exercising. People who have not been active, have health problems, are pregnant, or elderly may need special advice.

REASONS PEOPLE GIVE FOR NOT EXERCISING
People have many reasons for not exercising. Look for ways to overcome the ones that affect you.
• Not enough time or exercising is inconvenient: Find available time slots. Take exercise breaks at work. Walk for 10 to 15 minutes at a time.
• Lack of energy: Plan exercise time during the day or week when you do feel more energetic. Convince yourself that exercise will actually boost your energy level.
• It is not enjoyable, or it is boring: Watch television while you exercise. Do gardening or mow the lawn. Exercise with a friend. Join an exercise class.
• Fear of injury, or have had a recent injury: Learn how to warm up and cool down. Wear proper shoes for the activity. Pick activities that have little risk.
• Lack of confidence in being able to exercise: Exercise with friends who have the same skill level. Take a class to learn a new skill. Walking is the easiest exercise.
• Not able to maintain an exercise routine due to travel for work or other conflicting schedules: Walk in hotel halls and take stairs instead of elevators. Pack stretch bands and jump rope and use them in your room. Pick places to stay with pools or fitness rooms.
• Family or friends are not supportive or encouraging: Ask your family for support. Invite family or friends to exercise with you. Join a fitness class or hiking club.
• No place to walk nearby, such as a park or sidewalks, or the weather is bad: Always have activities that you can do indoors. Exercise to a video-tape. Walk in the mall. Ride an exercise bike.
• Family obligations take too much time: Exercise with the kids, such as walking or swimming. Plan on exercising when kids are at school, playing, or sleeping.

WHAT TO DO TO GET STARTED
• Plan on making exercise or physical activity a part of your everyday life. Do things you enjoy. Many people are getting their exercise doing things such as biking, skiing and tennis. Others prefer less active recreation such as walking, gardening, or golf.
• Children and adults should try to get at least 30 to 60 minutes of exercise a day. You can break this into shorter periods of 10 or 15 minutes during the day.

PARTS OF AN EXERCISE PLAN
• Endurance: Find an activity that makes you breathe harder, on most or all days of the week. That's called "endurance activity," because it builds your stamina.
• Muscle strength: Lack of use lets muscles waste away. Start lifting weights and increase the weight slowly. This will build bone mass and help avoid osteoporosis.
• Balance: Do things to help your balance. Stand on one foot, then the other, without holding onto anything for support. Walk heel-to-toe (the toes of the foot in back should almost touch the heel of the foot in front when you walk this way).
• Stretching: It won't build endurance or muscles, but keeps you limber and flexible, and reduces injuries.

SUGGESTIONS FOR BEING ACTIVE
• Walk, cycle, jog, or skate to work, school, stores, etc. Walk during breaks at work. Keep a comfortable pair of shoes handy in your office or car.
• Park the car farther away from where you want to go.
• Take the stairs instead of the elevator.
• Play actively with children or pets.
• Garden at home, or do home repair work.
• Exercise while watching television. Ride an exercise bike, walk in place, lift weights, or stretch.

CAUTIONS
• Don't overdo the activity. Listen to your body. A few muscle aches are to be expected, but not pain.
• Start off a new routine at an easy pace. Then increase your time and effort. If you can talk without any trouble at all, your activity is probably too easy. If you can't talk at all, it's too hard.
• Use the correct equipment, especially shoes.
• Take 3 to 5 minutes to warm up (e.g., start a walk at a slow pace, and then increase to a brisk pace.
• Be aware of any warning signs of heart problems: Severe sweating, chest and arm pain, and dizziness.
• Drink plenty of water to replace any lost fluids.

APPENDIX

KEGEL EXERCISES
(Pelvic Floor Exercises)

 GENERAL INFORMATION

DESCRIPTION

- Life's events can weaken pelvic muscles. Pregnancy, childbirth, and being overweight can do it. Luckily, when these muscles get weak, you can help make them strong again.
- Pelvic floor muscles are just like other muscles. Exercise can make them stronger. Women with bladder control problems can regain control through Kegel exercises (pelvic muscle exercises).

THE PELVIC MUSCLES

- Exercising your pelvic floor muscles for just 5 minutes, three times a day can make a big difference to your bladder control. Exercise strengthens muscles that hold the bladder and many other organs in place.
- The part of your body including your hip bones is the pelvic area. At the bottom of the pelvis, several layers of muscle stretch between your legs. The muscles attach to the front, back, and sides of the pelvis bone.
- Two pelvic muscles do most of the work. The biggest one stretches like a hammock. The other is shaped like a triangle. These muscles prevent leaking of urine and stool.
- You can make these pelvic floor muscles stronger with a few minutes of exercise every day.

DOING THE EXERCISES

- Find the right muscles. This is very important. Your doctor, nurse, or physical therapist will help make sure you are doing the exercises the right way.
- You should tighten the two major muscles that stretch across your pelvic floor. They are the "hammock" muscle and the "triangle" muscle. Here are three methods to check for the correct muscles.

   1. Try to stop the flow of urine when you are sitting on the toilet. If you can do it, you are using the right muscles.

   2. Imagine that you are trying to stop passing gas. Squeeze the muscles you would use. If you sense a "pulling" feeling, those are the right muscles for pelvic exercises.

   3. Lie down and put your finger inside your vagina. Squeeze as if you were trying to stop urine from coming out. If you feel tightness on your finger, you are squeezing the right pelvic muscle.
- Don't squeeze other muscles at the same time. Be careful not to tighten your stomach, legs, or other muscles. Squeezing the wrong muscles can put more pressure on your bladder control muscles. Just squeeze the pelvic muscle. Don't hold your breath.
- Repeat, but don't overdo it. At first, find a quiet spot to practice—your bathroom or bedroom—so you can concentrate. Lie on the floor. Pull in the pelvic muscles and hold for a count of 3. Then relax for a count of 3. Work up to 10 to 15 repeats each time you exercise. Healthy sphincter muscles can keep the urethra closed.
- Do your pelvic exercises at least three times a day. Every day, use three positions: lying down, sitting, and standing. You can exercise while lying on the floor, sitting at a desk, or standing in the kitchen. Using all three positions makes the muscles strongest.
- Be patient. Don't give up. It's just 5 minutes, three times a day. You may not feel your bladder control improve until after 3 to 6 weeks. Still, most women do notice an improvement after a few weeks.
- Exercise aids. You can also exercise by using special weights or biofeedback. Ask your health care provider about these exercise aids.

HOLD THE SQUEEZE UNTIL AFTER THE SNEEZE

- You can protect your pelvic muscles from more damage by bracing yourself.
- Think ahead just before sneezing, lifting, or jumping. Sudden pressure from such actions can hurt those pelvic muscles. Squeeze your pelvic muscles tightly and hold on until after you sneeze, lift, or jump.
- After you train yourself to tighten the pelvic muscles for these moments, you will have fewer accidents.

POINTS TO REMEMBER

- Weak pelvic muscles often cause bladder control problems.
- Daily exercises can strengthen pelvic muscles.
- These exercises often improve bladder control.
- Ask your health care provider or nurse if you are squeezing the right muscles.
- Tighten your pelvic muscles before sneezing, lifting, or jumping. This can prevent pelvic muscle damage.

R.I.C.E. THERAPY

 GENERAL INFORMATION

R.I.C.E. is an acronym (a word coined from first letters) for the most important elements—rest, ice, compression and elevation—in first aid for many injuries. This acronym appears in medical information in reference to athletic injuries. Use the word R.I.C.E. to jog your memory if you have injuries, such as contusions, sprains, strains, dislocations, or uncomplicated fractures.

REST
Stop using the injured part, and rest it (for about 48 hours) as soon as you realize an injury has taken place. Continued exercise or other activity could cause further injury, delay healing, increase pain, and risk bleeding. Use crutches to avoid bearing weight on injuries of the foot, ankle, knee, or leg. Use splints for injuries of the hand, wrist, elbow or arm. After medical care, the injured part may require immobilization with splints or a cast to keep the area at rest until it heals.

ICE
Ice helps stop internal bleeding from injured blood vessels. Sudden cold causes small blood vessels to contract. This contraction of blood vessels decreases the amount of blood that can collect around the wound. The more blood that collects, the longer the healing time. Ice can be safely applied in several ways using the following instructions:
- For injury to a small area, such as a finger, toe, foot, or wrist, immerse the injured area in a bucket of ice water. Use ice cubes to keep the water cold, as ice dissolves.
- For injury to a larger area, use ice packs. Avoid placing ice directly on the skin. Before applying the ice, place a towel, cloth, or one or two layers of an elasticized compression bandage (Ace bandage) on the skin to be iced. To make the ice pack, put ice chips or ice cubes in a plastic bag, or wrap them in a thin towel. Place the ice pack over the cloth. The pack may sit directly on the injured part, or it may be wrapped in place.
- Ice the injured area for about 20 minutes at a time.
- Repeat the icing four to eight times a day, while following the instructions below for compression and elevation. After 48 to 72 hours, you may add heat as a treatment. Or you might try both. Alternate five minutes of hot water with five minutes of ice water. Continue to ice the injured area until it is healed.

COMPRESSION
Compression decreases swelling by slowing the bleeding and limiting the accumulation of blood near the injured site. Without compression, fluid from adjacent normal tissues seeps into the injury area. The more blood and fluid that accumulate around an injury, the slower the healing. The following are instructions for safely applying compression to an injury:
- Use an elasticized bandage (Ace bandage) for compression, if possible. If you do not have one available, any kind of cloth will suffice for a short time. Wrap the injured part firmly, wrapping over the ice also. Begin wrapping below the injury site, and extend above the injury site.
- Be careful not to compress the area so tightly that the blood supply is impaired. Signs of deprived blood supply include pain, numbness, cramping, and blue or dusky-colored nails. Remove the compression bandage immediately if any of these symptoms appear. Leave the bandage off until all signs of impaired circulation disappear. Then rewrap the area—less tightly this time.

ELEVATION
Elevating the injured part to, or above, the level of the heart is another way to decrease swelling and pain at the injury site. Elevate the iced, compressed area in whatever way is most convenient. Prop an injured leg on solid objects or pillows. Elevate an injured arm by lying down and placing pillows under the arm or placing them on the chest with the arm folded across. The whole upper part of the body may be elevated gently with pillows or a reclining chair or by raising the head of the bed on blocks.

SAFE USE OF MEDICINE

LIST FOR SAFER DRUG USE
These suggestions for wise, safe use of medicine apply to all medicines.

INFORMATION YOU SHOULD PROVIDE
Always give the information listed in 1 and 2 below to your doctor, dentist, or other health care provider so that they can prescribe drugs properly:

    1. Your medical history: Tell the important facts of your medical history dealing with drugs. Include allergic reactions, side effects, or adverse reactions you have experienced in the past. Describe the allergic problems you have such as hay fever, asthma, eye watering and itching, throat irritation, and reactions to food. People who have allergies to common substances are more likely to develop side effects or adverse reactions to drugs.

    2. Drugs you are taking now: List all prescription and nonprescription drugs. Don't forget common ones such as laxatives; herbal, vitamin, or mineral supplements; skin, rectal, vaginal drugs; antacids; antihistamines; cold and cough remedies; aspirin and aspirin-containing pain pills; motion sickness remedies; weight-loss aids; salt and sugar substitutes; caffeine (in coffee, tea, cola drinks, and cocoa); oral contraceptives; sleeping pills; or "tonics."

INFORMATION TO KNOW BEFORE TAKING A DRUG
* Generic names and brand names of all the drugs you take. Write them down to help you remember. If a drug is a mixture of two or more generic ingredients, learn the names of each.
* Uses for each drug you take.
* How to take each drug—for example, with or without water, or with or without food.
* When to take it.
* What to do if you forget a dose.
* How each drug works in your body.
* Time lapse before drug works.
* Symptoms and treatment of overdose.
* Possible adverse reactions and side effects and what to do if they occur.
* Interactions with other drugs and other substances such as alcohol, food, beverages, cocaine, marijuana, and tobacco. When mixed, they can sometimes cause serious interactions.
* Know all warnings and precautions that apply to special circumstances, such as the following:

    1. Reasons (called contraindications) not to take the drug in the presence of some medical conditions.

    2. Special considerations for elderly patients, pregnant or breast-feeding women, infants, and children.

    3. Information about long-term use, exposure to sun and sunlight, driving, piloting aircraft, hazardous work, or flying in airplanes.

    4. Instructions before discontinuing the drug.

OTHER SAFETY TIPS
* Before taking any prescribed drug, discuss plans with the doctor that you may have for elective surgery, pregnancy, and breast-feeding.
* Don't hesitate to ask questions about a drug. We will be able to provide more information if we are familiar with you and your past medical history, especially regarding drugs.
* Never take a drug in the dark! It is always possible to take the wrong one. Recheck the label before each drug use.
* Notify our office about any new or unexpected symptoms you develop while taking a drug. You may need to change drugs or have a dose adjustment.
* Store all drugs out of children's reach. Keep drugs in a cool, dry place, such as a kitchen cabinet or bedroom. Avoid medicine cabinets in bathrooms—they get too moist and warm at times. Keep drugs in their original containers, tightly closed. Don't remove the labels! If directions call for refrigeration, keep the drug cool, but don't freeze it.
* Don't save leftover drugs to use later. Discard them on or before the expiration date shown on the label.
* Do not flush old drugs down the toilet or dispose in a drain. Doing so may result in traces of the drug seeping into the water supply. Throw the drugs in the trash, packaged in childproof containers and/or sealed plastic bags (out of the reach of children and pets). Another option is to check if local household hazardous-waste collection programs—where you're supposed to take motor oil and batteries—accept expired drugs.
* Don't take any drug prescribed for someone else.
* Prior to any surgery (including oral surgery or simple dental procedures), tell the doctor or dentist about all drugs you take or have taken in the past few weeks.
* If you become pregnant while taking any drug, tell your health care provider right away. Avoid all drugs when you are pregnant, if possible.

SEXUALLY TRANSMITTED DISEASES

 GENERAL INFORMATION

STD FACTS
- Sexually transmitted diseases (STDs) affect more than 12 million men and women in the United States each year. Many are teenagers or young adults.
- Using drugs or alcohol increases your chances of getting STDs. These substances can interfere with your judgment and your ability to use a condom correctly.
- Intravenous (IV) drug use puts a person at higher risk for human immunodeficiency virus (HIV) and hepatitis B, because IV drug users usually share needles.
- The more sexual partners you have, the higher your chance of being exposed to HIV or other STDs. This is because it is difficult to know if a person is infected, or has had sex with people who are more likely to be infected due to IV drug use or other risk factors.
- Sometimes, early in an infection, there may be no symptoms. Also, symptoms may be easily confused with other illnesses.
- You can not tell by looking at someone whether he or she is infected with HIV or another STD.
- Sexually transmitted diseases include HIV, chancroid, chlamydial infections, trichomoniasis, genital herpes, pubic lice, genital warts, gonorrhea, lymphogranuloma venereum, syphilis, viral hepatitis, scabies, candidiasis, molluscum contagiosum, and others.

STDs CAN CAUSE
- Pelvic inflammatory disease (PID). It can damage a woman's fallopian tubes and result in pelvic pain and being unable to have children.
- Tubal pregnancies (where pregnancy grows in the fallopian tube instead of the womb). It is sometimes fatal to the mother and always fatal to the fetus.
- Sterility—the inability to have children—in both men and women.
- Cancer of the cervix in women.
- Damage to major organs, such as the heart, kidney, and brain, if STDs go untreated.
- Death (e.g., with HIV infection).

RISKS
High-risk behaviors include having sex—vaginal, anal, or oral—with:
- A person who has an STD. This is the most risky behavior. If you know your partner is infected, avoid intercourse (including oral sex). If you do decide to have sex with an infected person, always be sure to use a new condom from start to finish, every time.
- Someone who has shared needles to inject drugs with an infected person.
- Someone with a past partner(s) who was/were infected. If your partner had sexual contact with a person infected with HIV, he or she could pass it on to you. This can happen even if the prior sexual contact was a long time ago—as long as 10 years. Your partner may seem perfectly healthy. HIV can be in the body a long time before a person feels sick.

PREVENTION
- Reduce the chance of being infected with HIV or other STDs. People who take part in risky sexual behavior should always use a condom.
- Use of a condom is also important for an uninfected pregnant woman. It can help protect her and her unborn child from STDs.

SEE A HEALTH CARE PROVIDER IF YOU HAVE ANY OF THESE STD SYMPTOMS
- Discharge from the vagina, penis, or rectum.
- Pain or burning during urination or intercourse.
- Pain in the abdomen (women), testicles (men), and buttocks and legs (both men and women).
- Blisters, open sores, warts, rash, or swelling in the genital or anal area, or the mouth.
- Persistent, flu-like symptoms. These include fever, headache, aching muscles, or swollen glands. These symptoms may precede STD symptoms.

ADDITIONAL RESOURCES FOR INFORMATION
- National AIDS Hotline (800) 342-2437; website: www.cdc.gov/hiv/dhap.htm.
- Sexually Transmitted Diseases Hotline (800) 227-8922.

APPENDIX

SKIN SELF-EXAMINATION

GENERAL INFORMATION

Skin self-exam means checking your own skin regularly for any abnormal growths or unusual changes. This helps you detect and treat skin cancer (or other skin abnormalities) as early as possible. Two types of skin cancer (basal cell carcinoma and squamous cell carcinoma) are almost always cured once correctly diagnosed. With melanoma (the most serious type of skin cancer), early diagnosis is essential to start treatment before it spreads.

The National Cancer Institute (NCI) and the American Academy of Dermatology (AAD) recommend that people should perform a skin self-exam once a month. It may take about 10 to 15 minutes. Along with your self-exam, always practice sun-protection care by using a sunscreen (SPF of 15 or higher) with both UVA and UVB protection. Wear protective clothing, and limit exposure time to the sun.

Get to know your skin, so you know what is normal for you. The first time you do the self-examination, locate all moles, warts, birthmarks, scars, spots, bumps, lumps, or other skin markings. It may be difficult to remember the color, shape, and size of each, so you may want to write down the information or draw a sketch of each area and abnormality.

HOW THE TEST IS PERFORMED
• The easiest time to do the exam may be after you take a bath or shower. Women may wish to perform their skin self-exam at the same time that they perform their monthly breast self-exam.
• Ideally, the room should have a full-length mirror and bright lights so that you can see your entire body well. Use a hand-held mirror also. It is very important to be able to examine all areas of your skin, including hard-to-see areas, such as the genitals, buttocks, scalp, and back.

WHEN YOU ARE PERFORMING THE TEST, LOOK FOR:
• New skin markings (e.g., moles, blemishes, colorations, bumps).
• Moles that have changed their size, texture, color, or shape.
• Moles or lesions that won't heal or that continue to bleed.
• Moles with ragged edges, differences in colors, or lack of symmetry.
• Observe and examine your entire body, both front and back, in the mirror.
• Check under your arms and both sides of each arm.
• Examine your forearms after bending your arms at the elbows, and then look at the palms of your hands and underneath your upper arms.
• Look at the front and back of both legs.
• Look at your buttocks and between your buttocks.
• Examine your genital area.
• Observe your face, neck, back of neck, and scalp. It is best to use both a hand mirror and full-length mirror, along with a comb, to see areas of your scalp.
• Look at your feet, including the soles and the space between your toes.
• Have a partner, friend, or relative help by examining hard-to-see areas. You may want to them to take photographs of your body (or certain moles) every six months to one year. Sometimes it is difficult to tell if a mole has grown or changed, or a new one has developed, and a photo may help.

STRESS, HOW TO COPE

 GENERAL INFORMATION

CAUSES OF STRESS
• There are numerous ways to reduce stress in your life; the correct answer is finding what works for you. A certain amount of stress is not always bad. It varies from person to person how much stress one can handle easily. Sometimes, stress can push us on to greater achievement. But excessive stress or chronic stress can be self-defeating. Many health professionals believe that stress has a role in almost any disorder. Stress can complicate an illness by preventing normal recovery, prolonging pain, and adding to disability.
• Reducing stress could be as simple has adding exercise to your daily routine or making new friends. To make the most of your life, limit your stress, and for that stress that you cannot avoid, learn to manage it.

TIPS FOR COPING
   Here are some tips that may help you reduce stress:
• Learn a meditation technique and practice it regularly—daily if possible. There are many methods available. Most of them include "tuning in to" and giving complete attention to a word, sound, sentence, or concept that you silently repeat to yourself. Don't try to banish other thoughts that enter your mind during your period of concentration, but don't focus on them enough to stop you from meditating. The purpose of meditation is to empty your mind of all disturbing thoughts for a given period of time to aid in mental relaxation. Mental relaxation, in turn, will help reduce stress.
• Take a short period of time away from any stressful situation you meet up with during a day. Practice a muscle-tensing and muscle-relaxing technique. Close your eyes. Take a series of deep breaths. Then start with the muscle groups in your face. Consciously tense them and hold the tension for a few seconds. Then consciously relax them. Continue through all major muscle groups in the body: neck, shoulders, hands, abdomen, back, and legs. You can use this technique to help you relax quickly any time you need to.
• Begin an exercise program. People who are physically fit are less likely to suffer the negative effects of stress, anxiety, or depression. One form of exercise is yoga. Yoga involves both stretching exercises and deep breathing techniques. However, any form of exercise is helpful in reducing the affects of stress on the body.
• Humor is another way of dealing with stress. Having the ability to find humor in a stressful situation and being able to laugh about it releases all the tension that is building inside. Even if the situation cannot be made light of, think of something else that will make you laugh.
• Healthy lifestyle changes can reduce the level of stress. A few suggestions include reducing caffeine intake, making new friends, eating healthy, and avoiding alcohol. Healthy lifestyle changes can help manage the stress as well as improve your overall well being.
• Get enough sleep. Avoid taking your problems to bed with you. At the end of the day, spend a few minutes going back over your entire day's experiences, event by event, as if you're replaying a tape. Release all negative emotions you have built up (anger, feelings of insecurity or anxiety). Relish all good energy or emotion (loving thoughts, praise, feeling good about your work or yourself). Reach a decision about undone events, and release mental or muscular tension. Now you're ready for a relaxing and emotionally healing sleep.
• Avoid self-medication or escape. Alcohol or other drugs of abuse can mask stress. They don't help deal with the problem.
• Set realistic goals for yourself. Reduce the number of events going on in your life and you may reduce the feeling of being overloaded.
• Don't overwhelm yourself by fretting about your entire workload. Handle each task as it comes, or selectively deal with matters in some priority.
• Do something for others to help get your mind off yourself.
• Avoid extreme reactions. Think about disliking something rather than hating it. Be a little nervous, not anxious. Don't be full of rage when anger will do the job. Don't be depressed when you can just be sad.
• Try to be positive. Give yourself messages as to how well you can cope rather than how horrible everything is going to be.
• Keep a stress diary. Write down stressful events, how they made you feel, what caused the event, and how you coped. On a scale of 0 (very relaxed) to 10 (extremely stressed), put down a number for your stress level.
• Research has shown that cognitive-behavioral therapy can be effective in reducing stress. Ask your health care provider about this option.

TESTICULAR SELF-EXAMINATION

GENERAL INFORMATION

This is an exam of the testicles to look for lumps that may be testicular cancer. The testicles are the male reproductive organs, and produce sperm and the hormone testosterone. They are located in the scrotum under the penis.

The exam should be performed on a monthly basis, especially if you have a family history of this cancer, have had a previous testicular tumor, or have an undescended testicle.

NORMAL TESTICLES
Each testicle should feel firm but not rock hard. One testicle may or may not be lower or slightly larger than the other. Normal testicles contain blood vessels and other structures that can make the exam confusing. Performing the self-exam monthly allows you to become familiar with your normal anatomy. Then, if you notice any changes from the previous exam, this will alert you to contact your health care provider. Always ask you health care provider if you have any doubts or questions.

HOW THE TEST IS PERFORMED
• Perform this test during or after a shower. This way, the scrotal skin is warm and relaxed. The test is best done while standing.

   1. Gently feel your scrotal sac to locate a testicle.

   2. Firmly, but gently roll the testicle between the thumb and fingers of both hands to examine the entire surface. Feel the testicle for lumps, swellings, or other changes in consistency.

   3. Repeat the procedure with the other testicle.

• Examine the epididymis for lumps. This is a rope-like cord that is located behind each testicle. This area is fairly tender, so be cautious with your touch.

• Examine the spermatic cord for lumps. This is the sperm-carrying tube that extends from the epididymis of each testicle.

ABNORMAL FINDINGS
A lump, swelling, or other change on the testicle, epididymis, or spermatic cord may be the first sign of testicular cancer. Therefore, if you find a lump, see a health care provider right away. Keep in mind that some cases of testicular cancer do not show symptoms until they reach an advanced stage.

CALL YOUR HEALTH CARE PROVIDER IF:
• You find a small hard lump (like a pea), have an enlarged testicle, or notice any other differences from your last self-exam.

• You can't find one or both testicles. The testicles may not have descended properly in the scrotum.

• There is a soft collection of thin tubes above the testicle. It may be a collection of dilated veins (varicocele).

• There is pain or swelling in the scrotum. It may be an infection or a fluid-filled sac (hydrocele) causing blockage of blood flow to the area.

• Acute pain in the scrotum or testicle is a surgical emergency. If you experience acute pain in the scrotum or testicle, seek immediate medical help.

Glossary

Introduction to the Glossary

The glossary contains brief definitions and/or descriptions of medical-related words and terminology. This includes easy-to-understand explanations about medical tests and medical abbreviations that are used throughout the book.

In addition, the glossary provides a brief description of some rare illnesses and disorders that are not covered in the other sections due to lack of space.

A

Abdominal Aorta—Section of the aorta that passes through the abdomen to supply blood to the lower part of the body.

Abscess—Swollen, inflamed, tender area of infection containing pus.

Accident Proneness—Tendency of some persons to have more accidents than normal. It may be due to a risk factor such as poor vision, but unconscious factors are often the cause.

Acetaminophen—Nonprescription medication used to relieve minor pain and to reduce fever. Its analgesic effects are similar to aspirin, but it does not reduce inflammation or swelling. It is less irritating to the stomach than aspirin.

Achalasia—Condition of the esophagus that disrupts normal swallowing.

Acquired Immune Deficiency Syndrome, Acquired Immunodeficiency Syndrome, AIDS—A disease of the human immune system that is caused by infection with HIV (human immunodeficiency virus).

Acupuncture—Method of anesthesia and treatment of pain developed by the Chinese. Needles are inserted through the skin to stimulate precise areas.

Acute—Beginning suddenly; also severe, but of short duration.

Addiction—Intense craving for substances such as alcohol, tobacco or narcotics, or a compulsive behavior such as gambling.

Adenoids—Infection-fighting tissue (part of the lymphatic system) in the upper throat, near the tonsils.

Adenoids, Enlarged—Adenoids that have swollen and impaired speech.

Adenovirus—Group of viruses that cause certain respiratory and eye infections.

Adhesions—Small strands of fibrous tissue that cause organs in the abdomen and pelvis to cling together abnormally, creating a risk of intestinal obstruction.

Adolescence—Time of life from the beginning of puberty until maturity.

Adrenal Glands—Two glands attached to the kidneys. Each has an outer layer (cortex) that produces steroid hormones and an inner layer (medulla) that produces adrenalin.

Adrenalin—Hormone produced by the adrenal glands that increases heart rate and prepares the body for crisis. Also called epinephrine.

Aging—The normal process of gradual physical and mental decline.

AIDS—*See Acquired Immune Deficiency Syndrome*.

Airways—Tubular passages that air passes through to the lungs: the trachea (windpipe), bronchi and bronchioles.

Alcoholic Cirrhosis—Widespread destruction of normal liver tissue caused by excessive intake of alcohol.

Alveoli—Lung cells at ends of the airways where oxygen enters the blood and waste gases leave the blood.

Ambulatory Medical Center—A health-care facility for patients who do not require prolonged bed rest or hospitalization.

Amniocentesis—The extraction and examination of a small amount of amniotic fluid in order to determine genetic and other disorders in the unborn child.

Amniotic Sac—The thin, transparent membrane filled with fluid in which the fetus lives until born.

Amphetamine Drugs—Habit-forming drugs that stimulate the brain and central nervous system, increase blood pressure, reduce nasal stuffiness or suppress appetite.

Amyloid Deposits—Abnormal protein material deposited in tissues, usually caused by diseases. These deposits cause impairment of certain organs.

Analgesics—Medications that relieve pain.

Anemia—Condition in which red blood cells or hemoglobin (oxygen-carrying substance in blood) is inadequate.

Anesthesia, General—Causing temporary loss of consciousness and inability to feel pain by use of inhaled gases or injected anesthetics.

Anesthesia, Local (Nerve Block)—Injection of the local anesthetic near the nerves of the surgical area.

Anesthesia, Local—Temporary prevention of pain by injecting medication (local anesthetic).

Aneurysm—Abnormal swelling or ballooning of a blood vessel.

Angina—Pain or pressure beneath the breastbone caused by inadequate blood supply to the heart.

Angiogram, Angiography—Study of arteries and veins by injecting material into them that x-rays can outline.

Anoscopy—Visual examination of the anus by means of a short tube called an anoscope, an optical instrument with lenses and a lighted tip.

Antacid—Medicine taken orally that reduces or neutralizes stomach acid.

Anti-inflammatory Drugs—Medications used to control inflammation not caused by infection.

Anti-arrhythmics—Medications used to treat heartbeat irregularities (arrhythmias).

Antibiotics—Medications that attack germs and fight infection.

Antibiotics, Cephalosporin—Class of antibiotics related to penicillin, capable of destroying more kinds of germs than penicillin.

Antibiotics, Erythromycin—Class of antibiotics that destroys germs similar to those destroyed by penicillin. Often used to treat infections in patients who are allergic to penicillin.

Antibodies—Proteins created in blood and body tissue by the immune system to neutralize or destroy sources of disease.

Anticancer Drugs—Medications that weaken or destroy cancerous tissues without harming healthy tissues.

Anticholinergic Drugs—Medications that reduce nerve impulses in the parasympathetic nervous system. They control some activities of the gastrointestinal system, heart, bladder and other organs.

Anticoagulants—Medications that slow or delay blood clotting.

Anticonvulsants—Medications that control seizures (convulsions), pain or conditions in which the brain or nerves are overly sensitive.

Antidepressants—Medications that help control depression.

Antiemetic Drugs—Medications that prevent or stop nausea and vomiting.

Antifungal Drugs—Medications used to treat fungus diseases.

Antigens—Germs or other sources of disease that antibodies (produced by the immune system) neutralize or destroy.

Antihelmintic Drugs—Medications used to treat worms in the intestines.

Antihistamines—Medications used to treat allergies.

Antihyperlipidemic Drugs—Medications that reduce fat (cholesterol) in the blood. They help prevent blood-vessel disease.

Antihypertensives—Medications used to reduce blood pressure.

Antimalarial Drugs—Medications used to prevent or treat malaria.

Antimetabolite Drugs—Medications that are used to treat some cancers and autoimmune diseases.

Antimicrobial Drugs—Same as *Antibiotics*.

Antinuclear Antibody—Substance that appears in the blood, indicating presence of an autoimmune disease.

Antiparkinsonian Drugs—Medications used to treat Parkinson's disease.

Antiprotozoal Drugs—Medications used in treatment of single-celled parasites (protozoa).

Antipruritic Drugs—Medications that reduce itching.

Antispasmodic Drugs—Medications that improve digestion and relieve intestinal cramps.

Antistreptococcal Titer—Blood test that measures body's response to infection by streptococcal bacteria.

Antithyroid Drugs—Medications used to counter the effects of an overactive thyroid gland.

Antiviral Drugs—Medications used to treat infections caused by viruses.

Anus—A muscular band at the end of the rectum that opens and expands to allow passage of feces.

Anus, Imperforate—Congenital abnormality of newborn infants in which the anus cannot pass feces.

Anxiety—Uncomfortable feeling that something unpleasant or dangerous will happen.

Aorta—Body's largest blood vessel, arising from the top of the heart. It carries blood from the heart to all parts of the body.

Aphrodisiac—Substance claimed to increase sexual arousal or pleasure.

Appendage—Body part that has a minor role (or no role at all) in normal body function. For example, the appendix is an appendage to the colon that seems to have no function.

Arteriogram, Arteriography—Studying arteries by injecting material into them that x-rays can outline.

Arteriosclerosis—Hardening of the arteries.

Arterial Doppler Studies—Measurement of blood flow through the arteries by means of doppler ultrasound.

Artery—Blood vessels that carry blood from the heart to the body.

Arthrograms—X-rays of the joints taken with an arthroscope.

Arthroscope—Slender optical instrument with a lighted tip that allows direct visual examination of some joints. It can also be used to correct some defects in joints.

Artificial Limbs—Mechanical substitutions for amputated arms or legs.

Ascending Colon—First part of the large colon (intestine) extending from the lower end of the small intestine.

Aspiration—1) Removal of accumulated pus or fluid with a needle. 2) Accidental inhalation of objects or fluids into the lungs.

Astigmatism—Visual impairment caused by abnormal eye shape.

Asymmetrical—Uneven in size, shape or position.

Atelectasis—Collapse of the expanded lung.

Atriums—Small chambers in the heart that pump blood into the ventricles. Also called auricles.

Atropine—Medication used to treat diseases of the eye, heart, gastrointestinal system and nervous system.

Audiogram, Audiometry—Test of hearing ability.

Autism—Mental illness of children in which they seem unaware of their surroundings.

Autoimmune Assays (ANA Tests)—Blood tests to identify autoimmune disease.

Autoimmune Disorder—Disease in which the immune system produces antibodies that attack the body's own tissues.

Autoimmune, Autoimmunity—Disease in which a person's immune system attacks its own tissues.

Autonomic Nervous System—Part of the nervous system that controls organs that function involuntarily, such as the heart, lungs, digestive system and blood vessels.

B

Bacteria—One-celled micro-organisms that can sometimes cause disease.

Balloon Angioplasty—Treatment for obstructed arteries, especially those supplying blood to the heart and brain. A small uninflated balloon is passed up the artery to the obstruction, and then expanded to release the obstruction.

Barium Enema—See *Barium X-rays*.

Barium X-Rays—Examining the gastrointestinal system by filling it with a barium solution that is detected by x-rays. Common barium tests are the barium swallow (upper GI series) and the barium enema (lower GI series).

Bartholin's Glands—Small glands in the lips of the vagina that secrete a lubricating fluid, especially during sexual arousal.

Behavior Therapy—Psychotherapy that focuses on ways to change the undesired behavior.

Belladonna—Medication derived from a plant used to treat some diseases of the gastrointestinal system. It is similar to atropine.

Benign—1) Tumor or growth that is neither cancerous nor located where it

might impair normal function. 2) Harmless.

Beta-Adrenergic Blockers (Beta-Blockers)—Medications that reduce heart or blood-vessel overactivity to improve blood circulation. Also used to prevent migraine headaches, high blood pressure and angina.

Bile Duct—A small tube that allows bile to pass from the gallbladder into the intestines.

Bile—A digestive juice produced in the liver and stored in the gallbladder. Bile empties into the small intestine for digestive processes.

Biliary Cirrhosis—Cirrhosis of the liver due to inflammation or obstruction of the bile ducts.

Bilirubin—A yellowish, red-blood-cell waste product in bile that the blood carries to the liver. It contributes to urine's yellowish color and can cause jaundice if it builds up in the blood.

Biopsy—Removal of a small amount of tissue or cells (such as fluid from a cyst) for laboratory examination that aids in diagnosis. The tissue sample may be removed by a variety of methods depending on the site to be biopsied.

Biopsy Needle—Instrument often used to perform a biopsy.

Biopsy, Skin—Removal of a sample of skin tissue for laboratory examination that aids in diagnosis. Skin biopsy is often required to confirm a clinical (visual) diagnosis. Removal techniques include shave excision, punch excision and elliptical excision.

Birth Canal—Passageway through the cervix and the vagina through which the baby passes during childbirth.

Bladder—An organ that holds fluids such as urine (urinary bladder) or bile (gallbladder).

Blood Cells, Red—Microscopic cells in the blood that carry oxygen to tissues of the body. One drop of blood contains about 200 million red cells.

Blood Cells, White—Microscopic cells in the blood that help fight infection by destroying germs. One drop of blood contains about 400,000 white cells.

Blood Chemistries—Tests that measure chemicals in the blood.

Blood Count—Counting red and white blood cells to aid in diagnosis of many diseases.

Blood Platelets—See *Platelet Count*.

Blood Studies—Examination of a blood sample to measure white blood cells, red blood cells, hemoglobin, hematocrit and chemical substances. See *Blood Chemistries*.

Blood Vessels—Arteries, veins and capillaries; the tubes in which blood circulates through the body.

Bone Bank—Facility where human bone is stored and made available for transplantation.

Bone Scan—Method of studying the bone structure or function by injecting into the bloodstream a medication that can be detected by a special scanning camera.

Bone Spurs—Abnormal and sometimes painful protrusions of bone with sharp points near joints or tendons.

Bronchial Tubes (Bronchi)—Hollow air passageways that branch from the windpipe (trachea) into the lungs. They carry oxygen into the lungs and pass waste gases (mostly carbon dioxide) out of the body.

Bronchioles—Small air passageways that serve the same purpose as bronchial tubes. Bronchioles are the smallest parts of the respiratory system.

Bronchodilator Drugs—Medications used to treat diseases of the bronchi that cause shortness of breath, such as asthma. The medicines help constricted tubes to relax.

Bronchogram—Diagnosing lung diseases by placing a material in the lung that x-rays can outline.

Bronchoscope, Bronchoscopy—An optical instrument with a lighted tip that is passed into the windpipe, then into the bronchi.

Bruising—Discoloration under the skin caused by injury or bleeding.

C

Calcification—A process in which calcium from the blood is deposited abnormally into tissues due to injury, infection or aging. Often it is part of healing and not a sign of active disease.

Calcium-Channel Blocker Drugs—Medication used to treat angina, hypertension and heartbeat irregularities.

Cancerous Growths—Extensions of cancerous tissues that invade nearby healthy tissues.

Cancers—Destructive tumors that can arise in almost all parts of the body. Cancer can destroy nearby healthy tissue and may spread to distant organs.

Capillaries—Microscopic vessels that supply all body cells and tissues with blood.

Carbohydrates, Complex—Starches, sugars, cellulose and gums. Complex carbohydrates are those contained in whole grains, fresh fruits and fresh vegetables. These are considered more nutritious than simple carbohydrates.

Carbohydrates, Simple—Refined carbohydrates (sugars) that have lower molecular weights than complex carbohydrates. They produce a quick rise in blood-sugar levels. Most nutrition counselors recommend that daily diets contain minimal amounts of refined sugars. So-called "junk foods" are frequently very high in simple carbohydrates.

Cardiac Catheter—A slender tube that is inserted into an artery or vein and then passed into the heart. It is used to examine the heart and nearby blood vessels by injecting material into the heart that x-rays can detect.

Cardiac Catheterization—Studying heart function with a cardiac catheter.

Cardiac Monitoring—see ECG

Cardiac Output—The volume of blood ejected from the left side of the heart in a one minute period.

Cardiopulmonary Resuscitation (CPR)—Emergency treatment for a patient whose heart has stopped (cardiac arrest).

Cardiovascular—Relating to the heart and blood vessels.

Cardiovascular Surgeon—Doctor specially trained to operate on the heart and blood vessels.

Cardiovascular System—System that supplies the body with blood. It consists of the heart and blood vessels (arteries, capillaries, veins).

Carotid Arteries—Large arteries that supply much of the blood to the brain.

Cartilage—Rubbery, dense connective tissue that permits smooth movement of joints. It also helps shape flexible parts of the nose and external ear.

Caruncle—Small, red protrusion of tissue near a body opening. The most common caruncles arise from the urethra or cervix.

CAT Scan—See *CT Scan.*

Catheter—A hollow tube used to introduce fluids into the body or to drain fluids away.

Catheterization—Any procedure in which a small flexible tube is inserted into the body for the purpose of withdrawing or introducing substances. It most often involves the passage of a small catheter through a vein in the arm or leg or the neck and into the heart for securing blood samples or to detect problems.

Caudal Anesthesia—Form of local (low-spinal) anesthesia used to reduce pain during childbirth and surgery on pelvic areas.

Cauterant—Chemical used to destroy abnormal or diseased cells on the skin.

Cauterization—Destruction of tissue by burning or searing it with a red-hot instrument, caustic chemicals or electricity.

Cautery—Destroying small areas of diseased tissue by burning with an electric needle or laser beam, freezing with low-temperature instruments or using a chemical that destroys tissue.

Cecum—The part of the intestinal tract at the beginning of the large colon (intestine).

Central Nervous System—System that controls the body's voluntary acts. It consists of the brain and spinal cord.

Cervical Spine—Bones in the neck at the top of the spinal column.

Cervix—Lower third of the uterus, which protrudes into the vagina.

Cesarean Section—Delivery of a baby through incisions in the mother's abdomen and uterus. It is performed when normal vaginal delivery would be dangerous for the mother or baby.

Chancre—Hard, slightly ulcerated, painless lesion that forms where syphilis enters the body, usually on the genital lips.

Chemocautery—Destruction of abnormal tissue by means of acids, caustics or poisons.

Chemotherapy—Treatment of cancer by injecting medications that kill cancer cells without harming healthy tissue. It is used to treat cancers that cannot be completely cured or treated with surgery or radiation.

Chiggers—Small red biting insects. Also called "red bugs."

Child—Person in the first 10 years of life.

Chiropractor—Practitioner of chiropractic treatment of disease, which involves massage and manipulations to restore normal body functions.

Chokes—Severe breathing difficulty experienced by scuba divers and others who go from high to normal air pressure too rapidly. Bubbles of nitrogen develop in the blood stream and obstruct blood supply to vital organs, sometimes resulting in severe injury or death.

Cholangiogram, Cholangiography— X-ray procedures to diagnose diseases of the bile system (liver, gallbladder, bile ducts). Special medications are used to make the bile system visible on x-rays.

Cholecystectomy—Surgical removal of the gallbladder.

Cholecystography—An x-ray of the gallbladder.

Cholera—Acute, severe, infectious disease causing extreme diarrhea and dehydration.

Choroiditis—Inflammation of the part of the eye that supports the retina and supplies blood to it.

Chromosome—Structures inside the nucleus of living cells that contain hereditary information. Defects in chromosomes cause many birth defects and inherited diseases.

Chronic—Long-term, continuing. Chronic illnesses are usually not curable, but they can often be prevented from worsening. Symptoms usually can be controlled.

Cinematography—Form of motion-picture photography used to record a fast-moving series of x-ray images.

Circulatory System—The system that provides blood to the body, consisting of the heart, arteries, veins and lymphatic system.

Cirrhosis—Chronic scarring of the liver, leading to loss of normal liver function.

Clinician—Health-care professional who has direct contact with patients. The word literally means "someone who is at the patient's bedside."

Clips—See *Skin Clips*.

Clot Retraction Test—Measurement of the time necessary for a tube of blood to form a clot. Abnormal results often indicate a defect in blood platelets, cells important in blood coagulation.

Clotting—Activity of the blood and blood vessels that cause blood to form a jellylike clot, usually near an injury. Clotting helps stop bleeding. The body's clotting mechanism is slowed or reduced ("thinning the blood") with anticoagulants to treat certain diseases.

Coagulation—Same as *Clotting*.

Cocaine—Medication applied directly to mucous membranes to control pain in the nose and throat. Used illegally as a mind-altering drug, it is addicting and dangerous.

Cognitive Therapy—Psychotherapy that is based on the idea that the way we think about the world and ourselves affects our emotions and behavior.

Colic, Colicky—A pain that recurs in a regular pattern every few seconds or minutes.

Collagen—A gelatinous protein from which body tissues are formed.

Colon—The last major portion of the gastrointestinal tract, where waste material is formed into feces and held for elimination. It is also known as the large intestine.

Colonoscope, Colonoscopy—Method of diagnosing diseases of the colon by visual examination of the inside of the colon through a flexible colonoscope, a fiber-optic instrument with a lighted tip.

Color-Blindness—Inability to recognize red and green, which appear to be gray. It is usually hereditary.

Colposcopy—Visual examination of the cervix by means of a colposcope, a slender optical instrument with a lighted tip.

Combined Immunodeficiency Disease—Serious inherited disease in which the immune system of infants is unable to defend against disease.

Complication—Undesirable event during disease or treatment that causes further symptoms and delay in recovery.

Compress—Cloth, sometimes soaked in warm water or coated with medication. It is applied to the skin to relieve discomfort.

Compression—Applying pressure to the surface of the body, usually to stop bleeding.

Compulsion, Compulsive—Intense, irrational urge to perform some action.

Condom—A thin sheath, usually of latex, applied to the penis before sexual intercourse. It is used to help prevent disease of the genitals and as a contraceptive.

Congenital—Abnormality of the body, present at birth, usually meaning a defect. Congenital defects may be inherited or caused by conditions occurring while the fetus grows in the uterus.

Congenital Hypoplastic Anemia—See *Hypoplastic Anemia*.

Conization of the Cervix—Removal of a cone of tissue from the cervix. Laboratory examination of the removed tissue identifies possible cancer.

Conjunctiva—The mucous membrane lining the outermost surface of the eye (white of the eye).

Connective Tissue—Body's supporting framework of tissue consisting of strands of collagen, elastic fibers and simple cells.

Contact Lenses—Small plastic lenses worn on the eyes to correct nearsightedness, farsightedness or astigmatism.

Contagious—Disease or condition that spreads from one person to another.

Convalescence—Recovery from an illness or surgery.

Copious—Large in amount.

Cornea—Clear thickened surface of the eye through which light passes. It has no blood supply and can be transplanted without danger of rejection.

Coronary—Referring to the blood vessels supplying the heart. Sometimes, it refers to a heart attack resulting from coronary-artery obstruction.

Coronary-Care Unit (CCU)—Area of a hospital equipped to care for patients who have suffered a heart attack or other life-threatening heart conditions.

Cortisone Drugs—Medications similar to natural hormones produced by the central core of the adrenal glands.

Cosmetic Surgery—Surgery to improve appearance.

Coxsackie Viruses—Group of viruses causing infections such as poliomyelitis, aseptic meningitis, herpangina and myocarditis.

CPR—See *Cardiopulmonary Resuscitation*.

Cranium—Bones that make up the skull.

Cryosurgery—Destruction of abnormal tissue by applying freezing temperatures, usually with liquid nitrogen.

Cryotherapy—The use of cold (below -200°F) temperatures in treatment.

CT Scan, CAT Scan (Computerized Axial Tomography)—A computerized x-ray procedure that provides exceptionally clear images of parts of the body. It aids in diagnosis of diseases that cannot be diagnosed by ordinary x-ray methods.

Culdocentesis—Piercing of the space deep in the vagina under the cervix, to obtain fluid. Laboratory examination of the removed fluid aids in diagnosis of ectopic pregnancy and other disorders.

Culdoscopy—Visual examination of the female pelvic organs using a slender instrument brought into the pelvic cavity by penetrating through the space deep in the vagina under the cervix.

Culture—Identification of bacteria, fungi and viruses. Material (pus, blood or urine) from an infected area is collected, placed on nutrient material, and kept warm (usually in an incubator) until the infecting agent has grown. The resulting growth is examined with a microscope.

Curettage—Scraping process frequently used to obtain tissue from the lining of the uterus for laboratory examination that aids in diagnosis.

Curette—Instrument with a sharp end used to scrape tissue from the inner lining of the uterus and to scrape away skin lesions.

Cyst—Sac or cavity filled with fluid or diseased matter.

Cyst Aspiration—Removal of cyst contents for examination, or drainage for relief of symptoms.

Cystography—An x-ray of the urinary bladder that is obtained by injecting a solution visible on x-rays into the bladder.

Cystoscopy—Visual examination of the inside of the urinary bladder by means of a cystoscope, a slender optical instrument with a lighted tip.

Cystourethroscope, Cystourethroscopy—An instrument used for examination of the posterior urethra and bladder.

Cytotoxic Drugs—Medications used to destroy cancerous cells with minimal harm to healthy cells.

D

DC Cardioversion—The restoration of normal rhythm of the heart by a brief electrical shock via two metal plates placed on the wall of the chest.

D & C—Same as *Dilatation and Curettage*.

Debilitating—Causing a general weakening or deterioration in health.

Defibrillation, Cardiac—Applying an electric current to the chest over the heart to interrupt fibrillation, a disturbance of heartbeat.

Dehydration—Loss of essential fluids from the tissues and blood of the body.

Dependence—Condition in which a person requires substances such as narcotics or alcohol to remain

comfortable. If the substances are not used, withdrawal symptoms develop.

Dermatome—Area of the skin to which feeling (sensation) is provided by a nerve to the spinal cord.

Descending Colon—The part of the colon in the left side of the abdomen that stores feces until they are passed from the body.

Desensitization—1) Reduction or prevention of allergic (hypersensitivity) reactions by administration of graded doses of allergen. 2) Treatment for phobias and other psychological disorders. A patient gradually increases the exposure to the source of fear while simultaneously learning to relax.

Diabetic Retinopathy—Degeneration of the retina that develops in patients with diabetes mellitus. It may cause vision impairment or blindness.

Diagnosis—Identifying disease. A complete diagnosis names the part of the body affected, the disease process (such as inflammation, cancer or allergy) and the cause of disease.

Dialysis—Removal of natural wastes from the bloodstream. It is used to treat patients with kidney failure.

Diaphragm—Thin, broad sheet of muscle separating the chest cavity from the abdominal cavity.

Diathermy—Treatment in which mild heat is generated within the body by high-frequency radio waves.

Digestive System—Organs in which food is processed for absorption into the blood stream. The major digestive organs are the mouth, esophagus, stomach, duodenum, small bowel (small intestine), colon (large intestine), and rectum. The liver, gallbladder and pancreas are also considered parts of the digestive system.

Digitalis—A drug used to treat congestive heart failure and some other heart diseases.

Dilatation and Curettage—A gynecological treatment or diagnostic procedure that involves the stretching (dilatation) of the cervix so that a spoon-shaped instrument (curet) can be inserted into the uterus to scrape away the lining (endometrium). The scrapings may be examined under a microscope to assess the condition of the uterus.

Dilate, Dilation, Dilatation—To widen, expand or open up.

Dilator—Instrument used to widen organs that have narrowed because of disease.

Discolored Teeth—A yellowish-brown discoloration of the teeth frequently occurring in infants whose mothers took tetracycline while pregnant. Children may also be affected if they take tetracycline before they have their permanent teeth.

Discomfort—Unpleasant physical or mental sensation.

Disease—Adverse change in health; sickness or ailment. A disease can be defined by the body part involved (for example, the heart or liver), by the abnormality present (cancer, infection, allergy, degeneration, etc.) or by its cause (bacteria, poisons, injury, etc.).

Disk—Same as *Intervertebral Disk*.

Disorder—Same as *Disease*.

Diuretics—Medications that force the kidneys to excrete more urine, sodium and potassium than normal, which helps eliminate excessive body fluid.

Diverticulum—Small pouch or sac that develops in the wall of tubular organs such as the esophagus or colon.

Dizziness—Sensation of faintness, lightheadedness or spinning (vertigo).

Donor—Person who gives to someone else. In transplantation surgery, the donor gives up an organ (such as a kidney) to be transplanted into the recipient.

Doppler Ultrasound—See *Ultrasound*; this is one of several methods of ultrasound.

Doppler Venous Studies—Measurement of blood flow through the veins by means of doppler ultrasound.

Dormant—Sleeping or inactive state of living things. Also, an inactive state of a disease.

Drainage—Passage of fluids out of the body through an opening or incision.

Dry Socket—A tooth socket in which after extraction a blood clot fails to form; a condition marked by pain associated with the occurrence of a dry socket.

Ductus Arteriosus—Small blood vessel connecting the aorta and the pulmonary artery, which is the main artery to the lung. The vessel is open during the time the fetus is in the uterus, but normally closes at birth.

Duodenum—First 12 inches of the small intestine.

Dupuytren's Contracture—Chronic condition in which scar tissue forms in the palms. In severe cases, it can impair use of the fingers.

Dwarfism—Condition of being undersized for one's age. It may be due to endocrine disorders, malnutrition or an inherited defect.

Dyspnea—Difficult or painful breathing.

E

Ear Canal—Passageway extending from the outer ear inward to the eardrum.

Ear, Nose and Throat (ENT) Specialist—A physician specially trained to treat diseases of the ears, nose and throat.

ECG (Electrocardiography)—Method of diagnosing heart diseases by measuring electrical activity of the heart with an electrocardiograph. The record produced is called an electrocardiogram.

Echocardiogram, Echocardiography—Studying the heart by examining sound waves created by an instrument placed on the chest. The waves reflected from the heart form an image (echocardiogram) on a monitor, aiding in diagnosis of heart diseases.

Echography—The use of ultrasound as a diagnostic aid.

Eclampsia—Convulsions or coma late in pregnancy in an individual affected with preeclampsia.

Ectopic Pregnancy—A gestation which occurs elsewhere than in the uterus, usually in a Fallopian tube or the peritoneal cavity.

Edema—Accumulation of fluid under the skin, in the lungs or elsewhere.

EEG (Electroencephalography)—Studying the brain by measuring electric activity ("brain waves") with an electroencephalograph. The record produced is the electroencephalogram.

EKG—See *ECG*.

Electrocardiography—See *ECG*.

Electrocautery—Destruction of tissue by heat applied with a controlled electric current.

Electroencephalography—See *EEG*.

Electrolyte—A chemical that is dissolved in the blood and all other body fluids. Electrolytes play an essential role in all body functions. The major electrolytes are: sodium, potassium, chloride, calcium, phosphorus, magnesium and carbon dioxide. Electrolytes come from food. They are regulated mostly by the kidneys and lungs.

Electrolyte Measurement—Laboratory test on blood or urine to identify and measure the electrolytes present.

Electrolyte Supplements—Electrolytes taken to correct or to prevent body-fluid or electrolyte imbalance.

Electromyography—Studying nerve and muscle disorders by recording electrical activity of muscles with an electromyograph. The record produced is the electromyogram.

Electroneuronography—A diagnostic procedure in which the nerve of a muscle under study is stimulated by application of an electric current.

Endemic—Disease that is constantly present in a community or group of people. Endemic disease may affect only a few people at any one time.

Endocrine System—System of organs that secrete hormones into the blood to regulate basic functions of cells and tissues. The endocrine organs are the anterior and posterior pituitary glands, thyroid and parathyroid glands, pancreas, adrenal glands, ovaries (in women) and testicles (in men).

Endocrinologist—Doctor specially trained in diagnosis and treatment of endocrine disorders.

Endometritis—Inflammation of the endometrium.

Endometrium—The mucous membrane lining of the uterus.

Endoscopy—Method of diagnosing diseases in hollow organs. An endoscope (an optical instrument with a lighted tip) is inserted into the organ, which allows visual examination of the cavity. Used in the abdomen, pelvis, lumen of the bronchial tubes or intestines.

Endotracheal Tube—Tube temporarily placed in the trachea (windpipe) of patients who are unable to breathe normally because of disease or surgery.

Enteric—Relating to the small intestine. Enteric-coated medicine is coated with a hard shell that dissolves when it reaches the small intestine.

Enteroscopy—Examination of the inside of the intestines with an endoscope, an optical instrument.

Enterostomy—Surgically created artificial opening for elimination of feces.

Enterostomy Nurse, Enterostomy Specialist—a professional who teaches patients how to care for an enterostomy.

Enzymes—Proteins manufactured by the body that regulate the rate of essential life processes (metabolism).

Epididymis—A system of ducts at the rear of the testes which holds sperm during maturation.

Epididymitis—Inflammation of the epididymis.

Epinephrine—Same as *Adrenalin*.

Episcleritis—Inflammation of tissues on the sclera (the white of the eye).

Epithelial Horn—Thick, rough lesion protruding from the skin. It may become cancerous if not removed.

Equine Virus—Virus that causes a serious form of encephalitis in horses and humans.

Ergot—Medication derived from a fungus that grows on rye plant. It is used to treat migraine headache and to increase strength of uterine contractions during and immediately after childbirth.

Esophageal Varices—Enlarged veins on the lining of the esophagus. They are subject to severe bleeding and often appear in patients with severe liver disease.

Esophagogram, Esophagoscopy—Method of diagnosing diseases of the esophagus by means of an esophagoscope, an optical instrument with lenses and a lighted tip.

Esophagus—Muscular tube connecting the throat and stomach.

Estrogen—Female sex hormone, primarily secreted by the ovaries. It can also be produced synthetically for use in estrogen replacement therapy.

Estrogen Receptor Value—Used in the study of breast-cancer cells to determine the best treatment.

Etiology—Cause or causes of a disease.

Eustachian Tubes—Slender passages between the throat and the middle ear that maintain normal air pressure in the middle ear.

Excise—To remove by cutting out.

Exploratory Laparotomy—Diagnosing abdominal disease by surgically opening the abdomen and examining its contents.

Extremities—Arms and legs.

Eye Bank—Facility where living corneas are stored and made available for transplantation.

Eyes, Crossed—Condition in which muscles controlling the eyes are unbalanced. The eyes point in different directions. Also called squint or strabismus.

F

Fallopian Tubes—Organs of the female reproductive tract through which an egg (ovum) passes from the ovary to the uterus. Tying these tubes (tubal ligation) accomplishes sterility.

Familial Polyposis—Inherited condition in which the lining of the intestines contains many polyps, some of which may become cancerous.

Family History—Information about illnesses that tend to occur within a family. This information is used to determine the likelihood of diseases occurring in other members of the family.

Farsightedness—Same as *Hypermetropia*.

Fascia—Sheet or band of tough, fibrous tissue that covers muscles and other body organs.

Fecal—Relating to feces, waste products eliminated through the lower intestinal tract.

Fecal-Oral—Pathway by which some fecal germs gain entry into the bloodstream. Sewage in drinking water, hand-to-mouth transmission after bowel movements or sexual contact can cause infection.

Feces—Body waste formed of undigested food that has passed through the gastrointestinal system to the colon. Feces are and stored in the colon until eliminated.

Fetal Monitoring—Measuring the heart rate of the fetus during labor.

Fetal-Scalp Electrodes—Fine wires attached to the scalp of a fetus to measure heart rate and rhythm during labor.

Fetal-Scalp Monitoring—Measuring the well-being of the fetus during labor by obtaining blood from the scalp or by measuring the heart rate of the fetus or contraction strength of the uterus.

Fever—Above-normal body temperature. Normal mouth temperature is 98.6°F (37°C). Normal rectal temperature is 99.6°F (37.6°C).

Fiber Optics—System of transmitting light and images through thread-like strands of glass. Fiber-optic instruments make some examinations and surgical procedures simple, safe and effective.

Fiber—A non-nutritious ingredient of many complex carbohydrates. Fiber increases bulk in the diet. Many nutritionists recommend including ample fiber in the diet. Experimental studies and clinical studies show that people who eat high-fiber diets are less likely to develop colon cancer, diverticulitis, atherosclerosis and gallbladder disease.

Fibrin—Protein formed by the action of blood clotting on fibrinogen.

Fibrinogen—Protein in the blood needed for blood clotting.

Fibrositis—Inflammatory conditions affecting connective tissue of muscles, joints, ligaments and tendons.

Fine Needle Biopsy—The use of a fine needle to remove cells or fluid from the body for microscopic laboratory examination.

First Molars—First permanent flat teeth, used for grinding food, which appear at about age 6 to 7.

Fissure—Break in the skin or inner lining of organs.

Fistula—Abnormal passage between two organs or between the body and the outside.

Flank—Area on the side of the body below the ribs and above the hip.

Fleas—Tiny biting insects. Most cause minor skin irritation; some carry and transmit serious diseases such as plague and typhus.

Flooding—A drastic form of psychotherapy used for treatment of phobias. A patient is suddenly confronted with the feared object or placed in the feared situation with no chance of escape. Having experienced the phobia at its fullest intensity, a person comes to realize that the dreaded thing is not dangerous.

Only a competent therapist should subject a phobic person to flooding.

Fluorescein-Dye Test—Method of diagnosis using fluorescein, a dye, to study tissues and germs. When these dyed tissues are exposed to ultraviolet light, they glow. Substances to which the dye does not cling do not glow.

Fluorescent Antibody Studies—Tests used to study some allergic and infectious conditions. When antibodies created by these conditions are present in the blood, they can be made to glow by using a dye and a microscope with ultraviolet light.

Fluoroscopy—Method of x-ray diagnosis in which moving organs (such as the heart or intestinal tract) can be studied in action.

Foley Catheter—Slender, flexible tube used to drain urine from the bladder of patients who are unable to urinate normally.

Forceps—Instrument with two blades and handles. It is used to grasp tissue, body parts or sterile materials. Also used to deliver babies when progress of labor is slow.

Fracture—Break; usually used to refer to a bone or tooth.

Frei Test—Test used to make a precise

diagnosis of lymphogranuloma, a sexually transmitted disease.

Friedreich's Ataxia—Rare, inherited nervous-system disease that causes loss of balance and coordination, awkward walking, speech difficulty and tremors.

Frozen Section—A study in a pathology laboratory of fresh tissue that was removed during surgery. The purpose is to determine if a suspicious area is or is not cancerous.

Fungus—Mold or yeast that may infect skin, internal surfaces (mouth, vagina) or tissues.

Fungus Infection—Infection caused by fungus.

Fusiform Bacteria—Bacteria shaped like slender rods.

G

Galactorrhea—1) Continued breast-milk flow after weaning. 2) Excess breast-milk flow during nursing.

Galactosemia—Inherited disease of infants in which milk cannot be digested. Milk should be eliminated from the infant's diet to prevent malnutrition, liver and kidney disease and mental retardation.

Gallbladder—Small organ under the liver that stores bile. For digestion, the gallbladder contracts to empty bile into the intestines.

Gamma Globulin—Protein in the blood manufactured by the immune system to help destroy or neutralize infection-causing germs. Gamma globulin derived and concentrated from blood of other humans is used to help create temporary immunity to some diseases.

Gammaglobulinemia—Extremely low levels in the blood of gamma globulin brought about by a disease of the immune system. The deficiency causes increased susceptibility to many infections by bacteria, viruses and fungi. Also called

hypogammaglobulinemia.

Gangrene—Death of tissue, usually due to partial or total loss of blood supply.

Gastrectomy—Removal of part or all of the stomach.

Gastroduodenoscopy—Examination of the stomach and duodenum by means of a gastroscope.

Gastroenterologist—Doctor who specializes in the diagnosis and treatment of diseases of the gastrointestinal system.

Gastrointestinal Series (Upper GI Series)—X-rays of the upper digestive system (esophagus, stomach and duodenum).

Gastrointestinal Tract—See *Digestive System*.

Gastroscope, Gastroscopy—Visual examination of the inside of the stomach by means of a gastroscope, an optical instrument with a lighted tip.

Gene—Basic unit of protein molecules in chromosomes of cells. Genes transmit inherited characteristics such as eye color, blood type, gender or body shape. Defective genes cause many kinds of birth defects and inborn diseases.

Gene, Dominant or Recessive—Dominant gene, if present in either the mother's egg or father's sperm, will transmit its characteristics to the newborn child. Recessive gene must be present in both parents before its characteristic will be transmitted.

General Surgeon—A doctor specially trained to perform operations.

Genetic Counseling—Counseling to help couples decide whether to have children or not when there is a risk of genetic disease being transmitted to the child.

Genetics—Science of determining inherited factors that result in the unique make-up of every human being; also, science that traces the appearance patterns to genetic (inherited) disease.

Genitourinary Tract—Body system that

forms, stores and eliminates urine. Also has a role in male and female reproductive functions. Organs include the kidneys, ureters, bladder, urethra, uterus, Fallopian tubes, ovaries, vagina, cervix, penis, scrotum and testicles.

Germs—Organisms that cause infection such as bacteria, viruses or fungi.

Gestation—Time spent in the mother's uterus by the fetus. Average gestation time for the human infant, from conception to delivery, is approximately 39 weeks.

Gigantism—Condition in which the body or a body part grows excessively, sometimes due to an overactive pituitary gland.

Glucagon—Hormone secreted by the pancreas that increases blood sugar. A synthetic form is sometimes used as emergency treatment for patients with diabetes who have temporarily low blood sugar.

Glucose—Major form of sugar in the blood, stored primarily in the liver. It provides energy to most tissues, organs and systems.

Glucose-Tolerance Test—Method of diagnosing diabetes mellitus or functional hypoglycemia. The patient drinks a measured amount of glucose (sugar). The blood and urine are tested at measured intervals for glucose content.

Gluten—Protein found in wheat and other foods that cannot be digested by some persons because of genetic disease. A gluten-free diet allows persons with the disorder to digest food and grow normally.

Glycosuria—Sugar in the urine.

Goiter—An enlargement of the thyroid gland that is visible as a swelling in the neck.

Gonads—Parts of the reproductive system that produce and release female eggs (ovaries) or male sperm (testes).

Growth Disorders—Conditions in children that result in underdevelopment or overdevelopment of the body. Diseases of the endocrine glands, nutritional problems or genetic abnormalities are frequently the causes.

Gynecologist—Doctor specially trained to treat diseases of the female reproductive system.

H

H-2 Blocker Drugs—Class of antihistamines that reduce the production of stomach acid for treatment of peptic ulcers.

Hallucinogens—Substances that produce hallucinations, apparent sights, sounds or other experiences that do not actually exist.

Hand Surgeon—Surgeon specially trained to treat hand diseases, injuries, infections and arthritic conditions.

Hangover—Unpleasant aftereffects of excessive consumption of alcoholic beverages. Symptoms include irritability, headache and nausea. Sometimes, the same feelings result from using certain medications.

Hashimoto's Thyroiditis—One of several kinds of inflammation of the thyroid gland.

Heart Catheterization—Same as *Cardiac Catheterization*.

Heart Tumors—Rare tumors that grow in the heart wall or in the heart chambers, interfering with normal heart function.

Heart-Lung Machine—Complex mechanical device that provides artificial function of a patient's heart and lungs for a short time during open-heart surgery and heart or lung transplantation.

Hematocrit—Blood test used to detect anemia and other blood disorders. It is expressed as the percentage of blood made up of red blood cells (remainder of the blood is made up of serum or plasma). Normal hematocrit range is approximately 35 to 45%, but it varies with age and sex.

Hematologist—Doctor specially trained to diagnose and treat diseases of the blood and blood-forming organs.

Hemochromatosis—Disease in which excessive iron accumulates in the liver, pancreas and skin, resulting in liver disease, diabetes mellitus and a bronzed skin color.

Hemoglobin, Hemoglobin Range—1) Component that carries oxygen to body tissues. 2) Blood test used to detect anemia and other blood disorders, expressed in grams per 100 cubic centimeters. The normal hemoglobin range is approximately 12 to 18 grams per 100 cubic centimeters and varies according to age and sex.

Hemothorax—blood in the pleural cavity.

Hepatitis—A disease or condition marked by inflammation of the liver.

Hirschsprung's Disease—Congenital defect of infants in which the colon cannot eliminate feces, resulting in severe constipation.

Histamine—Chemical in body tissues that dilates the smallest blood vessels, constricts the muscle around the bronchial tubes, stimulates stomach secretions and produces an allergic response.

HIV—*See Human Immunodeficiency Virus.*

Holter Monitor—Instrument that detects heartbeat-rhythm abnormalities 24 hours or longer. The device is portable for patients to carry wherever they go.

Hormones—Powerful substances manufactured by the endocrine glands and carried by the blood to body tissues and organs. Hormones determine growth and structure of many organs (such as during growth and maturation) and also control many vital body functions.

Host—Person or animal with an infection that has been received from another person, animal or plant, or the environment.

Human Immunodeficiency Virus—Any of a group of retroviruses that infect and destroy helper T cells of the immune system and weaken the body's natural abilities to fight infections and cancer. Also called the AIDS virus.

Hyaline-Membrane Disease—Serious condition of premature infants in which the lungs can't expand normally. Cause is unknown.

Hydatidiform Mole—Disease occurring during early pregnancy resulting in death of the fetus and an overgrowth of tissue within the uterus.

Hydramnios and Polyhydramnios—Condition in which amniotic fluid (fluid in the uterus that surrounds the fetus until birth) becomes excessive.

Hygiene—Personal self-care and cleanliness that reduces the risk of infections and diseases.

Hyoid Bone—V-shaped bone located just above the larynx.

Hyperalimentation—Method of supplying total nutritional needs of patients unable to eat normally. The method (usually intravenous or by tube through the nose into the stomach) provides nutrients containing essential proteins, fats, carbohydrates and vitamins.

Hyperbaric Chamber—Large, sealed room in which air pressure can be raised above normal levels. It is used primarily to treat patients with either decompression sickness or severe burns (sometimes).

Hypercalcemia—Presence of excessive calcium in the blood, occasionally a sign of malignancy.

Hyperlipoproteinemia—Condition in which excessive lipoproteins (cholesterol and other fatty materials) accumulate in the blood.

Hypermetropia—Seeing distant objects clearly while nearby objects appear blurred; also called farsightedness.

Hypersensitivity—Extreme sensitivity to any agent (drugs, pollens, chemicals, etc.)

that causes allergic reactions. Some reactions can be life-threatening, but most are less serious.

Hyperthyroidism—Excessive activity of the thyroid gland marked by increased metabolic rate, enlargement of the thyroid gland, rapid heart rate and high blood pressure.

Hypnotics—Medications that produce sleep.

Hypochondriasis—Mental illness in which a person is convinced that serious disease is present, despite examination that proves otherwise. The symptoms of the imagined disease seem real to the patient (often called a hypochondriac).

Hypogammaglobulinemia—An immunologically deficient state characterized by an abnormally low level of all classes of gamma globulin in the blood.

Hypoparathyroidism—Deficiency of parathyroid hormone in the body.

j**Hypoplastic Anemia (Aplastic Anemia)**—Group of anemias that decrease blood-producing bone marrow. This can be life-threatening.

Hypothalamus—Part of the brain that regulates body functions such as temperature, blood pressure, appetite and thirst.

Hypothyroidism—Deficient activity of the thyroid gland, marked by decreased metabolic rate and loss of vigor.

Hysteria—1) Condition in which a person becomes anxious and excitable and experiences impaired sensory and motor abilities. Sometimes, hysterical persons simulate conditions of diseases such as deafness or blindness. 2) Outbreak of uncontrolled emotions, such as fits of laughing or crying.

Hysterogram—An x-ray of the uterus.

Hysterosalpingography—Studying the uterus and Fallopian tubes by injecting material into the uterus that x-rays can detect. It is used primarily to determine if the passageway for the ovum (egg) is open all the way to the uterus. The x-ray image is the hysterosalpingogram.

Hysteroscope—An instrument with lens system and lighted tip used in direct visual examination of the cervix and cavity of the uterus.

Hysterotomy—Incision of the uterus to prepare for cesarean section delivery of a baby.

I

I-131 Uptake—Measuring thyroid activity with radioactive iodine and radiation emission counters.

Idiopathic—Condition caused by unknown factors.

Ileum—Part of the small intestine just above the large intestine (colon).

Ileus—Condition of the small intestine in which either an obstruction or paralysis prevents material from passing through the intestine.

Iliac Arteries—Large arteries in the inner pelvis that supply blood to the legs.

Immune System—Body's system of defense against infection.

Immune, Immunity—Resistance or protection against infection by the body's natural defenses. A person may be immune to one kind of infection but not immune to another. Some infections, such as measles, chickenpox or mumps, cause the body to become immune permanently to that infection.

Immunization—Producing immunity by giving a vaccine (orally or by injection) of germs that have been altered so they cannot produce significant disease. The vaccine causes the body's immune system to produce antibodies that create immunity.

Immunosuppressants—Drugs used in immunosuppression treatment to weaken the immune system and to inhibit immune response.

Immunosuppression—Prevention of the body from forming a normal immune response. It is used to treat diseases (especially when organs must be transplanted) where certain antibodies must be inactivated.

Impotence—Male's inability to achieve or to sustain an erection or to ejaculate sperm during sexual intercourse.

Incise, Incision—To cut open or cut into.

Incomplete Spontaneous Miscarriage—Naturally occurring miscarriage in which the fetus is expelled, but part of the placenta remains in the uterus. Excessive bleeding and infection can result unless the uterus is emptied, usually by dilatation and curettage of the uterus (D & C) or suction curettage.

Incubation Period—The time between exposure to an infecting germ and the appearance of symptoms indicating an infection. Also describes the period of bacterial growth in laboratory cultures.

Infant—Child between the ages of 2 weeks and 1 year.

Infection, Infectious—Disease caused by germs (bacteria, viruses, fungi) that enter the body and cause inflammation or other processes that have an adverse effect on health.

Inflammation, Inflammatory Process—Process by which the body attempts to overcome illness-producing causes such as germs, injuries such as burns, or diseases such as arthritis. The process causes increased body heat (fever or local warmth), swelling, pain and tenderness. If the inflammation is near the skin, redness results.

Inhalation—Breathing air into the lungs.

Inherited—Body characteristic that is transmitted from one generation to the next by chromosomes in the mother's egg and father's sperm. Some inherited characteristics such as brown eyes are normal; others such as Down's syndrome are disorders.

Ingestion—Taking in food, medicine, etc., by mouth.

Inoculation—Injection of infected material such as pus into a nutrient medium where the germs will grow, or incubate. They are then stained and analyzed through a microscope. Also describes any kind of immunization.

Insufflation Test—See *Rubin's Insufflation Test.*

Insulin—Hormone produced by the pancreas that helps regulate sugar in the blood and helps produce energy.

Intensive Care Unit (ICU)—Area of a hospital where patients who are seriously ill or recovering from serious surgery are given more care than is available in other hospital units. As soon as the condition improves, the patient is transferred from the ICU to a regular hospital unit.

Intermittent—Happening only occasionally or under certain conditions.

Internist—Doctor specially trained in nonsurgical diagnosis and treatment of diseases in adults.

Intervertebral Disk—Cartilage that connects adjacent vertebrae in the spinal column.

Intestinal Tract—All parts of the gastrointestinal tract except the mouth, esophagus and stomach. The intestinal tract organs are: duodenum, small bowel, ileum, cecum, appendix, ascending colon, transverse colon, descending colon, sigmoid colon, rectum and anus.

Intestine, Large—Last major portion of the gastrointestinal tract located just under the small intestine. It is also called the colon or large bowel. It processes waste material into feces, which are stored until eliminated from the body.

Intestine, Small—Longest section of the gastrointestinal tract, located just under the stomach and duodenum. It absorbs digested food into the bloodstream and passes waste material into the large intestine.

Intracardiac Pressures—Pressures occurring within the heart.

Intrauterine Death—Death of a fetus while inside the mother's uterus.

Intrauterine Device (IUD)—Birth-control method in which a small device placed permanently in the uterus prevents growth of fertilized eggs.

Intravenous—Within the vein. Fluids, medications and nutrients that cannot be taken orally are given intravenously by a needle placed in a large vein near the surface of the skin.

Intravenous Pyelogram (IVP)—See *Pyelogram, Intravenous*.

Intravenous Urography—Method of studying the kidneys and urinary tract by injecting into the bloodstream a medication that x-rays can detect.

IQ (Intelligence Quotient)—Supposedly a measure of a person's intelligence, rather than what one has learned. Recent research on intelligence raises questions about the accuracy and meaning of the I.Q. test.

Iridectomy—Surgery performed to treat some kinds of glaucoma.

Irrigation—Flooding with water or other liquid. It is used frequently to clean wounds or areas of the body that will undergo surgery.

Isolation, Reverse Isolation—Procedures to prevent spread of infection in a hospital. Isolation protects hospital staff and visitors from contracting a contagious disease from a patient. Reverse isolation protects a patient susceptible to infection because of immunosuppression from contracting infection from hospital staff or visitors.

IUD—See *Intrauterine Device*.

IVP—See *Pyelogram, Intravenous*.

J

Jaundice—Yellow skin and whites of the eyes, dark urine and light stools, symptoms of diseases of the liver and blood.

Joint—Structure that enables two or more bones to move easily in relation to each other. A joint consists of ligaments and cartilage that hold bones together.

Joint Capsule—Tough, fibrous tissue that surrounds a joint.

Joint Replacement—Replacement of diseased joints with mechanical joints. The wrist, hip and knee joints are among the most common joints replaced.

K

Ketoacidosis—Serious complication of diabetes mellitus in which the body produces acids that cause fluid and electrolyte disorders, dehydration and sometimes coma.

Klinefelter's Syndrome—Inherited disease of young males in which secondary sex characteristics are underdeveloped. The condition does not become evident until puberty. Mental deficiency and some female characteristics are present.

L

Laceration—Wound with jagged edges.

Lactiferous Ducts—Network of tubes in the female breast that collects milk and delivers it to the nipple.

Laminaria—Freeze-dried seaweed sometimes used to dilate the cervix when performing an abortion.

Laparoscope, Laparoscopy—Exploratory examination of the organs inside the abdominal cavity with a laparoscope, an optical instrument with a lighted tip. The laparoscope is inserted into the abdomen through a small incision. Visual examination can then be made of many abdominal organs.

Laparotomy—Exploratory surgery in the abdomen performed to diagnose and sometimes treat abdominal disease.

Laryngeal Nerve—Nerve located in the neck that controls the vocal cords and enables a person to speak.

Laryngoscopy—Examination of the inside of the larynx with a laryngoscope, an optical instrument.

Larynx—Structure of muscle and cartilage in the upper neck. It contains the vocal cords. Air passes through the larynx into the windpipe and then into the lungs. The "Adam's apple" is part of the larynx.

Laser Therapy—Using a laser beam to treat many diseases. Sharply focused laser light creates intense heat and is valuable in cutting tissue, destroying unwanted tissue and joining tissue together. It is most often used to treat retinal detachment, endometriosis or atherosclerosis.

Latent—Present but inactive; something that exists in an undeveloped form.

Laxatives—Medications used to treat constipation.

Lesion—General term for injury or damage to an organ or tissue.

Lethargy—Fatigue or lack of usual physical or mental energy.

Libido—Sexual desire.

Life Cycle—Growth and development from birth to death.

Ligaments—Strong, flexible cords of tissue near joints that hold bones together and permit bone motion.

Lipoproteins (High Density and Low Density)—Components of the fluid in blood that are measured to help predict the likelihood of atherosclerosis (hardening of the arteries).

Liquid Nitrogen—Nitrogen that has been cooled until it becomes a liquid. It is used most often in cryosurgery.

Local Anesthesia—See *Anesthesia, Local.*

Low-Residue Diet—Diet consisting of foods that are digested almost entirely, leaving minimal material to form feces.

Low-Spinal Anesthesia—Also called "saddle-block" anesthesia. An injection into the lower spinal canal provides anesthesia to the lower body.

Lower GI Series—Same as *Barium-Enema X-rays.*

Lumbar Puncture (Spinal Tap)—A diagnostic procedure in which a needle is inserted between 2 bones (vertebra) of the lower spine to collect spinal fluid for laboratory examination.

Lumbar Spine—Lower part of the spine, from the lowest ribs to the bottom of the spine.

Lung Function Studies—Tests to determine the effectiveness of a patient's respiration.

Lymph (or Lymphatic) System—Lymph channels and lymph glands considered as a single body system.

Lymph Channels—Tubes of tissue that carry lymph fluid away from tissues and back to the bloodstream. Lymph fluid is composed of proteins and water, varying in composition in different parts of the body.

Lymph Glands—Small collections of tissue (nodes) located along lymph channels in areas such as the elbow, armpit or groin. When infection is present, nearby lymph glands enlarge, become tender and destroy germs that enter lymph channels. Lymph glands also manufacture antibodies to help fight infection.

Lymphangiogram, Lymphangiography—Diagnostic method of studying the lymphatic system by infecting a material into the lymph channels that x-rays can detect. The image on x-ray film is the lymphangiogram.

Lymphatic Leukemia—Class of leukemias, involving primarily lymphatic cells, affecting children and adults.

Lymphedema—Painful swelling of soft tissues, caused by edema due to faulty lymphatic drainage. Swelling is often accompanied by decreased mobility in the affected limb, and by increased risk of infection.

Lymphocytes—One of several types of white blood cells that help fight infection.

Lymphosarcoma—Class of cancers of the lymphatic system.

M

Macular Degeneration of the Eye—Condition of the macula (area on the retina that provides detailed vision) in which impaired blood supply causes gradual vision loss.

Macule—General term for any discolored spot or patch on the skin, such as a freckle.

Malignant—Capable of causing great harm, including death. It usually refers to cancerous growth.

Magnetic Resonance Imaging—See *MRI*.

Mammogram, Mammography—Diagnostic method of studying the female breast by an x-ray technique that detects cancerous growths while they are still treatable. The image on x-ray film is the mammogram.

Manic-Depressive Illness—Mental illness in which behavior alternates between unrealistic enthusiasm and deep depression.

Manometer, Manometry—The measuring of pressure (of either liquid or gas) by means of a manometer.

MAO Inhibitors—See *Monoamine Oxidase Inhibitors*.

Marijuana—Mood-altering substance that is usually taken into the body by smoking. It is derived from Indian hemp or Cannabis leaves, stems and seed pods.

Marrow—Core of many bones, where most of the body's blood cells are produced.

Mastoiditis—Infection of the mastoid (bony area just behind the ear).

Mediators—Substances that: 1) help nerve impulses travel from one cell to the next; 2) participate in the allergic process.

Medic Alert—Nonprofit agency that maintains a medical-record system. Subscribers receive a bracelet or pendant that states their medical condition and provides a toll-free number for more information. The service can save the life of a person with a major medical condition who may not be able to provide medical history. For information write: Medic Alert Foundation, P.O. Box 1009, Turlock, CA 95381, (800) 344-3226.

Medical History—Essential facts about past and present medical conditions. Knowing your medical history enables your doctor to plan the best possible health care. Carry a card stating essential health details in your purse or wallet, and consider joining the Medic-Alert program (see above).

Meibomian Glands—Small glands on the inner eyelid. They secrete a fluid that helps the eyelids move easily over the surface of the eye.

Membrane—Thin tissue lining a body cavity, covering an internal organ or dividing a space.

Meninges—Three-layered membrane covering the brain.

Mental System (Mind)—Functions of the brain that provide the abilities to perceive surroundings, to have emotions, imagination, memory, will, and to process information.

Metastases—Cancerous cells or infectious germs that spread from their original location to other parts of the body.

Metatarsal Bones—Bones in the middle of the foot.

Midwife—Nurse with special training and experience in childbirth.

Mole—Skin lesion, often dark-brown or black.

Monoamine Oxidase (MAO) Inhibitors—Medications used to treat some forms of depression.

Motor Nerve—Nerve that transmits the stimulus that causes muscles to contract.

MRI (Magnetic Resonance Imaging)—A method of studying the body's internal structures that employs a strong magnetic field (rather than x-rays) and a computer to produce detailed pictures.

Mucous Membrane—Thin tissue lining internal cavities (nose, mouth, vagina) and tubular systems (respiratory and gastrointestinal) that produce mucus.

Mucus—Slippery liquid produced by the lining of internal cavities and tubular systems to protect tissue.

Muscle—Tissue that contracts, often with considerable force, when stimulated by the motor-nerve impulses.

Muscle Relaxants—Medications that relieve muscle spasms. They also can have significant side effects.

Muscle Tumors—Benign or cancerous tumors arising from muscle tissue.

Musculo-Skeletal System—The system of bones, muscles, ligaments and tendons that enable the body to move.

Myelogram, Myelography—Special x-ray of the spinal canal and spinal cord, requiring a spinal tap and injection of dye that is visible on x-ray film. Myelograms frequently are used to identify the location of ruptured disks.

Myoma—Tumor of the muscle.

Myopia—Disease of the eye in which close objects are clearly visible while distant objects are blurred. Also called nearsightedness.

Myringotomy—A surgical opening made through the eardrum to allow drainage of the middle ear cavity. It is usually performed on children.

N

Narcotics—Medications used to control severe pain. Narcotics should be used only when necessary because of their serious side effects: addiction; reduced breathing; nausea and vomiting; low blood pressure; reduced cough reflex; and constipation.

Nasogastric Tube—Slender tube passed through the nose into the stomach. It is used to drain away stomach secretions or to feed patients unable to eat normally.

Naturopathy—Health-care system relying on diet, sunshine, exercises, herbs and other nonmedicinal treatment.

Nausea—Unpleasant sensation of being about to vomit.

Nearsightedness—Same as *Myopia*.

Nebulizer—Device for administering medications used to treat asthma and similar conditions. It converts medication into a fine mist that is inhaled deeply into the lungs.

Necrosis—Death of living tissue.

Nerve-Block Local Anesthesia—See *Anesthesia, Nerve Block or Local*.

Nerve-Conduction Studies, Nerve Conduction Test—Diagnostic test that measures the rate at which an electrical impulse moves along a nerve. It is used to diagnose disorders of the peripheral nerves and muscle.

Nervous Breakdown—Nontechnical term for mental illness serious enough to interfere with daily activities.

Neuralgia—Severe, sharp pain along a nerve.

Neuritis—Inflammation of a nerve.

Neuromuscular System—Nerves and muscles acting together as a system to control body movements.

Neurological—Relating to the body's nervous system.

Neurologist—Doctor specially trained to diagnose and treat diseases of the nervous system.

Neuroma—Tumor arising from nerve tissue.

Neurosis—Mental illness in which anxiety is controlled by avoidance, blaming others, developing bodily complaints or other mechanisms.

Neurosurgeon—Doctor specially trained to diagnose and surgically treat diseases of the brain, spinal cord and nerves.

Nodes—See *Lymph Glands*.

Nodule—Small, rounded lump or firm swelling underneath the skin.

Nonsteroidal Anti-Inflammatory Drugs—Medications that control inflammation other than that caused by infection. Usually used to treat conditions of the joints and muscles and pain such as menstrual cramps or headache. "Nonsteroidal" means they are not steroid hormones such as cortisone, prednisone, dexamethasone and others.

Norwalk Virus—A type of virus that commonly causes epidemics of acute gastroenteritis with diarrhea and vomiting that lasts from 24 to 48 hours.

Nuclear Imaging—See *Radionuclide Scans*.

Nurse Practitioner (NP)—Registered nurse with additional medical training who can diagnose and treat common illness. Nurse practitioners usually work closely with a doctor, although in some states the practitioner can prescribe medicine and work independently of a physician.

Nutrient—Food or material containing elements needed to promote growth and development or to support life.

O

Obsessions—Unpleasant, frightening, senseless thoughts that won't go away despite reasoning.

Obstetrician-Gynecologist—Doctor specially trained to treat diseases of the female reproductive system and provide health care for pregnant mothers.

Occlusion—Closing or obstruction. Usually used to describe blockage in blood vessels. In dentistry, it means the way the teeth come together when the mouth is closed.

Occupational Therapy—Treatment for people disabled by accident or illness to relearn muscular control and coordination to cope with daily living tasks (dressing, eating, bathing, etc.) and if possible, to resume some form of employment.

Omentum—A fold of peritoneum which supports or connects abdominal structures.

Oncologist—Doctor specially trained to diagnose and treat cancer.

Operative Death Rate—Percentage of patients who die as a result of a certain surgery. It provides general measure of the risk of a surgery.

Ophthalmologist—Doctor specially trained to diagnose and treat diseases of the eyes.

Optic Neuritis—Inflammation of the nerve that conducts vision impulses from the eye to the brain.

Oral—Relating to the mouth.

Oral-Fecal—See *Fecal-Oral*.

Organic—Conditions or diseases resulting from change in body organs that can be measured or seen. Organic diseases are distinct from functional diseases in which no change can be observed in an organ that is not functioning normally.

Organic Psychosis—Mental illness that results from disease in the brain.

Orthodontia—Straightening teeth by applying temporary braces.

Orthopedic Surgeon (Orthopedist)—Doctor specially trained to diagnose and treat diseases of the muscles, bones and joints using surgical or mechanical means. A rheumatologist is an internist who diagnoses and treats similar conditions primarily with medications and other nonsurgical means.

Osteogenesis Imperfecta—Inherited condition in which the bones are brittle and easily broken.

Otolaryngologist—See *Ear, Nose and Throat Specialist*.

Ovary—Female sexual gland where eggs mature and ripen for fertilization.

Ovulation—Monthly process in which an egg leaves the ovary for possible fertilization by a sperm cell.

Ovum—Egg produced by the ovary.

P

Pain—Unpleasant sensation arising from stimulation of sensory nerves located in almost every part of the body. Disease, injury and strenuous activity can all cause pain.

Palate—Roof of the mouth, consisting of a bony front portion (hard palate) and a soft back portion (soft palate).

Palpitations—Irregular rapid heartbeat, noticeable to the patient.

Pancreas—Organ located on the back abdominal wall that produces and secretes digestive juices into the small intestine. It also produces and secretes insulin into the bloodstream to regulate the level of sugar and other nutrients.

Pancreatitis—Inflammation of the pancreas.

Pap Smear, Papanicolaou Smear—Test routinely done to screen for cancer of the cervix and uterus in an early and treatable stage.

Papule—Small, raised skin lesion. Papules may be red, brown, yellow, white or skin-colored. They may be flat-topped, pointed or dome-shaped.

Paranoia—Mental illness in which a person believes that he or she is being talked about or plotted against.

Parasite—Organism that lives within, upon or at the expense of another living organism. Human parasites include disease-causing agents such as amoebas or worms that infect the digestive system, or fungi that live on the skin.

Parasympathetic Nervous System—System of nerves that controls digestion, heartbeat, and relaxation or contraction of small muscles.

Parathyroid Glands—Small glands that control calcium levels in the blood and bones. They are located within or next to the thyroid glands at the base of the neck.

Passive Exercises—Exercises in which a therapist moves the arms and legs of a patient while the patient relaxes. These exercises keep the joints limber until the patient is able to move without assistance.

Patency—Blood vessels or any hollow organs that clog or become blocked are said to lose their patency.

Pathogenic—Disease-producing.

Pathological—Relating to an abnormal condition.

Pathological Examination—Laboratory study of abnormal tissue to establish or confirm a diagnosis.

Pediatrician—Doctor specially trained to care for children and adolescents, especially to foster normal growth and development.

Pediculicide—Medication that cures body lice (pediculosis). Usually applied to the skin.

Pelvic Examination—Examination of a woman's reproductive organs to diagnose pregnancy or detect diseases.

Pelvic Ultrasonography—Examination of a woman's reproductive organs that uses high-frequency sound waves to create an image. It is used to determine the age, size and position of a fetus in the uterus or to diagnose disease of the pelvic organs.

Pelvis—Lower part of the trunk of the body.

Penis—Male organ used for urination and sexual intercourse.

Perforation—Abnormal hole or opening.

Perforation, Intestinal—Complication of conditions such as ulcers, cancers, or injury to the digestive system. When this occurs, intestinal contents enter the abdominal cavity, causing severe inflammation.

Perfusionist—Medical professional who controls the heart-lung machine to sustain a patient's life during open-heart and lung-transplant surgery.

Perineum—Area between the vulva and anus in females and between the scrotum and anus in males.

Peripheral Nervous System—Nerves that connect to all parts of the body and carry information via electrical impulses to and from the brain and spinal cord.

Peripheral Vascular System—Network of arteries, veins and lymphatic channels supplying the head, arms and legs.

Perirectal—Skin and underlying tissue around the rectum.

Peristalsis—Rhythmic movements of hollow muscular organs (such as the intestines) that move contents (such as digestive material) in one direction.

Peritoneal Cavity—Space enclosed by the peritoneum.

Peritoneum—Very thin, two-layered tissue. One layer lines the outer surface of all the abdominal organs. The other layer lines the abdominal wall.

Peritonitis—Inflammation of the peritoneum.

Peritonsillar Abscess—Abscess forming in the back of the throat near the tonsils.

Pessary—Small ring-shaped device that is inserted into the vagina to help maintain the uterus in a normal position.

PET Scan—A sectional view of the body constructed by positron-emission tomography, which uses integrated x-ray and computing equipment.

pH Balance—Measure of blood's acidity or alkalinity. The pH is controlled by body fluids and electrolytes. Body tissues

cannot function normally if the pH varies from a limited range.

Phallus—Penis.

Phenothiazine Drugs—Medications used to slow and regulate mental-system activity. Usually used to treat anxiety and other mental conditions; also useful in producing sleep.

Phlebitis—Inflammation of a vein.

Phlebotomy—Removing blood from the blood vessels. This was once believed to cure many diseases; today, it is done to remove blood for diagnostic testing.

Phobia—Fear that cannot be overcome by reason.

Photochemotherapy—A treatment for some skin disorders that combines oral medication with exposure to ultraviolet light rays for set periods of time.

Physical Therapy—Treatment of diseases of the bone, muscular and nervous systems to help restore normal function after disease or injury.

Physician's Assistant (PA)—Someone trained to do some of the simpler tasks ordinarily performed by a doctor. The PA works under the direction of the doctor.

Pilocarpine—Medication used principally in eye drops to treat glaucoma.

Pituitary Gland—Small endocrine gland at the base of the brain that controls growth and regulates other endocrine glands.

Placenta—Disk-shaped organ that attaches and grows inside the uterus during pregnancy. It enables the fetus to receive nutrients from and transfer natural wastes to the mother's bloodstream. The umbilical cord connects the placenta to the fetus.

Placenta previa—An abnormal placement of the placenta in the lower uterine segment, so that it covers or adjoins the internal opening of the uterine cervix.

Plaque—1) Small raised area of abnormal material on a surface such as the skin or lining of a blood vessel. 2) Mixture of bacteria and calcium deposited on the teeth that can cause cavities and gum diseases.

Plasma—Liquid part of blood that remains when blood cells are removed.

Plastic and Reconstructive Surgeon (Plastic Surgeon)—Doctor specially trained to perform plastic and reconstructive surgery.

Plastic and Reconstructive Surgery—Special surgery to repair and change body parts to improve function or appearance. The face, hands, breasts and skin are areas most frequently treated.

Platelet Count—Platelets are blood cells (much smaller than red or white blood cells) that assist in the blood-clotting process. A drop of blood contains about 12.5 million platelets. A platelet count determines if the number of platelets is normal.

Plethysmography—A study that estimates the amount of blood flowing in vessels by measuring changes in the size of a body part.

Pleura—Thin tissue lining the lungs and chest cavity. Inflammation of the pleura (pleurisy) is a painful condition caused by lung diseases.

Pleural Effusion (Pleural Fluid Effusion)—Fluid that collects around the lungs, usually caused by inflammation of the lungs and pleura or congestive-heart failure.

Pneumonia—Infection and inflammation of the lungs.

Pneumothorax—A collection of air or gas in the lung which causes collapse of all or part of a lung.

Podiatrist—Health-care professional trained in the medical and surgical treatment of foot diseases.

Polyp—A growth, often on a stalk arising from dry mucous membranes, such as in the nose, cervix or colon.

Portal-Vein System—Veins that drain blood from the gastrointestinal system. The smaller veins empty into the portal vein, which transports blood into the liver.

Postmature Infant—Infant that spends 3 weeks or more beyond the normal 39 weeks of pregnancy in the womb.

Postoperative—Period of recuperation and return to normal health after surgery.

Postural Drainage—Exercises and body positions that promote drainage of fluid and secretions that collect in the lungs and airways.

Potassium—Electrolyte present in all body cells, blood and body fluids. Potassium is important in maintaining normal heart contractions and the strength and contractions of all muscles. Foods high in potassium include: dried apricots and peaches; whole-grain cereals; plain cocoa, dried lentils and peas; bananas; and molasses.

Precancerous—Characteristic of a growth that has the potential to become cancerous.

Predisposition—Tendency. For example, a person who gets many infections has a predisposition to infection.

Preeclampsia—A toxic condition of late pregnancy characterized by a sudden rise in blood pressure, excessive weight gain, generalized edema, protein in the urine, severe headache and visual disturbances.

Premature Labor—Labor beginning before the usual 39 weeks of pregnancy.

Presbyopia—Form of nearsightedness that normally accompanies aging.

Primary Disorder—Basic disease that may result in complications. Diabetes mellitus, for example, is a primary disorder that often causes secondary complications involving the kidneys, blood vessels and eyes.

Proctoscope, Proctoscopy—Method of examining the rectum and lower part of the colon with a proctoscope, an optical instrument with a lighted tip.

Prolapse—Pushing or falling out of a part or an organ from its normal position.

Prolapsed (Dropped) Uterus—Uterus that has moved from its normal position because of loose pelvic muscles and ligaments. In severe cases, it can protrude completely outside the vagina.

Prophylaxis—Measures taken to prevent an illness.

Prophylaxis, Dental—Regular care (including cleaning) of the teeth and gums that helps prevent tooth decay and gum inflammation.

Prostaglandins—Natural substances found in semen, menstrual fluid and many body tissues. They are involved in basic body functions such as inflammation, immune response and activities of the lungs, heart, kidneys, uterus and digestive system.

Prostate (Prostate Gland)—Male sex gland located at the base of the urinary bladder. It produces a fluid that is added to sperm to produce semen.

Prosthesis—Artificial device used as a substitute for a missing or badly functioning part of the body.

Prothrombin Time—Test to measure one of the components of the body's blood-clotting mechanism. It is used to diagnose clotting diseases and to control blood-thinning (anticoagulation) in treatment of some diseases of the heart and blood vessels.

Protozoa—One-celled organisms, the smallest type of animal life. Amoeba are protozoa. Some protozoa can cause disease.

Psychiatrist—Doctor specially trained to diagnose and treat mental illnesses.

Psychoanalysis—Treatment of some mental illness that involves a detailed understanding of how past events in a person's life may have resulted in mental disturbances.

Psychogenic—A symptom with an emotional origin instead of an organic one.

Psychologist—Health-care professional specially trained to diagnose and treat some kinds of mental illness.

Psychopathy—Psychological or mental illness.

Psychosis—Mental illness characterized by deranged personality, loss of contact with reality, and possible delusions, hallucinations or illusions.

Psychosocial—Influences of society on growth and development.

Psychosomatic Illness—Illness in which thoughts and emotions play an important role.

Psychotherapist—Professional specially trained to diagnose and treat some mental illnesses.

Puberty—Period in early adolescence when hormonal changes bring about full sexual maturity and capacity to reproduce.

Pubic Bone—One of the bones of the pelvis located above the genitals in both sexes.

Pulmonary—Relating to the lungs and breathing.

Pulmonary Angiography—Studies of the arteries and veins in the lungs.

Pulmonary Hypertension—Increased pressure in the blood vessels of the lungs.

Pulse—Heartbeat (contraction of the heart) as felt in an artery. Heart rate is often measured by counting the pulse felt in the artery in the wrist.

Pus—Thick fluid, usually green or yellow, that forms to fight local infection. Pus often collects in an enclosed sac, an abscess, at the site of an infection.

PUVA—A type of phototherapy used to treat some skin conditions. It combines the use of a psoralen drug that sensitizes the skin to sunlight with a controlled dose of ultraviolet light.

Pyelogram, Intravenous—Method of studying the kidneys and urinary tract by injecting into the bloodstream a medication that x-rays can detect.

Pyelogram, Retrograde—Method of studying the kidneys, similar to an intravenous pyelogram, but in which the medication detected by x-rays is placed in the urinary system by a catheter inserted through the bladder into the ureters.

R

Radiation Therapy or Treatment—Use of high-energy waves (generated by special x-ray machines, cobalt machines and other devices) to treat some forms of cancer. Radiation destroys cancerous tissue but does little harm to healthy tissue.

Radioactive Chromium Studies—Diagnostic method used to measure total blood in the body.

Radioactive Iodine Uptake and Scan—Same as *Thyroid Scan*.

Radioactive Studies—Same as *Radioisotope Studies*.

Radioactive Technetium 99 Scan—Radioisotope scan method used to diagnose some disorders of the heart, liver, spleen and other organs.

Radioisotope—Radioactive form of chemicals normally present in the body.

Radioisotope Scan—Scan of radioisotopes given orally or intravenously to a patient that become concentrated in organs such as the heart, lungs or brain. Instruments measure the radiation given off by the radioisotopes and create a photographic image of the organ being studied.

Radioisotope Studies—Radioisotopes are chemical elements that give off radiation. A radioisotope of a chemical element normally present in the body (such as carbon), if injected into the body, will mix with the nonisotopes. The body doesn't know the difference, but radiation from the isotopes can be detected with special instruments. Determining where radioisotopes go in the body allows diagnosis of diseases that cannot be detected otherwise.

Radioisotope Therapy—Treatment of some cancers with radioisotopes.

Radiologist—Doctor specially trained to use x-rays and other kinds of radiation in diagnosis and treatment.

Radionuclide Scan—Method of studying various body functions by means of photographs or videotape taken by special camera or a scanner after intravenous injection of radioactive chemical.

Rebound Phenomenon—A reversed response to the withdrawal of a stimulus. A common rebound phenomenon occurs when nose drops, which decrease congestion, wear off. The nasal congestion that develops on the rebound is greater than that which existed before the drops were administered.

Recovery Room—Specially equipped and staffed area of a hospital for observing and caring for a patient who has just undergone surgery. Postoperative patients usually remain in the recovery room until they are awake and their vital signs (blood pressure, pulse and respiration) are satisfactory.

Rectum—End of the large intestine, located in the pelvis below the sigmoid colon and above the anus.

Regenerate—Ability of some parts of the body to grow back to normal after being damaged.

Regurgitate—To vomit.

Relapse—Stage of illness in which the patient gets worse after having improved.

Remission—Stage of a chronic illness when the patient's condition improves.

Renal—Having to do with the kidneys.

Renal Dialysis—Mechanical and chemical method of removing normal wastes from the body of a patient whose kidneys cannot function adequately. It is also used to remove harmful poison or a drug overdose from the bloodstream.

Reproductive Organs, Female—Organs of a woman's body that enable her to become pregnant and deliver a baby. The major organs are the vagina, uterus, Fallopian tubes and ovaries.

Reproductive Organs, Male—Organs of a man's body that enable him to produce sperm and impregnate the woman. The major organs are the penis, testicles, seminal vesicles and prostate gland.

Reproductive System—Body system enabling impregnation and delivery of a baby. It also provides characteristic male or female appearance.

Resect—Surgical removal of a part of the body.

Respiratory-Distress Syndrome—A condition of newborn infants (often born prematurely) in which the lungs cannot supply adequate oxygen to the body.

Retained Placenta—Condition occurring immediately after childbirth in which part of the placenta remains attached to the uterus, creating a risk of serious bleeding or infection.

Retina—Light-sensitive part of the eye at the back of the eyeball on which the lens focuses images. The retina converts the image to impulses that go to the brain.

Retinal-Vein Occlusion—Condition in which a clot forms in the vein supplying the retina with blood.

Retinoblastoma—Cancerous tumor that forms in the eye of an infant.

Retrograde Pyelography—See *Pyelogram, Retrograde*.

Retrovirus—Group of viruses that cause HIV (human immunodeficiency virus) and some types of lymphoma and leukemia.

Rh Negative Blood—A subtype of red blood cells. Blood subtypes are inherited. The major subtypes are types A, B, O and Rh negative.

Rheumatologist—A specialist in internal medicine who subspecializes in medical diagnosis and treatment of rheumatic and arthritic disorders.

Rhinitis—Swelling of the nasal passages.

Rinne Test—Test using a tuning fork to diagnose hearing disorders.

Rotavirus—A type of virus that is often responsible for acute gastroenteritis in infants and for diarrhea in young children.

Rubin's Insufflation Test—Test used in diagnosing fertility problems in women. A harmless gas is introduced into the uterus to determine if there is a blockage in the Fallopian tubes.

S

Sacroiliac Region—Area of the lower back where the spine meets the pelvic bone.

Saline—Salt-containing solution similar to normal body fluid that is given intravenously to help correct fluid and electrolyte imbalances.

Salivary Glands—Glands located inside the mouth around the jaw that secrete saliva into the mouth.

Saphenous-Femoral Vein System—Network of large veins in the legs that helps return blood from the leg to the inferior vena cava, then to the heart.

Scale, Scaling—Flakes of dried skin that form as whitish skin lesions.

Schizophrenia—Mental illness characterized by a distorted sense of reality, bizarre behavior and fragmentation of the personality.

Sciatic Nerve—Large nerve that begins at the base of the spine and passes through the buttocks down the back side of the thigh and down the leg.

Sciatica—Painful condition resulting from irritation of the sciatic nerve.

Scleritis—Inflammation of the sclera (the white of the eye).

Scopolamine—Medication used to treat hyperactive or spastic conditions of the digestive system and to prevent motion sickness.

Scrotum—Organ of the male reproductive system that contains the testicles, blood vessels and the vas deferens.

Scurvy—Disease of bones, gums and blood vessels that is caused by a deficiency of vitamin C.

Second Molars—Permanent grinding teeth that appear at about age 11 to 13.

Secondary Infection—Infection that results from some other problem. It may occur after surgery or develop during antibiotic treatment of another infection.

Sedative—Medication used to produce relaxation or sleep.

Sedative-Hypnotics—Class of medications that help relieve anxiety and promote sleep.

Sedimentation Rate—Blood test measuring the rate that blood settles in a test tube. It identifies infection, inflammation or tissue damage.

Self-Care—Treatment that patients can administer for themselves.

Seminal Vesicles—Small sacs next to the prostate that help make and store seminal fluid and contract to eject semen.

Senile Dementia—Permanent loss of mental functions of older persons, resulting from conditions such as Alzheimer's disease and atherosclerosis (hardening of the arteries).

Senile Keratosis—Same as *Seborrheic Keratoses*. (See *Illness section*.)

Sensitivity Studies (Antibiotics)—Laboratory method of determining which antibiotic will most likely be successful in treating infections caused by bacteria.

Sensory—Ability to feel or experience sensations such as sound, light or pain.

Septic—Infected.

Serological Tests—Tests of serum (blood without cells) used to diagnose a variety of diseases, especially infections and autoimmune conditions.

Serum—Liquid portion of blood that remains after blood cells and blood clots have been removed.

Serum Alkaline Phosphatase—Material present in excessive amounts in the blood of patients with some bone and liver diseases.

Serum Electrolytes—Same as *Electrolytes*.

Sesamoid Bones—Small oval-shaped bones in the tendons of the hands and feet.

Sever's Disease—Painful condition of the heel bone of growing children.

Sexual Dysfunction—Inability to participate in sexual relations that are satisfactory for both partners.

Shave Biopsy—Procedure to diagnose skin disorders in which a thin layer of tissue from under a skin lesion is shaved away for laboratory examination.

Shock—Condition in which the blood pressure falls below the level needed to supply blood to the body. Signs and symptoms include weakness, paleness, rapid heartbeat, dry mouth, cold sweat and feelings of doom.

Sick-Sinus Syndrome—Form of heart-rhythm disorder (arrhythmia).

Sigmoid Colon—Lower part of the large colon (intestine) located in the pelvis just above the rectum.

Sigmoidoscope, Sigmoidoscopy—Same as *Proctoscope, Proctoscopy*.

Signs—Evidence of disease that can be observed and measured, in contrast to symptoms, which only patients can experience. For example, blood-pressure measurement or red tonsils are signs; headache or nausea are symptoms.

Silicone—Artificial compound used by plastic and reconstructive surgeons to reshape parts of the body, such as the breast.

Silver Nitrate—Chemical used for cautery.

Sims-Huhner Test—Test used in diagnosis of reasons for infertility in women in which the mucus from the cervix is examined, especially for presence of sperm after sexual intercourse.

Sitz bath—Sitting for a period of time in a bathtub that is filled with several inches of warm water. It provides temporary relief to certain types of infections, pain or swelling in the pelvic or buttocks area.

Skin Clips—Small U-shaped metal strips used instead of stitches to close skin that has been incised during surgery.

Skin Tests for Allergy—Diagnostic method used to determine whether a particular substance is causing allergic reactions. The test is carried out by introducing a small amount of the suspected material, such as pollen or dust, under the skin or on the skin. If inflammation results, the patient is allergic to the material.

Sleep Inducers—Medications used to produce sleep.

Sleep-Study Laboratory—Laboratory where persons are studied with sensitive instruments while asleep. Information from sleep study aids in diagnosis of sleep disorders.

Slow Viruses—Group of viruses that infect the brain but do not cause disease until many years afterward.

Small-Bowel Series—A test used to look for blockage in the small bowel, in which the patient swallows a radiopaque fluid (barium), which allows intermittent x-rays to be taken to follow the flow of the fluid through the esophagus, stomach, duodenum and then through the entire small intestine to the colon.

Soaks—Applying moisture—either plain water or water with dissolved medicines—to an inflamed area of the skin.

Soft Palate—Fleshy part of the roof of the mouth close to the throat.

Sonogram, Sonography—See *Ultrasound*.

Spasmodic—Sudden intermittent symptom, or intermittent muscle spasm.

Spastic, Spasticity—A description of muscles that are continuously contracting and in a state of excessive tension.

Speculum—Instrument used to examine the interior of openings such as the vagina, nose, ear or rectum.

Sperm—Male reproductive cells manufactured in testicles and ejaculated in semen.

Spherocytosis—Abnormally shaped red blood cells caused by some anemias. These cells are sphere-shaped, in contrast to the doughnut shape of normal red blood cells.

Spikes, Temperature—High but brief episodes of fever.

Spina Bifida—Congenital (inherited) disorder in which the base of the spine remains open, sometimes exposing the spinal cord and nerves.

Spinal Anesthesia—Method to provide anesthesia to the lower body by injecting an anesthetic into the fluid in the space that surrounds the lower spinal cord.

Spirometry—Test of lung (pulmonary) function.

Spleen—A large organ in the upper abdomen on the left side, located close to the left side of the stomach. It is the largest structure of the lymph system. The spleen causes disintegration of old red blood cells in adults, manufactures red blood cells in the fetus and newborn, and serves as an important reservoir of blood.

Splenic-Vein Thrombosis—Clot in the major vein that carries blood away from the spleen.

Splints—Rigid supports, made of metal, plastic or plaster, used to immobilize an injured or inflamed part of the body. Splints are used temporarily in the case of injury, following some surgical procedures on joints or ligaments, or occasionally in the case of arthritis.

Spore—Microscopic seed form of fungi. Spores are extremely hardy and survive extremes of temperature. If they enter the body of a susceptible person, they can cause fungal disease.

Sputum—Secretion of the lungs, coughed up in large amounts in some lung diseases.

Staphylococcus—Bacteria which frequently cause boils, abscesses, pneumonias, bone infections and infections in other tissues or organs.

Staples—Small U-shaped metal wires used in place of stitches to close incised skin after some surgeries, especially in the digestive system. Also used to close off some portions of the stomach during operations for extreme obesity.

Stenosis—Constriction or narrowing of a passage or opening.

Sterilized—1) Made completely free of all germs, usually by steam heat, toxic gas or chemicals. All instruments used in surgeries are sterilized, as is most other medical equipment. 2) Made unable to conceive children.

Steroids—Medications that resemble hormones produced by the cortex of the adrenal glands, ovaries and testicles.

Stethoscope—Instrument used to listen to the sounds produced by the heart, lungs, blood vessels and pregnant uterus.

Still's Disease—Form of arthritis in children similar to rheumatoid arthritis in adults.

Stimulant Drugs—Medications that increase the activity of the brain and nervous system.

Stomatitis—Inflammation of the mouth.

Stool—Feces.

Streptococcus—Bacteria that cause illnesses such as laryngitis, cellulitis of the skin, pneumonia, meningitis and others. If not treated, streptococcal infections may also cause serious heart and kidney diseases as complications that appear after the original infection has cleared.

Stricture—An abnormal narrowing of a bodily passage.

Subcutaneous—Under the skin.

Sublingual Salivary Glands—Small glands near the base of the tongue that secrete saliva into the mouth.

Submaxillary Salivary Glands—Small glands near the jaw that secrete saliva into the mouth.

Sulfonamides (Sulfa Drugs)—Class of drugs used to fight infections.

Sulfonylurea Drugs—Medications taken orally to treat some forms of diabetes mellitus.

Surgery—Treatment in which the body is restored to a healthy condition by physical methods (or operations) such as cutting, removing, replacing, straightening, repairing or joining.

Surgical Suite—Group of rooms used to perform surgery. In addition to operating rooms, where surgery takes place, there are supply areas, a recovery room, administrative rooms and a lounge for the staff to rest between surgeries.

Suture—Thread-like material used to hold tissues or skin edges together.

Symmetry, Symmetrical—Refers to the arrangement of the body in pairs, such as two arms, legs, kidneys, lungs, etc.

Sympathomimetics—Medications similar to adrenalin in their actions.

Symptoms—Effects of disease that only the patient can experience, such as pain, nausea, dizziness, anxiety, depression and others.

Synovial Membranes—Delicate tissue that lines the inside of joints.

Systemic—Conditions that affect most or all of the body, in contrast to conditions that affect only a limited area. For example, diabetes mellitus is a systemic condition; an abscess is a local condition.

T

Tartar—Hard deposit that forms on the teeth and causes inflammation of the gums.

Temperature Spike—See *Spikes, Temperature*.

Temporomandibular Joint—Joint that joins the jaw to the other head bones.

Tenderness—Condition that causes pain when pressure is applied.

Tendon—Tough cord of tissue at the end of muscles that attach to bone. Tendons transmit the force of muscle contraction to cause movement.

Testes or Testicles—Male sex glands that produce sex hormones and sperm.

Therapeutic Trial—Form of diagnosis and treatment where medication is used even though the diagnosis is not firmly established. If the patient improves after treatment with a medication known to be useful in treating a specific condition, the improvement suggests that the specific disease was present. Therapeutic trials are somewhat risky and are used only when other forms of diagnosis and treatment have failed.

Therapist—Health-care professional specially trained to provide therapy.

Thermogram, Thermography—Method of diagnosis that measures body heat. The area being studied is scanned by a heat-sensitive instrument capable of producing an image (thermogram) of areas of increased heat. They are useful in studying female breast tumors and some blood-vessel conditions.

Thiazide Diuretics—Class of medications that promote excretion of excess fluids by the kidneys.

Third Molars—Permanent grinding teeth that appear at about age 17 to 25.

Thoracic Duct—The largest channel of the lymphatic system, through which lymph fluid enters the vena cava.

Thoracic Spine—That part of the spinal column below the neck and above the back. Ribs attach to the thoracic spine.

Thoracic Surgeon—A surgeon who specializes in surgical treatment of disorders of the organs in the thorax (chest), including lungs, pericardium, heart, pleura (covering of lungs), bronchial tubes and large blood vessels.

Thyroglossal Duct—Small passageway, normally closed, located in the upper neck. It extends from the back of the tongue to just above the larynx. If an abnormally open duct becomes filled with fluid, a thyroglossal cyst results.

Thyroid Cartilage—Larynx (also called the voice box, or Adam's apple), made of semi-hard cartilage.

Thyroid Gland—Endocrine gland located in the lower neck next to the trachea that produces hormones that regulate the rate at which all body cells function. Thyroid hormones are also essential for normal growth and development.

Thyroid Scan—Method of examination of the thyroid gland in which a small amount of radioactive iodine introduced into the body collects in the thyroid gland. An instrument passed over the thyroid produces an image of the gland based on the concentration of the radioactive iodine.

Thrombocytopenia—A persistent decrease in the number of blood platelets, often associated with hemorrhaging.

TIA—See Transient Ischemic Attack.

Ticks—Small biting insects that may cause inflammation of the skin or serious infections such as Rocky Mountain spotted fever.

Tics—Brief, uncontrollable muscle spasms. Tics usually involve the face and the shoulders.

Tissue—Building blocks of body organs; living cells all of one type.

Tonsils—Lymphatic tissues that help fight infection located at the entrance of the throat. They frequently become infected, especially in children.

Topical—Medications applied to the skin, conjunctiva, or mucous membrane of the mouth, nose, vagina or rectum.

Tourette's Syndrome—A rare disorder of movement. It involves repetitive grimaces and tics, usually of the head and neck, sometimes arms, legs and trunk. Involuntary noises and foul language may occur.

Tourniquet—Cord or band wrapped around an arm or leg tightly enough to stop blood circulation temporarily.

Toxic, Toxicity—Harmful; capable of causing body damage.

Toxin—Poison. Usually refers to the chemicals produced by some living organisms that harm the human body.

Tracheostomy Tube—A tube which is connected to an artificial opening into the trachea through the neck, and through which breathing is performed.

Traction—Method of treating some conditions of bones, muscles and ligaments by exerting a steady pull on the affected parts. Some bone fractures and back pain due to a ruptured disk are treated this way.

Tranquilizer—Medication used to help diminish anxiety and to produce calmness.

Tranquilizers, Benzodiazepine—Class of tranquilizers commonly used to treat anxiety, nervousness or tension.

Transfuse—To give a patient blood, necessary in treatment of some conditions.

Transfusion—Process of introducing blood through a needle placed in the patient's vein.

Transfusion Reaction—Undesirable symptom or condition resulting from a blood transfusion.

Transient Ischemic Attack, TIA—A temporary decrease in the blood supply to part of the brain which temporarily interferes with normal brain function.

Transmission, Transmit—Passing a disease to another person.

Transplant, Transplantation—Living organ (such as kidney, cornea, heart, bone marrow or skin), removed from one person (donor), and placed in the body of another (recipient).

Transverse Colon—Middle part of the colon (intestine), lying horizontally in the middle or upper abdomen.

Trauma—Force that injures or damages any part of the body.

Tricyclic Antidepressant Drugs (Tricyclics)—Class of medications used to treat depression.

Trophoblastic Tumors—See *Hydatidiform Mole*.

Tube Feeding—Providing nutrients through a small tube placed in the stomach of patients who are unable to eat. The tube may pass through the nose to the stomach or be inserted through an incision in the stomach.

Tuberous Sclerosis—Rare inherited condition of the skin, nervous system and other organs of the body.

Tumor—Literally, a swelling; usually used to refer to a benign or cancerous growth.

Tympanogram—A test which measures the function of the tympanic membrane in the middle ear.

U

Ulceration—Wearing away of the surface or lining of an organ, exposing underlying tissue. Ulceration of the lining of the stomach exposes blood vessels, which may bleed. Ulceration may erode through the wall of an organ (perforation). Ulceration frequently affects the skin, if rubbed excessively or if diseased.

Ultrasonography, Ultrasound—Diagnostic method in which high-frequency (ultrasound) sound waves are transmitted into the body. Their reflections create images of body organs.

Ultrasound Treatment—Method of treatment in which high-energy sound waves are focused on the affected area, producing mild heat that helps relieve inflammation. It is especially useful in treatment of muscular symptoms.

Underlying—Beneath, below or more basic. Thus, losing weight may result from an underlying condition such as diabetes mellitus or cancer.

Upper Gastrointestinal Series—X-ray examination of the esophagus, stomach and duodenum accomplished by having the patient swallow barium solution that x-rays can detect.

Upper Respiratory System—Upper part of the breathing system, consisting of the nose, throat, larynx, trachea and bronchial tubes.

Uremia—A serious condition associated with kidney failure in which body wastes build up in the blood and body tissues.

Ureters—Slender muscular tubes that carry urine from the kidneys to the urinary bladder, where it is stored until eliminated from the body.

Urethra—Tubular passageway extending from the urinary bladder to the outside of the body.

Uric Acid—Chemical normally produced in the body from metabolism or breakdown of protein and eliminated in the urine. If the level of uric acid rises in the body as a result of disease, gout or kidney stones may result.

Urinalysis—Laboratory test performed on a urine sample that helps diagnose diseases of the kidney and other parts of the body.

Urinary Bladder—Muscular sac in the lower abdomen that stores urine brought to it from the kidneys by the ureters. The bladder stores urine until it can be eliminated through the urethra by contractions of the bladder muscles.

Urinary Studies—Laboratory or x-ray tests of the urinary tract.

Urinary Tract—Organs that produce, store and eliminate urine. The organs are the kidneys, ureters, urinary bladder and urethra.

Urography—See *Intravenous Urography*.

Uterus—Organ of the female reproductive system on the wall of which the fertilized egg (ovum) attaches and develops to form a fetus.

Uveitis—Inflammation of the parts of the eyes that make up the iris (the colored tissue encircling the clear center, the pupil).

Uvula—Soft tissue hanging down from the soft palate at the back of the throat.

V

Vaccination—Method of providing protection against disease (immunity) by giving a patient a small amount of the disease-causing germ that is weakened, killed or otherwise modified so that it cannot itself cause disease. Same as *Immunization*.

Vaccine—Medication used to provide immunity by vaccination. Vaccines are given mostly by injection or by mouth.

Vagus Nerve—Long cranial nerve, arising in the base of the brain and passing to the chest and abdomen. It helps regulate heart rate, breathing, swallowing, digestion and many other body functions.

Varicose—Swollen and twisting; usually used to describe varicose veins.

Vas Deferens—Tube that carries sperm manufactured by the testicles toward the prostate gland and seminal vesicles.

Vasculitis—Inflammation of blood vessels, the basis of many illnesses.

Vasoconstrictor Drugs—Medications that cause blood vessels to contract, tighten or become smaller.

Vasodilator Drugs—Medications that cause small arteries to widen, providing more blood to an area of the body where the blood vessels are constricted by spasm, narrowed or obstructed.

Vector—1) An imaginary line that represents both direction and quantity used to study electrocardiograms (ECG's). 2) An agent that transmits infectious germs from one organism to another.

Veins—Blood vessels that return blood from body organs to the heart and lungs. Veins are much thinner than arteries. Veins carry blood at a much lower pressure than do arteries.

Vena Cava—Largest vein in the body. It collects blood from the venous system and carries it to the heart.

Vena Cavography—Method of studying the vena cava by injecting into the bloodstream a medication that x-rays can detect.

Venereal—Related to sexual intercourse or sexual contact. Venereal diseases such as genital herpes, gonorrhea or syphilis are now usually referred to as sexually transmitted diseases (STD's).

Venography—Method of studying the veins by injecting into the bloodstream a medication that x-rays can detect.

Venous Stasis Ulcer—An open sore on the skin of the lower extremities, caused when normal outflow of blood in the legs is obstructed (as in deep venous thrombosis). The resulting pressure from the back-up of blood causes leaking and weeping of fluid into the surrounding tissues (edema), which then stretches the arteries and deprives the skin of oxygen. The skin then breaks down into open sores which leak serum and are prone to infection.

Venous System—Network of veins that extend from all body organs and transport blood back to the heart.

Ventricles—Chambers containing fluid. The ventricles of the heart pump blood; ventricles of the brain contain cerebrospinal fluid.

Ventricular Aneurysm—Ballooning of the wall of the heart resulting from a weakening of the heart muscle, a complication of scarring from a previous heart attack.

Vertebrae—Bones of the spine that form the vertebral column (backbone).

Vertebral Column—The spine; the bones of the back.

Virulent—Extremely dangerous or harmful. Virulent bacteria are ones capable of causing diseases.

Viruses—Small germs responsible for a variety of infectious illnesses. Viruses are not alive until they enter cells of the body, where they grow and reproduce, causing viral illnesses.

Visual Acuity—Clarity with which objects are seen.

Vitamins—Chemical substances found in food that are necessary for healthy body growth, function and tissue repair.

Vitreous—Clear fluid that fills much of the eye.

Vocal Cords—Two narrow bands of fibrous and muscular tissue in the larynx that vibrate to create the sounds of the voice.

Volvulus—Twisting of loops of intestines, which become closed off (obstructed) and may lose their blood supply.

Vulva—The external genitalia of the female including the clitoris and vaginal lips.

W

Warts—Small, often hard and rough skin growths caused by viruses that infect the skin.

Wasting of Body or Muscles—Severe loss of body tissues (other than surplus fat), especially muscles and vital organs, resulting in weakness, susceptibility to infection, bone fractures and sometimes death.

Weber Test—Hearing test performed with a tuning fork.

Wheezes—High-pitched sounds and whistles produced in the lungs where secretions have partially blocked air passages.

Wheal—A temporary skin elevation usually a result of an allergic reaction.

Whirlpool Treatment—Method of treating minor blood-vessel and musculo-skeletal diseases by immersion in a pool where jets of warm water enter and swirl under high pressure.

Wisdom Teeth—Same as *Third Molars*.

X

X-Rays—High energy, invisible waves capable of penetrating the body and creating shadows on photographic film. The shadows provide images of the body tissues through which the x-rays pass.

Xeroradiogram—Method of x-ray diagnosis, usually of the female breast, which uses a process similar to that used to produce photocopies.

Xerosis—Abnormal dryness.

Y

Yellow Fever—An acute disease caused by a virus spread by insect bites. Usually seen in Africa and South America.

Yersinia Infection—A type of foodborne bacteria that can cause gastroenteritis and diarrhea.

Z

Zoster—"Girdle," used to describe a form of virus infection (herpes zoster, shingles) that often produces bands of inflammation across the chest or abdomen.

Zygote—The fertilized egg before division.

Resources for
Additional Information

Websites & Other Resources for Information on Specific Health Problems & Medical Disorders

The following list provides names of organizations and support groups that offer medical information and assistance by telephone, mail or the internet. Toll-free numbers use prefixes of 800, 888, 877, 866 and 855.

If you are unable to find a listing for your disorder or problem, call the National Health Information Center at (800) 336-4797; website www.health.gov/nhic or the National Organization for Rare Disorders information line, (800) 999-6673; website www.raredisorders.org.

Acne Rosacea
National Rosacea Society
800 S. Northwest, Suite 200
Barrington, IL 60010
(888) 662-5874
www.rosacea.org

Aging
National Council on the Aging
409 Third St., S.W., Suite 200
Washington, DC 20024
(800) 373-4906

AIDS
HIV/AIDS Information Resources
P.O. Box 6003
Rockville, MD 20849
(800) 232-4636
www.cdc.gov/hiv/hivinfo.htm

Alcoholism
Alcoholics Anonymous
Grand Central Station
P.O. Box 459
New York, NY 10163
(212) 870-3400
www.aa.org

National Council on Alcoholism
20 Exchange Place, Suite 2902
New York, NY 10005
(800) 622-2255
www.ncadd.org

Allergies
American Academy of Allergy & Immunology
555 E. Wells St., Suite 1100
Milwaukee, WI 53202
(800) 822-2762
www.aaaai.org

Alopecia Areata
National Alopecia Areata Foundation
P.O. Box 150760
San Rafael, CA 94915
(415) 472-3780
www.naaf.org

Alzheimer's
Alzheimer's Association
225 N. Michigan Ave., Fl.17
Chicago, IL 60601
(800) 272-3900
www.alz.org

Amyotrophic Lateral Sclerosis
Amyotrophic Lateral Sclerosis Association
2700 Agoura Road, Suite 150
Calabasas, CA 91301
(800) 782-4747
www.alsa.org

Anorexia Nervosa
Anorexia Nervosa & Related Eating Disorders
P.O. Box 5102
Eugene, OR 97405
(503) 344-1144
www.anred.com

Anxiety
Anxiety Disorders Association of America
8730 Georgia Ave., Suite 600
Silver Spring, MD 20910
(240) 485-1001
www.adaa.org

National Institute of Mental Health (NIMH)
6001 Executive Blvd., Rm 8184,
MSC 9663
Bethesda, MD 20892.
(866) 615-6464
www.nimh.nih.gov

Arthritis
Arthritis Foundation
P.O. Box 7669
Atlanta, GA 30357
(800) 568-4045
www.arthritis.org

Asbestosis
American Lung Association
61 Broadway, 6th Floor
New York, NY 10006
(800) 548-8252
www.lungusa.org

Asthma
Asthma & Allergy Foundation of America
1233 20th St., NW, Suite 402
Washington, DC 20036
(800) 727-8462
www.aafa.org

National Jewish Medical & Research Center
  - Lung Line
1400 Jackson St.
Denver, CO 80206
(800) 222-5864
www.nationaljewish.org

Atelectasis— See Lung Disorders

Atherosclerosis— See Heart Disorders

Atrial Fibrillation— See Heart Disorders

Autism
Autism Society of America
7910 Woodmont Ave., Suite 300
Bethesda, MD 20814
(800) 328-8476
www.autsim-society.org

Bed Wetting
American Academy of Pediatrics
141 Northwest Point Blvd.
Elk Grove Village, IL 60007
(847) 434-4000
www.aap.org

American Enuresis Foundation
P.O. Box 54556
Tulsa, OK 74155

Birth Control & Family Planning
Planned Parenthood Federation of America
810 Seventh Ave.
New York, NY 10019
(212) 541-7800
www.plannedparenthood.org/pp2/porta

Birth Defects
March of Dimes
1275 Mamaroneck Ave.
White Plains, NY 10605
(888) 663-4637
www.marchofdimes.com

Blindness
American Council of the Blind
1155 15 St., NW, Suite 1004
Washington, DC 20005
(800) 424-8666
www.acb.org

American Foundation for the Blind (AFB)
11 Penn Plaza, Suite 300
New York, NY 10001
(800) 232-5463
www.afb.org

Brain Tumor
American Brain Tumor Association
2720 River Road
Des Plaines, IL 60018
(800) 886-2282
www.abta.org

Brain Disorders
Brain Research Foundation
5812 S. Ellis Ave., MC 7112, Rm. J141
Chicago, IL 60637
(773) 834-6751
www.brainresearchfdn.org

Breast Cancer
Y-ME National Breast Cancer Organization
212 W. Van Buren, Suite 1000
Chicago, IL 60607
(800) 221-2141
www.y-me.org

Bronchiectasis— See Lung Disorders

Bronchitis— See Lung Disorders

Bulimia— See Eating Disorders

Burns
World Burn Foundation
409 N. Camden Dr., Suite 106
Beverly Hills, CA 90210
(310) 858-1717
www.burnsurvivorsonline.com

Cancer
American Cancer Society
1599 Clifton Rd., NE
Atlanta, GA 30329
(800) 227-2345
www.cancer.org

National Cancer Institute
6116 Executive Blvd., Rm 3036A
Bethesda, MD 20892
(800) 422-6347
www.cancer.gov

Celiac Disease
Celiac Disease Foundation
13251 Ventura Blvd., Suite 1
Studio City, CA 91604
(818) 990-2354
www.celiac.org

Celiac Sprue Association
P.O. Box 31700
Omaha. NE 68131
(877) 272-4272
www.csaceliacs.org

Cerebral Palsy
United Cerebral Palsy Association
1660 L St., NW, Suite 700
Washington, DC 20036
(800) 872-5827
www.ucp.org

Cholecystitis or Cholangitis— See
Digestive Diseases

Chronic Fatigue Syndrome
Chronic Fatigue and Immune Dysfunction
   Syndrome (CFIDS) Association
P.O. Box 220398
Charlotte, NC 28222
(800) 442-3437
www.cfids.org

**Chronic Obstructive Pulmonary
Disease—** See Lung Disorders

Cirrhosis of the Liver— See Liver
Disorders

Colitis, Ulcerative
Crohn's & Colitis Foundation of America
386 Park Ave. South, 17th Floor
New York, NY 10016
(800) 932-2423
www.ccfa.org

Cor Pulmonale— See Heart Disorders

Coronary Artery Disease— See Heart
Disorders

Crohn's Disease
Crohn's & Colitis Foundation of America
386 Park Ave. South, 17th Floor
New York, NY 10016
(800) 932-2423
www.ccfa.org

Cystic Fibrosis
Cystic Fibrosis Foundation
6931 Arlington Rd.
Bethesda, MD 20814
(800) 344-4823
www.cff.org

Dementia— See Alzheimer's Disease

Dental Problems
American Dental Association
211 E. Chicago Ave.
Chicago, IL 60611
(312) 440-2500
www.ada.org

Depression
National Institute of Mental Health (NIMH)
6001 Executive Blvd., Rm 8184, MSC 9663
Bethesda, MD 20892
(866) 615-6464
www.nimh.nih.gov

Diabetes
American Diabetes Association
National Call Center
1701 North Beauregard St.
Alexandria, VA 22311
(800) 342-2383
www.diabetes.org

Digestive Diseases
National Digestive Diseases
   Information Clearinghouse
2 Information Way
Bethesda, MD 20892
(800) 891-5389

Diverticular Disease— See Digestive
Diseases

Domestic Violence
National Domestic Violence Hotline
(800) 799-7233
www.ndvh.org

National Coalition Against Domestic
Violence
P.O. Box 18749, Denver, CO 80218
(303) 839-1852
www.ncadv.org

Down Syndrome
National Down Syndrome Congress
1370 Center Dr.
Atlanta, GA 30338
(800) 232-6372
www.ndscenter.org

National Down Syndrome Society
666 Broadway
New York, NY 10012
(800) 221-4602
www.ndss.org

Drug Abuse
Cocaine Abuse Hotline
(800) 262-2463

National Institute on Drug Abuse
6001 Executive Blvd., Rm 5213
Bethesda, MD 20892
(301) 443-1124
www.drugabuse.gov

Eating Disorders
Anorexia Nervosa & Related Eating Disorders
P.O. Box 5102
Eugene, OR 97405
(503) 344-1144
www.anred.com

National Eating Disorders Association
603 Stewart St., Suite 803
Seattle WA 98101
(800) 931-2237
www.nationaleatingdisorders.org

Eczema
National Eczema Association
4460 Redwood Hwy, Suite 16-D
San Rapheal, CA 94903
(800) 818-7546
www.nationaleczema.org

Endocrine Disorders (Thyroid, Parathyroid, Pituitary, Sex Glands, Adrenals)
National Institute of Diabetes & Digestive
  & Kidney Diseases
9000 Rockville Pike
Bethesda, MD 20892
www.niddk.nih.gov

Endometriosis
Endometriosis Association
8585 N. 76 Pl.
Milwaukee, WI 53223
(800) 992-3636
www.endometriosisassn.org

Fertility Problems
Fertility Research Foundation
877 Park Ave.
New York, NY 10021
(212) 744-5500
www.frfbaby.com

National Infertility Association
7910 Woodmont Ave., Suite 1350
Bethesda, MD 20814
(888) 623-0744
www.resolve.org

Fibromyalgia
National Fibromyalgia Association
2200 N. Glassell St., Suite A
Orange, CA 92865
(714) 921-0150
www.fmaware.org

Food Allergy
Food Allergy & Anaphylaxis Network
11781 Lee Jackson Hwy., Suite 160
Fairfax, VA 22033
(800) 929-4040
www.foodallergy.org

Foot Disorders
American Podiatry Association
9312 Old Georgetown Rd.
Bethesda, MD 20814
(800) 366-8227

Gallstones— See Digestive Diseases

Glaucoma
Glaucoma Foundation
116 John St, Suite 1605
New York, NY 10038
(800) 452-8266
www.glaucomafoundation.org

Glaucoma Research Foundation
490 Post St., Suite 1427
San Francisco, CA 94102
(800) 826-6693
www.glaucoma.org

Gonorrhea— See Sexually Transmitted Diseases

Guillain-Barré
Guillain-Barré Syndrome Foundation
P.O. Box 262
Wynnewood, PA 19096
(610) 667-0131
www.guillain-barre.com

Head Injury
Brain Injury Association
8201 Greensboro Dr., Suite 611
McLean, VA 22102
(800) 444-6443
www.biausa.org

Headache
National Headache Foundation
820 N. Orleans, Suite 217
Chicago, IL 60610
(888) 643-5552
www.headaches.org

Hearing Disorders
National Association of the Deaf
814 Thayer Ave.
Silver Spring, MD 20910
(301) 587-1788
www.nad.org

American Speech-Language-Hearing
  Association
10801 Rockville Pike
Rockville, MD 20852
(800) 638-8255
www.asha.org

Dial a Hearing Screen Test (DAHST)
(800) 222-3277

National Hearing Aid Helpline
20361 Middlebelt Rd.
Livonia, MI 48152
(800) 521-5247

Heart Disorders
American Heart Association
7272 Greenville Ave.
Dallas, TX 75231
(800) 242-8721
www.americanheart.org

National Heart, Lung & Blood Institute
P.O. Box 30105
Bethesda, MD 20824
(301) 592-8573
www.nhlbi.nih.gov

Heartburn
National Heartburn Alliance
303 East Wacker Drive, Suite 440
Chicago, IL 60601
(877) 471-2081
www.heartburnalliance.org

Hemophilia
National Hemophilia Foundation
116 W. 32 St., 11 Floor
New York, NY 10001
(800) 424-2634
www.hemophilia.org

Herpes
National Herpes Resource Center
P.O. Box 13827
Research Triangle Park, NC 27709
(800) 230-6039
www.ashastd.org/hre

HIV— See AIDS

Hypertension— See Heart Disorders

Immunodeficiency Disease
Immune Deficiency Foundation
40 W. Chesapeake Ave., Suite 308
Towson, MD 21204
(800) 296-4433
www.primaryimmune.org

Impotence, Male Sexual
American Foundation for Urologic Disease
1000 Corporate Blvd., Suite 410
Linthicum, MD 21090
(800) 828-7866
www.afud.org

Incontinence
National Association for Continence
P.O. Box 1019
Charleston, SC 29402
(800) 252-3337
www.nafc.org

Simon Foundation for Continence
P.O. Box 815
Wilmette, IL 60091
(800) 237-4666
www.simonfoundation.org

Irritable Bowel Syndrome
Crohn's & Colitis Foundation of America
384 Park Ave. S., 11th Flr.
New York, NY 10016
(800) 932-2423
www.ccfa.org

Kidney Disorders
American Kidney Fund
6100 Executive Blvd., Suite 1010
Rockville, MD 20852
(800) 638-8299
www.kidneyfund.org

National Kidney Foundation
30 E. 33rd St.
New York, NY 10016
(800) 622-9010
www.kidney.org

Lead Poisoning
Environmental Protection Agency (EPA)
1200 Pennsylvania Ave., NW
Mail Code 7404T
Washington, DC 20460
(800) 424-5323
www.epa.gov/lead/

Leukemia
Leukemia & Lymphoma Society
1311 Mamaroneck Ave.
White Plains, NY 10605
(800) 955-4572
www.lls.org

Lice
National Pediculosis Association
50 Kearney Road
Needham, MA 02494
(781) 449-6487
www.headlice.org

Liver Disorders
American Liver Foundation
75 Maiden Lane
New York, NY 10038
(800) 465-4837
www.liverfoundation.org

Lung Disorders
American Lung Association
61 Broadway, 6th Floor
New York, NY 10006
(800) 548-8252
www.lungusa.org

National Heart, Lung & Blood Institute
P.O. Box 30105
Bethesda, MD 20824
(301) 592-8573
www.nhlbi.nih.gov

Lupus
Lupus Foundation of America, Inc.
2000 L St., NW, Suite 710
Washington, DC 20036
(800) 558-0121
www.lupus.org

Lyme Disease
American Lyme Disease Foundation, Inc.
Mill Pond Offices
293 Route 100
Somers. NY 10589
(914) 277-6970
www.aldf.com

Lyme Disease Foundation
P.O. Box 332
Tolland, CT 06084
(800) 886-5963
www.lyme.org

Marfan Syndrome
National Marfan Foundation
22 Manhasset Ave.
Port Washington, NY 11050
(800) 862-7326
www.marfan.org

Medical Identification
Medic Alert Foundation International
2323 Colorado Ave.
Turlock, CA 95382
(888) 633-4298
www.medicalalert.org

Menopause
National Institute on Aging
Building 31, Room 5C27
31 Center Dr., MSC 2292
Bethesda, MD 20892
(800) 222-2225
www.nia.nih.gov

North American Menopause Society
P.O. Box 94527
Cleveland, OH 44101
(440) 442-7550
www.menopause.org

Mental Health
National Mental Health Association
2001 Beauregard St., 12 Floor
Alexandria, VA 22311
(800) 969-6642
www.nmha.org

National Institute of Mental Health
6001 Executive Blvd., Rm 8184
MSC 9663
Bethesda, MD 20892.
(866) 615-6464
www.nimh.nih.gov

Movement Disorders
We Move
204 West 84th St.
New York, NY, 10024
(800) 437-6682
www.wemove.org

Multiple Sclerosis
National Multiple Sclerosis Society
733 3rd Ave.
New York, NY 10017
(800) 344-4867
www.nmss.org

Multiple Sclerosis Association
706 Haddonfield Rd.
Cherry Hill, NJ 08002
(856) 488-4500
www.msaa.com

Muscular Dystrophy
Muscular Dystrophy Association
3300 E Sunrise Dr.
Tucson, AZ 85718
(800) 572-1717
www.mdausa.org

Myasthenia Gravis
Myasthenia Gravis Foundation
1821 University Ave. W., Suite S256
St. Paul, MN 55104
(800) 541-5454
www.myasthenia.org

Myocarditis— See Heart Disorders

Narcolepsy
Narcolepsy Network
P.O. Box 294
Pleasantville, NY 10570
(888) 292-6522
www.nacolepsynetwork.org

Nephrosis— See Kidney Disorders

Nutrition & Dietetics
National Center for Nutrition & Dietetics
  Consumer Information
120 S. Riverside Plaza, Suite 2000
Chicago, IL 60606
(800) 366-1655
www.eatright.org

Department of Agriculture
Food Service & Inspection Service
Meat & Poultry Hotline
(888) 674-6854
www.fsis.usda.gov

Obesity
American Obesity Association
1250 24th St., NW, Suite 300
Washington, DC 20037
(800) 986-2373
www.obesity.org

Obsessive-Compulsive Disorder
Obsessive-Compulsive Anonymous
P.O. Box 215
New Hyde Park, NY 11040
(516) 739-0662

Obsessive-Compulsive Foundation, Inc.
676 State St.
New Haven. CT 06511
(203) 401-2070
www.ocfoundation.org

Osteoporosis
National Osteoporosis Foundation
1232 22 St., NW
Washington, DC 20037
(800) 223-9994
www.nof.org

Otosclerosis— See Hearing Problems

Pancreatitis— See Digestive Diseases

Parkinson's Disease
American Parkinson Disease Association
1250 Hylan Blvd., Suite 4B
Staten Island, NY 10305
(800) 223-2732
www.apdaparkinson.org

National Parkinson Foundation
1501 N.W. 9th Ave/Bob Hope Road
Miami, FL 33136
(800) 327-4545
www.parkinson.org

Pericarditis, Acute— See Heart Disorders

Phobias
Anxiety Disorders Association of America
8739 Georgia Ave., Suite 600
Silver Spring, MD 20910
(240) 485-1001
www.adaa.org

Pneumonia— See Lung Disorders

Porphyria
American Porphyria Foundation
P.O. Box 22712
Houston, TX 77277
(713) 266-9617
www.porphyriafoundation.com

Premenstrual Syndrome
National Women's Health Information
  Center
8550 Arlington Blvd., Suite 300
Fairfax. VA 22031
(800) 994 9662
www.4women.gov/faq/pms.htm

**Polymyalgia Rheumatica or Temporal
  Arteritis**— See Arthritis

Polymyositis— See Muscular Dystrophy

Prostate Disorders
Prostate Information Center
P.O. Box 9
Minneapolis. MN 55440
(800) 543-9632

Psoriasis
National Psoriasis Foundation
6600 SW 92 Ave., Suite 300
Portland, OR 97223
(800) 723-9166
www.psoriasis.org

Rape Crisis Syndrome
National Sexual Assault Hotline
(800) 656-4673
(connects callers to a nearby rape crisis center)
www.rainn.org

Women Organized Against Rape
1233 Locust St., Suite 202
Philadelphia, PA 19107
(215) 985 3333
www.woar.org

Rare Disorders
National Organization for Rare Disorders
55 Kenosia Ave., P.O. Box 1968
Danbury, CT 06813
(800) 999-6673
www.raredisorders.org

Raynaud's
Raynaud's Association
94 Mercier Ave.
Hartsdale, NY 10530
(800) 280-8055
www.raynauds.org

Reflex Sympathetic Dystrophy Syndrome
Reflex Sympathetic Dystrophy Syndrome
  Association
P.O. Box 502
Milford, CT 06460
(877) 662-7737
www.rsds.org

Renal Failure— See Kidney Disorders

Reye's Syndrome
National Reye's Syndrome Foundation
426 N. Lewis, P.O. Box 829
Bryan, OH 43506
(800) 233-7393
www.reyessyndrome.org

Rheumatic Fever— See Heart Disorders

Scleroderma
Scleroderma Foundation
12 Kent Way, Suite 101
Byfield, MA 01922
(800) 722-4673
www.scleroderma.org

Scoliosis
Scoliosis Association, Inc.
P. O. Box 811705
Boca Raton, FL 33481
(800) 800-0669
www.scoliosis-assoc.org

National Scoliosis Foundation
5 Cabot Pl.
Stoughton, MA 02072
(800) 673-6922
www.scoliosis.org

Seasonal Affective Disorder
National Organization for Seasonal
  Affective Disorder
P.O. Box 40133
Washington, DC 20016
(no telephone number available)
www.nosad.org

Seizure Disorders
Epilepsy Foundation of America
4351 Garden City Dr.
Landover, MD 20785
(800) 332-1000
www.efa.org

Sexually Transmitted Diseases
National Sexually Transmitted Diseases
  Hotline
(800) 227-8922
www.ashastd.org/nstd

Sickle Cell Disease
Sickle Cell Disease Association of America
16 S. Calvert St., Suite 600
Baltimore, MD 21202
(800) 421-8453
www.sicklecelldisease.org

Silicosis— See Lung Disorders

Sjögren's Syndrome
Sjögren's Syndrome Foundation
8120 Woodmont Ave.
Bethesda, MD 20814
(800) 475-6473
www.sjogrens.org

Skin Cancer
Skin Cancer Foundation
245 5th Ave., Suite 1403
New York, NY 10016
(212) 725-5751
www.skincancer.org

Skin Disorders
American Academy of Dermatology
P.O. Box 4014
Schaumber, IL 60168
(847) 330-0230
www.aad.org

Sleep Disorders
National Sleep Foundation
1522 K St., Suite 500
Washington, DC 20005
(202) 347-3472
www.sleepfoundation.org

Stroke
National Stroke Association
9707 E. Easter lane
Englewood, CO 80112
(800) 787-6537
www.stroke.org

American Heart Association
7272 Greenville Ave.
Dallas, TX 75231
(800) 242-8721
www.americanheart.org

Syphilis— See Sexually Transmitted
Diseases

Tay-Sachs Disease
National Tay-Sachs and Allied Disease
    Association
2001 Beacon St., Suite 204
Brighton, MA 02135l
(800) 906-8723
www.ntsad.org

Thyroid Disorders
Thyroid Foundation of America
One Longfellow Place, Suite 1518
Boston, MA 02114
(800) 832-8321
www.tsh.org

Tinnitus
American Tinnitus Association
P.O. Box 5
Portland, OR 97207
(800) 634-8978
www.ata.org

Tooth Problems
American Dental Association
211 E. Chicago Ave.
Chicago, IL 60611
(312) 440-2500
www.ada.org

Travel & Health
Centers for Disease Control Travel Health
    Traveler's Health Hotline
(888) 394-8747
www.cdc.gov/travel

Tuberculosis— See Lung Disorders

Tumors, Malignant— See Cancer

Ulcer, Peptic— See Digestive Diseases

Urinary Calculi— See Kidney Disorders

Vision
American Council of the Blind
1155 15 St., NW Suite 1004
Washington, DC 20005
(800) 424-8666
www.acb.org

Lighthouse International
111 E. 59 St.
New York, NY 10022
(800) 829-0500
www.lighthouse.org

National Eye Institute
2020 Vision Place
Bethesda, MD 20892
(301) 496-5248
www.nei.nih.gov

Wilm's Tumor— See Cancer

Websites for
General Health & Medical Information

This is a selected list of websites that provide general medical and health information. There are also many others (sponsored by different types of organizations) that are useful for valid and quality medical information, patient education materials, and helpful ideas for managing your health.

People looking for health and medical information have many choices on the World Wide Web. It is important to know the source and if it is reliable. Look at the web page address (also called the URL or Unifrom Resource Locator). The following types of addresses often have excellent websites:

1. Addresses that end in .gov are provided by the U.S. government.
2. Addresses that end in .org are normally provided by nonprofit organizations, such as the American Heart Association.
3. Addresses ending in .edu are provided by educational institutions such as universities or colleges.

Websites that advertise products (.com) can be good sources for medical information also, but should be read with some caution. It is often helpful to compare several different web resources on the same topic.

Information on the Web is not a substitute for your health care provider's instructions and advice. It can not replace the knowledge and experience that your health care provider can share with you.

American Dental Association
www.ada.org/public//index.asp
The American Dental Association provides information on topics about your teeth and oral health (such as Anxiety about dental visits).

CancerNet (National Cancer Institute)
www.cancernet.nci.nih.gov
A source of current cancer information for patients and anyone interested in learning more about cancer.

Centers for Disease Control (CDC) Division of Sexually Transmitted Diseases Prevention
www.cdc.gov/nchstp/dstd/dstdp.html
Provides information on specific diseases. A good starting point for reliable STD facts.

Family Doctor
www.familydoctor.org
The American Academy of Family Physicians provides information for general educational purposes for the whole family. All of the information has been written and reviewed by physicians and patient education professionals.

Healthfinder
www.healthfinder.gov
The U.S. Department of Health & Human services along with other federal agencies designed this web site as a gateway to consumer health information. It provides access to selected online publications, clearinghouses, databases, web sites, and support and self-help groups. It also links to government agencies and not-for-profit organizations that produce reliable information for the public.

Kids Health
www.kidshealth.org
Provides doctor-approved, up-to-date and accurate health information about children from before birth through adolescents.

Mayo Clinic
www.mayoclinic.com
Sponsored by the Mayo Clinic, this site offers general information about health and medical topics. New information is added daily.

Medem
www.medem.com
Medem is the web site project of several organizations—including the American Medical Association, the American Academy of Pediatrics, and the American College of Obstetricians and Gynecologists. It is a comprehensive and trusted source of health care content on the Internet.

Medlineplus
www.medlineplus.gov
A web site established by the National Library of Medicine, the world's largest biomedical library and creator of the Medline database. An alphabetical list of medical and health topics consists of hundreds of specific diseases, conditions and wellness issues. Health information in Spanish is also included.

National Health Information Center
www.health.gov/nhic
This site is run by the U.S. Department of Health and Human Services. It provides links to many organizations that have information about specific medical topics.

National Women's Health Information Center (NWHIC)
www.4woman.gov
A project of the Office on Women's Health in the U.S. Department of Health and Human Services (HHS). NWHIC is a gateway to women's health information resources that allows visitors to read and download a wide variety of materials developed by federal government agencies, and private sector resources.

EMERGENCY FIRST AID

This section lists basic steps in recognizing and treating immediate effects of emergencies.

If possible, take a course in first aid and learn technique, called cardiopulmonary resuscitation (CPR). This is a lifesaving procedure that is performed when someone's breathing or heartbeat has stopped. It combines rescue breathing which provides oxygen to the person's lungs and chest compression, which keeps the person's blood circulating.

ANAPHYLAXIS (Severe allergic reaction)

Symptoms

Itching, rash, hives, runny nose, wheezing, paleness, cold sweats, dizziness, low blood pressure, coma, cardiac arrest. Symptoms usually occur within 30 minutes after an insect sting or ingestion of certain foods or drugs.

Treatment

If Victim is Unconscious, Not Breathing

1. Yell for help. Don't leave victim.

2. Call or have someone call 911 (emergency) for an ambulance or medical help. The emergency operator may give you first-aid instructions to perform before emergency help arrives. These may include rescue breathing and/or chest compressions.

3. Check to see if the person is carrying special medication to inject to counter the effects of the allergic attack. If so, use it if you know how.

4. Clear the victim's mouth of foreign material, tilt jaw forward without moving the neck.

5. Chest compressions: If there is no pulse (no heartbeat), place one hand on top of the other between the person's nipples and push down on the chest 2 inches. Do this 15 times.

6. Rescue breathing: If chest compressions do not start heart beat, tilt the person's head back, pinch nose, cover the mouth with yours, and blow until you see the chest rise. Give 2 breaths.

7. Don't stop the 15 pumps and 2 breaths until emergency help arrives.

8. Don't try to make victim vomit. If vomiting does occur, save vomit to take to emergency room for analysis.

If Victim is Unconscious and Breathing

1. Call or have someone call 911 (emergency) for an ambulance or medical help.

2. Check to see if the person is carrying special medication to inhale, swallow or inject to counter the effects of the allergic attack. If so, use them if you know how.

3. If you can't get help immediately, take patient to nearest emergency room or other facility with adequate equipment and personnel to care for medical emergencies.

BLEEDING

Symptoms

Bleeding caused by any serious injury should be treated in an emergency facility. There is usually a lot of bright-red blood pumping from an injured artery, or darker blood if a large vein has been injured.

Treatment

1. Call or have someone call 911 (emergency) for an ambulance or medical help. Do not leave the victim. The emergency operator may give you first-aid instructions to perform before emergency help arrives.

2. Lay the person down. If possible, the head should be lower than the trunk of the body or the legs should be elevated. This helps increase blood flow to the brain. If possible, raise a bleeding arm or leg (if not broken) above the level of the victim's heart.

3. Use rubber gloves or plastic bags over your hands or other protection to avoid contact with victim's blood. Apply steady, firm pressure to the wound using a sterile bandage, clean cloth or your hand. Maintain pressure until the bleeding stops (or medical help arrives). Then wrap the wound securely with a bandage or dressing and tape it or tie it in place. Do not tie it so tightly that blood flow to the rest of the body area is cut off. If bleeding seeps through, add more absorbent material. Do not remove the first bandage.

3. If bleeding does not stop with the pressure method, try to stop the bleeding by applying pressure to the artery that that delivers blood to the area of the injury (continue to apply pressure to the bleeding site). Do not apply pressure for longer than 5 minutes to an artery.

BURNS

Symptoms

First- and second-degree burns are not usually life-threatening.

First-degree burns cause only red skin and mild swelling.

Second-degree burns cause blisters, pain and oozing.

Third-degree burns can be life-threatening if extensive. Skin turns white or appears charred.

Treatment for first- and most second- degree burns

1. Place the victim's burned area under cold running water for 15 minutes. If this is not possible, immerse the burn in cool water or cool it with cold compresses. Don't put ice directly on the burn and don't apply butter.

2. For more severe burns, cover the burn area with clean, moist gauze and seek medical help.

3. After cooling minor burns, you can apply an aloe lotion, a triple antibiotic ointment or a moisturizer to prevent drying and to ease some of the discomfort.

Treatment for more extensive burns

1. Keep victim lying flat and lightly covered to prevent shock. Elevate the feet and legs if possible. Wrap or cover the burned area with a clean, moist cloth. Call or have someone call 911 (emergency) for an ambulance or medical help.

2. Remove clothes and jewelry unless they are sticking to burned skin. Do not immerse the victim in a cold bath or apply any type of ointment.

Special instructions

Electrical Burns—Turn off the source of electricity if possible. If not, use a non-conductive material, such as a board or wooden chair, to pull the victim away from the electrical source. Don't use your bare hands. If the victim is not breathing, begin rescue breathing and chest compressions.

Chemical Burns of the Eye or Skin—Hold the victim's head or other burned area beneath a faucet. Turn on cool water at medium pressure. Rinse for at least 15 minutes, directing the water away from the unaffected area.

CHOKING

Symptoms

Choking is often caused by food or other foreign body lodged in the throat (airway). Symptoms include clutching at throat and is unable to speak; has trouble breathing or is unable to breathe; skin may turn blue, white or gray; loss of consciousness.

Treatment

1. If the victim can still talk, breathe or cough, don't interfere.

2. If the victim is unable to breathe, cough and talk, perform the Heimlich Maneuver as follows:

Heimlich Maneuver

1. Stand behind person, place both arms around his abdomen and clasp your hands just below the ribcage and above the navel. Make a fist with one hand, thumb side in. Grasp the fist with your other hand.

2. Give 3 or 4 quick forceful squeezes, pushing in and up until the object is coughed up. Keep your elbows away from your body. Be persistent. Continue the maneuver until the obstruction is relieved or medical help is available.

3. In the case of a collapsed person (who is conscious), extreme obesity or late pregnancy, lay the victim on their back and straddle them. Use chest thrusts by placing one hand on top of the other just above the navel and press upward.

4. If victim becomes unconscious, call 911 for emergency help. Lay victim down with head back. Use fingers sweep inside mouth to try and remove the foreign body. Use chest thrust as described above. If necessary, perform rescue breathing and chest compressions until help arrives.

5. If the victim is a child under 12 months, turn him or her upside down (such as over your knee). Pat firmly between the shoulder blades with the heel of your hand until the object is dislodged.

Note: If you are alone and are choking, perform thrusts on yourself or thrust your abdomen against back of a chair, sink edge or railing and push forcefully.

FRACTURES OR DISLOCATIONS

Symptoms

Extreme pain and tenderness in any injured area; change in appearance of injured part, such as swelling, protruding bone or blood under skin. An extremity, such as finger, arm or leg, may be bent out of normal alignment.

Treatment

1. Immobilize any injured area and don't move a broken limb unless absolutely necessary. Keep victim as warm and comfortable as you can. Control any bleeding. Call or have someone call 911 (emergency) for an ambulance or medical help.

2. If you must move a victim, improvise a splint from stiff rolled-up paper, scrap wood or metal. Pad the splint with clothing or blankets. The splint should extend beyond the joint on either end of the injury. Attach splint firmly to injured extremity with strips of cloth, twine or similar material to prevent movement (don't cut off the blood flow).

3. If leg, back or neck is severely injured and possibly fractured or dislocated, keep patient warm and still until ambulance arrives. Don't move the victim.

HEART ATTACK

Symptoms

Chest pain lasting more than 10 minutes that radiates into jaw or arm. Heavy sweating without obvious other cause. Weakness, nausea, pale skin. Irregular pulse.

Treatment

If Victim is Unconscious, Not Breathing

1. Yell for help. Don't leave victim.

2. Call or have someone call 911 (emergency) for an ambulance or medical help. You may be given first-aid instructions to perform before emergency help arrives. These may include rescue breathing and/or chest compressions.

3. Chest compressions: If there is no pulse (no heartbeat), place one hand on top of the other between the person's nipples and push down on the chest 2 inches. Do this 15 times.

4. Rescue breathing: If chest compressions do not start the heart beat, tilt the person's head back, pinch nose, cover the mouth with yours, and blow until you see the chest rise. Give 2 breaths.

5. Don't stop the 15 pumps and 2 breaths until emergency help arrives.

If Victim is Unconscious and Breathing

1. Call or have someone call 911 (emergency) for an ambulance or medical help.

2. Give the person an aspirin. If possible, get the person into a relaxed sitting position, with the legs up and bent at the knees, to ease the strain on the heart. Loosen tight clothing around the neck and waist.

3. If you can't get help immediately, take patient to nearest emergency room or other facility with adequate equipment and personnel to care for medical emergencies.

Index

Guide to the Index

Alphabetical entries in the index include titles and subtitles from the:
    Symptoms Section (these titles are shown in *italics*)
    Illness Section
    Surgery Section
    Appendix Section (including Diets)

A

Abdominal Aortic Aneurysm Repair 698
Abdominal Pain, Recurrent Attacks 3
Abdominal Pain, Sudden Attack 4
Abdominal Swelling 6
Abdominoperineal Resection 700
Abdominoplasty 1032
Abortion 702
Abruptio Placenta 126
Abscess Drainage Superficial 704
Acne 127
Acne Rosacea 128
Acne Vulgaris 127
Acquired Immunodeficiency Syndrome 381
Actinic Keratosis 418
Acute Respiratory Syndrome, Severe 594
Addison's Disease 129
Adenoidectomy 1020
Adenomatous Hyperplasia of the Uterus 293
Adhesions, Separation of 706
Adhesive Capsulitis 598
Adjustment Disorders 130
Adrenal Gland Removal 708
Adrenal Insufficiency 129
Adrenalectomy 708
Adult Acne 128
Adult Diet, Standard 1056
Agranulocytosis 131
AIDS & HIV 381
Alcoholism 132
Aldosteronism 384
Allergic Purpura 561
Allergic Rhinitis 348
Allergic Shock 142

Allergy/Food Sensitivity Diet 1057
Alopecia Areata 133
Altitude Illness 134
Alzheimer's Disease 135
Amebiasis 136
Amebic Dysentery 136
Amenorrhea, Primary 137
Amenorrhea, Secondary 138
Amniocentesis 710
Amputation 712
Amyotrophic Lateral Sclerosis 139
Anal Fissure 140
Anal Fissure Removal & Anal Sphincterotomy 714
Anal Fistula 141
Anal Fistula Repair 716
Anal Itching 550
Anaphylactoid purpura 561
Anaphylaxis 142
Anemia, Aplastic 143
Anemia During Pregnancy 144
Anemia, Folic-Acid Deficiency 145
Anemia, Hemolytic 146
Anemia, Iron-Deficiency 147
Anemia, Pernicious 148
Aneurysm 149
Aneurysm Repair 718
Angina Pectoris 150
Angioplasty, Coronary 720
Angle-Closure Glaucoma 336
Animal Bites 151
Ankle Pain 7
Ankles, Swollen 8
Ankylosing Spondylitis 613
Anorectal Abscess 152
Anorexia Nervosa 153
Anxiety and Nervousness 9

INDEX

Anxiety Disorder, Generalized 154
Aorto-Iliac Bypass Graft 722
Aortoiliofemoral Reconstruction 722
Aphthous Ulcers 201
Aplastic Anemia 143
Appendectomy 724
Appendicitis 155
Appetite Loss 11
Arm or Hand Pain 13
Arrhythmia 357
Arthritis, Infectious 156
Arthritis, Juvenile Rheumatoid 157
Arthritis, Psoriatic 556
Arthritis, Rheumatoid 158
Arthroplasty, Shoulder 726
Arthroscopy 728
Asbestosis 159
Ascariasis 581
Aseptic Meningitis 457
Asthma 160
Atelectasis 161
Atherosclerosis 162
Athlete's Foot 163
Atopic Dermatitis 252
Atrial Fibrillation 164
Atrioventricular Block 355
Atrophic Vaginitis 680
Attention-Deficit Hyperactivity Disorder
  (ADHD) 165
Atypical Pneumonia 525
Augmentation Mammoplasty 744
Autism 166
Autoeczematization 397
Autosensitization 397

B

B-12 Deficiency Anemia 148
Bacillary Dysentery 274
Back Pain, Low 167
Backache 14
Bacteremia 180
Bacterial Endocarditis 292
Bacterial Pneumonia 524

Bad Breath 21
Baker's Cyst Removal 730
Balanitis 168
Baldness, Pattern, 169
Bang's Disease 193
Bariatric Surgery (Gastric Bypass) 732
Barotitis Media 170
Barotrauma 170
Bartholin's Gland Abscess Drainage
  734
Basal-Cell Skin Cancer 603
Battering 269
Bed Sores 611
Bed-Wetting 171
Behavioral or Emotional Changes 16
Bell's Palsy 172
Bends 247
Benign Paroxysmal Positional Vertigo
  173
Bereavement 344
Bipolar Disorder 174
Bladder Infection, Female 175
Bladder Infection, Male 176
Bladder Injury 332
Bladder Tumor 177
Bladder (Urinary) Removal 736
Bland Diet 1059
Blastomycosis 178
Bleeding, Rectal 18
Blepharitis 179
Blepharoplasty 820
Blepharoptosis 557
Blood Poisoning 180
Blood-Transfusion Reaction 181
Body Lice 439
Boils 182
Bone Fracture 183
Bone Graft 738
Bone Marrow Aspiration & Biopsy 740
Botulism 184
Bowel, Lack of Control 19
Brain Attack 621
Brain or Epidural Abscess 185

INDEX

Brain Tumor 186
Breast Abscess 187
Breast Abscess Drainage 742
Breast Augmentation 744
Breast Biopsy by Excision 746
Breast Biopsy by Needle Aspiration 748
Breast Cancer 188
Breast Changes, Fibrocystic 318
Breast Pain or Lumps 20
Breast Reconstruction 750
Breast Reduction 752
Breast Self-Examination 1076
Breath, Bad 21
Breathing Difficulty 22
Bronchiectasis 189
Bronchiolitis 190
Bronchitis, Acute 191
Bronchitis, Chronic 192
Bronchogenic Carcinoma 444
Bronchoscopy 754
Brucellosis 193
Bruising or Blood Spots Under the Skin, Unexplained 24
Bruxism 660
Buerger's Disease 194
Bulimia Nervosa 195
Bunion 196
Bunion Removal 756
Burns 197
Burping or Gas 25
Bursitis 198

C

Calcium Imbalance 199
Callus or Corn 238
Candidiasis of Skin 200
Candidiasis, Vulvovaginal 688
Canker Sores 201
Car, Sea or Air Sickness 468
Carbon Monoxide Poisoning 202
Carbuncles 182
Carcinoid Syndrome 203

Cardiac Arrest 204
Cardiac Catheterization & Angiocardiography 758
Cardiomyopathy 205
Caries 659
Carotid Artery Endarterectomy 760
Carpal-Tunnel Syndrome 206
Carpal-Tunnel Syndrome Repair 762
Cataract 208
Cataract Extraction 764
Cat-Scratch Disease 207
Cavities 659
Celiac Disease 209
Cellulitis 210
Cerebral Palsy (CP) 211
Cerumen Impaction 284
Cervical Cancer 212
Cervical Dysplasia 213
Cervical Erosion 214
Cervical Polyps 215
Cervical-Rib Syndrome 643
Cervical Spondylosis 216
Cervical Sprain or Strain 692
Cervicitis 217
Cervix, Biopsy of 766
Cervix Cancer 212
Cervix, Cryosurgery of 768
Cervix, Electrocauterization of 770
Cesarean Section 772
Chalazion 218
Chalazion Removal 774
Chest Pain 26
Chickenpox 219
Child Abuse 220
Childhood Obesity 221
Chlamydia Infection 222
Cholangitis 223
Cholecystectomy, Open 826
Cholecystitis or Cholangitis 223
Cholelithiasis 325
Cholesterol, High 224
Chronic Fatigue Syndrome 225
Chronic Obstructive Pulmonary Disease 226

INDEX

Chronic Pelvic Pain 227
Circumcision 776
Cirrhosis of the Liver 228
Claudication 229
Cleft Lip Repair 778
Cluster Headache 350
Coccidioidomycosis 230
Cochlear Implant 780
Cold, Common 231
Cold Sores 371
Colic in Infants 232
Colitis, Ulcerative 233
Colon Cancer 426
Colonoscopy 782
Colorectal Cancer 426
Colostomy 784
Condom Usage 1077
Condylomata Acuminata 690
Confusion (Person Over Age 65) 28
Confusion (Person Under Age 29
Congestive Heart Failure 234
Conjunctivitis 235
Constipation 236
Constipation 30
Contact Dermatitis 253
COPD 226
Cor Pulmonale 237
Corn or Callus 238
Cornea Transplant 786
Corneal Abrasion and Ulcer 239
Coronary Artery Bypass Graft 788
Coronary Artery Disease 240
Coronary Atherosclerosis 240
Costochondritis 241
Cough 31
Cough with Blood 33
Coughing in Children 34
Coxa Plana 434
Crab Lice 439
Cramps, Menstrual 276
Craniotomy 790
Creeping Eruptions 428
Crohn's Disease 242

Croup 243
*Crying, Excessive (Infant 0 to 6
    Months) 35*
Cryosurgery 792
Cryptococcosis 244
Cryptorchidism 638
Culdocentesis 794
Curvature of the Spine 591
Cushing's Syndrome 245
Cutaneous Larva Migrans 428
Cutting Teeth 633
Cystectomy 736
Cystic Fibrosis (CF) 246
Cystitis in Men 176
Cystitis in Women 175
Cystitis, Interstitial 408
Cystoscopy 796

D

D&C 798
Dacryocystitis 632
Dacryostenosis 632
Deafness 353
Decompression Sickness 247
Decubitus Ulcers 611
Deep-Vein Thrombosis 647
Defibrillator, Implantation 800
Degenerative Joint Disease 487
Dehydration 248
Delayed Onset Muscle Soreness 249
Dementia 250
Dental Decay 659
Depression 251
Depression 36
Depression, Low-Grade 280
Dermatitis, Atopic 252
Dermatitis, Contact 253
Dermatitis, Herpetiformis 254
Dermatitis, Seborrheic 255
Dermatomyositis 533
Deviated Nasal Septum 478
Diabetes Feet & Skin Problems 256
Diabetes Hypoglycemia 257

INDEX

Diabetes Insipidus 258
Diabetes Type 1 259
Diabetes Type 2 260
Diaper Rash 261
Diarrhea (Infant 0 to 6 Months) 37
Diarrhea (Person Over 6 Months) 38
Diarrhea, Acute 262
Diarrhea, Chronic, Nonspecific of
   Childhood 263
Diets
  Adult Diet, Standard 1056
  Allergy/Food Sensitivity Diet 1057
  Bland Diet 1059
  Gluten-Restricted Diet 1051
  High-Fiber Diet 1063
  Lactose Intolerance Diet 1065
  Liquid Diet, Clear 1067
  Liquid Diet, Full 1068
  Low-Fat/Low-Cholesterol Diet 1069
  Low-Salt Diet 1071
  Weight Loss Diet 1073
  Weight Loss Suggestions 1075
Dilatation & Curettage of the Uterus
   798
Diphtheria 264
Discectomy 802
Discoid Lupus Erythematosus 445
Disk Removal, Ruptured 802
Disk, Ruptured 265
Dislocation or Subluxation 266
Disseminated Intravascular
   Coagulation 267
Diverticular Disease 268
Diverticulitis 268
Diverticulosis 268
Dizziness 39
Domestic Violence 269
Donovanosis 342
Down Syndrome 270
Drowning, Near 271
Drug Hypersensitivity 272
Ductus Arteriosus Closure 804
Dumping Syndrome 273

Duodenal Ulcer 672
Dysentery, Bacillary 274
Dysfunctional Uterine Bleeding 674
Dyshidrosis 275
Dyshidrotic Eczema 275
Dysmenorrhea 276
Dyspareunia 277
Dyspepsia 404
Dysphagia 278
Dysplastic Nevi 279
Dysthymia 280

E

Ear Infection, Middle 281
Ear Infection, Outer 282
Ear Plastic Surgery 932
Ear, Ringing or Buzzing Sounds 40
Earache 41
Eardrum, Ruptured 283
Earwax Blockage 284
Eclampsia 539
Ectopic Pregnancy 285
Ectropion & Entropion 286
Ectropion Repair 806
Eczema 252
Electric Shock 287
Electrocauterization 808
Electrocoagulation 808
Electrosurgery 808
Emphysema & COPD 226
Emphysema 288
Empyema 289
Encephalitis, Viral 290
Encopresis 291
Endocarditis 292
Endodontic Therapy 972
Endometrial Biopsy 810
Endometrial Carcinoma 675
Endometrial Hyperplasia 293
Endometriosis 294
Endovascular Surgery 812
Entamebiasis 136
Enterobiasis 513

INDEX

Entropion & Ectropion 286
Entropion Repair 814
Enuresis 171
Epicondylitis, Lateral 637
Epidermoid Cyst 593
Epidermoid Cyst Removal 978
Epididymitis 295
Epidural Hemorrhage 305
Epiglottitis, 296
Epilepsy 297
Episiotomy 816
Epistaxis 482
Erectile Dysfunction 401
Erectile Dysfunction 64
Erysipelas 210
Erythema Infectiosum 298
Erythema Multiforme 299
Erythema Nodosum 300
Erythroblastosis Fetalis 576
Esophageal Stricture 301
Esophagectomy 818
Esophagus Cancer 302
Essential Tremor 303
Exanthem Subitum 580
Exercise and Physical Fitness Benefits
    1079
Exophthalmos 304
Extradural Hemorrhage 305
Eye Contusion or Laceration 306
Eye, Foreign Body in 307
Eye Inflammation 411
Eye Pain; Swelling; Dryness; Itching;
    Tearing 42

F

Face Lift & Blepharoplasty 820
Face Pain 44
Facial Skin Problems 45
Failure to Thrive 308
Fainting 309
Faintness or Fainting 46
Fatigue or Tiredness 48
Fatty Liver 310

Febrile Seizure 311
Fecal Impaction 312
Female Athlete Triad 313
Female Sexual Dysfunction 595
Femoral Herniorrhaphy 854
Femoral Neck Fracture 378
Fertility Problems in Men 314
Fertility Problems in Women 315
Fetal Alcohol Syndrome (FAS) 316
Fever Blisters 371
Fever (Child 0 to 2 Years) 51
Fever (Child Over 2 Years) 52
Fever (Person Over Age 12) 53
Fever of Unknown Origin 317
Fibrocystic Breast Changes 318
Fibroid Tumor Removal 822
Fibromyalgia 319
Fibrositis 319
Fifth Disease 298
Fissure, Anal 140
Fistula, Anal 141
Flu 405
Fluid & Electrolyte Disorders 320
Folic-Acid Deficiency Anemia 145
Folliculitis 321
Food Allergy 322
Food Poisoning 323
Foot Problems 55
Fracture Reduction 824
Fracture Repair 824
Frostbite 324
Frozen Shoulder 598
Fulguration 808
Functional Hypoglycemia 393
Furuncles 182

G

Gallbladder Removal 826
Gallbladder Removal by Laparoscopy
    828
Gallstones 325
Gangrene 326
Gardnerella Vaginosis 681

INDEX

Gas 25
Gastric Carcinoma 616
Gastric Erosion 327
Gastric Ulcer 672
Gastritis 328
Gastroenteritis 329
Gastroenterostomy for Pyloric
    Obstruction 830
Gastroesophageal Reflux Disease 330
Gastrostomy 832
Gastrostomy, Percutaneous
Endoscopic 834
Genital Herpes 370
Genital Sores, Blisters, Warts or Boils
    57
Genital Warts 690
Genitourinary Injury 332
German Measles 582
Gestational Carbohydrate Intolerance
    331
Gestational Diabetes 331
Giant Cell Arteritis 532
Giant Urticaria 382
Giardiasis 333
Gilbert's Syndrome 334
Gilchrist's Disease 178
Gingivitis 335
Glaucoma, Angle-Closure 336
Glaucoma, Open-Angle 337
Glomerulonephritis 338
Glossitis 656
Gluten Enteropathy 209
Gluten-Restricted Diet 1051
Goiter 391
Gonorrhea 339
Gout 340
Granulocytopenia 131
Granuloma Annulare 341
Granuloma Inguinale 342
Granuloma, Pyogenic 343
Granulomatous Colitis 233
Granulomatous Ileitis or Ileocolitis 242
Graves' Disease 391

Grief 344
Guillain-Barré Syndrome 345
Gum Inflammation 503

H

Hair Growth in Women, Excessive 58
Hair Loss 59
Hair Transplant 836
Hallux Valgus 196
Hammertoe Correction 838
Hand, Foot & Mouth Disease 346
Hand Surgery 840
Hantaviral Pulmonary Syndrome 347
Hantavirus 347
Hardening of the Arteries 162
Hay Fever 348
Head Injury 349
Head Lice 439
Headache 60
Headache, Cluster 350
Headache, Migraine 351
Headache, Tension 352
Hearing Impairment or Loss 353
Hearing Loss 62
Heart Attack 354
Heart Block 355
Heart Bypass 788
Heart Failure, Congestive 234
Heart-Lung Transplantation 844
Heart Murmurs 356
Heart Rhythm Irregularity 357
Heart Transplantation 842
Heart Valve Disease 358
Heart Valve Replacement 846
Heartbeat Irregularity 63
Heartbeat, Rapid 359
Heartburn 360
Heartburn During Pregnancy 361
Heatstroke or Heat Exhaustion 362
Heel Bursitis 363
Heel Contusion 363
Heel Pain 363
Heel Spur 363

INDEX

Heel Spur Removal 848
Hemolytic Anemia 146
Hemophilia 364
Hemorrhoid Banding 850
Hemorrhoid Removal 852
Hemorrhoidectomy 852
Hemorrhoids 365
Hemothorax 520
Henoch-Schönlein purpura 561
Hepatitis, Viral 366
Hepatocellular Carcinoma 367
Hepatoma 367
Hernia 368
Hernia Repair, Femoral 854
Hernia Repair, Hiatal 856
Hernia Repair, Incisional 858
Hernia Repair, Inguinal 860
Hernia Repair, Umbilical 862
Herniated Disk 265
Herpangina 369
Herpes, Genital 370
Herpes Simplex 371
Herpes Zoster 372
Herpetic Whitlow 373
Herpetiformis, Dermatitis 254
Hiatal Hernia 374
Hiatal Herniorrhaphy 856
Hiccough 375
Hiccup 375
Hidradenitis Suppurativa 376
High Blood Pressure 390
High-Fiber Diet 1063
Hip Dislocation, Congenital 377
Hip Fracture 378
Hip Nailing for Hip Fracture 864
Hip Replacement, Total 866
Hirsutism 379
Histoplasmosis 380
HIV & AIDS 381
Hives 382
Hodgkin's Disease 383
Hordeolum 622
Human Immunodeficiency Virus 381

Hydrocelectomy 868
Hydrophobia 563
Hyperaldosteronism 384
Hyperbilirubinemia 334
Hypercalcemia 199
Hypercholesterolemia 224
Hyperemesis Gravidarum 385
Hyperhidrosis 386
Hyperlipidemia 387
Hypernephroma 388
Hyperparathyroidism 389
Hypertension 390
Hyperthyroidism 391
Hypertrophic Pyloric Stenosis 562
Hypocalcemia 199
Hypochondriasis 392
Hypoglycemia, Functional 393
Hypoparathyroidism 394
Hypopituitarism 514
Hypospadias Repair & Urethroplasty
    870
Hypothermia 395
Hypothyroidism 396
Hysterectomy (Abdominal) with
    Salpingo-Oophorectomy 872
Hysterectomy (Vaginal) 874

I

ID Reaction 397
Idiopathic Hypertrophic Subaortic
    Stenosis (IHSS) 398
Ileostomy 876
Immunodeficiency Disease 399
Impetigo 400
Impotence 401
Impotence, Male Sexual 64,
Incisional Herniorrhaphy 858
Incontinence, Stress 402
Incontinence, Stress, Operations 1000
Incontinence, Urge 403
Indigestion 404
Infectious Arthritis 156
Infectious Polyneuropathy 345

INDEX

Infective Endocarditis 292
Influenza 405
Ingrown Toenail 655
Inguinal Herniorrhaphy 860
Insect Bites & Stings 406
Insomnia 407
Insulin Resistance Syndrome 462
Interstitial Cystitis 408
Intestinal Obstruction 409
Intussusception 410
Iritis 411
Iron-Deficiency Anemia 147
Irritable Bowel Syndrome 412
Ischemic Heart Disease 240
Itching 65

J
Jet Lag 413
Jock Itch 652
Juvenile Rheumatoid Arthritis 157

K
Kaposi Sarcoma 414
Kegel Exercises 1080
Keloids 415
Keratitis 416
Keratoplasty 786
Keratoses, Seborrheic 417
Keratosis, Actinic 418
Keratosis Pilaris 419
Kidney Failure, Acute 570
Kidney Failure, Chronic 571
Kidney Infection, Acute 420
Kidney Infection, Chronic 421
Kidney Injury 332
Kidney, Polycystic 422
Kidney Removal 878
Kidney Stone Removal 880
Kidney Stones 423
Kidney Transplantation 882
Kidney Tumor 388
Knee Pain 66
Knee Replacement, Total 884
Kneecap Removal 886

L
Labyrinthitis 424
Laceration Repair 888
Lactase Deficiency 425
Lactose Intolerance 425
Lactose Intolerance Diet 1065
Laminectomy 802
Laparoscopic Cholecystectomy 828
Laparoscopy 890
Laparotomy 892
Large-Intestine Cancer 426
Large-Intestine Polyp 427
Larva Migrans, Cutaneous 428
Laryngeal Cancer 430
Laryngectomy 896
Laryngitis 429
Laryngoscopy 894
Laryngotracheobronchitis 243
Larynx Cancer 430
Larynx Removal 896
Laser In-Situ Keratomileusis 898
LASIK 898
Latex Allergy 431
Laxative Abuse 432
Lead Poisoning 433
Leg Pain 67
Legg-Calvé Perthes Disease 434
Legionella Pneumophilia
    Bronchopneumonia 435
Legionnaire's Disease 435
Leiomyomas 676
Leukemia, Acute 436
Leukemia, Chronic 437
Leukoplakia, Oral 438
Lice 439
Lichen Planus 440
Lipoma Removal 900
Lipomas 441
Liposuction 902
Liquid Diet, Clear 1067
Liquid Diet, Full 1068
Lithotripsy 904
Liver Cancer 367, 442

INDEX

Photosensitivity 510
Pica 511
Pilonidal Cyst Removal 952
Pilonidal Disease 512
Pink Eye 235
Pinworms 513
Pituitary Gland, Underactive 514
Pituitary Tumor 515
Pityriasis Alba 516
Pityriasis Rosea 517
Placenta, Abruptio 126
Placenta Previa 518
Plantar Fasciitis 519
Plantar Warts 689
Plasma Cell Myeloma 470
Pleural Effusion 520
Pleurisy 521
Pneumoconiosis 522
Pneumocystis Jiroveci Pneumonia 523
Pneumonectomy 910
Pneumonia Pneumocystis Carinii 523
Pneumonia, Atypical 525
Pneumonia, Bacterial 524
Pneumonia, Mycoplasma 525
Pneumonia, Viral 526
Pneumonia, Walking 525
Pneumothorax 527
Poison Ivy, Oak, Sumac 528
Polyarteritis Nodosa 529
Polycystic Kidney 422
Polycystic Ovarian Syndrome 530
Polycythemia 531
Polymyalgia Rheumatica & Giant Cell
    Arteritis 532
Polymyositis & Dermatomyositis 533
Polypectomy 962
Pompholyx 275
Popliteal Artery Embolectomy 954
Porphyria 534
Postmenopausal Bleeding 535
Postpartum Blues, Depression, &
Psychosis 536
Postpartum Infection 558

Postpartum Mood Disturbances 536
Post-Traumatic Stress Disorder 537
Potassium Imbalance 538
Preeclampsia & Eclampsia 539
Pregnancy-Induced Hypertension 539
Premature Ejaculation 540
Premature Labor & Premature Birth
    541
Premenopausal Abnormal Uterine
    Bleeding 674
Premenstrual Dysphoric Disorder 542
Premenstrual Syndrome 543
Presenile Dementia 135
Pressure Sores 611
Priapism 544
Prickly Heat 545
Procidentia 567
Proctitis 546
Progressive System Sclerosis 590
Proptosis 304
Prostate Cancer 547
Prostate Gland Removal, Suprapubic
    956
Prostate Gland Removal, Transurethral
    958
Prostate Hypertrophy 548
Prostatic Hypertrophy, Benign 548
Prostatitis 549
Pruritus Ani 550
Pruritus Vulvae 551
Pseudogout 552
Pseudomembranous Enterocolitis 553
Psittacosis 554
Psoriasis 555
Psoriatic Arthritis 556
Pterygium Excision 960
Ptosis 557
Puerperal Fever 558
Puerperal Infection 558
Pulmonary Edema 559
Pulmonary Embolism 560
Pulmonary Hypertension 237
Purpura, Allergic 561

Pyelonephritis, Acute 420
Pyelonephritis, Chronic 421
Pyloric Stenosis, Congenital 562
Pyoderma 400
Pyogenic Granuloma 343
Pyorrhea Treatment 950

R

Rabies 563
Radiation Sickness 564
Rape Trauma Syndrome 565
Rash with Fever 88
Rash without Fever 90
Raynaud Disease 566
Raynaud Phenomenon 566
Rectal Bleeding 18
Rectal or Colon Polyp Removal 962
Rectal Prolapse 567
Rectovaginal Fistula Repair 964
Red Measles 454
Reduction Mammoplasty 752
Reflex Sympathetic Dystrophy
   Syndrome 568
Regional Ileitis 242
Reiter's Syndrome 569
Renal Calculi 423
Renal Cell Carcinoma 388
Renal Failure, Acute 570
Renal Failure, Chronic 571
Respiratory Syncytial Virus 572
Respiratory Syndrome, Severe Acute
   594
Restless Leg Syndrome 573
Reticulum Cell Sarcoma 449
Retinal Detachment 574
Retinal Detachment Repair 966
Reye's Syndrome 575
Rh Isoimmunization 576
Rheumatic Fever 577
Rheumatoid Arthritis 158
Rhinoplasty & Septoplasty 968
R.I.C.E. Therapy 1081
Ringing in the Ear 40

Ringworm 578
Ringworm of the Feet 163
Rocky Mountain Spotted Fever 579
Root Canal Treatment 970
Rosacea 128
Roseola Infantum 580
Rotator Cuff Repair 972
Roundworms 581
Rubella 582
Rubeola 454
Ruptured Eardrum 283

S

Safe Use of Medicine 1082
Salivary Gland Infection 583
Salivary Gland Tumor 584
Salivary Gland Tumor Removal 974
Salmonella Infections 585
San Joaquin Valley Fever 230
Scabies 586
Scarlet Fever 587
Schizophrenic Disorders 588
Sciatica 167
Scleritis 589
Scleroderma 590
Scoliosis 591
Seasonal Affective Disorder 592
Seatworm 513
Sebaceous Cyst 593
Sebaceous Cyst Removal 976
Seborrheic Dermatitis 255
Seborrheic Keratoses 417
Seizure Disorder 297
Seizure, Febrile 311
Senility 250
Sentinel Node Biopsy 978
Septic Arthritis 156
Septic Shock 180
Septicemia 180
Septoplasty 970
Severe Acute Respiratory Syndrome
   594
Sexual Dysfunction, Female 595

INDEX

Sexual Dysfunction, Male 401
Sexual Intercourse, Painful for Man 79
Sexual Intercourse, Painful for Woman 80
Sexually Transmitted Disease 1083
Shigellosis 274
Shin Splints 596
Shingles 372
Shock 597
Shock Wave Treatment for Kidney Stones 904
Shoulder, Frozen 598
Shoulder Pain 81
Sickle Cell Anemia & Sickle Cell Trait 599
Sigmoid Colectomy 982
Sigmoid Colon Removal 980
Silicosis 600
Singer's Nodes 686
Singultus 375
Sinusitis 601
Sjögren's Syndrome 602
Skin, Bumps on 82
Skin Cancer, Basal Cell 603
Skin Cancer, Squamous Cell 604
Skin Graft 982
Skin Lesion Removal 984
Skin Lesions, Benign 605
Skin Problems (Child Under Age 2) 84
Skin Problems, Facial 45
Skin Problems (Person Over Age 2) 85
Skin Rash with Fever 88
Skin Rash without Fever 90
Skin Self-Examination 1084
Sleep Apnea 606
Sleep Disorders 607
Sleeping Problems 92
Slipped Disk 265
Slipped Femoral Epiphysis 434
Small-Bowel Neoplasms 608
Small-Bowel Resection 986
Small-Intestine Tumor 608
Snakebite 609

Sodium Imbalance 610
Sores, Pressure 611
Spastic Colon or Colitis 412
Speaking Difficulty 94
Spinal Cord Tumor 612
Spinal Meningitis 458
Spinal Tap 988
Spleen Removal 990
Splenectomy 992
Spondylitis, Ankylosing 613
Spontaneous Abortion 464
Sporotrichosis 614
Spousal Abuse 269
Sprains & Strains 615
Squamous Cell Skin Cancer 604
Squint Repair 1000
Stapedectomy 994
Stapes Removal 992
Steatosis 310
Stein-Leventhal Syndrome 530
Stem Cell Transplant 994
Stomach Cancer 616
Stomach Cancer Surgery 996
Stomach Flu 329
Stomatitis 617
Stool, Abnormal Appearance 95
Strabismus 618
Strabismus Surgery 998
Strains & Sprains 615
Strep Throat 619
Streptococcal Sore Throat 619
Stress 620
Stress, How to Cope 1085
Stress Incontinence 402
Stress Incontinence Operations 1000
Stroke 621
Stye 622
Subarachnoid Hemorrhage 623
Subconjunctival Hemorrhage 624
Subdural Hemorrhage & Hematoma 625
Substance Abuse 626
Suction Curettage 702

Suction Lipectomy 902
Sunburn 627
Sunstroke 362
Surgical Wound Infection 628
Swallowing Difficulty 96
Sweating, Excessive 97
Swelling or Lump 98
Swimmer's Ear 282
Swollen Ankles 8
Sympathectomy, Cervicodorsal 1002
Sympathectomy, Lumbar 1004
Syncope 309
Syndrome X 462
Syphilis 629
Systemic Lupus Erythematosus 446

T
Tachycardia 359
Tapeworm 630
Tay-Sachs Disease 631
Tear Duct Infection or Blockage 632
Tear Duct, Opening of 1006
Teething 633
Telogen Effluvium 634
Temporomandibular Joint Syndrome 635
Tendinitis 636
Tendon Repair 1008
Tennis Elbow 637
Tension Headache 352
Testicle Fixation 1010
Testicle Removal 1012
Testicle, Undescended 638
Testicles or Penis, Painful or Swollen 100
Testicular Cancer 639
Testicular Self-Examination 1086
Testicular Torsion 640
Tetanus 641
Thalassemia 642
Thoracic Outlet Syndrome 643
Threadworm 513
Throat, Sore 101

Thromboangiitis Obliterans 194
Thrombocytopenia 644
Thrombophlebitis, Superficial 645
Thrombosis & Embolus, Arterial 646
Thrombosis, Deep-Vein 647
Thrush 648
Thumb-Sucking 649
Thyroglossal Duct & Cyst Removal 1014
Thyroid Gland Removal 1016
Thyroid Nodule 650
Thyroid, Overactive 301
Thyroid, Underactive 396
Thyroidectomy 1016
Thyroiditis 651
Thyrotoxicosis 391
Tic Douloureux 669
Tick Typhus 579
Tietze's Syndrome 241
Tinea 578
Tinea Cruris 652
Tinea Pedis 163
Tinea Versicolor 653
Tinnitus 654
Tiredness or Fatigue 48
Toenail, Ingrown 655
Tongue, Cheek or Gum Biopsy 1018
Tongue Inflammation 656
Tongue, Sore 102
Tongue Tumor, Benign 469
Tonsil & Adenoid Removal 1020
Tonsillectomy 1020
Tonsillitis 657
Tooth Abscess 658
Tooth Decay 659
Tooth Eruption 633
Tooth Extraction 1022
Tooth Grinding 660
Tooth Replantation 1024
Tooth Transplantation 1026
Toothache 103
Torticollis 661
Torulosis 244

INDEX

Toxemia 539
Toxic Shock Syndrome 662
Toxic Synovitis 665
Toxoplasmosis 663
Tracheostomy 1028
Transient Ischemic Attack 664
Transient Synovitis Of The Hip 665
Trembling or Twitching 104
Trench Mouth 666
Trichinosis 667
Trichomoniasis 668
Trigeminal Neuralgia 669
Trisomy 21 270
Tubal Ligation 1030
Tuberculosis 670
Tummy Tuck 1032
Tympanic Membrane Perforation 283
Tympanoplasty 1034
Typhoid Fever 671

U

Ulcer, Duodenal 672
Ulcer, Gastric 672
Ulcer, Peptic 672
Ulcerative Colitis 233
Undescended Testicle 638
Undulant Fever 193
Ureter Injury 332
Ureterolithotomy 880
Urethra Injury 332
Urethral Caruncle Removal 1036
Urethritis 673
Urge Incontinence 403
Urinary Calculi 423
Urination, Frequent 105
Urination, Lack of Control 107
Urination, Painful 108
Urine, Abnormal Color 109
Urticaria 382
Uterine Bleeding, Dysfunctional 674
Uterine Cancer 675
Uterine Fibroids 676
Uterine Prolapse 677

Uterine Sarcoma 675
Uveitis 411

V

Vagina or Vulva Cancer 678
Vaginal Bleeding, Unexpected 110
Vaginal Discharge, Abnormal 111
Vaginal Itching 112
Vaginal Yeast Infection 688
Vaginismus 679
Vaginitis 680
Vaginitis, Nonspecific 681
Vaginosis, Bacterial 681
Vaginosis, Gardnerella 681
Vagotomy 1038
Valley Fever 230
Valvular Heart Disease 358
Varicella 219
Varicocele 682
Varicocele Removal 1040
Varicocelectomy 1040
Varicose Vein Removal 1042
Varicose Vein Sclerotherapy 1044
Varicose Veins 683
Vasectomy 1046
Vasectomy Reversal 1048
Venereal Warts 690
Verruca Vulgaris 689
Vesicovaginal Fistula Repair 1050
Vincent's Disease 666
Viral Encephalitis 290
Viral Hepatitis 366
Viral Meningitis 457
Vision Disturbance or Loss 113
Vitamin Deficiencies 684
Vitiligo 685
Vitrectomy 1052
Vocal-Cord Nodules 686
Voice Loss or Hoarseness 115
Vomiting (Infant 0 to 6 Months) 116
Vomiting, Recurrent Attacks 117
Vomiting, Sudden Attack 118
Vulva or Vagina Cancer 678

INDEX

Vulvovaginal Candidiasis 688
Vulvovaginitis 680
Vulvovaginitis Before Puberty 687

W

Walking Pneumonia 525
Warts 689
Warts, Genital 690
Weight Gain 120
Weight Gain, Slow (Child 0 to 5 Years)
    121
Weight Loss 122
Weight Loss Diet 1073
Weight Loss Suggestions 1075
Wens 593
West Nile Virus 691
Wheezing 124
Whiplash 692
Whooping Cough 693
Wilms' Tumor 694
Wilson Disease 695
Wryneck 661

Z

Zinc Deficiency 696